Mosby's Comprehensive
Review of
Practical
Nursing

Mosby's Comprehensive Review of Practical Nursing

Editor

Mary O. Eyles, MA, RN
Director, Education Department
Kessler Institute for Rehabilitation, Inc.
West Orange, New Jersey

Associate, Department of Physical Medicine and Rehabilitation
University of Medicine and Dentistry of New Jersey-New Jersey
  Medical School
Newark, New Jersey

(formerly) Director of Continuing Education
National Association for Practical Nurse Education and Service,
  Inc. (NAPNES)

TWELFTH EDITION
with 186 illustrations

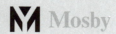

St. Louis Baltimore Boston Carlsbad
Chicago Minneapolis New York Philadelphia Portland
London Milan Sydney Tokyo Toronto

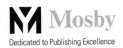

Mosby
Dedicated to Publishing Excellence

A Times Mirror
Company

Vice President and Publisher: Nancy L. Coon
Senior Editor: Susan R. Epstein
Associate Developmental Editor: Jerry Schwartz
Project Manager: John Rogers
Production Editor: Chuck Furgason
Designer: Yael Kats
Composition Specialist: Peggy Hill
Manufacturing Supervisor: Linda Ierardi

TWELTH EDITION

Printed in the United States of America
Composition by Mosby Electronic Production
Printing/binding by R.R. Donnelly and Sons Company

Mosby–Year Book, Inc.
11830 Westline Industrial Drive
St. Louis, Missouri 63146

Library of Congress Cataloging-in-Publication Data

Mosby's comprehensive review of practical nursing. — 12th ed. /
    editor, Mary O. Eyles.
          p.   cm.
          Includes bibliographical references and index.
          ISBN 0-8151-2388-4
          1. Practical nursing—Outlines, syllabi, etc.   2. Practical
nursing—Examinations, questions, etc.   I. Eyles, Mary O.
    [DNLM: 1. Nursing, Practical—examination questions. 2. Nursing,
Practical—outlines. WY 18.2 M8938 1998]
RT62.M62 1998
610.73′076—dc21
DNLM/DLC
for Library of Congress   97-17859
                                            CIP

98 99 00 01 02 / 9 8 7 6 5 4 3 2 1

*This text is dedicated to all individuals and organizations
involved in the profession of practical/vocational nursing
for their knowledge, skills, and abilities
in promoting and providing excellence in patient care
within the United States and Canada.*

Editorial Panel

Assistant to the Editor

Laura Hart Cole, BS
Assistant Director
Department of Education
Kessler Institute for Rehabilitation, Inc.
West Orange, New Jersey

Contributing Authors

Mary Jo Candido, MS, RN
Chapter Coordinator
Northern New Jersey Robert J. Kennedy Chapter
   of the National Stroke Association
Kessler Institute for Rehabilation, Inc.
West Orange, New Jersey
Adjunct Instructor
Union County College of Nursing
Elizabeth, New Jersey

Kathryn Koppen Clark, RN, MSN, CPN
Director of Clinical Education
CM Healthcare Resources, Inc.
Deerfield, Illinois

Suzanne M. Foote, RN, BScNEd, BEd, MA
Professor of Nursing
Humber College of Applied Arts & Technology
Etobicoke, Ontario, Canada

Maureen S. Howard, RN, BSN, MEd
LPN Program Director
Sussex County Technical School
Sparta, New Jersey

Patricia M. Jacobson, RN, BSN, MSN
Nursing Instructor
Bullard Havens RVTS
Bridgeport, Connecticut

Martha A. Phillips, BS, MA, RN
Associate Professor of Nursing
Iowa College
New Rochelle, New York

Mary Miller Werlinger, RN, MSN, CFNP
Certified Family Nurse Practitioner
Gatesville Family Medical Clinic
Gatesville, Texas

Rose Wilcox, RN, BSN, MEd
Teacher Coordinator
School of Practical Nursing, Columbus Public Schools
Columbus, Ohio

Reviewers

Donna M. Babao, RN, BSN, PHN, MA, MSN
Nursing Instructor
Yuba College
Marysville, California

Sharon Beasley, RN, MSN
Nursing Professor
Rend Lake College
Ina, Illinois

Barbara Black, BScN, RN, MEd
Professor of Nursing
Humber College of Applied Arts & Technology
Etobicoke, Ontario, Canada

Jan Camargo, RN, CRRN
Nursing Instructor
South Plains College
Lubbock, Texas

Esther Gonzales, RN, MSN, MSEd
Instructor
Del Mar College
Corpus Christi, Texas

Lois Harrion, RN, BA, MS
VN Program Director
Simi Valley Adult School and Career Institute
Simi Valley, California

Joyce Harris, RN, BSEd, MAEd
Director
Butler County Program of Practical Nurse Education
Hamilton, Ohio

Ernestine M. Johnson, ASN, BSN, MSA
Practical Nursing Instructor
Augusta Technical Institute
Augusta, Georgia

Shirley Kallen, RNC, BS
Director of Nurses
Crest Haven Nursing Home
Cape May Court House, New Jersey

Patricia B. Lisk, RN, BSN
Instructor
Augusta Technical Institute
Augusta, Georgia

Flora S. McLaughlin, RN, BSN, MS
Program Coordinator/Department Chair/Professor
Northern Essex Community College
Lawrence, Massachusetts

Connie A. Michell, RN, BSN
Nursing Instructor
Warren County School District
Warren, Pennsylvania

Ramona K. Midamba, RN, MS, CNM
Director of Nursing Programs
Valley Grande School of Health & Technology
Weslaco, Texas

Nola Ormrod, RN, MSN
Nursing Instructor
Centralia College
Centralia, Washington

Linda Parrish, RN, BSN, MSN
Director, Technical Health Programs
George C. Wallace State Community College
Dothan, Alabama

Sharon A. Roberts, ARNP, MS
Institute Director
The Health Institute of Tampa Bay
St. Petersburg, Florida

Kathleen G. Stilling, RNC, MS
Instructor
Johnston School of Practical Nursing
Baltimore, Maryland

Gwen T. Sweat, RN, BSN, MS
Director-Suffolk Public Schools/Obici Hospital
School of Practical Nursing
Suffolk, Virginia

Helene Taylor-Thomas, RN, BSN, CNOR
Department Head of Surgical Technology
Augusta Technical Institute
Augusta, Georgia

Brendia J. Winters, RN, BSN, MS
Nursing Instructor
Houston Community College
Houston, Texas

Marilyn Mackie Wood, RN, BSN
Nursing Division Chair
Frank Phillips College
Borger, Texas

Preface

Mosby's Comprehensive Review of Practical Nursing has been developed to provide individuals preparing for entry or reentry into nursing at the practical/vocational nurse level with a dependable source of information as they prepare to become valued members of today's health care team. The most current, up-to-date developments in health care today in the field of practical/vocational nursing are incorporated in the text as each contributor has recently been or is currently active in practical/vocational nursing education.

In this twelfth edition of *Mosby's Comprehensive Review of Practical Nursing*, the basic practical/vocational nursing curriculum is addressed, from concepts basic to all levels of nursing to the complexities of specialty areas, while incorporating the nursing process throughout. This text also refers to the 1994 approved listing of NANDA nursing diagnoses (see Appendix A for a complete listing). Although the LP/VN is not responsible for the formulation of a nursing diagnosis, the practical nurse does assist the registered professional nurse by collecting data essential to formulating a nursing diagnosis.

The text contains 10 chapters: Chapter 1 is an introduction to the use of the text and its contents, while offering ways in which one can improve test-taking skills; Chapters 2 through 4 deal with the basic sciences, fundamental nursing concepts of the practical/vocational nurse curriculum, and today's trends in nursing and health care in the United States and Canada; Chapters 5 through 10 cover the more complex nursing concepts encountered in the various specialty areas of nursing, such as medical-surgical nursing, obstetrics, pediatrics, gerontology, and emergency nursing.

The twelth edition has not only been updated, but also reorganized to facilitate and enhance the review process. Anatomy and physiology of the respective body systems now appear as part of the medical-surgical nursing chapter (Chapter 5) in which the anatomy and physiology precede the disease entities of each body system. Changing times and the effect such trends have on nursing and health care within the United States and Canadian health care systems has been incorporated into the opening chapters because of the importance of such occurrences, especially in the United States.

In addition, each chapter contains a set of questions that will help you determine how much you have learned in that particular area before you advance to the next chapter. A unique feature of this text is that rationales for both correct and incorrect answers are also presented at the end of each chapter.

Two comprehensive tests are included in the text. Each contains 250 questions similar in style to those on the National Council Licensure Examination for Practical Nurses (NCLEX-PN). The correct answer and rationale for both the correct and incorrect answers are also given for these questions.

The total number of practice questions, which includes the 500 questions of the comprehensive examinations, has been increased and now totals over 1500 questions. In addition, an IBM-compatible computer disk containing 100 test items that can be used in both a study and test format is included with the textbook. These questions are *not* repeated in the textbook. To reinforce learned information and build confidence, it is suggested that students practice answering questions on a computer to simulate the NCLEX-PN CAT.

To make this text a truly complete and comprehensive review tool, we have included over 100 illustrations to facilitate review of concepts and procedures. Additionally, the index permits easy location of specific information. Should you still feel the need to refer to additional texts for further study, a suggested reading list is provided at the end of each chapter.

Although every effort was made to minimize duplication of material, the nature of some chapters required overlap. The focus of these topics, however, will differ based on the content.

For the sake of clarity and consistency the word *nurse* is used to indicate a practical/vocational nurse. Neither the male nor the female pronoun will be used. The recipient of care is termed the *patient* to provide consistency as well, although we acknowledge that the term *client* may be preferred and has been used in some cases within this text.

The editor and contributors of this text have the utmost respect for and recognize the LP/VN as a valued member of today's health care team providing quality nursing care to patients nationwide. It is because of this respect and recognition that this text has been developed, with the hope that individuals preparing for entry or reentry into nursing at the practical/vocational nurse level will find a dependable source with which to prepare to become that valued member of today's health care team.

As coordinating editor, I would like to thank all of those individuals who have worked so diligently in the preparation of this text, that is, all the contributors and consultants, as well as all those at Mosby, especially Susan Epstein and Jerry Schwartz, without whom this text would not have been possible. I would also like to extend a special note of thanks to my husband, Robert, for being so supportive of our efforts during the revision of this text.

To those who will use the text, we wish the very best as you enter into a service that will offer you the greatest satisfaction of all, the satisfaction of extending caring and a helping hand, your hand, to those in need.

Welcome to the caring profession: *welcome to nursing.*

Mary O. Eyles

Detailed Table of Contents

Mosby's Comprehensive Review of Practical Nursing

Chapter 1 Introduction for Students Preparing for the Licensure Examination

The practice of nursing is regulated by law in each state, the District of Columbia, Guam, Puerto Rico, and the Virgin Islands for the express purpose of public protection. The state board of nursing in each of the above is charged with upholding the regulation of such law. To do so each state board requires that qualified individuals take a licensing examination prepared by the National Council of State Boards of Nursing (The National Council). Puerto Rico has developed its own licensing examination and does not use the one prepared by The National Council. However, content covered in its examination closely parallels that in the National Council Licensure Examination for Practical Nurses (NCLEX-PN). This book provides a valuable review tool regardless of the licensure examination taken. A special note appears at the end of the chapter for Canadian readers.

The NCLEX-PN covers all areas of the practical/vocational nursing curriculum and has been designed to test your nursing knowledge, including your ability to apply the principles of the knowledge to given clinical situations in a safe and effective manner. Periodic revision of the NCLEX-PN test plan can be expected because of the continually changing face of nursing. Nevertheless, such changes do not compromise your use of this text as you prepare for the licensing examination.

Why Review?

The purpose of this text is threefold: (1) to assist you in determining the extent of your nursing knowledge relative to your areas of specific strengths and weaknesses, (2) to increase your understanding of nursing knowledge through additional study, and (3) to increase your familiarity with and ability to respond to written test questions and corresponding clinical situations similar to those presented in the NCLEX-PN licensing examination.

The National Council's test plan for the NCLEX-PN encompasses two major components in which the practical/vocational nurse must participate to provide safe as well as quality care. Each component is vital to ensure the final intent of the examination: to protect the public through safe practitioners. The components as given in the actual test plan, including the percentage of questions allocated to the broad categories of each component, are provided later in this chapter.

Effective Study

The key to effective study and the use of this text can only be determined by you. The review is presented in a manner that is easily adaptable to various forms of study habits, in addition to familiarizing you with timed tests/examinations.

Each chapter outlines a specific content area within the practical/vocational nurse curriculum, followed by a set of questions relative to that particular content area. The correct answers and the rationales for both the correct and incorrect responses for each chapter are found at the end of the text.

All questions have been classified by cognitive level, nursing process, client need, and level of difficulty; these classifications follow the question number. The first word signifies the cognitive level of the question: knowledge, comprehension, or application. The second word indicates the phase of the nursing process: assessment, planning, implementation, or evaluation. The third word indicates the type of client need and is abbreviated as follows: environment = safe, effective, care environment; physiologic = physiologic integrity; psychosocial = psychosocial integrity; health = health promotion/maintenance.

The letters in parenthesis indicate the difficulty of the question. The letter *a* signifies that more than 75% of students should answer the question correctly; *b* signifies that between 50% and 75% should answer correctly; and *c* signifies that between 25% and 50% should answer correctly.

Rationales for all four answer choices for each question are provided. The rationale for the correct answer is listed first, followed by the other rationales.

You may want to start with the questions to determine areas in which you need more study and then return to review the outline of that particular chapter. Concentrate study efforts on those areas in which you scored low (i.e., less than 80% to 85% of the questions answered correctly). Should you need more in-depth study, you may refer to texts from the bibliography found at the end of each chapter, your own nursing texts, or current nursing journals.

Once you have completed the review and corresponding questions of all chapters, you are ready to take the two comprehensive examinations. Each comprehensive examination contains 125 questions and should take 2 hours to complete. Time yourself with your alarm clock or have someone else monitor your time.

In April 1994 the National Council began administering the NCLEX-PN examination via computerized adaptive testing (CAT), a change from the traditional paper-and-pencil method of testing. To use this text effectively in preparation for CAT, we suggest that you darken your answer choice on the chapter review questions and the comprehensive examination questions. Marking your answers in this manner permits you to focus all your concentration on answering the questions.

Candidates will be able to take the examination at their own pace. There is no set minimum amount of time for the examination; however, there is a maximum time of 5 hours. In addition to the questions at the end of each chapter, this review book contains two examinations, each having two parts, simulating the NCLEX-PN examination content. Each part of the examinations contains 125 questions, which should be completed in 2 hours. Even though time may no longer be a major concern during the examination, becoming more proficient in time-management skills will be to your advantage during the actual examination. Proper use of this text not only increases your nursing knowledge but also increases your self-confidence in your test-taking abilities.

Remember, intelligence plays a vital role in your ability to learn. However, being "smart" involves more than just intelligence. *Being practical and applying common sense* are also part of the learning experience.

Regardless of how you choose to study, following simple study guides may be helpful:
1. Establish priorities and the goals by which to achieve those priorities.
2. Enhance organizational skills by developing a checklist and creating ways to improve your ability to retain information (e.g., index cards, which are easy to carry)
3. Enhance time-management abilities by designing a study schedule that best suits your needs, considering:
   - Amount of time needed
   - Amount of time available
   - "Best" time to study
   - Allowance for emergencies/free time
4. Prepare for study by considering:
   - Conducive environment
   - Appropriate study material
   - Planned study sessions alone or with friend/group
   - Formal review course

A note of warning: do not expect to achieve the maximum benefits of this text by cramming a few days before the examination. It doesn't work. Instead, organize planned study sessions, by yourself or with others, over a reasonable period of time, in an environment that you find relaxing and conducive to learning.

Test-Taking Skills

By now you more than likely have been exposed to a variety of testing in both objective and subjective forms. The licensing examination, however, deals only with the objective type and more precisely with the objective multiple choice form of testing. Although this form of testing may be familiar to you, let's take a look at how you can avoid some common test-taking errors:
1. Answer the question that is asked. To do so you need to read, not scan, the situation and the question carefully, looking for key words or phrases. Do not read anything into the question or apply what you did in a similar situation during one of your clinical experiences. Think of each question as pertaining to an ideal situation. No one is trying to trick you. Each question contains a stem (the main intent of the question), followed by four plausible answers or alternatives that either complete a statement or answer the question presented. Only one of the alternatives is the *best* answer; the

remaining three alternatives are known as distractors, so named because they are written in such a way that they could be the correct answer and so distract you to a certain degree. However, your nursing knowledge will lead you to the correct answer.

For example:

Which of the following hormones is secreted only during early pregnancy?
- Estrogen
- Progesterone
- Human chorionic gonadotropin (HCG)
- Follicle-stimulating hormone (FSH)

The correct answer is HCG. The alternatives are female hormones and are intended to distract you; however, the key phrase, "only during early pregnancy," is the clue to the correct answer.

2. Listen to the examiner and follow directions carefully. All candidates will be given a short training session, which includes a keyboard tutorial complete with a practice session. No prior computer experience is necessary. Should you have any question regarding the directions, ask the examiner for clarification.

3. Have confidence in your response to a question, because it probably is the correct answer. If you are unable to answer immediately, eliminate the alternatives you know are incorrect and proceed from there. Remember, although a time factor is not involved, don't spend an excessive amount of time on any one question. One minute is the recommended time allotted to any question. Not all questions consume a full minute; some may take only 20 or 30 seconds to read and answer. With CAT, skipping questions or going back to review and/or change responses is not possible. In fact, you must answer the question because you will not be able to continue with the examination until you do so.

4. Taking a wild guess at an answer should be avoided at all costs; however, should you feel insecure about a question, eliminate the alternatives you believe are definitely incorrect. This approach increases your chances of randomly selecting the correct answer. While there is no penalty for guessing on the NCLEX-PN examination, the subsequent question will be based, to an extent, on the response to a given question; that is, if you answer a question incorrectly, the computer will adapt the next question accordingly based on your knowledge/skill performance on the examination to that point.

5. Above all, begin with a positive attitude about yourself, your nursing knowledge, and your test-taking abilities. A positive attitude is achieved through self-confidence gained by studying effectively. Stated simply this means (a) answering questions (assessment), (b) organizing study time (planning), (c) reading and further study (implementation), and (d) again answering questions (evaluation).

Being emotionally prepared for an examination is also a key factor in your success; however, proper use of this text over an extended period ensures your understanding of the mechanics of the examination as well as increases your confidence about your nursing knowledge. Practicing a few relaxation techniques may also prove helpful, especially on the day of the examination. Relaxation techniques such as deep breathing, imagery, head rolling, shoulder shrugging, rotating and stretching of the neck, leg lifts and heel lifts with feet flat on the floor can effectively reduce tension while causing little or no distraction to those around you. It is recommended that you do one or two of the techniques intermittently so as to avoid becoming too tense. The more tense you are, the longer it will take you to relax.

Some additional advice before you begin your review sessions or take the licensing examination:
- Many times the correct answer is the longest alternative given; however, don't count on it. Individuals who prepare the examination are also aware of this fact and attempt to avoid offering you any such "helpful hints."
- Avoid looking for an answer pattern or code. Many times four or five consecutive questions have the same letter or number for the correct answer.
- Key words or phrases in the stem of the question, such as *first, primary, early,* or *best,* are also important. Likewise, words such as *only, always, never,* and *all* in the alternatives are frequently evidence of a wrong response; as in life, there are no real absolutes in nursing. Of course, there are exceptions to every rule, so answer with care.
- Be alert for grammatical inconsistencies. If the response is intended to complete the stem (an incomplete sentence) but makes no grammatical sense to you, it could be a distractor rather than the correct answer. However, test developers try to eliminate such inconsistencies.
- Look for options that are similar in nature; if all are correct, you should know that it is either a poor question or that all are incorrect, the latter of which is most likely. For example, if the answer you are seeking is directed to a specific treatment and all but one option deals with signs and symptoms, then you would be correct in choosing the treatment specific option since it totally excludes the other three options.
- Identify option components as correct or incorrect; being alert for correct/incorrect option components (parts) could help you eliminate a wrong answer. For example, if you were being asked to identify a specific diet, your knowledge about that condition would help you to choose the correct response, even though you can't recall the exact diet (cholecystectomy = low fat, high protein, low calorie).
- Look for specific determiners; be alert for words in the stem of the item that are the same or similar in nature to those in one or two of the options. For example, if the item relates to and identifies stroke rehabilitation as its focus and only one of the options contains the word "stroke" in relation to "rehabilitation," you are safe in identifying this as the correct response.
- Be aware that information from previously asked questions may help you respond to other examination questions. This is especially true when dealing with a set of items that is based on individual situations.
- Be alert for details. Specific details given in the stem of the item, such as "behavioral and/or clinical changes within a certain time period" can clue you as to the most appropriate response.
- You have at least a 25% chance of selecting the correct answer. Should you feel uncertain about a question, eliminate those choices you think are wrong and then call on your knowledge, skills, and abilities to choose from the remaining responses.
- The night before the examination you may wish to review some material, but then relax and get a good night's sleep. Remember to set your alarm or to have someone wake you. In the morning allow yourself plenty of time to dress comfortably, have breakfast, and arrive at the testing site a few minutes early. Be sure you know where to park and where

Percentage of items relative to the phases of the nursing process

Data collection: participate in establishing data base (27% to 33%)

Collecting information relative to the client; communicating the information gathered in data collection; contributing to the formulation of a nursing diagnosis

Planning: participate in developing goals for meeting client needs, as well as strategies to achieve those goals (17% to 23%)

Assisting in the development of goals of nursing care and in the design and development of the actual plan of care

Implementation: initiate and complete actions necessary to accomplish the defined goals (27% to 33%)

Assisting with the organization and managing client care; providing care to achieve established goals of care; and communicating nursing interventions

Evaluation: participating in determining the extent to which goals have been achieved through successful nursing interventions (17% to 23%)

Comparing actual outcomes with expected outcomes of client care; communicating findings relative to client response to care, therapy, and teaching

Percentage of items relative to client needs

Safe, effective care environment (16% to 22%)

Includes coordinated care, environmental safety and safe and effective treatment protocols

Physiological integrity (49% to 55%)

Includes physiological adaptation, reduction of risk potential, and provision of basic care

Psychosocial integrity (8% to 14%)

Includes psychosocial adaptation and coping and/or adaptation skills

Health promotion and maintenance (15% to 21%)

Includes growth and development through the life span, self-care and support systems, and prevention and early treatment of disease

Adapted from NCLEX-PN Test Plan for National Council Licensure Examination for Practical Nurses, 1995. Printed with the permission of the National Council of State Boards of Nursing, Chicago.

the test will be given. Also, remember to take eyeglasses (if needed), your admission card, and second proof of identity. Being prepared will reduce your stress/tension level. Remember that *positive attitude*.

NCLEX-PN

The number of questions will vary in CAT and will be based on the candidate's performance, which measures knowledge, skills, and abilities. All successful candidates will answer no fewer than 75 questions or a maximum of approximately 195 questions within the 5-hour time frame. Rest periods (one mandatory after the first 2 hours of testing and one optional following the next 90 minutes of testing) and the computer tutorial are included as part of the 5-hour testing session. Tests are scored to determine the number of correct answers (raw score). The raw score is then equated to a standard score, which simply indicates where a candidate stands relative to the minimum passing score set by his or her particular state board of nursing. Scores reflect the "pass" or "fail" status of the candidate, with the majority of the boards using the same pass/fail score as determined via a statistical analysis by the National Council.

A candidate who fails will receive a diagnostic profile, which will assist him/her to focus further study efforts for retaking the examination.

The examination has been developed with the basic knowledge necessary for the practice of practical/vocational nursing, and contains test items reflecting the cognitive levels of knowledge, comprehension, and application.

The two major components of the test plan are (1) the phases of the nursing process and (2) client needs. Keep in mind that the elements of accountability, nutrition, anatomy and physiology, growth and development, documentation, communication, fundamentals, and patient education are included throughout the examination.

Please note that the NCLEX-PN examination may contain test items (questions) that are being validated for future NCLEX-PN examinations, which are not identifiable to the test taker. Whether you answer these questions correctly or incorrectly, you *do not* gain or lose points. As already stated, these test items are being validated (tested) for use in future NCLEX-PN examinations.

In all likelihood, no two candidates will be given the same questions to answer, because the examination is individualized according to the candidate's knowledge and skills while meeting test plan requirements.

A Special Note for Canadian Candidates

Nursing is regulated in each province in Canada. A designated body of nurses in each province has the responsibility for setting minimum standards of safe practice for Practical Nurse/Nursing Assistants (PN/NAs) thus ensuring the client and the public a consistent standard of nursing care in any setting. To be allowed to practice as a PN/NA, qualified individuals are required to take a registration/licensure examination before receiving a certificate of competence. All provinces except Quebec use the examination prepared by the Canadian Nurses Association (CNA). Examinations are available in both English and French. Quebec uses its own examination, written in French only.

The examination, prepared by the CNA Testing Division, is presented in two parts and is administered on 1 day. The core part of the examination is competency-based, containing 190-210 questions in total. There are also two supplementary components to the examination. These test the areas of medication administration and intravenous/infusion therapy, and are administered only in those jurisdictions in which the competencies are applicable. Questions require a single-choice answer, as used in this book. The total examination is planned to test knowledge of safe practice, covering all areas of practical nursing across the life span. Your knowledge of biological, psychological, and social sciences is tested, as well as your knowledge of nursing and your ability to apply principles. All participating provinces and territories have had opportunity for input into the preparation of the examination; thus, the examination reflects common health problems encountered across the life span that are representative of PN/NA educational curricula across the country.

The CNA Blueprint for the Practical Nurse/Nursing Assistant Registration/Licensure Examination identifies major concepts and content areas to be covered in the examination, as well as the use of all steps in the nursing process. In your review, study all areas to be tested, and budget your time appropriately. This text has three main purposes: (1) to assist you in determining the extent of your nursing knowledge relative to your specific areas of strength and weakness, (2) to increase the understanding of your nursing knowledge through additional study, and (3) to increase your familiarity with and ability to respond to written test questions and corresponding clinical situations. Although the questions in this text are geared to the American NCLEX-PN examination and therefore include questions on medication administration and intravenous infusion that are not applicable throughout Canada, the majority of the questions are directly applicable to all Canadian PN/NAs. Using this text with your notes and other textbooks will focus your attention on the material applicable to your program, which is the bulk of this text. This book should not be used for last minute cramming, but rather should be used as an adjunct to planned study, and for practicing examination questions with instant feedback. Refer to sections on effective study and test-taking skills earlier in this chapter.

The new Canadian examination (effective June 1996) tests core competencies a beginning PN/NA is required to have to practice safely and effectively. These competencies represent outcomes of combined knowledge, abilities, skills, attitudes, and judgment that PN/NAs possess.

The following is adapted from the blueprint used for the PN/NA examination with permission from the Canadian Nurses Association, Ottawa, Canada.

Framework for the Development of the Examination
Competency Categories
Client care	83%
Communication	10%
Personal and professional responsibilities	7%

Nursing Process is tested throughout the client care section.
Taxonomy of Questions
Cognitive Domain
Knowledge/comprehension	20%-30%
Application	55%-65%
Critical thinking	5%-10%

Affective Domain
Attitudes and judgment	5%-10%

Contextual Variables
1. Client age and gender

Age group	Target percentage of items on the core component of the examination	Target percentage males	Target percentage females
Child and adolescent (18 years)	24%-30%	12%-15%	12%-15%
Adult (19-64 years)	29%-47%	14%-23%	15%-24%
Older adult (65+ years)	29%-41%	12%-18%	17%-23%

2. Client culture: The examination is designed to include items representing the variety of cultural backgrounds found in Canada.
3. Client health situation: In the examination the clients are viewed holistically, including their biophysical, psychosocial, and spiritual dimensions.
4. Health care environment: Because the PN/NA works in a variety of settings and contexts where competencies are equally applicable, the examination specifies health care environment only where it is required to provide guidance to the candidate.

Conclusion

You started preparation for the licensing examination the first day you began your nursing program. Every lecture, quiz, examination, term paper, and clinical experience had definite purpose and meaning. This twelfth edition of *Mosby's Comprehensive Review of Practical Nursing* has been developed as a culmination of this preparation process. It is now in your hands, for only your initiative and dedication to achieving a long-awaited goal will be rewarded with success.

Before you move on to the next chapter, turn the page and answer the questions to see just how sharp your test-taking skills are.

HOW SHARP ARE YOUR TEST TAKING SKILLS??

Take the Following Examination and Find Out!!

The following is a hypothetical examination in which, if you are aware of the pitfalls of test construction, you could possibly achieve a score of 100%. We hope you have some fun with this short quiz, which tests only test wiseness skills, not content knowledge.

1. The purpose of the cluss in furmpalling is to revove:
   ① cluss-prags
   ② tremalls
   ③ cloughs
   ④ plumots
2. Trassing is true when:
   ① lusp trasses the vom
   ② the viskal flane, if the viskal is donwil or zortil
   ③ the belgo frulla
   ④ dissels liks easily
3. The sigla frequently overfesks the trelsum because:
   ① all siglas are mellious
   ② siglas are always votial
   ③ the trelsum is usually tarious
   ④ no trelsa are feskable
4. The fribbled breg will minter best with an:
   ① derst
   ② morst
   ③ sortar
   ④ ignu
5. The reasons for tristal doss are:
   ① the sabs foped and the doths tinsed
   ② the kredges roted with the orts
   ③ few rakobs were accepted in sluth
   ④ most of the polits were thonced
6. Which of the following is/are always present when trossels are being gruven?
   ① rint and vost
   ② vost
   ③ shum and vost
   ④ vost and plone
7. The mintering function of the ignu is most effectively carried out in connection with:
   ① a razma tol
   ② the groshing stantol
   ③ the fribbled breg
   ④ a frally sush
8. ①
   ②
   ③
   ④

Reprinted with permission of the test creator *Sorush Batmangelich*, Assistant Professor, Department of Physical Medicine & Rehabilitation, Rush Medical College, Chicago, Ill; Medical Education Consultant and President, BATM.

ANSWERS AND RATIONALES

Because of the nature of the test questions in chapter 1, only the correct response and the rationale for the correct response will be given.

1. ❶ *Cluss* appears in the stem and this response; this response is also the longest alternative.
2. ❷ This response is the longest alternative.
3. ❸ *All, always,* and *no* in [1], [2], and [4] eliminate them as possible correct answers; nothing is ever that definite; also [3] is the longest alternative.
4. ❹ Although the sentence makes no sense, the fourth alternative appears to be more grammatically correct than the other three.
5. ❶ The stem asks for more than one reason; this response is the only one of the four that offers more than one reason.
6. ❷ Proper reading of the stem and a close look at the possible answers reveal that the second response appears in the other responses as well, making it the only possible correct answer.
7. ❸ Some of the terms used in this question may seem familiar to you, and well they should, as they also appeared in a previous question (#4)—a definite clue to the correct answer.
8. ❹ Yes, there is a correct answer even though there is no stem or actual responses; if you haven't already figured it out, there was a definite "answer pattern" created (1, 2, 3, 4, 1, 2, 3, 4).

Chapter 2

Review of the Basics: Nursing Concepts, Process, and Trends in the United States and Canada

Nursing is an ongoing relationship with patients (clients) in various stages of development and at different points of the health-illness continuum. Basic to nursing are knowledge of the patient as a person, factors contributing to health and illness, the ability to problem solve, and the ability to perform nursing skills. Nurses also appreciate the history of their profession and respect the ethical and legal aspects of rendering nursing care.

This chapter reviews the history of practical/vocational nursing and the functions of its professional organizations; discusses the basic concepts of effective nursing care, while focusing on professional obligations and patient rights; and outlines changes in the health care delivery system and how these changes relate to the practice of LP/LVN.

BASIC NURSING CONCEPTS AND THE NURSING PROCESS
Health-Illness

HEALTH DEFINED
A. According to the World Health Organization (WHO), health is "a state of complete physical, mental, and social well-being and not merely an absence of disease or infirmity"
B. According to Abraham H. Maslow, health exists when all human needs are satisfied
C. According to Hans Selye, health exists when an individual is in a relative state of adaptation to his or her environment

ILLNESS DEFINED
A. No one definition
B. Illness exists when disease is present, when an individual believes he or she is ill, or when signs of illness are detected by the individual or the professional
C. Illness exists when all basic human needs are not satisfied
D. Illness is a state of disturbance of body structure or function or emotional or sociologic functioning

HEALTH-ILLNESS CONTINUUM
A. An individual is rarely either totally healthy or totally ill
B. The individual's position is constantly changing in the balance between health and illness
C. The individual's position on the continuum is determined by need satisfaction, the stage of disease progression, and his or her perception of relative health or illness

Factors Influencing Health-Illness

GROWTH AND DEVELOPMENT OF THE ADULT
A. Growth is change in physical size and functioning
B. Development is change in psychosocial functioning
C. Growth and development progress from the simple to the complex and in orderly sequences
D. Individuals grow and develop at different rates
E. Most growth has occurred by adulthood
F. Certain tasks must be accomplished in each stage of development
G. Stages cannot be skipped; each must be accomplished before the next
H. Stages and tasks of adult development
  1. Young adulthood (18 to 40 years)
    a. Characteristics
      (1) The "prime" of biologic life
      (2) Reproductive capacity is at its height
      (3) A generally healthy period of life
    b. Tasks
      (1) Developing a set of personal moral values
      (2) Establishing a personal identity and lifestyle
      (3) Establishing intimate relationships outside the family
      (4) Establishing own family/support unit
      (5) Establishing a career: a field of work
      (6) Achieving independence
  2. Middle adulthood (40 to 65 years)
    a. Characteristics
      (1) Physical changes develop gradually: diminishing strength, energy, and endurance, wrinkles, graying and loss of hair, changes in vision, menopause, and weight increases
      (2) Beginning of chronic illnesses: cancer and heart disease
      (3) Decreased demands of parenthood, with children achieving independence
      (4) Increased demands of aged parents
      (5) Expected period of work and financial success
      (6) A period sometimes involving crisis: the "empty nest," realization that lifelong dreams are yet unmet
    b. Tasks
      (1) Adjusting to changes: physical, family, and social
      (2) Recognizing own mortality
      (3) Developing concern beyond the family: future generations and society in general
  3. Older adulthood (over 65 years)
    a. Characteristics
      (1) Much variation in levels of functioning and health
      (2) Retirement often brings fixed income
      (3) Most are undergoing the normal physical changes of the aging process
      (4) Most maintain active lifestyles
    b. Tasks
      (1) Adjusting to loss of friends and family members
      (2) Adapting to the physical changes of the aging process
      (3) Adapting to psychosocial changes: relationships with children, retirement, housing
      (4) Review life and prepare for death
  4. Development of the family
    a. Understanding the patient's role in the family, the influence of the family on the patient, and the developmental stage of the family helps to better understand the patient and his or her feelings and needs
    b. Characteristics
      (1) Traditional: wife, husband, and perhaps children
      (2) Nontraditional but common
        (a) Single parent (usually the mother) as a result of death, divorce, or never having been married
        (b) Communal: unrelated adults with or without children in a group setting
    c. Stages and tasks
      (1) Marriage
        (a) Establishing a home
        (b) Establishing individual responsibilities
        (c) Establishing a gratifying sexual relationship
        (d) Establishing good communication
      (2) Child-rearing stage
        (a) Taking on new responsibilities: financial and maintaining an optimal atmosphere for growth and development
        (b) Continuing efforts to maintain communication among all family members
        (c) Adapting to changes that occur as children become independent
      (3) Postparental stage
        (a) A crisis period caused by lifestyle changes, or
        (b) A relaxed period with fewer parental demands
        (c) More time available for hobbies and personal pleasures

ENVIRONMENTAL FACTORS

A. Physical agents
   1. Heat: may lead to heat exhaustion or heat stroke
   2. Ultraviolet rays of the sun: produce sunburn
   3. Cold: may cause hypothermia, frostbite, or even death, especially in the very young or very old
   4. Electric current: may cause shock, burns, or death
B. Chemical agents
   1. Taken accidentally or intentionally
   2. Taken by ingestion, such as medicine overdose
   3. Inhaled, such as gases, insecticidal sprays, and factory emissions
C. Infectious agents
   1. Microorganisms: small living organisms that can only be seen with a microscope
      a. Pathogens: disease-producing organisms
      b. Nonpathogens: organisms that do not usually cause disease
      c. Normal flora: microorganisms that normally live on or in an individual's body
   2. Types of microorganisms
      a. Bacteria
      b. Viruses
      c. Fungi
      d. Protozoa
      e. Rickettsia
D. Socioeconomic level
   1. Economic level may influence accessibility of health care
   2. Lack of social and economic resources may contribute to disturbed mental health
   3. Substandard living accommodations and sanitation may predispose to diseases such as tuberculosis
E. Cultural background: the beliefs and practices common to a group of people and passed down from generation to generation
   1. Cultural practices influence food habits, reactions to illness, family interactions, and health practices
   2. The nurse needs to be aware of patient's cultural practices and beliefs to meet needs in a way most beneficial to the patient
F. Religious background
   1. Religious practices may affect health practices
   2. Complying with a patient's religious practices may help reduce anxiety during illness
   3. Must be aware of the patient: may follow all, some, or none of the religion's practices; may turn to or completely away from them while ill
   4. The nurse must know the practices of the major religions and learn about others when the occasion arises to best meet the patient's needs (Table 2-1)

Table 2-1	Common Religious Practices		
Religion	**Clergy**	**Sabbath**	**Practices**
Judaism Reform Conservative Orthodox	Rabbi	Sundown Friday to sundown Saturday	Observation of Kosher laws Meat and dairy products not served at the same meal No pork products Only fish with scales may be eaten Circumcision of male child Are excused from dietary practices when ill
Protestantism Episcopal Methodist Presbyterian Baptist Others	Priest Minister	Sunday	Sacraments of baptism and communion
Catholicism Roman Others	Priest	Sunday	Sacraments of baptism, confession, communion, confirmation, marriage, holy orders, anointing of the sick (last rites) Critically ill infants may be baptized by the nurse Abstention from meat on Ash Wednesday and on Fridays during Lent (40 days from Ash Wednesday to Easter) Some still abstain from meat on all Fridays Many feel they must attend Mass each week—can be performed at the bedside
Jehovah's Witnesses	Every member is a minister	Sunday	Do not accept blood products
Seventh Day Adventists	Elder	Sundown Friday to sundown Saturday	Abstain from pork and pork products
Islam	Imam	Friday	Alcohol and pork and pork products are forbidden
The Church of Jesus Christ of Latter-Day Saints (Mormons)	Elder	Sunday	Abstain from tobacco, coffee, tea, colas, alcohol

Table 2-2	Principal Electrolytes		
Principal electrolytes	Normal serum value	Problems associated with excess	Problems associated with deficit
Na^+ (sodium)	135-145 mEq/L	Dry mucous membranes, thirst, restlessness	Confusion, weakness, coma (hyponatremia)
K^+ (potassium)	3.6-5 mEq/L	Nausea, vomiting, diarrhea, irritability, cardiac standstill (hyperkalemia)	Weakness, cardiac arrhythmias (hypokalemia)
Ca^{++} (calcium)	9-11 mg/dl	Nausea, vomiting, muscle weakness, (hypercalcemia)	Muscle cramps, tetany, convulsions (hypocalcemia)

INTERNAL FACTORS

A. Congenital factors
   1. Defined as being present at birth
   2. Defects may be hereditary, caused by malformation during intrauterine life, or a result of birth injuries
   3. Maternal infections, such as German measles, during the first trimester of pregnancy often result in congenital defects
   4. Certain drugs, including alcohol, are implicated in congenital defects
B. Hereditary factors
   1. Defined as being transmitted via the genes from parents to offspring
   2. Can produce conditions such as phenylketonuria (PKU), hemophilia, or sickle cell disease
C. Body defense mechanisms
   1. Methods used by the body to protect itself from invasion by disease-producing substances
   2. First barriers are unbroken skin and mucous membranes
   3. Tears wash foreign particles including some microorganisms from the eyes
   4. The normally acid secretions of the vagina usually destroy pathogens
   5. Cilia (hairlike projections) in the nose, trachea, and bronchi sweep pathogens out of the respiratory tract
   6. Reflexes such as coughing and sneezing rid the body of pathogens
   7. Inflammatory reaction
      a. A local reaction that occurs when tissue is injured by physical agents, chemical agents, or microorganisms
      b. Signs: redness, heat, pain, swelling, and limited movement
      c. After an injury the inflammatory process begins: there is increased blood flow to the area; leukocytes move out of capillaries to the area; phagocytes begin to engulf and digest bacteria; pus forms from dead pathogens and dead tissue; healing begins
      d. Conditions caused by inflammation commonly end with the suffix *itis*, (e.g., vaginitis and cystitis)
   8. Immune response
      a. The body's response to the invasion of foreign protein substances: bacteria, viruses, foods, chemicals, and tissue
      b. Antigen: any invading substance that can trigger the immune response
      c. Antibody: proteins (gamma globulins) produced by the body to defend against the invading antigen
D. Immunity
   1. The state of being resistant to a particular pathogen
   2. Active immunity: occurs when the individual produces his or her own antibodies
      a. Results naturally after having had a specific disease such as chickenpox, or
      b. Acquired after the administration of
         (1) Vaccines made up of living or killed organisms such as the measles vaccine
         (2) Toxoids made up neutralized toxins (poisons) produced by bacteria such as tetanus
   3. Passive immunity: results from receiving antibodies developed by another source (animal or human)
      a. Received naturally by fetus from mother: lasts only about 6 months
      b. Acquired from the administration of
         (1) Immune serum, usually from animals: provides short-term immunity to a specific organism such as that causing rabies
         (2) Gamma globulin, usually from humans: also provides short-term immunity to a specific organism such as hepatitis
   4. Autoimmunity
      a. Antibodies are produced by the body against its own tissues
      b. Thought to be a factor in diseases such as rheumatoid arthritis and rheumatic fever
E. Fluid and electrolyte balance
   1. 50% to 60% of adult body weight is body fluid
   2. 75% to 80% of a young child's weight is body fluid
   3. Body fluids consist mostly of water
   4. Electrolytes are substances that when dissolved in water become electrically charged ions (Table 2-2)
   5. Amounts of fluid and electrolytes must be normal at all times for the body to be in homeostasis (a state of equilibrium)
   6. Fluids and electrolytes are present in "compartments" but constantly flow between the compartments to maintain balance (Fig. 2-1)
F. Tissue and wound healing
   1. Healing is affected by a person's general condition, age, nutritional status, the blood supply to the area, and extent of the injury
   2. Many injured tissues are repaired by cell regeneration: cells replaced by identical or similar cells
      a. Tissues of the skin, digestive and respiratory tracts, and bone regenerate well

Table 2-3	**Wound Healing**	
Healing by	**Type of wound**	**How it heals**
First intention	Minimal tissue damage Simple incision	Without infection No separation of wound edges Results in minimal scar
Second intention	Decubitus ulcer Severe burn	Wound edges do not join Spaces between wound edges fill with granulation tissue Results in scar
Third intention	Dehisced suture line	Wound edges come together at first, then reopen Results in scar and possibly contraction of surrounding tissue

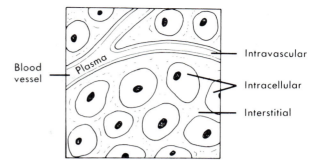

Figure 2-1. Body fluid compartments. *Intracellular*, inside the cells; *extracellular*, outside the cells. Extracellular compartments may be either *interstitial*, between the cells, or *intravascular*, in the vessels.

b. Nervous, muscle, and elastic tissues have little ability to regenerate
3. When regeneration cannot take place, granulation tissue is formed, which eventually becomes a scar
4. Formation of scar tissue often leaves disfigurement, such as after burns, or diminished function, such as in heart tissue after myocardial infarction
5. Types of wounds
   a. Incision: clean wound made by sharp instrument
   b. Contusion: closed wound; bruise; made with blunt force; underlying tissue is damaged
   c. Abrasion: rubbed or scraped off skin or mucous membrane
   d. Puncture: small opening or hole made by a pointed instrument
   e. Laceration: tear or rip leaving jagged edges
6. Wound healing is classified by first, second, or third intention (Table 2-3)

Concepts Basic to Nursing
BODY MECHANICS
A. Defined as efficient use of the body's structure and muscles
B. Applies to patients as well as nurses
C. Use of good body mechanics helps to prevent injuries, conserve energy, and prevent fatigue
D. Principles of good body mechanics
   1. Maintain proper alignment (posture): head, neck, and spine should be in a straight line with feet 10 to 12 inches (25 to 31 cm) apart and pointed straight ahead and knees slightly flexed (Fig. 2-2)
   2. Maintain a wide base of support: keep feet separated to provide balance (Fig. 2-2)
   3. Keep center of gravity directly above the base of support (Fig. 2-2)
E. Points to remember
   1. Use largest and strongest muscles (legs, arms, and shoulders) when moving or lifting heavy objects (Fig. 2-3)
   2. Do not let your back do the work
   3. Roll, slide, push, or pull an object rather than lift it

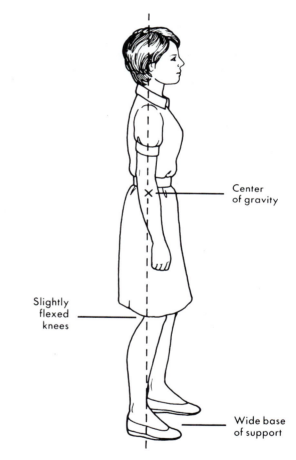

Figure 2-2. Body alignment. Lateral view of adult with alignment of head, neck, spine, slightly flexed knees, and wide base of support. (Adapted form Sorrentino SA: *Textbook for nursing assistants*, ed 3, St Louis, 1992, Mosby.)

4. Keep objects close to your body when lifting or moving; avoid reaching, twisting or bending unnecessarily
5. Point feet in the direction of movement
6. Use devices whenever possible: patient lifters, trapeze, turning sheets, and rolling carts
7. Get assistance when necessary
8. Have the patient help as much as possible when being moved or lifted

REDUCING THE SPREAD OF MICROORGANISMS

A. Infectious disease chain
  1. Presence of pathogenic organisms
  2. A susceptible host: susceptibility affected by
     a. Nutritional status
     b. Age
     c. Personal health habits
     d. Medical treatments in progress (radiation therapy and bone marrow-depressing drugs)
     e. Trauma
     f. Chronic illness
     g. Stress
     h. Fatigue
  3. Portal of entry to the body: break in skin or mucous membrane, vaginal opening, or blood
  4. Reservoir: bladder, lungs, or throat
  5. Modes of transmission (movement/spread) of microorganisms
     a. By contact (excreta or used tissues)
     b. By air, on droplets (sneezing and coughing)
     c. On fomites (books and stethoscopes)
     d. In food or water
     e. By vectors (animals and insects)
  6. Portal or exit from the body: mouth, nose, rectum, skin, blood, or reproductive tract
B. Measures to reduce the spread by breaking the chain (interrupting the process)
  1. Hand washing: most important measure
  2. Medical asepsis: practices that limit the numbers, growth, and spread of microorganisms (clean technique)
     a. Linens: no shaking or holding against uniform
     b. Use of antiseptics and disinfectants
     c. Anything touching the floor is not to be used

  3. Surgical asepsis: practices that eliminate microorganisms and their spores from sterile items or areas (sterile technique)
     a. Used in operative procedures, delivery room, and caring for patients with breaks in skin and for procedures that enter sterile body cavities (e.g., bladder, lung, and vein)
     b. General principles
        (1) Sterile items become nonsterile (contaminated) when touched by anything that is not sterile
        (2) Sterile field that becomes wet is considered nonsterile
        (3) Sterile items out of eyesight or below waist level are considered nonsterile
        (4) Nurses need to develop a sterile conscience (self-judgment of whether aseptic practices have been broken) and act accordingly
     c. Means of sterilization
        (1) Steam under pressure: autoclave
        (2) Boiling
        (3) Liquid chemicals
        (4) Gas
  4. Isolation and barrier techniques (protective asepsis): practices that limit the transfer of microorganisms either from the infected person or to a highly susceptible person
     a. Category-specific isolation
        (1) Enteric: to reduce spread of pathogens via feces (e.g., hepatitis A)
        (2) Respiratory: to reduce spread of pathogens through the air (e.g., pneumonia)
        (3) TB isolation: to reduce exposure in health care settings; gown and particulate respirator mask, patient in negative air pressure isolation room
        (4) Strict: to reduce spread of pathogens by air or contact (e.g., chickenpox)

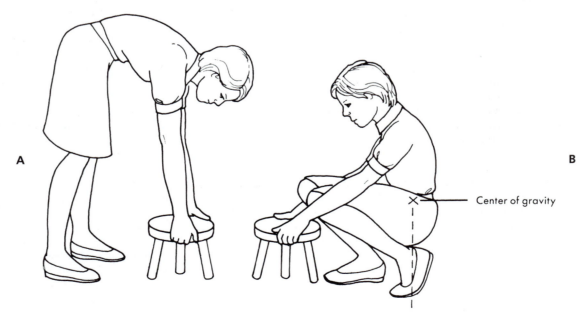

Center of gravity

Figure 2-3. **A,** Lifting with poor body mechanics: using back muscles. **B,** Lifting with good body mechanics: using leg muscles with object close to body. (Adapted from Sorrentino SA: *Textbook for nursing assistants*, ed 3, St Louis, 1992, Mosby.)

(5) Drainage/secretion: to reduce spread of pathogens by contact with the infected person or contaminated articles (linens) (e.g., draining wounds)

(6) Universal blood and body fluid (universal precautions): used by everyone to prevent transmission by direct or indirect contact with blood or body fluids (e.g., AIDS)

(7) Care of severely compromised patients: to protect a highly susceptible person (with lowered resistance) from becoming infected (e.g., leukemia)

b. Disease-specific isolation: each disease receives its specific protective measures

C. Types of infections
   1. Nosocomial: acquired as a result of hospitalization
   2. Local: confined to a relatively small, specific area (e.g., a wound)
   3. Systemic: infection spreads throughout body

COMMUNICATION

A. Definition: exchange of messages between two or more people, including information, thoughts, and feelings
B. Purposes in nursing
   1. To establish a meaningful, helping relationship between nurse and patient
   2. To transmit information between health care workers
C. Means
   1. Verbal
   2. Written
   3. Nonverbal
D. Guidelines
   1. Verbal communication
      a. Introduce self, stating name and title
      b. Be sincerely interested in the patient
      c. Be an attentive, active listener
      d. Stand or sit close to the patient
      e. Allow the patient to express thoughts and feelings freely without fear of being judged
      f. Clarify what has been said to ensure understanding
      g. Ask open-ended questions rather than questions resulting in yes or no answers: "what has happened to change your mind?"
      h. Use incomplete sentences: "you are afraid that …"
      i. Report information accurately and thoroughly
      j. Report abnormal findings immediately
      k. Maintain confidentiality
   2. Written communication
      a. Record information clearly, concisely, and accurately
      b. Nurses' notes are part of a legal document
         (1) Use pen
         (2) Use only standard abbreviations
         (3) Do not erase or obliterate errors (Fig. 2-4)

(4) Leave no blank spaces
(5) Sign the note at the time it is written
(6) Date and time each entry

c. Formats for nurses' notes
   (1) Narrative—in paragraph form
   (2) SOAP: **S**ubjective data, **O**bjective data, **A**ssessment, **P**lan (Fig. 2-5)
   (3) PIE: **P**roblem, **I**ntervention, **E**valuation
   (4) Focus charting: Data (assessment); Action (planning/implementation); Response (evaluation)
   (5) Charting by exception: used with flow sheets, pertinent data charted at beginning shift, only changes in treatments or patient condition noted after that; must include details on patient status for accurate monitoring

3. Nonverbal communication
   a. Exchanging messages by body posture, movements, gestures, and touch
   b. Often a more accurate expression of what is being thought or felt than verbal expression

Basic Human Needs

A. Definition: described by the psychologist Abraham Maslow as those needs that must be met for humans to function at their highest possible level
B. Used by many nurses as a systematic guide for assessment
C. Premises
   1. There is a hierarchy of needs; lower level needs must be met before higher level ones can be addressed
   2. People will usually be able to meet their own needs
   3. When people are unable to meet their own needs, intervention is required
   4. In caring for the whole person, the nurse is involved in helping to meet the basic needs as well as in dealing with signs and symptoms of disease
D. Hierarchy of needs (Fig. 2-6)
   1. Physiologic: oxygen, water, food, elimination, rest and sleep, activity, sexuality, and relief of pain
   2. Safety and security: protection from injury, maintenance of body defenses, structure and order in both the environment and relationships, and freedom from anxiety
   3. Love and belonging: not just romantic love but a feeling of affection (the need for caring relationships)
   4. Esteem: a feeling of worth and value to both self and others
   5. Self-actualization: reaching one's fullest potential

4/18/92	Went for ~~chest~~ @ leg x-ray via wheelchair
4 PM	Mary Jones, L.P.N.

Figure 2-4.   Correcting an error in a nurse's note.

4/18/92	PROBLEM #6 — Drainage on Cast, Ⓛ
4 PM	lateral aspect of knee
	S — "I have no pain or numbness"
	O — Toes pink, warm, mobile. VS stable
	A — Normal postoperative drainage
	P — Mark area of drainage. Reassess patient and cast q ½ hr.
	Elaine Stevens, L.P.N.

Figure 2-5.   **A,** Nurse's note in SOAP format.

Continued

NURSE'S RECORD

ADDRESSOGRAPH

000-123
Doe, Jane   Room 348ᴬ
female - 60
Dr. Pearson-Bennett

Great Plains Regional Medical Center

Code: ✓ = Yes	0 = No	⊗ = Refer to Nurse's Notes

DATE:	12/4/94	/

	DIET Cl Liq	APPETITE

CODE for 23:00 to 7:00		A = Awake		S = Sleeping		C = Comatose	
23:00 A	24:00 S	1:00 S	2:00 S	3:00 A	4:00 S	5:00 S	6:00 A

		100%
B	Cl Liq	100%
D		
S		

G = Good	F = Fair	P = Poor

	OBSERVATIONS:	23-7	7-15	15-23
SYSTEMS	CardioVascular, Regular	✓	✓	
	G.I., soft	✓	✓	
	G.U., voiding	✓	⊗	
	Catheter care	0	0	
	Neuro., no deficit	✓	✓	
	Resp., Regular	✓	✓	
	Skin Assessment	✓	✓	
	O₂	0	0	
	Telemetry	0	0	
ROUTINE	Bath	0	BB	
	Oral Care	✓	✓	
	Back Care	✓	✓	
	Side Rails up	✓	✓	
	Call Light in reach	✓	✓	
	Bed in Lo Position	✓	✓	
	Turn every 2°	✓	✓	
	Safety Reminder Device	0	0	
IVs	Location	RT Hand	RT Hand	
	Site Care			
	Tubing Change	✓	✓	
	Site Evaluation q 8 hours	✓	✓	
	Labels Dated	✓	✓	
	Flow Meter	✓	✓	
	Discontinued	0	0	
	Site Change	0	0	
	IV to Heparin Lock	IV	IV	
OTHER	Egg Crate			

INITIALS:	FE FE	JC JC	/

NURSE'S NOTES: 0600   awake and alert. Skin pink, arm and dry. T-tube draining dark green liquid. IV infusing in lt. antecubital area @ 20 gtts/minute. No evidence of erythema or edema. Sleeping well for 2 hour intervals. Has obtained relief from pain since 11p.m. medication. Ambulated to bathroom, voided 100 ml of dark amber urine c/o slight vertigo and assisted to bed. Dressings dry and intact. ⁓⁓⁓⁓⁓⁓⁓⁓⁓ F Ellefson R.N.

0700-1100   0700   alert and oriented x3. Skin pink, warm & dry. 99⁸-88-22. Denies incisional discomfort. Coughs well c̄ splinting of incision. Cough non-productive, lungs clear, bowel sounds hyperactive. Abdominal dressing dry and intact. T-tube draining dark green liquid, 30 ml drainage in bag. IV infusing @ 20 gtts/minute in lt. antecubital space, no erythema or edema @ site J. Christensen. LPN

0900   ambulated to bathroom with 1 assist. c/o burning on urination ⊗ Voided 100 ml of dark, amber, cloudly urine. T. 101² (0), c/o feeling hot and flushed.
1100   Dr. Pearson-Bennett notified. Fluids encouraged. #16 Fr. Catheter inserted s̄ difficulty. 300 ml of dark, amber, cloudy urine obtained. Specimen to laboratory for C & S. IV antibiotic started after catheterization by G Johnston RN Oral fluids taken well. A bd. dressings changed-incision approximated. Staples intact - no erythema noted. T-tube in place. T. 100 (0). Resting comfortably.
⁓⁓⁓⁓⁓⁓⁓⁓⁓ J. Christensen. LPN

SIGNATURES:	G. J. Garnet Johnston. RN FE Francis Ellefson RN
	J.C. Jessica Christensen. LPN

Figure 2-5, cont'd.   **B,** Narrative charting. (Courtesy Great Plains Regional Medical Center, North Platte, Neb.)

DATE	12/7	
TIME	FOCUS	NURSES NOTES
1400	post-op pain	Ambulating in hall c̄ moderate assist. I.V. infusing
		@ 20 gtts/min. Still feels warm, main concern is
		incisional pain, splinting is helpful. Positioned in
		bed c̄ pillows for support. Medicated for pain.
		Practiced relaxation breathing exercises. *J. Christensen LPN*
1400	pain/fever	States, "I am more comfortable and relaxed now." Skin warm
		and dry. T. 99⁶ (O). c/o some burning on urination,
		less than in a.m. Taking fluids well. Urine light
		yellow and less cloudy. ～～～～～ *J. Christensen LPN*

Figure 2-5, cont'd.   **C,** Focus charting nurse's notes.

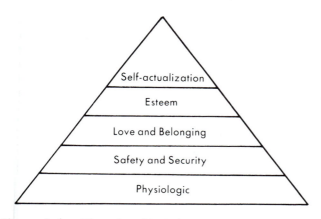

Figure 2-6.   Hierarchy of basic human needs as described by Maslow.

The Nursing Process

A. Definition: a set of predetermined steps used by nurses to identify and to help solve patient problems
B. Purposes
   1. To provide planned, coordinated, and individualized patient care
   2. To communicate problems and approaches among all those providing patient care
C. The process: names of steps differ slightly according to various sources but include the following

1. Assessment: gathering and organizing of data; statement of patient problems (unmet needs); the nursing diagnosis
2. Planning: setting goals to be accomplished and constructing a plan of action to accomplish the goals
3. Implementation: carrying out the nursing actions to accomplish the goals and solve the problem (meet the need)
4. Evaluation: determining whether the goal was accomplished and the problem solved

Assessment: A Continuous Process

A. Sources of data
   1. Patient
   2. Family or significant others
   3. Patient's chart
      a. Physician's order sheet
      b. Nurses' notes
      c. Laboratory reports
         (1) Blood chemistry
            (a) Electrolytes: see fluid and electrolyte balance
            (b) Creatinine: assesses kidney function
         (2) Complete blood count (CBC): assesses adequacy of the various blood cells: red, white, and platelets
         (3) Blood sugar (BS) or glucose: fasting (FBS) or postprandial (after meals)
      d. X-ray reports
         (1) Chest x-ray examination: assesses condition of lungs and size of heart

(2) Upper gastrointestinal (UGI) series: assesses condition of esophagus, stomach, and duodenum with barium sulfate used as the contrast medium

(3) Barium enema (BaE): assesses condition of colon with barium sulfate used as the contrast medium

(4) Gallbladder series (GBS): assesses condition of the gallbladder with radiopaque dye

 e. Electrocardiogram (ECG) reports: assesses the electrical activity of the heart

 f. Biopsy reports: assesses a tissue specimen for cell changes

 g. Progress notes of other health care workers

(1) Physician

(2) Social worker

(3) Dietician

(4) Physical therapist

(5) Occupational therapist

(6) Respiratory therapist

4. Nursing report

B. Subjective versus objective data

 1. Subjective data

  a. Information reported by the patient

  b. Information that is not observable by another person

EXAMPLES

Pain

Nausea

Anxiety

Dizziness

Ringing in the ears (tinnitus)

Numbness

 2. Objective data

  a. Information gathered through the senses: sight, hearing, smell, and feel

  b. Information gathered with a measuring instrument: thermometer, sphygmomanometer, and scale

EXAMPLES

Vital signs

Weight, height

Hematuria

Wheezing

Edema

Cyanosis

C. Methods of gathering data

 1. Formal interviewing (communication with patient or family or significant others): usually on patient's admission to the hospital

  a. Gather data on age, occupation, reason for hospitalization, medications, allergies, previous hospitalizations, previous illnesses, prostheses, valuables, and special diet

  b. Gather data on difficulty with activities of daily living (ADLs), sleep, elimination, activity, eating, and any special needs

 2. Listening

 3. Observation of the patient and attached equipment

  a. Use and orderly approach

(1) Head-to-toe

(2) System-by-system

(3) Basic human needs

  b. Look for signs and symptoms of disease or change in disease

4. Physical examination

 a. Methods

(1) Inspection

(2) Palpation

(3) Percussion

(4) Auscultation

 b. Assisting with the physical examination

(1) Be sure that the patient understands the examination and why it is being done

(2) Gather equipment

(3) Position patient appropriately (Fig. 2-7)

(4) Drape covers to provide for privacy

(5) Assist as necessary

(6) After the examination make the patient comfortable and safe, following orders, if any

(7) Chart the procedure and patient's reactions; note specimens obtained

 c. The practical nurse's role in assisting with diagnostic examinations

(1) Explain procedure to the patient

(2) Explain and carry out specific requirements

 (a) Nothing by mouth (NPO) or special meals

 (b) Clothing

 (c) Positioning

 (d) Medications

(3) Chest x-ray examinations: no metal objects in view of x-ray (zippers, bra fastenings, necklaces, and pins)

(4) Blood studies: see agency's procedure manual for requirements of various studies

(5) UGI series: nothing by mouth after midnight (NPO p̄ MN), medication or enema to eliminate barium after the x-ray examination

(6) BaE: low-residue meal evening before, NPO p̄ MN, medications or enema to clear colon before and after x-ray examination

(7) Excretory urogram or intravenous pyelogram (IVP): NPO p̄ MN, medications to clear colon before x-ray examination; uses iodine-based dye; notify physician if patient is allergic to iodine or shellfish

(8) GBS: fat-free meal evening before, NPO p̄ MN, oral ingestion of dye tablets; dye is iodine based; check patient for iodine or shellfish allergy

(9) Lumbar puncture: signed consent form is required; empty bladder and bowel before procedure; patient lies curled on side with head almost touching knees; nurse faces patient holding shoulders and knees; patient remains flat in bed after procedure

5. Measurement of vital signs: to assess functioning of cardiovascular and respiratory systems

 a. Temperature

(1) Normal ranges

 (a) Axillary: 96° to 98° F

 (b) Oral: 97° to 99° F

 (c) Rectal: 98° to 100° F

 (d) Tympanic: 97° to 99° F

(2) Oral temperature

 (a) Mercury thermometer left in place 2 to 4 minutes or according to agency policy

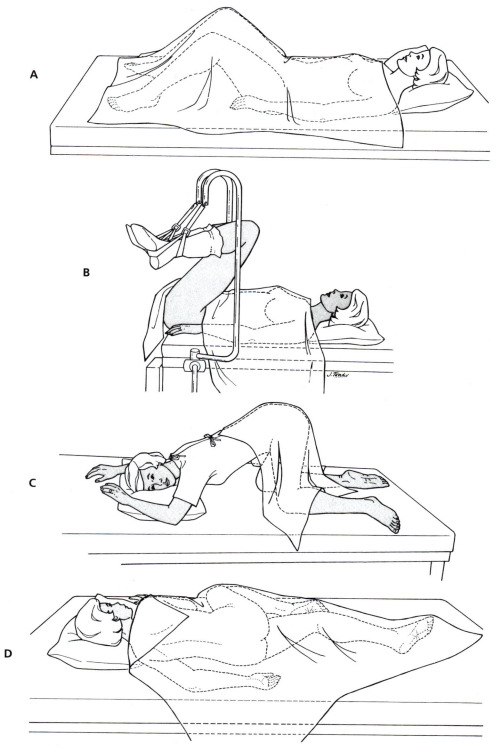

Figure 2-7.   Positioning and draping for the physical examination. **A,** Dorsal recumbent position. **B,** Lithotomy position. **C,** Knee-chest position. **D,** Sims' position. (Adapted from Sorrentino SA: *Textbook for nursing assistants*, ed 3, St Louis, 1992, Mosby.)

(b) Electronic thermometer left in place until final reading is indicated

(c) Wait 10 minutes if the patient has been eating, smoking, drinking a hot or cold beverage, or chewing gum

(d) Contraindications
- Patient is receiving oxygen
- Patient is irrational or unconscious
- Patient is under 5 years of age
- Patient is breathing through the mouth
- Patient is prone to seizures
- Patient recently had oral surgery or mouth trauma
- Patient is on suicide precautions

(3) Rectal temperature

(a) Mercury thermometer held in place 3 to 4 minutes or according to agency policy

(b) Electronic thermometer held in place until final reading is indicated

(c) Lubricate before inserting; insert 1½ inches (3.75 cm)

(d) Contraindications
- Rectal or perineal surgery
- Diseases of the rectum
- Diarrhea

(4) Axillary temperature

(a) Mercury thermometer held in place 10 minutes

(b) Electronic thermometer held in place until final reading is indicated

(c) Pat dry the axilla before inserting; hold arm close to side

(5) Tympanic temperature

(a) Press "On" button and apply disposable cover on probe tip

(b) Seal ear opening with probe; seal outer ear opening in infants

(c) Press "Scan" button and read temperature after beeper sounds

(d) Discard probe cover and replace thermometer in recharger

(e) Contraindications
- Recent exposure to cold air
- Inflammatory ear condition

b. Pulse: the beat of the heart heard at the apex or felt at specific sites as a wave of blood flows through an artery

(1) Observe rate, rhythm, and strength

(2) Normal adult range: 60 to 80 beats/min varies greatly among individuals; rate is more rapid for children

(3) If rate or rhythm is irregular, take pulse apically and count for one full minute

(4) Variations

(a) Bradycardia: slow heart rate—under 60 beats/min

(b) Tachycardia: fast heart beat—over 100 beats/min

(c) Irregular: intervals between beats are uneven

(d) Thready: weak pulse—easily obliterated

(e) Bounding: very strong pulse—difficult to obliterate

(5) Sites: felt with fingertips at places where an artery crosses over muscle or bone close to the skin and at the apex of the heart

(a) Temporal
(b) Carotid
(c) Brachial
(d) Radial
(e) Femoral
(f) Popliteal
(g) Pedal
(h) Apical: heard with stethoscope

(6) Apical-radial pulse: to detect a difference between rates at the two sites (the pulse deficit)

(a) Requires two people: one taking the radial pulse and one taking the apical pulse

(b) Must be counted simultaneously for 1 full minute

(c) Apical rate can never be lower than the radial rate

c. Respiration: the process of inhaling and exhaling air into and out of the lungs; one inhalation plus one exhalation equals one respiration

(1) Observe rate, rhythm, and depth; normal adult range is 14 to 20 respirations per minute; varies greatly with activity level; rate is higher for children

(2) Patient must not be aware that respirations are being observed

(3) Variations

(a) Apnea: absence of breathing
(b) Tachypnea: rapid breathing
(c) Stertorous: noisy breathing—snoring
(d) Cheyne-Stokes: rhythmic repeated cycles of slow shallow respirations increasing in depth rate, then gradually becoming slower and more shallow, followed by a period of apnea; often precedes death
(e) Dyspnea: difficulty breathing
(f) Orthopnea: breathing is possible only while in an upright position
(g) Kussmaul's: paroxysms of dyspnea often preceding diabetic coma

(4) Count respirations for 1 full minute if rate is abnormal or rhythm is irregular

d. Blood pressure (BP): force exerted by the blood against the walls of the arteries (measured in millimeters [mm] of mercury [Hg])

(1) Normal adult range is 60 to 80 mm Hg diastolic, 90 to 120 mm Hg systolic, varies among individuals and with activity

(2) Can be measured at brachial artery or popliteal artery

(3) Be sure cuff is proper size for the individual

(4) Terminology

(a) Systolic: pressure in the arteries during contraction of the heart

(b) Diastolic: pressure in the arteries during relaxation of the heart

(c) Hypotension: lower than normal blood pressure—under 100/60

(d) Hypertension: higher than normal blood pressure—140/90

(e) Pulse pressure: difference between systolic and diastolic pressures

(f) Pulse oximetry: Noninvasive continuous monitor of blood oxygen saturation

    (1) Normal adult range 95% to 100%

    (2) Report readings under 90%, indicate hypoxia. SaO_2 under 70% is life-threatening

    (3) Clip-on or adhesive probe attaches to finger, toe, earlobe, or bridge of nose

    (4) Uses light for reading, do not block light on probe. Area being assessed should be clean, dry, and without nail polish

    (5) Rotate clip q4h, adhesive

    (6) Check abnormal readings with arterial blood gases

6. Measurement of weight and height

  a. Weight

    (1) Should be done before breakfast

    (2) Should be done in same amount of clothing each day; shoes should be off

    (3) Can use results in establishing medication dosages, gain or loss of body fluid, and nutritional status

    (4) Can use standing, chair, or stretcher scale; be sure scale is balanced

  b. Height

    (1) Have patient be in bare feet, standing on a paper towel

    (2) Have patient stand tall

    (3) Can use in determining some medication dosages and anesthesia requirements

7. Collection of specimens

  a. General guidelines

    (1) Follow your agency's procedure for collection, container, labels, requisitions, and recording

    (2) Label all specimen containers correctly and send with a laboratory requisition

    (3) Send specimens to the laboratory promptly

    (4) Wear protective gloves

    (5) Wash hands thoroughly after handling specimen

  b. Urine specimens

    (1) Urinalysis: routine examination of urine

      (a) Patient and container need only be clean

      (b) Often collected as part of admission procedure

    (2) Culture and sensitivity

      (a) Clean-catch, midstream: genitalia and meatus are cleansed; specimen is taken after stream has started but before voiding is completed

      (b) Catheterized specimen: by using sterile technique and equipment

    (3) 24-hour specimens: first voiding is discarded and time is noted; all urine for the next 24 hours is collected; see agency policy for type of container and storage methods

    (4) Sugar and acetone testing

      (a) Urine should be obtained 30 to 60 minutes before meal or at designated time

      (b) Double-voided specimen gives more accurate results

        ▪ Have patient empty bladder

        ▪ Collect specimen as soon as patient can void again

        ▪ May need additional fluids to produce specimen

      (c) Test specimen with Tes-tape, Clinitest, Clinistix, or Keto-diastix; follow manufacturer's directions precisely for accurate results

      (d) Report results immediately to medication nurse

      (e) Record results in proper place

    (5) Specimens from indwelling catheter

      (a) Closed drainage system must be maintained

      (b) Specimens must be obtained from specimen "port" with needle and syringe by sterile technique

  c. Stool specimens

    (1) Collect in clean bedpan

    (2) Use tongue depressor or wooden spatula to transfer stool to specimen container

    (3) Types of testing

      (a) For blood: occult (guaiac, Hematest); patient must be on a red meat–free diet 3 days before test

      (b) For culture and sensitivity: use sterile container

      (c) For ova and parasites: stool must still be warm when it reaches the laboratory

  d. Sputum specimens

    (1) Best collected in the morning before breakfast

    (2) Patient first rinses mouth with water

    (3) Instruct patient to take deep breath, cough deeply, and expectorate into container

    (4) Specimen must be from the lung, not just mouth saliva

  e. Blood specimen: capillary puncture e.g., blood glucose testing. May be finger stick for child/adult, heel stick for infant. May require agency certification

    (1) Explain procedure to patient; warn that it does hurt

    (2) Assemble equipment: gloves, alcohol swab, lancet, collector, gauze or cotton ball, and adhesive bandage

    (3) Wash hands; don gloves

    (4) Enhance blood supply by applying warmth; do not milk site

    (5) Puncture side of nondominant finger or side of heel

    (6) Puncture with lancet; wipe away first drop of blood; collect sample

    (7) Apply pressure to site; apply bandage

  f. Blood specimen: venipuncture; requires puncture of vein for collection of several ml of blood for variety of laboratory tests; agency certification usually required

    (1) Explain procedure to patient; procedure hurts

    (2) Assemble equipment: gloves, tourniquet, alcohol swabs, sterile gauze pads, tape, a sharps container, appropriate vacuum tubes, vacuum adaptor, and double-ended needle

(3) Wash hands, don gloves

(4) Hyperextend arm for ease of access to antecubital vein; apply tourniquet; have patient make fist

(5) Clean site with alcohol; pull skin taut from below site; insert needle (bevel up) at 5° angle

(6) Once needle "pops" into vein, slide vacuum tube onto needle; remove and replace tubes as each fills

(7) Remove final tube; loosen tourniquet; lay gauze over puncture site, remove needle and apply pressure to site

(8) Immediately discard needle into sharps container; label tubes before leaving patient's side

  g. Other specimens

(1) Vomitus: may be tested for blood

(2) Gastric analysis: examination of stomach contents; obtained by aspirating from nasogastric tube

(3) Wound drainage: if infection is suspected

D. Statement of patient problems requiring nursing intervention

1. Identifying unmet basic human needs resulting in a problem for the patient

2. Identifying problems arising from the patient's signs and symptoms

3. Actual problems: those that the patient is currently having

4. Potential problems: those that may develop and should be prevented from occurring (see the example below)

E. Nursing diagnosis: the practical nurse assists the registered nurse in formulating nursing diagnosis

PLANNING PATIENT CARE

A. Definition: process of setting priorities, determining patient-centered goals, and deciding on nursing actions to achieve the goals; ends with writing of the nursing care plan

B. Setting priorities

1. Problems that are life threatening are of highest priority

2. When no single problem seems more important than the others, the patient may help determine priorities

C. Determining goals/expected outcomes

1. Stated in terms of patient behavior so that achievement can easily be evaluated

2. Whenever possible patients should be involved in setting goals

3. Long-term goals are those hoped for in the future, usually set by the registered nurse

4. Short-term goals are those sought immediately or in the near future

D. Decisions about which nursing measures to use are based on sound knowledge of current nursing practice, principles, rationales, and judgment

E. Written nursing care plan provides continuity of patient care (see the example below)

IMPLEMENTATION OF NURSING MEASURES

A. Principles

1. Preparation

  a. Nurse: must know how, when, and why measure is to be performed, checking for a physician's order when necessary

  b. Patient/family/significant others

(1) To reduce anxiety, patients need to know what measure is to be performed and why, as well as what is expected of them

(2) May need special preparation for the specific measure: positioning, medications, attire

  c. Have all necessary equipment ready and in working order

2. Performance

  a. Nurse must have knowledge of and ability to perform measure and to seek help when necessary

  b. Medical asepsis is always followed: surgical asepsis and universal precautions are followed as required

  c. Work must be organized to conserve nurse's and patient's energy and to meet patient's need for security

  d. Assessment of patient's response to the measure is ongoing

3. Aftercare

  a. Patient made safe and comfortable

  b. Equipment cleaned and returned to proper place or disposed of

  c. Evaluation of results of the measure and whether it helped achieve the goal

4. Reporting and recording

  a. Significant observations immediately

  b. When the measure was performed and the results

EXAMPLE: Actual and potential unmet basic needs and problems

Situation: At 7 AM, Mrs. Clayton tells the nurse that she has a productive cough. She states that it began at about 3 AM and continues.

Actual problem: productive cough
Actual unmet need: rest and sleep
Potential unmet need: oxygen
Potential problem: decreased oxygen

EXAMPLE	Nursing care plan for 39-year-old woman 4 days after cesarean section	
Problem	**Goal**	**Nursing actions**
Constipation × 4 days	Will have a stool today and at least every other day thereafter	Encourage walking Encourage fluids to at least 250 ml/day Encourage eating roughage and fruits Give prn laxative Record bowel movements (BMs) in nurses' notes every shift Teach patient relationship of activity, fluids, and fiber to stool elimination

EVALUATION OF PLAN OF CARE

A. Criteria for evaluation
   1. Has the need been met?
   2. Is the problem solved or being solved?
   3. Has the goal/expected outcome been achieved?
B. Revision of the nursing care plan
   1. Based on evaluation of effectiveness
   2. Practical nurse collaborates with the registered nurse in revising problem list, goals, and nursing measures

Measures to Meet Oxygen Needs

A. Assessment: color, level of consciousness, vital signs, presence of cough (productive or nonproductive), nature of sputum (amount, consistency, and color), and energy level
B. General measures
   1. Encourage exercise and activity to help expand lungs, providing better oxygenation
   2. Bedridden patients must be turned and positioned every 2 hours (q2h) to prevent pooling of secretions in the lungs
   3. Encourage coughing and deep breathing at least q2h for inactive or bedridden patients to help with oxygenation and bringing up secretions
   4. Ensure adequate fluid intake to keep secretions thin, thus easier to expectorate
C. Use of nebulizer (aerosol)
   1. Method of delivering medications directly to the respiratory tract
   2. Nebulizer breaks liquids into a mist of droplets, which are inhaled
D. Incentive spirometer: to improve inspiratory volume
   1. With lips sealed around a mouthpiece, the patient takes a deep breath, holds it for 3 seconds, and slowly exhales
   2. The spirometer indicates with a light or small plastic balls reaching an indicated level whether the patient has inhaled the desired volume
E. Intermittent positive pressure breathing therapy (IPPB)
   1. Forces the patient to inhale more deeply, allowing better oxygenation and loosening of secretions
   2. May be attached to oxygen or compressed air
   3. Humidity is provided, usually by normal saline solution
   4. Medications may be added
   5. Patient should be sitting up during treatment and encouraged to cough up secretions after treatment
F. Chest physical therapy
   1. Postural drainage: use of various positions so that gravity can assist in removal of secretions (Fig. 2-8)
   2. Percussion is a manual technique of striking the chest wall over the affected area with cupped hands in a rhythmic motion
   3. Vibration is a manual compression and tremorlike motion with hands or mechanical device against chest wall of affected area done during exhalation
   4. Nurse positions patient so affected areas are vertical and gravity can assist in drainage
   5. Position also depends on diagnosis and condition

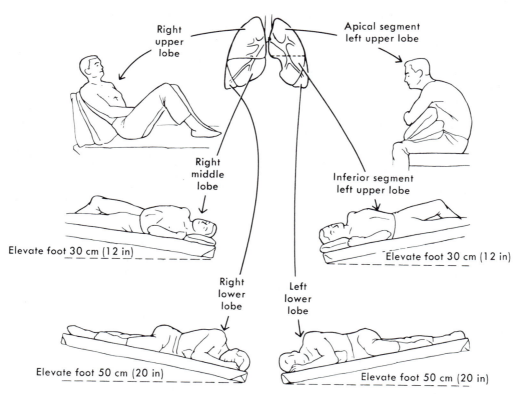

Right upper lobe

Apical segment left upper lobe

Right middle lobe

Elevate foot 30 cm (12 in)

Inferior segment left upper lobe

Elevate foot 30 cm (12 in)

Right lower lobe

Left lower lobe

Elevate foot 50 cm (20 in)

Elevate foot 50 cm (20 in)

Figure 2-8.   Positions for postural drainage. (From Phipps WJ, Long BC, Woods NF, editors: *Medical-surgical nursing: concepts and clinical practice*, ed 4, St Louis, 1991, Mosby.)

6. Schedule before or at least 2 hours after meals. Provide emesis basin and tissues; oral hygiene after treatment
7. This therapy is contraindicated in patients with lung abscess or tumors, pneumothorax, and diseases of the chest wall

G. Suctioning: oral, nasopharyngeal, or tracheal
   1. To remove accumulated secretions blocking airway or to obtain sputum specimen
   2. Usually a sterile procedure
   3. Introduce catheter gently; do not apply suction while introducing catheter
   4. Suction intermittently for no more than 10 seconds
   5. Slowly withdraw catheter by rotating motion while suctioning continues
   6. Unless there are copious amounts of secretions, wait 30 seconds between suctionings
   7. Repeat procedure until all excess secretions are removed
   8. Administer oxygen before and between suctionings if needed

H. Administration of oxygen
   1. Safety precautions
      a. Caution patients and visitors that smoking is prohibited
      b. Post warning sign on door or bed: NO SMOKING—OXYGEN IN USE
      c. Do not use heating pads, electric blankets, or electric razors
      d. Do not use woolen blankets
      e. Secure oxygen tanks so they do not tip over
   2. Physician's order is required for method of administration, rate of oxygen flow, or concentration
   3. Oxygen must always be humidified
   4. Nasal cannula: prongs fit into nares
      a. Turn oxygen on and check flow through prongs before positioning on patient
      b. Adjust strap after placing cannula on patient
      c. Periodically check that there is sufficient water in humidity source
      d. Periodically check patient's nares and behind ears for pressure
      e. Periodically assess patient for changes in condition
   5. Oxygen by mask: simple; Venturi (delivers oxygen in precise concentrations)
      a. Proceed as with nasal cannula
      b. Fit mask snugly to face and adjust strap
      c. Periodically assess patient and equipment as with nasal cannula

I. Care of patient with a tracheostomy
   1. Tracheotomy: opening into the trachea
   2. Tracheostomy: tube inserted into tracheal opening
   3. Tube is either metal or plastic, which is usually cuffed (Figs. 2-9 and 2-10)
   4. Tube is held securely in place with cotton ties around the neck (Fig. 2-11)
   5. Ties are changed with extreme caution to prevent patient from coughing out tube
   6. A gauze dressing is placed under the tube to absorb secretions and must be changed at least every shift
   7. Inner cannula is removed, cleaned with peroxide and pipe cleaners, and rinsed with normal saline at least once a shift by sterile technique; commercially prepared kits are available

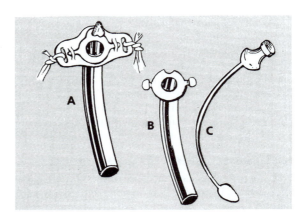

Figure 2-9. Metal tracheostomy tube. **A,** Outer cannula. **B,** Inner cannula. **C,** Obturator. (From Harkness GA, Dincher JR: *Medical-surgical nursing: total patient care,* ed 9, St Louis, 1996, Mosby.)

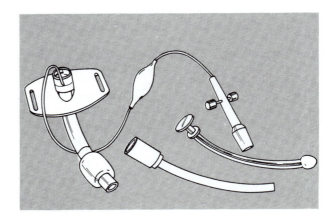

Figure 2-10. Cuffed tracheostomy tube. (From Harkness GA, Dincher JR: *Medical-surgical nursing: total patient care,* ed 9, St Louis, 1996, Mosby.)

8. Skin around stoma is cleansed with peroxide, rinsed with saline, and assessed at least once a shift
9. Patient is often apprehensive and needs frequent reassurance
10. Tube must be suctioned frequently

J. Medication classifications: refer to Chapter 3 for more detailed information on drugs that affect the respiratory system
   1. Respiratory stimulants
   2. Respiratory depressants
   3. Those acting on mucous membranes: administered orally or as spray or vapor
      a. Mucolytics
      b. Expectorants
   4. Bronchodilators

MEASURES TO MEET FLUID NEEDS

A. Assessment: daily weights, comparison of intake and output, appearance of urine, presence of edema, fluid preferences, and skin turgor
B. Fluid excess (edema)

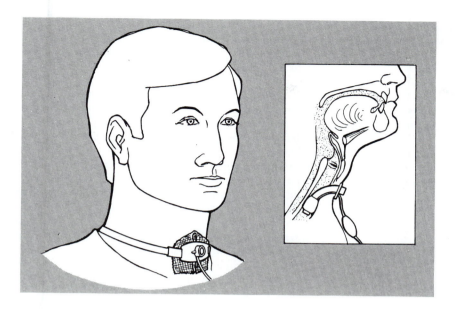

Figure 2-11. Tracheostomy tube in place. (From Harkness GA, Dincher JR: *Medical-surgical nursing: total patient care*, ed 9, St Louis, 1996, Mosby.)

1. Associated with heart and kidney disease: body unable to rid itself of excess fluid
2. Can result from excessive intravenous (IV) fluids
3. Observed as edema as well as weight gain and reduced urine output
4. Sites of edema: eyes, fingers, ankles, and sacral area
C. Fluid deficit (dehydration)
  1. Associated with inadequate fluid intake, diarrhea, excessive perspiration, vomiting, bleeding, and increased urine output
  2. Observed as dry skin and mucous membranes, thick mucus, poor skin turgor, behavioral changes, or changes in vital signs
D. Measuring intake and output
  1. Measure all fluids taken in: IV, tube feedings, and obvious fluids such as water, milk, ice cream, gelatin, custard, and soup
  2. Measure all fluids leaving the body: urine, vomitus, diarrhea, gastric secretions, and blood
  3. Know capacity of agency's fluid containers
  4. Set measuring containers on level surface to read measurements accurately
  5. Record and total amounts in appropriate places
E. Administering IV fluids
  1. Assess site of needle insertion
    a. Infiltration: fluid entering subcutaneous tissues instead of vein; area is pale, cool, and swollen
    b. Phlebitis: inflammation of vein; area is red, warm, and swollen
  2. Assess tubing: no kinks; no leakage along entire length of tubing; tubing should be labeled and changed every 48-72 hours or per agency policy
  3. Assess rate of flow
  4. Assess container
    a. It must match physician's order
    b. Check that the amount absorbed is on schedule
F. Medication classifications—diuretics: refer to Chapter 3 for more detailed information

Measures to Meet Nutritional Needs

A. Assessment: weight/height ratio, weight changes, skin and mucous membranes, food preferences, meal patterns, ability to eat, and appetite
B. Preparing for meals
  1. Environment
    a. Control odors, noise, and unpleasant sights; remove soiled equipment and linens
    b. Avoid stressful situations before and during mealtime
  2. Patient
    a. Provide oral hygiene and opportunity for elimination and hand washing
    b. Position comfortably, preferably in sitting position
  3. Meal tray
    a. Ensure correct tray for correct patient
    b. Arrange tray to be accessible to patient
    c. Assist in opening containers, removing covers, and cutting and preparing food
    d. Serve trays first to patients able to feed themselves
C. Assisting the patient to eat
  1. Place napkin across chest
  2. Explain what foods and liquids are on the tray
  3. Prepare foods and feed in order of patient's preference
  4. Encourage the patient to assist as much as possible
  5. Do not rush: allow time to chew and swallow
  6. Talk with the patient during meal
  7. Provide opportunity for hand washing and oral care
D. Gastric gavage (tube feeding)
  1. Used when patient is unable to eat, swallow, or take in adequate quantities of food
  2. Blended foods and fluids (commercially or agency prepared) are passed to the stomach through a nasogastric tube either intermittently or by slow continuous drip
  3. Check amount, frequency, and type ordered by physician
  4. Feeding must be at room temperature before administering
  5. Placement of tube must be checked before feeding begins
    a. By aspirating stomach contents with a syringe

b. Inject 10 cc of air into tube while simultaneously listening with a stethoscope over the stomach to hear a whoosing sound

6. Place patient in sitting position

7. Administer feeding slowly: 200 ml during 30- to 45-minute period

8. Feeding should be followed by ordered amount of water

9. Clamp tube after completion of feeding to prevent air entering stomach

10. If nausea, vomiting, diarrhea, or cramps occur, rate may be too fast or patient may be intolerant of feeding or volume

11. Tube may be left in place between feedings or removed after each feeding as ordered by physician

12. Have patient remain in sitting position for 45 minutes to help prevent aspiration

E. Medication classifications: refer to Chapter 3 for more detailed information

1. Vitamin supplements

2. Mineral supplements

Measures to Meet Urinary Elimination Needs

A. Assessment: intake/output ratio, color, odor, amount, and consistency of urine, frequency of urination, and continence

B. Common problems of urination

1. Incontinence: inability to control voiding
   a. Requires frequent skin care and linen change
   b. May be reduced with scheduled toileting

2. Retention: inability to void
   a. If adequate amounts of fluid have been taken in, no more than 8 hours should pass between voidings, except during sleeping hours
   b. Palpation of bladder can determine distention of full bladder

3. Anuria: no urine being produced by the kidneys

4. Dysuria: difficult or painful urination ("burning")

C. Assisting with urination

1. Offer bedpan or urinal at regularly scheduled times

2. Keep bedpan or urinal and toilet tissue within easy reach for patients who can assist themselves

3. Keep call signal within easy reach

4. Provide privacy

5. Hearing the sound of running water or having warm water poured over the perineum may induce voiding

6. Provide opportunity for hand washing after urination

D. Care of patient with retention catheter

1. Presence of indwelling catheter greatly predisposes patient to urinary tract infection

2. Opening a closed urinary system is to be avoided

3. Drainage container must be kept below level of the bladder but must not touch the floor

4. Drainage tubing must be free of kinks and catheter taped to patient's leg allowing slack

5. Drainage container is emptied at end of shift or if container becomes nearly full; urine is measured, assessed, and amount recorded

6. Catheter care is given at least once per shift and after every bowel movement
   a. Meatus and catheter are cleansed with soap and water; from meatus down catheter and away from body
   b. Removal of crusts and secretions from meatus and catheter may require use of hydrogen peroxide

c. A bacteriostatic ointment is often ordered to be applied to the meatus

7. Unless contraindicated, fluid intake should reach 2000 to 3000 ml/24 hr

E. Catheterization

1. "Straight": catheter removed at end of procedure; often ordered to relieve urine retention or to measure residual urine after voiding

2. Indwelling, retention or Foley: catheter is left in place in bladder

3. Assemble equipment: sterile catheterization tray or disposable kit containing catheter, basin, container with lid (for specimen, if ordered), cotton balls, antiseptic solution, lubricant, sterile gloves, and drape

4. For indwelling catheterization, add Foley catheter, syringe, solution for inflating balloon, drainage bag with tubing, and tape for securing catheter

5. After explaining procedure to patient and ensuring privacy, place female in dorsal recumbent position and male in supine position

6. Place equipment between patient's legs; using sterile technique open package, don gloves, and place drape

7. For female patient, while holding labia apart, cleanse vulva and meatus well going from front to back toward vagina; use cotton ball for one stoke only before discarding

8. For male patient, cleanse around penis from meatus toward base using each cotton ball once around

9. Insert catheter into meatus (3 to 4 inches [7.5 to 10 cm] in female and 6 to 8 inches [15 to 20 cm] in male) until urine flows; drain urine (no more than 750 ml at one time to prevent bleeding or shock); remove catheter ("straight") or inflate balloon and connect drainage tubing (indwelling)

F. Intermittent bladder irrigation (hand bladder irrigation)

1. To rid bladder and catheter of clots or mucus; to instill antibiotic or other solutions

2. Open technique
   a. Assemble equipment: sterile solution (type and amount as ordered), sterile container for solution, bulb syringe, and basin for return flow
   b. Disconnect catheter from drainage tube over empty basin; protect ends from contamination
   c. Allow solution to flow in by gravity or gentle pressure; drain by gravity or gentle solution; repeat until returns are clear or ordered amount of solution has been used
   d. Subtract amount of solution used from amount of returns; record output

3. Closed technique
   a. Assemble equipment: 20- to 30-ml syringe with needle, alcohol swabs, solution ordered, and clamp
   b. Draw solution into syringe by sterile technique
   c. Clamp tubing distal to needle entry point
   d. Cleanse resealable rubber entry port on drainage tubing with alcohol swab
   e. Insert needle into port
   f. Inject fluid into catheter
   g. Remove needle
   h. Release clamp and allow fluid to drain into drainage bag
   i. Observe fluid return

j. Repeat until ordered amount of solution has been used

k. Empty drainage bag, subtracting amount of irrigant from total; record urine output

G. Continuous bladder irrigation (through and through or three-way irrigation)

1. To prevent clot formation; to reduce obstruction of catheter; to circulate antibiotic or other solutions continuously in bladder

2. Equipment: patient has three-way catheter or needs sterile Y tube connector attached to regular two-way catheter's drainage channel; large bottle or bag of solution, with tubing attached, hanging from IV pole

3. With three-way catheter: using sterile technique

a. Remove plug from irrigating channel; protect plug and tubing from contamination

b. Insert solution tubing into irrigating channel

4. With two-way catheter: using sterile technique

a. Attach single end of sterile Y tube connector to catheter

b. Attach drainage tubing to one end of Y

c. Attach solution tubing to other end of Y

5. Start solution flow at rate ordered by physician

6. Observe fluid return through drainage tubing

7. Replace solution bottle or bag as it becomes nearly empty

8. Empty drainage container as it becomes nearly full and when solution container is replaced

9. Subtract amount of irrigant solution from total amount of drainage to record actual urine output

H. Removal of indwelling catheter

1. Assemble equipment: syringe without needle, underpad, basin, urinal or bedpan, toilet tissue, and protective gloves

2. After explaining procedure and ensuring privacy, place pad under patient

3. Remove tape from catheter and patient's leg

4. Put on protective gloves

5. Place basin under patient's meatus

6. Insert syringe into balloon channel; fluid will return on its own

7. After all fluid has returned, gently pull on catheter to remove it

8. If resistance is met, stop and obtain assistance

9. Assist patient to wash perineum

10. Teaching

a. Patient should continue to drink fluids

b. Burning on urination may occur during first few voidings

c. Complete continence and normal voiding pattern may take awhile to return

d. Patient should void into bedpan or urinal so that urine can be assessed

11. Encourage relaxation: anxiety may inhibit ability to void

12. Continue to assess bladder distention, intake/output ratio, and patient complaints until normal patterns of elimination are achieved

I. Medication classifications

1. Cholinergics: to induce bladder contraction (bethanechol [Urecholine] and neostigmine [Prostigmin])

2. Anticholinergics: to reduce bladder spasms and urinary frequency (methantheline [Banthine] and flavoxate hydrochloride [Urispas])

Measures to Meet Bowel Elimination Needs

A. Assessment: the patient's pattern of elimination; amount, color, consistency, odor, and shape of stool; patient's activity level; amount and type of food and fluid intake; passage of flatus; abdominal distention

B. Common problems of elimination

1. Constipation: passage of dry, hard feces

2. Diarrhea: frequent passage of liquid or unformed stools

3. Impaction: formation of a hardened mass of stool in the lower bowel forming an obstruction to the passage of normal stool; often characterized by the frequent seepage of small amount of liquid stool

4. Abdominal distention: swollen abdomen caused by retention of flatus in the intestines

C. General nursing measures

1. Encourage intake of roughage in the diet: fresh fruits and vegetables and whole grain breads and cereals

2. Encourage intake of adequate amounts of fluids unless contraindicated: 2000 to 3000 ml/day

3. Encourage maximum amount of physical activity

4. Encourage patient to respond to the urge to defecate

5. Position patient comfortably and provide adequate time and privacy for elimination

6. Provide access to call signal and toilet tissue

7. Provide opportunity for hand washing after elimination

D. Rectal tube

1. To assist in expelling flatus

2. Assemble equipment: rectal tube with flatus bag or waterproof pad, lubricant, glove, and tape

3. After explaining procedure and providing privacy, position patient in side-lying (Sims') position

4. With gloved hand insert lubricated tube 2 to 4 inches (5 to 10 cm) into rectum

5. Tape tube to patient's buttock and leave in place no longer than 20 to 30 minutes

6. Note passage of flatus or stool; report and record findings

E. Rectal suppository

1. To stimulate peristalsis and aid stool elimination; to soothe painful rectum or anus

2. Assemble equipment: suppository as ordered, glove, bedpan, and toilet tissue

3. Suppository begins to melt at room temperature, providing its own lubrication

4. Separate buttocks and with gloved index finger insert pointed end of suppository into anus

5. Gently insert 3 to 4 inches (7.5 to 10 cm) into rectum

6. Hold buttocks together until initial urge to defecate has passed

7. Best results occur within 30 minutes

F. Commercially prepared prefilled enema

1. To promote bowel or flatus movement

2. Assemble equipment: enema (usually 120 ml), underpad, bedpan, toilet paper, and gloves

3. After explaining procedure and providing privacy, place patient in side-lying (Sims') position

4. With gloved hand insert prelubricated tip of enema to the hub and squeeze container until most of solution is instilled

5. Encourage patient to retain solution until urge to defecate is felt

6. Place call signal, bedpan, and toilet tissue within easy reach
7. If patient uses toilet, instruct not to flush so that results can be assessed

G. Oil-retention enema
   1. To soften and lubricate stool, promoting easier passage
   2. Often followed by cleansing enema
   3. Equipment and administration are the same as for commercially prepared enema above
   4. Encourage patient to retain oil 30 to 60 minutes

H. Cleansing enemas
   1. To relieve constipation or flatus or to cleanse the bowel before diagnostic procedures, surgery, or childbirth
   2. Solutions used as ordered by physician
      a. Tap water: can cause fluid and electrolyte imbalance
      b. Soap solution: 5 ml of liquid soap to 1000 ml of water; can irritate mucous membranes of bowel
      c. Saline solution: can cause fluid and electrolyte imbalance
   3. Assemble equipment: disposable enema kit containing enema bag, tubing with clamp, liquid soap, and lubricant; waterproof underpad; solution at a temperature no greater than 105° F; bedpan and toilet tissue; IV pole; protective gloves
   4. After explaining procedure and providing privacy, place patient in side-lying (Sims') position (usually left)
   5. Put on protective gloves.
   6. Insert lubricated tubing about 3 to 5 inches (7.5 to 12.5 cm) into rectum
   7. With bottom of enema bag hanging 12 inches (30 cm) above anus or 18 inches (45 cm) above mattress, slowly administer 500 to 1000 ml of solution
   8. If patient complains of cramping or has difficulty retaining solution
      a. Slow administration rate, or
      b. Temporarily stop flow
      c. Encourage slow, deep breathing through the mouth
   9. After fluid has been administered, assist patient to bathroom or onto bedpan or commode; instruct patient not to flush toilet so that results can be assessed
   10. If enemas are ordered "until clear," repeat procedure until returns are clear of stool (or of barium after barium enema)
   11. Observe patient during procedure for signs of weakness or fatigue, which would necessitate stopping the procedure to allow rest

I. Digital removal of fecal impaction
   1. Breaking up the hard fecal mass and removing it
   2. Assemble equipment: gloves, waterproof underpad, lubricant, and bedpan
   3. Liberally lubricate gloved index finger
   4. With patient in side-lying (Sims') position gently insert finger into hardened mass of stool
   5. Gently break off small pieces of the stool, bringing them out and placing them in the bedpan
   6. Assess patient for signs of weakness and fatigue; this is an uncomfortable, tiring procedure and may need to be intermittently stopped
   7. Assist patient to bedpan: disimpaction may induce defecation

J. Colostomy irrigation
   1. To regulate the discharge and drainage of fecal contents and flatus
   2. Time of irrigation depends on physician's order and patient's own established routine; when colostomy has become regulated, irrigation may be only done every other day; some patients never irrigate their colostomy
   3. Assemble equipment
      a. Irrigating appliance (types vary)
      b. Irrigating container (enema bag)
      c. Tubing and catheter (may be part of enema kit)
      d. Irrigating solution: usually 500 to 1000 ml of tap water or physiologic saline solution at 100° F
      e. Lubricant
      f. Drainage bag (may be part of irrigating appliance) and bedpan if not using on toilet
      g. Waterproof underpad if being performed in bed
      h. Fresh colostomy appliance, dressing, or stoma pad
      i. IV pole
      j. Protective gloves
   4. After explaining procedure and ensuring privacy, place patient on toilet (most convenient) or in bed in side-lying (Sims') position
   5. Put on protective gloves
   6. Raise irrigation container 18 inches (45 cm) above stoma, clear catheter of air, lubricate catheter, introduce catheter through irrigating appliance, and insert catheter into stoma 2 to 6 inches (5 to 15 cm); do not advance if resistance is met
   7. Allow solution to flow slowly and remove catheter; return is usually completed within 45 to 60 minutes
   8. When return is completed, remove irrigating appliance, wash and dry abdomen, and apply fresh colostomy appliance, dressing, or stoma pad as indicated
   9. Record character and amount of returns, patient's tolerance, and degree of assistance provided by patient

K. Medication classifications: refer to Chapter 3 for more detailed information on drugs that affect the gastrointestinal (GI) system
   1. Stool softeners
   2. Laxatives/cathartics
   3. Antidiarrhetics

Measures to Meet Rest and Sleep Needs

Rest and sleep are necessary for restoring physical and mental well-being, reducing stress and anxiety, and maintaining the ability to attend to and concentrate on activities of life

A. Assessment: normal number of hours of sleep, usual bedtime, usual bedtime habits or practices, sleep difficulties, daytime fatigue, usual methods of obtaining rest, and sleep medications being used

B. Physician's orders for rest must be clarified: is bed rest ordered to provide rest for a damaged heart, the entire body, or an injured part such as a foot?

C. Providing for rest and sleep
   1. Promote relaxation: provide diversions, pain relief, clean, wrinkle-free bed, a noise-free and odor-free room, and easy access to bedside equipment and call signal; give a relaxing back rub
   2. Reduce patient's anxiety level by allowing time for the patient to talk about stressful or fear-producing situations
   3. If possible, position patient in usual sleeping position with amount of covers desired

4. Plan and organize care to allow the patient uninterrupted rest and sleep periods
5. Give sleeping medication if ordered and if required by the patient

D. Medication classifications: refer to Chapter 3 for more detailed information
   1. Sedatives: to reduce anxiety
   2. Hypnotics: to induce sleep

Measures to Meet Activity and Exercise Needs

Physical activity is necessary for proper functioning of all body systems as well as for promotion of emotional well-being; immobility can lead to physical as well as emotional disability

A. Assessment: posture, ability to walk, ability to turn and move in bed, usual activity level, and skin condition
B. Patient's activity and exercise level is ordered by the physician
   1. Bed rest (BR): patient is confined to bed
   2. Bathroom privileges (BRP): although confined to bed, patient may perform urinary and bowel elimination in the bathroom
   3. May dangle: although confined to bed, patient may sit on edge of bed with legs and feet hanging down over side of bed and supported by footstool
      a. Often accompanied by orders for frequency and duration of dangling time (e.g., dangle every shift for 10 minutes)
      b. Provide footstool
      c. Assess vital signs
      d. Stay with patient to assess tolerance and assist back to bed
   4. Allow to chair: although patient may sit in chair, he or she is not permitted to ambulate any farther
   5. Out of bed (OOB) ad lib: can and should perform as much activity out of bed as desired
   6. Encourage patients to perform as much activity as orders permit
C. Dangers of immobility
   1. Atelectasis: collapse of lung caused by reduced depth and rate of respirations or obstruction of lungs by excessive secretions
   2. Hypostatic pneumonia: caused by pooling of lung secretions and the resulting congestion
   3. Thrombus formation: caused by reduced rate of blood flow through the veins and prolonged coagulation time
   4. Constipation: caused by slowed peristaltic action
   5. Contractures: permanent shortening of muscles leading to joint immobility
   6. Skin breakdown and decubitus ulcer formation caused by prolonged pressure and reduced circulation to an area
   7. Development of urinary tract infections and kidney stones caused by stasis of urine and demineralization of bones
D. Measures to prevent dangers of immobility
   1. Coughing and deep breathing
      a. Performed q2h
      b. Patient should be in semi-Fowler's position and take 10 deep breaths followed by deep cough to raise secretions
   2. Turning and repositioning q2h
   3. Range-of-motion (ROM) exercises: to maintain full range and flexibility of joint movement
      a. Performed 8 to 10 times on each joint at least qd

b. Passive range-of-motion (PROM): performed for the patient
c. Active range-of-motion (AROM): performed by the patient
d. Each joint is put through all its possible movements (Fig. 2-12)
   4. Maintain adequate fluid intake (2000 to 3000 ml/day)
   5. Provide for adequate nutritional intake
   6. Frequent skin care, keeping skin clean, dry, and lubricated
E. Devices used to help prevent dangers of immobility
   1. Footboard: to prevent plantar flexion (footdrop)
      a. Soles of patient's feet are flat against board and in good alignment
      b. Board should be padded
   2. Bed cradle: to keep weight of bed covers off a body part
   3. Alternating pressure mattress: to constantly change pressure on body parts in contact with the mattress
      a. Only one layer of loosely pulled linen should be between mattress and patient
      b. Keep pins and other pointed objects away from this mattress
   4. Sheepskin: provides a soft surface, reducing skin abrasion
   5. Special beds such as the CircOlectric allow patient's position to be changed more readily
   6. Venodixie boots: prevent thrombophlebitis
   7. Antiembolism stockings

Measures to Meet Pain Relief Needs

Individuals (including nurses) vary in their perception of and response to pain. Pain is often intensified in the presence of anxiety and fatigue.

A. Assessment: intensity, onset, duration, quality, and location of pain, patient's nonverbal responses to pain: behavior, change in vital signs, and nausea; factors associated with the pain: activity and visitors; pain relief measures
B. Therapeutic relationship may help reduce anxiety, thus reducing pain level
C. Altering contributing factors: relieving constipation and nausea; eliminating environmental disturbances such as bright lights, odors, and noise
D. Providing diversional activities: television, radio, and visitors
E. Repositioning, back rub, and tightening linens
F. Application of heat or cold if ordered
G. Relaxation
   1. To reduce muscle tension
   2. First need
      a. A comfortable position
      b. A quiet environment
      c. Focus on something outside the body, such as a word to repeat, an object to look at, or something to imagine
   3. Techniques
      a. Exercises in which various muscle groups are alternately tensed and relaxed
      b. Exercises in which various muscle groups are alternately stretched and relaxed
      c. Breathing techniques similar to those used in the Lamaze method of childbirth
      d. Biofeedback: learning to control normally autonomic body functions
         (1) Muscle tension is monitored
         (2) Subject receives feedback as to the success of attempts to control functions

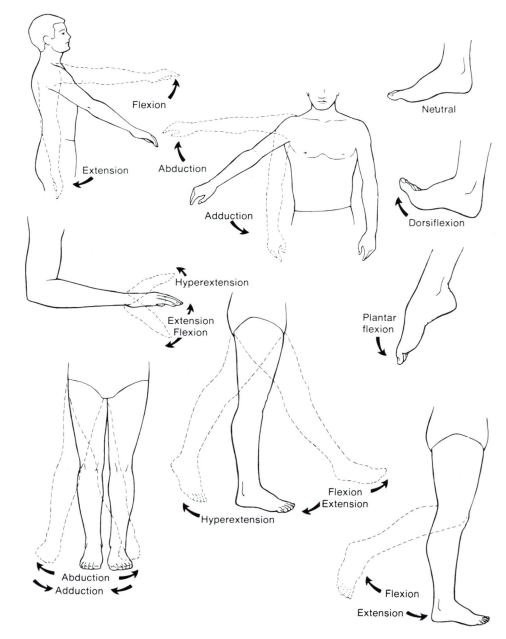

Figure 2-12. Range-of-joint motions. (From Harkness GA, Dincher JR: *Medical-surgical nursing: total patient care*, St Louis, 1996, Mosby.)

H. TENS: Transcutaneous electrical nerve stimulation; small, battery-operated device that provides continuous mild electric current to skin
1. Clean skin with alcohol before applying electrodes on or around pain site
2. No tingling indicates controls are too low; pain or muscle spasm indicates controls are too high
I. Medication classifications: refer to Chapter 3 for more detailed information
1. Placebo: inactive substance administered to satisfy the patient's need for a drug
   a. Pain relief after administration is probably a result of anxiety reduction

b. That relief is felt after placebo does not mean there was no pain
2. Analgesics
   a. Narcotics
   b. Nonnarcotics

Measures to Meet Safety and Hygiene Needs

Individuals are usually capable of meeting these needs themselves, but in strange environments and in times of stress and illness, help is often needed. Individuals need protection from injury, maintenance of intact skin and mucous membranes and of body alignment, and structure and order in their environment

A. Assessment
  1. Protection from injury: level of consciousness, ability to move, knowledge of environment and equipment, and patient's medications
  2. Maintenance of intact skin and mucous membranes and alignment: personal hygiene, condition of skin, mucous membranes, and joints, and posture
  3. Structure and order in the environment: arrangement of personal belongings, cleanliness of patient's unit, environmental conditions, and potential hazards
B. Measures to protect from injury
  1. Bed side rails: use whenever bed is above its lowest level; use for patients who are unconscious, disoriented, or confused or for children
  2. Call signal: should always be within patient's reach; patient should know how to use it
  3. Restraints (patient protectors/patient protective devices)
     a. Require physician's order to place and remove unless there is an emergency and patient is in immediate need of protection
     b. Used to restrict movement of the individual or of one or more extremities
     c. Explain to patient and family why restraint is being used
     d. Remain quiet and calm while applying restraint to reduce patient's fear and stress
     e. Apply restraint securely enough to provide protection but loosely enough to permit circulation and lung expansion
     f. Periodically check pulses and skin integrity
     g. Continue to provide patient with all necessary nursing care including turning, fluids, hygiene, and opportunity for elimination
     h. Secure restraint to bed frame rather than to bed rail
     i. Types of restraints
        (1) Sheet around waist to secure patient in chair
        (2) Jacket or vest, mitts, ankle and wrist restraints
        (3) Safety belts
     j. Measures to avoid restraints
        (1) Reorientatiom measures
        (2) Alarms and monitors
        (3) Specialized chairs
  4. Reduce environmental hazards
     a. Proper care of hospital equipment
        (1) Equipment should be stored properly
        (2) All apparatus, equipment, and furnishings should be kept in good repair
        (3) All apparatus, equipment, and furnishings should be used correctly
     b. Prevention of fire
        (1) Proper care and use of electrical equipment
        (2) Minimization of smoking in bed
        (3) Observance of oxygen safety measures
     c. Prevention of accidents
        (1) Keep floor dry, clean, and free of litter
        (2) Place rubber tips on crutches, canes, and walkers
        (3) Dispose of dressings and needles properly
        (4) Have frequent fire drills
        (5) Lock wheels on beds, wheelchairs, and stretchers
        (6) Maintain good lighting
     d. Protect from microorganisms and pests
        (1) Hand washing and maintenance of medical asepsis
        (2) Proper disinfection and sterilization
        (3) Minimize food storage in patient unit
  5. Transferring patient from bed
     a. Protect from falling by using transfer belt and having patient wear sturdy shoes rather than slippers
     b. Two or three people may be required to transfer helpless or heavy patients
     c. Be sure bed and stretcher wheels and wheelchairs are in locked position
     d. Make use of lifting devices such as Hoyer lift
     e. Use good body mechanics
C. Measures to promote and maintain intact skin and mucous membranes
  1. Bed making: dry, tight, wrinkle-free bed helps maintain skin integrity as well as provide for comfort
     a. Assemble equipment: sheets, spread, blanket, pillow, and pillow covering
     b. Care of soiled linens
        (1) Always place on a surface above floor or in individual laundry bags
        (2) Deposit in linen hamper (disposable "linens" are available and are used especially for patients with communicable diseases)
     c. Types of bed making
        (1) Closed bed is made in preparation for new patient
        (2) Open bed is occupied but patient is out of bed
        (3) Occupied bed is made with patient in it
        (4) Fracture or orthopedic bed is made from head to foot
        (5) Postanesthetic or recovery bed is made to receive patient easily from stretcher (Fig. 2-13)
     d. Bed positions
        (1) Low Fowler's: head is raised (gatched) 18 to 20 inches (45 to 50 cm) above flat bed level
        (2) Semi-Fowler's: head is raised 45 degrees and knee is gatched 15 degrees
        (3) High Fowler's: head of bed is raised to a 90-degree angle
        (4) Trendelenburg's: head is lower than the level of the feet (no gatch)
  2. Daily bath
     a. Clean, dry, intact, and healthy skin and mucous membranes are first line of defense against microorganisms
     b. Bath time is also important for establishing relationship with patient and for assessment
     c. Some patients do not desire, need, or require complete bath each day
     d. Bed bath: given to patient who is restricted to bed or helpless in bathing self
     e. Assisted bath: patient bathes as much of self as possible; may need assistance with back, feet, legs, and perineum
     f. Tub bath or shower: for patient who is capable of doing so; must have physician's order
     g. Commercial sponge bath packets: contain moisturizing cleansing agent; warm in microwave; decreases heat loss, skin drying, exposure and task time
  3. Skin care
     a. Use soap sparingly; rinse well with warm water; pat skin dry

b. Lotions prevent dry skin

c. Gently massage bony prominences with lotion to promote circulation

d. Use deodorant or antiperspirant as necessary

e. Avoid heavy use of powder, which can cake, causing skin irritation

4. Mouth care

   a. Routine mouth care: use of toothbrush, mouthwash, or substitutes

   b. Special mouth care: more frequent routine care plus the judicious use of glycerin and lemon swabs or hydrogen peroxide if ordered

   c. Care of dentures

     (1) Clean dentures over towel-lined basin of water to reduce chance of breakage if dropped

     (2) Hold dentures with gauze or cloth to prevent dropping

     (3) Clean with tepid water; hot water may change shape

     (4) Store dentures in denture cup with tepid water in drawer of bedside stand when not in patient's mouth

5. Hair care

   a. Comb or brush daily; groom as desired

   b. If tangled

     (1) Use 95% alcohol for oily hair

     (2) Use mineral oil for dry hair

     (3) Start at ends working toward scalp

     (4) Hold hair close to head to prevent pulling

   c. Braid long hair if not objectionable to patient

   d. Shampoo as often as necessary and as patient's condition permits

   e. Give pediculosis (lice) treatment as ordered by physician

     (1) Commercial preparations are available

     (2) Use fine-toothed comb to remove nits (eggs)

     (3) Patient may be isolated to avoid spread

6. Nail care: daily and as indicated; must have physician's order to cut nails; extreme care must be used with patients with diabetes or circulatory problems

   a. Scrub under nails as necessary

   b. Cut nails even with tips of fingers and toes

   c. Round fingernails to curve with fingertips

   d. Cut toenails straight across

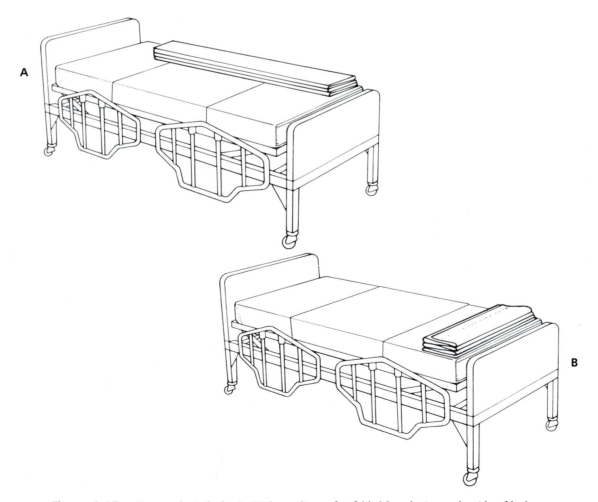

Figure 2-13. Postanesthetic beds. **A,** With top linens fan folded lengthwise to the side of bed. **B,** With top linens fan folded from the head of the bed to the foot. (Adapted from Sorrentino SA: *Textbook for nursing assistants,* ed 3, St Louis, 1992, Mosby.)

7. Decubitus (pressure) ulcer care: assess areas over all bony prominences, such as sacrum, heels, elbows, hips and shoulder blades, and along edges of casts and braces
   a. Contributing factors
      (1) Crumbs or food particles in the bed
      (2) Exposure to moisture such as urine
      (3) Wrinkles in sheets
      (4) Unrelieved pressure for longer than 2 hours
      (5) Conditions that restrict movement
      (6) Poor nutritional or fluid balance states
   b. Treatment
      (1) "An ounce of prevention is worth a pound of cure"—turn and reposition q2h
      (2) Identify high-risk patients
      (3) Report and initiate care for beginning signs of redness, whiteness, or breaks in skin
      (4) Use devices such as sheepskin, egg-crate mattress, alternating-pressure mattress, water mattress, or Clinitron bed
      (5) Avoid use of waterproof underpads
      (6) Use special cleansing agents and dressings as ordered by physician or as indicated by agency policy
8. Use turning sheet to move and turn patient with minimum of friction, which may cause abrasions

D. Measures to maintain body alignment
   1. Encourage good posture while sitting, standing, and lying
   2. Bed lying positions
      a. Supine: lying on back
      b. Prone: lying on abdomen with head turned to the side
      c. Side-lying (Sims'): lying on side with upper hip and knee sharply flexed
   3. Reposition patient at least q2h
   4. Guidelines for proper positioning
      a. Normal body curves must be supported by small pillows or pads: use "bridging" techniques
      b. Joints that are normally flexed need support
      c. Bony prominences need to be protected from pressure
      d. Use devices such as sandbags or rolls to keep joints and body parts positioned
      e. Periodically check patient for discomfort or difficulties
      f. Ensure that patient can reach call signal

E. Measures to promote structure and order in the patient's environment
   1. Physical factors
      a. Lighting
         (1) Lighting should be indirect except for reading or for procedures
         (2) General lighting should be diffused
         (3) Sunlight promotes healing and feeling of well-being
      b. Waste disposal: trash, human excretions, and soiled dressings and linens should be discarded according to agency's procedures
   2. Esthetic factors
      a. Sound
         (1) Music therapy promotes rest and relaxation
         (2) Noise causes fatigue and anxiety
      b. Decor
         (1) Pastel colors (yellow or pink) are soothing and relaxing

(2) Harsh colors (red or black) overstimulate senses
(3) Flowers and pictures enhance environment
   c. Odors
      (1) Foul or strong odors should be eliminated by means of room deodorizer or removal of causative agent
      (2) Mild, fragrant odors reduce antiseptic smell and patient embarrassment
   d. Privacy: curtains, screens, and proper draping should be used as indicated to reduce embarrassment and protect patient dignity
3. Care of the environment: varies according to agency policy
   a. Responsibilities of housekeeping and ancillary services (central supply and maintenance)
      (1) Daily damp dusting and floor cleaning
      (2) Scrubbing, disinfecting, sterilizing, and storing of equipment after patient transfer, discharge, or death
      (3) Repairing or replacing defective equipment or furnishings
   b. Responsibilities of the nursing personnel
      (1) Place bedside table, call signal, phone, and personal articles within patient's reach
      (2) Straighten and damp dust bedside unit (includes care of flowers)
      (3) Care for patient belongings (clothing, valuables, glasses, dentures, and prostheses)
      (4) Prevent cross-infection between patients

Other Therapeutic Nursing Measures
WOUND CARE
A. Cleaning the wound
   1. Commonly used antiseptics
      a. 70% alcohol
      b. Povidone-iodine (Betadine)
   2. Hydrogen peroxide to remove dry and crusted secretions
   3. Always clean from innermost to outermost aspect of wound
B. Wound irrigation
   1. To remove secretions or excessive discharge from surfaces or body cavities or to apply moist heat
   2. May use clean or sterile technique depending on area to be irrigated
   3. Assemble equipment: may vary according to area to be irrigated (disposable kits are available)
      a. Container to hold irrigating solution
      b. Container for return flow of solution
      c. Irrigating solution
      d. Irrigator: usually bulb syringe or large plunger-type syringe
      e. Protection for patient and linens
      f. Gloves and eye protectors (protection from spray)
      g. Replacement dressing if indicated
C. Dressing changes
   1. Dressing: material placed on a wound or incision to protect, absorb drainage, or promote healing
   2. Dressings are classified by method of application
      a. Clean
      b. Sterile
      c. Moist or dry
   3. Disposable kits or hospital-assembled kits

4. Types of dressing material
   a. Gauze
   b. Petrolatum gauze
   c. Telfa
5. Material for securing dressings
   a. Tape: in various widths
      (1) Adhesive
      (2) Paper
      (3) Nonallergic
   b. Montgomery straps
   c. Bandages and binders
6. Nurse may be responsible for changing dressing or assisting physician in changing dressing
7. Initial change of postoperative dressing is done by physician unless an order specifies otherwise
8. Dressings that are not to be changed should be reinforced with additional material if drainage seeps through

D. Care of patient with wound infection
   1. Infection may be local (confined to wound) or systemic (generalized throughout body), often depending on the causative organism
   2. Signs of local infection result from increased circulation and accumulation of waste in the area
      a. Redness, heat, pain, and swelling
      b. Purulent drainage
      c. Loss of function
      d. Changes in vital signs
   3. Signs of systemic infection
      a. Increase in temperature, pulse, and respirations (TPR); possible decrease in blood pressure
      b. Nausea and vomiting
      c. General malaise
      d. Loss of appetite
   4. Basic principles of treatment
      a. Physical and mental rest
      b. Elevation and rest of infected part
      c. Application of heat or cold
   5. Special treatment may include
      a. Chemotherapy (sulfonamides and antibiotics)
      b. Incision and drainage of wound
      c. Debridement: removal of foreign, infected, or necrotic tissue
   6. Infection control committee investigates and follows up infections occurring in an agency

BANDAGES

A. Applied to give support, immobilize a part, apply pressure, or hold dressings
B. Types of bandages
   1. Strips or rolls of gauze, cotton flannel, or elastic material
   2. Many widths, depending on purpose and part to be bandaged
C. Types of basic turns in bandaging
   1. Circular
   2. Spiral
   3. Spiral reverse
   4. Recurrent
   5. Figure-of-eight
D. Safety factors
   1. Apply in direction from distal to proximal
   2. Apply tight enough to serve purpose but loose enough to permit circulation (presence of pulse)
3. Do not fasten over bony prominence, area of pressure, or a wound
4. Part being bandaged should remain in functional position

BINDERS

A. Purposes
   1. Support: abdomen or chest
   2. Hold dressings in place
   3. Apply pressure
B. Types
   1. Straight
   2. Tailed: T-binder, four-tailed, or scultetus (many-tailed)

ANTIEMBOLISM STOCKINGS

A. Purposes
   1. To help maintain circulation
   2. To prevent thrombi or phlebitis formation
B. Application and maintenance
   1. Exact size is obtained by measuring calf or leg length and circumference
   2. Be sure legs are clean and dry before applying
   3. Apply with patient lying down; stockings should fit evenly and smoothly; no wrinkles
   4. Periodically check foot and leg for redness, irritation, swelling, and presence of pulse
   5. Stockings should be removed daily for bathing and skin inspection purposes. Occasional laundering is necessary

APPLICATION OF HEAT AND COLD

A. Physiologic principles
   1. Cold applications (by constricting blood vessels) prevent or reduce swelling, stop bleeding, decrease suppuration, and reduce pain
   2. Heat applications (by dilating blood vessels) increase supply of oxygen and nutrients to body cells and increase amount of toxins and excess fluids carried away
B. Types of cold applications
   1. Dry: ice bag, ice cap, ice collar, and hypothermic devices
   2. Moist: cold packs and compresses
C. Nursing observations
   1. White, mottled skin
   2. Frostbite
   3. Numbness
   4. Lowered body temperature
D. Guidelines
   1. Caps and bags are two-thirds filled and air is removed
   2. Containers are closed securely
   3. Caps and bags are always covered
   4. Application is removed every half hour for 1 hour
   5. Ice is replaced frequently
   6. These treatments are contraindicated or used only with great care in patients with poor circulation or impaired sensation
   7. Physician's order is always required
E. Types of heat applications
   1. Dry: hot water bottle, sunlight, heating pad, and incandescent, ultraviolet, and infrared lights
   2. Moist: warm compresses, hot soaks, hot packs, and K pad units
F. Nursing observations
   1. Redness
   2. Swelling

3. Pain
4. Change in vital signs
5. Loss of function in part
G. Guidelines
1. Always requires physician's order
2. Carefully observe body parts that are very sensitive and burn easily (eyes, neck, and inner aspect of arm)
3. Bottles and pads are always covered
4. Never allow patient to lie on heating device
5. Check for faulty electric wiring
6. Never use safety pins with electric devices
7. Check body temperature frequently
8. Check distance of heating bulbs from body area; should be at least 18 inches (45 cm) away
9. Wring out compresses well to prevent burn; if area is infected, use compresses only once and discard
10. Agency policy may require application of a thin layer of petrolatum to area receiving heat
H. Special baths
1. Hot (sitz) or cold (Fig. 2-14)
2. Medicated

Measures for Eye, Ear, and Throat Disorders
EYE TREATMENTS
A. Hot compresses
1. Assemble equipment: sterile basin of solution as ordered, gauze pad, heating device, paper bag, and protective gloves

2. Put on protective gloves
3. Apply thin layer of petrolatum over lid
4. Wring out gauze pad with hands if clean technique or with two pairs of forceps if sterile technique and allow pad to stop steaming; apply compress slowly until patient is accustomed to heat, or allow patient to apply compress if able
5. Try to keep compress on eyelid only; if lid is inflamed, compress may be placed on lid and cheek; if eyeball is inflamed, compress may be placed on lid and brow
6. Change compresses every 30 to 60 seconds for 15 to 20 minutes as ordered
7. If discharge is present, use clean pad each time compress is applied
8. Use two sets of equipment if both eyes are involved
B. Irrigation
1. Assemble equipment: basin of sterile solution as ordered at 95° to 100° F, medicine dropper or ear syringe, basin for return flow, cotton balls to protect uninvolved eye and to dry treated eye, and face towel to protect bed; separate irrigating tip is needed for each eye
2. Direct flow of solution into conjunctival sac from inner angle to outer angle of eye; position patient toward affected side (Fig. 2-15)

EAR TREATMENT: IRRIGATION
A. Assemble equipment: sterile ear syringe, solution as ordered at 105° to 108° F, basin for return flow, and towel to protect bed

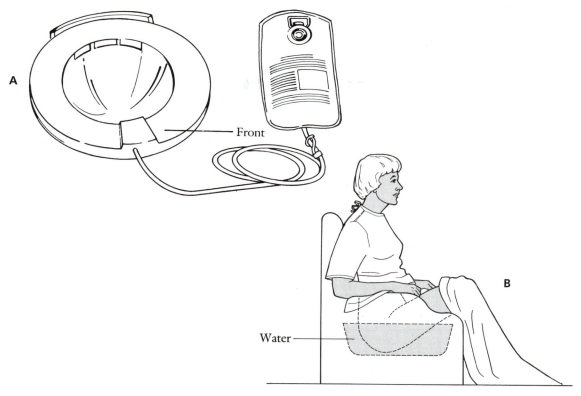

A — Front

Water

B

Figure 2-14. Sitz baths. **A,** Disposable. **B,** Built-in. (Adapted from Sorrentino SA: *Textbook for nursing assistants,* ed 3, St Louis, 1992, Mosby.)

B. Position patient: patient may lie down, but sitting position is preferred, with head tilted slightly so affected ear is downward; patient may hold basin for return flow, if able

C. Retract pinna, in direction according to age, to expose orifice of external canal; direct flow gently against side of canal; interrupt irrigation if pain or dizziness occurs and notify physician

Throat Treatments

A. Throat swab
   1. Assemble equipment: sterile applicators, tongue blade, medication as ordered, tissue wipes, flashlight, and paper bag
   2. When swabbing throat, avoid stimulating gag reflex by not touching uvula
B. Throat culture
   1. Assemble equipment: sterile culture tube, applicator, and tissue wipes
   2. After touching sides and back of throat with applicator, put applicator in culture tube without contaminating inside of tube by breaking off top of applicator that was touched by fingers
C. Throat irrigation
   1. Assemble equipment: irrigating container, solution as ordered at 110° F, tubing with rubber tip on end, tissue wipes, basin for return flow, towel to protect patient; protective gloves
   2. Put on protective gloves
   3. Have patient tilt head forward over basin and breathe through nose; discourage deep breathing
   4. Have patient do treatment if able
   5. Hold container slightly above patient's mouth; direct flow toward affected area
      a. Irrigation may be interrupted for patient's comfort
      b. Flow should not be directed toward uvula or base of tongue
   6. Tilt patient's head to one side and then the other to facilitate results

Measures for Gastrointestinal Disorders

GASTRIC INTUBATION

A. Purposes
   1. To administer gavage feedings
   2. To obtain specimens (gastric analysis and cytology)
   3. To irrigate or cleanse (lavage)
   4. For decompression (suction)
B. Tube locations
   1. Nose to stomach: nasogastric
   2. Mouth to stomach: orogastric
   3. Artificial opening into stomach: gastrostomy
C. Insertion of tube
   1. Is not always a licensed practical/vocational nurse (LP/VN) responsibility: refer to your agency's policy
   2. Assemble equipment: flashlight, tongue blade, stethoscope, cup of water, irrigating syringe, water-soluble lubricant, 12- to 18-gauge French tube, gloves, and towel to protect patient's clothing
   3. If rubber tube is used, it should be chilled first
   4. Place patient in semi-Fowler's position with towel protecting clothing

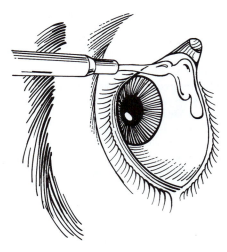

Figure 2-15.   Irrigation of the eye. The nurse turns the patient's head toward the eye that is to be irrigated. Solution flows from the inner canthus to the outer canthus of the eye. The irrigator is held less than 4 inches (10 cm) away from the eye. The patient may assist by retracting the lower eyelid and collecting irrigating solution with absorbent material. (From Elkin et al: *Nursing interventions and clinical skills*, St Louis, 1996, Mosby.)

   5. Approximate distance of tube insertion is the length from tip of nose to ear lobe to xiphoid process
   6. Apply water-soluble lubricant to tip of tube; if intubation is for cytology study, tube is lubricated with water or saline solution
   7. With gloved hands hold tube 3 inches (7.5 cm) from tip, place into nostril or mouth, and advance
   8. Have patient flex neck and take repeated shallow breaths when tube passes into pharynx (about 3 inches [7.5 cm])
   9. Have patient swallow while advancing tube
D. Checking placement of tube
   1. Check back of throat with tongue blade and flashlight to see if coiling has occurred
   2. Aspirate stomach contents; may need to advance tube if no stomach contents are obtained
   3. While injecting 5 ml of air, use stethoscope to listen for air entering stomach
   4. Observe patient's respirations and note ability to speak; respirations may be labored or patient will be unable to speak if tube is in trachea or lungs
E. Securing tube (Fig. 2-16)
   1. Anchor with strip of tape; secure to nose and cheek if nasogastric; avoid resting tube on side of nares to avoid irritation or necrosis
   2. Tube may be looped through a rubber band and attached to patient gown with safety pin for added security
F. Removal of tube
   1. Clamp tube
   2. Remove anchoring tape
   3. Put on protective gloves
   4. Draw tube through towel so it is wiped of secretions
   5. Have patient inhale and exhale slowly
   6. Pull tube with one continuous, rapid motion
   7. Have basin ready if patient vomits

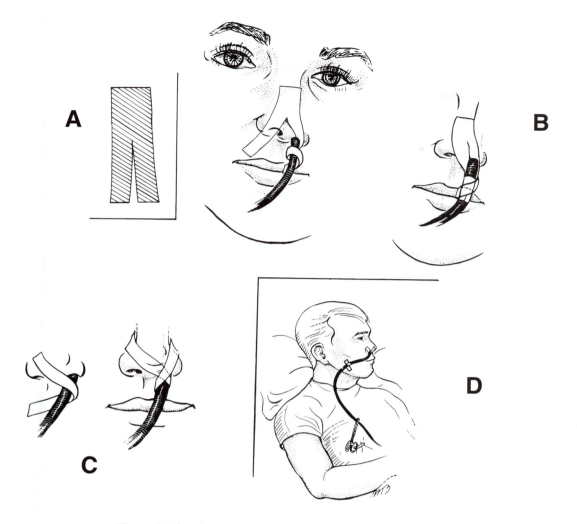

Figure 2-16.   Securing the nasogastric tube. **A**, A length of adhesive tape is split for use in anchoring the tube to the nostril. **B**, The unsplit portion is affixed to the nose: one of the split portions is wrapped around the tube, and then the other portion is wrapped around the tube. **C**, A narrow strip of tape may be used to secure the tube. **D**, The tube is taped to the nostril and cheek and clamped or connected to suction. (From Dison N: *Clinical nursing techniques*, ed 4, St Louis, 1975, Mosby.)

SUCTION AND IRRIGATION

A. Nasogastric or GI tubes (Levin, Cantor, Miller-Abbott, or Salem sump) may be connected to mechanical suction apparatus

B. Suction
1. Rate is ordered by physician or according to agency policy
2. May be intermittent or continuous
3. Collection container is emptied and rinsed; amount of drainage is measured and recorded at end of shift and when container becomes nearly filled

C. Irrigation
1. Check orders for frequency, solution type, amount, and method of aspiration (force or gravity)
2. Assemble equipment: solution as ordered, container for solution, basin for return flow, irrigating syringe (bulb or plunger type), and protective pad
3. Fill syringe and free it of air
4. Instill solution into tube slowly and gently
5. Allow solution to return by aspirating or by gravity
6. Remove syringe and reconnect to suction if ordered

D. Patients with indwelling tubes should be given frequent mouth and nose care

E. Accurate measurement of intake and output (subtracting irrigating solution) is essential

Measures for Vaginal Care

PERINEAL CARE

A. Assemble equipment: solution as ordered, cotton balls for cleansing and drying, gloves, perineal pad with belt, and bedpan

B. With gloved hands put patient on bedpan; pour solution over vulva, clean with cotton balls; dry vulva; make patient comfortable

C. If using bottle method, fill bottle with warm water and squeeze solution over vulva; dry, wiping from urinary meatus toward anus and wiping only once with each cotton ball

VAGINAL IRRIGATION (DOUCHE)
A. Assemble equipment: irrigating container with solution as ordered, tubing with douche tip, clamp, cotton balls for drying, gloves, perineal pad with belt, bedpan, and bed protection
B. Have patient void; place on bedpan, or patient may administer to self in bathroom if able
C. Insert tip down and back into vagina
D. Give irrigation under low pressure; have solution flowing before inserting douche tip; rotate douche tip until prescribed amount is used
E. If patient is on bedpan, raise head of bed slightly to allow fluid to drain into bedpan

Measures for Patients Undergoing Surgery
PREOPERATIVE PREPARATION
A. Psychosocial aspects
   1. Nurse assesses patient's knowledge and expected results of surgery
   2. Anxiety may interfere with learning
   3. Extremely frightened patients may respond poorly to surgery
   4. Planned, individualized, simple explanations will enhance patient cooperation and reduce anxiety
   5. Nurse assesses and responds to patient's religious needs
   6. Common preoperative fears
      a. Fear of mutilation
      b. Fear of death
      c. Fear of change in family role
      d. Fear of pain
   7. Family or significant others must understand measures taken to prepare patient
   8. Family or significant others should participate in explanations and encouragement
B. Physical preparation
   1. Explain preoperative tests (CBC, ECG, urinalysis, x-ray examinations)
   2. Explain, demonstrate, and have patient practice any special postoperative exercises that will need to be done (turning, deep breathing, and pumping feet)
   3. Follow preoperative orders as prescribed by physician (enema, diet, and medications)
   4. Prepare appropriate skin area (see agency procedure manual)
   5. Care for valuables
   6. Follow and complete preoperative checklist
      a. Informed consents for surgery and anesthesia signed and witnessed
      b. Nail polish, prostheses, jewelry, and makeup removed
      c. Patient dressed in hospital gown only
      d. Hygienic measures performed (bath with mouth care and voiding or catheterization)
      e. Vital signs checked and recorded and abnormalities reported
      f. Identification and allergy bracelets in place
C. Observations and procedures recorded

D. After patient leaves for operative procedure, prepare postoperative bed and unit

POSTOPERATIVE CARE
A. Immediate care
   1. Ensure and maintain patent airway
   2. Maintain adequate circulation
   3. Observe for complications at operative site and in general (hemorrhage, shock, swelling, and severe pain)
   4. Assess and secure dressing, drainage, and IV tubings
   5. Assess mental status (orientation)
   6. Position patient properly; keep patient warm
   7. Assess vital signs as often as ordered or more frequently as condition warrants
   8. Follow physician's orders
   9. Report signs of restlessness, excessive drainage, or abnormal reactions
   10. Support patient and family by briefly answering questions and offering explanations
B. Routine care
   1. Follow physician's orders
   2. Assess and record vital signs frequently during first 24 hours; report changes immediately
   3. Assess dressing or surgical site frequently
   4. Give oral hygiene as needed
   5. Have patient turn, deep breathe, and, unless contraindicated, cough and exercise legs at least q2h
   6. Assess and record intake and output (patient may need order for catheterization if he or she does not void within 6 to 8 hours after surgery)
   7. Help patient with passive or active exercises unless contraindicated
   8. Encourage and assist patient to ambulate as much as orders permit
   9. Perform daily assessment
      a. Lungs: breath sounds and cough
      b. Circulation: pain in legs or chest and IV site
      c. GI tract: nausea, vomiting, distention, bowel sounds, and passage of flatus
      d. Urine: amount, color, odor, and frequency
      e. Mental status: withdrawal, confusion, anxiety, or restlessness
   10. Offer pain medication

Measures Related to Radiation Therapy
A. Radiation
   1. Radiate: to send out rays (light, heat, or roentgen)
   2. Radiation is used in diagnosis and therapeutic treatment of various conditions (especially for malignancies)
   3. Types of radiation
      a. Alpha rays: harmless; do not travel far
      b. Beta rays: more penetrating; stop at person's body surface
      c. Gamma rays: very penetrating
B. Types of therapy
   1. Infrared lamp
   2. Ultraviolet
   3. Diatherapy
   4. Roentgen ray (x-ray: low voltage, external)
   5. Betatron, cobalt, cesium (high voltage, external)
   6. Internal radiation

a. Implants (skin surface, intratumor, intracavitary)
b. Liquid forms of radioisotopes
c. Injection (intracavitary, systemic)

C. Radiation therapy and the nurse
1. Internal implant
   a. Explain procedure and precautions to patient and family or significant others
      (1) Patient needs to know that he or she will be in isolation and how many days isolation is likely to last
      (2) Patient should know that nursing personnel and visitors will be spending a minimal amount of time at the bedside and yet will be available when needed
   b. Ensure good fluid intake
   c. Have patient move about as little as possible
   d. Assess for signs of radiation reactions (nausea, vomiting, or skin irritation)
   e. Communicate frequently with patient from doorway without entering room
   f. Use precautions at all times
2. Radiation precautions with implant
   a. RADIATION IN USE sign with directions posted on patient's door
   b. No staff member or visitor spends more than 1 hour per day with patient; care must be well organized
   c. Pregnant women and children should not enter the patient's room
   d. Check placement of implant q4h
   e. Wear gown and gloves while handling excreta, secretions, and utensils
   f. Wash contaminated gloves with soap and water before removing
   g. Wash hands with soap and water
   h. If implant becomes dislodged, call radiologist immediately—do not touch implant
3. Nursing care for specific situations
   a. Therapy involving mouth
      (1) Oral hygiene with brushing teeth (or dentures) should be done 3 times a day (tid)
      (2) Smoking should be discouraged
      (3) Teeth should be assessed for change in condition; if changes observed, notify physician
      (4) Male patient should not shave if jaw is being treated
   b. Uterine therapy
      (1) Bed rest is maintained to prevent displacement of implant
      (2) Bedpan is inspected for loss of implant before contents are discarded
      (3) Foley catheter with continuous irrigation may be ordered to reduce bladder irritation
      (4) Vaginal irrigation may be ordered after removal of implant
   c. Radioactive gold administered intraperitoneally
      (1) Leakage on dressings appears bright red and may be confused with blood
      (2) Dressings should be wrapped in newspaper and disposed of in special container
4. External radiotherapy
   a. Explain procedure to patient and family or significant others
   b. Never remove skin markings
   c. Avoid washing the marked area
   d. Do not apply ointments, creams, or powders to marked area
   e. Encourage good fluid intake and nutrition
   f. Observe for radiation reactions

Measures Concerning Patient's Departure

A. Transferring patient
1. Patient may be transferred from one service to another, from one floor to another, or from one agency to another
2. Physician's order is required
3. Transfer patient ambulatory, by wheelchair, or on stretcher; follow agency's policy
4. Explain transfer to patient; be sure all personal belongings are transferred with patient
5. Avoid transferring during mealtime or change of shift to reduce confusion
6. Make proper charting notations; notify significant others

B. Discharging patient
1. Written order by physician is required
2. Nurse's responsibilities
   a. Gather and check with patient all personal belongings
   b. Make sure patient understands all instructions regarding diet, medications, treatments, and follow-up appointments
   c. Notify family as necessary
   d. Accompany patient to exit
   e. Make proper charting notations
3. Discharge planning
   a. Begins after initial nursing assessment and is included on care plan
   b. Nursing interventions are directed toward eventual discharge of patient
   c. Planning consists of teaching patient and family or significant other
      (1) Cause of illness
      (2) Drugs, treatments, and diet
      (3) Health care follow-up
      (4) Functions within limitations

Caring for the Dying

A. Signs of approaching death
1. Patient is pale with pinched expression of anxiety
2. Eyes are glazed and dull; pupils do not react to light
3. Mouth remains partially open unless patient attempts to speak; speech is mumbled and often confused
4. Muscle tone becomes flaccid
5. Skin is cool and clammy and may be mottled; this is caused by diminished circulation; body temperature is often elevated
6. Respirations are rapid and shallow, often progressing to Cheyne-Stokes
7. Pulse becomes weak and thready
8. Patient may be diaphoretic, thirsty, and incontinent of urine and feces

B. Five stages in the process of reaction to a terminal illness or to dying: refer to Chapter 6 for more detailed information relative to death and dying
1. Denial
2. Anger
3. Bargaining

4. Grief/depression
5. Acceptance
C. Nursing care of dying patient
1. Give symptomatic nursing care
2. Give good personal hygiene
3. Turn patient frequently
4. Give treatments and medications as long as possible or until discontinued
5. Carry out desires of patient, family, or significant others as far as possible
6. Be available to provide emotional support and privacy to patient, family, or significant other
7. Remember that hearing may be the last sense to fail
D. Spiritual needs of patient
1. Fulfill needs as requested by patient, family, or significant other
2. Continue to adhere to patient's individual religious beliefs
E. Care of body after death (postmortem care)
1. Lower head of bed
2. Leave one pillow under head to prevent congestion of blood in vessels of face
3. Close eyes
4. Place dentures in mouth immediately and close mouth
5. Clean body; follow agency's policy for removal of drains, IV needle and tubing, dressings, and tubes
6. Straighten body and place in natural position
7. Allow viewing of body by family or significant other if they desire
8. Wrap in shroud and label with tags according to agency policy
9. Gather, pack, label, and care for patient's personal belongings
10. Record observations, procedures, disposition of valuables, and time of death; complete records

TRENDS IN NURSING
Practical/Vocational Nursing in the United States
HISTORY
A. Practical/vocational nursing evolved to provide better use of nursing personnel and to ease the shortage of nurses
B. The first school to train practical/vocational nurses was the Ballard School in New York City, founded in 1893. This 3-month program taught care of chronic invalids, elderly persons, and children
C. In 1907 the Thompson School was founded in Brattleboro, Vermont. The Household Nursing Association School of Attendant Nursing was founded in Boston in 1918.
D. In the 1940s there were about 50 approved programs; during the 1950s the number of schools of practical/vocational nursing grew. Most programs were extended to 12 months, and placed emphasis on integrating class instruction with clinical experience.
E. In 1956 Public Law 911 appropriated millions of dollars for the improvement and expansion of practical/vocational nurse training. The United States Office of Education established a practical nurse education service.
F. Today more than 1,000 practical/vocational nursing schools are located in hospitals, colleges, and vocational-technical schools providing instruction to over 50,000 students each year. Practical/vocational nurses are the nation's second largest group of health care providers.

EDUCATION
A. Practical/vocational nursing programs must meet requirements and be approved by the state board of nursing
B. Practical/vocational nursing schools of high standards may voluntarily apply for national accreditation by the National League for Nursing
C. Admission requirements to practical/vocational nursing programs vary, but generally applicants must
1. Be at least 17 years of age
2. Have a high school diploma or equivalent
3. Have good physical and mental health
4. Be of good moral character
D. The curriculum incorporates content and concepts from the biologic and physical sciences, behavioral sciences, and principles and practices of nursing
E. The curriculum includes nursing theory and clinical practice, which provide the students with learning opportunities to meet physical and psychosocial needs of mothers and infants, children, medical-surgical patients, the elderly, and patients with long-term illnesses
F. Graduates receive a diploma or certificate and are eligible to take the practical/vocational nurse licensing examination
G. Practical/vocational nursing is the entry level into the practice of nursing

ROLE RESPONSIBILITIES
A. The licensed practical/vocational nurse (LP/VN) has a vital and effective role as a member of the health care team
B. The LP/VN provides direct nursing care to patients whose conditions are stable under the supervision and direction of a registered nurse or physician
C. The LP/VN assists the registered nurse with the care of patients whose conditions are unstable and complex
D. The LP/VN, adhering to the nursing process, observes, assesses, records, reports, and performs basic therapeutic, preventive, and rehabilitative procedures
E. LP/VNs work in acute and long-term care hospitals, nursing homes, physician's offices, ambulatory care facilities, home health agencies, community agencies, and industries
F. To identify the abilities of the beginning practitioner in practical/vocational nursing, see the statement by the National Association for Practical Nurse Education and Service in the box on p. 39.

CONTINUING EDUCATION
A. Each LP/VN is responsible for maintaining competency and increasing level of knowledge
B. The rapid growth of nursing and medical knowledge and advances in technology require nurses to keep up to date
C. The LP/VN must take advantage of learning opportunities through in-service programs where employed; attending seminars and workshops available through institutions, school, official, or voluntary organizations; and reading professional journals
D. Membership in nursing organizations provides continuing education opportunities, usually at a lower cost to their members

HEALTH CARE TEAM
A. Members of the health care team vary depending on the patient's needs and goals
B. Constant team members are

1. Physicians: diagnose and prescribe
2. Nurses: plan and carry out nursing care
3. Patient and family: participate in planning care
C. Other team members include physical therapists, social workers, occupational therapists, respiratory therapists, dieticians, clergy, and others
D. Successful nursing care depends on the interaction and cooperation of all members of the team
E. The LP/VN collaborates with team members

DELIVERY OF NURSING CARE

A. Functional method: each nursing team member is assigned specific tasks (e.g., obtaining and recording all vital signs, administering all medications)
B. Team nursing: a group of patients are cared for by a team consisting of professional nurses, practical/vocational nurses, nurses' aides, and student nurses
C. Primary nursing
   1. One nurse assigned to patient from admission to discharge, usually registered nurse
   2. Total responsibility for care on all shifts
   3. Coordinates care with other health workers, for example, LP/VN, aide

Legislation Related to Practice of LP/VN

NURSE PRACTICE ACT
A. Nursing is subject to laws passed by the state's legislature
B. Laws pertaining to nursing are in the state's nurse practice act
C. The nurse practice act varies from state to state. Some states define the practice of nursing, whereas others describe what a nurse may or may not do in the practice of nursing
D. The nurse practice act also provides for some type of nursing board to regulate nursing practice and procedures for
   1. Approval of nursing schools and curriculum requirements
   2. Licensure and renewal
   3. Grounds for suspension and revocation of licensure
E. The LP/VN must practice nursing within the legally defined scope of her state's nurse practice act

STATE BOARDS OF NURSING
A. Administer the state nurse practice act
B. Membership on the board varies from state to state, usually consists of RNs, LP/VNs, and consumers appointed by the governor
C. In most states, both professional and practical/vocational nursing practice are under the same board; some states have two boards, one for each
D. Functions
   1. Enforces established educational requirements of schools of nursing
      a. Surveys program to determine if preestablished standards are being met
      b. Approves new programs that meet standards
      c. Withholds or withdraws approval from programs that do not meet standards
   2. Controls licensure
      a. Administers the official licensure examination
      b. Grants license to authorized applicants
      c. Renews license

d. Denies, suspends, or revokes license for cause
   3. Conducts investigations and hearings relating to charges of unsafe nursing practice
   4. Interprets the nurse practice act based on past practice, standard of care, and information from other states

National Association for Practical Nurse Education and Service, Statement of Practical/Vocational Nursing Entry Level Competencies

Assessment
Uses basic communication skills in a structured care setting
Obtains specific information from patients through goal-directed interviews
Participates in the identification of physical, emotional, spiritual, cultural, and overt learning needs of patients by collecting appropriate data
Analyzes data collected in relation to patients' pathophysiology

Planning
Determines priorities and plans nursing care accordingly
Formulates and/or collaborates in developing written nursing care plans
Participates in developing preventive or long-term health plans for patients and/or families

Implementation
Protects the rights and dignity of patients and families
Uses basic communication skills in a structured care setting
Safely performs therapeutic and preventive nursing procedures, incorporating fundamental biologic and psychologic principles in giving individualized care
Observes patients and communicates significant findings to the health care team
Conducts incidental teaching and supports and reinforces the teaching plan for a specific patient and/or family

Evaluation
Evaluates, with guidance if necessary, the care given and makes necessary adjustments
Records evaluations of the results of nursing actions
Identifies own strengths and weaknesses and seeks assistance for improvement of performance

Professional responsibilities
Recognizes the LP/VN's role in the health care delivery system and articulates that role with those of other health care team members
Maintains accountability for own nursing practice within ethical and legal framework
Serves as a patient advocate
Accepts role in maintaining and developing standards of practice in providing patient care
Participates in nursing organizations
Seeks further growth through educational opportunities

LICENSURE

A. Protects the public from unqualified practitioners
B. A license is mandatory to practice nursing
C. Permits use of title LPN or LVN
D. Qualifications vary from state to state but most require
   1. Graduation from an approved program in practical/ vocational nursing
   2. Proof of moral character
   3. Attaining a minimum score on the nationally administered examination
E. License must be renewed for a small fee at regular intervals
F. Many states require LP/VN to submit proof of continuing education before license will be renewed
G. License may be revoked or suspended for acts of misconduct or incompetence such as drug addiction or conviction of a felony
H. Licensure by endorsement occurs when a state board of nursing reviews the credentials of a nurse licensed in another state and determines that the nurse meets the qualifications of their state

EXAMINATION

A. As of 1994, all states administer the National Council of State Boards of Nursing (NCSBN) examination as a computer adaptive test (CAT). This test, the National Council Licensure Examination for Practical Nurses (NCLEX-PN), is used to determine if the LP/VN candidate is prepared to practice nursing safely. It tests knowledge of nursing care and ability to apply that knowledge in a clinical situation
B. Testing occurs in over 1,200 computer testing sites throughout the nation. Candidates schedule a testing date following graduation. Testing occurs throughout the year, 6 days per week, 15 hours per day. Each examinee sits at an individual computer terminal and answers questions on the screen. The candidate's answer to each question determines the next question to be presented. No two persons receive the same test
C. The test stops when the candidate's ability level has been estimated at a predetermined degree of accuracy. There is a minimum number of questions which must be answered, and a maximum time allotment for the test (5 hours). Some candidates will complete the test in less than 5 hours

Ethical Principles: Code of Ethics

A. Principles established by professional group as a means of self-regulation
B. Each LP/VN is responsible for upholding the professional standards of conduct and ethics

Legal Implications for the LP/VN

RESPONSIBILITIES

A. Function within the scope of state nurse practice act
B. Maintain standards of care (see the standards of practice for the LP/VN in the box to the right)
C. Function according to employer or agency policy
D. Apply the skills and knowledge that a prudent LP/VN with comparable training would apply in a similar situation
E. Maintain complete and accurate patient records
F. Maintain confidentiality

ILLEGAL ACTIONS

A. Torts—civil law

Standards of Practice for the LP/VN

The LP/VN provides individual and family-centered nursing care

Follow principles of nursing process in meeting specific needs of patients of all ages in the areas of safety, hygiene, nutrition, medication, elimination, psychosocial, cultural, and respiratory needs

Apply appropriate knowledge, skills, and abilities in providing safe, competent care

Apply principles of crisis intervention in maintaining safety and making appropriate referrals when necessary

Use effective communication skills
- Communicate effectively with patients, family, significant others, and members of the healthcare team
- Maintain appropriate written documentation

Provide appropriate health teaching to patients and significant others in the areas of
- Maintenance of wellness
- Rehabilitation
- Use of community resources

Serve as a patient advocate
- Protect patient's rights
- Consult with appropriate others when necessary

The LP/VN fulfills the professional responsibilities of the practical/vocational nurse

Know and apply the ethical principles underlying the profession

Know and follow the appropriate professional and legal requirements

Follow the policies and procedures of the employing institution

Cooperate and collaborate with all members of the health care team to meet the needs of family-centered nursing care

Demonstrate accountability for own nursing actions

Maintain current knowledge and skills in the area of employment

Adapted from Standards of Practice for LP/VN.

Adopted in 1985 by the National Association for Practical Nurse Education and Service.

---

   1. An act or wrong committed by one person against another that results in injury or damage
   2. Can be either the commission or omission of an act
   3. Acts of negligence include
      a. Professional misconduct
      b. Performing care incorrectly
      c. Illegal or immoral conduct
      d. Examples include
         (1) Administration of wrong medication
         (2) Administration of medication or treatment to wrong patient
         (3) Failure to ensure safety through use of side rails or restraints as ordered by the physician
         (4) Failure to prevent injury while applying heat
      e. Gross negligence: patient's life is endangered or lost— often results in criminal action

B. Intentional torts
1. Legal liability exists even if no damage occurs to the other person
2. May not be covered by malpractice insurance
3. Assault and battery
   a. Assault
      (1) Definition: threat or attempt to make bodily contact with another person without that person's consent with intent to injure
      (2) Example: threatening to restrain or physically punish patient if he or she does not cooperate
   b. Battery
      (1) Definition: act of making unauthorized contact
      (2) Example: nurse actually restrains patient
4. False imprisonment
   a. Definition: unwarranted restriction of another person by force or threat of force
   b. Examples: detaining patient in hospital against his or her will; unwarranted use of restraints
   c. Patient who wishes to leave hospital against advice of physician may be asked to sign a release; cannot detain patient if he or she refuses to sign
5. Invasion of privacy
   a. Definition: unauthorized disclosures about a patient even if information is true
   b. Examples
      (1) Release of patient's medical information
      (2) Exposure of patient during procedures or transportation
6. Defamation
   a. Definition: attack on the name, business, or professional reputation of another through false and malicious statements to a third person
   b. Types
      (1) Slander: oral statement
      (2) Libel: written statement

OTHER LEGAL ASPECTS
A. Good Samaritan laws
1. Laws that give certain persons legal protection when giving aid at the scene of an accident; not all states cover nurses
2. Purpose: to encourage people to give assistance at the scene of an emergency
3. These laws do not make it legally necessary for a nurse to assist
4. When nurses do assist, they are expected to use good judgment in deciding whether an emergency exists
5. The LP/VN is expected to give a standard of care that a reasonable LP/VN with comparable training would give in similar circumstances
B. Child abuse
1. All states have laws that require reporting known or suspected cases of child abuse
2. The laws grant immunity from civil suits to those who are required to report child abuse
C. Narcotics
1. The Federal Controlled Substances Act of 1970 is a federal law that regulates the manufacture, sale, prescription, and dispensing of narcotics and other harmful drugs
2. Violation of the law by a nurse is a felony and will result in revocation of the LP/VN license

D. Wills
1. A legal declaration of how a person (testator) wishes to dispose of his or her property after death
2. For a will to be valid, the testator must be of sound mind and acting without force
3. No legal reason for the nurse not to witness a will; the witness is only witnessing the person's signature, not the contents of the will
4. A beneficiary of the will must not witness it
E. Malpractice insurance
1. Professional liability policies cover liability arising out of the rendering of or failure to render professional service
2. Policy is safeguard against suits for damages; can be expensive to prove innocence
3. Can be purchases from nursing organizations, bargaining organizations, and private insurance companies
4. Provides monetary award of damages within specified limits of the policy, also legal fees, court costs, and payment of bond
5. Employer's insurance only protects employee while on duty

Patient's Rights
BILL OF RIGHTS
A. Patients have the right to courteous, individual care given without discrimination as to race, color, religion, sex, marital status, national origin, or ability to pay
B. A patient's bill of rights is a statement of what the patient can expect from the institution
C. The following is paraphrased from the Patient's Bill of Rights adopted by the American Hospital Association. The patient should
1. Be given considerate and respectful care
2. Obtain from the physician complete current information concerning diagnosis, treatment, and prognosis in terms he or she can be reasonably expected to understand
3. Receive from the physician information necessary to give informed consent prior to the start of any procedure or treatment
4. Be allowed to refuse treatment to the extent permitted by law and be informed of the medical consequences of that action
5. Be given every consideration of privacy concerning his or her own medical care program
6. Expect that all communications and records pertaining to his or her care be treated as confidential
7. Expect that within its capacity a hospital must make reasonable response to the request of a patient for services
8. Obtain information as to any relationships of the patient's hospital to other health care and educational institutions insofar as his or her care is concerned
9. Be advised if the hospital proposes to engage in or perform human experimentation affecting the patient's care or treatment
10. Expect reasonable continuity of care
11. Examine and receive an explanation of the bill regardless of the source of payment
12. Know what hospital rules and regulations apply to the patient's conduct

STANDARD OF CARE

A. Patients are entitled to a safe, competent standard of nursing care no matter who administers it (RN, LP/VN, student)

B. The LP/VN is accountable for her own actions and must ensure that the patient receives qualified care

C. If the LP/VN thinks that the patient assignment is beyond her ability, the LP/VN must discuss the matter with the registered nurse before carrying it out

D. Standard of care is established by
   1. State nurse practice act
   2. Institution's job description
   3. Hospital policies and procedures
   4. Patient's nursing care plan

PATIENT ADVOCATE

A. An advocate acts on behalf of another person and stands up or speaks up on behalf of that person

B. Patient has the right to information needed to make informed decisions freely and without pressure

C. The responsibility of the LP/VN is to
   1. Maintain standard of care
   2. Support patients in the decisions they make
   3. Inform physician when the patient apparently does not understand what is going to happen to him or her
   4. Observe and speak out regarding instances of incompetent, unethical, or illegal practice by any member of the health care team
   5. Know hospital policy regarding procedure to follow when patients' rights are being violated

D. Many hospitals employ a patient representative who serves as a liaison between patient and institution and who has the power to act to resolve patients' problems

CONSENT FORMS

A. Before any procedure can be performed, the patient must give written consent, except in extreme emergency when failure to treat may be considered negligence

B. Patient must be fully informed of the extent of the proposed procedure, risks and benefits, alternatives, and their consequences

C. Consent must be obtained by the physician, whose duty it is to advise the patient

D. Consent may be withdrawn by the patient prior to the procedure

PATIENT'S MEDICAL RECORDS

A. The chart is a legal document

B. Provides a written account of the patient's hospitalization

C. May be used as evidence in courts of law; records only information related to patient's health problem

D. Information contained in records must be held in confidence

E. Only authorized persons should have access to patient's records

F. Most states consider medical records the property of the hospital, and the contents the property of the patient

Nursing Organizations

A. Membership
   1. LP/VN has the responsibility to join a professional organization and support practical/vocational nursing by becoming an active member
   2. Membership provides
      a. Fellowship and interaction with other LP/VNs
      b. Opportunity to enhance and strengthen role of LP/VN
      c. Means to keep current on issues relating to practical/vocational nursing
      d. A voice in planning policies of the association
      e. Continuing education opportunities

B. National Association for Practical Nurse Education and Service (NAPNES)*
   1. NAPNES was organized in 1941 to promote the development of sound practical/vocational nursing education and to promote advancement and recognition of the LP/VN as a member of the health team
   2. Membership includes
      a. Regular members: LP/VNs, practical nursing educators, other registered nurses, general educators, physicians, hospital and nursing home administrators, practical nursing students, and interested lay persons
      b. Student members: students in state-approved schools of practical/vocational nursing
      c. Agency members: hospitals, nursing homes, schools of practical nursing, alumni groups, civic organizations, and other institutions or groups in harmony with NAPNES' objectives
   3. Functions and activities listed by NAPNES
      a. Serves as clearing house for information about practical/vocational nursing, including information about functions and roles of LP/VNs
      b. Publishes *Journal of Practical Nursing,* a monthly magazine
      c. Prepares publications useful to faculties in schools of practical/vocational nursing
      d. Sponsors workshops and seminars for LP/VNs and practical nursing educators in conjunction with state LP/VN associations, universities, and national organizations
      e. Engages in activities aimed at protecting and strengthening position of LP/VNs and cooperates with state LP/VN associations in activities of this kind
      f. Provides consultation to state LP/VN constituencies on matters relating to their organization and programs
      g. Sponsors "national certification" in pharmacology and long-term care for LP/VNs.

C. National Federation of Licensed Practical Nurses (NFLPN)†
   1. NFLPN was organized in 1949 to foster high standards in practical nursing and to promote practical nursing
   2. Membership limited to LP/VNs and student practical/vocational nurses
   3. Affiliate membership is available to individuals who are not LP/VNs or students but are interested in the work of NFLPN
   4. There are state associations in many states
   5. Functions of the NFLPN
      a. Provides leadership for LP/VNs employed in the US
      b. Fosters high standards of practical/vocational nursing education and practice
      c. Encourages every LP/VN to make continuing education a priority

*1400 Spring Street, Suite 310, Silver Spring, MD 20910.
†PO Box 18088, 3948 Browning Place, Raleigh, NC 27619.

National League for Nursing Statement Supporting Practical/Vocational Nursing and Practical/Vocational Nursing Education*

The Executive Committee of the Council of Practical Nursing Programs of the National League for Nursing believes that practical/vocational nursing is a vital component of the occupation of nursing and supports those who elect practical/vocational nursing as a permanent career choice. The minimal educational credential for entry into practical/vocational nursing is a diploma or certificate.

Nursing is an occupation that exists on a continuum, and education for nursing can be developed at different levels of knowledge and skills required to fulfill identified yet different nursing roles. The nursing profession has an obligation to society to develop sound and efficient patterns for nursing education that meet the varied nursing needs of society and permit educational options for those who wish them.

Practical/vocational nurses are involved in the nursing process. Practical/vocational nurses, with the supervision and direction of a registered nurse or physician, utilize the nursing process to give direct care to patients whose conditions are considered to be stable. This care encompasses observation, assessment, recording, reporting to appropriate persons, and performing basic therapeutic, preventive, and rehabilitative procedures. When patients' conditions are unstable and complex, the practical/vocational nurse assists and collaborates with the registered nurse in the provision of care.

The practical/vocational nurse is prepared for employment in health care settings in which the policies and protocols for providing patient care are well defined and in which supervision and direction by a registered nurse or physician are present. These settings may be acute or long-term care hospitals, nursing homes, home health agencies, and ambulatory care facilities.

Practical/vocational nurses function within the definition and framework of the regulations set forth by the nurse practice act of the state in which they are employed. The practice of practical/vocational nursing requires licensure, which is the responsibility of the board of nursing in each state, in order to protect the public and safeguard nursing practice.

Education of the practical/vocational nurse is characterized by its consistent emphasis on the clinical practice experience necessary to meet common nursing problems. The curriculum—based on concepts from the physical and biologic sciences that underlie nursing measures and the behavioral science concepts necessary to individualize care—is a planned sequence of correlated theory and clinical experience.

On completion of the program of study in practical/vocational nursing, the graduate demonstrates the specific competencies related to assessment, planning, implementation, and evaluation of nursing care as identified by the Council of Practical Nursing Programs.

The licensed practical/vocational nurse is responsible for maintaining and updating her or his competencies. Adequate orientation and continuing inservice education are responsibilities of the employing agency. However, the practical/vocational nurse must take advantage of other opportunities for continuing self-improvement and, if desired, career advancement.

Opportunities for career mobility without undue penalty must exist in the system of nursing education to provide for changing career goals.

*Issued in 1982, reaffirmed in 1987.

---

d. Achieves recognition for LP/VNs and advocates the effectiveness of LP/VNs in every type of health care facility
e. Interprets the role and function of the LP/VN for the public
f. Represents practical/vocational nursing through relationships with other national nursing, medical, and allied health organizations, legislators, government officials, health agencies, educators, and other professional groups
g. Serves as the central source of information on the new and changing aspects of practical/vocational nursing education and practice
D. National League for Nursing (NLN)*
1. The NLN was organized in 1952 by combining the National League for Nursing Education and six other national nursing organizations

2. Membership includes
a. Individual membership; anyone interested in nursing; registered nurses, LP/VNs, student nurses, consumers
b. Agency membership: hospitals, nursing homes, public health agencies, schools of nursing
3. Functions are
a. Defining and furthering good standards for all nursing service
b. Defining and promoting good standards for institutions giving nursing education on all levels
c. Helping to extend facilities to meet these services when necessary
d. Helping in proper distribution of nursing education and nursing service
e. Working to improve organized nursing services in hospitals, public health agencies, nursing homes, and other agencies; accrediting community public health nursing services; developing criteria and other self-evaluation tools

*350 Hudson St, New York, NY 10014.

f. Working to improve nursing education programs; acting as an accrediting agency for all levels of nursing education

g. Constructing, processing, and providing preadmission, achievement, and qualifying tests

h. Gathering and publishing information about trends in nursing, personnel needs, community nursing services, and schools of nursing

4. Official journal is *Nursing and Health Care*

5. In 1984 the NLN Council of Practical Nursing Programs adopted a resolution that recognized the NFLPN as the official organization for LP/VNs

E. National Council of State Boards of Nursing (NCSBN)*
1. Established in 1978 to strengthen and coordinate the credentialing of nurses nationally
2. Membership open to any state board of nursing; presently composed of 53 state boards
3. Maintains a liason with national organizations that represent nursing
4. Controls the NCLEX, which prepares the LP/VN and RN licensure examinations

F. American Nurses Association (ANA)†
1. National organization for registered nurses formed in 1896 as the Nurses Association Alumnae; renamed ANA in 1911
2. Concerned with standard of nursing practice and promoting general welfare of the professional nurse
3. Membership limited to registered nurses
4. Publishes *American Journal of Nursing (AJN),* a monthly magazine

G. Alumni associations
1. Organization of graduates from the LP/VN's respective school
2. Membership provides a means of
   a. Keeping informed of school's progress
   b. Offering suggestions to improve programs
   c. Providing continuing education
   d. Facilitating social activities with classmates and other graduates
   e. Offering scholarships to future students

Trends in Delivery of Health Care

A. Traditionally the health care focus was on diagnosis and treatment of disease

B. Trends
1. Emphasis on prevention of illness and maintenance of health
2. Decrease in length of hospital stay
3. Rise in home health care

C. Reason for changes in delivery of health care
1. Technologic advances: scientific knowledge has provided early diagnosis and effective treatment of diseases
2. Consumer movement: the public has exerted pressure for the right to health at an affordable price through legislative action
3. Population change: life expectancy has significantly increased with an increase in the number of elderly and a declining birth rate
4. Nature of disease pattern is changing: decrease in acute diseases with an increase in chronic and degenerative diseases
5. Continuing scrutiny of health care costs

D. Related health problems
1. Growing technology and use of complex scientific equipment has caused
   a. Increase in cost of health care; even a short hospitalization can be financially crippling
   b. Fragmentation of care caused by increased number of health workers required by technology
2. Increased population has caused health problems related to air, noise, and water pollution with overcrowding and unsanitary living conditions
3. Aging population: more likely for elderly persons to become ill and to develop chronic and degenerative diseases
4. Uneven distribution of health care facilities and resources available to
   a. Elderly, poor, and minorities
   b. Rural areas and inner cities
5. Cost capitation: managed care strategy that provides a fixed payment for all members (patients) for each pay period (usually a year); profit attained by keeping patients out of expensive care setting; focuses on health promotion for cost containment. Risk for patient related to denied payment for expensive, high-tech treatments

Disease Prevention and Maintenance of Health
BARRIERS TO PREVENTIVE HEALTH CARE

A. High cost
1. Preventive measures not always covered under insurance plan
2. Lower economic group unable to finance cost

B. Inconvenience
1. Clinics usually open during day
2. Difficult to get appointment with physician

C. Unpleasantness of diagnostic or treatment measures accompanied by fear of pain

D. Fear of findings causes many to seek care only after symptoms are acute

Levels of Health Care

A. Primary
1. Promotion of health and prevention of disease including
   a. Immunization against infectious diseases
   b. Health education such as nutrition counseling
   c. Physical fitness program
   d. Research to find cause of disease
2. Primary care takes place in prenatal centers, well-baby centers, schools, and health maintenance organizations

B. Secondary
1. Early diagnosis and treatment to stop progress of disease
2. Prevention of complications
3. The largest and most expensive segment of the health care delivery system
4. Secondary care usually takes place in hospitals, but also occurs in clinics and physicians' offices

C. Tertiary
1. Rehabilitation after illness to return the patient to a level of maximum functioning

---

*676 N St Clair, Suite 550, Chicago, IL 60611.
†600 Maryland Avenue, SW, Suite 100 West, Washington, DC 20024.

2. Involves assessing patient's strengths and weaknesses, assisting the patient to increase strengths and cope with limitations, assisting with rehabilitation measures, and encouraging self-care
3. Agencies providing tertiary care are rehabilitation hospitals, skilled nursing homes, and hospices
4. Other groups involved with rehabilitation are special interest groups such as Alcoholics Anonymous and Reach to Recovery

ROLE OF LP/VN
A. To act as a role model by promoting personal health
1. Assess own health status through regular physical and dental examinations
2. Observe basic principles of personal hygiene and avoid products known to be harmful to health such as tobacco and drugs
3. Provide for adequate rest, sleep, and nutrition
4. Participate in primary care programs
5. Obtain treatment of any infection or injury
B. LP/VN functions within the health care system
1. Promote health: patient teaching
2. Prevention of disease: provide safe environment for patients; encourage and participate in screening programs
3. Discovery and treatment of disease by assisting physician with patient's physical examination, making observations, collecting specimens and data, and performing procedures as ordered
4. Rehabilitation: assist patients with rehabilitation procedures

Health Care Agencies

A. The LP/VN should know what resources are available, what services they provide, and how to make use of the services
B. International agency
1. WHO is an agency of the United Nations established in 1948
2. WHO assists nations to strengthen and improve their health services by providing advisory service in disease control
C. Official agencies in the United States—federal, state, and local—are supported by tax dollars and are accountable to the public
1. Department of Health and Human Services (DHHS)
a. Administration of federal programs relating to health is under the jurisdiction of the DHHS
b. The DHHS has five divisions
(1) Social Security Administration (SSA): administers the national system of health, old age, survivor, and disability insurance
(2) Health Care Financing Administration created in 1977 to oversee the Medicare and Medicaid programs
(3) Office of Human Development Services: administers programs on aging, children, youth and families, and native Americans
(4) Public Health Service (PHS): involved with improving and protecting the health and environment of the United States; the major components of the PHS include
(a) Centers for Disease Control

(b) Food and Drug Administration
(c) Health Resources and Services Administration
(d) National Institutes of Health
(e) Alcohol, Drug Abuse, and Mental Health Administration
(5) Family Support Administration
2. State health departments
a. Supported by tax funds from the state
b. Functions vary among the states; usually responsible for licensing of hospitals, nursing homes, and undertakers; health education materials; vital statistics; and communicable disease control
3. Local health department functions also vary; the general functions include
a. Keeping vital statistics
b. Reporting communicable disease
c. Maternal and child health service
d. Environmental sanitation; inspecting food establishments
D. Voluntary agencies
1. Depend on voluntary contributions for funds
2. Concerned with prevention and solution of specific health problem
3. Provide funds for research and educational projects
4. National organizations function through state or local chapters; examples of voluntary agencies are
a. The American Cancer Society
b. The American Diabetes Association
c. The American Heart Association
d. The American Red Cross
e. The National Society for the Prevention of Blindness
E. Health service providers: presently a realignment of services is shifting care from acute hospital setting to ambulatory and home care
1. Hospitals
a. Short-term facilities provide acute care for patients undergoing treatment for health problems
b. Long-term facilities provide service over an extended period for patients with chronic or long-term health problems; rehabilitation as well as recreational and occupational therapy are stressed
2. Nursing homes, also called long-term or extended-care facilities; the federal government has established two categories of nursing homes
a. Skilled nursing facility (SNF), which provides 24-hour nursing service for the recuperating resident who no longer needs intensive nursing but still requires skilled nursing
b. Intermediate care facility (ICF), which provides regular nursing care, but not around the clock, for residents not capable of living by themselves
3. Hospices
a. Care provided to assist the terminally ill patient to achieve the highest possible quality of life
b. The goal is to maintain the patient in his or her own environment
c. Care is provided in the home by home care nurses
4. Home care
a. Provides continuity and comprehensive health service for individuals who do not need to be hospitalized but who require more than ambulatory care

b. Services provided vary from homemaker services to skilled nursing care
c. Estimated skilled nursing care may be provided at one third of the cost of hospitalization
5. Ambulatory care: care provided on outpatient basis
6. Geriatric day-care centers: patients are cared for during the day at the center and returned home during the evening
F. Financing health care
1. Health maintenance organizations (HMOs)
a. Provide comprehensive health services to participants on a prepaid basis
b. Emphasize primary care to prevent costly illness and hospitalization
c. Do not cover illness outside service area
2. Related health insurance plans/organizations
a. Preferred provider organization (PPO): network of health care agencies that offer insurance plan enrollees services at reduced rates; costs more to go to outside providers
b. Exclusive provider organization (EPO): PPO insurance plan that does not reimburse for services of providers outside the network.
c. Point of service (POS): plan that uses a primary care physician to refer patients to additional services within the plan; unauthorized use of services costs more
3. Medicare and Medicaid are government-supported health insurance programs created in 1965 by an amendment to the Social Security Act
a. Medicare, title XVIII, provides medical care to the elderly receiving Social Security benefits regardless of their need, to people with permanent disabilities, and to those with end stages of renal disease
b. Medicaid, title XIX, was designed to defray expenses that Medicare did not provide for the elderly in need; it also provides services for the poor; program is jointly sponsored with matching funds from federal and state governments; today the states contribute a larger share than the federal government
4. Diagnosis-related groups (DRGs)
a. Originally established to determine Medicare reimbursement for health care, it averaged costs of care based on diagnosis. Presently being phased out in preference to managed care
b. Serves as incentive for efficient, economical care because hospital knows in advance what the payment will be based on the patient's diagnosis. If treatment costs less, hospital keeps the difference; if treatment cost exceeds payment, hospital must absorb the cost
c. Has caused early discharges, decreased acute care census, and reevaluation of need for in-hospital care for many diagnoses

Practical Nursing in Canada
HISTORY
A. There has always been a person working as an assistant to the professional nurse
B. During and following World War II there was a shortage of nurses; to meet this need, hospitals began a variety of short courses on the job

C. In response to these many and varied short courses, the Canadian Nurses Association developed a syllabus for a course to be used as a guide by provincial nursing associations, with the aim of standardizing courses
D. The title for graduates suggested by the CNA was "nursing assistant"
E. In 1940 Ontario was the first province to pass legislation protecting the title "certified nursing assistant"
F. In 1941 the Registered Nurses Association of Ontario opened a demonstration school in London, Ontario, to determine the feasibility of training an auxiliary group; the course lasted 6 months and had a grade 8 admission requirement
G. Following the war, arrangements were made through the Department of Veterans Affairs, the national and provincial nursing associations, and the departments of health and education in each province to organize courses to meet the needs of people released from the armed services
H. Standardized courses developed across the country were offered to the public in such places as hospitals, secondary schools, and technical/vocational schools, as well as independent schools
I. Each province assumed responsibility for supervising the course of instruction, evaluating the programs, and registering/licensing the graduates, plus designating their title: this accounts for the variation in title, program lengths, and responsibilities of the nursing assistant across the country
J. In 1971 the Ontario Association for Nursing Assistants began discussions with the other provinces to form a national organization
K. In 1975 the Canadian Association of Practical Nursing Assistants was incorporated; all provinces are affiliated except Quebec
L. There are currently approximately 84,000 practical nursing/nursing assistants in Canada

EDUCATION
A. Practical nursing/nursing assistant (PN/NA) programs must meet requirements of the registering/licensing body in each province/territory
B. There is no national accreditation body for nursing in Canada
C. Admission requirements vary from province to province and the territories; a high school diploma or its equivalent is usually required
D. The curriculum incorporates content and concepts from the biologic and psychosocial sciences, as well as principles and practice of nursing
E. The curriculum includes nursing theory and clinical practice, which provide the students with learning opportunities to meet physical, psychosocial, and spiritual needs of patients across the lifespan
F. Graduates receive a diploma or certificate and are eligible to take the certification/licensing examination in their jurisdiction

RESPONSIBILITIES OF THE CANADIAN PRACTICAL NURSE/NURSING ASSISTANT
A. The PN/NA has a vital and effective role as a member of the health care team
B. The PN/NA provides direct nursing care to patients whose conditions are stable under the supervision and direction of

a registered nurse, registered psychiatric nurse in certain provinces, or physician

C. The PN/NA aids the registered nurse with the care of patients whose conditions are unstable and complex

D. The PN/NA using the nursing process observes, assesses, records, reports, and performs basic therapeutic, preventive, and rehabilitative procedures

E. The PN/NA works in acute and long-term care hospitals, nursing homes, physicians' offices, ambulatory care facilities, home health agencies, public health agencies, community agencies, and industry

F. The PN/NA uses the nursing process, that is, assessment, planning, implementation, and evaluation in delivering nursing care in all settings

G. The PN/NA practices within the legal and ethical boundaries for the province/territory

CONTINUING EDUCATION

A. Each PN/NA has the responsibility to maintain competency and increase level of knowledge

B. The rapid growth of medical knowledge and advances in technology make it necessary that PN/NAs keep up-to-date

C. The PN/NA must take advantage of learning opportunities through in-service programs where employed; attending seminars and workshops available through institutions and school, official, or voluntary organizations; and reading professional journals

D. Membership in nursing organizations provides continuing education opportunities, usually at a lower cost to their members

LEGISLATION RELATED TO THE PRACTICE OF PRACTICAL NURSING IN CANADA

A. Legislation
1. Nursing is subject to legislation passed by each province/territory
2. Laws pertaining to nursing are specific to each province/territory
3. The regulating body is designated through legislation in each province/territory
4. Each province/territory designates a body to approve and review nursing schools

B. Regulatory body: each province/territory has either an independent body such as a council or a college or a professional association responsible for the practice of its members

C. Registration/licensure
1. Each province/territory determines the title held by the PN/NA in that jurisdiction
2. Registration/licensure ensures the public of a minimum standard of safe nursing care
3. Registration protects the title of the registrant only; licensure also protects the practice of nursing
4. Licenses are usually renewed annually
5. Licenses may be revoked or suspended for acts of misconduct, negligence, or incompetence as outlined in legislation

D. Examination
1. All provinces and territories except Quebec purchase the Canadian Nurse Association examinations
2. The CNA examination for PN/NAs is held three times a year, in March, June, and October
3. All provinces and territories administer the examination on the same day
4. Passing scores are determined by each province or territory; 350 is generally required
5. Quebec administers its own examinations

CANADIAN NURSING ORGANIZATIONS

A. Membership
1. The PN/NA has the responsibility to join a professional organization and support PN/NAs by becoming an active member
2. Membership provides
   a. Fellowship and interaction with other PN/NAs
   b. Opportunity to enhance and strengthen role of PN/NA
   c. Means to keep current on issues relating to the PN/NA
   d. A voice in planning policies of the association
   e. Continuing education opportunities
   f. Malpractice insurance (most provinces)

B. Canadian Association of Practical Nursing Assistants (CAPNA)
1. CAPNA was formed in 1971 and incorporated in 1975. CAPNA is a voluntary association currently representing members of associations from all provinces and the territories with the exception of Quebec. It can be accessed through each organization
2. Membership includes
   a. Association member: a member of any provincial or territorial association of PNs/NAs which belongs to CAPNA
   b. Affiliate member: individual PNs/NAs from province or territories that do not belong to CAPNA are entitled to membership upon payment of the prescribed annual fee
3. CAPNA objectives are
   a. To promote the concept of health
   b. To promote the high standards and uniformity of nursing education to achieve reciprocity
   c. To interpret and promote the Practical Nurse/Nursing Assistant role on the health team
   d. To safeguard the interest, professional identity, and practice of the Practical Nurse/Nursing Assistant
   e. To promote and encourage an attitude of mutual understanding and unity among all provincial and/or territorial associations
   f. To safeguard and promote the autonomy and self-governance of the Practical Nurse/Nursing Assistant
   g. To promote nursing research that facilitates the provision of quality nursing care for the people of Canada.
   h. To participate in the provision and development of an effective, efficient, client-centered interdisciplinary approach to the delivery of health care services.

SUGGESTED READING

Barnie DC, Currier J: What's that GI tube being used for? *RN* 58:(8) 45-49, 1995.

Becker BG, Fendler DT: *Vocational and personal adjustments in practical nursing*, ed 7, St. Louis, 1994, Mosby.

Carroll P: Safe suctioning prn, *RN* 57:(5) 32-37, 1994.

Christensen BL, Kockrow EO: *Foundations of nursing*, ed 2, St. Louis, 1995, Mosby.

Clayton BD, Stock YN: *Basic pharmacology for nurses,* ed 10, St. Louis, 1993, Mosby.

Cole G: *Fundamental nursing concepts and skills,* ed 2, St. Louis, 1996, Mosby.

Cooper KM: Measuring blood pressure the right way, *Nursing 92* 4:75, 1992.

Cunningham D: Improving your teaching skills, *Nursing* 23:(12) 24J, 1993.

Dowd SB: Radiation safety and the nurse, *Journal of Practical Nursing* 12: 31-33, 1990.

Dunham-Taylor J, Penny Marquette R, Pinczuk JZ: Surviving capitation, *AJN* 96:(3) 26-29, 1996.

Eisenberg PG: A nurse's guide to tube feeding, *RN* 57:(10) 62-70, 1994.

Ernst DJ: Flawless phlebotomy: becoming a great collector, *Nursing* 25:(10)54-57, 1995.

Glass CA, Grap MJ: Ten tips for safer suctioning, *AJN* 95:(5) 51-53, 1995.

Grossman D: Cultural dimensions in home health nursing, *AJN* 96:(7) 33-36, 1996.

Kuehl PG: Immunizations for special situations, *Journal of Practical Nursing* (3):52-61, 1992.

McDevitt MJ: A (TENS) tion!, *Nursing* 25:(12) 46-47, 1995.

Metzler DJ, Harr J: Positioning your patient properly, *AJN* 96:(3) 33-37, 1996.

Morris JJ: *Canadian nurses and the law,* Markham and Vancouver, 1991, Butterworth's Canada

Parisi SB: What to do after a med error, *Nursing* 24:(6) 59, 1994.

Perry AG, Potter PA: *Clinical nursing skills and techniques,* ed 3, St. Louis, 1994, Mosby.

Spyr J, Preach MA: Pulse oximetry: understanding the concept of knowing the limits, *RN* 53:(5) 38-45, 1990.

Stolley JM: Freeing your patients from restraints, *AJN* 95:(2) 26-31, 1995.

Tammalleo AD: Charting by exception: there are perils, *RN* 57:(10) 71-72, 1995.

Thomas DO: Fever in children: friend or foe?, *RN* 58:(4) 42-48, 1995.

Trombley J: Listen up! Don't trust tympanic thermometers?, *Nursing* 26:(2) 58-59, 1996.

Wheeler SR: Helping families cope with death and dying, *Nursing* 26:(7) 25-30, 1996.

REVIEW QUESTIONS

Answers and rationales begin on p. 58.

1. Your female patient has a radium cervical implant. The nurse knows that care for this patient must be carefully planned because:
   ① The patient's hospital stay will be limited
   ② The nurse must limit patient contact time
   ③ Patients receiving this type of therapy are easily fatigued
   ④ Patient discomfort levels increase with excessive activity

2. When approaching families of potential organ donors, the nurse remembers that:
   ① This request will intensify the family's grief
   ② Culture can affect the family's response to death
   ③ The family has no legal rights to the patient's body
   ④ A living will is necessary for family to allow organ donation

3. When considering purchasing liability insurance, the nurse should keep in mind that professional liability coverage:
   ① Costs the same in all health care settings
   ② Protects the nurse from prosecution for criminal acts
   ③ Does not cover acts outside the scope of nursing practice
   ④ Provides coverage to the nurse for his/her entire professional career

4. The nurse determines the effectiveness of nasotracheal suctioning by:
   ①. Encouraging the patient to cough
   ② Assessing the rate and character of respirations
   ③ Providing mouth care at the end of the procedure
   ④ Noting the characteristics of the respiratory secretions

5. You are the home care nurse for a 40-year-old wheelchair-bound quadriplegic who lives with his elderly mother in a small, cluttered apartment. The patient's mother is quite frail, suffers from arthritis, and has cataracts. Which of the following instructions would promote safety for this family?
   ① Take all medications as ordered
   ② Remove the throw rugs from your floors
   ③ Request that the agency provide a home health aide
   ④ Range of motion exercises would benefit both of you

6. Your patient, 60 years old, is an alert, hypertensive female who lives alone in a senior citizens housing complex. She has been having difficulty sleeping at night and asks you for suggestions in managing this problem. Your best response would be:
   ① "As we age, we need less sleep"
   ② "Call your doctor for a prescription"
   ③ "Drink a glass of warm milk at bedtime"
   ④ "Take a 20-30 minute walk each day"

7. You have just medicated your patient with Flurazepam (Dalmane) 30 mg PO at h.s. Which of the following measures will promote the purpose of this medication?
   ① Tightening his bed linens
   ② Raising the side rails of his bed
   ③ Placing the call bell within reach
   ④ Instructing patient about the drug's side effects

8. Your 59-year-old female patient has arrived at the physician's office complaining of severe back pain. Which of the following questions would be most important to ask when gathering information for the physician?

① Are you allergic to any drugs?
② Can you point to where the pain is?
③ How have you treated the pain at home?
④ Are you experiencing any other symptoms?

9. Your patient is being prepared for sealed internal radiation therapy of her cervical cancer. You can help reduce her anxiety by emphasizing that:
   ① Pain medication will be offered regularly
   ② Visitors will be limited during this treatment
   ③ The nurse will be available whenever needed
   ④ The client will not be radioactive during this treatment

10. Your male patient has just left the physician after receiving instructions concerning his scheduled cholecystectomy. As the office nurse, you will question the patient as a review of the physician's instructions because:
   ① Repetition increases learning
   ② Physicians use very technical terms
   ③ Patient anxiety may have interfered with understanding
   ④ Preop checklists require teaching reinforcement by the nurse

11. When performing a throat culture, the nurse swabs the sides of the throat before the back in order to:
   ① Delay stimulating the gag reflex
   ② Stimulate production of secretions
   ③ Avoid contamination of the culture site
   ④ Obtain adequate specimens for culture

12. One hour after the nurse applies an elastic bandage to the patient's sprained ankle, the patient complains of tingling and burning in her toes. The nurse should:
   ① Palpate for pedal pulses
   ② Reapply the bandage less snugly
   ③ Instruct her to elevate the affected foot
   ④ Encourage her to wiggle her toes every two hours

13. During a surgical dressing change, the nurse notes that there is copious purulent drainage along the reddened incision site. These symptoms most likely indicate:
   ① Local infection
   ② Systemic infection
   ③ Necrosis of the wound
   ④ Nosocomial wound contamination

14. When performing wound irrigations, the nurse is best protected by:
   ① Raising the bed to a workable height
   ② Explaining the procedure to the patient
   ③ Hand washing before and after the procedure
   ④ Donning appropriate personal protective equipment

15. Which of the following patients is most at risk for decubitus formation?
   ① A 20 year old with an L4 injury confined to a wheelchair.
   ② A 6 year old in skeletal traction for a fractured right femur.
   ③ An ambulatory 90-year-old patient with Alzheimer's disease.
   ④ A seventy-five-year-old male on bedrest following total knee replacement.

16. Use of a footboard on the bed of an immobilized patient serves the following function:
    ① Prevents footdrop
    ② Assists patient to move about in the bed
    ③ Maintains patient position at the head of the bed
    ④ Relieves pressure of bedding on the lower extremities

17. The night following gastric resection, your patient complains of severe thirst. Because this patient has a nasogastric tube hooked up to low suction you would:
    ① Call the physician for an order allowing ice chips
    ② Instill approximately 100 ml of normal saline into his tube
    ③ Explain that he must remain NPO until the tube is removed
    ④ Assist the patient in brushing his teeth and rinsing his mouth

18. Which of the following behaviors is more likely to place the nurse at risk for a lawsuit?
    ① Responsiveness to client complaints
    ② Flexibility dealing with patient, family, and staff
    ③ Reliance upon institutional malpractice insurance
    ④ Delegation of nursing duties to ancillary personnel

19. In a managed care environment, the nurse has an ethical responsibility to the patient to:
    ① Provide only allowable services
    ② Assume the role of patient advocate
    ③ Interpret insurance coverage for the patient
    ④ Determine level of care based upon insurance benefits

20. Your 68-year-old patient has been a resident of the nursing home for a week. He states that he has been unable to sleep since admission, and is now considering asking his physician for sleeping pills. Your first response would be:
    ① "What helped you to sleep before you came here?"
    ② "It's not unusual to have difficulty sleeping in a new setting"
    ③ "Medications can often cause confusion in someone your age"
    ④ "I'm certan your doctor will find an appropriate medication for you"

21. When performing an intermittent bladder irrigation, the nurse discontinues instilling fluid if:
    ① Irrigant returns are clear
    ② Irrigant returns are bloody
    ③ The returns equal the fluid instilled
    ④ The patient complains of bladder spasm

22. Your patient has returned to the unit following TURP. He has an indwelling Foley catheter hooked up to bedside drainage. You note that the bedside drainage unit is filled with red urine and numerous large clots. The abdomen is distended, and the bladder can be palpated above the symphysis pubis. Your first action would be to:
    ① Change the patient's position
    ② Notify the surgeon of your findings
    ③ Check the chart for bladder irrigation orders
    ④ Document your observations on the flow sheet

23. Your male patient has just been admitted in acute respiratory distress. The physician has prescribed nasal oxygen at 3 L and has ordered that a Foley catheter be inserted. In light of this patient's condition, the most appropriate position for the catheterization procedure would be:
    ① Supine
    ② Dorsal recumbent
    ③ High Fowler's with knees flat
    ④ High Fowler's with knees gatched

24. Bacterial contamination of indwelling catheters in home care patients can often be avoided by:
    ① Scheduling weekly catheter changes
    ② Administration of prophylactic antibiotics
    ③ Daily cleansing of meatus and catheter with soap and water
    ④ Thorough cleansing of the meatus with appropriate antiseptic solution

25. You are caring for a 48-year-old fresh post-op hysterectomy patient on your unit. The patient has an indwelling Foley catheter. An IV of dextrose 5% in Ringer's lactate is infusing at 100 ml/hour in her left arm. She may receive Demerol 175 mg. IM q4h for pain. The patient is complaining of a sense of urinary urgency and lower abdominal pressure. Your first nursing measure for this patient would be to:
    ① Check when this patient was last medicated for pain
    ② Request that the physician change the IV flow rate order
    ③ Determine that urine is draining into the bedside drainage unit
    ④ Assure the patient that catheters often cause this type of discomfort

26. Your patient, 89 years old, is recovering in the same-day surgery unit, after undergoing cataract repair to the left eye. When you bring the lunch tray to this patient you would:
    ① Offer to feed the patient
    ② Remove all hot fluids from the tray
    ③ Describe the tray in clock fashion to the patient
    ④ Place the tray so that the patient does not have to strain to reach it

27. You have been assigned to care for a 30-year-old African-American admitted to the hospital with status asthmaticus. The patient is very dyspneic and uncomfortable today. Because he is dark-complexioned, you can best determine if he is cyanotic by:
    ① Examining his oral mucosa
    ② Monitoring his vital signs hourly
    ③ Observing his lips and nail beds
    ④ Placing a pulse oximeter probe on his finger

28. Your patient, an alert, 79-year-old diabetic, has resided in an assisted living facility since her right leg was amputated 3 years ago. She has called you to her room today because she has been vomiting during the night and is now feeling weak and lightheaded. An important nursing assessment for this patient would be to:
    ① Take her blood pressure
    ② Perform a glucometer test
    ③ Instruct her to remain in bed today
    ④ Have her maintain a clear fluid diet today

29. The physician has ordered Ringer's lactate IV at a rate of 100 ml per hour. The IV was started at 7:00 this evening. When you make rounds at 11:00 P.M., you note that 200 ml fluid has infused into the patient. You would first:
    ① Notify the physician that the IV has infiltrated
    ② Note the amount on the patient's intake and output record
    ③ Check the tubing and infusion site for possible obstructions
    ④ Change the rate of flow until the correct amount has infused

30. The volume of a client's Foley catheter bedside drainage unit is most accurately measured by:
    ① Holding the drainage bag up at eye level
    ② Approximating output from the markings on the drainage unit
    ③ Emptying the urine into a bedpan and noting what level it reaches
    ④ Pouring the urine into a measuring container on a flat eye-level surface

31. The nurse addresses an important comfort measure for the new tracheostomy patient by:
    ① Providing a pad and pencil within reach
    ② Having tissues easily available to the patient
    ③ Reassuring the patient that nurses are always nearby
    ④ Arranging to have telephone service discontinued postoperatively

32. Your patient, an 88-year-old female admitted for COPD, is receiving nasal oxygen at 2 L and has been placed on bedrest. During the evening, the patient complains that her feet are cold. Your best response would be to:
    ① Offer the patient cotton socks
    ② Bring the patient a woolen blanket
    ③ Place a hot water bottle under the patient's feet
    ④ Assure the patient that this is a common complaint for her diagnosis

33. You have been assigned to perform colostomy care for a 45-year-old recent hemicolectomy patient. You can best determine how the patient tolerated the procedure by:
    ① Noting all objective signs and symptoms during the procedure
    ② Asking the patient if anything is bothering him during the procedure
    ③ Questioning the patient regarding his well-being at the end of the treatment
    ④ Observing the patient's verbal and nonverbal actions throughout the procedure

34. The chief reason that the nurse explains procedure steps and purpose to the patient prior to performing a treatment is:
    ① It diminishes the likelihood of malpractice suits
    ② Patient anxiety is decreased with understanding
    ③ It allows the patient the opportunity to refuse the treatment
    ④ It provides the nurse with an opportunity to mentally review the procedure

35. Which instruction is most appropriate for a COPD patient with copious bronchial secretions?
    ① Decrease your fluid intake to solidify bronchial secretions
    ② Tracheal suctioning is the best method for removing heavy secretions
    ③ Try to drink several glasses of juice or water daily to loosen secretions
    ④ You'll find it easier to breathe if you sit up straight during postural drainage treatments

36. When contributing to a plan of care for a patient with high risk for injury due to debilitating illness, the nurse is aware that:
    ① This patient has a potential problem
    ② This is not a recognized nursing diagnosis
    ③ The statement is based on subjective data
    ④ The care plan addresses an actual problem

37. When contributing to the nursing care plan, the practical nurse knows that an example of a short-term goal is:
    ① Assist patient in range of motion exercises
    ② Patient will transfer from bed to chair this week
    ③ Patient will return to previous level of functioning
    ④ Physical activity will improve muscle tone and function

38. The physician has ordered a urine sugar and acetone level. The best approach for obtaining this specimen would be to:
    ① Have the patient collect a midstream specimen
    ② Instruct the patient in the procedure for a clean-catch specimen
    ③ Discard the first voiding of the day and collect all following urines for 24 hours
    ④ Discard the first voided urine and collect the specimen as soon as the patient can void again

39. Measure of a diabetic's blood glucose control is best determined by:
    ① Regular evaluation of glucose tolerance tests
    ② Home blood glucose monitoring several times daily
    ③ Daily monitoring of sugar and acetone content in the urine
    ④ Measurement of sugar and acetone in double-voided specimens

40. When instructing a patient in the procedure for collecting stools for occult blood, the nurse explains to the patient that:
    ① Diarrhea stools are unacceptable sources for this examination
    ② The specimen should be kept warm until delivery to the laboratory
    ③ Small samples should be taken from two separate areas of the stool
    ④ The specimen should only be obtained from stool areas containing blood.

41. Your 72-year-old patient is taking diuretics for congestive heart failure. As part of his home care directions you would instruct him to weigh himself:
    ① Each morning upon arising
    ② One hour after taking his medication
    ③ If he notices an increase in pedal edema
    ④ Whenever he develops shortness of breath

42. Arterial oxygen saturation in respiratory patients can be determined quickly and noninvasively by:
    ① Attaching the patient to a pulse oximeter
    ② Monitoring incentive spirometer capacity
    ③ Observing the patient for circumoral cyanosis
    ④ Drawing arterial blood gas levels from the patient

43. When evaluating a patient for possible pulse deficit, the nurse will need:
    ① The assistance of a second nurse
    ② An understanding of systolic murmur
    ③ The cooperative assistance of the patient
    ④ The availability of an electocardiagraph machine

44. After positioning a female patient for gynecological examination, the nurse knows to perform the following for primary patient comfort:
    ① Loosen any tight or constricting clothing
    ② Place an appropriate drape across the patient
    ③ Place a trochanter roll under the lumbar curvature
    ④ Elevate the patient's upper torso to sitting position

45. Your patient, a 60-year-old female, is in Bucks running traction for right hip fracture. The nurse understands that pulses would be most significant when measured over which site?
    1. Pedal
    2. Apical
    3. Radial
    4. Carotid

46. When measuring patient temperature via a tympanic thermometer, the nurse should:
    1. Place the patient in the side-lying position
    2. Gently pull the pinna down and back for insertion
    3. Insert the thermometer while pulling the pinna up and back
    4. Question the patient regarding recent eating, drinking, or smoking

47. When preparing a patient for X-ray examination, the nurse takes care to instruct the patient to:
    1. Remove all undergarments for better visualization
    2. Fast from food and fluids 12 hours prior to the exam
    3. Layer clothing to avoid chilling during the examination
    4. Remove all pins and jewelry in the path of the X-ray exam

48. When preparing a patient for sigmoidoscope exam, the nurse knows that the patient will be most comfortable in which position?
    1. Sims'
    2. Lithotomy
    3. Knee-chest
    4. Trendelenburg

49. While documenting the care of your home care patient, you realize that you mistakenly omitted significant observations from yesterday's notes. You would:
    1. Rewrite the notes after discarding the original
    2. Include yesterday's observations in today's note
    3. Document the observations in a dated addendum
    4. Write error with your initials after drawing a line through the notes

50. You are providing hospice care for a 63-year-old female with terminal bone cancer. Tonight she is weeping and states, "I can't take any more of this. I wish you would just give me something to end it all." Your best response would be:
    1. "You can't take any more of this?"
    2. "I'll get you something for the pain"
    3. "It would be unethical for me to do something like that"
    4. "I'm sure you'll feel much better after you've had some sleep"

51. Your 93-year-old female patient required a Foley catheter following hip surgery. Lab tests now indicate that she has a *Pseudomonas* urinary tract infection. In light of this patient's medical history, the nurse would suspect that this is a (an):
    1. Superinfection
    2. Nosocomial infection
    3. Autoimmune response
    4. Antibiotic resistance response

52. A mother has made an appointment to see the pediatrician because her child, who has chickenpox, has developed a high fever and ear pain. As the office nurse, you would:

1. Immediately bring the child into a closed examination room
2. Suggest that the child see the physician in the emergency room
3. Have the child wear a face mask if he must be near any other patients
4. Tell the mother to avoid letting the child touch any toys in the waiting room

53. When moving heavy physical therapy equipment onto a patient's bed, nurses know that they can best avoid personal injury by:
    1. Carrying the equipment close to the body
    2. Sliding equipment from the floor to the bed
    3. Using the back muscles to do the major lifting
    4. Holding the equipment at arm's length from the body

54. A young child is brought to the emergency room after falling from his bike. The child's upper and lower extemities are covered with multiple areas of scraped skin. You would document these as:
    1. Incisions
    2. Abrasions
    3. Contusions
    4. Lacerations

55. A 3-month-old female infant arrives at the pediatric clinic with chief presenting symptoms of vomiting, diarrhea, and fever of 102° for 36 hours. You would immediately place her in an examining room to be seen by the pediatrician because:
    1. She should not be exposed to other illnesses
    2. Fever in children is a symptom of serious illness
    3. Fluid loss is potentially life-threatening in children
    4. The waiting room should have a pleasant environment

56. Which of the following breakfasts would be appropriate to serve to a postpartum mother observing Kosher diet rules?
    1. Oatmeal, poached egg, whole wheat toast with jelly, grapefruit, tea
    2. Blueberry pancakes with syrup, pork sausage, fresh orange, coffee
    3. Creamed chipped beef on toast, corn flakes, yogurt, sliced melon, milk
    4. Scrambled eggs and bacon, bagel and cream cheese, orange juice, tea

57. When collecting a patient's psychosocial history, the nurse questions religious affiliation because:
    1. Religion may affect health practices
    2. It determines whether the patient should receive last rites
    3. Certain religious denominations offer social supports to ill members
    4. The patient may wish to have specific clergy notified of hospitalization

58. When considering a patient's state of health, the nurse is aware that:
    1. Wellness is essentially a state of mind
    2. Illness is a more common occurrence than wellness
    3. Genetics fix one's position on the wellness-illness continuum
    4. One's position on the wellness-illness continuum is constantly changing

59. During the past decade health care trends have caused nursing care to be:
    ① Greatly diminished in scope
    ② More focused on treatment of illness
    ③ Less concentrated in the acute care setting
    ④ Based on technology rather than treatment

60. Your home care patient has a glass rectal thermometer for measuring temperatures. Following the temperature procedure, you would clean this equipment by:
    ① Soaking the thermometer in alcohol between uses
    ② Scrubbing it with an alcohol and water solution
    ③ Washing it in hot soapy water, then soaking it in alcohol
    ④ Washing it with a wet soapy tissue, and rinsing in cool water

61. As a professional, the nurse is ethically bound to:
    ① Regularly file for relicensure
    ② Maintain active membership in professional nursing organizations
    ③ Keep abreast of changing trends and technologies within the field
    ④ Campaign for political programs which guarantee nursing employment

62. Nurses completing incident reports following medication errors should take care to:
    ① Correct the error as quickly as possible
    ② Notify the patient and his family of the error
    ③ Document completion of the incident report on the patient's chart
    ④ Note the medication administered as well as notification of the physician

63. When purchasing liability insurance, the nurse knows that liability insurance:
    ① Protects the nurse from being sued for malpractice
    ② Is more of a concern for the higher levels of nursing practice
    ③ Provides legal protection in cases of criminal conduct by the nurse
    ④ Safeguards the nurse from the monetary costs of malpractice lawsuits

64. Licensing laws regulate the practice of nursing to:
    ① Protect the public from injury
    ② Guarantee the best possible nursing care
    ③ Ensure that every nurse has good moral character
    ④ Support nurse employment by limiting the competition

65. Your home care patient is scheduled for 24-hour skilled nursing care. The nurse assigned to relieve you at the end of your shift has failed to arrive. Your most appropriate action would be to:
    ① Notify the home care agency before going home
    ② Remain with the patient until relieved by another nurse
    ③ Instruct family members in appropriate nursing care before leaving
    ④ Report the nurse to the state board of nursing for disciplinary action

66. You are a home care nurse for a formerly active 80 year old who recently suffered a severely disabling CVA. You note that the patient is often angry and critical of the nurses providing care. When planning care for the patient, you must remember that:

① You are not required to work in abusive settings
② The patient is still dealing with the loss of his physical health
③ You have an ethical responsibility to accept all patient behaviors
④ The patient will become less critical as the level of care improves

67. When the practical nurse provides patient care in a patient's home, he/she functions under what form of supervision?
    ① No supervision; as self-employed nurse
    ② The directives of the state board of nursing
    ③ The owner of the employing home care agency
    ④ The direction of a physician or registered nurse

68. You have been assigned to help teach a patient regarding the use of a new blood glucose monitor. You are unfamiliar with the equipment. Your best approach would be to:
    ① Refuse the assignment since you are unprepared
    ② Have the charge nurse explain the equipment to you
    ③ Use a different, more familiar monitor for teaching the patient
    ④ Have the patient demonstrate what he knows concerning the monitor

69. Your patient, 44 years old, is preparing for discharge after incision and drainage of an infected hand wound. You have been assigned to review his instructions concerning home care of his wound. You find the patient sitting in his room watching TV. Your best approach to ensure his understanding of these instructions would be to say:
    ① "This should only take us a few minutes if you listen carefully"
    ② "Would you mind if I turn off your TV while we discuss your wound care?"
    ③ "I can see that you're busy right now, so I'll come back later if I have time"
    ④ "Wound care can be very complicated, so we may be practicing this for a while"

70. Your patient, 64 years old, is receiving tap water enemas until clear as preparation for a colonoscopy. Which of the following is a critical instruction concerning the procedure for this patient?
    ① "Please don't flush the toilet after expelling the enema"
    ② "You must hold the enema fluid as long as possible for best result"
    ③ "We must continue giving you enemas until no more stool is expelled"
    ④ "The enemas remove stool so that the doctor can see inside your colon"

71. To ensure optimum evacuation, patients receiving sodium phosphate (Fleet) enemas should be encouraged to:
    ① Expel the enema immediately following instillation
    ② Retain the enema solution for at least five minutes
    ③ Receive the enema while seated on the commode
    ④ Rest quietly in bed immediately following enema instillation

72. During the bed bath procedure, the nurse reduces the chance of infection by:
    ① Thoroughly rinsing and drying all skin folds
    ② Applying clean gloves before beginning the bath
    ③ Using separate wash cloth sections for each eye

④ Changing the bath water after bathing each extremity

73. The rules and regulations governing the practice of nursing in the United States are made by:
① Each state's legislative body
② Each state's board of nursing
③ The National Council of State Boards of Nursing
④ The Joint Commission of Accreditation of Health Care Organizations

74. When first ambulating a patient, the nurse encourages the patient to dangle at the bedside to:
① Increase joint flexibility
② Assess the patient's ability to move unassisted
③ Prevent the complication of orthostatic hypotension
④ Align the patient's extremities for optimum ambulation

75. Your patient has spent several weeks in traction for a leg fracture. During his morning bath he confides in you that he keeps hearing voices in his room although he knows he is alone. Your best response would be:
① "Tell me more about these voices"
② "Have you ever had this happen before?"
③ "Ignore them. You've been alone in this room too long"
④ "That's interesting, but tell me more about how your leg is feeling"

76. A 60-year-old patient has arrived at the physician's office complaining of ear pain, vertigo, and impaired hearing. The physician has ordered a normal saline ear irrigation to loosen embedded ear wax. Following this procedure, the nurse would take care to:
① Retract the pinna of the ear
② Determine the patient's tolerance of movement
③ Encourage the patient to remain supine for several hours
④ Thoroughly dry the ear canal with cotton-tipped applicators

77. Your 34-year-old female patient has been admitted to the hospital unit with a fever of unknown origin. Her physician has ordered urine and blood specimens for culture as well as a broad-spectrum antibiotic. You would:
① Obtain the specimens before beginning antibiotic therapy
② Ask the physician to clarify which procedure should be performed first
③ Begin the antibiotic therapy immediately before obtaining the specimens
④ Obtain the blood, start the medication, and tell the patient to call when she is able to void

78. When instructing a patient in the proper procedure for obtaining a clean-catch urine specimen, the nurse tells the patient to place the container lid:
① On a dry, sterile surface
② Face down on a level bathroom surface
③ Face up on any clean bathroom surface
④ Outside of the bathroom until the specimen is collected

79. When applying sterile gloves, the nurse is careful to:
① Handle only the outside of each glove
② Pick the first glove up by the inside of the cuff
③ Keep the gloves on the sterile field throughout the procedure
④ Insert his/her fingers under the outside cuff to apply the first glove

80. Which of the following observations would indicate that the nurse should withhold a tube feeding?
① Oozing at the gastrostomy site
② Absence of an adequate gag reflex
③ Presence of more than 100 ml of residual feeding
④ Absence of residual feeding when the gastrostomy tube is suctioned

81. Patients receiving gastrostomy tube feedings may experience gastric bloating and diarrhea if:
① The feeding formula is changed
② The feeding is delivered by electronic pump infusion
③ The patient does not remain upright for 1 hour post-infusion
④ The gastrostomy tube is not adequately flushed following each feeding

82. When administering a tap water enema, if the patient complains of the urge to defecate early in the procedure, the nurse should:
① Readjust the tube location while maintaining fluid flow
② Lower the enema bag while instructing the patient to breathe deeply
③ Reassure the patient that the discomfort should pass in a few minutes
④ Immediately discontinue the procedure to allow patient bowel evacuation

83. The nurse knows that a patient undergoing NG suction will soon have his tube removed when:
① The patient no longer compains of nausea
② Bowel sounds are heard in all four quadrants
③ Scant drainage is present on the surgical dressing
④ There is no gastric drainage into the suction container

84. Your patient is an elderly male who underwent emergency resection of the colon two days ago. He is receiving intravenous fluids and has a nasogastric tube hooked up to low wall suction. You note that the patient is hiccoughing and complaining of nausea. You would first:
① Irrigate the tube to assess for blockage
② Call the physician for medication orders
③ Retape the tube to decrease throat irritation
④ Position the client to diminish the risk of emesis aspiration

85. During a sterile dressing change, the nurse should dispose of soiled dressings:
① In the dirty utility room
② In the patient's bedside trash
③ On the sterile waterproof barrier
④ In a waterproof container away from the sterile field

86. When cleansing an open wound, the nurse should:
① Apply constant pressure
② Forcefully irrigate all wound areas
③ Scrub encrusted areas thoroughly
④ Work from cleanest to dirtiest areas

87. Which of the following should the nurse carefully document following surgical dressing changes?
① The specific location of the wound
② The characteristics of the suture line
③ The type of antibiotic cleansing solution
④ The patient's emotional response to the surgical procedure

88. When dealing with body fluids, the nurse is best protected by:
① Hand washing before applying and after removing gloves

② Avoiding procedures which involve exposure to body fluids

③ Reviewing the client's chart for AIDS screening tests results

④ Wearing protective gloves whenever client contact is involved

89. When preparing to apply clean gloves, the nurse performs a thorough hand washing both before and after the procedure because:
① Hand washing is a standard of universal precaution
② This action best protects the nurse from the patient's pathogens
③ Gloved hands are an excellent environment for growth of pathogens
④ Minute holes in the gloves could allow the passage of some microbes

90. When the nurse performs a skin puncture blood collection on a newborn infant, he/she takes special care to:
① Pierce only the center of the fingertip
② Limit punctures to the soles of the feet
③ Avoid piercing the center of the infant's heel
④ Avoid puncturing fingers on the dominant hand

91. During venipuncture, the tourniquet should be released:
① As soon as an appropriate vein is palpated
② Before withdrawing the needle from the patient's vein
③ After application of a bandage to the venipuncture site
④ As soon as blood begins flowing into the specimen tube

92. Placing the patient's arm in a downward position during venipuncture helps to:
① Dilate blood vessels for better access
② Diminish patient discomfort during the procedure
③ Prevent backflow of any chemical additives in the blood tubes
④ Prevent any unnecessary arm movement during the procedure

93. Blood specimen tubes should be labelled with the patient's name and date:
① Before the venipuncture procedure
② Upon receipt of the physician's order
③ Before leaving the venipuncture patient's side
④ Before delivery of the specimen tubes to the laboratory

94. During venipuncture, the nurse should palpate the vein following:
① Application of the tourniquet
② Cleansing the site with alcohol
③ Insertion of the needle through the skin
④ Withdrawal of the venipuncture needle from the vein

95. Which of the following lab studies is a priority nursing assessment when caring for patients receiving TPN infusions?
① Blood glucose
② Complete blood count
③ Hemoglobin and hematocrit
④ Erythrocyte sedimentation rate

96. When changing the dressing of a new PEG (gastric) tube insertion site, the nurse always cleanses the exit site:
① With a vigorous back and forth sweeping motion
② Circularly, from the center of the exit site outward
③ Downward, from the side farthest away to the side closest

④ Upward, through the center of the site, then down each side

97. You would suspect circulatory overload in an IV patient if you observed the following symptoms:
① Bounding pulse, dyspnea, and cough
② Pain, edema and erythema at the infusion site
③ Pain, edema, and a palpable venous cord at the infusion site
④ Fever, chills, and purulent discharge from the IV insertion site

98. Leakage of IV fluid with resultant necrosis of surrounding tissue is termed:
① Embolus
② Phlebitis
③ Infiltration
④ Extravasation

99. Shortly after your patient's IV ampicillin piggyback begins infusing, she complains of itching. You note that her back and abdomen are covered by large, red, macular wheals. You would:
① Discontinue the IV immediately and notify the physician
② Discontinue the IV, and set up for a restart in opposite arm
③ Replace the piggyback with the original IV and notify the physician
④ Reassure her regarding this reaction and apply ointment to the rash

100. When performing venipuncture, the bevel of the needle should be:
① Facing toward the vein
② Facing away from the vein
③ At a 90-degree angle to the vein
④ At a 60-degree angle to the vein

101. When caring for patients with active tuberculosis, the nurse maintains isolation measures by:
① Keeping the patient room door closed at all times
② Maintaining sterility of all equipment entering the room
③ Double bagging all items removed from the patient's room
④ Donning a gown, mask, and gloves whenever entering the patient's room

102. Shaking out bed linens while making the patient's bed can result in:
① The airborne spread of pathogens
② Removal of any foreign objects from the bedding
③ Drier, smoother sheets for greater patient comfort
④ Possible injury to the nurse due to poor body mechanics

103. After cleaning feces from an incontinent patient the nurse should:
① Change gloves before continuing other aspects of patient care
② Scrub his/her hands thoroughly to remove all fecal contamination
③ Remove isolation gown, mask, and gloves in the prescribed manner
④ Delay removal of gloves until all aspects of patient care are completed

104. A 14-month-old baby is being treated by the pediatrician for bilateral otitis media. Her mother has asked you how she should treat her daughter's fever. As the office nurse, you may suggest that she:
    ① Sponge bathe the baby with alcohol.
    ② Place the baby in a tub of cool water
    ③ Give the baby a bath in tepid tub water
    ④ Call the physician as soon as any fever develops

105. Your male patient, 49 years old, has undergone complicated abdominal surgery and is now receiving TPN via a central venous catheter. During his A.M. care, the patient suddenly becomes dyspneic, anxious, and cyanotic. You find the connector to his TPN infusion disconnected. Your first action would be to:
    ① Initiate the hospital's protocol for respiratory emergency
    ② Reconnect the TPN ports after swabbing them with alcohol
    ③ Place the patient on his left side with his head below chest level
    ④ Place the patient in high Fowler's position to assist his respiratory efforts

106. When a patient has died, the nurse should schedule postmortem care:
    ① Before family viewing of the body
    ② Following transport of the body to the morgue
    ③ As quickly as possible to decrease tension on the unit
    ④ After allowing the family the opportunity to view the body

107. Your patient has just undergone a lumbar puncture. As you position him in bed, he asks why he must remain flat in bed for several hours. Your best response would be:
    ① "You are less likely to fall if you remain quiet today"
    ② "It is easier for the nurses to check for any complications this way"
    ③ "This position prevents any increased blood loss from the spine area"
    ④ "This position allows your body to readjust pressure around your brain"

108. A 70-year-old man is a patient in a rehabilitation center for treatment following a CVA. He is scheduled for ROM exercises every 4 hours during the day. To maintain maximum muscle tone for this patient, the nurse should:
    ① Move each of his joints to the point of resistance
    ② Encourage him to skip the exercises if he is tired
    ③ Move all of his joints through the full range of prescribed exercises
    ④ Only assist him with those movements he is unable to perform on his own

109. If drains are present when changing a surgical dressing, the nurse should:
    ① Irrigate the wound with the prescribed solution
    ② Rinse each drain with half-strength peroxide to maintain patency
    ③ Apply petroleum jelly to each drain to diminish friction along the suture line
    ④ Remove one layer of dressing at a time to avoid dislodging the drains

110. Your patient wants to know why wet-to-dry dressings are being used to treat his stasis leg ulcer. Your best response would be that this treatment:
    ① Increases circulation to the wound
    ② Cleans the wound by removing dead tissue and debris
    ③ Promotes the absorption of drainage by capillary action
    ④ Decreases pain by lowering edema along wound edges

111. When preparing a feeding pump for a patient's tube feeding, the nurse knows that the pump should be filled with:
    ① The full day's supply of formula
    ② One full can of formula each time
    ③ Eight hours worth of feeding each time
    ④ No more than a 2-hour supply each time

112. Which of the following would you carefully document following irrigation of a patient's nasogastric suction tube?
    ① Period of time patient retained the irrigant
    ② Character of irrigation returns
    ③ Amount of residual fluid returned
    ④ Type of irrigant solution

113. Which of the following is a significant lab value to monitor on patients receiving nasogastric (NG) suctioning?
    ① Arterial blood gases
    ② Chemistry profile
    ③ Hemoglobin
    ④ CBC

114. Which of the following is a critical nursing measure when caring for patients undergoing nasogastric (NG) suctioning?
    ① Mouth care every two hours
    ② Thorough skin care to the nares
    ③ Turn and position every two hours
    ④ Maintain accurate intake and output record

115. When performing a patient's surgical dressing change, the nurse knows that the correct application of sterile gloves:
    ① Prevents the spread of nosocomial infection to other patients
    ② Assures the patient that the staff is maintaining proper asepsis
    ③ Protects the nurse from contamination from the infected wound
    ④ Helps prevent infection of the wound by opportunistic hospital organisms

116. Your client, a 20-year-old HIV-positive female, is receiving treatment in the hospital for MRSA pneumonia. What type of infection control measure would you employ in caring for this patient?
    ① Enteric precautions
    ② Protective isolation
    ③ Respiratory isolation
    ④ Universal precautions

117. A 16-year-old female has just returned to your unit following a tonsillectomy. Which of the following routes would be most appropriate for measuring her body temperature?
    ① Oral
    ② Rectal
    ③ Axillary
    ④ Tympanic

118. Passive range of motion exercises are performed to:
    ① Strengthen bones
    ② Enhance muscle tone
    ③ Prevent muscle atrophy
    ④ Prevent joint contractures

119. An elderly, inactive nursing home resident is continuously seeping small amounts of liquid stool. This may be an indication of:
    ① Incontinence
    ② Flatulence
    ③ Impaction
    ④ Diarrhea

120. While assisting an elderly nursing home resident with her bath, you observe that her skin is dry and that she has been scratching. A priority in planning her care would be to:
    ① Avoid bathing her
    ② Call the physician
    ③ Avoid the use of soap
    ④ Apply a medicated lotion

121. Before beginning a new tube feeding via a nasogastric tube, the nurse must first:
    ① Measure and replace any residual feeding
    ② Warm the feeding to approximately 105°
    ③ Check for correct tube placement in the stomach
    ④ Dislodge encrusted formula with a warm water flush

122. You have requested an aide to assist you in moving your paralyzed patient up in bed. Which of the following is an appropriate instruction to the aide for this procedure?
    ① Stand one step back from the bed while lifting
    ② Keep your back straight, and your knees flexed
    ③ Keep your knees straight, and your back flexed
    ④ Keep your feet close together for balance

123. While caring for your bedridden patient, you note that she has developed a reddened area on her sacrum. The best method for treating the area is
    ① Turning and positioning the patient q2h
    ② Placing a sheepskin on the patient's bed
    ③ Providing an alternating pressure mattress
    ④ Performing range-of-motion exercises q2h

124. When monitoring a patient receiving IV therapy, which of the following observations may indicate fluid excess?
    ① Poor skin turgor
    ② Thick, tenacious sputum
    ③ Weight loss of 5 pounds
    ④ Wedding ring is too tight

125. When considering the need for application of restraints on an elderly confused patient, the nurse knows that restraints:
    ① Provide patients with a sense of security
    ② Should only be applied with a physician's order
    ③ Are applied loosely on elderly patients to prevent skin abrasion
    ④ Must be tied to side rails to allow faster removal in an emergency

126. When preparing a nasal cannula oxygen set-up, the nurse attaches the oxygen flowmeter to a container of sterile distilled water to:
    ① Decrease the danger of oxygen combustion
    ② Increase the patient's level of oxygen absorption
    ③ Remove any particle contaminants from the tubing
    ④ Prevent drying the patient's nasooropharyngeal mucosa

127. Your patient refuses his morning care today and states that he does not like to bathe in the morning; he prefers an evening shower. Your response should be:
    ① "The staff is too busy to provide for an evening shower"
    ② "The staff will do its best to provide for an evening shower"
    ③ "Bathing in the morning makes one feel more refreshed"
    ④ "Hospital routine requires nurses to provide for bathing in the morning"

128. A 70-year-old male patient recovering from myocardial infarction continuously refuses to cooperate with treatments or comply with the physician's orders. You find yourself increasingly frustrated by this patient's behavior. Your next action should be to:

① Call the physician
② Call the patient advocate
③ Consult with the nursing staff
④ Request a psychiatric consult

129. Assessments of a patient's cultural background may help the nurse to understand his/her:
    ① Immune response
    ② Reaction to illness
    ③ Socioeconomic level
    ④ Body defense mechanisms

130. Which of the following is the responsibility of the provincial regulatory bodies?
    ① Setting and administering examinations
    ② Reporting acts of criminal negligence to the police
    ③ Passing laws pertaining to the practice of nursing
    ④ Establishing minimum levels of safe nursing practice

131. Which of the following descriptions best reflects the role of the Canadian Practical Nurse/Nursing Assistant?
    ① Able to work independently in all settings
    ② Works under the direct supervision of an RN
    ③ Works as an integral part of the health care team
    ④ Cares for only those clients whose condition is stabilized

132. Which of the following is registration intended to protect?
    ① The public
    ② The individual registrant
    ③ The title of the registrant
    ④ The level of nursing practice

133. Which of the following regulates Canadian registration/licensure?
    ① Federal legislation
    ② Provincial legislation
    ③ Municipal legislation
    ④ Professional associations

134. Which of the following is registration/licensure designed to protect?
    ① The public
    ② The practice of nursing
    ③ Level of the practitioner
    ④ Individual registrants

135. Which of the following organizations is responsible for admission requirements to practical nursing/nursing assistant programs?
    ① Individual educational institution
    ② Provincial professional associations
    ③ Provincial licensing bodies
    ④ The Canadian Association of Practical Nursing Assistants (CAPNA)

136. Which of the following organizations offers malpractice insurance to practical nurses/nursing assistants?
    ① CAPNA
    ② Provincial licensing bodies
    ③ Provincial professional associations
    ④ Private insurance companies

137. Which of the following statements best describes membership in CAPNA?
    ① It is voluntary and optional for PNs/NAs
    ② It is mandatory in each province/territory
    ③ It is included with membership in affiliated organizations
    ④ It is automatic with registration/licensure

ANSWERS AND RATIONALES

1. Comprehension, planning, environment (a)
   - ❷ When caring for patients receiving internal radiation therapy, staff members should spend no more than 1 hour per day in the room to limit personal radiation exposure.
   - ① The length of the hospital stay allows sufficient time to care for and instruct patients receiving internal radiation therapy.
   - ③ Minor fatigue during radiation therapy is common but does not warrant special care planning required by patient contact limits.
   - ④ Patients receiving internal radiation therapy are kept on bed rest to decrease the possibility of dislodging the implant.

2. Comprehension, implementation, psychosocial (b)
   - ❷ Practices surrounding death and dying are influenced by culture.
   - ① This request may intensify or diminish family grief, depending on the family's beliefs and practices.
   - ③ Under the Uniform Anatomical Gifts Act, the family has the legal right to allow organ donation when the patient is unable to express his/her wishes.
   - ④ A living will outlines the patient's desires concerning medical care if incapacitated; it does not specify organ donation.

3. Knowledge, planning, environment (b)
   - ❸ Liability insurance only covers nurses in the performance of their professional duties.
   - ① Malpractice insurance costs vary from setting to setting, depending on the level of liability.
   - ② Liability insurance protects against financial damages from malpractice lawsuits.
   - ④ Liability insurance coverage only extends through the specified term of the policy.

4. Comprehension, implementation, physiologic (b)
   - ❷ Clear breath sounds indicate an open airway.
   - ① Encouraging the patient to cough diminishes the need for suctioning.
   - ③ Mouth care following the procedure contributes to patient comfort.
   - ④ Noting characteristics of respiratory secretions assists in determining the presence of respiratory infection.

5. Application, planning, environment (b)
   - ❷ Loose rugs and floor clutter increase the risk of falling for patients with impaired vision or mobility.
   - ① No indication that either patient is receiving prescribed medications.
   - ③ Home health aide will assist with ADLs, not environmental safety.
   - ④ Range of motion exercises maintain joint flexibility in immobile clients.

6. Application, planning, health (b)
   - ❹ Increased physical activity promotes more normal sleep patterns.
   - ① The response does not recognize patient need for solution to problem.
   - ② Sleep medication is contraindicated in the elderly.
   - ③ Warm milk is a comfort measure but not a proven sleep inducer.

7. Application, planning, environment (b)
   - ❶ Comfort and rest are promoted by smooth, wrinkle-free bedding.
   - ② Raising side rails is an important safety measure for the patient with diminished level of alertness.
   - ③ Availability of the call bell is an important safety measure for the patient with diminished level of alertness.
   - ④ The informed patient can make better decisions regarding his or her care.

8. Application, assessment, physiologic (b)
   - ❷ Assessing the exact location of pain assists in determining cause and treatment.
   - ① Drug allergies will help the physician determine the treatment of pain, but diagnosis must first occur.
   - ③ This may help the physician determine treatment, but diagnosis must first occur.
   - ④ This may be related, but the exact characteristics of the pain must first be determined.

9. Application, implementation, psychosocial (b)
   - ❸ Isolation increases the patient's fear of abandonment.
   - ① Pain management is not a common need related to this treatment.
   - ② Visitor limitation causes isolation and increases the patient's fear of abandonment.
   - ④ The patient and the patient's secretions are radioactive during treatment.

10. Application, assessment, health (b)
    - ❸ Anxiety often interferes with the patient's ability to listen to or comprehend instructions.
    - ① The patient needs to understand rather than memorize instructions.
    - ② Too broad a statement concerning physician's instructions.
    - ④ A poor reason for the nursing action. Interventions are enacted by the nurse because of understood principles.

11. Comprehension, implementation, physiologic (b)
    - ❶ Stimulating the gag reflex may result in vomiting.
    - ② Secretions will originate in the bronchial tree and the mouth, not the throat.
    - ③ Contamination of the culture site is not a consideration with this procedure.
    - ④ The size of the specimen is not a concern with a throat culture.

12. Application, assessment, physiologic (b)
    - ❶ This gathers more information concerning neurovascular status before determining interventions.
    - ② There is not enough information to determine whether this is the problem.
    - ③ Elevating the affected foot diminishes edema but does not address the presenting problem.
    - ④ Toe movement assists in neurovascular assessment of the foot, but does not address the presenting problem.

13. Application, assessment, physiologic (a)
    - ❶ Symptoms of local infection include edema, erythema, and purulent drainage.
    - ② Symptoms of systemic infection include general symptoms of GI upset, malaise, fever, increased pulse, and respirations.
    - ③ Necrotic wounds are not reddened.
    - ④ There is not sufficient information for this assumption.

14. Comprehension, implementation, physiologic (b)
    ❹ Wound irrigation presents the danger of splashing or spraying. Goggles, gown, and mask should be applied.
    ① The bed should be at a workable height for all nursing procedures.
    ② Explaining the procedure encourages patient cooperation.
    ③ Hand washing is indicated before and after all patient contact.
15. Comprehension, planning, environment (b)
    ❶ Individuals with spinal cord injuries suffer from immobility complicated by impaired sensory function.
    ② Patients in skeletal traction retain skin sensation and can assist with relieving pressure points.
    ③ Ambulatory patients are at low risk for decubitus formation.
    ④ Immobility is short term. Skin sensation is not limited.
16. Comprehension, planning, environment (a)
    ❶ Footboards keep the patient's foot in dorsal flexion.
    ② Footboards are not mobility aids.
    ③ Gatching the knee of the bed will assist in maintaining the patient at the head of the bed.
    ④ Bedding pressure is not a common problem for the immobilized patient.
17. Application, implementation, physiologic (b)
    ❹ Mouth care relieves dryness discomfort secondary to mouth breathing.
    ① An inappropriate action. The condition does not warrant immediate medical attention.
    ② This causes a potential for electrolyte imbalance.
    ③ The response does not address patient discomfort.
18. Comprehension, planning, environment (b)
    ❹ Delegation of nursing duties to unskilled staff places the patient at risk for injury and the nurse at risk for malpractice suit.
    ① A warm and caring demeanor prevents lawsuits.
    ② A warm and caring manner prevents lawsuits.
    ③ Institutional malpractice insurance protects against costs of malpractice damages, not against the possibility of lawsuit.
19. Application, implementation, health (b)
    ❷ In all care situations, the nurse assumes a role protective of the patient's best interests.
    ① Allowable services may not always meet the patient's needs.
    ③ The nurse is not the representative of the insuring agency.
    ④ Level of care is based upon patient needs, not allowable benefits.
20. Application, assessment, psychosocial (b)
    ❶ Further assessment of the problem will help determine planning and implementation of care.
    ② Reassuring, but doesn't address the problem.
    ③ Does not address the patient's complaint.
    ④ Communication block. Nurse is not offering self.
21. Application, implementation, physiologic (b)
    ❹ Bladder pain may indicate complication, allergy, or bladder distention. Requires further assessment before resuming procedure.
    ① This is a desirable outcome of the procedure.
    ② Irrigation may be ordered because of blood in urine.

③ Returns may be lower than instillation because of patient positioning.
22. Application, implementation, physiologic (b)
    ❸ Bladder irrigation can relieve catheter obstruction and prevent blood clots from forming in the bladder.
    ① Position change will not relieve an obstruction to catheter drainage.
    ② Bloody drainage is an expected sequela to TURP.
    ④ The nurse is expected to act on these observations.
23. Application, implementation, environment (b)
    ❸ This addresses the patients' orthopnea while still allowing for efficient completion of procedure.
    ① This does not address the patient's respiratory distress.
    ② This is an inadequate position for respiratory distress and does not allow optimum visualization for the procedure.
    ④ Gatched knees interfere with efficient performance of catheterization.
24. Application, implementation, health (b)
    ❸ This reduces bacterial counts at the entry point to the bladder.
    ① Multiple invasive procedures predispose the patient to infection.
    ② Unnecessary antibiotic medication predisposes to the development of resistant organisms.
    ④ Antiseptic solutions are irritating to mucosa.
25. Application, assessment, physiologic (b)
    ❸ Urinary urgency and lower abdominal pressure are symptoms of a full bladder. This may be caused by malfunction of the Foley catheter equipment.
    ① The cause of the pain must first be determined before medication.
    ② This is not related to the patient's discomfort.
    ④ This response fails to address the patient's discomfort.
26. Application, implementation, environment (b)
    ❸ This allows the patient to independently and safely feed herself.
    ① This denies the patient's independence and individuality.
    ② This denies the patient full nourishment. It is unnecessary if safety is observed.
    ④ This does not address the patient's impaired vision.
27. Application, assessment, physiologic (b)
    ❶ Cyanosis is a blue tinge to the skin or oral mucosa indicating poor oxygenation.
    ② Vital signs (temperature, pulse, respirations, and blood pressure) indicate cardiopulmonary status.
    ③ Because of skin pigmentation, cyanosis is difficult to ascertain on the lips or nail beds of dark-skinned clients.
    ④ Pulse oximetry measures the arterial oxygenation levels of the extremities.
28. Application, assessment, physiologic (b)
    ❷ Blood glucose levels are a significant assessment for diabetics, especially during illness.
    ① This is an assessment for cardiovascular function. It is not as significant as blood glucose levels for this patient.
    ③ This nursing implementation addresses vertigo and safety.
    ④ This nursing intervention addresses nausea and hydration.

29. Application, implementation, physiologic (c)
    ❸ A delayed infusion of IV solution is often caused by obstruction of the rate of flow. The action allows for further assessment of the problem.
    ① Not enough information has been gathered to make this assumption.
    ② These data indicate further action on the nurse's part.
    ④ Changing the rate of flow places the patient at risk for injury.

30. Knowledge, implementation, environment (b)
    ❹ The most accurate measurement of fluid level is at eye level, in a firm container on a level surface.
    ① The flexibility of the drainage bag interferes with accurate measurement.
    ② Approximation is not an accurate measure.
    ③ Bedpan markings are approximations.

31. Application, implementation, psychosocial (b)
    ❶ This enables the patient to communicate his needs.
    ② This is a secondary comfort measure. Communication of needs would be a primary patient concern.
    ③ The presence of the nurse is more important than reassurance.
    ④ The patient should determine what services he wishes continued.

32. Comprehension, implementation, environment (b)
    ❶ This provides a warm, absorbent covering for the feet without combustion danger.
    ② Wool creates sparking. This is dangerous in an oxygen-rich environment.
    ③ The poor circulation and sensation of the elderly place them at high risk for injury with heat application.
    ④ This does not address patient's discomfort.

33. Comprehension, evaluation, physiologic (b)
    ❹ A full assessment includes both subjective and objective data.
    ① Objective signs do not address cues that the patient himself can provide when evaluating progress.
    ② Limiting data collection to subjective information ignores the observable, measurable symptom not offered by the patient.
    ③ Data must be gathered throughout the procedure to fully determine their effect upon the patient

34. Comprehension, planning, environment (b)
    ❷ Knowledge of the procedure diminishes patient fear, which improves patient cooperation and promotes the expected outcome of the procedure.
    ① Competent nursing practice reduces the likelihood of malpractice suits.
    ③ Procedures are not explained to avoid them, although this may be a secondary aspect of patient teaching.
    ④ The nurse must review the procedure before explaining it to the patient to provide complete information.

35. Application, implementation, health (b)
    ❸ Increased fluid intake decreases the tenacity of respiratory secretions, making sputum removal easier.
    ① Low hydration makes respiratory secretions tenacious and difficult to expel.
    ② Tracheal suctioning is invasive and should only be employed if the patient is unable to expel secretions independently.
    ④ Postural drainage relies on gravity to assist with expulsion of secretions. Affected lung areas vary and must be vertical for this to occur.

36. Comprehension, planning, environment (c)
    ❶ High-risk nursing care plans address the needs of patients more vulnerable to developing a health problem.
    ② High-risk nursing problems are NANDA-approved nursing diagnoses.
    ③ There is no indication of how this statement was formulated. Subjective data include information supplied by the patient, which cannot be easily measured.
    ④ Actual problems represent conditions that presently exist. This statement describes a condition that might occur.

37. Application, planning, environment (b)
    ❷ This is an expected outcome of the nursing action that should occur within a short period of time.
    ① This is a nursing intervention. It outlines the actual nursing activity.
    ③ This is a long-term goal, outlining the overall purpose of the nursing actions.
    ④ This is the rationale; it explains why the action is being implemented.

38. Knowledge, assessment, environment (a)
    ❹ The second voiding is the best measure of how much glucose the kidneys are clearing at that time.
    ① A midstream voiding reduces the number of tissue and skin bacterial contaminants in the urine specimen.
    ② A clean-catch specimen reduces the number of tissue and skin bacteria contaminants in the urine specimen.
    ③ Urine sugar and acetone is not a 24-hour specimen.

39. Comprehension, assessment, health (b)
    ❷ Frequent and regular home blood glucose monitoring best determines the stability of the patient's blood sugar.
    ① The glucose tolerance test is a diagnostic procedure for diabetes. It does not measure how well the diabetic is controlling the disease.
    ③ Sugar and acetone urine testing is not as accurate a blood glucose measure because of the delay of processing blood glucose through the kidneys and bladder.
    ④ Double voiding provides a more accurate urine test but is still less accurate than blood glucose monitoring.

40. Knowledge, implementation, environment (a)
    ❸ This procedure increases the likelihood of detecting occult blood in the stool.
    ① Diarrhea stools are acceptable sources provided they are not contaminated with urine.
    ② Stools for ova and parasites must be kept warm and delivered to the laboratory immediately.
    ④ Occult blood is hidden or unseen blood.

41. Application, implementation, health (b)
    ❶ Weight should be measured at the same time each day, in the same clothing.
    ② There is not enough information to assume this. The patient may be taking medication several times a day or at irregular intervals.
    ③ Daily weights are a more accurate measurement of fluid retention
    ④ Daily weights will indicate early fluid retention, avoiding symptoms of advancing congestive failure.

42. Knowledge, assessment, environment (b)
    ❶ Pulse oximeters measure oxygen saturation by a noninvasive light-beam scan through finger, toe, earlobe, or tip of nose.

② Incentive spirometers encourage sustained inspiratory effort in patients at risk for pulmonary complications.

③ Circumoral cyanosis is a visual, nonspecific measurement of arterial oxygenation.

④ The arterial blood gas procedure is invasive.

43. Comprehension, planning, environment (b)

❶ The pulse deficit examination requires one nurse to take the radial pulse while the second nurse takes the apical pulse at the same time.

② Pulse deficit does not determine systolic murmur.

③ The assistance of a second nurse is more necessary than patient cooperation.

④ The electrocardiograph is a diagnostic tool that measures electrical currents in the heart; it is not needed to measure pulse deficit.

44. Comprehension, implementation, psychosocial (a)

❷ This diminishes patient exposure and minimizes embarassment

① Most clothing is removed for a gynecological exam.

③ This may hyperextend lumbar curvature. Ignores patient's sense of vulnerability because of exposure.

④ This may interfere with visualization during exam. It also ignores patient's sense of exposure.

45. Application, implementation, physiologic (b)

❶ Pedal pulses indicate the level of perfusion to the foot. Traction treatment has the potential for impairing circulation to the affected extremities.

② The apical pulse is the standard auscultatory site for measuring the rate, regularity, and strength of the heartbeat.

③ The radial pulse is the standard palpation site for measuring heartbeat. It also indicates perfusion to the hand.

④ The carotid pulse measures blood flow to the brain.

46. Comprehension, implementation, environment (a)

❸ Pulling the pinna up and back straightens the ear canal ensuring an effective seal.

① Tympanic temperature can be taken effectively while patient is seated or even standing.

② Pulling the pinna down and back does not straighten the ear canal for an effective seal as is desired.

④ Eating, drinking, and smoking affects the accuracy of oral thermometers.

47. Comprehension, implementation, environment (b)

❹ Metal objects will interfere with X-ray visualization.

① There is not enough information to assume that undergarments are contraindicated.

② There is not enough information to assume that this is a fasting examination.

③ Clothing may interfere with the examination in some instances.

48. Comprehension, implementation, environment (b)

❶ A side-lying position with flexion of the anterior leg allows full visualization of the anus with patient comfort.

② This position causes unnecessary client exposure, causing patient discomfort.

③ The knee-chest position interferes with full chest expansion and can lead to respiratory difficulty for some patients.

④ The Trendelenberg position does not allow adequate visualization of the anus, and may impair full lung expansion.

49. Application, implementation, environment (b)

❸ A dated addendum can be added to the chart if appropriately noted.

① The chart is a legal document. No part of the chart may be discarded or altered.

② Addendums to the chart must be dated for clarity of information.

④ If vital information was omitted from the notes, they were not in error. The omission should be added as an addendum.

50. Application, implementation, psychosocial (b)

❶ A reflective statement that encourages further communication.

② This does not respond to the patient's statement. It changes the subject and impairs communication.

③ This response diminishes the patient's individuality. It impairs communication by not allowing the patient to express concerns.

④ This is false reassurance. It impairs communication.

51. Comprehension, evaluation, physiologic (b)

❷ A nosocomial infection is an infection acquired during the course of or as a result of medical treatment.

① A superinfection is the illness produced by growth of a resistant organism during antibimicrobial therapy.

③ An autoimmune response is the immune reaction of the body against its own tissues.

④ Antibiotic resistance is the continued growth of pathogenic organisms during antibiotic medication therapy.

52. Application, implementation, environment (b)

❶ Chickenpox is spread by both droplet and direct contact mechanisms. This measure limits any patient contact with susceptible hosts.

② This places emergency room patients at risk for contracting illness.

③ Chickenpox is spread by both droplet and direct contact. The mask only addresses one mode of infection.

④ Chickenpox is spread by both droplet and direct contact. This measure only addresses one mode of infection.

53. Knowledge, planning, physiologic (b)

❶ Carrying the object close to the body places it over the base of support, diminishing the strain on back muscles.

② Sliding the equipment from the floor to the bed is unwieldy and disrupts the bedding.

③ Leg muscles, which are stronger, should be involved in the lift effort to limit the danger of injury.

④ Holding the equipment at arm's length places it out of the base of support and strains arm and back muscles.

54. Application, assessment, physiologic (a)

❷ An abrasion is a scrape, the result of friction rubbing away the skin surface.

① An incision is a surgical cut in the skin.

③ A contusion is closed skin injury; a bruise.

④ A laceration is an irregular tear in the skin.

55. Application, planning, physiologic (b)

❸ Children have a much higher percentage of fluid to body mass than adults, making dehydration a serious complication.

①,④ The gravity of the patient's illness is the chief reason for rapid assessment by the physician.

② Fever is a common symptom in children because of their immature temperature regulatory control.

56. Application, implementation, psychosocial (b)
   ❶ This provides a well-balanced meal while observing kosher dietary practices.
   ②,④ A kosher diet forbids pork and pork products.
   ③ A kosher diet does not allow mixing meat with dairy products.

57. Knowledge, planning, health (b)
   ❶ Religious beliefs influence the patient's choice of treatment form, as well as the patient's beliefs about the cause of illness.
   ② Last rites is a religious practice concerning the sick or dying limited to the Roman Catholic religion.
   ③,④ This is not the primary reason for gathering this information. The nurse needs to understand the patient's health practice beliefs to plan care.

58. Comprehension, assessment, physiologic (b)
   ❹ The wellness-illness continuum is the ever-changing condition of a person's health through the lifespan.
   ① Wellness is a function of one's physical, mental, and social well-being.
   ② Wellness and illness exist on a continuum.
   ③ Genetics may influence wellness, but does not determine an individual's permanent status on the wellness-illness continuum.

59. Comprehension, evaluation, environment (a)
   ❸ The movement toward cost reduction has shifted health care delivery out of hospitals and into long-term care, home care, and skilled nursing facilities.
   ① The scope of nursing practice has increased with technological advances in health care.
   ② The focus of all health care delivery has moved to wellness promotion rather than illness treatment.
   ④ Nursing care remains patient-centered. Treatment is more technology-based but still involves direct contact with the patient by the nurse.

60. Knowledge, implementation, environment (a)
   ❹ The wet soapy tissues remove fecal matter. Rinsing with cool water prevents thermometer breakage.
   ① The alcohol will be ineffective if fecal matter has not been removed from the thermometer.
   ② Alcohol may not remove fecal matter from the thermometer
   ③ Washing the thermometer with hot water risks thermometer breakage and may seal fecal matter to the thermometer.

61. Application, planning, environment (c)
   ❸ Maintaining skill levels guarantees safe, effective nursing practice.
   ① Regular relicensure is a legal requirement for nursing practice.
   ② Maintenance of membership in professional nursing organizations helps the nurse to keep abreast of changes in the field.
   ④ This action promotes professionalism, but is not a moral issue.

62. Application, implementation, environment (b)
   ❹ This clarifies the error and the corrective measure.
   ① An incident report is completed after error is corrected.
   ② The family is not notified unless they have power of attorney.
   ③ An incident report is an internal record and is never documented in the patient's chart.

63. Knowledge, assessment, health (a)
   ❹ Liability insurance pays damages, when indicated, should the nurse be sued for malpractice.
   ① Competent nursing practice is the best protection from malpractice lawsuits.
   ② Health care providers at every level are at high risk for lawsuit.
   ③ Criminal acts are covered by criminal law. Malpractice is a matter of civil law.

64. Comprehension, implementation, environment (b)
   ❶ Licensing laws are public safety measures guaranteeing minimum standards for nursing practice.
   ② Licensing laws establish minimum standards.
   ③ Moral character is a subjective measure that can only be minimally established by licensing law.
   ④ Licensing laws do not limit the numbers of applicants to nursing practice.

65. Application, implementation, environment (b)
   ❷ This measure guarantees continuity of nursing care.
   ① Failing to provide required skilled care constitutes patient abandonment.
   ③ This does not guarantee continuous skilled nursing care and constitutes patient abandonment.
   ④ There is too little information to determine any unethical action.

66. Comprehension, planning, psychosocial (b)
   ❷ Anger is part of the grieving process.
   ① Anger and criticism are expressions of the patient's needs. They are not necessarily indicators of abuse.
   ③ Acceptance of patient behaviors is made possible by understanding underlying causes.
   ④ Quality of care does not necessarily determine patient behaviors.

67. Knowledge, implementation, environment (b)
   ❹ The LP/VN functions in home care settings under the direct supervision of a physician or registered nurse.
   ① The LPN/VN functions in all health care settings under the direct supervision of the physician or registered nurse.
   ② The state board of nursing administers the Nurse Practice Acts. It is not involved in direct supervision.
   ③ The owner of the home care agency may not be a physician or registered nurse and can, therefore, not supervise the nursing activities of the LP/VN.

68. Application, planning, environment (c)
   ❷ Networking with fellow nurses is an important measure for guaranteeing quality care.
   ① The nurse has a responsibility to update skills and knowledge necessary for patient care.
   ③ This action fails to meet the patient's need to understand the equipment he will use.
   ④ The nurse will have no point of reference for determining if the patient's knowledge is correct.

69. Application, implementation, psychosocial (b)
   ❷ Instruction should take place in a distraction-free environment. Asking permission to turn off the TV recognizes the individuality of the patient and makes him more receptive to instruction.
   ① This is a belittling approach toward the patient; fails to establish teaching environment.
   ③ Self-care teaching is an important aspect of this patient's care.

④ This does not establish a teaching environment; prejudices the patient.

70. Application, planning, physiologic (b)
    ❶ Results of the procedure determine whether additional enemas are needed.
    ② This increases the effectiveness of any enema, but answer #1 is more specific to this particular procedure.
    ③ This increases patient understanding of the procedure, but answer #1 is more specific to an order for enemas until clear.
    ④ This increases patient understanding of the procedure, but answer #1 is more specific to an order for enemas until clear.

71. Application, planning, physiologic (a)
    ❷ Retention of the enema increases its effectiveness.
    ① The enema may be expelled before it has been fully effective.
    ③ The position does not allow adequate visualization of procedure and risks injury to the rectal wall.
    ④ This ignores the patient's need to evacuate the enema.

72. Knowledge, implementation, physiologic (a)
    ❸ Using separate washcloth sections prevents spread of organisms from one eye to the other.
    ① Rinsing and drying skin folds reduces skin irritation.
    ② Clean gloves are a useless protective mechanism if hands are immersed in bath water.
    ④ Changing bath water after bathing each extremity maintains the warmth of bath water.

73. Knowledge, implementation, environment (b)
    ❶ Each state passes nurse practice acts that define and determine the scope of nursing within that state.
    ② Each state's board of nursing administers the nurse practice acts
    ③ The National Council of State Boards of Nursing is a professional association composed of the state boards of nursing. It administers the licensing examination for nursing.
    ④ The JCAHO is a professional association organized to promote standards for health care delivery

74. Comprehension, implementation, health (b)
    ❸ Bed rest often causes pooling of blood in the lower extremities resulting in poor blood flow to the brain when patient arises.
    ① Range of motion exercises improve joint flexibility.
    ② Assessment of the patient's ability is ongoing throughout the ambulation procedure.
    ④ Although this can take place during dangling, the chief purpose is to balance patient's blood pressure.

75. Application, assessment, psychosocial (b)
    ❶ Further assessment of the patient's complaint is necessary before determining action.
    ② This encourages a *yes* or *no* answer. Answer #1 allows for more information.
    ③ This discourages communication by diminishing the importance of the patient's complaint, and fails to allay the patient's fears.
    ④ This discourages communication by changing the topic, and fails to allay the patient's fears.

76. Application, implementation, physiologic (b)
    ❷ Vertigo is a common side effect of this treatment.
    ① The pinna of the ear is retracted during the procedure.

③ Most patients can resume activity shortly after treatment.
④ Use of cotton-tipped applicators in the ears can lead to injury.

77. Application, implementation, physiologic (b)
    ❶ Culture specimens can be inaccurate if obtained while the patient is receiving antibiotics.
    ② There is no need for clarification; this is a standard nursing function.
    ③ Antibiotics will interfere with microbial growth on the specimen cultures.
    ④ Antibiotics will interfere with microbial growth on the urine culture.

78. Application, implementation, environment (b)
    ❸ Placing the lid face up maintains the sterility of the lid interior, preventing contamination of the specimen container.
    ① A dry, sterile surface is not readily available in a bathrooom setting.
    ② Placing the lid face down contaminates the lid interior with organisms on the surface, thus contaminating any specimen placed in the container.
    ④ Placing the lid outside the bathroom places the sterile field outside of vision range, increasing the risk for contamination.

79. Comprehension, implementation, environment (b)
    ❷ Handling the glove on the inside guarantees that your bare, unsterile hand will not contaminate the sterile exterior of the glove.
    ①,④ Contamination occurs if your nonsterile hand touches the sterile exterior of the glove.
    ③ Keeping the gloves on the sterile field throughout the gloving procedure risks contamination of the field.

80. Application, assessment, physiologic (b)
    ❸ This may indicate delayed gastric emptying. Further feedings could induce vomiting.
    ① Gastrostomy site oozing is a common occurrence that requires skin integrity measures but does not indicate a need to withhold feedings.
    ② An absence of the gag reflex is an indicator for tube feeding.
    ④ No residual feeding return usually indicates full absorption of the feeding.

81. Comprehension, evaluation, physiologic (b)
    ❶ The most common cause of GI discomfort in a tube feeding patient is formula intolerance.
    ② Electronic pump infusion is a common, nonirritating delivery route for tube feedings.
    ③ Remaining upright for 1 hour after feeding reduces the likelihood of regurgitation or reflux.
    ④ Failing to correctly flush the tube after each feeding eventually leads to tube blockage.

82. Application, implementation, physiologic (a)
    ❷ This measure should relax the patient, allow the colon to adjust to the fluid flow, and allow the patient to retain more enema fluid for better results.
    ① Maintaining fluid flow will increase the urge to defecate.
    ③ This is a false reassurance.
    ④ Allowing the patient to evacuate too soon deceases the effectiveness of the procedure.

83. Application, planning, health (b)
    ❷ Bowel sounds indicate the return of GI function. The NG tube is in place to empty stomach contents until the GI tract can resume drainage itself.
    ① The patient should not be nauseated if the NG tube is operating effectively. This does not mean that the patient no longer needs GI suction.
    ③ Drainage indicates wound healing progress, not GI function return.
    ④ Absence of gastric drainage may indicate a problem with the NG suction rather than return of GI function.

84. Application, assessment, physiologic (c)
    ❶ Hiccoughing and nausea are indications of accumulated gastric secretions. The most likely cause for this would be something interfering with gastric suction.
    ② Full assessment of the patient's condition must be made before contacting the physician. Function of the GI suction must first be ascertained.
    ③ Throat irritation is not the most likely cause of the GI symptoms.
    ④ Clearing any blockage to the GI suction will most likely diminish nausea, making measures for possible emesis unnecessary.

85. Application, implementation, environment (a)
    ❹ This prevents contamination of the environment with wound drainage.
    ① The nurse cannot leave the patient's bedside during a sterile procedure.
    ② Leaving soiled dressing materials in the bedside trash creates odor problems and the potential for spread of pathogens.
    ③ This contaminates the sterile field.

86. Comprehension, implementation, physiologic (b)
    ❹ This prevents bacterial spread into the wound.
    ① Pressure on a wound diminishes bleeding. It would interfere with wound cleansing.
    ② Forceful wound irrigation disrupts healing tissue.
    ③ Scrubbing disrupts healing tissue.

87. Application, evaluation, environment (b)
    ❷ Healing, as well as complications, is best determined by inspection of the actual wound.
    ① This is unnecessary unless there is more than one wound present.
    ③ An antibiotic cleanser cannot be used without a physician's order.
    ④ Although this is important, it is not directly relevant to the dressing change procedure.

88. Application, implementation, physiologic (a)
    ❶ Studies have demonstrated that this measure best reduces the number of organisms on the nurse's hands in any situation involving exposure to body fluids.
    ② Nursing entails exposure to body fluids. Management of infection potential is the one measure for diminishing risk.
    ③ It is illegal and unethical to limit care based upon the patient's diagnosis.
    ④ Not all patient contacts involve exposure to body fluids.

89. Comprehension, implementation, environment (b)
    ❸ The warm, dark, moist environment of gloves promotes microbial growth. The nurse's hands may be more contaminated with organisms following removal than before application of gloves if hand washing is not observed.
    ① Universal precautions require hand washing before and after any client contact for a variety of reasons. This is a nonspecific answer to the question.
    ② Gloving is the nurse's best protection against the patient's pathogens.
    ④ This measure only addresses the potential for patient contamination of the nurse.

90. Knowledge, implementation, physiologic (b)
    ❸ Bony structures of the heel are just below this site, which places the child at risk for osteomyelitis.
    ① The newborn fingertip is too small, with inadequate blood vessels.
    ② There is inadequate skin depth at this site.
    ④ Newborn fingers are too small, with inadequate blood vessels.

91. Knowledge, implementation, physiologic (b)
    ❹ Once blood begins to enter the specimen tube, the tourniquet is released to allow unrestricted blood flow.
    ① Releasing the tourniquet causes the vein to recede, hindering access.
    ② Keeping the tourniquet on during the blood draw lengthens the procedure and promotes venispasm.
    ③ This would promote bruising at the venipuncture site.

92. Comprehension, implementation, physiologic (c)
    ❸ Chemical additives have a greater potential for backflow into the patient's vein if they rest against the tube stopper.
    ① Tourniquet application dilates the blood vessels for access.
    ② The nurse's personal approach and skill of technique prevents patient discomfort.
    ④ Preventing unnecessary arm movement prevents vein injury and patient discomfort.

93. Knowledge, planning, environment (b)
    ❸ The specimen tubes should be labeled as soon as the blood has been obtained.
    ① Labeling tubes before the procedure may be wasteful if the venipuncture is unsuccessful.
    ② Loose labeled specimen containers create a potential for donor error.
    ④ Unlabeled specimen tubes may be mislabed with the wrong patient's name.

94. Knowledge, implementation, physiologic (b)
    ❶ The tourniquet slows blood return in the vein, causing it to dilate for better access.
    ② Palpating the vein after cleansing the site with alcohol contaminates the venipuncture site.
    ③ Palpating the vein helps the nurse to determine where to insert the needle.
    ④ After withdrawing the needle from the vein, the nurse should apply direct continuous pressure to the site for hemostasis.

95. Application, assessment, health (c)
    ❶ Blood glucose measurements often determine the adequacy of the TPN solution concentration and flow rate.
    ② Complete blood count is a blood test measuring the various cell components of the blood. It is not a priority assessment for TPN therapy.
    ③ Hemoglobin and hematocrit tests measure blood volume and oxygen-carrying capacity. TPN is a nutritional IV therapy.

④ Erythrocyte sedimentation rate is a blood test that indicates inflammatory conditions such as rheumatic fever or endocarditis. There is no link to TPN therapy.

96. Application, implementation, physiologic (b)
    ❷ Surgical tube sites are cleansed concentrically, from the cleanest area outward, to minimize contamination of the wound.
    ① Scrubbing the site disrupts wound healing and can contaminate the wound.
    ③ This brings distal organisms into the surgical site.
    ④ This is not an effective measure for cleansing ostomy sites; there is a potential for missing areas under the ostomy tube.

97. Comprehension, assessment, physiologic (b)
    ❶ Bounding pulse, dyspnea, and cough are symptoms of congestive heart failure, seen when the heart can no longer manage excessive IV fluid volumes.
    ② These are symptoms of IV infiltration.
    ③ These are symptoms of phlebitis caused by IV.
    ④ These are symptoms of infection originating at the IV infusion site.

98. Knowledge, assessment, physiologic (a)
    ❹ Extravasation is seen when irritating or desiccating IV fluid leaks into surrounding tissue at the infusion site.
    ① An embolus is a foreign object or quantity of gas that travels through the bloodstream until it becomes lodged in a blood vessel. IV therapy can cause this complication.
    ② Phlebitis is the inflammation of a vein. As a complication of IV therapy, it demonstrates as pain, palpable cord, and redness at the infusion site.
    ③ Infiltration is the leakage of IV fluid into tissues surrounding the infusion site.

99. Application, implementation, physiologic (c)
    ❸ Symptoms of allergic reaction; action removes the allergen while preserving the IV line.
    ① This causes the patient undue risk and pain if the IV must be restarted.
    ② This causes the patient undue risk and pain. If allergic reaction worsens, an IV line may be needed quickly.
    ④ The nurse cannot apply ointment without a physician's order.

100. Knowledge, implementation, physiologic (b)
     ❷ When performing venipuncture, the bevel of the needle faces up toward the nurse and is inserted at a 15-degree angle.
     ① The procedure is more traumatic and painful if the sharpest portion of the needle does not pierce the skin first.
     ③ Intramuscular injections are inserted at a 90-degree angle.
     ④ Subcutaneous injections are inserted at a 60-degree angle.

101. Application, implementation, environment (b)
     ❶ An open door allows transport of pathogens on air currents.
     ② Protective isolation requires introduction of only sterile items into the patient's room.
     ③ The measure is specific for contaminated items that could spread pathogens via contact as well as droplet route.

④ A mask is needed whenever entering the patient's room. Additional equipment may not be needed depending upon the degree of patient contact.

102. Knowledge, implementation, environment (b)
     ❶ Shaking linen releases organisms into the air and increases air currents.
     ② Foreign objects can be removed from bedding more safely by hand.
     ③ Pulling sheets taut while making the bed creates a dry, smooth sheet surface.
     ④ Proper body alignment during bed making prevents poor body mechanics.

103. Comprehension, implementation, environment (b)
     ❶ Clean gloves should be applied whenever handling organic matter, and removed before performing other facets of patient care.
     ② The nurse is best protected by applying clean gloves when handling body substances. Thorough hand scrubbing is not as effective a protection.
     ③ Isolation gowning is not necessary when caring for simple fecal incontinence.
     ④ Failing to remove gloves after this procedure contaminates the patient and the environment with fecal pathogens.

104. Knowledge, implementation, physiologic (a)
     ❸ Bathing in tepid water is an effective fever-reducing measure
     ① Alcohol is a volatile chemical that can be inhaled by the client with neurological results.
     ② Placing the client in cool water is uncomfortable and causes shivering, which may actually raise body temperature.
     ④ Fever is a normal body response to infection that can usually be managed at home.

105. Application, assessment, physiologic (c)
     ❸ The symptoms indicate an air embolism. Placing the patient in this position prevents embolism movement from the right atrium.
     ① Despite the respiratory symptoms, this is a circulatory emergency. The patient needs to be positioned to prevent further injury.
     ② TPN ports should be reconnected after the patient is positioned.
     ④ Placing the patient in high Fowler's position allows embolism dispersal to vital organs. It will not diminish patient distress.

106. Knowledge, planning, psychosocial (a)
     ❶ Cleansing and preparing the body before family viewing decreases the stress of the situation.
     ② Postmortem care is always completed before the body is moved.
     ③ Family and patient needs are the priority of unit function.
     ④ The family will be less stressed if the patient's body is clean and has a more normal appearance.

107. Comprehension, implementation, physiologic (b)
    ❹ It takes approximately 4 to 6 hours for spinal fluid pressure to stabilize following lumbar puncture. Fewer neurological side effects occur if bed rest is maintained during this period.
    ① Falling may occur because of vertigo, but this explanation is not as inclusive as answer #4.
    ② The nursing staff's convenience is not a reason for positioning the patient.
    ③ Although the position may limit spinal fluid leakage from the site, there should be scant or no blood loss with this procedure.

108. Application, implementation, health (b)
    ❹ Muscle tone is maintained through active contraction and relaxation.
    ① Moving joints to the point of resistance prevents joint injury, but the passive activity does not maintain muscle tone.
    ② Fatigue is expected in relation to this exercise. Avoiding activity increases loss of tone.
    ③ Passive range of motion maintains joint flexibility but does not maintain muscle tone.

109. Knowledge, planning, physiologic (b)
    ❹ Drains are often caught between dressing layers and can be inadvertently removed if care is not used during the dressing change.
    ① Wounds should not be irrigated without a specific physician's order.
    ② Drains should not be rinsed without a physician's order.
    ③ Petroleum jelly is an inappropriate treatment for drains or surgical suture lines.

110. Comprehension, planning, physiologic (b)
    ❷ The drying and subsequent removal of wet-to-dry dressings creates mechanical debridement of wounds.
    ① This is not the chief effect of this wound treatment. Application of moist heat or increased client activity would increase circulation.
    ③ Wet-to-damp dressings promote absorption of wound secretions.
    ④ Wet-to-dry dressings have no effect on wound edema.

111. Knowledge, implementation, environment (a)
    ❸ Formula hang time should not exceed 8 hours because bacteria will multiply in the feeding once it is opened and kept at room temperature.
    ① One day's supply of formula may require 16 to 20 hours of infusion time, providing an environment for bacterial growth.
    ② More than one can of formula can be hung for efficiency provided the solution is not open at room temperature for more than 8 hours.
    ④ A 2-hour time frame is inefficient and unnecessary.

112. Application, implementation, physiologic (b)
    ❷ The character of the irrigation returns indicates any problems or abnormalities related to the treatment.
    ① The irrigant should not be retained during this procedure.
    ③ Residual fluid would be obtained and measured during a GI tube feeding, not during a GI suction irrigation.
    ④ The standard solution for NG suction is normal saline. Only use of a different solution would be documented.

113. Application, assessment, physiologic (b)
    ❷ GI suction depletes the body of sodium and potassium. Significant loss of these electrolytes can be life-threatening.
    ① Arterial blood gases gauge oxygenation levels, more appropriate to cardiac or respiratory conditions.
    ③ Hemoglobin measures the protein-iron compound of blood used to carry oxygen. It is unrelated to GI suction although it may be significant if GI bleeding is present.
    ④ CBC is a complete blood count. Although it reflects many body conditions and illnesses, it is not specific to GI suction.

114. Application, implementation, physiologic (b)
    ❹ An accurate intake and output record is necessary for correct calculation of the patient's fluid replacement needs.
    ① Mouth care is an important comfort measure for the patient undergoing GI suction, but it is not as critical as I&O.
    ② Thorough skin care of the nares is important for skin integrity, but fluid balance is more critical.
    ③ Turning and positioning the patient may promote better GI drainage and will prevent decubitus formation, but fluid balance measures are more acute.

115. Knowledge, implementation, environment (b)
    ❹ Hospitals frequently host large numbers of resistant organisms that can infect susceptible patients. Sterile gloves ensure that no organisms are present on the dressing equipment.
    ① The action protects the spread of nosocomial infection specifically to this patient.
    ② Although the measure may reassure the patient, this is not its chief purpose.
    ③ Gloves will protect the nurse, but sterile gloves chiefly protect the patient.

116. Comprehension, planning, environment (b)
    ❸ MRSA pneumonia is spread by droplet infection. It requires respiratory isolation to prevent transmission to others.
    ① Enteric precautions control pathogens contained in urine or fecal matter.
    ② Protective isolation is not usually employed in caring for AIDS patients. Careful hand washing has been found to be the most effective infection control measure.
    ④ Universal precautions should be employed with all patients regardless of HIV status.

117. Application, implementation, environment (b)
    ❹ Tympanic thermometers measure core body temperatures noninvasively.
    ① Throat surgery forces oral breathing after surgery, causing an inaccurate temperature reading.
    ② Rectal thermometer reading is uncomfortable and embarrassing to the patient.
    ③ Axillary thermometer readings are too reliant upon placement and environmental factors for accuracy.

118. Knowledge, implementation, physiologic (b)
    ❹ Range of motion exercises provide joint motion and flexibility.
    ① Bone strength increases with weight-bearing exercises.
    ② Muscle tone is increased with resistance exercises.
    ③ Active muscle contraction and relaxation are needed to prevent muscle atrophy.

119. Knowledge, assessment, physiologic (b)
    ❸ Impacted, hardened stool allows only liquid feces from the upper colon to pass through the rectum.
    ① Incontinence is the inability to control the passage of stool.
    ② Flatulence is an accumulation of gas in the intestines.
    ④ Diarrhea is the frequent passage of loose, watery stools.

120. Application, planning, physiologic (b)
    ❸ Soap has a drying effect on the skin of the elderly.
    ① The patient must be cleaned.
    ② There is no indication that this is a medical issue.
    ④ This requires a physician's order. Nursing interventions should be tried first.

121. Comprehension, implementation, physiologic (a)
    ❸ Because of the danger of aspiration, fluids should not be introduced into a nasogastric tube until correct placement has been verified.
    ①,② Although this is part of a tube-feeding procedure, the primary step is verification of tube location.
    ④ Fluid should never be introduced into a nasogastric tube until placement in the stomach is verified.

122. Knowledge, implementation, environment (b)
    ❷ This is appropriate body alignment for lifting.
    ① This nurse must stand close to the object being lifted.
    ③ The back and arms do most of the work.
    ④ The nurse needs a wide base of support to maintain balance.

123. Application, implementation, physiologic (a)
    ❶ This is the most easily applied measure for prevention of decubiti.
    ② Although this can reduce friction on pressure points, it is not as effective as regular position change.
    ③ This, also, can relieve pressure on bony prominences but only in the supine position.
    ④ This measure addresses joint mobility, not skin integrity.

124. Application, assessment, environment (a)
    ❹ The tightness of the ring may be caused by peripheral edema secondary to fluid overload.
    ① Poor skin turgor is a symptom of dehydration.
    ② In fluid overload, the sputum would be frothy and possibly blood-tinged.
    ③ Weight would increase in response to fluid retention.

125. Knowledge, implementation, environment (a)
    ❷ Legal constraints make restraints a medically ordered procedure.
    ① Restraints often increase patient restlessness and powerlessness.
    ③ Too loose application increases patient injury risk.
    ④ Side rails cannot be lowered in an emergency if restraints are tied to them.

126. Knowledge, implementation, physiologic (b)
    ❹ Oxygen has a drying effect on mucous membrane.
    ① Ventilating oxygen through water will not reduce its combustibility.
    ② The patient's level of oxygen absorption is related to liter flow, not humidity.
    ③ Particle contamination is not a factor in oxygen therapy.

127. Application, implementation, psychosocial (a)
    ❷ This response recognizes the patient's need for self-determination.

① This response fails to value the patient's needs.
③ This response imposes the nurse's values on the patient.
④ An inflexible response that fails to recognize patient individuality.

128. Comprehension, planning, physiologic (b)
    ❸ Consultation with peers is an important aspect of problem-solving in patient care planning.
    ① An inappropriate problem for the physician. The problem deals with nursing care approaches to care delivery.
    ② The nurse is the patient's advocate in this setting.
    ④ The patient's behavior is not indicative of a psychiatric problem.

129. Comprehension, assessment, health (a)
    ❷ Life experience affects the level of one's response to stressors.
    ① Immune response is a physiological effect. The only influence culture has on this is in terms of health practices or nutrition. Answer #2 is more specific to this.
    ③ One cannot assume a specific socioeconomic level based upon patient's race, creed, or culture.
    ④ Body defense mechanisms are the same as immune response; see answer #1 rationale.

130. Knowledge, legal and professional (a)
    ❹ Provision of safe care is the responsibility of each province.
    ① Other than in Alberta and Quebec, certification/registration/licensing examinations are set by CNAT.
    ② Laws are passed by the provincial legislature.
    ③ Regulatory bodies decide whether there is negligence in the individual practice of nursing and are completely autonomous from the court system.

131. Comprehension, legal and professional (a)
    ❸ All members of the health care team work together.
    ① An RN has responsibility for a team in most settings.
    ② The RN is responsible for the direction, not the supervision, of the PN/NA.
    ④ The PN/NA cares for a variety of patients with different degrees of responsibility, depending on the complexity of care required.

132. Knowledge, legal and professional (a)
    ❸ The purpose of registration is to prohibit those not registered from using the title.
    ① The standards of care set by the regulatory bodies protect the public.
    ② Each registrant is responsible for his/her own practice.
    ④ Licensure protects the actual acts within the practice of nursing.

133. Knowledge, legal and professional (a)
    ❷ Health care delivery is the responsibility of the provinces.
    ① Federal legislation applies to matters of national or international nature, e.g., testing new drugs.
    ③ Regulatory bodies are provincial, not local or municipal.
    ④ Professional associations are provincial, not local, and have a lobbying function only with regard to legislation.

134. Comprehension, legal and professional (a)
- ❷ Licensure protects the practice of nursing through legislation, which provides mechanisms for charging those practicing without a license.
- ① It is the role of the licensing body to protect the public by setting and ensuring implementation of minimum standards of safe practice.
- ③ Licensure indicates the level of the practitioner.
- ④ The individual registrant is protected while providing safe care within the minimum standards of practice of the licensing body.

135. Knowledge, legal and professional (a)
- ❸ Provincial licensing bodies are responsible for setting admission requirements for their own jurisdiction.
- ① Educational institutions may only set admission requirements for general interest courses.
- ② Provincial professional associations may make recommendations regarding, but do not set, admission requirements.
- ④ CAPNA is a voluntary professional association representing provincial professional associations, and as such has nothing to do with admission requirements.

136. Knowledge, legal and professional (a)
- ❸ Malpractice insurance is not mandatory in Canada, and is offered as a reason to join voluntary professional associations.
- ① CAPNA is the professional voice for PNs/NAs in Canada and has nothing to do with the practice of individual members.
- ② The role of the licensing bodies is to protect the public; therefore it would be seen as conflict of interest to provide malpractice insurance
- ④ Private insurance companies do not provide malpractice insurance for PNs/NAs; it is handled through the provincial associations.

137. Knowledge, legal and professional (a)
- ❸ Every member of each affiliated provincial/territorial association is a member of CAPNA upon payment of association fees.
- ① Membership is voluntary and optional to individuals in provinces *not* affiliated with CAPNA, or in provinces where the professional association and licensing body are not the same.
- ② Membership is not mandatory in any province/territory.
- ④ Membership in CAPNA is only automatic with membership in affiliated provincial/territorial associations.

Chapter 3 Pharmacology

This chapter covers two major areas: (1) administration of medications and (2) pharmacologic aspects of nursing care. The nursing process as it applies to drugs and drug administration is explained and integrated throughout the text.

Calculation of dosage and intravenous infusion rate, principles of medication administration, procedures and sites for medication administration, blood transfusion administration, and pediatric drug administration are reviewed.

The major classifications of drugs are presented as to their action, adverse effects, and nursing process application. Commonly used clinical drugs are listed with generic name and brand name.

The role of the licensed practical/vocational nurse (LP/VN) in the administration of medications is determined by the state nurse practice acts and agency policy. However, knowledge of drugs has a significant impact on the quality of nursing care provided each patient by the LP/VN.

Pharmacology and the Nursing Process

A. Assessment: systematic collection and interpretation of data
B. Management
  1. Planning: defining objectives, setting priorities, selecting the best approach
  2. Implementation: plan is carried out
C. Evaluation: determination of effectiveness of the plan and making necessary modification

NURSING ASSESSMENT

A. Assessing the patient
  1. Variables
    a. Age
    b. Body build
    c. Pathologic conditions
    d. Diet and fluid intake
    e. Concurrent drug use
    f. Allergies
    g. Health-illness values
    h. Understanding of disease and drugs
    i. Cognitive function
    j. Physical abilities and disabilities
  2. Medication history
    a. Prescription and nonprescription drugs
    b. Caffeine-containing products
    c. Alcohol
    d. Tobacco
    e. Street drugs
B. Assessing the drug
  1. Medication order
    a. Accuracy
    b. Legibility
    c. Need for clarification
  2. Types of medication orders
    a. Routine or standard
    b. Prn order: given on a "when necessary" basis
    c. Single order: to be given only once
    d. Stat order: to be given only once and immediately
    e. Standing order: established for all patients with a specific condition

NURSING MANAGEMENT

A. Planning
  1. Goal setting: statement of expected outcomes of actions taken in relation to the problem
  2. Establishing priorities: weighing the importance of one problem against the others
  3. Selecting the best approach: identifying the approach most likely to succeed with minimal risk and high acceptability to the patient
B. Implementation
  1. Proper administration technique
  2. Measures to support the therapeutic effect
  3. Observation for desired therapeutic response
  4. Observation for adverse effects
  5. Teaching patients
  6. Accurate recording
C. Institutional level management: drug distribution systems
  1. Floor stock
  2. Individual patient medication system: a supply of medication is dispensed and labeled for a particular patient
  3. Unit dose: individual doses of each medication ordered

D. Individual patient care management
  1. Approach to patient
    a. "Therapeutic use of self" attitude of nurse
    b. Consistency of approach
    c. Informed consent for patient
    d. Compliance and right to refuse
  2. Patient teaching: explain drug dose, side effects, food-drug interactions, and so forth
    a. Identify need for teaching
    b. Establish realistic teaching goals
    c. Select teaching methods
    d. Implement teaching
    e. Evaluate effeetiveness of teaching
  3. Patient observation: establish observational parameters—vital signs, laboratory studies, etc.—to evaluate effects of drugs
  4. Supportive therapy: nursing actions can complement drug therapy or minimize unpleasant, adverse reactions
  5. Documentation of medications (form is set by agency policy)
    a. Information must be complete and accurate
    b. Documentation must be done immediately after administration
    c. Legal implications: if drug administration is not documented, it is assumed not to have been administered
    d. Data should include
      (1) Observations relevant to therapeutic effects
      (2) Actions taken to prevent or treat adverse reactions
      (3) Time when a drug is discontinued
      (4) Reason(s) for discontinuation of drug
      (5) Reasons for refusal/noncompliance of patient
E. Dosage form and route
  1. Factors influencing route of administration
    a. Specific chemical and physical properties of the drug
    b. Pathologic condition of the patient
    c. Adequacy of medication compliance
  2. Dose: amount of the drug to be given at one time
  3. Dosage: regulation of the frequency, size, and number of doses
  4. Dosage form: final product administered to the patient
    a. Tablet: solid dosage form made by compression of a powdered drug
      (1) Enteric-coated tablet: tablet coated with material to prevent dissolution in stomach; disintegrates in small intestine to prevent stomach irritation
      (2) Press-coated or layered tablet: tablet with a second layer of material pressed on or around it, which allows incompatible ingredients to be separated and to dissolve at different rates
      (3) Sublingual tablet: dissolves under the tongue
      (4) Buccal tablet: dissolves between the cheek and gum
      (5) Troche or lozenge: Dissolves in mouth over a long period of time
    b. Capsule: gelatin shell containing a drug; it dissolves quickly in stomach or small intestine
    c. Caplet: coated tablet in the shape of a capsule
    d. Timed release or sustained action: slow, continuous dissolution for an extended time, allowing larger doses to be given fewer times

e. Solution: a liquid, usually water, in which one or more compounds are dissolved
   (1) Oral solutions: may contain flavoring
   (2) Intravenous solutions: must be sterile and particle free
   (3) Other injectable solutions: need only be sterile
   (4) Solutions for external use

f. Syrup: medication dissolved in a concentrated solution of a sugar to which flavors may have been added

g. Elixir: clear fluid that serves as a vehicle for drugs; contains primarily water, alcohol, glycerine, and a sweetener

h. Tincture: alcohol or water-alcohol solutions of a drug

i. Suppository: solid dosage form that dissolves after insertion into a body cavity such as rectum, vagina, or urethra

j. Suspension: a liquid in which fine drug particles are suspended; shake vigorously before use; not for intravenous use
   (1) Emulsion: an aqueous medium in which microscopic oil particles are dispersed
   (2) Lotion: a suspension for external application

k. Ointment: semisolid mixture of a drug, which is rubbed onto the skin

l. Cream: semisolid mixture of a drug in a thick emulsion, which is rubbed into the skin

m. liniment: an oily liquid used on the skin

n. aerosol spray: a liquid, powder, or foam deposited in a thin layer on the skin by air pressure

o. extract: a concentrated form of a drug made from vegetables or animals

p. spirit: a concentrated alcoholic solution of a volatile substance

q. paste: a preparation similar to an ointment, but thicker and stiffer, that penetrates the skin less than an ointment

r. powder: a finely-ground drug or combination of drugs

5. Dosage route: means of access to the site of action or systemic circulation.
a. Oral: drug is ingested and absorbed from stomach or small intestine; convenient, economical; can irritate stomach; may be destroyed by digestive juices

b. Sublingual: drug dissolved under tongue and absorbed through mucous membrane of mouth; can irritate oral mucosa

c. Buccal: drug dissolved between cheek and gum and absorbed through mucous membrane of the mouth

d. Rectal: drug inserted into rectum and absorbed through rectal mucous membrane; may be used in unconscious or vomiting patient

e. Lungs: drug inhaled as a gas or aerosol; useful for drugs intended to act directly on the lung

f. Subcutaneous: drug injected under the skin into subcutaneous fascia; sterile procedure

g. Intramuscular: drug injected into muscle mass; relatively rapid absorption due to good blood supply; sterile procedure

h. Intravenous: drug injected into vein for immediate effect; permits direct control of blood drug concentrations; sterile procedure

i. Intradermal: drug injected directly under skin; sterile procedure

j. Vaginal: drug inserted into the vagina and absorbed through the mucous membrane

k. Intraarterial: drug injected directly into an artery

l. Intraarticular: drug injected directly into a joint

m. Intraspinal (intrathecal): drug injected directly into spinal canal

n. Ophthalmic: drug applied to the eye in form of drops or ointments; must be sterile

o. Otic or aural: drugs applied in the ear

p. Nasal: drugs applied to the nasal cavity by dropper or atomizer

q. Transdermal: patch applied to skin that provides controlled release of medication

NURSING EVALUATION

A. Therapeutic goals: evaluate therapeutic effectiveness of drugs

B. Diagnostic goals: observe for potential adverse reactions

C. Teaching goals: verify patient's knowledge of drug or ability to perform a skill necessary for administration of the drug

D. Patient compliance: evaluate adherence by the patient to a prescribed plan of treatment

Sources of Drugs

A. Animals
B. Plants
C. Microorganisms
D. Synthetic chemical substances
E. Food substances

Drug Legislation

A. Food, Drug, and Cosmetic Act: 1938 (amended 1952, 1962)
  1. Contains detailed regulations to ensure that drugs meet standards of safety and effectiveness
  2. Requires physician's prescription for legal drug purchase

B. Controlled Substances Act: 1970
  1. Defines drug dependency and drug addiction
  2. Classifies drugs according to potential abuse and medical usefulness
  3. Establishes methods for regulating manufacture, distribution, and sale of controlled substances
  4. Establishes education and treatment programs for drug abuse

C. Controlled substances schedule

Schedule I: Drugs that have a high potential for abuse and are not approved for medical use in the United States (e.g., cocaine)

Schedule II: Drugs that have a high potential for abuse but have a currently accepted medical use in the United States; abuse may lead to severe psychologic or physical dependence (e.g., morphine sulfate)

Schedule III: Drugs that have a lower potential for abuse than those in schedules I and II; abuse may lead to high psychologic or low-to-moderate physical dependence (e.g., aspirin [Empirin] with codeine)

Schedule IV: Drugs that have some potential for abuse; abuse may lead to limited psychologic or physical dependence (e.g., diazepam [Valium])

Schedule V: Drugs that have the lowest potential for abuse; products that contain moderate amounts of controlled substances that may be dispensed by the pharmacist without a physician's prescription but with some restrictions such as amount, record keeping, and other safeguards (e.g., Robitussin A-C)

Principles of Drug Action

MECHANISMS OF DRUG THERAPY

A. Dissolution: disintegration of dosage form; dissolution of an active substance
B. Absorption: the process that occurs between the time a substance enters the body and the time it enters the bloodstream
C. Distribution: the transport of drug molecules within the body to receptor sites
D. Metabolism: biotransformation; the way in which drugs are inactivated by the body
E. Excretion: elimination of a drug from the body

VARIABLES THAT AFFECT DRUG ACTION

A. Dosage
B. Route of administration
C. Drug-diet interactions: food slows absorption of drugs; some foods containing certain substances react with certain drugs
D. Drug-drug interactions
   1. Additive effect: occurs when two drugs with similar actions are taken together
   2. Synergism (potentiation): a total effect of two similar drugs that is greater than the sum of the effects if each is taken separately
   3. Interference: occurs when one drug interferes with the metabolism or elimination of a second drug, resulting in intensification of the second drug
   4. Displacement: occurs when one drug is displaced from a plasma protein-binding site by a second, causing an increased effect of the displaced drug
   5. Antagonism: a decrease in the effects of drugs caused by the action of one on the other
E. Age
   1. Fetus: metabolism and elimination mechanisms immature
   2. Newborn: organ systems not fully developed
   3. Children: depends on age and developmental stage
   4. Elderly adults: physiologic changes may alter a drug's actions in the body
F. Body weight: affects drug action mainly in relation to dosage
G. Pregnancy: influence on drug interactions can be pronounced
H. Pathologic condition: disease processes are capable of altering drug mechanisms (e.g., patients with kidney disease have increased risk of drug toxicity)
I. Psychologic considerations: attitudes and expectations influence patient response (e.g., anxiety can decrease effect of analgesics)

ADVERSE REACTIONS TO DRUGS

A. Idiosyncratic reaction: unusual, unexpected reaction usually the first time a drug is taken
B. Allergic reactions: stimulate antibody reactions from the immune system of body
   1. Urticaria (hives)
   2. Anaphylaxis: severe allergic reaction involving cardiovascular and respiratory systems; may be life threatening
C. Gastrointestinal effects
   1. Anorexia
   2. Nausea, vomiting
   3. Constipation
   4. Diarrhea
   5. Abdominal distention
D. Hematologic effects
   1. Blood dyscrasia
   2. Bone marrow depression
   3. Blood coagulation disorders
E. Hepatotoxicity
   1. Hepatitis
   2. Biliary tract obstruction or spasms
F. Nephrotoxicity: renal insufficiency or failure; kidney stones
G. Drug dependence
   1. Physiologic: physical need to relieve shaking; pain
   2. Psychologic: need to relieve feeling of anxiety; stress
H. Teratogenicity: ability of a drug to cause abnormal fetal development

TOLERANCE AND CROSS TOLERANCE

A. Tolerance: acclimation of the body to a drug over a period of time so that larger doses must be given to achieve the same effect
B. Cross tolerance: tolerance to pharmacologically related drugs

SOURCES OF DRUG INFORMATION

A. Resource people
   1. Pharmacists
   2. Physicians
   3. Registered nurses
B. Poison control centers
C. Published sources of information
   1. *United States Pharmacopeia (USP)* and *National Formulary (NF)*
      a. Official reference books
      b. Establish legally binding standards to which drugs must conform
      c. Revised every 5 years with periodic supplements
   2. Package insert: Food and Drug Administration (FDA)—approved label for drug products in the United States
   3. *Physicians' Desk Reference (PDR)*
      a. Published annually with interim supplements
      b. Contains information supplied by manufacturers
      c. Is most useful for finding drugs according to brand name
   4. American Hospital Formulary Service
      a. Contains data on almost every drug available in the United states
      b. Kept current by periodic supplements
   5. Pharmacology textbooks; drug reference books/cards
   6. Nursing journals

NURSING PROCESS

A. Nursing assessment: obtain data on patient regarding problems related to
   1. Route of administration
   2. Elimination or metabolism
   3. Baseline laboratory data
   4. Patient teaching needs
B. Nursing management
   1. Proper timing of dosage
   2. Ways to improve effectiveness of the drug
   3. Instruction of patient concerning drugs

C. Nursing evaluation
   1. Effectiveness of drug
   2. Presence of side effects, adverse reactions
   3. Effectiveness of patient teaching
   4. If therapy is ineffective, examine possible causes such as drug interactions

Administering Medications

CALCULATION OF DOSAGE

A. Practical nurse responsibility
   1. Abide by the guidelines of the health care agency
   2. Check for accuracy in dosage calculation before preparing and administering drug
   3. Check calculations with another knowledgeable person
   4. Measure doses exactly as prescribed by physician
B. Systems of measurement
   1. Household system: measurements commonly used in the home; not as accurate as other systems; following are examples:
      a. 1 teaspoon (tsp or t) = 60 drops (gtt)
      b. 3 or 4 tsp = 1 tablespoon (tbsp or T)
   2. Apothecary system: an older system but one that continues to be used in dosage calculations
      a. Common units of measurements
         (1) Weight: grain (gr)
         (2) Volume
            (a) 60 minims ($\mathfrak{m}$) = 1 dram (dr or 3)
            (b) 8 dr = 1 ounce (oz or $\overline{3}$)
      b. Notations in this system use lowercase Roman numerals; quantities less than 1 are expressed as common factors: exception: one half is written as $\overline{ss}$
   3. Metric system: international decimal system
      a. Common units of measurement
         (1) Weight: unit is expressed in terms of the gram (g)
            (a) Prefix kilo indicates 1000
            (b) Prefix milli indicates $1/1000$
            (c) 1 g = 1000 milligrams (mg)
         (2) Volume: unit is expressed in terms of the liter (L)
            (a) Prefix milli indicates $1/1000$
            (b) 1 L = 1000 milliliters (ml)
      b. Notations in this system use Arabic numbers; fractions are expressed as decimals
   4. Equivalents between systems: a given quantity considered to be of equal value to a quantity expressed in a different system; some common approximate equivalents are
      a. 1 kilograms (kg) = 2.2 pounds (lb)
      b. 1 g = 15 gr
      c. 60 mg = 1 gr
      d. 1 cubic centimeter (cc) = 1 ml
      e. 1000 ml = 1 quart (qt)
      f. 30 ml = 1 oz
      g. 1 ml = 15 or 16 $\mathfrak{m}$
      h. 1 tsp = 4 or 5 ml
      i. 1 ml = 15 or 16 gtt
C. Mathematics of conversion within and between systems; ratio and proportion method:
   1. Household

EXAMPLE: 3 tsp = gtt
teaspoons : drops :: teaspoons : drops
1 : 60 :: 3 : x
x = 180
Answer: 3 tsp = 180 gtt

   2. Apothecary system

EXAMPLE: 3 oz = _____ dr
ounces : drams :: ounces : drams
1 : 8 :: 3 : x
x = 24
Answer: 3 oz = 24 dr

   3. Metric system

EXAMPLE: 250 mg = _____ g
milligram : gram :: milligram : gram
1000 : 1 :: 250 : x
1000 x = 250
x = 0.25
Answer: 250 mg = 0.25 g

   4. Conversion between systems

EXAMPLE: gr $1/6$ = _____ mg
grains : milligrams :: grains : milligrams
1 : 60 :: $1/6$: x
$1x$ = 60 × $1/6$
x = 10
Answer: gr $1/6$ = 10 mg

D. Dosage calculations: The dose for oral tablets, capsules, and liquids or solutions for injections can be calculated by using the following formula:

$$\frac{\text{Desired dose (D)}}{\text{Dose on hand (H)}} \times \text{Quantity (Q)} = \text{Amount to be given}$$

EXAMPLE: Give 500 mg of tetracycline (Achromycin) using capsules containing 250 mg

$$\frac{D}{H} \times Q = \frac{500 \text{ mg}}{250 \text{ mg}} \times 1 \text{ capsule} =$$

Answer: 2 capsules

EXAMPLE: Physician orders digoxin 0.125 mg to be given orally; stock bottle is labeled "Digoxin 0.25 mg" scored tablets

$$\frac{D}{H} \times Q = \frac{0.125 \text{ mg}}{0.25 \text{ mg}} \times 1 \text{ tablet} =$$

Answer: 0.5 tablet or $1/2$ tablet

EXAMPLE: Erythromycin suspension 750 mg is ordered orally. The bottle is labeled 250 mg/5 ml

$$\frac{D}{H} \times Q = \frac{750 \text{ mg}}{250 \text{ mg}} \times 5 \text{ ml} =$$

Answer: 15 ml

EXAMPLE: Morphine sulfate gr $1/4$ is to be given by subcutaneous injection; the vial is labeled "Morphine Sulfate gr $1/2$/ml"

$$\frac{D}{H} \times Q = \frac{\text{gr } 1/4}{\text{gr } 1/2} \times 1 \text{ ml} =$$

Answer: 0.5 ml

EXAMPLE: Penicillin 600,000 units is to be given by intramuscular injection; the vial is labeled "Penicillin 300,000 units per ml"

$$\frac{D}{H} = Q = \frac{600,000 \text{ units}}{300,000 \text{ units}} \times 1 \text{ ml} =$$

Answer: 2 ml

NOTE: This formula can be used with any system of measurement. When two systems are involved, it is necessary to convert to the system of measurement of the dose on hand.

EXAMPLE: Codeine sulfate gr $\overline{ss}$ is ordered by mouth; on hand are codeine sulfate tablets labeled 30 mg

STEP 1: conversion between systems
grain : milligram :: grain : milligram
1 : 60 :: ½ : x
x = 60 × ½
x = 30
Answer: codeine gr s̄s̄ = 30 mg

STEP 2: Formula
$$\frac{D}{H} \times Q = \frac{30 \text{ mg}}{30 \text{ mg}} \times 1 \text{ ml} =$$
Answer: 1 tablet

CALCULATION OF DRIP RATE FOR INTRAVENOUS INFUSION

A. Information that must be known
   1. Volume of solution to be infused
   2. Length of time over which this volume is to be infused
   3. Number of drops per milliliter delivered by the administration set being used
B. The drip rate may be calculated as follows:
   1. Find the volume of fluid to be administered per hour
$$\frac{\text{Milliliters of fluid to be infused}}{\text{Number of hours for infusion}}$$
= Milliliters of fluid per hour

   2. Find the volume of fluid to be administered per minute
$$\frac{\text{Milliliters of fluid per hour}}{60 \text{ min/hr}}$$
= Milliliters to run per minute

   3. Multiply the milliliters of fluid to run per minute by the number of drops per milliliter delivered by the infusion set; this gives the number of drops that should fall in the drip chamber per minute

   Milliliters per minute × Drops per milliliter
   = Drops per minute

   EXAMPLE: Administer 1000 ml of dextrose 5% in water (D5W) over 8 hours using an infusion set that delivers 10 gtt per minute
$$\frac{1000 \text{ ml}}{8 \text{ hr}} = 125 \text{ ml/hr}$$
$$\frac{125 \text{ ml/hr}}{60 \text{ min/hr}} = 2.1 \text{ ml/min}$$

   2.1 ml/min x 10 gtt/ml =
   Answer: 21 gtt/min

   EXAMPLE: Administer 250 ml of dextrose 5% in water over 8 hours using a microdrip infusion set that delivers 60 gtt per minute
$$\frac{250 \text{ ml}}{4 \text{ hrs}} = 62.5 \text{ ml/hr}$$
$$\frac{62.5 \text{ ml/hr}}{60 \text{ min/hr}} = 1.04 \text{ ml/min}$$

   1.04 ml/min × 60 gtts/ml = 62.4 gtt/min
   Answer: 62 gtt/min
C. If the administration rate has been ordered as milliliters per hour, step 1 above is omitted
D. Alternate formula to calculate drip rate:
$$\frac{\text{Milliliters to administer} \times \text{Drops per milliliter}}{\text{Hours to run} \times = 60 \text{ min/hr}}$$
= Drops per minute

EXAMPLE: Administer 1000 ml of D5W over 8 hours using an infusion set that delivers 10 gtt/min
$$\frac{1000 \text{ ml} \times 10 \text{ gtt/ml}}{8 \text{ hr} \times 60 \text{ min/hr}} =$$
Answer: 21 gtt/min

E. Adjust the flow rate to the number of drops per minute as calculated; assess the fluid volume at hourly intervals to see that the fluid is being administered at the desired rate; the calculated drip rate is an approximation of the actual flow rate; the type of solution, additives, position of the patient or infusion tubing, height of the reservoir, and volume of fluid in the container can influence the actual drip rate; the practical nurse should verify computations with another knowledgeable person before readjusting the drip rate to ensure volume delivery for the prescribed time

METHODS OF ADMINISTERING MEDICATIONS

A. Nurse's responsibilities
   1. Knowledge of drug
      a. Its actions
      b. Ranges of dosage
      c. Methods of administration
      d. Common use
      e. Adverse reactions
      f. Contraindications
      g. Patient education
   2. Assess patient regarding history of allergies or sensitivities to drugs
   3. Be aware of and follow agency's policy regarding procedure by which the medication order is checked
   4. Know agency's system of medication distribution
      a. Cards
      b. Kardex/Medex
      c. Computer printout sheet
   5. Know occasions when drugs may be withheld
      a. Fasting for diagnostic tests or surgery; illness
      b. Required laboratory blood work before medication administration
      c. Specific guidelines for certain drugs, for example, apical pulse rate before cardiotonics or blood pressure (BP) readings before antihypertensive agents
   6. Position the patient to properly administer medications; assist as needed
   7. Observe the "5 rights" of medication administration
      a. *Right patient*
      b. *Right drug*
      c. *Right dose*
      d. *Right route*
      e. *Right time*
   8. Inform patient of any anticipated change in normal body functions such as drowsiness, nausea, or change in color of urine
   9. Report patient noncompliance or adverse reactions to other responsible person, that is, registered nurse or physician
   10. Be aware of and follow procedure for controlled substances
   11. Remain with patient until medication is taken
   12. Never leave medications at patient's bedside unless specifically ordered

13. Ensure accuracy in drug calculation; when in doubt, verify with other responsible person, that is, registered nurse or pharmacist
14. Check expiration date on all medication labels and orders
15. Accurately document medications given and, if omitted or refused, document reason
16. Document effectiveness of medication
17. Be aware of and follow agency procedure in event of medication error
18. Acknowledge and respect patient's request to refuse medication

B. Safety measures in preparing medications
1. Environment
   a. Quiet
   b. Free from distractions
   c. Good lighting
2. Do not leave prepared medications unattended; keep in a locked area
3. Read each label three times
   a. When reaching for the container
   b. Immediately before pouring the medication
   c. When replacing or discarding the container
4. Transport drugs for administration by using trays or carts that allow the identifying information and the medication container to be kept together safely
5. Do not allow tray or cart to be left out of sight during administration
6. Make positive identification of patient before administering the medication, preferably by checking the patient's identification bracelet; having patient state his or her name; having second person identify patient
7. Remain with the patient until patient takes the medication
8. Document necessary supplemental information according to agency policy, for example, pulse rate, blood pressure, site of application or injection

C. Oral administration of medications
1. General information
   a. Simplest and most convenient route
   b. Liquid preparations
      (1) Pour into a container placed on a flat surface
      (2) Read at eye level
      (3) Measure amount by using the bottom of meniscus
   c. Irritating drugs should be dissolved or diluted and given with food or immediately after a meal
   d. Distasteful oral medications can be disguised, for example, by having patient suck on a piece of ice for a few minutes to numb taste buds, by storing oily medications in a refrigerator, by having patient use a straw, or by mixing medication with a small amount of fruit juice, milk, applesauce, or gelatin; always inform patient that a food vehicle contains the medication
   e. For patients who have difficulty taking liquid medications from a cup a medication extractor resembling a syringe or a syringe with the needle removed may be used; this allows for accurate measurement of certain liquids in amounts measured in minims, because the syringe or extractor is calibrated in cubic centimeters and minims; device can be placed directly in patient's mouth; must be done carefully and administered slowly to avoid choking or aspiration
   f. For patients who have difficulty swallowing tablets, some tablets may be crushed to facilitate swallowing; be aware of contraindications for crushing of certain medications, for example, enteric coated tablets, or of opening capsules containing timed-release medications
   g. Liquid medications that are harmful to teeth, for example, liquid iron preparations, should be administered with a straw placed at the back of the tongue
2. Specific procedure is described in Table 3-1

D. Parenteral administration of medications: administration by a route other than through the enteral or gastrointestinal (GI) tract, such as intradermal, subcutaneous, intramuscular, or intravenous routes
1. General information: maintain surgical aseptic technique in preparation and administration; it is preferable to use prepackaged, disposable sterile needles and syringes
2. Selection of syringe and needle: thick or oily solutions require a large lumen; short needles are used for children and adults with little adipose tissue; obese individuals may require longer needles to ensure delivery of medications to proper tissue level (Table 3-2)
3. Putting the drugs into the syringe
   a. Manufacturer prefilled syringes or cartridges: contain the name and dose of the drug and the intended parenteral route; should not be given by any route other than the one specified
   b. Rubber-capped vials: single or multidose container; solution or powder form; dry form of drug dissolved according to label instructions; to remove the drug
      (1) Remove the soft metal cover on top of the vial
      (2) Using friction; wipe the rubber cap with a pledget soaked with antiseptic solution
      (3) Fill syringe with air equal to amount of solution to be withdrawn to increase pressure within the vial and to facilitate withdrawal of solution
      (4) Insert needle into the rubber cap while holding the needle in a slightly lateral position to prevent a piece of the stopper from entering the vial
      (5) Inject the air and remove prescribed amount of solution while holding the syringe in a vertical position
   c. Glass ampules: prescored or unscored tops; constricted neck ampules require that solution be in base of ampule
      (1) Quickly snap finger on the stem to move the solution into the base of the ampule
      (2) Use a saw-toothed file for unscored ampules to scratch the glass on opposite sides of the stem, where it will be broken
      (3) Hold the ampule in one hand
      (4) Protecting the fingers of the other hand with a sterile, dry gauze pledget, break off the stem of the ampule; check solution for fragments of glass
      (5) Insert needle into the opened ampule, avoiding needle contamination by not touching the rim of the ampule with the needle
      (6) Keep needle under solution and withdraw the prescribed amount of the solution
4. Skin preparation
   a. Heavily soiled skin in area of intended injection site should be washed with soap and water

Table 3-1	Administration of Oral Medications	
Suggested action		**Rationale**
Wash hands before and practice medical asepsis while preparing and administering medication		Careful hand washing and separate medication cups prevent cross-contamination between nurse and patients
Check the order and read label three times while preparing the drug		Frequent checking prevents errors and ensures accuracy
Pour tablets and capsules into the cap of a stock container and then transfer proper amount into medication cup		Pouring medications into the nurse's hand contaminates the tablet or capsule
Pour liquids from the side of the bottle opposite the label		Liquid that may spill onto the label makes reading the label difficult
Transport medications to patient's bedside carefully		Prevents accidental or deliberate disarrangement of medications
Keep medications in sight at all times		For safety reasons
Identify patient carefully		Illness and different environment can often cause confusion
Assist patient to an upright position as necessary		Proper positioning facilitates swallowing
Offer sufficient water or other permitted fluids		Liquids allow for ease in swallowing and help to dissolve solid drugs
Remain with patient until each medication is swallowed		Patient may discard unwanted medications or may accumulate them with intent to harm himself or herself
Document each medication administered, promptly and according to agency's policy; report/document medications not taken		The patient's chart is a legal record; prompt documentation avoids the possibility of repeating administration of the same drug
If patient's intake is being measured, record the amount of fluid taken with the medication		All fluids taken are to be recorded for determining total intake

Table 3-2	Selection of Syringe and Needle	
Type of injection	**Syringe size**	**Needle size**
Intradermal	1 ml calibrated in tenths or hundreths of a milliliter or in minims	26 or 27 gauge, ½ or ¾ inch
Subcutaneous	2, 2½, or 3 ml calibrated in 0.1 ml	25 gauge, ½ or ⅝ inch
Intramuscular	2-5 ml calibrated in 0.2 ml	10 or 22 gauge, 1½ inch
Insulin (subcutaneous)	Insulin syringe 1-2 ml calibrated in units	25, 26, or 27 gauge, ½ or ⅝ inch

     b. Antiseptic-soaked gauze or pledget is then used to disinfect injection site and thus prevent injection of harmful organism into body tissue
       (1) Wipe in a circular motion, starting at point of injection and moving outward to carry debris away from injection site
       (2) Use firm pressure and friction when wiping to help remove soil
5. Reduce discomfort
     a. Use sharp needle
     b. Use appropriate gauge
     c. Select site free of irritation or nodules from previous injections
     d. Numb skin receptors: cold compresses or ice cube over injection site
     e. Hold tissue taut or compress tissue to form a pad, depending on type of injection
     f. Be sure there is no solution on the needle
     g. Help patient to relax
     h. Insert needle without hesitation
     i. Aspirate when appropriate
     j. Inject solution slowly
     k. Remove needle quickly
     l. Massage area after injection unless contraindicated with certain medications or certain routes (i.e.: intradermal; z-track)
6. Care of equipment after injections: use needle disposal unit; follow agency policy
7. Injection sites
     a. Intradermal injection: solutions injected directly under the epidermis into the dermis, (10- to 15-degree angle)
       (1) Absorption occurs slowly through the capillaries
       (2) Common site: inner aspect of the forearm
     b. Subcutaneous injection: solutions injected into the subcutaneous layer of the skin (45- to 90-degree angle)
       (1) Common sites
         (a) Outer aspect of upper arm
         (b) Thigh
         (c) Lower abdomen
         (d) Upper back
       (2) Suggested procedure for subcutaneous injection is described in Table 3-3

Table 3-3	Administration of Subcutaneous Injection	
Suggested action	**Rationale**	
Verify physician's order and read medication three times; check expiration date	Ensures accuracy and prevents errors	
Obtain and assemble equipment maintaining sterile technique	Prevents contamination	
Draw the drug into syringe and protect needle with sterile needle cover	Exposure to air or contact with moist surface contaminates needle	
Identify patient by identification bracelet and by having patient state name, if possible	Prevents potential medication error	
Select appropriate injection site and cleanse area with antiseptic pledget, using firm, circular motion moving outward from injection site	Friction helps to clean skin and decreases possibility of introducing bacteria into body	
Grasp the tissue surrounding the injection site and hold it to form a cushion pad	Ensures placement of medication into subcutaneous tissue and helps prevent deposition of medication into muscle tissue	
Inject the needle quickly at an angle of 45 to 90 degrees, depending on the quality and amount of tissue and length of needle	Ensures placement of medication into subcutaneous tissue	
After needle is in proper tissue level, release grasp of the tissue	Reduces discomfort of injection	
Aspirate to determine whether needle is in a blood vessel	Prevents discomfort and possible serious reaction if medication is injected into vein	
If there is no blood return, inject solution slowly	Reduces discomfort by reducing pressure in subcutaneous tissue	
Withdraw needle quickly	Reduces discomfort	
Massage area gently, unless contraindicated with certain medications	Helps to distribute the solution and hasten absorption of the medication	

c. Intramuscular injection: solutions injected into the muscular layer of tissue (90-degree angle)
   (1) Common sites
      (a) Dorsogluteal site
      (b) Ventrogluteal site
      (c) Vastus lateralis muscle
      (d) Deltoid muscle
      (e) Posterior triceps muscle
      (f) Rectus femoris muscle
   (2) Suggested procedure for intramuscular injection is described in Table 3-4
d. Z-track injection: technique used to prevent damage to and staining of the skin and subcutaneous tissues; common site is the upper outer quadrant of the gluteal region
e. Intravenous infusion: administration of a large amount of fluid into a vein
   (1) Purposes
      (a) To restore or maintain electrolyte balance
      (b) To supply drugs for immediate effect
      (c) To replace nutrients and vitamins
      (d) To replace blood loss
   (2) Nurse practice acts and agency policy dictate who may administer intravenous infusions
   (3) Nurse's responsibilities for intravenous infusion
      (a) Verifying physician's order
      (b) Calculating rate of flow
      (c) Monitoring rate of flow
      (d) Assessing patient for adverse reactions
         ■ Infiltration
         ■ Circulatory overload
         ■ Thrombophlebitis

f. Hyperalimentation: total parenteral nutrition (TPN), that is, an intravenous infusion containing sufficient nutrients to sustain life; provides amino acids, glucose, vitamins, and electrolytes for those patients unable to ingest nutrients normally for extended periods and for whom standard infusions are inadequate
g. Blood transfusion: infusion of whole blood from a healthy person into a recipient's vein
   (1) Blood is typed and cross matched before administration to determine compatibility
   (2) Nurse's responsibility for blood transfusion
      (a) Check and double-check
         ■ The labels
         ■ The numbers
         ■ The Rh factor
         ■ Compatibility
      (b) Stay with patient for at least the first 5 minutes after transfusion is started
      (c) Monitor rate of transfusion
      (d) Assess patient for signs of adverse reactions
         ■ Hemolytic reaction: stop transfusion immediately, keep vein open with slow drip normal saline solution, and notify physician; indications include
            □ Headache
            □ Sensations of tingling
            □ Difficulty in breathing
            □ Pain in lumbar region or legs
         ■ Allergic reactions: stop transfusion immediately and notify physician; indications include

Table 3-4	Administration of Intramuscular Injection	
Suggested action		**Rationale**
Verify physician's order and read medication label three times; check expiration date		Ensures accuracy and prevents errors
Obtain and assemble equipment, maintaining sterile technique		Prevents contamination
Draw the drug into syringe; create small air bubble in the syringe; protect needle with sterile needle cover		Air bubble forces medication out of needle shaft when injected; exposure to air or contact with most surfaces contaminates needle
Identify patient by identification bracelet and by having patient state name, if possible		Prevents potential medication error
Have the patient assume appropriate position according to site selected		Helps to relax muscles and eases discomfort
Select appropriate injection site and cleanse area with antiseptic pledget, using firm, circular motion moving outward from injection site		Friction helps to clean the skin, thus decreasing possibility of introducing bacteria into body tissue
Press down and hold tissue taut over the injection site		Ensures needle reaches muscle layer
Hold syringe at 90-degree angle and quickly thrust needle into the tissue		Minimizes discomfort
Aspirate to determine whether needle is in a blood vessel		Prevents discomfort and possible serious reaction if medication injected into vein
If there is no blood return, inject medication slowly, followed by the air bubble		Reduces discomfort and allows medication to disperse into the tissue; air bubble clears medication from needle
Withdraw needle quickly		Reduces discomfort
Massage area gently, unless contraindicated with certain medications		Helps to distribute the solution and hasten absorption of the medication

      □ Pruritus
      □ Hives (urticaria)
      □ Difficulty in breathing
   ■ Febrile reactions resulting from contaminant in the blood: usually occurs late in the transfusion or after it is completed; indications include
      □ Flushed skin
      □ Elevated temperature
      □ Chills, muscular spasms
      □ General malaise
      □ Signs of systemic infection
   ■ Circulatory overload can lead to pulmonary edema; indications include
      □ Increased pulse rate
      □ Dyspnea
      □ Respiratory distress
      □ Moist coughing
      □ Expectoration of blood-tinged mucus
   ■ Anticoagulant reaction: indications include
      □ Tingling in the fingers
      □ Muscular cramping
      □ Convulsions
  h. Blood extracts: specific components of whole blood that meet specific needs of the patient
    (1) Packed red blood cells (RBCs)
    (2) Plasma
    (3) Human albumin
    (4) Fibrinogen
    (5) Gamma globulin
E. Percutaneous administration

1. Description: application of medication for absorption through mucous membrane or skin
2. Common sites
  a. Instilling solution into the ear, eye, nose, mouth, or vagina
  b. Applying topical creams, powders, ointments, or lotions onto the skin
  c. Using aerosolized liquids/gases to medicate nasal passages, sinuses, or lungs

Pediatric Drug Administration
GENERAL RULES
A. Pediatric drug therapy should be guided by the child's age, weight, and level of growth and development
B. The nurse's approach to the child should convey the impression that he or she expects the child to take the medication
C. Explanation regarding the medication should be based on the child's level of understanding
D. The nurse must be honest with the child regarding the procedure
E. It may be necessary to mix distasteful medication or crushed tablets with a small amount of honey, applesauce, or gelatin
F. Never threaten a child with an injection if he refuses an oral medication
G. All medications should be kept out of the reach of children, and medications should never be referred to as candy

CALCULATING THE PEDIATRIC DOSE
Safe dosage ranges of drugs are less well defined for children than for adults. Not all drug dosage ranges for children are listed in the literature. It is not the nurse's responsibility to

determine the dose of a drug for the infant or child, but at times it may be necessary to verify or calculate a dose as a fraction of the adult dose. The following methods may be used:

A. Body surface area: considered most accurate; requires a nomogram—a device for rapid estimation of body surface area

$$\text{Child's dose} = \frac{\text{Body surface area (in square meters)}}{1.73 \text{ sq m}^2} \times \text{Adult dose}$$

B. Clark's rule: based on weight and used for children at least 2 years old

$$\text{Child's dose} = \frac{\text{Weight (in pounds)}}{150} \times \text{Adult dose}$$

C. Young's rule: based on age and used for children at least 2 years old

$$\text{Child's dose} = \frac{\text{Age (in years)}}{\text{Age (in years)} + 12} \times \text{Adult dose}$$

D. Fried's rule: used for children less than 2 years old

$$\text{Child's dose} = \frac{\text{Age (in months)}}{150} \times \text{Adult dose}$$

IDENTIFYING THE PATIENT
A. Check the child's identification bracelet
B. Ask the older child his name

ORAL MEDICATION
Verify, calculate, and document all medications
A. Infants
  1. Draw up liquid medication in a dropper or a syringe without the needle
  2. Elevate infant's head and shoulders; hold infant in a feeding position
  3. Depress the chin with the thumb to open infant's mouth
  4. Using the dropper or syringe, direct the medication toward the inner aspect of the infant's cheek and release the flow of medication slowly
  5. Release the thumb and allow the infant to swallow
  6. Liquid medication can also be measured into a nipple and the infant allowed to suck the medication through the nipple
  7. Crushed tablets can be mixed with a small amount of honey or applesauce and fed slowly with a teaspoon
B. Toddlers
  1. Draw up medication in a syringe or measure into a medication cup
  2. Elevate the child's head and shoulders
  3. Place the syringe in the child's mouth and slowly release the medication, directing it toward the inner aspect of the cheek, or allow the child to hold the medicine cup and drink it at own pace; offer praise
C. School-age children
  1. When the child is old enough to take medicine in tablet or capsule form, direct him or her to place the medicine near the back of the tongue and to immediately swallow fluid such as water or juice
  2. Offer the child praise after he or she has taken medication

INTRAMUSCULAR INJECTION
A. Infants
  1. Common site: largest muscle group is the quadriceps femoris, located in the anterolateral thigh; largest mus-

cle of this group is the vastus lateralis, situated on the anterior surface of the midlateral thigh
    a. Place infant in supine position
    b. Compress muscle tissue at upper aspect of thigh, pointing the nurse's fingers toward the infant's feet
    c. Needle is inserted at a 90-degree angle; maximum length of needle for an infant is 1 inch (2.5 cm)
  2. Alternate site: rectus femoris muscle, located on the anterolateral surface of the upper thigh; needle is inserted at a 45-degree angle and is directed toward the knee
B. Toddlers and school-age children: common sites are
  1. Dorsogluteal muscle; upper outer quadrant; gluteal muscle does not develop until child begins to walk; should be used for injections only after the child has been walking for a year or more
  2. Ventrogluteal muscle: a dense muscle mass; the disadvantage is that the site is visible to the child
  3. Deltoid muscle may be used for older, larger children
  4. Lateral and anterior aspect of thigh: upper outer quadrant of thigh

ADMINISTRATION OF INJECTIONS
A. Infants
  1. Place infant in a secure position to avoid movement of the extremity
  2. Usually, have a second person to secure the infant
  3. Hold, cuddle, and comfort the infant after the injection
B. Toddlers and school-age children
  1. Have syringe and needle completely prepared before contact with the child
  2. Keep needle outside of child's visual field
  3. Explain, according to the child's developmental age, the reason for an injection and where it will be given; do not say "it won't hurt"
  4. Inspect injection site before injection for tenderness or undue firmness
  5. Have a second person available to help secure the child and offer comfort during the procedure
  6. Allow the child to express fears
  7. Perform the procedure quickly and gently
  8. Praise the child for his or her behavior after the injection

Central Nervous System
DEPRESSANTS
A. Characteristics of drug-induced central nervous system (CNS) depression
  1. Mild: disinterest in surroundings, inability to focus on a topic or to initiate talking or movement, slowed pulse and respirations
  2. Moderate or progressive: drowsiness or sleep, decreased muscle tone and ability to move, diminished acuity of all sensations—touch, vision, hearing, heat, cold, or pain
  3. Severe: unconsciousness or coma, loss of reflexes, respiratory failure, death
B. Analgesics: drugs used to relieve pain; unresponsive to non-narcotic analgesics (Table 3-5)
  1. Narcotic analgesics (opioids: morphine, prototype)
    a. Actions
      (1) Raises pain perception threshold
      (2) Reduces fear and anxiety
      (3) Induces sleep

Table 3-5	Composition of Oral Narcotic Preparations	
Name	**Narcotic**	**Other components**
Empirin compound no. 1	Codeine phosphate 8 mg	Aspirin
2	Codeine phosphate 16 mg	Phenacetin
3	Codeine phosphate 32 mg	Caffeine
4	Codeine phosphate 65 mg	
Fiorinal with codeine no. 1	Codeine phosphate 7.5 mg	Aspirin
2	Codeine phosphate 15 mg	Phenacetin
3	Codeine phosphate 30 mg	Caffeine
4	Codeine phosphate 60 mg	Butalbital
Percodan	Oxycodone hydrochloride	Aspirin
		Phenacetin
		Caffeine
Darvon compound	Propoxyphene hydrochloride	Aspirin
Darvon compound-65		Phenacetin
		Caffeine
Darvon with ASA	Propoxyphene hydrochloride	Aspirin
Darvon-N with ASA	Propoxyphene napsylate	Aspirin
Darvocet-N	Propoxyphene napsylate	Acetaminophen
Percobarb	Oxycodone hydrochloride	Aspirin
		Phenacetin
		Caffeine
		Hexobarbital
Percocet	Oxycodone hydrochloride	Acetaminophen
Phenaphen with codeine no. 1	Codeine phosphate 8 mg	Aspirin
2	Codeine phosphate 16 mg	Phenacetin
3	Codeine phosphate 32 mg	Phenobarbital
4	Codeine phosphate 65 mg	Hyoscyamine sulfate
Tylenol with codeine no. 1	Codeine phosphate 7.5 mg	Acetaminophen
2	Codeine phosphate 15 mg	Acetaminophen
3	Codeine phosphate 30 mg	Acetaminophen
4	Codeine phosphate 60 mg	Acetaminophen

    (4) Depresses respiratory and cough centers in medulla

    (5) Inhibits gastric, billiary, and pancreatic secretions; depressing gastrointestinal tract

    (6) Stimulates release of antidiuretic hormone, resulting in decreased urine volume

    (7) Induces hypotension

    (8) Slows heart rate

    (9) Causes pupillary constriction

  b. Agents

Examples	**Comments**
Alpharodine hydrochloride (Nisentil)	Not given orally; schedule II drug
Anileridine hydrochloride (Leritine)	Schedule II drug
Butorphanol tartrate (Stadol)	Currently not classified as a controlled drug
Codeine sulfate	Schedule II drug
Codeine phosphate	
Hydromorphone hydrochloride (Dilaudid)	Schedule II drug
Levorphanol tartrate (Levo-Dromoran)	Schedule II drug

Examples	**Comments**
Meperidine hydrochloride (Demerol)	Schedule II drug
Methadone hydrochloride (Dolophine, Methadose)	Also used as a replacement drug for opiate dependence or to ease withdrawal; schedule II drug
Morphine sulfate	Poor oral absorption; schedule II drug
Nalbuphine hydrochloride (Nubain)	Currently not classified as a controlled drug
Oxycodone hydrochloride (Percodan)	Schedule II drug
Oxymorphone hydrochloride (Numorphan)	Schedule II drug
Pentazocine hydrochloride (Talwin)	Schedule IV drug; oral preparation
Pentazocine lactate (Talwin)	Schedule IV drug; oral parenteral preparation
Propoxyphene hydrochloride (Darvon)	Schedule IV drug
Propoxyphene napsylate (Darvon-N)	Schedule IV drug

c. Adverse reactions and contraindications
  (1) Nausea and vomiting
  (2) Constipation
  (3) Urinary retention
  (4) Pruritus
  (5) Hypotension
  (6) Morphine can cause respiratory depression, so is used cautiously for patients with impaired respiratory function; it is not used for patients with head injury as it will obscure CNS evaluation
d. Dependency: develops rapidly
  (1) There is a distinct physical reaction when the drug is suddenly stopped and the body readjusts to functioning in the absence of the drug (abstinence syndrome); symptoms include
    (a) Runny nose
    (b) Gooseflesh
    (c) Tearing
    (d) Yawning
    (e) Muscle twitching and abdominal cramping
    (f) Insomnia
    (g) Nausea and vomiting
    (h) Diarrhea
  (2) Methadone hydrochloride is used for detoxification and maintenance
e. Acute toxicity: usual cause of death is respiratory depression; treated with support to respiration and with a narcotic antagonist such as levallorphan tartrate (Lorfan), nalorphine hydrochloride (Nalline), or naloxone hydrochloride (Narcan)

2. Nonnarcotic analgesics/antiinflammatory analgesics
  a. Action: sensitization of peripheral pain receptor
  b. Agents
    (1) Acetylsalicylic acid (aspirin): effective in management of low-intensity pain
      (a) Adverse reactions
        ▪ Gastric irritation
        ▪ Ulceration and gastric bleeding
        ▪ Intoxication (salicylism): tinnitus, reversible hearing loss, hyperventilation, fever, metabolic acidosis, vomiting, hypokalemia, convulsions, coma, and death
      (b) Drug interactions with aspirin
        ▪ Anticoagulants: increase likelihood of bleeding
        ▪ Alcohol: increases likelihood of gastrointestinal irritation and bleeding
    (2) Acetaminophen (Datril, Tylenol): effective in management of low-intensity pain; does not produce gastric irritation or alter platelet function and bleeding times as does aspirin; does not interact with oral anticoagulants; prolonged use or frequent high doses can cause liver and kidney damage
    (3) Nonsteroidal antiinflammatory drugs (NSAIDs): effective in treatment of osteoarthritis, degenerative joint disease, rheumatic diseases
      (a) Adverse reactions
        ▪ Heartburn/indigestion
        ▪ Nausea/vomiting
        ▪ Constipation or diarrhea
        ▪ Fluid retention
        ▪ Hypertension

        ▪ Dizziness
        ▪ Blurred vision
        ▪ Skin rash
      (b) Drug interactions vary because of the chemical makeup of the various NSAIDs
      (c) Agents: the following are examples

      Ibuprofen (Motrin, Nuprin, Advil)   Phenylbutazone (Azolid)
      Indomethacin (Indocin)   Piroxicam (Feldene)
      Meclofenemate sodium (Meclomen)

3. Nursing assessment: determine character, location, onset, contributing factors, duration of pain, time of last dose: presence of head injury; hepatic or renal failure
4. Nursing management
  a. Determine the most effective way to manage the pain: drug versus nondrug measure (i.e., positioning, turning)
  b. Obtain vital signs
    (1) Be alert to hypotension/hypertension
    (2) Analyze rate and character of respiration
    (3) Withhold drug and notify physician in presence of respiratory depression: respiratory rate of 10 or less respirations per minute or a decrease of 8 or more respirations per minute from baseline data
  c. Caution patient to remain quiet after drug administration to decrease possible nausea and vomiting
  d. Implement safety measures: use side rails and advise patient to remain in bed if there are changes in mental status, alterations in judgment, or unsteadiness
  e. Initiate intake and output records to determine effectiveness of bladder function
  f. Determine efficacy of bowel activity
  g. Patient instruction concerning
    (1) How to take drug
    (2) Safe storage in the home
    (3) Avoidance of driving
    (4) Danger of simultaneous administration of alcohol or other CNS depressant with narcotics
5. Nursing evaluation
  a. Subjective interviewing: ask if patient is comfortable
  b. Objective observations
    (1) Decreased restlessness and anxiety
    (2) Ability of the patient to function

C. Narcotic antagonists
  1. Action: reverses CNS and respiratory depression caused by overdose of narcotics
  2. Agents

Examples	Comment
Levallorphan tartrate (Lorfan)	If effects of the narcotic persist, repeat doses may be necessary
Naloxone hydrochloride (Narcan)	
Naltrexone hydrochloride (Trexan)	

  3. Adverse reactions and contraindications
    a. Arrhythmias
    b. Hypertension
    c. Hypotension

d. Nausea/vomiting
e. Return of severe pain
4. Failure to improve indicates need to investigate other causes of CNS and respiratory depression

D. Anesthetics: provide a pain-free experience during an operative procedure along with a relaxed state of mind and sense of security
1. General anesthetics: provide loss of pain sensation, loss of consciousness, loss of memory, and loss of voluntary and some involuntary muscle activity
   a. Inhalation agents: the following are examples

Cyclopropane	Methoxyflurane
Ether	(Penthrane)
Halothane	Nitrous oxide

   b. Intravenous agents: the following are examples

Droperidol (Inapsine)	Methohexital sodium
	(Brevital)
Droperidol-Fentanyl	Thiamylal sodium
citrate (Innovar)	(Surital)
Ketamine hydrochloride	Thiopental sodium
	(Pentothal)

2. Regional anesthetics: provide loss of sensation and motor activity in localized areas of the body
   a. Types
      (1) Topical
      (2) Infiltration
      (3) Peripheral nerve blocks
      (4) Spinal
      (5) Epidural
      (6) Caudal
   b. Agents: the following are examples

Carbocaine	Pontocaine
Novocain	Xylocaine
Nupercaine	

3. Nursing assessment
   a. Preoperative: obtain health history including allergies, psychologic status, physiologic baseline data; inform patient about surgical procedure
   b. Intraoperative: implement safety measures in presence of explosive or flammable agents
   c. Postoperative: determine vital signs and respiratory function
4. Nursing management
   a. Preoperative: prepare patient physically and psychologically; initiate measures to prevent complications: deep breathing and bed exercises; administer preoperative medications; initiate safety measures and provide quiet environment
   b. Intraoperative: maintain quiet during stage 2 anesthesia; position patient properly and pad pressure points adequately; transfer patient from operating table in a smooth, coordinated manner to avoid severe hypotension
   c. Postoperative: preserve quiet atmosphere; maintain airway, control pain using careful nursing judgment; prevent complications by encouraging deep breathing, coughing
5. Nursing evaluation
   a. Preoperative: effects of preoperative medication

b. Intraoperative: ongoing evaluation of patient's status, usually the responsibility of the anesthesiologist
c. Postoperative: concerned with pulmonary complications, thrombophlebitis, infection, or other complications, postanesthesia nausea, vomiting, hypotension, tachycardia

E. Anticonvulsants: drugs used to control seizures
1. Action: not completely understood; thought to depress neuron excitability and to modify the ability of brain tissue to respond to stimuli that initiate seizure activity
2. Agents

	Examples	**Adverse Reactions**
a.	Long-acting barbiturates Mephobarbital (Mebaral) Phenobarbital (Luminal) Primidone (Mysoline)	Sedation, drowsiness, tolerance, nystagmus, ataxia, anemia, congenital malformations in fetus; sudden withdrawal can induce convulsions
b.	Hydantoins Ethotoin (Peganone) Mephenytoin (Mesantoin) Phenytoin (Dilantin)	Nystagmus, ataxia, slurred speech, tremors, nervousness, drowsiness, fatigue, overgrowth of the gums (gingival hyperplasia), occasional folic acid or vitamin D deficiency; congenital malformations in fetus
c.	Succinimides Ethosuximide (Zarontin) Methsuximide (Celontin) Phensuximide (Milontin)	Gastrointestinal irritation, dizziness, drowsiness, headache, fatigue
d.	Oxazolidinediones Trimethadione (Tridione)	Serious allergic dermatitis, kidney and liver damage, vertigo, photophobia, spontaneous abortion, congenital malformations
e.	Benzodiazepines Clonazepam (Clonopin) Diazepam (Valium)	Drowsiness, ataxia, personality changes
f.	Miscellaneous Acetazolamide (Diamox)	Loss of appetite, drowsiness, confusion
	Carbamazepine (Tegretol)	Drowsiness, dizziness, ataxia, double vision, gastrointestinal upset
	Lidocaine hydrochloride (Xylocaine)	Depressed heart action
	Paraldehyde	Bronchopulmonary irritation, thrombophlebitis at intravenous injection site
	Valproic acid (Depakene)	Gastrointestinal distress, sedation

3. Nursing assessment: observe course of the seizure; assist in case finding; assess baseline data with concentration on areas known to be affected by the drug, e.g., pheny-

toin (Dilantin): assess mouth, teeth, and gums for development of gingival hyperplasia
4. Nursing management: instruct patient concerning
    a. Drug characteristics
    b. Importance of taking medication even when patient is seizure free; awareness that reaching a therapeutic level may take time
    c. Impairment of absorption of the anticonvulsant when taken with milk or antacids
    d. Wearing or carrying identification indicating seizure activity and drugs and dosages being taken
    e. Reducing gastric irritation by taking drug with meals
    f. Good gum massage and oral care after each meal
5. Nursing evaluation: continued medical follow-up; blood level tests

F. Skeletal muscle relaxants: drugs used to treat muscle spasticity
1. Action: Inhibits nerve impulse transmission by blocking polysynaptic pathways in the spinal cord
2. Agents

Examples	Adverse Reactions
a. Drugs to treat spasticity Baclofen (Lioresal)	Drowsiness incoordination, gastrointestinal upset
Dantrolene sodium (Dantrium)	Liver damage
Diazepam (Valium)	Drowsiness, incoordination
b. Drugs to treat muscle spasm Carisoprodol (Rela, Soma) Chlorphenesin carbamate (Maolate) Chlorzoxazone (Paraflex) Cyclobenzaprine hydrochloride (Flexeril) Dantrolene (Dantrium) Diazepam (Valium) Methocarbamol (Delaxin, Robaxin) Meprobamate (Miltown, Equanil) Orphenadrine citrate (Flexon, Norflex)	Drowsiness, dizziness

3. Nursing assessment: obtain baseline data, focusing on spasticity, including degree, aggravating factors, associated pain, and interference with activities of daily living (ADLs); observe baseline liver function studies
4. Nursing management: monitor for drug effectiveness and side effects; institute safety measures if drowsiness occurs; teach patient to avoid alcohol and CNS depressants
5. Nursing evaluation: at regular intervals, assess the continuing degree of spasticity

G. Antiparkinsonian drugs: drugs used in the management of Parkinson's disease
1. Action: restores action of the neurotransmitter dopamine to the basal ganglia of the brain or blocks the effects of excessive action of acetylcholine

2. Agents

Examples	Adverse Reactions
a. Anticholinergics Benztropine mesylate (Cogentin) Biperiden (Akineton) Cycrimine hydrochloride (Pagitane hydrochloride) Ethopropazine hydrochloride (Parsidol) Procyclidine hydrochloride (Kemadrin) Trihexyphenidyl hydrochloride (Artane, Pipanol, Tremin)	Dry mouth, constipation, urinary retention, blurred vision; impairment of recent memory, confusion, insomnia, and restlessness
b. Antihistamines Chlorphenoxamine hydrochloride (Phenoxene) Diphenhydramine hydrochloride (Benadryl) Orphenadrine citrate (Disipal)	Sedation
c. Other drugs Amantadine hydrochloride (Symmetrel)	Dry mouth, constipation, urinary retention, blurred vision
Levodopa (Dopar, Larodopa)	Nausea, vomiting, anorexia, orthostatic hypotension, GI bleeding, cough, hoarseness, dyspnea, blurred vision, increased sex drive
Carbidopa-levodopa (Sinemet)	Same as Levodopa

H. Sedatives, hypnotics, antianxiety drugs
1. Sedatives: small dose to calm an anxious patient
2. Hypnotics: larger dose to induce sleep
3. Antianxiety drugs (minor tranquilizers): drugs used to treat anxiety
4. Barbiturates: classified according to duration of action: ultra short acting, short acting, intermediate acting, and long acting
    a. Action: produce CNS depression ranging from sedation to anesthesia
    b. Adverse reactions
        (1) Mild withdrawal symptoms: rebound REM sleep, nightmares, daytime agitation, and a "shaky" feeling—dosage must be decreased gradually
        (2) Acute overdose: depression of medullary centers regulating respiration and cardiovascular system—tachycardia, hypotension, loss of reflexes, marked depression of respiration
    c. Agents: the following are examples

Amobarbital (Amytal, Tuinal)	Pentobarbital (Nembutal)
Butabarbital sodium (Butalan, Butisol Sodium)	Phenobarbital (Luminal)
	Secobarbital (Seconal)

5. Benzodiazepines
   a. Action: produce CNS depression
   b. Adverse reactions: daytime sedation, motor incoordination, dizziness, headaches; schedule IV substances
   c. Agents: the following are examples

Chlordiazepoxide hydrochloride (Librium)	Flurazepam hydrochloride (Dalmane)
Clorazepate dipotassium (Tranxene)	Lorazepam (Ativan)
Diazepam (Valium)	Oxazepam (Serax)
	Prazepam (Verstran, Centrax)

6. Miscellaneous
   a. Action: produce CNS depression; generally short acting
   b. Agents

Examples	Adverse Reactions
Chloral betaine (Beta-Chlor)	Gastric irritation; schedule IV substance
Chloral hydrate (Noctec)	Gastric irritation; schedule IV substance
Ethchlorvynol (Placidyl)	Muscular weakness; schedule IV substance
Glutethimide (Doriden)	Dilated pupils, dry mouth; schedule III substance
Hydroxyzine hydrochloride (Vistaril)	Dry mouth, hypotension, blurred vision, urinary retention
Meprobamate (Equanil, Miltown)	Schedule IV substance
Methaqualone (Quaalude, Sopor, Parest)	Paresthesia, peripheral neuropathy; schedule II substance
Methyprylon (Noludar)	Schedule II substance

7. Nursing assessment: give special attention to vital signs, level of consciousness, sleep patterns
8. Nursing management: observe for signs of CNS depression; identify nondrug solutions to sleep problems; monitor safety aspects of patient care
9. Nursing evaluation: review purpose for which drug is given and observe effectiveness; instruct patient concerning self-medication, medical follow-up, and drug-dependence potential

I. Alcohol
1. Action: produces CNS depression: sedation, disinhibition, sleep, anesthesia; vasodilation; gastric irritation
2. Effects of an acute overdose: death, accidents, hangover, upset stomach, thirst, fatigue, headache, depression, anxiety; chronic toxicity can lead to liver, esophagastrointestinal and cardiovascular disorders
3. Withdrawal symptoms after chronic use: tremors, anxiety, tachycardia, increased blood pressure, diaphoresis, anorexia, nausea, vomiting, insomnia, hallucinations, seizures, delirium tremens
4. Withdrawal therapy: one of the benzodiazepines; restoration of normal metabolic functions, and vitamin B_1, B_{12}, and folic acid
5. Aversion therapy: disulfiram (Antabuse) given to detoxified patient who wishes to avoid drinking again; produces unpleasant reaction in presence of alcohol: flushing, throbbing in head and neck, respiratory difficulty, nausea, copious vomiting, diaphoresis, fainting, dizziness, blurred vision, confusion

PSYCHOTHERAPEUTIC AGENTS
A. Antidepressants: Characteristic of drug-induced prevention or relief of depression
   1. Tricyclic antidepressants
      a. Action: primarily used to relieve symptoms of endogenous depression; also used to treat mild exogenous depression
      b. Agents: the following are examples

Amitriptyline hydrochloride (Elavil)	Imipramine hydrochloride (Tofranil)
Clomipramine hydrochloride (Anafranil)	Nortriptyline hydrochloride (Aventyl hydrochloride, Pamelor)
Doxepin hydrochloride (Adapin, Sinequan)	

   2. Monoamine oxidase (MAO) inhibitors
      a. Action: relieve symptoms of severe reactive or endogenous depression that has not responded to tricyclic antidepressant therapy, electroconvulsive therapy, or other modes of psychotherapy
      b. Agents: the following are examples

      Isocarboxazid (Marplan)
      Phenelzine sulfate (Nardil)
      Tranylcypromine sulfate (Parnate)

   3. Nursing assessment: obtain complete health history, history of insomnia, fatigue, or loss of motivation; observe motor movements, facial expression, and posture; assess for any feelings of suicide
   4. Nursing management: administer medication with food to avoid gastric distress
   5. Nursing evaluation: observe for adverse effects such as drowsiness
   6. Patient teaching: stress compliance of taking medication as ordered; instruct patient to avoid using alcohol with sleeping pills and hay fever or cold medications because doing so increases the effects of these medications

B. Antipsychotic drugs
   1. Phenothiazines/thioxanthenes
      a. Action: primarily to reduce or relieve symptoms of acute and chronic psychoses, including schizophrenia, schizoaffective disorders, and involutional psychoses
      b. Agents: the following are examples

Chlorpromazine (Thorazine)	Trifluoperazine hydrochloride (Stelazine)
Promazine hydrochloride (Sparine)	Triflupromazine hydrochloride (Vesprin)
Thioridazine hydrochloride (Mellaril)	

   2. Nursing assessment: obtain complete health history, current use of medications, and possibility of pregnancy; obtain history of emotional unrest, agitation, paranoid ideation, delusions, and inability to cope with reality
   3. Nursing management: administer medication with food or milk to avoid or reduce gastric distress

4. Nursing evaluation: observe for adverse effects such as urinary retention, change in vision, sore throat with fever, muscle spasms, trembling or shaking of hands, skin rash, yellow tinge to skin or eyes, uncontrollable movements of the tongue.

C. Antimanic drugs: used to treat manic-depressive psychoses in the acute manic phase; also used to prevent recurrent episodes of mania in the manic-depressive patient
   1. Agent: Lithium carbonate (Lithane, Carbolith)
   2. Nursing assessment: obtain complete health history, possibility of pregnancy, and medications currently being taken; observe for restlessness, hyperactivity, aggressiveness
   3. Nursing management: ensure adequate fluid and electrolyte balance
   4. Nursing evaluation: monitor serum lithium levels to avoid drug toxicity and reduce side effects
   5. Patient teaching: stress compliance of taking medication as ordered; instruct patient to wear medical identification tag

STIMULANTS

Stimulants are medically accepted only for treatment of narcolepsy, hyperkinetic behavior in children, and obesity. Occasionally they are used for depression in the elderly and to reverse respiratory depression from CNS depressants.

A. Amphetamines
   1. Action: increase the release and effectiveness of catecholamine neurotransmitters in the brain and peripheral nerves and create increased alertness and sensitivity to stimuli
   2. Adverse reactions
      a. Gastrointestinal system: vomiting, diarrhea, abdominal cramps, dry mouth, anorexia
      b. Central nervous system: restless behavior, tremor, irritability, talkativeness, insomnia, mood changes, excessive aggressiveness, confusion, panic, increased libido
      c. Autonomic nervous system: headache, chilliness, palpitation, pallor or facial flushing
      d. Children: growth retardation
   3. Agents: the following are examples

Amphetamine sulfate
Dextroamphetamine sulfate (Dexedrine, Ferndex)
Methamphetamine hydrochloride (Desoxyn)
Methylphenidate (Ritalin)
Pemoline (Cylert)

   4. Nursing assessment: obtain thorough history of patient's presenting problem; obtain vital signs, weight, and height in children
   5. Nursing management: monitor height, weight, and vital signs; inquire about relief of subjective symptoms such as insomnia, agitation, headache, and irritability; begin preparation of patient and family for long-term management; teach patient that last daily dose should be taken at least 6 hours before retiring
   6. Nursing evaluation: success of goals of therapy evaluated
      a. Hyperkinesis: less hyperactivity and a more normal attention span
      b. Narcolepsy: ability to remain awake and alert during specified appropriate time periods

B. Appetite suppressants: used to help control obesity
   1. Action: exert an anorectic effect on the appetite-control center in the brain
   2. Agents

Examples	Adverse Reactions/ Comments
Amphetamine sulfate (Benzedrine)	See Amphetamines
Benzphetamine (Didrex)	See Amphetamines
Caffeine	Nervousness, jitteriness, gastrointestinal bleeding, nausea, vomiting, excessive CNS stimulation, and convulsions
Caffeine sodium benzoate injection	Same as caffeine
Dextroamphetamine sulfate (Dexedrine)	See Amphetamines
Diethylpropion hydrochloride (Propion, Tenuate)	Dry mouth, constipation; schedule IV drug
Doxapram hydrochloride (Dopram)	Dizziness, apprehension, disorientation
Fenfluramine hydrochloride (Pondimin)	Sedation and depression; schedule IV drug
Mazindol (Sanorex)	Insomnia, dizziness, agitation; schedule III drug
Methamphetamine hydrochloride (Desoxyn, Obedrin-LA)	See Amphetamines
Nikethamide (Coramine)	Hypertension, tachycardia, tremors, flushing, increased body temperature, convulsion
Phendimetrazine tartrate (Bacarate)	Gastrointestinal distress; schedule III drug
Phenmetrazine hydrochloride (Preludin)	Schedule II drug; see Amphetamines
Phentermine hydrochloride (Adipex-P, Fastin, Tora)	Insomnia; schedule IV drug
Phenylpropanolamine hydrochloride (Acutrim, Control, Diadax, Dexatrim)	Blood pressure increases
Theophylline	Increased heart rate, nervousness, jitteriness, nausea, vomiting, excessive CNS stimulation, and convulsions

   3. Nursing assessment: obtain vital signs and weight; discuss usual eating habits and establish reasonable goals for losing weight
   4. Nursing management: promote weight reduction; monitor for adverse reactions; offer support
   5. Nursing evaluation: instruct patient concerning medication and its potential for drug abuse; assess achievement of goal—weight loss

C. Respiratory stimulants (analeptics): used to stimulate respiration when it has been depressed by drugs, asphyxiation, or electric shock
  1. Action: stimulates central nervous system medullary centers controlling respiration, vasomotor tone, and vagal tone
  2. Agents: see Amphetamines
  3. Nursing assessments: check respiratory rate and depth of respirations; may measure vital capacity and arterial blood gas levels
  4. Nursing management: monitor vital signs with focus on respirations; keep suction machine at bedside
  5. Nursing evaluation: observe whether patient is breathing at a rate and depth nearing normal and whether short-term hospitalization is necessary

Autonomic Nervous System
CHOLINESTERASE INHIBITORS (CHOLINERGIC AGENTS)
A. Description: drugs that produce a physiologic response similar to that of acetylcholine released on nerve stimulation
B. Action
  1. Direct-acting cholinergic stimulants: mimic the action of acetylcholine
  2. Indirect-acting cholinergic stimulants: inhibit the enzyme cholinesterase, which acts to limit acetylcholine action
C. Effects
  1. Vasodilation
  2. Lowered blood pressure
  3. Slowing of heart rate
  4. Salivation
  5. Perspiring
  6. Increased tone and movement in the gastrointestinal and genitourinary systems
  7. Increased tone and contractility in striated muscles
D. Adverse reactions: heart block, arrhythmias, hypotension, hypertension, nausea, vomiting, cramps, diarrhea, heartburn, muscle weakness, increase in intraocular pressure
E. Agents: the following are examples

Ambenonium chloride (Mytelase Chloride, Mysuran)
Demecarium bromide (Humorsol)
Echothiophate iodide (Phospholine iodide)
Edrophonium chloride (Tensilon)
Isoflurophate (Floropryl)
Neostigmine bromide (Prostigmin)
Pyridostigmine bromide (Mestinon)

F. Nursing assessment: history of lung disease, hyperthyroidism, prostate enlargement
G. Nursing management: monitor vital signs; insert rectal tube to relieve flatus
H. Nursing evaluation: observe for adverse reactions, bowel activity, intake and output records

PARASYMPATHETIC BLOCKING AGENTS (PARASYMPATHOLYTIC OR CHOLINERGIC BLOCKING AGENTS)
A. Action: prevent acetylcholine released by nerve stimulation from exerting its effects
B. Effects:
  1. Gastrointestinal: slows peristalsis
  2. Heart: increases rate

  3. Secretions: depresses all body secretions including perspiration and respiratory, salivary, pancreatic, and gastric secretions
  4. Eye: dilates pupils (mydriasis); paralyzes ciliary muscles; increases intraocular pressure
C. Adverse reactions: dry skin, delirium, tachycardia, convulsions, mydriasis, hypertension, dry mouth, urinary retention
D. Agents

Examples	Clinical Uses
Atropine sulfate	Adjunct to anesthesia, antispasmodic, cardiac stimulant
Cyclopentolate hydrochloride (Cyclogyl)	Mydriatic, cycloplegic
Homatropine hydrobromide	Mydriatic, cycloplegic
Scopolamine hydrobromide (Hyoscine)	Sedative-hypnotic, adjunct to anesthesia, antiemetic, mydriatic, cycloplegic
Isopropamide iodide (Darbid)	Antispasmodic
Methantheline bromide (Banthine)	Antispasmodic
Propantheline bromide (Pro-Banthine)	Antispasmodic
Benztropine mesylate (Cogentin)	Antiparkinsonian agent
Procyclidine hydrochloride (Kemadrin)	Antiparkinsonian agent
Trihexyphenidyl hydrochloride (Artane)	Antiparkinsonian agent

E. Nursing assessment: monitor vital signs; tachycardia; bowel functions; stimulation or depression of central nervous system; elevation in temperature; respiratory status; history of urinary difficulty, familial history of glaucoma
F. Nursing management: maintain oral hygiene for dry mouth; initiate methods to prevent abdominal distention and constipation, and safety measures in presence of blurred vision
G. Nursing evaluation: establish intake and output records when these drugs are given to elderly males; observe for effectiveness of drug

NEUROMUSCULAR BLOCKING AGENTS
A. Action: act at the striated neuromuscular junction to produce paralysis of the voluntary muscles
B. Effects
  1. Produce muscular relaxation for insertion of endotracheal tubes during surgical interventions
  2. Protect against violent thrashing that occurs with electroconvulsive therapy
  3. Alleviate spasms that accompany tetanus
C. Adverse reactions: paralysis of respiration, which may be reversed with neostigmine or Tensilon
D. Agents: the following are examples

Decamethonium bromide (Syncurine)
Pancuronium bromide (Pavulon)
Succinylcholine chloride (Anectine)
Tubocurarine chloride (Tubarine)

E. Nursing assessment: elicit medical history: asthma, myasthenia gravis remission; potassium blood levels
F. Nursing management: cardiopulmonary resuscitation skills—have resuscitative equipment available; monitor vital signs
G. Nursing evaluation: observe for early signs of flaccid paralysis in muscles of face, neck, eyes
H. Know that patient may appear to be asleep, but can still hear

SYMPATHOMIMETIC DRUGS: ADRENERGIC STIMULANTS
A. Actions
  1. Act directly on adrenergic receptors to produce either excitation or inhibition of a particular effector organ
  2. Act indirectly by releasing the stored catecholamines norepinephrine and epinephrine
B. Major effects
  1. Excitation of the heart, both its rate and force of contraction
  2. Excitation and constriction of smooth muscle in blood vessels
  3. Inhibition and relaxation of smooth muscles in bronchi, gastrointestinal tract, and skeletal muscle blood vessels
  4. Metabolism: release of fatty acids from adipose tissue and increased gluconeogenesis in muscle and liver
  5. Excitation of functions controlled by central nervous system, for example, respiration
  6. Suppression of appetite
  7. Lessening of fatigue
C. Adverse reactions: anxiety, apprehension, headache, arrhythmias, cerebral hemorrhage, heart failure, pulmonary edema
D. Agents

Examples	Clinical Indications
Dopamine hydrochloride (Intropin)	Hypotension
Ephedrine hydrochloride (Bronkotabs)	Bronchospasms, nasal decongestion, allergy
Epinephrine bitartrate (Medihaler-Epi)	Acute or chronic bronchial asthma, allergic disorders, acute hypersensitivity to drugs
Epinephrine hydrochloride (Adrenalin Chloride)	Cardiac arrest, heart block, acute asthma, adjunct to local anesthesia, acute hypersensitivity to drugs Ophthalmic use: control hemorrhage, decrease intraocular pressure
Isoproterenol hydrochloride (Isuprel)	Bronchodilation, cardiac stimulant
Isoproterenol sulfate (Medihaler-Iso)	Bronchodilation
Mephentermine sulfate (Wyamine)	Maintain blood pressure during anesthesia
Metaraminol bitartrate (Aramine)	Hypotension
Naphazoline hydrochloride (Privine)	Nasal decongestion
Norepinephrine bitartrate (Levophed, Noradrenalin)	Shock, cardiac arrest
Nylidrin hydrochloride (Arlidin)	Peripheral vascular disease

E. Nursing assessment: obtain history of hyperthyroidism, diabetes, hypertension, emotional lability, heart disease
F. Nursing management: monitor vital signs; check infusion rate often; observe for infusion infiltration; record bowel and urinary activity; teach patient to keep fluid intake to at least 2,000 ml/day to reduce viscosity of secretions.
G. Nursing evaluation: monitor effect on blood pressure, pulse rate, and regularity of heart rate; observe for therapeutic and adverse effects

ADRENERGIC RECEPTOR BLOCKERS AND NEURON BLOCKERS
A. Action: interfere with peripheral adrenergic activity by blocking alpha and beta receptors, by depleting peripheral neural stores of norepinephrine, and by inhibiting peripheral sympathetic activity through an action on the central nervous system
B. Adverse reactions: postural hypotension, miosis, inhibition of ejaculation, headache, intense vasoconstriction, diarrhea, nausea, disturbances of vision, insomnia, depression
C. Agents

Examples	Clinical Indications
Clonidine (Catapres-TTS)	Chronic hypertension
Ergoloid mesylate (Hydergine)	Mental and emotional complaints of the elderly
Guanethidine monosulfate (Ismelin)	Hypertension
Methyldopa (Aldomet)	Hypertension
Metoprolol tartrate (Lopressor)	Chronic hypertension, angina prophylaxis
Nadolol (Corgard)	Chronic hypertension, angina prophylaxis
Phenoxybenzamine hydrochloride (Dibenzyline)	Peripheral vascular disease
Phentolamine mesylate (Regitine)	Hypertension secondary to pheochromocytoma, adrenal tumor surgery
Prazosin hydrochloride (Minipress)	Chronic hypertension
Propranolol hydrochloride (Inderal)	Chronic hypertension, angina prophylaxis, cardiac dysrhythmias, migraine headaches
Reserpine (Serpasil)	Chronic hypertension
Timolol maleate (Timoptic)	Glaucoma
Tolazoline hydrochloride (Priscoline)	Peripheral vascular disease

D. Nursing assessment: ascertain if patient has history of ulcer disease, diabetes, ulcerative colitis, emotional depression, renal problems, coronary heart disease, predisposition to asthma, or congestive heart failure
E. Nursing management: aim instruction toward patient compliance; administer medications with meals or milk; maintain safety measures in presence of postural hypotension; monitor vital signs
F. Nursing evaluation: observe for therapeutic and adverse reactions; observe for changes in sleep patterns and appetite and depression or suicidal tendencies; observe for interactions with other arrhythmias or channel blockers; may cause additive

effect; interaction with insulin or hypoglycemic agents could alter insulin requirements and mask signs of hypoglycemia

GANGLIONIC AGENTS

A. Action: reduces sympathetic tone, particularly in the cardiovascular system
B. Adverse reactions: postural hypotension, pupillary dilation, blurring vision, dry mouth, constipation
C. Agents

Examples	Clinical Indications
Mecamylamine hydro-chloride (Inversine)	Hypertensive crisis, chronic hypertension
Trimethaphan camsylate (Arfonad)	Hypertensive crisis

D. Nursing assessment: obtain baseline vital signs; assess factors contributing to hypertension such as diet, weight, exercise, and lifestyle
E. Nursing management: instruction aimed at patient compliance
F. Nursing evaluation: observe for therapeutic effects and adverse reactions

Respiratory System

ANTIHISTAMINES

A. Action: blocks histamine effects at the receptor site
B. Adverse reactions: sedation, drowsiness, dry mouth, blurred vision, urinary retention, constipation; can also stimulate the nervous system, especially in children, causing insomnia, irritability, and nervousness
C. Agents

Examples	Clinical Indications
Brompheniramine maleate (Dimetane)	Colds, allergies
Carbinoxamine maleate (Clistin)	Colds, allergies
Chlorpheniramine maleate (Chlor-Trimeton, Teldrin, Chlortab)	Colds, allergies
Cyproheptadine hydro-chloride (Periactin)	Pruritus
Dexchlorpheniramine maleate (Polaramine)	Colds, allergies
Dimethindene maleate (Forhistal)	Colds, allergies
Diphenhydramine hydro-chloride (Benadryl)	Allergic reactions, motion sickness, mild parkinsonism
Meclizine hydrochloride (Bonine)	Motion sickness
Methdilazine hydrochloride (Tacaryl)	Pruritus
Promethazine hydrochloride (Phenergan, Promine, Remsed, Zipan)	Sedation, pruritus, motion sickness, nausea, vomiting
Trimeprazine tartrate (Temaril)	Pruritus
Tripelennamine hydrochloride (Pyribenzamine)	Colds, allergies

D. Nursing assessment: obtain vital signs; assess respiratory and cardiovascular status; ascertain if patient has history of allergy and extent and type of rash if present.
E. Nursing management: monitor respiratory response, vital signs, urinary and bowel function
F. Nursing evaluation: observe for therapeutic effects and adverse reaction; instruct patient on dangers of operating machinery and to wear medical identification tag in presence of allergies

NASAL DECONGESTANTS

A. Action: sympathomimetic agents (see the Autonomic Nervous System) when applied to nasal mucosa or taken orally constrict the smooth muscle of arterioles in the nasal mucosa and thus reduce blood flow and edema
B. Adverse reactions: rebound nasal congestion if used too frequently; nervousness, irritability
C. Agents: the following are a few examples of the numerous preparations available

Afrin	Neo-Synephrine
Allerest	Privine
Contac	Sine-Off
Coricidin	Sinutab
Dristan	Sudafed

D. Nursing assessment: obtain history of irritants or environmental conditions contributing to symptoms and such objective data as respiratory rate and vital signs
E. Nursing management: instruct patient regarding medication use
F. Nursing evaluation: monitor for therapeutic effects and adverse reactions

EXPECTORANTS, ANTITUSSIVES, MUCOLYTIC DRUGS

A. Definitions
   1. Expectorant: increases output of respiratory tract fluid that coats the bronchi and trachea
   2. Antitussive: suppresses cough
   3. Mucolytic: breaks up viscous mucus to allow for ease in expectoration of drainage
B. Adverse reactions
   1. Expectorants: nausea, drowsiness; iodide base drugs: skin rash, metallic taste, fever, skin eruptions, mucous membrane ulcerations, salivary gland swelling
   2. Antitussives: nausea, dizziness, constipation
   3. Mucolytics: gastrointestinal upset
C. Agents: the following are examples
   1. Expectorants: Robitussin, iodinated glycerol (Organidin), potassium iodide
   2. Antitussives: codeine, hydrocodone bitartrate, dextromethorphan hydrobromide (Romilar), Benylin, benzonatate (Tessalon)
   3. Mucolytics: acetylcysteine (Mucomyst), Alevaire
D. Nursing assessment: obtain history relevant to cough, vital signs, and such objective data as character and quantity of secretions
E. Nursing management: monitor symptoms, vital signs, and amount of secretions with mucolytics
F. Nursing evaluation: instruct patient regarding drugs, how/when to take them and when they should be discontinued; encourage patients with persistent coughs to seek follow-up treatment

BRONCHODILATORS

A. Action: act on bronchial cells to dilate the bronchioles
B. Adverse reactions: CNS stimulation, increased heart rate, muscle tremors, headache, nausea, epigastric pain, bronchospasms
C. Agents: the following are examples

Aminophylline	Isoetharine mesylate
Dyphylline	(Bronkometer)
(Dilin, Protophylline)	Isoproterenol hydrochloride
Ephedrine sulfate	(Iprenol, Isuprel
(Slo-Fedrin)	hydrochloride)
Epinephrine (Sus-Phrine)	Metaproterenol sulfate
Epinephrine bitartrate	(Alupent, Metaprel)
(AsthmaHaler,	Oxtriphylline (Choledyl)
Medihaler-Epi,	Terbutaline sulfate
Primatene Mist)	(Brethine, Bricanyl)
Epinephrine hydrochloride	Theophylline
(Adrenalin Chloride)	(many preparations)
Isoetharine hydrochloride	
(Bronkosol)	

D. Nursing assessment: obtain relevant history and vital signs; note amount and characteristics of secretions
E. Nursing management: monitor vital signs and lung sounds, closely monitor intravenous drugs; teach patient to increase fluid intake to 2,000–3,000 ml/day
F. Nursing evaluation: observe for therapeutic effects; instruct patient regarding drug knowledge and usage

Cardiovascular System

DRUGS TO IMPROVE CIRCULATION

A. Action: vasoconstriction (direct- and indirect-acting sympathomimetic amines cause release of norepinephrine, which stimulates alpha receptors and thus produces vasoconstriction)
B. Adverse reactions: headache, anxiety, palpitation, nausea, vomiting, insomnia, tremors
C. Agents: the following are examples

Dobutamine hydrochloride	Metaraminol bitartrate
(Dobutrex)	(Aramine)
Dopamine hydrochloride	Methoxamine hydrochloride
(Intropin)	(Vasoxyl)
Epinephrine hydrochloride	Norepinephrine bitartrate
(Adrenalin Chloride)	(Levarterenol bitartrate;
Isoproterenol hydrochloride	Levophed)
(Isuprel Hydrochloride)	Phenylephrine hydrochlo-
Mephentermine sulfate	ride (Neo-Synephrine
(Wyamine)	hydrochloride, Isophrin)

D. Principal clinical use: treatment of cardiogenic and anaphylactic shock; to maintain blood pressure in life-threatening situations and during anesthesia
E. Nursing assessment: obtain pulse, respirations, and blood pressure; note level of consciousness
F. Nursing management: use infusion-control device to monitor intravenous administration; monitor vital signs frequently
G. Nursing evaluation: observe for therapeutic effects

VASODILATOR DRUGS (ANTIANGINAL DRUGS)

A. Action: dilate arterioles and veins to lower blood pressure, which reduces workload on the heart and decreases the heart's oxygen demand; increases circulation to cardiac muscle

B. Adverse reactions: flushing, headache, dizziness
C. Agents: the following are examples

Amyl nitrite (Vaporole)	Nitroglycerin (Nitro-Bid)
Erythrityl tetranitrate	Nitroglycerine lingual aerosol
(Cardilate)	(Nitrolingual Spray)
Isosorbide dinitrate	Nitroglycerin ointment,
(Iso-Bid, Isordil,	2% (Nitrol)
Sorbide, Sorbitrate)	Pentaerythritol tetranitrate
Mannitol hexanitrate	(Peritrate)
(Nitranitol)	Trolnitrate phosphate
	(Metamine)

D. Nursing assessment: obtain vital signs and history relevant to onset and duration of pain
E. Nursing management: observe and monitor for additional angina attacks; instruct patient about prescribed drugs
F. Nursing evaluation: observe for therapeutic effects

VASODILATOR DRUGS FOR PERIPHERAL VASCULAR DISEASE

A. Action: work directly on vascular smooth muscle to cause relaxation or stimulate beta receptors in blood vessels to produce vasodilation
B. Adverse reactions: gastrointestinal upset, flushing, hypotension, dizziness, increased heart rate, headache
C. Agents: the following are examples

Cyclandelate	Nylidrin hydrochloride
(Cyclospasmol)	(Arlidin, Rolidrin)
Ergoloid mesylates	Papaverine hydrochloride
(dihydrogenated ergot	(many trade names)
alkaloids; Hydergine)	Tolazoline hydrochloride
Isoxsuprine hydrochloride	(Priscoline)
(Vasodilan)	

D. Nursing assessment: obtain history of onset and course of vascular disease; assess blood pressure, pulses, including peripheral pulses, mental status, and color and temperature of affected extremities
E. Nursing evaluation: observe for therapeutic and adverse effects
F. Nursing management: monitor presenting signs and symptoms; instruct patient regarding medications

ANTIHYPERTENSIVES

Several subgroups of drugs can lower blood pressure
A. Action
  1. Adrenergic drugs
    a. Beta-1 adrenergic receptor antagonists (beta-blockers): reduce cardiac output; reduce renin release from kidney (blocks response to sympathetic impulses)
    b. Alpha-1 adrenergic receptor antagonists: prevent norepinephrine from constricting blood vessels to increase resistance to blood flow
  2. Centrally-acting antihypertensive drugs that inhibit the activity of the sympathetic nervous system: decrease sympathetic tone and activate alpha receptors in the medulla that decrease heart rate and cardiac output
  3. Vasodilators: relax arteriolar smooth muscle
  4. Vasodilators in hypertensive emergencies: rapidly relax smooth muscle
B. Adverse reactions: bradycardia, hypotension, nasal congestion, reflex tachycardia, dry mouth, fluid retention, arthralgia, depression, drowsiness

C. Agents: the following are examples

1. Beta adrenergic
   receptor antagonists
   Metoprolol tartrate
   (Lopressor)
   Nadolol (Corgard)
   Propranolol hydro-
   chloride (Inderal)
2. Alpha adrenergic
   receptor antagonists
   Phenoxybenzamine
   hydrochloride
   (Dibenzyline)
   Phentolamine
   mesylate (Regitine)
   Prazosin hydrochloride
   (Minipress)
3. Drugs interfering with
   norepinephrine
   Deserpidine (Harmonyl)
   Guanethidine mono-
   sulfate (Ismelin)
   Rauwolfia serpentina
   (Raudixin)
   Reserpine (Serpasil,
   Sandril)
4. Centrally acting anti-
   hypertensive drugs
   Clonidine
   hydrochloride
   (Catapres)
   Methyldopa (Aldomet)
5. Vasodilators
   Hydralazine
   hydrochloride
   (Apresoline)
   Minoxidil (Loniten)

6. Vasodilators:
   hypertensive
   emergencies
   Diazoxide (Hyperstat)
   Sodium nitroprusside
   (Nipride)
   Trimethaphan
   camsylate
   (Arfonad)

D. Nursing assessment: obtain vital signs and additional baseline data, such as weight, diet, and serum electrolyte levels for electrolyte imbalances
E. Nursing management: monitor vital signs, intake and output, weight, blood studies; instruct patient regarding drugs
F. Nursing evaluation: observe for therapeutic effects and adverse reactions
G. Patient teaching: stress the importance of knowing acceptable ranges of blood pressure and pulse; taking medication as ordered; preventing orthostatic hypotension; and reporting asthmalike signs and symptoms

DIURETICS

A. Action: increase the excretion of sodium ion and thus increase urine flow
B. Agents

Examples	Adverse Reactions
1. Ethacrynic acid (Edecrin)	Dehydration, thrombosis, emboli, electrolyte imbalance
Furosemide (Lasix)	Acute dehydration, sodium and potassium depletion, calcium loss, dermatitis, blood dyscrasias
2. Thiazide diuretics Bendroflumethiazide (Naturetin) Benzthiazide (Aquatag, Urazide) Chlorothiazide (Diuril) Chlorthalidone (Hygroton) Cyclothiazide (Anhydron)	Fluid and electrolyte imbalance, increased calcium serum levels, gastrointestinal irritation, dizziness, headache, paresthesias, blood dyscrasias, allergy, hypotension

Examples

Hydrochlorothiazide
(Esidrix, HydroDiuril)
Hydroflumethiazide
(Saluron)
Methyclothiazide (Enduron)
Metolazone (Zaroxolyn)
Polythiazide (Renese)
Trichlormethiazide
(Diurese, Naqua)

3. Carbonic anhydrase inhibitors

Examples

Acetazolamide (Diamox)
Ethoxzolamide (Cardrase, Ethamide)

4. Potassium-sparing diuretics

Examples	**Adverse Reactions**
Spironolactone (Aldactone)	Hyperkalemia, fatal cardiac dysrhythmias, endocrine alterations, blood dyscrasias
Triamterene (Dyrenium)	

C. Nursing assessment: perform total patient assessment with emphasis on presenting signs and symptoms, vital signs, and laboratory blood studies
D. Nursing management: to foster drug therapy such as by restriction of fluid and diet; monitor weight, intake and output, and vital signs
E. Nursing evaluation: observe for therapeutic effects and adverse reactions; instruct patient regarding drugs and diet, prevention of orthostatic hypotension

CARDIOTONIC DRUGS (CARDIAC GLYCOSIDES)

A. Action: act directly on myocardial cells to increase contractility and thus cardiac output; slows heart rate
B. Adverse reactions: anorexia, nausea, vomiting, bradycardia, weakness, fatigue, visual dimming, double vision, altered color vision, mood alterations, hallucinations, dysrhythmias
C. Toxic reactions, contusion, heart block, PVCs
D. Agents: the following are examples

Digitoxin
(Crystodigin)

Digoxin
(Lanoxin)

E. Nursing assessment: obtain baseline data, weight, vital signs, electrocardiogram (ECG) results
F. Nursing management: monitor vital signs, weight, fluid intake and output, serum electrolyte level, especially potassium; instruct patient regarding drugs, eating foods high in potassium
G. Nursing evaluation: observation for therapeutic effects and adverse reactions

DRUGS TO CONTROL DYSRHYTHMIAS

A. Action: slow conduction through atrioventricular (AV) node; block effects of vagal nerve stimulation; block beta adrenergic stimulation; suppress automaticity; increase electrical threshold for stimulation

B. Agents

Examples	Adverse Reactions
Atropine	Dry mouth, cycloplegia, mydriasis, fever, urinary retention
Bretylium tosylate (Bretylol)	Anginal attacks, bradycardia, hypotension
Deslanoside (Cedilanid-D)	Bradycardia, premature ventricular beats, atrioventricular tachycardia, anorexia, nausea, vomiting
Digitoxin (Crystodigin, Purodigin)	
Digoxin (Lanoxin)	
Disopyramide phosphate (Norpace)	Dry mouth, constipation, urinary retention, blurred vision
Lidocaine (Xylocaine without epinephrine)	Muscle twitching, respiratory depression, convulsions, coma
Phenytoin (Dilantin)	Bradycardia, cardiac arrest, nausea, dizziness, drowsiness
Procainamide hydrochloride (Pronestyl)	Hypotension, decreased cardiac output, gastrointestinal distress
Propranolol hydrochloride (Inderal)	Bradycardia, lowered cardiac output, bronchospasm
Quinidine sulfate (Cin-Quin, Quinora)	Peripheral vasodilation, hypotension, gastrointestinal distress
Quinidine gluconate (Duraquin)	
Quinidine polygalacturonate (Cardioquin)	

C. Nursing assessment: obtain baseline data, history of subjective and objective symptoms, vital signs
D. Nursing management: monitor vital signs; instruct patient regarding drugs; maintain therapeutic blood levels by administering around the clock
E. Nursing evaluation: observe for therapeutic effects and adverse reactions

ANTICOAGULANTS
A. Action: inhibit the aggregation of platelets; interfere with any of the steps leading to the formation of fibrin
B. Adverse reactions: hemorrhage, hematuria, melena, rashes, depression of bone marrow
C. Agents: the following are examples

1. Antiplatelet drugs
   Aspirin
   Dipyridamole (Persantine)
2. Heparin sodium (Liquaemin Sodium, Panheprin, Lipo-Hepin)
3. Coumarins
   Dicumarol
   Phenprocoumon (Liquamar)
   Warfarin sodium (Coumadin, Panwarfin)
4. Indanediones
   Anisindione (Miradon)

D. Nursing assessment: obtain baseline data relevant to general condition of the patient, history of problems with clots, and blood coagulation studies: prothrombin time (PT), partial thromboplastin time (PTT), platelet count, and clotting times

E. Nursing management: monitor blood coagulation studies carefully; use infusion monitoring device for constant infusions of heparin; have drug antidotes readily available
F. Nursing evaluation: observe for therapeutic effects and adverse reactions
G. Patient teaching: stress home safety factors to prevent tissue trauma and bleeding; advise to avoid foods high in vitamin K; avoid aspirin, dextran, dipyridamole, and nonsteroidal antiinflammatory drugs that increase risk of bleeding; instruct patient to observe excreta for signs of bleeding
H. Drug interactions
   1. Drugs potentiating response: clofibrate (Atromid S), disulfiram (Antabuse), neomycin sulfate, phenylbutazone (Butazolidin), salicylates, sulfisoxazole (Gantrisin)
   2. Drugs diminishing response: barbiturates, cholestyramine (Questran), ethchlorvynol (Placidyl), glutethimide (Doriden), griseofulvin (Grifulvin-V)
I. Antidotes
   1. Heparin: protamine sulfate
   2. Coumarins: vitamin K

THROMBOLYTIC DRUGS
A. Action: promote the digestion of fibrin to dissolve the clot
B. Agents: enzymes urokinase and streptokinase
C. Adverse reaction: hemorrhage
D. Special considerations: reserved for use in acute pulmonary embolism, deep vein thrombosis, or peripheral arterial occlusion; posttreatment: treated with heparin
E. Nursing assessment: obtain baseline data relevant to size, location, and symptoms of clot; vital signs and peripheral pulses for adequate circulation to extremities
F. Nursing management: used only in acute care setting; monitor laboratory blood studies and for signs of clot dissolution
G. Nursing evaluation: observe for therapeutic effects and adverse reactions

HEMOSTATIC AGENTS
A. Action: inhibit the dissolution of blood clots
B. Adverse reactions: nausea, cramps, dizziness, tinnitus, thrombophlebitis, flushing, vascular collapse
C. Agents

Examples	Clinical Indications
1. Systemic agents	Used in special surgical situations
Aminocaproic acid (Amicar)	
Menadiol sodium diphosphate (Synkayvite)	Correction of secondary hypoprothrombinemia, correction of severe vitamin K deficiency
Menadione sodium bisulfite (Hykinone)	
Phytonadione; vitamin K (AquaMEPHYTON, Konakion, Mephyton)	Oral anticoagulant overdose emergency
2. Local hemostatic agents	Control bleeding in wound or at operative site
Absorbable gelatin sponge (Gelfoam)	

D. Nursing assessment: obtain baseline data relevant to type, location, and amount of bleeding, appropriate laboratory blood studies, and general condition of patient

E. Nursing management: monitor appropriate laboratory blood studies

F. Nursing evaluation: observe for therapeutic effects and adverse reactions

DRUGS THAT LOWER BLOOD LIPID LEVELS

A. Action: in general these drugs lower blood lipid concentrations

NOTE: no present proof that lowering blood lipid concentrations will reverse or halt atherosclerosis

B. Adverse reactions: bloating, nausea, constipation, muscle cramps, impotence, flushing, weight loss, insomnia, water retention

C. Agents: the following are examples

Cholestyramine resin (Questran)	Lovastatin (Mevacor)
Colestipol hydrochloride (Colestid)	Niacin; nicotinic acid (Nicobid, Niac, Nicolar)

D. Nursing assessment: obtain baseline data relevant to weight, serum cholesterol and triglyceride levels, blood pressure, and dietary history

E. Nursing management: observe for any new symptoms; instruct patient regarding drugs; restrict intake of fats, cholesterol, and alcohol; stop smoking; follow recommended exercise program

F. Nursing evaluation: observe for adverse effects; monitor blood levels for therapeutic effects

DRUGS THAT TREAT NUTRITIONAL ANEMIAS

A. Action: supplement or replace essential vitamins and minerals

B. Agents

Examples	Adverse Reactions
1. Iron salts Ferrous sulfate (Feosol, Fer-In-Sol, Fero-Gradumet, Mol-Iron)	Acute toxicity: acute nausea and vomiting, metabolic acidosis, extensive liver and kidney damage
Ferrous gluconate (Fergon, Ferralet Plus, Entron)	Chronic toxicity: bronze coloration of skin, development of diabetes mellitus, heart failure
Ferrocholinate (Chel-Iron, Kelex) Ferrous fumarate (Ferranol, Feostat) Iron dextran injection (Imferon)	
2. Antidote for iron toxicity Deferoxamine mesylate (Desferal)	
3. Vitamin B$_{12}$ Cyanocobalamin (Betalin 12 Crystalline, Redisol, Rubramin PC, Sytobex)	Virtually free of adverse reactions

Examples	Adverse Reactions
Hydroxocobalamin (alphaRedisol)	
4. Folic acid for anemia Folic acid (Folvite) Leucovorin calcium	Nontoxic

C. Nursing assessment: obtain baseline data for vital signs, weight, dietary history, blood studies, and presence of neurologic symptoms

D. Nursing management: monitor blood studies, vital signs

E. Nursing evaluation: observe for therapeutic effects and adverse reactions; instruct patient regarding medications; use z-track techniques when injecting iron to avoid staining of skin

F. Patient teaching: expect dark or black stools and the possibility of gastrointestinal distress; nutritionally balanced diet

Gastrointestinal System

DRUGS THAT INCREASE TONE AND MOTILITY

A. Action: cholinomimetic action to stimulate or restore intestinal tone or urinary bladder tone

B. Adverse reactions: salivation, skin flushing, sweating, diarrhea, abdominal cramps

C. Agents: bethanechol chloride (Urecholine); neostigmine methylsulfate (Prostigmin)

D. Nursing assessment: obtain baseline data regarding vital signs, bowel sounds, fluid intake and output, bowel activity

E. Nursing management: stay with patient at least 15 minutes after administration to observe for adverse reactions; monitor vital signs, fluid intake and output, bowel activity

F. Nursing evaluation: observe for therapeutic effects and adverse reactions

DRUGS THAT DECREASE TONE AND MOTILITY (ANTICHOLINERGICS)

A. Action: inhibit gastric secretion and depress gastrointestinal motility

B. Adverse reactions: dry mouth, mydriasis, blurred vision, tachycardia, constipation, and acute urinary retention

C. Agents: the following are examples

Atropine sulfate	Homatropine methylbromide (Homapin)
Belladonna extract	
Belladonna tincture	Oxyphencyclimine hydrochloride (Daricon)
Dicyclomine hydrochloride (Bentyl, Di-Spaz)	Propantheline bromide (Pro-Banthine)
Diphemanil methylsulfate (Prantal)	Thiphenamil hydrochloride (Trocinate)
Glycopyrrolate (Robinul)	Tridihexethyl chloride (Pathilon)

D. Nursing assessment: obtain baseline data for vital signs; frequency and character of stools and presence of occult blood in stools; ability to empty bladder

E. Nursing management: monitor vital signs

F. Nursing evaluation: observe for therapeutic effects and adverse reactions; instruct patient regarding medication

DRUGS TO TREAT ULCERS

A. Action
  1. Antacids: neutralize gastric hydrochloric acid

2. Anticholinergic drugs: see drugs under the Autonomic Nervous System

3. Antihistamines: block the histamines' receptors and decrease gastric acid production

B. Adverse reactions: constipation, diarrhea; can interfere with absorption of some drugs: tetracycline, digoxin, quinidine

C. Agents (antacids): the following are examples

Aluminum hydroxide (Amphojel)

Calcium carbonate (Dicarbosil, Tums)

Dihydroxyaluminum aminoacetate (Robalate)

Dihydroxyaluminum sodium carbonate (Rolaids)

Magnesium hydroxide (Milk of Magnesia)

Aluminum hydroxide } Calcium carbonate } (Camalox) Magnesium hydroxide }

Aluminum hydroxide Magnesium hydroxide } (Maalox)

Aluminum hydroxide Magnesium trisilicate } (Trisogel)

Aluminum hydroxide gel Magnesium hydroxide Simethicone } (Maalox Plus, Mylanta, Gelusil)

Aluminum phosphate gel (Phosphaljel)

Magaldrate (Riopan)

D. Agents (Histamine H$_2$-receptor antagonists): the following are examples

Cimetidine (Tagamet)

Famotidine (Pepcid)

Nizatidine (Axid)

Ranitidine hydrochloride (Zantac)

E. Nursing assessment: obtain baseline data relevant to vital signs, level of consciousness, character and quality of emesis and stool, appropriate laboratory blood studies, abdominal pain, frank bleeding, and occult bleeding

F. Nursing management: monitor vital signs, fluid intake and output, level of consciousness, and character of stools and vomitus; teach that antacids decrease absorption of many drugs including iron, tetracyclines; teach not to take antacids for more than 2 weeks without consulting a physician.

G. Nursing evaluation: observe for therapeutic effects and adverse reactions

ANTIEMETICS

A. Action: control nausea and vomiting by reducing stimulation of labyrinthine receptors; dopamine antagonists, which act on the chemoreceptor trigger zone in the medulla

B. Adverse reactions: drowsiness, blurred vision, dilated pupils, dry mouth, extrapyramidal symptoms

C. Agents: the following are examples

1. Anticholinergics
Scopolamine hydrobromide

2. Antihistamines
Dimenhydrinate (Dramamine)
Diphenhydramine hydrochloride (Benadryl)

Hydroxyzine pamoate (Vistaril)
Meclizine hydrochloride (Antivert, Bonine)
Promethazine hydrochloride (Phenergan)

3. Miscellaneous drugs
Benzquinamide hydrochloride (Emete-con)
Diphenidol hydrochloride (Vontrol)
Trimethobenzamide hydrochloride (Tigan)

4. Dopamine antagonists
Chlorpromazine hydrochloride (Thorazine)
Fluphenazine hydrochloride (Prolixin)
Haloperidol (Haldol)
Perphenazine (Trilafon)
Prochlorperazine (Compazine)
Promazine hydrochloride (Sparine)
Triflupromazine hydrochloride (Vesprin)

D. Nursing assessment: obtain baseline data regarding vital signs, character and quantity of any emesis, presence of bowel sounds, fluid intake and output

E. Nursing management: monitor vital signs and fluid intake and output

F. Nursing evaluation: observe for therapeutic effects and adverse reactions

ANTIDIARRHETIC AGENTS

A. Action: decrease tone of small and large bowel; depress smooth muscle contraction; decrease release of acetylcholine; absorb toxins

B. Adverse reactions: respiratory depression, constipation, impaction

C. Agents: the following are examples

Bismuth subsalicylate (Pepto-Bismol)
Codeine phosphate
Codeine sulfate
Diphenoxylate hydrochloride with atropine sulfate (Diphenatol, Lomotil, Lofene)

Loperamide hydrochloride (Imodium)

D. Nursing assessment: obtain baseline data relevant to vital signs, fluid and solid intake and output, nature, and character of stools, skin turgor, fluid and electrolyte balance

E. Nursing management: monitor vital signs, intake and output, frequency and character of stools

F. Nursing evaluation: observe for therapeutic effects and adverse reactions

LAXATIVES

A. Action: retain water to keep stools large and soft; stimulate motility in large intestine; inhibit reabsorption of water; attract water by osmosis; soften feces

B. Adverse reactions: loss of bowel tone, dehydration, hypokalemia, hyponatremia, malabsorption of fat-soluble vitamins

C. Agents: the following are examples

1. Bulk-forming agents
Gum karaya
Plantago seed (psyllium)

Psyllium hydrocolloid (Effersyllium)
Psyllium hydrophilic mucilloid (Metamucil)

2. Stimulant cathartics (irritants)
   Bisacodyl (Bisco-Lax, Dulcolax)
   Cascara sagrada
   Castor oil
   Glycerin suppositories
   Phenolphthalein (Ex-Lax, Feen-A-Mint, Phenolax)
   Senna concentrate (Senokot)
   Senna pod
3. Saline cathartics
   Magnesium hydroxide (Milk of Magnesia)
   Magnesium sulfate (Epsom salt)
   Monosodium phosphate (Sal Hepatica)
   Sodium phosphate with sodium biphosphate (Phospho-Soda)
4. Lubricants
   Mineral oil (Agoral Plain, Petrogalar Plain)
5. Fecal softeners
   Docusate calcium (dioctyl calcium sulfosuccinate; Surfak)
   Docusate sodium (dioctyl sodium sulfosuccinate; Colace, Comfolax, D-S-S)
6. Osmotic agents
   Glycerin (Sani-supp)
   Lactulose (Chronulac, Duphalac, Enulose)

D. Nursing assessment: obtain baseline data relevant to vital signs, intake and output, presence of bowel sounds, bowel habits, dietary history, medications
E. Nursing management: monitor diet and fluid intake; instruct patient regarding drugs, and to increase fiber in diet and increase fluid intake
F. Nursing evaluation: observe for therapeutic effects and adverse reactions

Endocrine System

DRUGS AFFECTING PITUITARY GLAND

A. Action
   1. Antidiuretic hormone (ADH): increases renal tubule's permeability and thus its ability to reabsorb water
   2. Oxytocin: promotes uterine contractions during last stages of labor when cervix is fully dilated
   3. Growth hormone: anabolic agent that increases cell size and cell numbers and stimulates linear growth
   4. Gonadotropic hormone (GTH): regulates maturation and function of male and female sexual organs
   5. Adrenocorticotropic hormone (ACTH): stimulates adrenal cortex to release its hormone
B. Adverse reactions: hyponatremia, water retention, glycosuria, vasoconstriction, nausea
C. Agents

Examples	Clinical Indications
Desmopressin acetate (DDAVP)	Diabetes insipidus
Lypressin (Diapid)	Diabetes insipidus
Posterior pituitary extract (Pituitrin)	Smooth muscle contraction
Vasopressin (Pitressin)	Short-term maintenance of unconscious patient

D. Nursing assessment: obtain baseline data relative to excesses or deficiencies of specific hormone

E. Nursing management: monitor fluid intake and output, laboratory values; instruct patient regarding medications
F. Nursing evaluation: observe for therapeutic effects and adverse reactions

DRUGS AFFECTING ADRENAL GLANDS

A. Action: replace the body's normal amount of hormones; block inflammatory responses; antineoplastic; antagonize autoimmune responses
B. Adverse reactions: impaired glucose tolerance or hyperglycemia; fat deposition; muscle weakness or wasting; peptic ulcer; growth inhibition; mood changes or psychosis; osteoporosis; sodium retention; potassium loss
C. Agents: dosage is individualized to patient and diagnosis; the following are examples

Betamethasone valerate (Valisone)
Cortisone acetate (Cortone)
Desoxycorticosterone acetate (Doca, Percorten)
Dexamethasone (Decadron, Hexadrol)
Fludrocortisone acetate (Florinef)
Hydrocortisone (cortisol; Cortef, Cortril, Hydrocortone)
Hydrocortisone acetate (Cortef)
Methylprednisolone (Medrol, Wyacort)
Methylprednisolone acetate (Depo-Medrol)
Methylprednisolone sodium succinate (Solu-Medrol)
Prednisolone (Delta-Cortef, Paracortol)
Prednisolone sodium phosphate (Hydeltrasol)
Prednisone (Meticorten, Delta-Dome)
Triamcinolone (Aristocort, Kenacort)
Triamcinolone acetonide (Kenalog)
Triamcinolone hexacetonide (Aristospan)

D. Nursing assessment: obtain baseline data relevant to vital signs, weight, glycosuria
E. Nursing management: monitor vital signs, weight, serum electrolyte levels, sugar concentrations in blood and urine, signs of masked infection; instruct patient regarding medications, additive hypokalemia
F. Nursing evaluations: observe for therapeutic effects and adverse reactions

DRUGS AFFECTING THYROID GLAND

A. Action
   1. Hypothyroidism: replace the body's normal amount of hormone
   2. Hyperthyroidism
      a. Control the symptoms of hyperthyroidism
      b. Inhibit the synthesis of thyroid hormones
      c. Inhibit iodine uptake by thyroid gland
      d. Inhibit thyroid hormone release and symptoms
      e. Suppress continued uptake of iodine
      f. Destroy surrounding tissue by emission of low energy radiation
B. Adverse reactions to drugs for hyperthyroidism: agranulocytosis; skin rash, nausea, vomiting, twitching muscles, bronchospasm, iodism, symptoms of hyperthyroidism
C. Adverse reactions to drugs for hypothyroidism: dysrhythmias, hypertension, headache, insomnia, irritability, vomiting, weight loss

D. Agents: the following are examples

1. Hypothyroidism
   a. Natural thyroid hormones
      Thyroglobulin (Proloid)
      Thyroid (Delcoid, Thyrar, Thyrocrine)
   b. Synthetic thyroid hormones
      Levothyroxine sodium (Eltroxin, Levoid, Synthroid)
      Liothyronine sodium (Cytomel)
      Liotrix (Euthroid, Thyrolar)
   c. Adenohypophyseal hormone
      Thyroid-stimulating hormone (TSH) (thyrotropin; Thytropar)
      Protirelin (Thypinone)

2. Hyperthyroidism
   a. Thioamides
      Methimazole (Tapazole)
      Propylthiouracil
   b. Beta adrenergic blocker
      Propranolol hydrochloride (Inderal)
   c. Iodine
      Potassium or sodium iodide (Lugol's solution)
   d. Radioactive iodine (^{131}I)

E. Nursing assessment: obtain baseline data relevant to vital signs, weight, level of energy, symptoms of hypofunctioning or hyperfunctioning of gland and serum thyroid levels
F. Nursing management: monitor vital signs, weight; instruct patient regarding medications, compliance with therapy
G. Nursing evaluation: observe for therapeutic effects and adverse reactions

DRUGS AFFECTING PARATHYROID GLAND
A. Action: maintain blood calcium levels in the blood
B. Adverse reactions: nausea, local irritation at injection sites, drowsiness, gastrointestinal complaints, hypertension, facial flushing
C. Agents: the following are examples
   Calcitonin (Calcimar)
   Calcitriol (Rocaltrol)
   Parathyroid hormone
D. Nursing assessment: obtain baseline data relevant to vital signs and blood calcium levels
E. Nursing management: monitor vital signs, blood calcium levels; teach avoidance of spinach, whole grains, and rhubarb and maintaining adequate intake of calcium and vitamin D
F. Nursing evaluation observe for therapeutic effects (i.e., decreased muscle cramping) and adverse reactions; instruct patient regarding medications

Female Reproductive System
ESTROGENS
A. Action: replace or supplement natural body hormones; alter cell environment in neoplastic processes
B. Adverse reactions: breast tenderness, increased risk of breast and endometrial cancer, nausea, vomiting, anorexia, malaise, depression, salt and water retention
C. Agents: the following are examples

Chlorotrianisene (TACE)
Diethylstilbestrol (DES) (Stilbestrol)
Ethinyl estradiol (Estinyl)
Estradiol (Estrace)
Estrone (Theelin, Femogen)
Estrogen, conjugated (Premarin)

PROGESTINS
A. Action: suppress endometrial bleeding; withdrawal of drug induces tissue sloughing
B. Adverse reactions: edema, breast tenderness, depression, midcycle bleeding
C. Agents: the following are examples

Medroxyprogesterone acetate (Depo-Provera, Provera)
Megestrol acetate (Megace)
Norethindrone (Norlutin, Ortho-Novum)

FERTILITY DRUGS
A. Action: stimulate ovulation by pituitary or ovarian mechanisms
B. Adverse reactions: relatively rare
C. Agents: the following are examples

Clomiphene citrate (Clomid)
Menotropins (Perganol)
Human chorionic gonadotropin (HCG) (Antuitrin S, Follutein)

CONTRACEPTIVE DRUGS
A. Action: suppress ovulation; induce changes in cervical mucus, making uterine entry by sperm difficult; produce changes in endometrium, making implantation difficult
B. Adverse reactions: thromboembolitic diseases, stroke, hypertension
C. Agents: the following examples contain varying amounts of progesterone and estrogen

Brevicon
Enovid
Norlestrin
Ortho-Novum
Ovrette
Ovulen

OXYTOCIC DRUGS
A. Action: induce contraction of the myometrium
B. Adverse reactions: fetal or maternal cardiac dysrhythmias, acute hypertension, nausea, water intoxication, uterine hypertonicity with fetal or maternal injury
C. Agents: the following are examples

Dinoprost tromethamine (Prostin F2 Alpha)
Dinoprostone (Prostin E2)
Ergonovine maleate (Ergotrate)
Methylergonovine maleate (Methergine)
Oxytocin (Pitocin, Syntocinon)

UTERINE RELAXANTS
A. Action: stimulation of beta-2 adrenergic receptors produces relaxation of uterine muscle
B. Adverse reactions: heart palpitations, nausea, vomiting, trembling, flushing, and headache
C. Agents: Ritodrine, Terbutaline (Brethine)

NURSING PROCESS

A. Assessment: obtain baseline data relevant to vital signs, weight, current problem; elicit history of previous pregnancies and deliveries, fetal heart tones
B. Management: inform of possible side effects and benefit; monitor vital signs, weight; with oxytocics: maternal and fetal monitoring; infusion monitoring device
C. Evaluation: observe for therapeutic effects and adverse reactions; instruct patient regarding medications

Male Hormones
ANDROGENS

A. Action: replace or supplement normal body hormone; relieve postpartum breast engorgement; alter cell environment in neoplastic disease in females
B. Adverse reactions: female masculinization; premature closure of epiphyses in children; nausea, vomiting, diarrhea, mood swing
C. Agents: the following are example

Danocrine (Danazol)	Testosterone
Fluoxymesterone	(Delatestryl)
(Halotestin)	(Testaqua, Oreton)
Methyltestosterone	
(Android)	

ANABOLIC STEROIDS

A. Action: increase nitrogen retention and protein formation; stimulate red blood cell formation and increase bone deposition
B. Adverse reactions: increased libido; priapism (continuous erection), female masculinization, precocious sexual development in children, premature epiphyseal fusion
C. Agent: the following are examples

Ethylestrenol (Maxibolin)	Nondrolone phenpropionate
Methandrostenolone	(Durabolin)
(Dianabol)	Oxandrolone (Anavar)
Methandriol	Stanozolol (Winstrol)

NURSING PROCESS

A. Assessment: obtain baseline data relevant to vital signs, weight, height (children), current problem
B. Management: monitor vital signs, weight, height, (children); review possible effects with patient
C. Evaluation: observe for therapeutic effects and adverse reaction; instruct patient regarding medications

The Eye
ANTICHOLINERGIC DRUGS

A. Action: cause mydriasis (dilated pupils) and cycloplegia (blurred vision)
B. Adverse reaction: dry mouth and skin, fever, thirst, confusion, hyperactivity
C. Agents: the following are examples

Atropine sulfate (Atropisol, Isopto Atropine)	Scopolamine hydrobromide (hyoscine hydrobromide; Isopto Hyoscine)
Cyclopentolate hydro-chloride (Cyclogyl)	
Homatropine hydrobromide (Isopto Homatropine, Homatrocel)	Tropicamide (Mydriacyl)

ADRENERGIC DRUGS

A. Action: cause mydriasis
B. Adverse reactions: rare
C. Agents: the following are examples

Phenylephrine hydrochloride (Alconefrin, Mydfrin, Neo-Synephrine Hydrochloride)

DRUGS USED TO TREAT GLAUCOMA

A. Action: cause miosis (pupil constriction); reduce resistance to outflow of aqueous humor; decrease production of aqueous humor
B. Adverse reactions: blood vessel congestion causing increased intraocular pressure, ocular pain, headache, tachycardia or bradycardia, hypertension, diaphoresis, anorexia, gastrointestinal upset, lethargy, depression, diuresis, dehydration
C. Agents: the following are examples

Acetazolamide (Diamox)	Glycerin (Glyrol, Osmoglyn)
Carbachol (Isopto Carbachol)	Isoflurophate (Floropryl)
Demecarium bromide (Humorsol)	Isosorbide (Ismotic)
	Mannitol (Osmitrol)
Dichlorphenamide (Daranide, Oratrol)	Physostigmine sulfate (Eserine)
Echothiophate iodide (Phospholine Iodide)	Pilocarpine hydrochloride (Isopto Carpine, Pilocar)
Epinephrine bitartrate (Epitrate, Primatene Mist Suspension)	Timolol maleate (Timoptic)
	Urea (Ureaphil, Urevert)

NURSING PROCESS

A. Nursing assessment: obtain history of eye-related symptoms such as difficulty in driving or ambulating; examine eyes for signs of infection, exudate, tearing, or drying; assess for eye pain
B. Nursing management: advise patient about effects of drugs such as blurred vision and photophobia; instruct patient regarding drugs (i.e., do not skip doses); teach proper administration of eye medication
C. Nursing evaluation: observe for therapeutic effects and adverse reactions

Drugs Used to Control Muscle Tone
ACETYLCHOLINESTERASE INHIBITORS (ANTICHOLINERGIC AGENTS)

A. Action: allow the accumulation of acetylcholine at neuro-muscular junctions and thus ensure muscle contractility; drugs are not used during pregnancy or with patients who have hyperexcitability of muscular symptoms
B. Adverse reactions: muscle cramps, fasciculations (rapid, small contractions), weakness; excessive salivation, perspiration, nausea, vomiting
C. Agents: the following are examples

Ambenonium chloride (Mytelase)	Neostigmine bromide (Prostigmin)
Edrophonium chloride (Tensilon)	Pyridostigmine bromide (Mestinon, Regonol)

D. Nursing assessment: obtain baseline data relevant to vital signs, ability to swallow, muscle strength, eyelid ptosis, gait, reflexes

E. Nursing management: monitor disease symptoms and vital signs; have suction and intubation equipment at bedside
F. Nursing evaluation: observe for therapeutic effects and adverse reactions

Neuromuscular Blocking Agents

A. Action: produce muscle paralysis
B. Adverse reactions: hypotension, bronchospasm, tachycardia, bradycardia, cardiac dysrhythmias, respiratory distress
C. Agents: the following are examples

Decamethonium bromide (Syncurine)	Succinylcholine chloride (Anectine Quelicin, Sucostrin)
Gallamine triethiodide (Flaxedil)	Tubocurarine chloride (Tubarine)
Pancuronium bromide (Pavulon)	

D. Nursing assessment: obtain baseline data relevant to pulse, respiration, and blood pressure
E. Nursing management: monitor vital signs; continually assess respiratory status, lung sounds, rate and depth of respirations; have suction and intubation equipment at bedside
F. Nursing evaluation: observe for therapeutic effects: sufficient muscle relaxation to allow procedure to be done; observe for adverse reactions: cough and inability to breathe unassisted and to handle secretions

Diabetes Mellitus

INSULIN

A. Action: restores the cell's ability to use glucose and to correct the metabolic changes that occur with diabetes mellitus
B. Adverse reactions: Table 3-6; allergic reactions, insulin resistance, injection-site lipoatrophy
C. Agents: Table 3-7 lists insulin preparations

NURSING PROCESS

A. Assessment: obtain baseline data relative to nonfunctioning of the pancreas, vital signs, weight, blood glucose level, urine glucose level, and ketone level.
B. Management: Teach patient to follow recommended diabetic diet and use exchange system when planning meals; teach how to maintain serum and urine glucose levels, signs and symptoms of hypoglycemia and hyperglycemia and actions patient should take, to carry sugar and ID describing drug regimen in case of hypoglycemic reaction; teach importance of regular exercise, care of feet and nails, contacting physician if unable to eat, self-administration of insulin, rotation of injection sites
C. Evaluation: Serum glucose levels, absence of signs and symptoms of hypo/hyperglycemia.

Oral Hypoglycemic Agents

A. Action: stimulate release of insulin from pancreas
B. Adverse reactions: gastrointestinal distress, muscle weakness, paresthesias, skin reactions, hypoglycemia
C. Agents

Examples	Duration of Action
Tolbutamide (Orinase)	6 to 12 hours
Acetohexamide (Dymelor)	12 to 24 hours
Tolazamide (Tolinase)	12 to 24 hours
Glyburide (Micronase)	up to 24 hours
Chlorpropamide (Diabinese)	up to 24 hours
Glipizide (Glucotrol)	up to 24 hours

NURSING PROCESS

A. Nursing assessment: obtain baseline data relevant to vital signs, weight, blood and urine glucose levels, and other signs and symptoms of the disease

Table 3-6	Hyperglycemia and Hypoglycemic Reactions	
	Hyperglycemia: ketoacidosis, diabetic coma, too little insulin	**Hypoglycemia: insulin reaction, too much insulin**
Onset	Gradual—days	Minutes to hours
Causes	Neglect of therapy, untreated diabetes, intercurrent disease or infection, increase in emotional or psychologic stress	Insulin overdose, omission or delay of meals, excessive exercise before meals
Signs and symptoms	Thirst, headache, excessive urination, nausea, vomiting, abdominal pain, dim vision, coma, flushed face, Kussmaul breathing—rapid, deep—air hunger, dehydration, acetone breath, soft eyeballs, normal absent reflexes	Nervousness, hunger, weakness, cold clammy sweat, nausea, dizziness, double or blurred vision, behavioral changes, stupor, convulsions, pallor, shallow respirations, normal eyeballs, Babinski's reflex may be present
Urine glucose	Positive	Negative or low
Urine acetone	Positive	Negative
Blood glucose	High (above 250 mg)	Low (below 60 mg)
Blood CO_2	Low	Usually normal
Treatment	Insulin, fluid replacement, electrolyte replacement, close observation	Glucose, glucagon, close observation
Response to treatment	Slow	Rapid

Table 3-7	Insulin Preparations		
	Onset of action	Peak action	Duration of action
Rapid acting			
Insulin injection (Regular insulin)	Within 1 hr	2-4 hr	6-8 hr
Prompt insulin zinc suspension (Semilente Iletin, Semilente Insulin)	1.5-2 hr	4-7 hr	12-16 hr
Intermediate acting			
Globin zinc insulin injection	2-4 hr	10-14 hr	14-22 hr
Isophane insulin suspension (NPH Iletin, NPH Insulin)	1-2 hr	10-16 hr	18-30 hr
Insulin zinc suspension (Lente Iletin, Lente Insulin)	1-2 hr	10-16 hr	18-30 hr
Long acting			
Protamine zinc insulin suspension (Protamine Zinc Iletin, Protamine Zinc Insulin, PZI)	6-8 hr	14-24 hr	24-36 hr or longer
Extended insulin zinc suspension (Ultralente Iletin, Ultralente Insulin)	5-8 hr	16-18 hr	24-36 hr or longer

B. Nursing management: monitor vital signs, blood and urine glucose levels, and other appropriate laboratory results; instruct patient regarding medication and administration; teach that stress, fever, trauma, infection, surgery may increase requirements and the need to temporarily switch from oral hypoglycemic to insulin; teach signs and symptoms of hypoglycemia and steps to correct
C. Nursing evaluation: observe for therapeutic effects and adverse reactions

Prevention and Treatment of Infections (Antimicrobials/Antiinfectives)

PENICILLINS AND CEPHALOSPORINS

A. Action: bacteriocidal by interfering with the synthesis of the bacterial cell wall
B. Adverse reactions: allergies—rash, anaphylaxis; convulsions with high parenteral doses; gastrointestinal distress—nausea, vomiting, and diarrhea
C. Agents: the following are examples

1. Penicillins
   Amoxicillin (Amoxil, Larotid, Polymox, Trimox)
   Ampicillin (Amcill, Omnipen, Polycillin, Principen)
   Carbenicillin disodium (Geopen)
   Cloxacillin sodium (Cloxapen, Tegopen)
   Dicloxacillin sodium (Dycill, Dynapen)
   Methicillin sodium (Celbenin, Staphcillin)
   Nafcillin sodium (Nafcil, Unipen)
   Oxacillin sodium (Bactocill, Prostaphlin)
   Penicillin G potassium (Pentids, Pfizerpen)
   Penicillin G benzathine (Bicillin)
   Penicillin G procaine (Crysticillin, Duracillin, Wycillin)
   Penicillin V (Pen Vee K, V-Cillin, Veetids)
   Ticarcillin (Ticar)
   Ticarcillin with Clavulanate (Timentin)

2. Cephalosporins
   Cefaclor (Ceclor)
   Cefamandole nafate (Mandol)
   Cefazolin sodium (Ancef, Kefzol)
   Cefoxitin (Mefoxin)
   Cephalexin (Keflex)
   Cephaloridine (Loridine)
   Cephalothin sodium (Keflin)
   Cephapirin sodium (Cefadyl)
   Cephradrine (Anspor, Velosef)

D. Clinical indications
   1. Wound and skin infections
   2. Respiratory infections
   3. Prophylaxis for patients with rheumatic fever or congenital heart disease
   4. Gram-positive infections caused by streptococci and some staphylococci
   5. Gram-negative infections caused by *Haemophilus influenza, Escherichia coli,* and *Neisseria gonorrhoeae*
E. Patient teaching
   1. Importance of compliance and completing full therapeutic course
   2. Signs and symptoms of super infection
      a. Vaginal irritation, itching, discharge
      b. Black tongue, furry overgrowth
      c. Loose, foul-smelling stools

ERYTHROMYCIN, CLINDAMYCIN (PENICILLIN SUBSTITUTES)

A. Action: bacteriostatic or bacteriocidal (dosage related) by inhibiting protein synthesis
B. Adverse reactions: abdominal discomfort, cramping, nausea, vomiting, diarrhea, urticaria, anaphylaxis, colitis, liver dysfunction, deafness (vancomycin), permanent kidney damage (systemic bacitracin, vancomycin)
C. Agents: the following are examples

1. Erythromycins
   Erythromycin (E-Mycin, Ilotycin, Robimycin, RP-Mycin)
   Erythromycin estolate (Ilosone)
   Erythromycin ethyl-succinate (E.E.S.)
   Erythromycin stearate (Erythrocin)
2. Clindamycins/Lincomycins
   Clindamycin (Cleocin)
   Lincomycin hydrochloride (Lincocin)
3. Penicillin substitutes
   Bacitracin
   Novobiocin sodium (Albamycin)
   Spectinomycin hydrochloride (Trobicin)
   Vancomycin hydrochloride (Vancocin)

D. Clinical indications
   1. See clinical indications for penicillins
   2. Used for patients allergic to penicillin

TETRACYCLINES AND CHLORAMPHENICOL

A. Action: bacteriostatic by preventing the start of protein synthesis (tetracyclines) or inhibiting protein synthesis (chloramphenicol)

B. Adverse reactions
  1. Tetracyclines: nausea, vomiting, stomach pain, diarrhea, superimposed infections, impaired kidney functions, jaundice, delayed blood coagulation, brown discoloration of teeth in children under 8 years of age
  2. Chloramphenicol: bone marrow toxicity, aplastic anemia, allergies, gastrointestinal irritation, headache, mental confusion, depression

C. Agents: the following are examples

Chloramphenicol (Chloromycetin)
Chlortetracycline hydrochloride (Aureomycin)
Demeclocycline hydrochloride (Declomycin)
Doxycycline hyclate (Vibramycin, Doxychel)
Methacycline hydrochloride (Rondomycin)
Minocycline hydrochloride (Minocin, Vectrin)
Oxytetracycline hydrochloride (Terramycin, Oxlopar)
Tetracycline hydrochloride (Achromycin, Panmycin Hydrochloride, Sumycin, Tetracyn)

D. Clinical indications
  1. Gram-negative and gram-positive infections
  2. Severe acne vulgaris
  3. Used for patients allergic to penicillin

AMINOGLYCOSIDES AND POLYMYXINS

A. Action
  1. Aminoglycosides: inhibit early stages of protein synthesis
  2. Polymyxins: alter bacterial cell membrane permeability

B. Adverse reactions: eighth cranial nerve damage, renal damage, respiratory paralysis

C. Agents: the following are examples

  1. Aminoglycosides
    Amikacin sulfate (Amikin)
    Gentamicin sulfate (Garamycin)
    Kanamycin sulfate (Kantrex)
    Neomycin sulfate (Mycifradin, Neobiotic)
    Streptomycin
    Tobramycin sulfate (Nebcin)
  2. Polymyxins
    Colistimethate sodium (Coly-Mycin M)
    Colistin sulfate (Coly-Mycin S)
    Polymyxin B sulfate (Aerosporin)

D. Clinical indications
Drugs are potentially dangerous and are used only in cases of severe infections, such as gram-negative bone and joint infections and septicemia

SULFONAMIDES, TRIMETHOPRIM, NITROFURANTOINS, NALIDIXIC ACID

A. Action: block bacterial synthesis of folic acid; inhibit bacterial enzymes required for proper metabolism of sugar; interfere directly with DNA synthesis

B. Adverse reactions
  1. Sulfonamides, trimethoprim, nitrofurantoins: allergies, nausea, vomiting, diarrhea, stomatitis, blood dyscrasias, renal calculi, and hematuria
  2. Nalidixic acid: convulsions, mental instability, headache, dizziness, visual disturbances, photosensitivity

C. Agents: the following are examples

  1. Sulfonamides
    Sulfadiazine
    Sulfameter (Sulla)
    Sulfamethizole (Microsul, Thiosulfil, Forte)
    Sulfamethoxazole (Gantanol)
    Sulfamethoxazole-phenazopyridine (Azo Gantanol)
    Sulfamethoxazole-trimethoprim (Bactrim, Septra)
    Sulfamethoxypyridazine acetyl (Midicel)
    Sulfasalazine (Azulfidine, Salazopyrin)
    Sulfisoxazole (Gantrisin, Rosoxol, Sulfalar)
    Sulfisoxazole-phenazo-pyridine hydro-chloride (Azo Gantrisin, SK-Soxazole, Azosul)
  2. Sulfonamides: topical agents
    Mafenide (Sulfamylon)
    Nitrofurantoin (Furadantin, Furalan, Nephronex)
    Nitrofurantoin macrocrystals (Macrodantin)
    Nalidixic acid (NegGram)
    Silver sulfadiazine (Silvadene)
    Sulfacetamide sodium (Sulamyd)
    Sulfisoxazole diolamine (Gantrisin Ophthalmic)
    Trimethoprim (Proloprim, Trimpex)

D. Clinical indications
  1. Used to treat acute and chronic urinary tract infections
  2. Other uses include trachoma, chancroid, toxoplasmosis, acute otitis media, and prophylactic therapy in cases of recurrent rheumatic fever
  3. Treatment of ulcerative colitis
  4. Prophylaxis for patients scheduled for bowel surgery (To prevent renal calculi, teach patient to maintain fluid intake of 2,000 to 3,000 ml/day.)

DRUGS USED TO TREAT TUBERCULOSIS AND LEPROSY

A. Action: alter several metabolic processes in mycobacteria

B. Adverse reactions: peripheral neuropathies, visual disturbances, gastrointestinal distress, ototoxicity, headache

C. Agents: the following are examples

  1. First-line antitubercular drugs
    Ethambutol hydro-chloride (Myambutol)
    Isoniazid (Isotamine, Niconyl, Nydrazid)
    Para-aminosalicylic acid (PAS) (aminosalicylic acid, Teebacin acid)
    Rifampin (Rifadin, Rimactane)
    Streptomycin
  2. Second-line antitubercular drugs
    Capreomycin (Capastat)
    Cycloserine (Seromycin)
    Ethionamide (Trecator S.C.)
    Pyrazinamide
  3. Antileprosy agents
    Clofazimine (Lamprene)
    Dapsone (Avlosulfon)
    Rifampin (Rifadin, Rimactane)
    Sulfoxone sodium (Diasone)

D. Patient teaching: stress importance of long-term compliance and follow-up visits with the physician; report any adverse reactions promptly; refrain from using alcohol; refrain from taking other medications without the knowledge and permission of the physician; wear a medical identification tag indicating medication being taken.

ANTIFUNGAL DRUGS
A. Action: selectively damages the membranes of fungi
B. Adverse reactions: renal damage, anemia, nausea, diarrhea
C. Agents: the following are examples

1. Systemic agents
   Amphotericin B
     (Fungizone)
   Flucytosine (Ancobon)
   Hydroxystilbamidine
     isethionate
   Miconazole
     (Monistat-IV)
2. Topical agents
   Acrisorcin (Akrinol)
   Amphotericin B
     (Fungizone)
   Candicidin (Vanobid)
   Clioquinol (Vioform)

   Clotrimazole
     (Gyne-Lotrimin,
     Lotrimin)
   Griseofulvin
     (Fulvicin-P/G,
     Grifulvin V, Grisactin)
   Haloprogin (Halotex)
   Miconazole nitrate
     (MicaTin, Monistat)
   Nystatin (Mycostatin,
     Nilstat)
   Tolnaftate (Aftate,
     Tinactin)
   Undecylenic acid—zinc
     undecylenate (Desenex,
     Ting, Cruex)

D. Patient teaching: proper administration of vaginal tablets, use of condom by sexual partner to avoid reinfection

DRUGS USED TO TREAT VIRAL DISEASES
A. Action: selective toxicity in various processes of virus reproduction
B. Adverse reactions: ataxia, slurred speech, lethargy, local irritation, anorexia, nausea, vomiting, diarrhea, dizziness, headache, anemia and bone marrow depression (zidovudine), bone marrow depression (ganciclovir), visual haze, irritation, burning of eyes, photophobia (idoxuridine)
C. Agents: the following are examples

Acyclovir (Zovirax)
Amantadine (Symmetrel)
Ganciclovir (DHPG)
Idoxuridine (Dendrid,
   Herplex Liquifilm,
   Stoxil)

Methisazone
Vidarabine (Vira-A)
Zidovudine*
   (AZT, Retrovir)

ANTIPROTOZOAL AND ANTHELMINTIC AGENTS
A. Action: destroy the protozoa and helminths at various stages of development
B. Adverse reactions: gastrointestinal distress, flatulence, vision changes, irritability, hemolysis, skin eruptions, blood dyscrasias
C. Agents: the following are examples

1. Amebic infestations
   Chloroquine phosphate
     (Aralen)
   Diloxanide (Furamide)

   Emetine hydrochloride
   Iodoquinol (Yodoxin)
   Metronidazole (Flagyl)

2. Malaria
   Amodiaquine
     hydrochloride
     (Camoquin)
   Chloroquine hydro-
     chloride (Aralen)
   Primaquine
     phosphate
   Quinine
3. Others
   Povidone-iodine
     (Betadine, Proviodine)
   Quinacrine
     hydrochloride

4. Anthelmintics
   Mebendazole (Vermox)
   Niclosamide
     (Yomesan)
   Piperazine citrate
     (Antepar)
   Pyrantel pamoate
     (Antiminth)
   Pyrvinium pamoate
     (Povan)

NURSING PROCESS
A. Nursing assessment: obtain history of allergies; evaluate baseline data relevant to signs and symptoms of infection, vital signs, pertinent laboratory tests, appearance of wounds, incisions, or lesions, amount and description of drainage, swelling, erythema, subjective symptoms of pain or pressure
B. Nursing management: obtain culture for specimens before starting antibiotics; maintain supportive measures such as rest, comfort, nutrition, fluids and electrolyte balance; maintain proper administration regarding route, time, and dosage; monitor vital signs and laboratory results
C. Nursing evaluation: observe for therapeutic effects and adverse reactions; instruct patient regarding medications to ensure compliance

Neoplastic Diseases
SPECIFIC ANTINEOPLASTIC AGENTS
A. Action: selective toxicity during various stages of the cell cycle
B. Agents

Examples	Adverse Reactions
Asparaginase (Elspar)	Central nervous system depression
Bleomycin sulfate (Blenoxane)	Pulmonary toxicity, skin reactions
Busulfan (Myleran)	Bone marrow and kidney toxicity
Calusterone (Methosarb)	Mild virilism, edema, hypercalcemia, nausea, vomiting
Carmustine (BiCNU)	Bone marrow suppression, nausea
Chlorambucil (Leukeran)	Bone marrow suppression
Cisplatin (Platinol)	Renal damage, nausea and vomiting, ototoxicity, neurotoxicity, and anaphylactic reactions
Cyclophosphamide (Cytoxan)	Hemorrhagic cystitis, bladder fibrosis
Cytarabine (Cytosar-U)	Bone marrow suppression
Dacarbazine (DTIC-Dome)	Bone marrow suppression
Dactinomycin (Cosmegen)	Bone marrow suppression, gastrointestinal irritation, skin reactions

*Used in treatment of AIDS; prevents replication of HIV virus, thus delaying disease progression.

Examples	Adverse Reactions
Diethylstilbestrol diphosphate (Stilphostrol)	Risk of thromboembolic disease, edema, mood changes
Doxorubicin hydrochloride (Adriamycin)	Bone marrow suppression, gastrointestinal distress, alopecia
Dromostanolone propionate (Drolban)	Mild virilism, edema, hypercalcemia
Estradiol (Progynon)	Risk of thromboembolic disease, edema, mood changes
Etoposide	Bone marrow suppression
Floxuridine (FUDR)	Gastrointestinal and hematologic toxicity
Fluorouracil (5-FU, Adrucil)	Gastrointestinal and hematologic toxicity
Hydroxyurea (Hydrea)	Bone marrow suppression
Lomustine (CeeNU)	Myelosuppression, nausea
Mechlorethamine hydrochloride or nitrogen mustard (Mustargen)	Bone marrow suppression
Medroxyprogesterone (Depo-Provera)	Menstrual irregularities, rashes, and thromboembolic diseases
Megestrol acetate (Megace)	Thromboembolic disease
Melphalan (Alkeran)	Leukopenia, anemia, menstrual irregularities
Mercaptopurine (Purinethol)	Hematologic toxicity, immunosuppression
Methotrexate	Gastrointestinal toxicity, bone marrow suppression, immunosuppression
Mitomycin (Mutamycin)	Bone marrow suppression, gastrointestinal irritation, alopecia, renal toxicity
Mitotane (Lysodren)	Gastrointestinal disturbances, skin reactions
Plicamycin (mithramycin; Mithracin)	Gastrointestinal, skin, liver, and kidney toxicity
Polyestradiol phosphate (Estradurin)	Risk of thromboembolic disease, edema, mood changes
Prednisone (Deltasone, Panasol, Meticorten)	Cushing's syndrome
Procarbazine hydrochloride (Matulane)	Bone marrow suppression, gastrointestinal disturbances
Tamoxifen citrate (Nolvadex)	Hot flashes, nausea, vomiting
Teniposide	Bone marrow suppression
Testolactone (Teslac)	Pain and irrigation at injection site, hypercalemia
Thioguanine	Hematologic toxicity
Thiotepa	Bone marrow toxicity
Vinblastine sulfate (Velban)	Peripheral neuropathy and bone marrow suppression
Vincristine sulfate (Oncovin)	Alopecia, abdominal pain, peripheral neuropathy

C. Nursing assessment: obtain baseline data regarding possible adverse reactions of drugs; evaluate condition of hair, skin, nails, weight, vital signs and necessary blood laboratory studies (especially WBC, RBC, and platelet count)
D. Nursing management: monitor weight, vital signs, and laboratory studies; institute regular inspection of mouth; maintain good medical asepsis; use infusion monitoring device for IV administration; provide patient/family teaching and psychologic support; check hydration status
E. Nursing evaluation: observe for therapeutic effects and adverse reactions

Nutrients, Fluids, and Electrolytes
Substances required for human nutrition include water, carbohydrates, proteins, fats, vitamins, and minerals; necessary to maintain health, prevent illness, and promote recovery from illness.

NUTRITIONAL PRODUCTS: ORAL AND TUBE FEEDINGS
A. Nutritionally complete formulas
  1. Action
    a. Provide United States Recommended Dietary Allowance for protein, minerals, and vitamins
    b. Provide 1 calorie per milliliter (Sustagen: 1.84 cal/ml)
  2. Agents: the following are examples

Compleat-B	Osmolite
Ensure	Sustacal
Isocal	Sustagen
Meritene	

B. Nutritional agents for limited use
  1. Vital H.N.: contains easily digested forms of protein, carbohydrate, and fat; used for critically ill patients
  2. Lofenalac: a low-phenylalanine preparation used for infants and children with phenylketonuria (PKU)
  3. MBF (Meat Base Formula): hypoallergenic infant formula for those who are allergic to milk or have galactosemia
  4. Neo-Mull-Soy, Pro Sobee, Isomil: soybean products used as hypoallergenic, milk-free formulas
  5. Pregestimil: infant formula containing easily digested protein, fat, and carbohydrate; used in infants with diarrhea or malabsorption syndromes
  6. Vivonex: nutritionally complete diet containing amino acids as its protein
C. Nutritionally incomplete supplements
  1. Amin-Aid: source of protein for patients with renal insufficiency
  2. Casec: carbohydrate calories supplement
  3. Lipomul: unsaturated fat supplement
  4. Liprotein: high caloric and protein oral supplement for use in burn or debilitated patients
  5. Lonalac: milk substitute for sodium-restricted diets
  6. Probana: iron-free, high-protein formula for infants and children with diarrhea or malabsorption syndromes
D. Complete infant formulas
  1. May be used alone for bottle-fed babies or to supplement breast-fed babies, similar to human breast milk; iron deficient
  2. Preparations: Enfamil and Similac are examples

INTRAVENOUS FLUIDS
A. Dextrose injection: contains 2.5%, 5%, 10%, 20%, 40%, 50%, 60%, and 70% dextrose, the 20% to 50% solutions

are used for calories in total parenteral nutrition (TPN) and administered through a central or subclavian catheter

B. Dextrose and sodium chloride injection: most commonly used concentrations are 5% dextrose in 0.25% or 0.45% sodium chloride

C. Amino acid solution (Aminosyn): contains essential and non-essential amino acids; most often used with dextrose in TPN

D. Liposyn, Intralipid: concentrated calories and essential fatty acids; most often used as part of TPN

VITAMINS

A. General information
   1. Group of substances that act as coenzymes to help in the conversion of carbohydrate and fat into energy and to form bones and tissues; necessary for metabolism of fat, carbohydrate, and protein; normally obtained from foods
   2. Subclassified as
      a. Fat soluble: A, D, E, K
      b. Water soluble: B complex, C

B. Agents
   1. Fat-soluble vitamins: the following are examples

   Vitamin A
      (Alphalin,
      Aquasol A)
   Vitamin E
      (Tocopherol,
      Aquasol E)

   Vitamin K
      Menadiol sodium
      diphosphate (Synkayvite)
   Phytonadione
      (Mephyton,
      AquaMEPHYTON)

   2. Water-soluble vitamins: the following are examples
      a. B-complex

   Calcium
      pantothenate
      (B_5)
      (Pantholin)
   Cyanocobalamin
      (B_{12})
      (Rubramin PC,
      Betalin 12)
   Folic acid
      (Folvite)

   Niacin
   Pyridoxine hydrochloride
      (B_6)
      (Hexa-Betalin)
   Riboflavin
      (Riobin-50, B_2)
   Thiamine hydrochloride
      (B_1)
      (Betalin S)

      b. Vitamin C: ascorbic acid

MINERALS AND ELECTROLYTES

A. General information: basic constituents of living tissues and components of many enzymes; function to maintain fluid, electrolyte, and acid-base balance; maintain muscle and nerve function; assist in transfer of materials across cell membranes and contribute to the growth process

B. Agents: the following are examples

   Deferoxamine mesylate
      (Desferal)
   Ferrous gluconate (Fergon)
   Ferrous sulfate (Feosol)
   Iron dextran injection
      (Imferon)
   Magnesium sulfate
   Potassium bicarbonate—
      potassium citrate
      (K-Lyte)

   Potassium chloride
      (Kay Ciel, K-Lor)
   Potassium gluconate
      (Kaon)
   Sodium bicarbonate
   Sodium polystyrene
      sulfonate (Kayexalate)

Multiple Mineral-Electrolyte Preparations

   Normosol-R
   Pedialyte (oral)
   Plasma-Lyte 56

   Plasma-Lyte 148
   Polysal M
   Ringer's lactate

NURSING PROCESS

A. Nursing assessment: obtain baseline data with emphasis on presenting signs and symptoms, vital signs, and laboratory blood studies

B. Nursing management: perform nursing actions to foster drug therapy; monitor diet and laboratory blood studies

C. Nursing evaluation: observe for therapeutic effects specific to type of nutrient supplement; instruct patient regarding medications and diet

SUGGESTED READING

Albanese AA, Nutz PA: *Mosby's 1998 nursing drug cards,* St Louis, Mosby (revised annually).

Brown M, Mulholland JL: *Drug calculations: process and problems for clinical practice,* ed 4, St Louis, 1992, Mosby.

Clark JF, Queener SF, Karb VB: *Pharmacologic basis of nursing practice,* ed 4, St Louis 1992, Mosby.

Clayton BD, Stock YN: *Basic pharmacology and the nursing process,* ed 10, St Louis, 1993, Mosby.

Dison N: *Simplified drugs and solution for nurses,* ed 10, St Louis, 1991, Mosby.

Edmonds MW: *Introduction to clinical pharmacology,* ed 2, St Louis, 1995, Mosby.

Gahart BL: *Intravenous medications,* ed 8, St Louis, 1992, Mosby.

Lilley LL, Aukers RS, Albanese JA: *Pharmacology and the nursing process,* St Louis, 1996, Mosby.

McHenry LM, Salerno E: *Mosby's pharmacology in nursing,* ed 19, St Louis, 1995, Mosby.

Physicians' desk reference, Montvale NJ, Medical Economics (published annually).

Skidmore-Roth L: *Mosby's 1998 nursing drug references,* St Louis, Mosby (published annually).

REVIEW QUESTIONS

Answers and rationales begin on p. 111.

1. If 8 dr of a drug is ordered by the doctor, the nurse will safely administer:
   ① ½ oz
   ② 1 oz
   ③ 1½ oz
   ④ 2 oz

2. A 76-year-old patient suffers from CHF and dependent edema. Her feet and legs often swell to twice their normal size. The patient takes 80 mg of furosemide (Lasix) each morning. The nurse knows it would be most important to report:
   ① A 3-pound weight loss
   ② Pitting edema in the right foot
   ③ Confusion
   ④ Intake less than output

3. A 62-year-old patient has an attack of acute angina. The nurse knows that the treatment of choice will be:
   ① Calcium channel blockers
   ② Beta adrenergic blockers
   ③ Nitrates
   ④ Narcotic analgesics

4. A 56-year-old patient takes heparin each evening. Which of the following will the nurse assess in regard to drug overdose?
   ① Dypsnea
   ② Polyuria
   ③ Hematuria
   ④ Frequency of urination

5. The patient suffering from salicylate (aspirin) poisoning is most likely to complain that:
   ① "My head hurts all the time."
   ② "My stools are hard and tarry."
   ③ "I'm beginning to have diarrhea."
   ④ "I hear ringing in my ears."

6. If 125 ml of a drug is ordered by the doctor, the nurse will safely administer:
   ① 0.125 L
   ② 1.25 L
   ③ 12.5 L
   ④ 1250 L

7. A poisonous effect of a drug, either from a regular dose or an overdose is referred to as a(an):
   ① Side effect
   ② Untoward effect
   ③ Toxic action
   ④ Idiosyncratic action

8. The physician orders IV administration of 1 g of Kefzol in 100 ml of D5W in 20 minutes q6h. The drip factor is 15 gtt/ml. The nurse regulates the IV at:
   ① 25 gtt/min
   ② 50 gtt/min
   ③ 75 gtt/min
   ④ 100 gtt/min

9. The action of a drug in the body other than the main effect for which the drug was given is called a(an):
   ① Side effect
   ② Idiosyncratic action
   ③ Synergistic action
   ④ Antagonistic action

10. In relation to drugs, the term *blood level* refers to the:
    ① Metabolism of the drug
    ② Excretion of the drug
    ③ Amount of the drug in the circulating fluids
    ④ Effect of the drug on the red blood cells

11. Fluoxetine (Prozac) has been ordered for a 49-year-old man who suffers from depression. In teaching him about his new medicine, the nurse will tell him that:
    ① It should be taken at bedtime
    ② A feeling of euphoria will occur within 24 hours
    ③ It will take 2 to 3 weeks before the effects of the drug will be felt
    ④ It should be taken with meals.

12. KCL (potassium chloride) is ordered for a 65-year-old patient taking Lasix. Before administering the medication the nurse will:
    ① Be sure the patient has been NPO since 12 midnight
    ② Dilute it in 3 to 8 oz of cold water or juice
    ③ Crush the controlled release tablet and mix it with water
    ④ Partially dissolve the effervescent tablet

13. A 20-year-old male patient is taking ciprofloxacin (Cipro) for a UTI. He also takes Theophylline for asthma. In teaching him about his medication, the nurse knows:
    ① Fluids should be restricted while on Cipro
    ② The patient should not be started on Cipro until the culture results are obtained
    ③ Theophylline levels may be elevated and can become toxic
    ④ The two medications should be given at alternate times

14. Tromethamine (Toradol) has been ordered IM to control pain in a patient who has had gallbladder surgery. The nurse will know to take the following precaution when administering Toradol:
    ① Keep bed down, side rails up, call bell within reach
    ② Check blood sugars qid
    ③ Have oxygen ready in case of an emergency
    ④ Numb the injection site because of severe pain

15. The nurse is going to give a subcutaneous injection to a 42-year-old patient. The needle length and gauge the nurse will use is:
    ① 19 gauge: 1½ inch
    ② 22 gauge: 1 inch
    ③ 24 gauge: 1 inch
    ④ 25 gauge: ⅝ inch

16. While the nurse administers the daily dose of furosemide (Lasix) to the patient, the opportunity arises for patient teaching. Which of the following will the nurse be sure to stress?
    ① "Take the medicine at bedtime"
    ② "You may need sodium and potassium supplements"
    ③ "Weigh yourself twice a day"
    ④ "Change positions slowly to prevent dizziness"

17. A 9-year-old patient was recently started on methylphenidate (Ritalin) for ADD. On his follow-up office visit his mother reports to the nurse that he is having difficulty sleeping. The nurse knows:
    ① Ritalin needs to be given early in the day because insomnia is a side effect.
    ② Children with ADD are frequently hyperactive and this is probably why he can't sleep.
    ③ The patient may be taking in too much caffeine each day.
    ④ The patient may need an increase in his Ritalin dose.

18. A 29-year-old patient is being discharged on metoclopramide (Reglan). In his discharge teaching the nurse will stress that:
    ① The drug may cause drowsiness
    ② The drug is best taken after meals
    ③ Nausea and vomiting are common side effects
    ④ If a dose is missed, skip it and get back on schedule with the next dose

19. A 19-year-old patient has been given naloxone HCL (Narcan) to overcome a narcotic overdose. The nurse knows that the expected action of the drug is to:
    ① Induce hypertension
    ② Induce hypotension
    ③ Reverse CNS/respiratory depression
    ④ Prevent arrhythmias

20. When administering a buccal tablet the nurse will tell the patient to:
    ① Chew the tablet
    ② Swallow the tablet with water
    ③ Let the tablet dissolve under the tongue
    ④ Let the tablet dissolve between the cheek and the gum

21. If 500 mg of a drug is ordered by the doctor, the nurse will safely administer:
    ① 500 g
    ② 0.5 g
    ③ 0.05 g
    ④ 0.005 g

22. A 64-year-old patient with CHF takes a digitalis preparation every day. Before administering the medication the nurse will:
    ① Weigh the patient
    ② Check the patient's apical pulse
    ③ Take the patient's blood pressure
    ④ Monitor the patient's clotting time

23. Theophylline (Theolair) has been prescribed for a 48-year-old patient with asthma. You are teaching her about the medication. Which of the following statements by the patient indicates she has correct understanding of the medication's action?
    ① "This medication should relieve the tightness when I breathe."
    ② "I'm so fortunate to be on a medication that will cure my asthma."
    ③ "My mucus should be a lot thinner with this medication."
    ④ "This medication should help my runny nose."

24. An 80-year-old patient is known to often be noncompliant with his medical regimen. When he refuses to take his medication, the nurse will
    ① Leave the medication at the bedside in case the patient changes his mind
    ② Document the patient's refusal and reason for refusal
    ③ Warn the patient that his doctor will be told of his refusal
    ④ Give the medication to his visitors so that they will urge the patient to comply

25. A 44-year-old female patient had a laminectomy 4 days ago. She is complaining of pain every 2 hours. The doctor has ordered meperidine HCL (Demerol) every 4 hours in steadily increasing doses over the past 4 days. In conferring with the doctor regarding her care, the nurse will express her concern that the patient is developing a(an):

① Addiction to Demerol
② Dependence on Demerol
③ Tolerance to Demerol
④ Hypersensitive reaction to Demerol

26. A 76-year-old patient has congestive heart failure (CHF). The patient is on furosemide (Lasix), Digoxin, and potassium (Micro-K) and is complaining of abdominal discomfort and visual disturbances described as: "People look like they have yellow-green skin." It is time for all three medications. The nurse will hold the:
    ① Lasix and Digoxin and notify the doctor
    ② Lasix and Micro-K and notify the doctor
    ③ Three drugs and notify the doctor
    ④ Digoxin and notify the doctor

27. A 72-year-old patient with osteoarthritis has been taking nabumetone (Relafen) for 6 weeks. She complains to the nurse that she feels a gnawing feeling in her stomach that doesn't go away for any length of time and that it seems to be getting worse. The nurse calls the doctor and he discontinues the drug. The nurse will:
    ① Tell the patient that nabumetone (Relafen) can cause ulcers
    ② Observe the patient for continuance of her symptoms
    ③ Give the patient other NSAIDS with food
    ④ Monitor the patient for the presence of occult blood in the stools

28. The process by which drugs are inactivated by the body is:
    ① Absorption
    ② Distribution
    ③ Metabolism
    ④ Excretion

29. A patient asks for medication to relieve pain postoperatively. Subjective evidence that the medication she has been given is effective is that the patient:
    ① Is beginning to fall asleep
    ② Is talking with her visitors
    ③ States: "I feel so much better now."
    ④ Is walking around her room

30. The nurse knows that preparations that supply slow, continuous dissolution of a medication over an extended period of time are known as:
    ① Enteric coated
    ② A tablet within a tablet
    ③ Sustained action
    ④ Lozenges

31. When taking a patient's medical history, the most important thing a nurse will determine is:
    ① The names of all medications kept in the patient's home
    ② The patient's dislike of injections
    ③ If the patient takes nonprescription vitamins
    ④ The patient's known allergies to medication

32. The patient is to receive an IV of lactated Ringers at 75 ml/hr. The drip factor is 20 gtt/ml. The nurse will run the IV at:
    ① 5 gtt/min
    ② 15 gtt/min
    ③ 25 gtt/min
    ④ 35 gtt/rnin

33. The patient will be taught to take his iron preparation:
    ① At bedtime
    ② Before breakfast
    ③ With meals
    ④ Between meals

34. A patient is receiving temazepam (Restoril) 0.015 g po at bedtime for insomnia. The label indicates 15 mg tablets. How many tablets will the nurse give?
    ① 1
    ② 1.5
    ③ 2
    ④ 2.5

35. When chest pain is not relieved by nitroglycerin, the dose should be repeated in:
    ① 1 minute
    ② 5 minutes
    ③ 10 minutes
    ④ 30 minutes

36. The 70-year-old patient is receiving aminophylline. The nurse knows the medication will act to:
    ① Dilate blood vessels increasing capillary permeability
    ② Increase contraction of the bronchi and alveoli
    ③ Decrease contraction of the smooth muscle
    ④ Decrease the amount of mucous secretion from the bronchi

37. The nurse will caution a patient on antihypertensive medication to avoid sudden changes in position, especially from a supine to an upright position, because:
    ① A thrombus might become dislodged
    ② Severe nausea might result
    ③ Postural hypotension might occur
    ④ Increased diuresis will occur

38. The patient is receiving meperidine hydrochloride (Demerol) 100 mg q4h for relief of pain. The nurse will monitor the patient closely for:
    ① Decreased blood pressure
    ② Increased respirations
    ③ Increased heart rate
    ④ Decreased respirations

39. Some adrenergic drugs can be used to stop bleeding and relieve nasal and ocular congestion by causing:
    ① Constriction of blood vessels
    ② Vasodilation of blood vessels
    ③ Astringent action on mucous membranes
    ④ A rise in arterial blood pressure

40. An adverse reaction to atropine sulfate that may be serious for patients with underlying heart disease is:
    ① Delirium
    ② Tachycardia
    ③ Constipation
    ④ Dry mouth

41. A 31-year-old patient who is experiencing nausea and vomiting has an elevated temperature. The nurse will give the antipyretic:
    ① Orally
    ② Rectally
    ③ Sublingually
    ④ Topically

42. Adverse reactions associated with the use of acetylsalicylic acid (aspirin) include
    ① Vomiting, petechiae, tinnitus
    ② Constipation, polyphagia, hematuria
    ③ Hypertension, anaphylactic shock, tachycardia
    ④ Bradycardia, hypotension, dermatitis

43. When a medication is ordered for "swish and swallow," the nurse will tell the patient to:

    ① Thoroughly rinse the mouth and then swallow
    ② Swallow immediately followed by 60 ml of water
    ③ Thoroughly rinse the mouth and spit out the remains
    ④ Gargle deep in the throat and then swallow

44. Drugs that relieve pain are classified as:
    ① Sedatives
    ② Hypnotics
    ③ Analgesics
    ④ Antipyretics

45. The nurse will watch a patient receiving a cholinergic drug for which of the following side effects?
    ① Increased peristalsis
    ② Decreased peristalsis
    ③ Increased urine output
    ④ Decreased urine output

46. The nurse knows that anticholinergic drugs would not be ordered for a patient with:
    ① Hypertension
    ② Diabetes mellitus
    ③ Cardiac failure
    ④ Glaucoma

47. The nurse gives the 59-year-old patient atropine sulfate as a preoperative medication. The nurse will tell the patient that he will not be allowed out of bed because:
    ① There is depression of the central nervous system
    ② Vertigo might occur because of dilation of the pupils
    ③ One effect of the drug is the development of postural hypertension
    ④ Diaphoresis may predispose to a chill

48. The patient has just returned from the postoperative recovery room and is complaining of pain. The most appropriate nursing action will be to first:
    ① Call the physician
    ② Administer the pain medication as ordered
    ③ Ask the patient to describe the pain and its location
    ④ Check when the medication was given last

49. A nursing measure requiring the use of the anticholinesterase agent neostigmine bromide (Prostigmin) is:
    ① Inserting a Foley catheter
    ② Inserting a rectal tube
    ③ Encouraging oral fluids
    ④ Assisting the patient to ambulate

50. The patient with glaucoma should *not* receive:
    ① Atropine sulfate
    ② Morphine sulfate
    ③ Meperidine hydrochloride (Demerol)
    ④ Hydroxyzine hydrochloride (Vistaril)

51. Spironolactone (Aldactone) is often prescribed for children with congestive heart failure because it is a(an)
    ① Potassium-sparing diuretic
    ② Loop diuretic
    ③ Thiazide carbonic anhydrase inhibitor diuretic
    ④ Osmotic diuretic

52. Estrogen (Premarin) is contraindicated in patients with a history of:
    ① Allergies
    ② Ulcers
    ③ Breast cancer
    ④ Obesity

53. In an attempt to stop a spontaneous abortion, the physician has ordered terbutaline (Brethine), a uterine relaxant for the patient. Adverse reactions the nurse will be alert for are:
    ① Heart palpitations, nausea, vomiting, headache
    ② Drowsiness, incoordination, gastrointestinal upset
    ③ Sedation, dry mouth, blurred vision, urinary retention
    ④ Anxiety, apprehension, headache, cerebral hemorrhage
54. When administering medication to a patient, an important step the nurse must take to prevent cross-contamination between nurse and patients is to:
    ① Check the order with another nurse
    ② Wash hands before preparing medication
    ③ Identify patient carefully
    ④ Remain with the patient until the medication is swallowed
55. The patient tells the nurse that she is bothered by a "ringing in the ears." The nurse knows that this is a:
    ① Sign of aspirin toxicity
    ② Sign of ear infection
    ③ Side effect of headache
    ④ Side effect of diarrhea
56. To obtain fastest absorption and action from a medication, the nurse knows it should be administered:
    ① By mouth
    ② Intramuscularly
    ③ Subcutaneously
    ④ Intravenously
57. When a patient experiences an unexpected effect of a medication, it is referred to as an:
    ① Untoward effect
    ② Idiosyncratic effect
    ③ Unexpected effect
    ④ Antagonistic effect
58. Diazepam (Valium) is given for treatment of status epilepticus. The nurse knows its expected action is to:
    ① Decrease anxiety
    ② Relieve pain
    ③ Lower neuron excitability
    ④ Induce sleep
59. An assessment the nurse would take before giving a digitalis preparation is the patient's
    ① Blood pressure
    ② Pulse rate
    ③ Temperature
    ④ Hydration status
60. When administering an intramuscular injection, the nurse will aspirate after insertion of the needle to:
    ① Avoid injecting the drug directly into the bloodstream
    ② Ease the patient's discomfort
    ③ Facilitate absorption into the bloodstream
    ④ Avoid injuring organs
61. When teaching self-administration of a diuretic, the nurse will tell the patient to:
    ① Take the diuretic at bedtime
    ② Cut down on fluid intake
    ③ Take the diuretic after rising
    ④ Stop taking the diuretic when feeling better
62. When the blood level of a drug is ordered and the lab results indicate the level is above normal, the nurse knows that the:
    ① Dose of medication is correct for the patient
    ② Patient is not absorbing the drug properly
    ③ Patient is not excreting the drug properly
    ④ Drug is being given by the wrong route
63. An elderly patient states that his medication costs too much for his fixed income. The nurse will tell him to ask his doctor to write prescriptions for which of the following forms of the medication?
    ① Generic name
    ② Brand name
    ③ Chemical name
    ④ Official name
64. Before administering medication through a nasogastric tube, the nurse will make sure that the
    ① Tube is in the esophagus
    ② Tube is in the stomach
    ③ Pill will dissolve
    ④ Pill is enteric coated
65. When administering a bulk-forming laxative such as psyllium husk (Metamucil) the nurse will give it:
    ① At bedtime
    ② With meals
    ③ With a full glass of water
    ④ With an antacid
66. The nurse expects a placebo to be effective because of the:
    ① Production of endorphins in the brain
    ② Nurturing attitude of the nurse
    ③ Action of the active drug in the placebo
    ④ Patient's ability to metabolize the placebo
67. A 28-year-old patient with hyperthyroidism is placed on phenobarbital to achieve which of the following effects?
    ① Sedation
    ② Control of seizures
    ③ Vasoconstriction
    ④ Vasodilation
68. The nurse will administer thyroid drugs:
    ① In a single dose, usually before breakfast
    ② In divided doses, before meals
    ③ In divided dose, after meals
    ④ As the patient's energy level decreases
69. When a mydriatic eye medication is being administered the nurse will observe for:
    ① Decreased drainage
    ② Constriction of the pupil
    ③ Dilation of the pupil
    ④ Decreased intraocular pressure
70. The nurse knows that an 80-year-old patient on medication would be prone to which of the following?
    ① Developing a tolerance to medication
    ② Metabolizing medications more rapidly
    ③ Developing more frequent adverse reactions
    ④ Experiencing more cumulative effects
71. The nurse will do a daily assessment of the integrity of the oral mucosa when the patient is receiving:
    ① Antibiotics
    ② Cancer drugs
    ③ Antiparkinsonian drugs
    ④ Vitamins
72. Which of the following instructions is essential for the patient to understand when he is sent home on antitubercular drugs?
    ① Eat foods high in calcium to improve the absorption of the drug
    ② Continue the drug regimen as ordered by the physician

③ Perform postural drainage each morning before taking the medication

④ Have those with whom you work take the medication also

73. A major adverse reaction the nurse will observe for in a cancer patient receiving antineoplastic drugs is:
① Bone marrow depression
② Oliguria
③ Lethargy
④ Photosensitivity

74. When a 23-year-old mother asks about giving an antibiotic ordered by the physician for her child after signs and symptoms of the infection have disappeared, the nurse will tell her to:
① Discard what is left
② Finish what is left of the drug
③ Save what is left
④ Call the physician

75. The law that regulates the manufacture, distribution, advertisement, and labeling of drugs to ensure safety and effectiveness is the:
① Harrison Narcotic Act
② Consumer Protection Act
③ Controlled Substance Act
④ Federal Food, Drug and Cosmetic Act

76. When preparing narcotics and other controlled substances for administration the nurse will:
① Confirm the dosage with another nurse
② Sign for the drugs on separate record forms
③ Be sure the order sheet has been signed by two physicians
④ Have a witness during preparation

77. A dialysis patient is placed on 1,000 ml fluid restriction per 24 hours. The best way for the nurse to regulate the fluid intake with the least effect on the patient would be to allow the patient:
① 400 ml on 7-3 shift, 400 ml on 3-11 shift, and 200 ml on 11-7 shift
② 350 ml on 7-3 shift, 350 ml on 3-11 shift, and 300 ml on 11-7 shift
③ To drink as much as he wants on 7-3 shift
④ To drink only what comes on meal trays

78. A 49-year-old patient is admitted with deep vein thrombosis. He is on complete bed rest and a standard heparin drip. The nurse will know to report the following as a complication of the therapy:
① Orange urine
② Coffee-ground emesis
③ Ringing in the ear
④ Abdominal cramping

79. The name given to a drug that is designated and patented by the manufacturer is the:
① Official name
② Generic name
③ Chemical name
④ Brand name

80. The study of drugs is called:
① Pharmacokinetics
② Pharmacology
③ Pharmacy
④ Pharmadynamics

81. The parental route of medication administration that allows for the fastest absorption is the:

① Intradermal route
② Subcutaneous route
③ Intramuscular route
④ Intrastitial route

82. When the appearance, odor, or color of a medication changes, the nurse will:
① Disregard this and give the medication as ordered
② Have the registered nurse give the medication
③ Withhold the medication and consult with the pharmacist
④ Understand that this is a normal occurrence when dealing with chemicals

83. The nurse is teaching a 36-year-old patient about her medications and tells her that enteric-coated drugs are made to dissolve:
① In the stomach
② Under the tongue
③ In the intestine
④ Between the cheek and the gum

84. When assessing the patient's medication history, the nurse should:
① Only be interested in prescribed medication being taken
② Know the names of all medications kept in patient's home
③ Record all nonprescription and prescription drugs being taken
④ Only be interested in nonprescription drugs being taken

85. When the nurse is administering medications, the patient informs the nurse that the tablet usually received is a different color. The nurse will:
① Insist that the patient take the tablet she poured
② Have the patient take the tablet and then recheck the order
③ Leave the medication at the bedside and recheck the order
④ Recheck the order before giving the drug

86. You are administering a medication to a 49-year-old patient who has been on your unit for 1 week. The most accurate way to verify the patient's identification is to:
① Call the patient by the name on the drug card or Kardex
② Ask the patient to state her name
③ Rely on your memory
④ Check the patient's identification bracelet

87. For accurate drug administration the nurse will read the drug label:
① Two times
② Three times
③ Four times
④ Five times

88. A 65-year-old patient is receiving morphine for postoperative pain. The nurse will closely monitor the patient for:
① Accelerated rate and depth of respirations
② Depressed rate and depth of respirations
③ Increased pulse rate
④ Increased temperature

89. To instill ear drops in the adult patient, the ear canal is opened by pulling the ear:
① Up and back
② Down and back
③ Up and forward
④ Back and forward

90. A patient who had received an overdose of insulin would be exhibiting which of the following symptoms?
① Hyperpnea, drowsiness, fever
② Pallor, fatigability, dizziness
③ Nervousness, anxiety, diaphoresis
④ Flushed skin, nausea, vomiting

91. Emergency treatment of hyperinsulinism consists of administering:
① Glucose intravenously
② Insulin hypodermically
③ Epinephrine (Adrenalin) intramuscularly
④ High caloric liquids by gavage feedings

92. A drug used as a substitute for morphine or heroin in the management of addiction is:
① Meperidine
② Narem
③ Methadone
④ Talwin

93. The most serious reaction to anticoagulant therapy is:
① Rapid fall in blood pressure
② Formation of thrombi in major blood vessels
③ Hemorrhage
④ Infection

94. Doses of warfarin sodium (Coumadin) are ordered on the basis of measurement of the patient's:
① Clotting time
② Prothrombin time
③ Bleeding time
④ Capillary fragility testing

95. When teaching the patient about adverse reactions of corticosteroid treatment, the nurse will tell the patient that a common adverse reaction is:
① Bradycardia, mental dullness
② Anorexia, polyuria
③ Tachycardia, insomnia
④ "Moon face," obese trunk

96. The nurse will know that the patient understands teaching done about self-administration of oral corticosteroids when the patient states she will take the medication:
① Before meals
② With or after meals
③ At bedtime
④ With orange juice

97. A patient who is in the 40th week of pregnancy is receiving an IV administration of oxytoxin (Pitocin). The nurse knows the drug is expected to:
① Produce rhythmic contractions of uterine muscle fibers
② Relax smooth muscle fibers of the cervix
③ Initiate vigorous sustained contractions of the abdominal muscles
④ Produce relaxation of vaginal walls and perineal muscles

98. The daughter of a diabetic patient is learning to administer insulin to her mother at home. The nurse will teach the daughter to:
① Give the insulin intramuscularly
② Use a 1½ inch needle
③ Rotate injection sites
④ Massage insulin into tissues

99. An intermediate-acting insulin is being used to attempt to regulate a diabetic patient on insulin. The nurse knows that an example of an intermediate-acting insulin is:

① Insulin injection (Regular Insulin)
② Prompt insulin zinc suspension (Semilente)
③ Insulin zinc suspension (Lente Insulin)
④ Extended insulin zinc suspension (Ultralente Insulin)

100. When teaching self-administration of eye drops to a patient, the nurse will stress that the correct method for instilling eye drops is to drop the medication on the:
① Eyeball itself
② Inner canthus of the eye
③ Lower conjunctival sac
④ Outermost point of the eye

101. The patient who understands proper self-administration of cimetidine (Tagamet) will take the medication:
① With a liquid antacid preparation
② After meals and at bedtime
③ With meals and at bedtime
④ Only when the patient has gastric distress

102. An example of a long-acting insulin is:
① Prompt insulin zinc suspension (Semilente)
② Isophane insulin suspension (NPH)
③ Insulin zinc suspension (Lente)
④ Extended insulin zinc suspension (Ultralente)

103. When injecting the patient on blood and body fluid precautions, the Centers for Disease Control and Prevention (CDC) recommends that the nurse:
① Wear two pair of gloves
② Wear a mask
③ Wear a gown
④ Wash the injection site with povidine-iodine (Betadine)

104. The physician has ordered meperidine hydrochloride as a postsurgical medication. The nurse knows the brand name is:
① Dilaudid
② Demerol
③ Dilantin
④ Diamox

105. An important nursing consideration in the administration of diuretics is to:
① Limit the patient's intake of fluids
② Withhold the diuretic if the pulse rate is below 60 beats/min
③ Give in the early morning if ordered daily
④ Delay administration if BP is below 110/80

106. Foods to avoid when patients are receiving an MAO-inhibitor drug include:
① Aged cheese, coffee, chocolate
② Poultry, bananas, eggs
③ Green leafy vegetables, raisins, milk
④ Pork, pickles, whole-wheat bread

107. The major action of amitroptyline hydrochloride (Elavil) is to decrease:
① Euphoria
② Depression
③ Confusion
④ Hallucinations

108. Which of the following is effective in the treatment of status epilepticus?
① Diazepam
② Hydroxyzine
③ Meprobamate
④ Chlordiazepoxide

109. A 72-year-old patient is exhibiting signs of digoxin toxicity. The nurse will:
① Give the drug if the apical rate is above 60 beats/min and report to the physician
② Omit the drug, take the apical rate, and report to the physician
③ Administer an antacid with the digoxin
④ Administer oxygen by nasal cannula with the digoxin

110. To assess the therapeutic effectiveness of a parkinsonian drug, the nurse will observe the patient's:
① Increased sleep patterns
② Increased ability to ambulate and speak
③ Decreased emotional stability
④ Decreased caloric and nutritional intake

111. A sedative hypnotic has been ordered for a 53-year-old patient. The nurse knows a major adverse reaction to watch for is:
① Hypertension
② Hypotension
③ Respiratory depression
④ Hypothermia

112. The nurse is charting objective evidence of the therapeutic effect of an antianxiety drug which is:
① Crying, facial grimaces, rigid posture
② Anger, aggressive behavior
③ Decreased blood pressure, pulse, respiration
④ Verbal statements of worry, feeling ill, resting poorly

113. The nurse has administered a sedative to an 82-year-old patient. An important nursing action that she will now implement is:
① Apply a Posey jacket restraint
② Leave the overhead light in the room on
③ Raise the side rails on the bed and tell the patient not to get out of bed unassisted
④ Check the patient every half hour to determine the effectiveness of the medication

114. When administering pentobarbitol (Nembutal) to a patient, the nurse knows it will act to:
① Allay apprehension and induce sleep
② Relieve moderate to severe pain
③ Depress the cough center in the brain
④ Increase blood pressure and decrease respirations

115. The medication that is the drug of choice to treat a 26-year-old patient with AIDS is:
① Acetylsalicylic acid (ASA)
② Azidothymidine (AZT)
③ Pralidoxime chloride (PAM)
④ Tripelennamine (PBZ)

116. A 66-year-old patient with pain associated with angina pectoris is given sublingual nitroglycerin. The nurse knows this medication will:
① Dilate blood vessels and increase circulation
② Inhibit the pain sensors in the brainstem
③ Increase respirations and cause drowsiness
④ Dull nerve endings in the myocardium

117. The process that occurs from the time a drug is taken into the body to the time it enters the circulatory or lymphatic system is called:
① Absorption
② Distribution
③ Metabolism
④ Excretion

118. The doctor has ordered secobarbitol (Seconal) 100 mg hs for a 27-year-old patient. The apothecary equivalent for this dose is:
① gr v
② gr iss
③ gr iii
④ gr 1/150

119. If 7.5L of a medication is ordered by the physician, the nurse will safely administer:
① 75 ml
② 0.075 ml
③ 750 ml
④ 7500 ml

120. A 3-year-old patient has been receiving high dosages of metaclopramide (Reglan) for side effects associated with chemotherapy. You are reinforcing home care instructions related to adverse medication effects. Which of the following symptoms should be reported to the health care provider immediately?
① Mild sedation and fatigue
② Rigidity and tremors
③ Constipation and dry mouth
④ Headache and insomnia

121. If the nurse is unable to read the doctor's order or if the order seems erroneous, the nurse will:
① Administer what seems to be the correct order
② Ignore the order because it is not clear
③ Question the order before the drug is given
④ Verify the order with another nurse

122. The physician's order reads to administer 3 liters of 5%D/0.45% normal saline IV over 24 hours. The drip factor is 60 gtt/ml. The nurse will regulate the IV at:
① 25 gtt/min
② 100 gtt/min
③ 125 gtt/min
④ 150 gtt/min

123. The position of choice for instilling nose drops in an adult patient is:
① Lying on the right side
② Lying down or sitting with the neck hyperextended
③ Lying down or sitting with the neck flexed
④ Lying on the left side

124. The patient is to receive an IV of 5%D/0.33 normal saline at 1000 ml/8 hr. The drip factor is 10 gtt/ml. The nurse will run the IV at:
① 7 gtt/min
② 14 gtt/min
③ 20 gtt/min
④ 28 gtt/min

125. Early signs of digoxin toxicity are:
① A sustained pulse rate above 60 beats/min.
② Nausea and vomiting
③ Diarrhea and rectal bleeding
④ Elevated respiration and blood pressure

126. Toxic effects of digitalis occur more rapidly when body stores of which of the following ion are depleted?
① Sodium
② Potassium
③ Calcium
④ Chloride

127. Digitalis preparations must not be given without the specific direction of the physician whenever the:
    ① Systolic blood pressure is above 100
    ② Rectal temperature is subnormal
    ③ Pulse rate is below 60 beats/min
    ④ Patient is flushed and perspiring

128. The patient is to receive 50 mg of meperidine hydrochloride (Demerol) for pain. The charge nurse states that she drew up the medication for you and hands you the syringe. Which of the following actions is the most appropriate?
    ① Place the syringe in the medication drawer for the patient
    ② Recheck the physician's order before administering
    ③ Check the patient's chart for allergies to medication
    ④ Refuse to give the medication

129. Drugs absorbed into the bloodstream and circulated to various parts of the body are said to have a:
    ① Systemic effect
    ② Local effect
    ③ Palliative effect
    ④ Curative effect

ANSWERS AND RATIONALES

1. Knowledge, implementation, environment (a)
   ❷ Correct equivalent.
   ①,③,④ Incorrect equivalent.

2. Comprehension, evaluation, physiologic (c)
   ❸ Confusion may be a sign of fluid and electrolyte imbalance.
   ① Not unusual with diuretic therapy.
   ② May be a sign of congestive heart failure (CHF).
   ④ Not unusual with diuretic therapy.

3. Knowledge, evaluation, physiologic (b)
   ❸ Dilates coronary arteries in acute angina.
   ① Used in long-term management.
   ② Used for chronic angina.
   ④ Used for severe physical pain.

4. Comprehension, assessment, physiologic (b)
   ❸ Could indicate free bleeding into the urinary system.
   ① Does not affect respiratory system.
   ② Amount of urine not significant.
   ④ Frequency of urination not affected.

5. Comprehension, assessment, environment (a)
   ❹ Tinnitus is the most common side effect of salicylate poisoning.
   ① Symptom of increased intracranial pressure.
   ② Side effect of iron ingestion.
   ③ Symptom of gastric distress.

6. Knowledge, implementation, environment (a)
   ❶ Correct equivalent.
   ②,③,④ Incorrect equivalent.

7. Knowledge, evaluation, environment (a)
   ❸ Definition.
   ①,② Undesired effect of drug.
   ④ Unusual or unexpected effect.

8. Knowledge, implementation, environment (b)
   ❸ Correct calculation.
   ①,②,④ Incorrect calculation.

9. Knowledge, assessment, environment (a)
   ❶ Correct definition.
   ② Unusual or unexpected effect.
   ③ Two drugs taken together produce a greater effect than each taken alone.
   ④ Decreased results.

10. Knowledge, assessment, environment (a)
    ❸ Correct definition.
    ① Inactivation of the drug in the body.
    ② Elimination of the drug from the body.
    ④ Adverse reaction of the drug.

11. Application, implementation, physiologic (b)
    ❸ The action of the drug takes 2 to 3 weeks while blood levels are building.
    ① It should be taken in the morning so that the effects of the drug are the strongest during waking hours.
    ② The action of the drug does not occur in 24 hours; takes 2 to 3 weeks while blood levels are building.
    ④ Not necessary.

12. Application, implementation, environment (c)
    ❷ KCL is diluted to decrease GI upset.
    ① Should be given with or after meals.
    ③ Never crush controlled release tablets.
    ④ Fully dissolve effervescent tablets before administering.

13. Application, implementation, physiologic (c)
    ❸ Cipro can increase Theophylline levels.
    ① Fluids should be forced.
    ② Cipro should be started while results are pending.
    ④ The two medications can be given together.

14. Application, implementation, environment (b)
    ❶ These precautions must be taken because Toradol causes drowsiness.
    ① Toradol affects blood coagulation, not blood sugar.
    ③ Dypsnea and asthma are not common side effects.
    ④ Injection is painful but does not require anesthesia.

15. Knowledge, planning, environment (a)
    ❹ Correct size needle to reach subcutaneous tissue.
    ①,②,③ Too long; could pass through subcutaneous tissue to underlying muscle, bone.

16. Application, implementation, physiologic (b)
    ❹ Orthostatic hypotension is a side effect of diuretic use.
    ① Is taken in the morning so as not to disturb sleep.
    ② May require potassium supplement.
    ③ Monitor weight each week.

17. Comprehension, evaluation, physiologic (b)
    ❶ Insomnia is a common side effect. Doses are usually administered at breakfast and lunch.
    ② The patient may be hyperactive but this is not the best answer.
    ③ Caffeine is a CNS stimulant and should be limited, but this is not the best answer.
    ④ Ritalin can be addicting so dose should not be increased; it would increase his insomnia.

18. Application, implementation, physiologic (c)
    ❶ It may cause drowsiness. Machinery should not be operated until the patient's response is known.
    ② Effectiveness of the drug is not affected by food.
    ③ It is used to treat nausea.
    ④ If a dose is missed, it should be taken as soon as that is realized, unless it is time for the next dose.

19. Comprehension, assessment, physiologic (b)
    ❸ Desired action of drug for which it is administered.
    ① Hypertension is a possible side effect for which the patient must be monitored.
    ② Hypotension is a possible side effect for which the patient must be monitored.
    ④ Arrhythmias are a possible side effect for which the patient must be monitored.

20. Comprehension, planning, physiologic (a)
    ❹ The tablet is prepared to dissolve between the cheek and the gum.
    ① A buccal tablet should not be chewed.
    ② A buccal tablet is not dissolved in the stomach.
    ③ Sublingual tablets are taken this way.

21. Knowledge, implementation, environment (a)
    ❷ Correct equivalent.
    ①,③,④ Incorrect equivalent.

22. Application, implementation, physiologic (b)
    ❷ Check the apical pulse one full minute and hold medication if it is less than 60.
    ① Should be weighed every week.
    ③ Pulse is more significant.
    ④ Digitalis level, not clotting time, is monitored.

23. Comprehension, evaluation, physiologic (c)
    ❶ Theophylline is a bronchodilator that will relax the smooth muscle of the bronchi; air flow will be enhanced. Subjective complaints of "tightness" will be relieved.
    ② Theophylline provides symptomatic relief only; it does not cure.
    ③ Theophylline is not a muccolytic; it does not thin mucus.
    ④ Theophylline does not dry up secretions; it works on smooth muscle.

24. Application, implementation, environment (a)
    ❷ Immediate documentation of refusal and reason for refusal must be done to avoid medication errors.
    ① Medication is never left at the bedside except when specifically ordered.
    ③ Inappropriately used as a threat to gain compliance.
    ④ Medication is never left at the bedside except when specifically ordered.

25. Application, implementation, physiologic (b)
    ❸ Tolerance is when increasingly larger doses are needed to provide the same effect.
    ① Addiction is rare when a narcotic is administered to a patient during a short hospital stay.
    ② Dependence occurs when a drug is stopped and physical symptoms occur.
    ④ The patient is not demonstrating allergic symptoms.

26. Evaluation, implementation, physiologic (c)
    ❶ The symptoms are typical of digitalis toxicity. The patient could be dehydrating, so administration of Lasix could complicate the problem.
    ② The patient could be dehydrating, so administration of Lasix could complicate the problem. The Micro-K is given to replace potassium loss and should be administered.
    ③ The symptoms are typical of digitalis toxicity. The patient could be dehydrating, so administration of Lasix could complicate the symptoms. The Micro-K is given to replace potassium loss and should be administered.
    ④ This answer is partially correct, but Lasix needs to be held along with the Digoxin because administration of either will increase symptoms.

27. Comprehension, evaluation, physiologic (c)
    ❷ The nabumetone (Relafen) may not be the cause. If the symptoms get worse, another cause must be looked for.
    ① Nabumetone (Relafen) can irritate the gastric mucosa but this is not the priority; ulcers are more frequently caused by bacteria.
    ③ Nabumetone (Relafen) and all NSAIDS should be administered with food. The nurse may have given the nabumetone (Relafen) with food and the patient may still have developed the symptoms.
    ④ Testing for blood could be done but is a medical action; observation of continuance of symptoms is a more important priority.

28. Knowledge, assessment, physiology (a)
    ❸ Definition of metabolism.
    ① Time drug enters the body and time it enters the bloodstream.
    ② Transport of drugs in the body.
    ④ Elimination of drugs from the body.

29. Comprehensive, evaluation, physiologic (b)
    ❸ Subjective evidence is stated by the patient to the nurse.
    ①,②,④ This is objective evidence.

30. Comprehension, assessment, physiologic (a)
    ❸ Releases a small amount at a time over a long period.
    ① Coated to dissolve in the intestine.
    ② Outer portion dissolves in stomach; inner pill dissolves in intestine.
    ④ Circular or oblong disks.

31. Application, assessment, physiologic (b)
    ❹ To prevent administration of a drug to which the patient is allergic.
    ① Not necessary to know.
    ② Good to know to allay patient's fears, but not most important.
    ③ Good to know as part of complete patient history, but not most important.

32. Knowledge, implementation, environment (a)
    ❸ Correct calculation.
    ①,②,④ Incorrect calculation.

33. Comprehension, implementation, physiologic (a)
    ❸ Drug is irritating to the GI tract; taking the drug with meals decreases irritation.
    ① Taking the drug at bedtime could irritate the GI tract.
    ② Taking the drug before breakfast could irritate the GI tract.
    ④ Taking the drug between meals could irritate the GI tract.

34. Comprehension, planning, environment (b)
    ❶ Correct calculation.
    ②,③,④ Incorrect calculation.

35. Knowledge, implementation, physiologic (a)
    ❷ Correct procedure.
    ① One minute is not enough time to give the drug to work.
    ③ Ten minutes is too long to wait to repeat the dose.
    ④ Thirty minutes is too long to wait to repeat the dose.

36. Comprehension, evaluation, physiologic (c)
    ❷ Correct action.
    ① Action of histamine.
    ③ Action of beta-antagonist.
    ④ Action of decongestant.

37. Comprehension, implementation, physiologic (b)
    ❸ Adverse reaction.
    ① Adverse reaction of antifibrinolytics.
    ③ Adverse reaction of antineoplastics.
    ④ Expected action of diuretics.

38. Application, evaluation, physiologic (b)
    ❹ Demerol is a CNS depressant, thereby decreasing respiration.
    ① Should always be monitored, but not an expected reaction to Demerol.
    ② Is a CNS depressant; would decrease respirations.
    ③ Is a CNS depressant; would decrease heart rate.

39. Application, assessment, physiologic (a)
    ❶ Action of drug.
    ② Constricts blood vessels.
    ③ Does not act on mucous membranes.
    ④ Has no effect on blood pressure.

40. Comprehension, evaluation, environment (b)
    ❷ Can increase heart rate.

① Serious symptom, not related to adverse reaction of atropine.
③ Caused by lack of bulk in diet.
④ Expected reaction of atropine; would have no effect on heart disease.

41. Knowledge, planning, physiologic (b)
❷ Optimal absorption.
①,③ Patient is vomiting; would not retain medication.
④ Poor absorption.

42. Knowledge, assessment, environment (b)
❶ Common side effects.
② Unrelated reactions, not adverse reactions to aspirin.
③ Hypotension occurs with-anaphylactic shock, tachycardia.
④ Dermatitis is a skin disorder, unrelated to bradycardia, hypotension.

43. Knowledge, implementation, environment (b)
❶ Correct procedure.
② Water would dilute medication.
③ Should be swallowed for expected effectiveness of medication.
④ Medication is to treat mouth infection, not throat.

44. Knowledge, assessment, physiologic (a)
❸ Lower pain perception.
① Produce relaxation and decrease anxiety.
② Produce sleep.
④ Reduce fever.

45. Knowledge, assessment, physiologic (c)
❶ Common side effect.
② Common side effect of abdominal surgery.
③ Expected effect of a diuretic.
④ Expected effect of dehydration.

46. Knowledge, assessment, environment (b)
❹ Can increase intraocular pressure.
① Has no adverse effect on hypertension.
② Has no adverse effect on diabetes.
③ Not applicable to cardiac failure.

47. Comprehension, implementation, environment (a)
❸ Could cause patient injury.
① Not action of atropine.
② Dilation of pupils does not cause vertigo.
④ Decreases diaphoresis.

48. Application, assessment, health (b)
❸ Identifying the location and intensity of the pain ensures that the problem is not a complication; provides information maintaining quality of care.
① Not appropriate action.
②,④ Not until intensity and site have been assessed.

49. Application, implementation, physiologic (b)
❷ Increases gastrointestinal muscle tone and motility.
①,③ Does not facilitate action of drug.
④ Patient remains in bed with rectal tube.

50. Knowledge, assessment, physiologic (a)
❶ Dilates pupils and increases intraocular pressure.
② Can receive morphine safely.
③ Can receive Demerol safely.
④ Can receive Vistaril safely.

51. Knowledge, assessment, health (c)
❶ Action of drug.
② Loop diuretics deplete potassium.
③ Used for open-angle glaucoma.
④ Used for acute renal failure.

52. Knowledge, assessment, health (b)
❸ Increase risk of breast cancer.
① Allergies are not affected by Premarin.
② Ulcers are not affected by Premarin.
④ Obesity is not affected by Premarin.

53. Application, evaluation, physiologic (c)
❶ Adverse reaction of uterine relaxants.
② Adverse reaction of skeletal muscle relaxants.
③ Adverse reactions of antihistamines.
④ Adverse reactions of adrenergic stimulants.

54. Application, implementation, environment (a)
❷ Prevent cross-contamination.
① Does not prevent cross-contamination.
③,④ Important, but does not prevent cross-contamination.

55. Comprehension, evaluation, physiologic (a)
❶ Ringing in the ear or tinnitus occurs with aspirin toxicity.
② Earache is a sign of ear infection.
③,④ Side effects of headache do not include ringing in the ear.

56. Comprehension, planning, physiologic (b)
❹ Medication administered directly into the bloodstream.
① Absorption from the stomach is an additional step before entering the bloodstream.
② Absorption from muscle is an additional step before entering the bloodstream.
③ Absorption from the subcutaneous tissue is an additional step before entering the bloodstream.

57. Knowledge, assessment, physiologic (a)
❷ Not generally known to be a side effect.
① Unexpected, not usual side effect.
③ Not a medical term.
④ Diminishes action of medication.

58. Comprehension, evaluation, physiologic (b)
❸ Diminishes seizure activity.
① Is an action Diazepam produces, but not the reason it is given for status epilepticus.
② Is not an action of Diazepam.
④ Is not an action of Diazepam.

59. Application, implementation, physiologic (b)
❷ The medication will be withheld if the patient's apical pulse is below 60.
① Assessment of blood pressure is important, but would have no bearing on the administration of the medication.
③ Assessment of temperature is important, but would have no bearing on the administration of the medication.
④ Assessment of hydration status is important, but would have no bearing on the administration of the medication.

60. Comprehension, implementation, physiologic (b)
❶ The medication is not safe for direct intravenous administration.
② This action will nor relieve any discomfort patient may have.
③ This action will not facilitate absorption.
④ There are no organs at intramuscular sites.

61. Comprehension, implementation, physiologic (b)
❸ Major diuresis will occur during waking hours.
① Frequent urination caused by the diuretic would disturb the patient's sleep.
② Salt intake, not fluid intake, should be cut down.
④ Should be stopped only by physician's order.

62. Comprehension, assessment, physiologic (b)
    ❸ Blood levels build when the drug is not being excreted.
    ① The dose may have to be adjusted because of the elevated blood level.
    ② The drug is being absorbed but not excreted.
    ④ The route of administration has no bearing on an elevated blood level.

63. Comprehension, implementation, psychosocial (a)
    ❶ Are often the least expensive.
    ② Are often the most expensive.
    ③,④ Prescriptions are not written in this form.

64. Application, implementation, physiologic (b)
    ❷ Essential to know the tube is in the stomach and not in the lungs.
    ① Does not indicate correct placement in the stomach.
    ③ Not applicable.
    ④ Pill made to dissolve in intestine.

65. Knowledge, implementation, physiologic (a)
    ❸ To prevent possible obstruction as a result of thickening and expansion of the drug.
    ① Will not prevent unwanted side effects.
    ② Fluid, not food, is necessary to prevent undesired effects.
    ④ Gastric distress is not a side effect.

66. Knowledge, evaluation, physiologic (a)
    ❶ Therapeutic effect.
    ② Not applicable to the effect of the drug.
    ③ There is no active drug in a placebo.
    ④ Metabolism of the placebo is not necessary to produce the desired effect.

67. Knowledge, assessment, physiologic (a)
    ❶ Sedation is part of therapy.
    ② Does not control seizures.
    ③ Does not cause vasoconstriction.
    ④ Does not cause vasodilation.

68. Application, implementation, environment (b)
    ❶ Allows peak drug activity during daytime hours.
    ②,③,④ Not applicable to effect of drug.

69. Application, evaluation, environment (a)
    ❸ Mydriatic action.
    ① Antiinfective action.
    ② Miotic action.
    ④ Osmotic action.

70. Comprehensive, assessment, physiologic (c)
    ❹ Elderly metabolize drugs more slowly because of declining body function, thus prolonging the half-life of the drug resulting in drug accumulation.
    ① Age does not make a difference in tolerance
    ② Elderly metabolize drugs more slowly.
    ③ Age does not cause more frequent adverse effects

71. Comprehension, assessment, environment (a)
    ❷ Cancer drugs can affect the integrity of the oral mucosa.
    ① Antibiotics do not affect the oral mucosa.
    ③ Antiparkinsonian drugs do not affect the oral mucosa.
    ④ Vitamins do not affect the oral mucosa.

72. Comprehension, evaluation, environment (b)
    ❷ Compliance to the drug regimen is essential because of the survival of the causative microorganism.
    ① Not applicable.
    ③ Not necessary.
    ④ Should not be done.

73. Knowledge, evaluation, physiological
    ❶ Major adverse reaction.
    ② Sign of kidney disease.
    ③ Not a major adverse reaction; can be caused by depression.
    ④ Caused by pupil dilation by medication.

74. Knowledge, implementation, health (a)
    ❷ To prevent further infection or superinfection.
    ① Should take until completed, to prevent further infection or superinfection.
    ③ Should take until completed, to prevent further infection or superinfection, and taken only by the person the medication is prescribed for.
    ④ Only if the infection continues.

75. Knowledge, environment (a)
    ❹ Definition of the law.
    ① Replaced by Controlled Substance Act.
    ② No such act.
    ③ Regulates distribution of narcotics and other drugs of abuse.

76. Application, implementation, environment (a)
    ❷ Is a regulation of the Controlled Substance Act.
    ① Not necessary, unless order is unclear.
    ③ Not appropriate; orders are signed by one physician.
    ④ Not necessary.

77. Application, implementation, physiologic (c)
    ❶ The patient will have an adequate intake on the 7 to 3 and 3 to 11 shifts, so will not be adversely affected. On the 11 to 7 shift the intake is more restricted because the patient will be asleep and not miss the fluid intake. The 200 ml will be enough to take medications if ordered.
    ② Patient will not need as much fluid intake on the 11 to 7 shift because he will be sleeping.
    ③ Patient may drink all 1,000 ml on the 7 to 3 shift and would have to do without it for the rest of the day.
    ④ The trays for patients with restricted fluid have very little liquids on them. Patient will feel deprived if no other fluids are allowed. Also, fluids must be allowed for medication intake.

78. Application, implementation, physiologic (b)
    ❷ The most common complication of heparin is bleeding.
    ① Orange urine results from therapy with pyridium, a drug used to treat the pain associated with urinary tract infections.
    ③ Tinnitus is a side effect associated with salicylate poisoning.
    ④ These are vague general complaints not specific to heparin therapy.

79. Knowledge, assessment, environment (a)
    ❹ Correct definition.
    ① Name as listed in official publications.
    ② Name given by developer of the drug.
    ③ Chemical composition of the drug.

80. Knowledge, assessment, environment (a)
    ❷ Study of drugs.
    ① Study of the processes a drug undergoes in the body.
    ③ Place where drugs are stored and dispensed.
    ④ Study of movement of drugs in the body.

81. Knowledge, planning, physiologic (a)
    ❸ Muscle tissue has a greater blood supply.
    ① Slow absorption from beneath the surface of the skin, not vascular.
    ② Slow absorption from tissue, not vascular.
    ④ Slow absorption; route seldom used.

82. Knowledge, implementation, environment (a)
    ❸ It may cause harmful effects or potency may be decreased.
    ①,②,④ These actions do not demonstrate nursing responsibility and proper knowledge of the process regarding administration of medications.

83. Knowledge, implementation, physiologic (a)
    ❸ Special coating prevents the drug from dissolving in the stomach before reaching the intestine.
    ① Will not dissolve in stomach because of special coating.
    ② Sublingual form.
    ④ Buccal form.

84. Knowledge, assessment, environment (a)
    ❸ All medications currently being taken by the patient, prescription and nonprescription, are important when getting a medication history.
    ① A complete medication history would include nonprescription drugs.
    ② Not necessary; need to know only those the patient takes.
    ④ A complete medication history would include prescription drugs.

85. Application, implementation, environment (a)
    ❹ To promote safety and prevent errors.
    ①,② Unsafe before rechecking the order.
    ③ Medication is never left at the bedside unless specifically ordered.

86. Application, implementation, environment (a)
    ❹ Most reliable, accurate method.
    ① Sleepy or drugged patient may answer to any name.
    ② Can be done, but this is not the most accurate method.
    ③ Memory is unreliable.

87. Knowledge, implementation, environment (a)
    ❷ When removing the container, while measuring the drug, and before returning or discarding the container.
    ① Not enough times for accuracy.
    ③ No need for checking more than 3 times.
    ④ Can be done, but 3 times is sufficient.

88. Application, implementation, physiologic (b)
    ❷ Adverse reaction of morphine.
    ① Morphine has an opposite effect on rate and depth of respiration.
    ③ Morphine has no effect on pulse rate.
    ④ Morphine has no effect on temperature.

89. Application, implementation, physiologic (a)
    ❶ Straightens the canal and promotes maximum contact of medication with tissue.
    ② Is proper procedure for children.
    ③ Would block entrance to ear canal.
    ④ Procedure would not allow access to ear canal.

90. Application, assessment, physiologic (a)
    ❸ Early signs of hyperglycemia.
    ① Signs of infection.
    ② Signs of anemia.
    ④ Signs of gastrointestinal distress.

91. Knowledge, assessment, physiologic (a)
    ❶ Glucose reverses the effects of too much insulin.
    ② Given for hyperglycemia.
    ③ Facilitates increase in blood glucose, but is not an appropriate treatment.
    ④ Is not an emergency treatment.

92. Knowledge, assessment, physiologic (a)
    ❸ Used in addiction management.
    ① Is a narcotic-analgesic used to control pain.
    ② Is a narcotic-antagonist used to reverse CNS and respiratory depression.
    ④ Is a narcotic agonist-antagonist used to control pain.

93. Comprehension, evaluation, environment (a)
    ❸ Major adverse reaction.
    ① Serious symptom of shock.
    ② Given to prevent formation of thrombi.
    ④ Not caused by anticoagulant therapy.

94. Knowledge, assessment, physiologic (a)
    ❷ Dosage individualized according to blood coagulation.
    ① Laboratory test for platelet activity.
    ③ Laboratory test for time of actual bleeding.
    ④ Laboratory test for strength of capillary walls.

95. Knowledge, implementation, physiologic (b)
    ❹ Caused by abnormal fat deposits.
    ① Medication has no effect on heart or mental sharpness.
    ② Medication has no effect on appetite, voiding.
    ③ Medication has no effect on heartbeat, sleep patterns.

96. Knowledge, evaluation, environment (a)
    ❷ Considered to be ulcerogenic.
    ① Can irritate stomach, must be taken with meals.
    ③ Can irritate stomach when not taken with meals.
    ④ With antacid, not orange juice, to prevent stomach irritation.

97. Comprehension, assessment, physiologic (a)
    ❶ Stimulates uterine contractions.
    ② Acts on uterine muscle fibers.
    ③ Unwanted action.
    ④ Contracts uterine muscle fibers.

98. Application, implementation, physiologic (b)
    ❸ Rotating sites enhances absorption of the drug and prevents hardening of the tissue at the site of injection.
    ① Insulin is given subcutaneously.
    ② Needle too long for subcutaneous injection.
    ④ Not done with insulin injection.

99. Knowledge, assessment, physiologic (b)
    ❸ Peaks in 10 to 16 hours.
    ① Fast-acting insulin.
    ② Not applicable.
    ④ Long-acting insulin.

100. Knowledge, implementation, environment (a)
    ❸ Proper procedure.
    ①,②,④ Part of dose will be wasted.

101. Knowledge, planning, physiologic (a)
    ❸ Inhibits daytime and nocturnal gastric acid secretion as well as gastric acid stimulated by food.
    ① Tagamet *is* an antacid.
    ② After meals gastric acid has already been produced.
    ④ Given to prevent gastric distress.

102. Knowledge, planning, physiologic (a)
    ❹ Peaks in 14 to 24 hours.
    ① Rapid-acting insulin.
    ②,③ Intermediate-acting insulin.

103. Application, implementation, health (a)
    ❶ Correct procedure.
    ② A mask is not a barrier for blood and body fluid.
    ③ A gown is not a barrier for blood and body fluids.
    ④ Injection sites are cleansed with alcohol to protect the patient from infection.

104. Knowledge, assessment, environment (a)
    ❷ One brand name.
    ① Brand name of hydromorphone.
    ③ Brand name of phenytoin.
    ④ Brand name of acetazolamide.

105. Application, implementation, environment (a)
    ❸ To allow for diuresis during patient's normal waking hours.
    ① Normal fluid intake is appropriate.
    ② Diuretics do not affect pulse rate.
    ④ Desired action of medication; administration should not be delayed.

106. Comprehension, planning, environment (b)
    ❶ Can produce drug-diet interactions.
    ②,③,④ Are not restricted.

107. Knowledge, assessment, physiologic (a)
    ❷ Antidepressant.
    ① Not an action of Elavil.
    ③,④ Undesired symptom; not an action of Elavil.

108. Knowledge, assessment, physiologic (a)
    ❶ Given intravenously to control seizures.
    ② Is an antianxiety agent.
    ③ Is a sedative/hypnotic agent.
    ④ Is used to treat alcohol withdrawal.

109. Application, implementation, physiologic (b)
    ❷ Correct actions.
    ①,③ Drug should be withheld.
    ④ Withhold drug. Oxygen would not be administered without a physician's order.

110. Application, evaluation, physiologic (a)
    ❷ Therapeutic effect.
    ① Sleep patterns are not affected by antiparkinsonian drugs.
    ③ Emotional stability is not affected by antiparkinsonian drugs.
    ④ Diet and nutrition are not affected by antiparkinsonian drugs.

111. Comprehension, assessment, physiologic (b)
    ❸ Depresses the medulla oblongata.
    ①,② Sedative hypnotics do not affect blood pressure.
    ④ Sedative hypnotics do not affect body temperature.

112. Application, evaluation, physiologic (c)
    ❸ Decreases physiologic manifestations.
    ①,④ Signs of anxiety.
    ② Paradoxical reaction.

113. Application, implementation, environment (a)
    ❸ Safety precautions.
    ① Must have physician's order.
    ② Not conducive to sedation.
    ④ Patient must be checked to determine effectiveness of medication but not at this frequency.

114. Knowledge, assessment, physiologic (a)
    ❶ Action of the drug.
    ② Analgesic action.
    ③ Antitussive action.
    ④ Adverse reaction.

115. Knowledge, planning, physiology (a)
    ❷ Most promising.
    ① Antipyretic, analgesic.
    ③ Miotic.
    ④ Antihistamine.

116. Application, evaluation, physiology (b)
    ❶ Action of drug.
    ② Has no effect on brainstem.
    ③ Does not affect respiration or alertness.
    ④ Acts on the myocardial blood vessels, not nerve endings.

117. Knowledge, assessment, physiology (a)
    ❶ Definition.
    ② Transport of drugs in the body.
    ③ Inactivation of drugs in the body.
    ④ Elimination of drugs from the body.

118. Knowledge, implementation, environment (a)
    ❷ Correct equivalent.
    ①,③,④ Incorrect equivalent.

119. Knowledge, implementation, environment (a)
    ❹ Correct equivalent.
    ①,②,③ Incorrect equivalent.

120. Application, evaluation, environment (c)
    ❷ Children on high doses of Reglan are particularly prone to the extrapyramidal effects of the drug. Presence of these symptoms should be reported immediately so that the dose can be adjusted or a new drug prescribed.
    ①,③,④ Common side effects. Need not be reported.

121. Application, implementation, environment (a)
    ❸ Proper procedure to clarify order.
    ① Unsafe; nurse must be sure of order.
    ② Not appropriate; must be clarified with physician, then administered.
    ④ Unsafe; nurse must clarify with physician.

122. Knowledge, implementation, environment (b)
    ❸ Correct calculation.
    ①,②,④ Incorrect calculation.

123. Knowledge, implementation, environment (a)
    ❷ Best anatomical position.
    ① Nose drops would not be retained.
    ③ Flexion of neck prevents administration.
    ④ Nose drops would not be retained.

124. Knowledge, implementation, environment (b)
    ❸ Correct calculation.
    ①,②,④ Incorrect calculation.

125. Comprehension, evaluation, environment (a)
    ❷ Early sign.
    ① Normal range.
    ③ Possible signs of colitis.
    ④ Possible signs of stress or other problems.

126. Knowledge, assessment, physiology (b)
    ❷ Hypokalemia can increase risk of toxicity.
    ① Sodium intake is usually limited for heart patients.
    ③ Calcium is stored in bone, not depleted by digitalis.
    ④ Chloride depletion has no effect on digitalis toxicity.

127. Comprehension, implementation, environment (a)
    ❸ Could lead to adverse reactions.
    ① Blood pressure measurement is not a reason for withholding the digitalis preparation.
    ② Body temperature is not a reason for withholding the digitalis preparation.
    ④ Symptoms have no relation to digitalis therapy.

128. Application, implementation, environment (a)
   ❹ According to state nurse practice acts, the nurse who draws up the medication is responsible for giving the drug.
   ① Never leave medication with a patient without a physician's order.
   ② For safety reasons, the nurse who draws up the medication is the only nurse who may give it.
   ③ Allergies have no bearing on the situation; refuse to give the medication.

129. Knowledge, assessment, physiologic (a)
   ❶ Correct definition.
   ② Act at site of application.
   ③ Relieve symptoms.
   ④ Cure disease.

Chapter 4 Nutrition

Nutrition is the combination of processes by which the body uses food for growth, energy, and maintenance. Nutrition is also the study of food and its relation to health and disease. Increasing emphasis is being placed on the role of balanced nutrition in the preventon of many chronic illnesses. The nurse plays an especially important role in the nutritional aspects of patient care. Because of close and continual contact with the patient, the nurse is able to evaluate and monitor the patient's nutritional status and inform the dietician or appropriate dietary person about the patient's nutritional needs and acceptance of the nutritional plan of care. Good nutrition is essential to good health throughout the life cycle, and the nurse is in an excellent position to encourage sound nutritional practice for each patient and the patient's family.

Health Promotion

A. Goal: to increase the level of health of individuals, families, groups, and communities, which requires a lifestyle change that will lead to new positive health behaviors.
B. In 1990, the U.S. Department of Health and Human Services issued a national report, *Healthy People 2000*, that outlined national health promotion and disease prevention objectives for Americans to be achieved by the year 2000. Nutrition is the key to these goals.

Principles of Nutrition

A. Functions of food
   1. Provides energy
   2. Builds and repairs body tissues
   3. Regulates and controls the body's chemical processes, which are essential for providing energy and building tissues
B. Evidence of good nutrition (Table 4-1); persons receiving less than desired amounts of nutrients have a greater risk of physical illness, are limited in physical work and mental capacity, and have lower immune system function than persons receiving adequate nutrients
C. Primary causes of nutritional deficiency
   1. Dietary lack of specific essential nutrients caused by
      a. Anorexia (resulting from a variety of causes)
      b. Alcoholism (and the resulting lack of proper nutrition)
      c. Poor food habits or eating nutritionally deficient foods
   2. Inability of the body to use a specific nutrient properly as a result of
      a. Diseases of the digestive tract such as ulcerative colitis
      b. Faulty absorption in digestive tract (such as the way in which the excessive use of mineral oil impedes the absorption of fat-soluble vitamins)
      c. Metabolic disorders such as diabetes
      d. Drug interactions and/or toxicity
D. Classification of nutrients
   1. Nutrients are chemical substances that are present in food and needed by the body to function
   2. Six prime nutrients
      a. Carbohydrates
      b. Fats
      c. Proteins
      d. Vitamins
      e. Minerals
      f. Water

Table 4-1	Clinical Signs of Nutritional Status	
Features	**Good**	**Poor**
General appearance	Alert, responsive	Listless, apathetic; cachexia
Hair	Shiny, lustrous; healthy scalp	Stringy, dull, brittle, dry, depigmented
Neck glands	No enlargement	Thyroid enlarged
Skin, face, and neck	Smooth, slightly moist, good color, reddish-pink mucous membranes	Greasy, discolored, scaly
Eyes	Bright, clear; no fatigue circles	Dryness, signs of infection, increased vascularity, glassiness, thickened conjunctivae
Lips	Good color, moist	Dry, scaly, swollen, angular lesions (stomatitis)
Tongue	Good pink color; surface papillae present; no lesions	Papillary atrophy, smooth appearance; swollen, red, beefy (glossitis)
Gums	Good pink color; no swelling or bleeding; firm	Marginal redness or swelling; receding, spongy
Teeth	Straight, no crowding; well-shaped jaw; clean, no discoloration	Unfilled cavities, absent teeth, worn surfaces; mottled, malpositioned
Skin, general	Smooth, slightly moist; good color; good turgor	Rough, dry, scaly, pale, pigmented, irritated; petechiae, bruises
Abdomen	Flat	Swollen
Legs, feet	No tenderness, weakness, swelling; good color	Edema, tender calf; tingling, weakness
Skeleton	No malformations	Bowlegs, knock-knees, chest deformity at diaphragm, beaded ribs, prominent scapulae
Weight	Normal for height, age, body build	Overweight or underweight
Posture	Erect, arms and legs straight, abdomen in, chest out	Sagging shoulders, sunken chest, humped back
Muscles	Well developed, firm	Flaccid, poor tone; undeveloped, tender
Nervous control	Good attention span for age; does not cry easily; nor irritable or restless	Inattentive, irritable
Gastrointestinal function	Good appetite and digestion; normal, regular elimination	Anorexia, indigestion, constipation or diarrhea
General vitality	Endurance; energetic; sleeps well at night; vigorous	Easily fatigued; no energy; falls asleep in school; looks tired, apathetic

From Williams SR: *Basic nutrition and diet therapy*, ed 9, St Louis, 1992, Mosby.

3. Individual nutrients have many specific metabolic functions. No nutrient ever works alone. In addition, the lack of one nutrient may inhibit the absorption or utilization of another nutrient

E. Culture and nutrition
   1. Food habits are among the oldest and most deeply rooted aspects of many cultures
   2. In many cultures foods take on significance in life events
   3. If possible cultural preferences should be considered when planning any dietary modifications

Assimilation of Nutrients

DIGESTION AND ABSORPTION

A. Digestion: the process of changing foods to be absorbed and used by cells; mechanical digestion and chemical digestion occur simultaneously
   1. Mechanical digestion (chewing, swallowing, peristalsis) breaks food into small pieces, mixes it with digestive juices, and moves it along the digestive tract
   2. Chemical digestion occurs through the action of enzymes, which break large food molecules into smaller molecules
      a. Carbohydrate digestion begins in the mouth and occurs primarily in the small intestine; carbohydrates are reduced to simple sugars (monosaccharides), such as glucose, for absorption
      b. Protein digestion begins in the stomach and is completed in the small intestine; proteins are broken down into amino acids for absorption
      c. Fat digestion begins in the stomach but occurs primarily in the small intestine; fats are reduced to fatty acids and glycerol for absorption

B. Absorption: the process by which end products of digestion (fatty acids, glycerol, amino acids, and glucose) are absorbed from the small intestine into circulation (blood and lymph) to be distributed to the cells

METABOLISM

A. Use of food by the body cells for producing energy and for building complex chemical compounds
B. Consists of two processes
   1. Catabolism: the breakdown of food molecules into carbon dioxide and water, which releases energy; carbohydrates are primarily catabolized for energy
   2. Anabolism: the process by which food molecules are built up into more complex chemical compounds; proteins are primarily anabolized (used for building)

ENERGY

A. Energy is required for the metabolic processes of catabolism and anabolism; energy needs of the body are based on three factors
   1. Physical activity: the type of activity and how long it is performed
   2. Basal metabolism: the energy required for the body to sustain life while in a resting state (1 calorie per kilogram of body weight per hour)
   3. Thermic effects of food: energy required for the digestion, absorption, and metabolism of foods
B. Measurement of energy
   1. The calorie (or kilocalorie) is the unit used to measure the energy value of food
   2. Fuel values of basic nutrients

a. Carbohydrate: 4 calories per gram
b. Fat: 9 calories per gram
c. Protein: 4 calories per gram
3. Total number of calories needed per day
   a. Moderately active man: 20.5 calories per pound (0.45 kg) of ideal weight
   b. Moderately active woman: 18 calories per pound (0.45 kg) of ideal weight

DRUGS AND NUTRITION

A. Drugs affect taste, appetite, intestinal motility, absorption, metabolism, and excretion of nutrients, as well as causing nausea and vomiting. Many of these interactions may compromise nutritional status and health.
B. If a nutrient binds with a medication, decreased solubility of both the nutrient and drug can result
C. People at greatest risk of undesirable drug-nutrient interaction are those taking medication for long periods, those taking two or more medications, and those not eating well. Elderly people fall into the high-risk category

Nutrients

CARBOHYDRATES

A. Classification
   1. Monosaccharides: single sugars, which require no digestion and are easily absorbed into the bloodstream (e.g., glucose, fructose, and galactose)
   2. Disaccharides: double sugars, which must be broken down before absorption (e.g., sucrose [table sugar], lactose, and maltose)
   3. Polysaccharides: complex carbohydrates composed of many sugar units (e.g., starches, glycogen, and dietary fiber)

B. Functions
   1. Provide energy (glucose is the only form of energy that can be utilized by the CNS)
   2. Protein-sparing effect allows protein to be used for tissue building rather than energy
   3. Essential for complete metabolism of fats (incomplete fat metabolism leads to buildup of ketones and acidosis)

C. Sources
   1. Polysaccharides (complex carbohydrates): bread, cereal, pasta, rice, corn, baked goods
   2. Disaccharides (double sugars): table sugar, sugar cane, molasses
   3. Monosaccharides (simple carbohydrates): fruit, honey, milk

D. Digestion and metabolism
   1. Carbohydrate digestion primarily occurs in the small intestine. It is acted upon by 3 enzymes: sucrase, lactase, and maltase.
   2. Carbohydrates must be broken down into monosaccharides before being absorbed
   3. Monosaccharides are carried to the liver, where glucose is released to the cells
   4. Excess glucose is stored as glycogen to be used when needed or converted to fat and stored as fat tissue
   5. Insulin regulates the use of glucose for use by the cells, thereby lowering blood sugar
   6. The hormone glucagon regulates the conversion of glycogen back to glucose, causing an increase in blood glucose

E. Excess carbohydrates in diet may lead to
   1. Obesity

2. Tooth decay and gum disease
3. Malnutrition (if empty calorie foods such as candy and soft drinks are eaten/drunk extensively)
F. Dietary considerations
  1. Approximately 50% to 60% of total caloric intake may come from carbohydrates (mainly starches)
  2. Encourage the intake of whole grain bread and cereal products; if refined cereal products are used, they should be enriched
  3. Reduce the dietary intake of simple sugars (which provide empty calories) and substitute starches as sources of carbohydrates
G. Dietary fiber
  1. Definition: the total amount of naturally-occurring material in foods, mostly plants, that is not digested by the human digestive system and therefore is not absorbed
  2. Two categories of dietary fiber: soluble and insoluble based on the solubility in water

PROTEIN

A. Composed of amino acids
  1. Essential amino acids: amino acids the body cannot manufacture and therefore must be supplied in the diet; there are eight essential amino acids
  2. Nonessential amino acids: those the body can manufacture and therefore are not as important in the diet
B. Functions
  1. Build and repair body tissue (primary function)
  2. Furnish energy if there is insufficient carbohydrate or fat for this purpose
  3. Maintain normal circulation of tissue and blood vessel fluids through the action of plasma protein
  4. Aid metabolic functions by combining with iron to form hemoglobin; used to manufacture enzymes and hormones
  5. Aid body defenses by manufacturing lymphocytes and antibodies
C. Digestion and metabolism
  1. Digestion of protein begins in the stomach, where it is acted upon by the enzyme pepsin. It is completed in the small intestine by three enzymes: trypsin, chymotrypsin, and carboxypeptidase
  2. Protein must be broken down into amino acids to be absorbed and distributed to the cells
  3. End products of protein metabolism are hydrogen, oxygen, nitrogen, water, uric acid, and urea
D. Types and sources
  1. Complete proteins: foods that contain all eight essential amino acids in amounts capable of meeting human requirements (e.g., mainly animal sources, such as meats, fish, poultry, eggs, milk, and cheese)
  2. Incomplete proteins: foods that lack one or more of the essential amino acids (e.g., mainly plant sources, such as cereal grains, nuts, legumes, and lentils)
  3. Complementary proteins: foods that, when eaten together, supply the amino acid that is missing or in short supply in the other food (e.g., peanut butter with bread, beans with rice, and baked beans with brown bread) A rule of thumb is that a grain and a legume eaten together supply all the essential amino acids.
E. Dietary considerations
  1. The recommended daily protein intake for adults is 0.8 g/kg of body weight (15% of total caloric intake)
  2. Dietary proteins are not stored in the body as amino acids. Proteins are the main components needed to build and repair body tissues. If the right amount and the right kinds are not available, the nitrogen is broken off and the remainder of the protein is used for energy or stored as fat. The need for cell building and maintenance is continuous. For a supply of proteins to be available on a regular basis, a source of complete proteins should be eaten at every meal
  3. Increased protein is necessary during periods of growth, illness, injury, or stress; after surgery; and when bed rest is prescribed (especially for the elderly)
  4. Kwashiorkor, a protein deficiency disease, is seen in many underdeveloped countries
  5. Marasmus is overt starvation caused by a deficiency of calories from any source

FATS (LIPIDS)

A. Functions
  1. Supply energy for body activities when CHO is not available; all body tissues except brain and nervous cells can use fat for energy; most concentrated form of energy yields 9 calories per gram
  2. Act as insulation to maintain body temperature and protect organs from mechanical injury
  3. Carry fat-soluble vitamins A, D, E, and K and aid in their absorption
  4. Provide a feeling of fullness and satisfaction after eating because of their slow rate of digestion
  5. Furnish the essential fatty acid, linoleic acid, which is found primarily in vegetable oils; called essential because it cannot be synthesized in the body and is vital to body functioning
B. Types
  1. Saturated fats: those whose structure is completely filled with all the hydrogen it can hold; they are usually from animal sources and are usually solid at room temperature (e.g., fats in meat, dairy products, and eggs; coconut oil, palm oil, and chocolate are also highly saturated)
  2. Unsaturated fats: those whose chemical structure has one or more places where hydrogen can be added; they are less dense, usually liquid at room temperature, (with the exception of margarine) and are chiefly from plant sources (e.g., vegetable oils such as cottonseed, soybean, corn oil)
    a. Monounsaturated fats have one place for hydrogen to be added
    b. Polyunsaturated fats have two or more places for hydrogen to be added
    c. Hydrogenation: the process of adding hydrogen to a liquid or polyunsaturated fat and changing it to a solid or semisolid state (however, hydrogenation reduces the polyunsaturated fat content and therefore possibly reduces its health value)
C. Digestion and metabolism
  1. Digestion of fat begins in the stomach, where gastric lipase acts on emulsified fats
  2. Major portions of fat digestion occur in the small intestine, where bile emulsifies fats (breaks it into small droplets); pancreatic lipase changes the emulsified fats into fatty acids and glycerol, the end products of fat digestion.

3. Fats are carried as lipoproteins to body cells, where they are either broken down for use as energy or stored as adipose tissue
D. Sources
  1. Visible fats: those readily seen (e.g., butter and margarine, salad oils, shortening, and fat in meats)
  2. Invisible fats: those in which the fat is less obvious (e.g., milk, avocado, cheese, and lean meat)
E. Cholesterol: a complex fat-related compound
  1. A normal component of blood and of all body cells, especially brain and nerve tissue
  2. Necessary for normal body functioning as structural material in cells, in the production of vitamin D, and in the production of a number of hormones
  3. Supplied by food (mainly animal sources); some synthesized within the body, mainly in the intestinal walls and liver, in response to need
  4. Blood cholesterol levels are affected by a variety of factors including diet, heredity, emotional stress, and exercise; saturated fats tend to raise blood cholesterol, whereas polyunsaturated fats are recommended for lowering cholesterol levels
  5. Cholesterol is carried to and from body cells by special carriers called *lipoproteins*
    a. High-density lipoprotein (HDL), or "good" cholesterol, carries cholesterol away from the arteries and back to the liver for removal from the body
    b. Low-density lipoprotein (LDL), or "bad" cholesterol, tends to circulate in the bloodstream and form plaque on the inner walls of arteries
  6. Risk is classified according to total cholesterol level as follows
    a. Desirable—below 200 mg/dl
    b. Borderline high—200 to 239 mg/dl
    c. High—above 240 mg/dl
  7. If the total cholesterol level is borderline high or high, then the levels and ratio of LDL and HDL should be evaluated
  8. High cholesterol levels predispose individuals to atherosclerosis and other serious health problems
  9. Foods high in cholesterol: organ meats, animal fat, egg yolk, and shellfish
F. Dietary considerations
  1. The *Dietary Guidelines for America 1990* recommended that daily intake of fats for adults should not be more than 30% of the total caloric intake; no more than 10% of the intake should be from saturated fat
  2. To decrease dietary fat
    a. Use leaner cuts of meat and more poultry; trim fats from all meats
    b. Use fewer eggs or egg substitute products
    c. Use low-fat milk products
    d. Limit use of fat in cooking as much as possible
    e. Decrease frequency of red meat use
G. Effects of excess fat intake
  1. Obesity
  2. Consumption may predispose to serious conditions such as heart disease, diabetes, and stroke
  3. Increased surgical risk

VITAMINS
A. Definitions

1. Vitamins: organic compounds needed in small amounts for growth and maintenance of life
2. Precursor (or provitamin): substances that precede and can be changed into active vitamins (e.g., carotene is the precursor of vitamin A)
3. Hypervitaminosis: the excess of one or more vitamins
4. Synthetic: man-made vitamins
5. Enriched: the addition of nutrients to a food often in amounts larger than might be found naturally in that food
6. Fortified: the replacement in food of nutrients lost during processing
B. Characteristics
  1. Contain no calories
  2. Essential to life because they generally cannot be synthesized by the body and are necessary for cell metabolism
  3. Functions include tissue building and regulation of body functions
  4. Needed in minute amounts (milligrams [mg] or micrograms [μg]); the safety of taking megadoses is debatable
  5. Well-balanced diet should provide adequate vitamins to fulfill body requirements
C. Classified on basis of solubility (Table 4-2)
  1. Fat-soluble vitamins: A, D, E, and K
    a. Sufficient fats needed in diet to carry fat-soluble vitamins
    b. Stored in body, so deficiencies are slow to appear
    c. Absorbed in the same manner as fats so anything that interferes with absorption of fats interferes with absorption of fat-soluble vitamins (mineral oil, an indigestible substance, carries fat-soluble vitamins with it out of the body)
    d. Fairly stable in cooking and storage
  2. Water-soluble vitamins: C and B complex (Table 4-2)
    a. Not stored in body; deficiency can occur if vitamins are not consumed in the daily diet.
    b. Easily destroyed by air and in cooking

MINERALS
A. Definition: Inorganic elements essential for growth and normal functioning (Table 4-3)
B. Types
  1. Major minerals, or macrominerals, are found in the largest amounts in the body and are needed in large amounts (100 mg or more per day); they are calcium, phosphorus, potassium, sodium, chlorine, magnesium, and sulfur
  2. Microminerals, or trace elements, are needed in small amounts (e.g., iron, zinc, copper, and iodine)
C. Characteristics
  1. Found in all body tissues and fluids
  2. Occur naturally in foods (especially unrefined foods)
  3. Do not furnish energy, but regulate body processes that furnish energy
  4. Remain stable in food preparation
D. Functions
  1. Constitute bones and teeth (calcium and phosphorus)
  2. Transmit nerve impulses and aid in muscle contraction
  3. Control water balance (sodium and potassium)
  4. Maintain acid-base balance
  5. Synthesize essential body compounds (e.g., iodine for thyroxine)
  6. Act as catalysts for tissue reactions (e.g., calcium needed for blood clotting)

		Table 4-2	Vitamins	

Vitamin	Sources	Functions	Deficiency symptoms
Fat-soluble vitamins			
A (retinol) Precursor: carotene	Fish liver oils Liver Green, leafy vegetables Yellow vegetables (corn, carrots, and sweet potatoes) Yellow fruits (apricots and peaches) Egg yolk Whole milk	Regenerates visual purple (necessary for good vision) Formation of bones and teeth Maintains skin and mucous membranes	Night blindness Retardation of skeletal growth Dry, scaly skin Dry mucous membranes Susceptibility to epithelial infection Xerophthalmia (corneal cells become opaque, slough off, could lead to blindness)
D (calciferol)	Sunshine Fish liver oils Fortified milk	Regulates calcium and phosphorus absorption and metabolism Essential for normal formation of bones and teeth	Lowered levels of calcium and phosphorus in blood Soft bones Rickets Malformed teeth
E (tocopherol)	Wheat germ Vegetable oils Dark green, leafy vegetables	Inconclusive at present Preserves integrity of RBCs Antioxidant (protects materials that oxidize easily) Protects structure and function of muscle	Increased hemolysis (breakdown) of red blood cells (RBCs) Anemia Breakdown of vitamin A and essential fatty acids
K (menadione)	Synthesis by intestinal bacteria Green, leafy vegetables Pork liver	Formation of prothrombin (necessary in blood clotting)	Prolonged clotting time (bleeding tendencies) Hemorrhagic diseases
Water-soluble vitamins			
C (ascorbic acid)	Citrus fruits Tomatoes, broccoli, strawberries, green peppers, cantaloupes, potatoes	Formation and maintenance of capillary walls and collagen formation Aids in absorption of iron	Scurvy (deficiency disease) Sore gums Tendency to bruise easily Poor wound healing Anemia
B_1 (thiamine)	Wheat germ Whole or enriched grains Legumes Pork and organ meats	Maintains carbohydrate metabolism Maintains muscle and nerve functioning Maintains appetite	Beriberi (deficiency disease) Anorexia, fatigue, nerve disorders, irritability
B_2 (riboflavin)	Milk Organ meats Green leafy vegetables Enriched bread and cereals	Maintains healthy eyes Maintains color and structure of lips Metabolism of nutrients	Sensitivity to light, dim vision Inflammation of lips and tongue Loss of appetite and weight
B_6 (pyridoxine)	Red meats (especially organ meats) Whole grain cereals Pork, lamb, veal	Synthesis and metabolism of proteins Hemoglobin synthesis Maintenance of muscles and nerves	Nausea and vomiting, anorexia, anemia, irritability, CNS dysfunction, kidney stones, dermatitis
B_{12} (cobalamin)	Found only in animal products Organ and muscle meats Dairy products	Protein metabolism Production of RBCs Normal functioning of nervous system	Pernicious anemia (resulting from lack of intrinsic factor needed for B_{12} absorption)
Niacin (nicotinic acid) Precursor: tryptophan	Meats (especially organ meats) Poultry and fish Peanut butter	Essential for normal functioning of digestive and nervous systems Essential for growth and metabolism	Pellagra (deficiency disease) Nervous disorders Diarrhea and nausea Dermatitis
Folic acid (folacin)		Essential in formation of all body cells, especially RBCs Protein metabolism	Anemia (macrocytic) Gastrointestinal disturbances Glossitis Stomatitis

Table 4-3	Major Minerals and Microminerals (Trace Elements)		
Vitamin	**Sources**	**Functions**	**Deficiency symptoms**
Major minerals			
Calcium (Ca): absorption aided by vitamin D	Milk and milk products Cheese Some green, leafy vegetables (turnips, collards, kale, broccoli)	Bone and tooth formation Blood clotting Muscle (including heart muscle) contraction Nerve transmission Cell wall permeability	Poor bone and tooth formation Rickets (deficiency disease) Stunted growth Osteoporosis Poor blood clotting Tetany
Phosphorus (P): absorption with Ca aided by vitamin D	Milk and cheese Meat Egg yolk Whole grains (Diet adequate in protein and Ca should be adequate in P)	Functions as calcium phosphate in the calcification of bones and teeth Energy metabolism Regulation of acid-base balance Cell structure and enzyme activity	Poor bone and tooth formation Retarded growth Rickets (deficiency disease) Weakness Anorexia
Sodium (Na)	Salt Baking powder and soda Dairy products Meat, fish, and poultry	Regulation of acid-base balance Fluid balance Nerve transmission and muscle contraction Glucose absorption	Nausea and vomiting Apathy Exhaustion Abdominal and muscle cramps
Potassium (K)	Meat, fish, and poultry Whole grain breads and cereals Fruits (oranges, bananas)	Regulates nerve conduction and muscle contraction Necessary for regular heart rhythm Fluid and acid-base balance Cell metabolism	Abnormal heartbeat Muscle weakness Nausea and vomiting
Chlorine (Cl)	Table salt (NaCl)	Formation of hydrochloric acid and maintenance of gastric acidity Maintenance of acid-base balance, osmotic pressure, and water balance	Deficiency results from fluid loss through vomiting, diarrhea, and heavy sweating
Magnesium (Mg)	Green, leafy vegetables Legumes Milk Whole grains	Component of bones and teeth Enzymes essential in general metabolism Conduction of nerve impulses Muscle contraction	Tremors leading to convulsive seizures
Sulfur (S)	Protein foods Meat Milk Eggs Cheese Nuts and legumes	Component of all body cells; important in building connective tissue Component in several B vitamins and several amino acids Energy metabolism	None documented
Microminerals			
Iron (Fe): absorption enhanced by vitamin C	Organ meats (especially liver) Egg yolk Green, leafy vegetables Lean red meats Dried fruits (apricots, raisins)	Synthesis of hemoglobin General metabolic activities	Anemia
Iodine (I)	Iodized salt Saltwater fish	Normal functioning of thyroid gland	Goiter
Zinc (Zn)	Oysters Liver High-protein foods	Component of enzymes Assists in regulation of cell growth Protein synthesis	Impaired wound healing Poor taste sensitivity Retarded sexual and physical development
Copper (Cu)	Liver Cocoa Nuts Raisins	Aids in absorption of iron Component of hemoglobin Component of enzymes	Unknown at present, although secondary conditions may develop

WATER

A. Water makes up 50% to 65% of the weight of an average adult
   1. Intracellular: fluid within cells composed of water plus concentrations of potassium and phosphates: contains minerals, potassium, magnesium, and phosphorus
   2. Extracellular: all body fluids outside cells including interstitial fluid, plasma, and watery components of body organs and substances; contains minerals, sodium chloride
B. Functions
   1. Essential component of all tissues and fluids
   2. Transportation of nutrients from the digestive tract to the bloodstream and from cell to cell; also removal of waste products from cells to outside the body
   3. Lubrication of joints
   4. Maintenance of stable body temperature (as temperature increases, sweating occurs, evaporates, and cools the body)
   5. Solvent for all the body's chemical processes
C. Overall water balance in the body
   1. Intake: under ordinary conditions, adults need 2 to 3 L of liquid per day—5 to 6 glasses of which should be water
      a. Ingested fluids such as water, soups, and beverages
      b. Water in foods that are eaten
      c. Water formed from cell oxidation (when nutrients are burned)
   2. Output: averages 2600 ml daily
      a. Normal routes of excretion: primarily the kidney but also the skin, lungs, and feces
      b. Abnormal and extensive losses can occur from vomiting and diarrhea, open or draining wounds, fever, extensive burns, hemorrhage, and anything that causes excessive perspiration
D. Additional fluids are required
   1. By infants
   2. During fever or disease process
   3. In warm weather
   4. During heavy work or extensive physical activity

CELLULOSE

A. Definition: a polysaccharide that makes up the framework of plants; provides bulk (fiber or roughage) for the diet; cannot be broken down by the human digestive system and therefore is not absorbed
B. Function: to absorb water, provide bulk, and stimulate peristalsis
C. Found in the stalks and leaves of plants, in the skins of fruit and vegetables, and in the outer covering of seeds and cereals (refined cereals have most of the fiber removed and provide little bulk)

Nutritional Guidelines

RECOMMENDED DIETARY ALLOWANCES (RDA)

A. Developed by the Food and Nutrition Board of the National Academy of Science
B. Suggested levels of essential nutrients (proteins, vitamins, and minerals) known from current research to be adequate to meet nutritional needs of most healthy individuals
C. Used as a guideline for most federal, state, and local feeding programs but not to be used as requirements for individuals with specific nutritional deficiencies

U.S. Dietary Goals or Dietary Guidelines

A. Developed by the U.S. Department of Agriculture, U.S. Department of Health and Human Services
B. Seven factors to discourage excesses in the diet
   1. Eat a variety of foods (for a variety of nutrients)
   2. Maintain ideal weight (obesity is linked to several chronic diseases such as hypertension and diabetes)
   3. Avoid too much fat, saturated fat, and cholesterol (which contributes to increased risk of cardiovascular disease)
   4. Eat foods with adequate starch and fiber (better sources of fuel than simple sugars; contain more essential nutrients and add more bulk to the diet)
   5. Avoid excessive sugar
   6. Avoid excessive sodium
   7. If you drink alcoholic beverages, do so in moderation (alcohol is high in calories but low in nutrients; also heavy drinking contributes to many chronic liver and neurologic disorders)

NUTRITIONAL ASSESSMENT

A. Two phases: screening and assessment. Purpose: to screen for nutritional risks and apply specific assessment techniques to determine an action plan
B. Components of nutritional assessment; anthropometric measurements, biochemical tests, clinical observations, dietary and personal histories. All components work together to determine the best action plan for the individual in the healthy population and the sick population within the context of their personal, social, and economic background

FOOD GUIDE PYRAMID (FIG. 4-1)

A. Emphasizes grains, fruits, and vegetables as the foundation of a balanced diet and downplays meats, dairy products, and fats; fats, oils, and sweets are recommended sparingly
B. Specific guidelines
   1. Breads, cereals, rice, pasta: six to eleven servings daily (1 serving equals 1 slice of bread, 1 oz of ready-to-eat cereal, or ½ cup of cooked cereal, rice, or pasta); nutrients primarily supplied are iron, B complex vitamins, and carbohydrates (starches); refined products contain fewer vitamins, whereas the enriched, fortified, or restored products contain many more vitamins
   2. Fruits: two to four servings daily (1 serving equals 1 medium apple, banana, or orange or ½ cup of cooked, chopped, or canned fruit); nutrients primarily supplied are vitamins A and C and fiber
   3. Vegetables: three to five servings daily (1 serving equals 1 cup of raw, leafy vegetables or ½ cup of other vegetables cooked, chopped, or raw); nutrients primarily supplied are vitamins A and C and fiber
   4. Milk, yogurt, cheese: two to three servings daily (1 serving equals 1 cup of milk or yogurt or 1½ oz of natural cheese); nutrients primarily supplied are calcium, protein, and riboflavin
   5. Meat, poultry, fish, dry beans, eggs, and nuts: two to three servings daily (1 serving equals 2 to 3 oz of cooked lean meat, poultry, or fish; ½ cup of cooked dry beans, or 1 egg; 2 tbsp of peanut butter equals 1 oz of lean meat); nutrients primarily supplied are protein, iron, and B vitamins

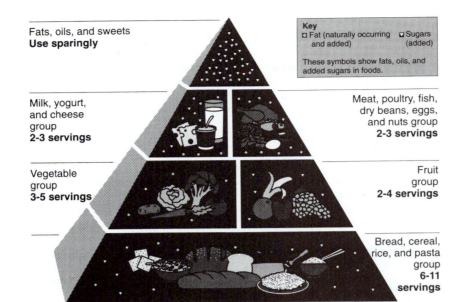

Figure 4-1.   Food guide pyramid: a guide to daily food choices. (Courtesy U.S. Department of Agriculture, Washington, DC, 1992.)

Food Management
ECONOMIC CONSIDERATIONS IN MENU PLANNING
A. Plan menus in advance
1. Take advantage of specials to prepare balanced meals
2. Shop from a list to avoid impulse buying
B. Choose foods wisely
1. Buy foods in season and in good supply
2. Buy in quantity if adequate storage is available (larger quantities may cost less per unit)
3. Buy sale items only if they can be used
4. Use unit pricing to find the best buys among brands
5. Know grades and brands of foods; grading of canned goods has no bearing on nutritive value; generic labeling can save up to 25% of name brand items
6. Purchase staple and canned goods when on sale
7. Remember that cost per serving rather than per pound is important, especially in buying meat
8. Compare labels for weights and ingredients
9. Buy less expensive forms of food (margarine is less expensive than butter)
10. Limit purchase of empty-calorie foods
11. Decrease the cost of protein in the diet by using small amounts of meats, fish, and poultry and by using lower grades and less expensive cuts of meat; also legumes, peanut butter, eggs, and cheese are good sources of less expensive protein
12. Try to avoid convenience foods (any food bought partially prepared and ready to eat with little home preparation); they are usually more expensive than those prepared entirely at home and are less nutritionally balanced, containing high proportions of fat, calories, and sodium
C. Care for foods after purchase
1. Store foods properly to avoid spoilage and loss of nutrients
2. Consume leftover foods quickly

STORAGE AND PREPARATION OF BASIC FOODS
A. Milk
1. Store milk refrigerated in covered container; powdered milk should be stored in a cool, dry place; refrigerate powdered milk after reconstituting
2. Cook over low heat; avoid scorching
B. Cheese
1. Refrigerate well wrapped or in tight containers
2. Most palatable if served at room temperature; cook at low temperatures for a short time
C. Eggs
1. Refrigerate promptly; if cracked, use only in foods that will be well cooked
2. Cook at lower temperatures to prevent discoloration, curdling, or toughness
D. Cereals and breads
1. Store in cool, dry place; bread retains freshness best at room temperature, but molds faster; bread freezes well
2. Cook cereals according to directions; overcooking reduces vitamin content
E. Meat, fish, and poultry
1. Store in refrigerator for a short time or freeze for longer storage
2. Less expensive meats, although nutritionally equivalent to more expensive ones, require longer cooking at lower temperatures
F. Fruits and vegetables
1. Store ripe fruits and vegetables in the refrigerator (fruits ripen best at room temperature)
2. Cook only until tender, using as little water as possible (cooking liquids contain valuable nutrients and should be used if possible); raw fruits and vegetables are especially nutritious

TYPES OF MILK

A. Skim: fat and vitamin A removed (may have vitamins A and D added); contains all other nutrients of whole milk

B. Homogenized: fat particles evenly dispersed so cream does not separate

C. Pasteurized: heated to a specific temperature to destroy pathogenic bacteria (but nutrients are not affected)

D. Condensed: water removed and sugar added so carbohydrate content is increased; low in calcium and vitamins and high in sugar compared with whole milk

E. Evaporated: heated above the boiling point so that more than half the water evaporates

F. Low fat: contains 0.5% to 2% fat; lower in calories than whole milk but comparable in nutrient value

G. Powdered or dry: water removed; least expensive form of milk on the market; when reconstituted, it has the same nutrient value as the milk from which it was made

Nutrition Throughout the Life Cycle

INFANT NUTRITION

A. Infants require more protein and calories per pound of body weight than adults do because they have more body surface in proportion to weight and because of their growth and activity

B. Breast-feeding is the recommended method of feeding if possible; provides more vitamin C and more easily digested protein and sugar than cow's milk; also provides the infant with antibodies against disease and assists in establishing the mother-child bond; in addition, breastfed babies experience fewer allergies and intolerances as well as easier digestion

C. Bottle-feeding is an acceptable alternative if close mother-child contact is maintained; most mothers use a commercially prepared formula such as Enfamil; a soy-based product such as Isomil can be used if the infant is allergic to milk products. At no time during the first year of life should an infant be fed regular whole cow's milk. Its concentration may cause GI bleeding or renal discomfort. Skim milk or low-fat milk provides infants with too little energy and linoleic acid

D. The American Academy of Pediatrics recommends breast milk supplemented by vitamin D and fluoride from birth, and iron supplements after 4 months of age

E. Introduction of solid foods varies among pediatricians, most favoring a delay until the infant is at least 6 months of age
   1. Infant cereal is usually given first (often with added iron to supplement a possible lack in the infant's diet; prenatal iron reserves last 5 to 6 months)
   2. Fruits, vegetables, and egg yolk are frequently given next (because of possible allergic reactions, egg white is delayed until late in the first year)
   3. Solid foods should be introduced one at a time and at 4- to 5-day intervals to observe for any allergic reactions
   4. Adding sugar or salt to infant's food is undesirable
   5. Infants can choke on small foods such as berries, corn, popcorn, or candy
   6. Infants should not receive honey, because honey contains botulism spores, which could harm the infant (even though quantities are too low to harm older children and adults)

PRESCHOOL CHILDREN

A. Growth rate is slower and more erratic, and food intake will vary accordingly

B. A variety of foods should be offered
   1. "Finger foods" such as carrot sticks are enjoyed
   2. Serve small amounts because too large a serving can discourage a child from eating
   3. Avoid refined sweets
   4. Do not coax a child to eat; if a food is refused, offer it at a later date
   5. Nutritious snacks are a viable alternative for a child who is a poor eater

C. Teach healthy eating habits; avoid rewarding good behavior with food

SCHOOLCHILDREN (5 TO 10 YEARS OF AGE)

A. Gradual increase in growth at this age (approximately equal for boys and girls)

B. Proper nutrition is important to proper mental and physical development (adequate breakfast is important for alertness during class)

C. Children are usually good eaters at this age and should be encouraged by the examples set at home and at school; promote healthy eating

ADOLESCENTS

A. Tremendous growth spurt occurs at puberty (age of sexual maturity)
   1. For girls, usually between 10 and 13 years of age
   2. For boys, between 13 and 16 years of age

B. Diets are influenced by peers, with much empty-calorie foods being consumed

C. Boys gain mostly lean muscle tissue; they consume large amounts of food to meet energy requirements

D. Girls gain more fat tissue; their diets may be more influenced by a desire to remain thin; frequently require iron supplements to meet their needs; adequate nutrition during adolescence helps avoid complications during pregnancy; promote healthy eating along with exercise

ADULTS

A. Adequate nutrition throughout the life span is important in avoiding many serious illnesses

B. Proper nutrition is based on guidelines set by U.S. government agencies (such as the food pyramid)

C. Persons who consume a balanced diet usually do not need vitamin supplements

GERIATRICS

A. Physiologic changes affect nutrition of the elderly
   1. Aging slows the basal metabolic rate (BMR); combined with decreased activity the result is decreased energy requirements and decreased number of calories needed
   2. Taste may be adversely affected by gradual diminishment of the senses of smell, sight, and taste
   3. Loss of teeth may affect proper chewing, food intake, or enjoyment
   4. Reduced saliva makes swallowing more difficult and digestion less efficient
   5. Decreased movement of wastes through intestines contributes to constipation

6. Marginal deficiencies of ascorbic acid, thiamin, riboflavin have occurred in some elderly patients
7. Decreased absorption and use of nutrients results from decreased digestive juices and gastric motility reduction

B. Economic and social considerations
   1. Decrease in income among the elderly, combined with an increase in the amount spent for medical care, leaves less for adequate nutrition; tendency is to eat less protein (which is expensive) and more carbohydrates (which are cheaper and easier to prepare)
   2. Loss of spouse, friends, or mobility results in isolation, depression, and often decreased will to obtain adequate nutrition

C. Planning diets
   1. Diet should be well balanced in protein, vitamins, and minerals (especially calcium and iron) to allow for diminished absorption
   2. Calories sufficient to maintain energy and activity (reduced from those previously required)
   3. Soft bulk in diet to prevent constipation (cooked fruits and vegetables)
   4. Increased fluid intake required to eliminate metabolic wastes
   5. Meals should be light and easily digested, that is, contain only a small amount of fats; frequent small meals may be easier to digest than three large meals
   6. Individual preferences should be respected and the diet built around them; make changes slowly
   7. Meals eaten with others are often more appetizing than those eaten alone

PREGNANCY

A. A well-balanced diet with increased amounts of essential nutrients is important to the well-being of the mother and baby
   1. A protein increase of 20% or 60 g/day over the normal diet is recommended to allow for growth of the baby, placenta, maternal tissues, and increased circulating blood volume, amniotic fluid, and storage
   2. An increase in calories meets increased energy demands and allows protein to be used for tissue building
   3. Increased amounts of the following: calcium, phosphorus, and vitamin D are needed both for the mother and for the bones and teeth of the baby; iron for hemoglobin and prenatal storage for the baby; iodine for thyroxine for the mother's increased BMR; and vitamins A, B complex, and C
   4. Weight should not be severely restricted; a gain of 30 lb is considered healthy
   5. Severe restriction of salt is unfounded

B. Vomiting (morning sickness)
   1. Lower fat intake with more high-carbohydrate foods
   2. Fluids between instead of with meals
   3. Dry toast or crackers on awakening

LACTATION

A. A baby requires 2 to 2½ oz (60 to 75 ml) of breast milk per pound (488 g) of body weight (1 oz [30 ml] = 20 calories); there is an increased maternal need for all nutrients during lactation
B. Diet of a lactating mother should be high in protein and calories

C. Increased fluids are also required; at least 6 cups (1.5 L) of milk in some form is recommended

Diet Therapy

NURSING RESPONSIBILITIES

A. Nutritional assessment: assess physical characteristics of patient; individualize care to allow for patient differences
B. Evaluate the patient's tolerance to diet and provide feedback to other health team members
C. Assist patient in learning about required dietary changes; reinforce information and answer questions
D. If possible, incorporate patient's preferences to increase compliance with the nutritional care plan
E. Prepare the patient for mealtime; assist as necessary
F. See that each person receives the correct tray unless foods are being withheld
G. Serve and remove tray promptly
H. Teach patients the value of proper nutrition and urge compliance with the nutritional care plan

PURPOSES

A. To increase or decrease weight
B. To allow a particular organ or system to rest (e.g., a low-fat diet in gallbladder disease)
C. To regulate the diet to correspond with the body's ability to metabolize a specific nutrient (e.g., diabetes)
D. To correct conditions caused by deficiencies
E. To eliminate harmful substances from the diet (e.g., caffeine, cholesterol, and alcohol)
F. To nourish the body

DIET MODIFICATIONS

A. Calories may be increased or decreased
B. Nutrients may be adjusted (high or low protein)
C. Certain foods may be omitted or added
D. Modifications in texture (consistency-soft diet)
E. Frequency of meals: more than the standard three

STANDARD HOSPITAL DIETS (MODIFICATIONS IN CONSISTENCY)

A. Clear liquid (surgical liquid)
   1. Temporary diet of clear liquids, nonresidue, nonirritating, nongas-forming; inadequate in protein, vitamins, minerals, and calories
   2. Used postoperatively to replace fluids, before certain tests, and to lessen amount of fecal matter in colon
   3. Includes water, coffee, tea, fat-free broth, pulp-free fruit juices (apple), gelatin, and ginger ale

B. Full liquid diet
   1. Foods liquid at room or body temperatures; may be adequate if carefully planned, although frequently deficient in iron
   2. Used postoperatively as a transition between clear and soft diet, in infections and acute gastritis; in febrile conditions; and for patients unable to chew or swallow or with an intolerance to food for other reasons
   3. Includes all clear liquids, milk, creamed soups, ice creams, sherbets, plain puddings, and thin, strained cereal

C. Soft diet
   1. Normal diet modified in consistency to have limited fiber; easily digested; nutritionally adequate

2. Used between full liquid and regular, for chewing difficulties, and in gastrointestinal disorders
3. Includes tender meats and tender, well-cooked vegetables (those with a great deal of fiber should be pureed or omitted); fruits (no fiber) and plain cakes are allowed; no spicy or coarse foods are allowed

D. Regular (general or house) diet
   1. Adequate, well-balanced diet designed to appeal to most people
   2. Used for those not requiring a modified or therapeutic diet
   3. Includes all foods from the four basic food groups

ADDITIONAL MODIFIED (OR THERAPEUTIC) DIETS

Table 4-4 lists diets; foods allowed and omitted; and when the diets are used.

Diets for Specific Disease Conditions

DIABETES MELLITUS

A. Classification
   1. IDDM (type I), or insulin dependent: onset is usually before the age of 20; difficult to manage and requires both dietary restrictions and insulin injections
   2. NIDDM (type II), or maturity onset: usually develops after age 35; frequently controlled by diet alone; insulin or oral hypoglycemics or both may also be needed

B. Diet is determined by age, sex, body build, weight, and activity; maintenance requirements are the same as for a nondiabetic patient
   1. Calories: sufficient to maintain ideal body weight (approximately 30 cal/kg ideal weight)
   2. Protein: 10% to 20% of daily caloric intake
   3. Carbohydrates: 50% to 60% of total calories (obtain greatest portion from complex carbohydrates such as starches, and the least from simple sugars)
   4. Fats: moderately controlled; 30% or less of total calories and <10% from saturated fat
   5. High-fiber foods, which decrease postprandial blood glucose levels, are encouraged

C. Exchange system is used for planning the diabetic diet
   1. Based on simple grouping of common foods according to equivalent nutritional values
   2. Six basic food groups or food exchanges; each food within the group contains approximately the same food value as other foods within the same group
      a. Milk: equal to 1 cup (240 ml) whole milk
      b. Vegetables: variety of low-carbohydrate vegetables
      c. Fruit: fresh or canned without sugar
      d. Bread: starchy items (breads, pasta, cereals, and vegetables equal to 1 slice bread)
      e. Meat: protein food equal to 1 oz (28 g) lean meat
      f. Fat equal to 1 tsp (5 ml) margarine
   3. Total exchanges per day is determined by individual nutritional needs based on nutritional standards (Table 4-5 shows a sample diet based on the exchange system)
   4. Advantages of exchange system
      a. Is easy to understand
      b. Allows diabetic patients more freedom to choose foods they like
      c. Allows choice of foods that fit into their economic status
      d. Can be used for other types of diets
      e. Does not require dietetic or specialized diabetic foods

SURGERY

A. Surgery increases the nutritional demands on the body
   1. Protein: increased for tissue repair, to prevent tissue breakdown, and to help replace blood and fluid losses
   2. Carbohydrates: increased to meet body demands for energy and to spare protein for tissue building
   3. Vitamins: especially important in wound healing; vitamin C cements cells, and builds connective tissue and capillaries

B. Types of feeding available postoperatively
   1. Intravenous: immediately administered to supply essential water, electrolytes, and vitamins; intended only as short-term for fluid and electrolytes supplement
   2. Parenteral hyperalimentation (total parenteral nutrition [TPN]): administered through a larger central vein such as the superior vena cava because the TPN solution is hypertonic (high osmolarity) and must enter the body in a region of high blood flow so that the solution is rapidly diluted; provides a higher percentage of water, glucose, amino acids, fats, vitamins, minerals, and electrolytes; requires surgical insertion, careful monitoring, and special care; may also be indicated preoperatively or for debilitated patients whose intake does not meet body requirements
   3. Oral feedings: most patients should begin oral feedings as soon as bowel sounds return; provide nutrients essential to recovery; progress from clear liquid onward

BURNS

A. Rate of tissue breakdown and loss of other body nutrients is greater with serious burns than with any other disease process

B. Increase of fluids and nutrients is required
   1. Increased energy requires 3000 to 5000 calories
   2. Protein increase of 50% above normal
   3. Vitamin C requirements greatly increased for wound healing
   4. B vitamins increased for higher metabolic rate
   5. Increased fluids to replace lost body fluids and help eliminate waste products

C. Intravenous dextrose, electrolytes, and plasma are given initially; a high-protein, high-calorie diet is given when oral foods can be taken

D. Victims of extensive burns may require parenteral hyperalimentation to meet their extensive nutritional requirements

CANCER

A. The National Cancer Institute and the American Cancer Society have issued the following guidelines for cancer prevention based on information available in 1991:
   1. Eat a variety of foods
   2. Maintain a desirable body weight
   3. Eat a variety of both fruits and vegetables every day
   4. Eat more high-fiber foods, such as whole-grain breads and cereals, legumes, vegetables, and fruits
   5. Reduce fat intake to < or = 30% of total calories
   6. If you drink alcohol, use in moderation
   7. Limit consumption of salt-cured, smoked, and nitrite-preserved foods

B. Diet for the patient with cancer must supply enough protein, fats, carbohydrates, vitamins, minerals, and fluids to meet increased energy demands, prevent weight loss, and rebuild body tissues during treatment; energy and protein needs may increase up to 20%; dietary supplements may be given to supply all necessary nutrients

Table 4-4	**Modified or Therapeutic Diets**		
Diet	**Condition**	**Foods allowed**	**Purpose of diet**
High calorie	Underweight (10% or more) Anorexia nervosa Hyperthyroidism	Emphasis on increase in calories Easily digested foods (carbohydrates) recommended Full meals with high-calorie snacks	To meet the increased metabolic needs of the body or provide increased calories for weight gain
Low calorie	Overweight	Fruits and vegetables especially recommended	To reduce the caloric intake below what the body requires so weight loss will occur
High protein	Children who need additional protein for growth Following surgery Pregnancy and lactation Conditions that cause protein loss Extensive burns	Added amounts of poultry, meat, fish, milk, cheese, and eggs Nonfat dry milk added to soups and baked goods	To increase the intake of high-protein foods for maintaining and rebuilding tissues and correcting protein loss
Low protein	Liver disease Kidney diseases leading to renal failure	Fruits and vegetables Severely limited in amounts of meats, fish, poultry, eggs, and dairy products	To limit the end products of protein metabolism to avoid disturbing the fluid, electrolyte, and acid-base balances
High residue	Constipation (atonic) Diverticulitis (when inflammation has ceased)	Increased whole grain cereals Increased fruits and raw vegetables Fibrous meats	Mechanically stimulates the gastrointestinal tract
Low residue	Before and after bowel surgery Ulcerative colitis Diverticulitis (during inflammatory stage) Diarrhea	Soft cheeses Tender meats Refined cereals and breads Pureed fruits and vegetables Plain puddings	To soothe and be nonirritating to gastrointestinal tract
Low fat	Gallbladder disease Obesity Cardiovascular disease	Vegetables and fruits Skim milk Sherbet Increased carbohydrates and proteins	To lower fat content in diet (may be deficient in fat-soluble vitamins)
Low cholesterol	Cardiovascular disease	Lean meats and fish Poultry without the skin Liquid vegetable oils Skim milk	To decrease the blood cholesterol levels or maintain them at acceptable levels
High iron	Anemias	Regular diet with high-iron foods Liver and organ meats Red meats Dried fruits Egg yolks	To correct an iron deficiency
Sodium restricted	Kidney disease Cardiovascular disease Hypertension	Natural foods without salt Milk and meat in limited quantities	To control or correct the retention of sodium and water in the body by controlling sodium intake
High carbohydrate	Preparation for surgery Liver disease Kidney disease	Emphasis on carbohydrate foods Full meals with high carbohydrate snacks	To provide increased energy and spare protein for tissue building
Low carbohydrate	Dumping syndrome Hyperinsulinism Diabetes mellitus (although severe restriction of carbohydrates is currently considered unwarranted)	Proteins Only enough carbohydrate to maintain health and perform activities	To decrease the amounts of glucose in the bloodstream (increased blood glucose causes increased amounts of insulin to be produced by the body)
Lactose restricted	Lactose intolerance	Avoid Foods containing lactose, such as milk, cheese, and ice cream	To eliminate or cut down on lactose—a substance certain individuals cannot metabolize

Table 4-5	1800-Calorie Diet Translated into Food Exchanges	
Exchange group	**Total exchanges for the day**	
Milk	2	
Vegetables	2	
Fruit	5	
Bread	9	
Meat	8	
Fat	7	

Sample diet	Food	Exchange list
Breakfast	Black coffee	Free
	2 eggs	2 meat
	2 pieces toast with butter	2 bread
		2 fat
	Cereal with milk	1 bread
		1 milk
	and plain blueberries	1 fruit
Lunch	Turkey sandwich (3 oz or 84 g)	2 breads
		3 meat
	with mayonnaise (2 tsp or 10 ml)	2 fat
	with tomatoes	1 vegetable
	Sponge cake	1 bread
	with strawberries	1 fruit
	and whipped cream	2 fat
Supper	Roast beef (3 oz or 84 g)	3 meat
	Mashed potatoes, butter	3 bread
		1 fat
	Carrots and butter	1 vegetable
		1 fat
	Applesauce	1 fruit
	1 small apple	1 fruit
Snack	Raspberries (1 cup or 224 g) in	1 fruit
	light cream (2 tbsp or 30 ml)	1 fat
	Milk (8 oz or 240 ml)	1 milk

C. When the GI tract cannot be used, nutritional support may be given by total parenteral nutrition (TPN)

D. Nutritional factors most likely are involved in the development of some cancers. Excesses as well as deficiencies have been implicated. Further evaluation is needed

E. No one food causes cancer, and no one food can prevent it. Diet is considered to be one of the most important environmental/lifestyle factors in the etiology and prevention of cancer in the United States.

AIDS

A. Nutritional support is vital in all stages of the acquired immune deficiency virus. Weight loss is a major symptom in HIV infection. Malnutrition itself contributes to the suppression of immune function

B. Good nutritional care is essential to: help preserve lean body mass; maintain weight and strength; improve body's response to medication

C. Nutritional status of individuals with AIDS can be com-

promised by: decreased oral intake, anorexia, nausea, vomiting, dyspnea, fatigue, neurological disease, disorders of mouth and esophagus

D. Techniques to help with food intake: small meals, readily available snacks, ensure adequate hydration, high caloric, high protein diet, give drugs after meals

E. General goals of nutrition intervention are to:
   1. Preserve optimal somatic and visceral protein status
   2. Prevent nutrient deficiencies or excesses known to compromise immune function
   3. Minimize nutrition-related complications that interfere with either intake or absorption of nutrients
   4. Enhance the quality of life
   5. Educate individuals about the importance of consuming a well balanced diet

CARDIOVASCULAR DISEASE

A. Cardiovascular diseases are the primary causes of death in the United States; research has shown that diet may be a risk factor in determining whether a person develops heart disease

B. Objectives in dietary treatment of heart disease
   1. Provide an adequate diet
   2. Prevent gas- and bulk-forming foods from distending stomach and exerting pressure against the heart
   3. Maintain patient's weight as near to ideal as possible to reduce workload of heart
   4. Prevent edema by lowering sodium intake
   5. Reduce the risk of atherosclerosis by reducing circulating blood lipids (low-saturated fat, low-cholesterol diet)

C. Sodium restriction
   1. Component of many diets used in cardiovascular diseases
   2. Helps reduce excess edema and is thought to reduce the risk of hypertension
   3. Sources of sodium
      a. Naturally present in foods, especially animal products such as meat, poultry, fish, milk, and eggs; fruits have little sodium
      b. Sodium added to foods in the form of table salt and preservatives in processed foods; most canned, packaged, and frozen foods have sodium added
      c. Water supplies may have a high-sodium content; water softeners add a significant amount of sodium to a diet
      d. Nonprescription medicines and home remedies such as baking soda, alkalizers for indigestion, cough medicines, and laxatives may contain large amounts of sodium
   4. Sodium-restricted diets limit the intake of sodium to a level prescribed by the physician
      a. Mild sodium-restricted diet (2 to 3 g) contains about half of the salt previously used; no additional salting of processed foods; no salty foods allowed
      b. 1000 mg sodium diet (moderate)
      c. 500 mg sodium diet (strict)
      d. 250 mg sodium diet (severe)

PEPTIC ULCER TREATMENT

A. Current advances in drug therapy to decrease acid secretion and promote healing have decreased the need for a highly restrictive bland diet

B. These bland diets have been shown to be ineffective and lacking in nutrients to support the healing process. Therapy is based on an individual's response to food choices; avoidance of foods that cause gastric stimulation is recommended

CHRONIC RENAL FAILURE

Renal patients require strict monitoring for protein, water, and electrolyte balance. Specific nutritional therapy varies greatly depending on the patient's age and the stage of the disease. Enough protein should be supplied to repair and maintain tissues and avoid the use of protein for energy. The BUN (blood urea nitrogen level) and creatinine clearance level are monitored to assist in regulating protein levels

Common Types of Food Poisoning

STAPHYLOCOCCAL FOOD POISONING

A. Caused by *Staphylococcus aureus* bacteria; quite resistant to heat
B. Involves foods such as custard, potato, macaroni, egg, chicken salad, cheese, ham, and salami
C. Exhibited by symptoms such as abdominal cramps, diarrhea, and vomiting; lasts 1 to 2 days; usually mild and attributed to other causes
D. Prevented by keeping foods above 140°F (60°C) or below 40°F (4°C); toxin is destroyed by boiling for several hours or heating in a pressure cooker at 240°F (138.5°C) for 30 minutes

CLOSTRIDIAL FOOD POISONING

A. Perfringens
   1. Caused by *Clostridium perfringens,* spore-forming bacteria that grow in the absence of oxygen
   2. Involves foods such as stews, soups, and gravies made from poultry and red meat
   3. Exhibited by symptoms such as nausea without vomiting, diarrhea, and acute inflammation of the stomach and intestine; usually lasts 1 day
   4. Prevented by storing foods properly and keeping foods above 140°F (60°C) or below 40°F (4°C)
B. Botulism
   1. Caused by *Clostridium botulinum,* spore-forming bacteria that grow and produce toxins in absence of oxygen (anaerobic)
   2. Involves canned low-acid foods, especially home-canned foods such as meats, corn, peas, green beans, asparagus, and mushrooms
   3. Exhibited by symptoms such as inability to swallow; double vision, and progressive respiratory paralysis; fatality rate is high if untreated
   4. Prevented by pressure cooking canned foods for specified length of time; any can or jar with a bulging top should be discarded

SALMONELLOSIS

A. Caused by *Salmonella,* bacteria widespread in nature that live in the intestinal tracts of humans and animals; transmitted by eating infected food or by contact with people who are infected or are carriers of the disease; also transmitted by insects or rodents
B. Involves poultry, red meats, dairy products, and eggs
C. Exhibited by symptoms such as severe headache, vomiting, diarrhea, abdominal cramps, and fever; usually last 2-7 days
D. Prevented by heating foods to 140°F (60°C) for 10 minutes or higher temperatures for less time

E. COLI

A. Caused by pathogenic *Escherichia coli,* some types are normally found in human intestinal system.
B. Pathogenic *E. coli* found in raw ground beef
C. Bacteria attacks intestinal wall and spreads to body
D. Exhibited by symptoms such as bloody diarrhea, cramps, fever, chills, dehydration, kidney problems; can be fatal
E. Prevented by using well-cooked meats and sanitary food handling

Food: Fads and Facts

MEAT EATERS VERSUS VEGETARIANS

A. Problems exist when too large a portion of the diet consists of meat
   1. Excess calories tend to be consumed; meat (and the fat therein) is high in calories, and because of the taste the tendency is to eat more than is required
   2. When a large portion of the meal is meat, a smaller portion of fruits and vegetables is consumed; therefore less fiber and fewer of the nutrients in fruits and vegetables are consumed
B. Vegetarians also can have nutritional deficiencies
   1. Calories may be insufficient despite large amounts of foods being consumed
   2. Protein can be lacking; incomplete protein must be supplemented with complementary proteins
   3. Strict vegetarians may need supplements of cobalamin, because it is found only in animal proteins
C. The ideal diet combines both types of diet with a variety of foods
   1. Meat eaters should eat smaller servings of leaner meats with more fruits, vegetables, and cereals
   2. Vegetarians should improve the quality of their diet by adding dairy products such as eggs and milk (if no dairy products are taken, complementary proteins should be carefully selected)

INFLUENCES ON FOOD CHOICES

Personal food habits develop as a result of lifestyle, cultural heritage, and social and economic factors

NUTRITIONAL LABELING AND EDUCATION ACT OF 1990

This regulation has increased consumer access to safe products and knowledge of what nutrients are in food; The Nutrition Facts Panel must include the quantities of energy, fat, and other specific nutrients

SMOKING

If a woman of childbearing age is a smoker and has poor dietary intake, a vitamin C supplement of 100/mg day is needed

VITAMIN C

A. Current research indicates that the effects of megadoses of vitamin C on the common cold are minimal
B. Effects of vitamin C on cancer still require further study

VITAMIN E

A. Claims list vitamin E as a "cure-all," especially in prolonging virility in males, preventing miscarriages, and curing muscular weakness
B. Current research has not established the validity of these claims; however, the amounts usually taken in supplements have caused no damage

SUGGESTED READING

Eschleman MM: *Introductory nutrition and diet therapy,* ed 3, Philadelphia, 1996, JB Lippincott.

Grodner: *Foundation and clinical applications of nutrition: a nursing approach,* St. Louis, 1996, Mosby.

Mahan/Stump: *Krause's food, nutrition and diet therapy,* ed 9, Philadelphia, 1996, WB Saunders.

Physicians' desk reference, Montvale, NJ, Medical Economics (published annually).

Pipes PL, Trahms CM: *Nutrition in infancy and childhood,* ed 5, St Louis, 1993, Mosby.

Poleman CR: *Nutrition: essentials and diet therapy,* ed 6, Philadelphia, 1991, WB Saunders.

Williams SR: *Basic nutrition and diet therapy,* ed 9, St Louis, 1992, Mosby.

Williams, SR: *Nutrition and diet therapy,* ed 7, St Louis, 1993, Mosby.

REVIEW QUESTIONS

Answers and rationales begin on p. 139.

1. Preoperatively, which diet would be given to a patient scheduled for a cholecystectomy to prevent further recurrence of her abdominal discomfort?
   ① Broiled fish, boiled potatoes, canned peaches, and skim milk
   ② Lamb, mashed potatoes, ice cream, and coffee
   ③ Hamburger, french fries, and milkshake
   ④ Avocado salad, cookies, and chocolate milk

2. Which of the following recommendations should the nurse recognize as incorrect according to the U.S. dietary guidelines?
   ① Eliminate sugars in your diet
   ② If you must drink alcohol, do so in moderation
   ③ Use salt only in moderation
   ④ Choose plenty of fruits

3. Which of the following recommendations should the nurse make to a 15-year-old high school student who tells her that her typical diet for the day is:

   Breakfast orange juice, toast with butter, 1 egg
   Lunch   hamburger on a roll, milk, apple, ice cream
   Dinner   fish, green beans, diet coke
   Snacks   yogurt, cookies, milk, pear

   ① Increase intake of dairy products
   ② Increase vegetables
   ③ Decrease intake of sweets
   ④ Decrease intake of saturated fats

4. Which of the following vegetables would supply a vitamin that might be lacking in a diet used in the treatment of gallbladder disease?
   ① Oranges and cantaloupe
   ② Sweet potatoes and carrots
   ③ Oranges and bananas
   ④ Raisins and prunes

5. Which of the following meals should the nurse recognize as appropriate for a patient on a moderate sodium restriction?
   ① Corned beef, cabbage, bread, and fresh fruit
   ② Barbecued chicken, fresh corn, and fresh fruit
   ③ Lobster, baked potatoes, and canned peaches
   ④ Macaroni and cheese and cookies

6. A home care nurse is scheduled to make 4 visits today. Which of the following patients in her practice should not be advised to increase protein in their diet?
   ① An elderly gentleman who lives alone and primarily eats vegetables
   ② A recovering alcoholic showing evidence of cachexia
   ③ A teenager who tells the nurse that she is on a grapefruit only diet
   ④ A person on home dialysis with an elevated blood urea nitrogen level

7. A postoperative patient will be on intravenous (IV) fluids for the first several days. What remark made by the patient indicates that she is probably ready to be started on oral feedings?
   ① "I can't wait to see some real food rather than this IV bottle!"
   ② "My stomach is feeling a little distended. Do you think it's because I haven't had anything in it for so long?"
   ③ "My stomach is really rumbling—I don't know why—there's nothing in it!"
   ④ "I'm so glad I don't have any more nausea—what a nuisance that was!"

8. A nurse is teaching a class on proper nutrition to homemakers. One of the students asks the nurse how to supply protein to her family of six when meat is so expensive and they have a limited income. Which of the following menu suggestions should the nurse make to assist this student?
   ① "Pasta is great and it will fill them up."
   ② "Try peanut butter with bread or beans with rice."
   ③ "Don't worry, we really eat too much protein anyway."
   ④ "Satisfy their appetites with vegetables."

9. A postoperative patient has progressed to a full liquid diet. Which of the following meals meets the specifications for a full liquid diet?
   ① Cottage cheese, custard, and coffee
   ② Pureed sweet potatoes, ground beef, and tea
   ③ Banana, baked squash, and custard
   ④ Cream of tomato soup, ice cream, and coffee with cream and sugar

10. A nurse is assisting a physician performing physical exams in a clinic. Which of the following signs should the nurse recognize as a potential clinical sign of poor nutrition?
    ① Complaints of chronic constipation
    ② Feeling of fatigue after exercise
    ③ Sleeping 8 to 10 hours every night
    ④ Smooth reddish-pink mucous membranes

11. Which of the following menus best meets a postoperative patient's needs for a vitamin especially important in tissue healing?
    ① Baked chicken, white rice, and sliced peaches
    ② Liver, mashed potatoes, and carrots
    ③ Roast pork, egg noodles, and baked squash
    ④ Swiss steak in tomato sauce, mashed potatoes, and strawberries

12. Which of the following patients would most benefit from using a jejunostomy tube for supplemental feedings?
    ① A 2-day postoperative or appendectomy patient with positive bowel sounds
    ② A postoperative gastrectomy patient
    ③ A patient with gastric ulcerative disease
    ④ A patient with a fractured hip who is reluctant to eat

13. A patient stops a nurse one day and states her confusion over what she hears about vitamin C. When discussing this vitamin with her, the nurse should include:
    ① Vitamin C is fat soluble and readily stored in the body
    ② Vitamin C has been proven to reduce significantly the incidence and severity of colds
    ③ Deficiency symptoms include night blindness and dry, scaly skin
    ④ Improper storage and cooking can result in food losing its vitamin C

14. A home health care nurse is caring for a patient who is recovering from a mild heart attack. The partner says, "He loves to eat milk, meat, and cheese, especially when his family comes for dinner. How am I ever going to get him to change?" The most appropriate response for the nurse should be:
    ① I will explain all the dangers of not changing his lifestyle
    ② His family will understand the importance of his maintaining his health
    ③ Do the best that you can; his heart attack was mild. He does not have to worry all that much
    ④ Make changes gradually; incorporate small portions of his favorite foods in moderation

15. A neighbor asks a nurse for help in following a recently prescribed low-sodium diet. Which of the following suggestions should the nurse make to assist her neighbor?
    ① Canned vegetables are preferable because their sodium is lost in processing
    ② You will be fine; just do not eat too much meat
    ③ Read your labels carefully. Many foods have hidden sodium
    ④ Check with your health care provider to obtain a list of permitted foods

16. Which of the following statements should indicate to the nurse that a mother understands the dietary needs of her teenage diabetic child?
    ① "Lots of fruit is good, because fruit has natural sugar."
    ② "She can eat my baked goods if I use a sugar substitute."
    ③ "I am definitely going to start serving more pasta and whole grains."
    ④ "I am definitely not going to let her hang around with her friends at fast food places anymore."

17. A home health care nurse is interviewing and assessing a family with a newborn. There are also two toddlers living in the household. Which of the following foods on the kitchen counter would be of most concern to the nurse?
    ① a big bag of popcorn
    ② apples
    ③ chocolate cake
    ④ whole milk

18. A nurse is teaching a class for newborns. A question is asked about when it is appropriate to introduce solid food into the baby's diet. The most appropriate answer to this question should be:
    ① A baby really only needs breast milk for the first year or so
    ② Check with your pediatrician; they all have different opinions
    ③ Check with your pediatrician; however, generally cereals are introduced first at about 5 to 6 months
    ④ Check with your pediatrician; however, generally fruits are introduced first at about 5 to 6 months

19. A patient returns to the med-surg unit after undergoing a total gastrectomy. After 5 days the patient is placed on total parenteral nutrition. The nurse should understand that this means:
    ① A short-term supplementation via nasogastric tube until full oral feedings can be resumed
    ② A long-term method of feeding using different points along the gastrointestinal tract
    ③ Full nutritional support for longer periods of time via a large central vein
    ④ A short-term supplementation via tube placed in a peripheral vein

20. A newly diagnosed HIV patient is angry and withdrawn. He verbalizes to the nurse that he does not understand why she is even bothering to tell him about nutrition, when he is going to die anyway. What should the nurse say at this point?
    ① When you are ready to listen we will talk again
    ② I will leave written material here for you to look at
    ③ Eating well is a way you can maintain your immune system
    ④ I know you feel you have lost control over your life

21. A nurse is teaching a class for cardiac patients. Which of the following statements would best indicate to the nurse that at least one of the patients has understood her presentation?
    ① "If I decrease my fat intake and watch my portion size, this will be a start to improving my health"
    ② "If we could just eliminate cholesterol from the body it would help to solve the problem of coronary artery disease"
    ③ "I have to have some cholesterol in my diet because it has specific functions in the body"
    ④ "I hate to exercise, but I suppose I have to try"

22. A patient has been diagnosed with a peptic ulcer. Which of the following instructions would be most beneficial concerning diet therapy?
    ① Eat a very bland diet; this means no caffeine or spicy foods
    ② Include a lot of dairy products in your diet
    ③ Eat a well-balanced diet and remember to take your medications
    ④ Eat 6 small meals a day, because this will decrease stomach discomfort

23. A patient has had diverticulosis for 5 years. She seems confused about the type of diet to follow. A nurse tells her that current evidence suggests the best diet for diverticulosis is a:
    ① High-fiber diet
    ② Bland diet
    ③ Low-fiber diet
    ④ Low-fat diet

24. An 84-year-old woman is in the health care provider's office complaining of fatigue, anorexia, and indigestion. Which of the following groups of vitamins might be prescribed if the health care provider suspects a deficiency?
    ① A, D, and E
    ② C and B complex
    ③ C and B_{12}
    ④ B_6 and B_{12}

25. A nurse is counseling a 23-year-old woman who is trying to eat a healthier diet. She says she is trying to quit smoking, but is having a hard time doing so. Which of the following vitamins should the nurse recommend as a supplement?
    ① Vitamin A
    ② Vitamin K
    ③ Vitamin C
    ④ Vitamin B

26. A patient has come to the physician's office with a complaint of irregular heartbeat. Following laboratory studies, hypokalemia was diagnosed and he was advised to increase his dietary intake of potassium. He asks the nurse: "What foods are high in potassium?" The nurse's answer should include:
    ① Apricots, oranges, and bananas
    ② Fish liver oils and fortified milk
    ③ Wheat germ and dark green, leafy vegetables
    ④ Dairy products

27. A patient, whose blood pressure has been elevated, tells the nurse that the physician has recommended that he reduce his intake of dietary sodium. The nurse advises the patient to:
    ① Increase canned and processed meats in his diet
    ② Increase dairy products in his diet
    ③ Limit fresh fruits and vegetables
    ④ Substitute spices, herbs, or lemon juice for salt in seasoning his food

28. A nurse in a prenatal clinic is counseling a patient who wants to lose weight. The patient wants to try a high-protein, high-carbohydrate diet. What should the nurse explain to her to promote a safe weight loss plan?
    ① Some fats are needed in any weight loss diet because they perform specific functions in the body
    ② Fats should be eliminated from the diet as much as possible to prevent heart disease
    ③ This diet is dangerous; you could give yourself serious metabolic problems
    ④ This is a healthy diet because protein builds new cells and carbohydrates supply energy

29. A patient confides to a nurse that she is desperate to lose 10 pounds before she goes to a class reunion in 2 weeks. She says that she is going to try eating a fruit diet with lots of water. The best response for the nurse should be:
    ① All nutrients are needed to supply a healthy diet
    ② It is all right for a short period but be certain to take vitamins
    ③ Eat a variety of foods from all levels of the food pyramid; watch your portions and increase exercise
    ④ The fruit will supply you with energy and the water will help circulation

30. The patient has been told by her physician that she has a lactose intolerance. In discussing dietary adjustments the nurse advises the patient to avoid:
    ① Foods containing seeds and nuts
    ② Milk and milk products
    ③ Highly seasoned foods
    ④ Citrus fruits

31. A neighbor asks a nurse for advice on cooking healthy meals for her family. Which of the following should the nurse emphasize?
    ① Raw fruit and vegetables contain more nutrients than cooked vegetables
    ② The more expensive the meat, the more nutrients it contains
    ③ The higher the grade on canned goods, the more nutritious the contents
    ④ Refined cereal products are more nutritious than fortified cereal products

32. A nurse is working in a prenatal clinic. Which of the following patients should she be most concerned about for the potential of nutritional complications?
    ① A patient in her third trimester who has gained 39 pounds
    ② A woman in her third trimester with complaints of heartburn
    ③ An underweight adolescent who confesses to eating erratically
    ④ A 36-year-old primigravida in her second trimester who is slightly anemic

33. A high school student asks the school nurse whether or not he should drink a "special electrolyte solution" because he is in training to make the track team. His specialty is the high jump. The best reply for the nurse should be:
    ① "Yes. Absolutely. They help to replace minerals lost when you sweat."
    ② "For nonendurance events, water is the best solution to prevent dehydration."
    ③ "No, you need a sugar solution to add energy for endurance."
    ④ "Make certain it has vitamins to increase energy."

34. A patient is a newly diagnosed noninsulin dependent diabetic (NIDDM). The nurse should know that this patient is most likely:
    ① A young child of normal weight
    ② An overweight middle-aged individual
    ③ An individual who recently lost 50 pounds over the course of the past year
    ④ An underweight anorexic individual

35. A patient is recovering from burns over 40% of his total body surface area. A high protein high carbohydrate diet is essential for recovery because;
    ① The vitamins supplied will promote healing and supply energy
    ② Extra carbohydrates will assist in counteracting the negative nitrogen balance caused by massive trauma
    ③ Extra calories are needed to allow the person to be active in the rehabilitation process
    ④ Protein is needed for tissue healing and carbohydrates will allow protein to be used for this purpose

36. A patient tells the nurse that she is going on a completely vegetarian diet, which includes no meat or dairy products. In what nutrient would this patient be particularly deficient if she continues on this diet?
    ① Iron
    ② B complex vitamins
    ③ Protein
    ④ Fat-soluble vitamins

37. The nutritional requirements of elderly persons differ from those of younger people. In particular, they will require:
    ① Increased fats
    ② Fewer vitamins and minerals
    ③ Decreased fluid intake
    ④ Fewer calories

38. A patient has been taking a diuretic for the past 3 months. Of the following statements made by the patient, which would alert the nurse to a possible dietary deficiency caused by the diuretic?
    ① "My eyes seem especially sensitive to that light."
    ② "I seem to bruise so easily these days."
    ③ "Every once in awhile my heart feels like it's skipping beats!"
    ④ "I feel so terribly nervous. Do you think I need a tranquilizer?"

39. A patient tells the nurse that she uses mineral oil as a base for her salad dressing. The nurse's best response to this statement should be:
    ① "Why don't you try a vegetable oil instead? Mineral oil can hinder the absorption of some important vitamins."

② "That's a good idea! Mineral oil doesn't add any calories to your diet."

③ "That's a good idea! It even fits into your mother's bland diet."

④ "I would use another type of oil. Mineral oil is high in calories with very few vitamins."

40. A patient is on a bland diet. Her choice of which of the following menus would indicate a good understanding of what a bland diet contains?
① Roast beef, tomato salad, and coffee
② Hamburger, french fries, and coke
③ Steak, baked potatoes, salad, and iced tea
④ Baked filet of sole, baked potato, canned peaches, and milk

41. A mother of a 2-week-old infant is nervous about his feedings. The nurse's advice to her should include:
① Begin infant cereal at 1 month of age
② Do not give honey to the baby until he is at least 1 year old
③ Add sugar or salt to foods if he finds something unpalatable
④ Delay giving egg yolk to the baby until he is 1 year old because this portion of the egg causes most instances of allergic reactions

42. A patient who has a history of family allergies asks what foods she can feed her 4-month-old son Benjamin that would be least likely to cause an allergic reaction. The nurse's most appropriate response would be to suggest:
① Scrambled eggs
② Cow's milk
③ Wheat cereal
④ Rice cereal

43. A young schoolteacher has recently learned that she is pregnant. Her question concerns how she can eliminate morning sickness. The nurse's suggestions to her might include:
① Eat dry toast or crackers when you wake in the morning
② Drink liquids with your meals
③ Increase fat products within your diet
④ Decrease the carbohydrates within your meals

44. A patient has decided to decrease her intake of red meat, but is concerned that she will also be decreasing her intake of iron. The nurse suggests that she can increase her intake of iron by eating additional:
① Yellow vegetables, such as carrots and sweet potatoes
② Milk and dairy products
③ Refined cereal products
④ Dried fruits, such as raisins and apricots

45. The absorption of iron, especially iron from nonmeat sources, can be enhanced significantly if iron is ingested with:
① Milk and dairy products
② Fish liver oils
③ Citrus juices
④ Green, leafy vegetables

46. The diabetic diet is based on the exchange system. In using this system the patient should be instructed that:
① Dietetic or diabetic foods should be used as much as possible
② Only foods listed in the same exchange can be substituted

③ Food exchanges are not particularly important as long as you stay within your recommended calories
④ Substitution within a food exchange for meal planning can only be done by a physician or dietician

47. When visiting friends, a diabetic patient was offered half a cup of blackberries. Since she does not care for blackberries, what would she be able to substitute for them?
① Ice milk
② Pineapple juice
③ Cheddar cheese
④ Pecans

48. For dinner one evening a diabetic patient fries an egg in 1 teaspoon of margarine, has a biscuit with 1 teaspoon of butter, and drinks a cup of black coffee. Out of which exchange lists has she selected her meal?
① One milk, two bread, and one fat exchange
② One meat, one milk, one fruit, and one fat exchange
③ One bread, one meat, and one vegetable exchange
④ One meat, one bread, and two fat exchanges

49. A diabetic patient remarks that in the late afternoon she frequently becomes shaky and feels very nervous. What would the nurse suggest to her as a readily available source of carbohydrate that could get her over this hypoglycemic episode?
① Crackers
② Oranges
③ Bread and butter
④ Cereal

50. A patient is admitted with a diagnosis of chronic renal failure. Which of the following dinner selections would be best suited for this patient?
① Apple juice, 1 oz roast chicken, asparagus, sliced tomatoes, fruit cup, and tea with sugar
② Ground round steak, asparagus, bread and butter, fruit cup, and milk
③ Hamburger with tomato on a bun, potato chips, and a glass of chocolate milk
④ Liver, cottage cheese with peach half, deviled eggs, and coffee with cream and sugar

51. A postoperative patient has just begun a clear liquid diet. Which of the following selections would she be allowed?
① Cream-of-mushroom soup, jello, and tea
② Chicken broth, lime sherbet, and apple juice
③ Beef bouillon, raspberry ice, and tea
④ Beef bouillon, orange juice, and cherry jello

52. A 35-year-old banker is hospitalized with ulcerative colitis. The acute flare-up of his condition has passed, and the nurse should expect him to be placed on a diet:
① Low in residue and high in vitamins and protein
② High in residue and high in vitamins and protein
③ Low in fat and calories
④ Low in sodium and carbohydrates

53. A patient is admitted with a diagnosis of suspected myocardial infarction. He complains about the soft diet ordered by the physician. The nurse explains to the patient that the purpose of this diet is to:
① Reduce the number of calories in his diet
② Decrease peristalsis within the digestive tract
③ Decrease irritation to the digestive tract
④ Reduce the workload on the heart

54. A patient has a problem with atonic constipation probably caused by poor eating habits coupled with his dependence on laxatives. Which of the following menus would be best suited to helping him overcome constipation?
    ① Ground beef patty, boiled potato, baked squash, and milk
    ② Beef stew with carrots and onions, coleslaw, rye bread, and tea
    ③ Macaroni and cheese, peach halves, vanilla ice cream, and milk
    ④ Baked chicken, macaroni, cooked carrots, custard, and coffee

55. The National Institute of Health, the American Heart Association, and the U.S. Surgeon General have issued similar dietary recommendations. Each has stated that the average person should:
    ① Decrease total calories in the diet
    ② Increase carbohydrates to approximately 30% of total caloric intake
    ③ Decrease dietary fat, especially polyunsaturated fats
    ④ Decrease total dietary fats, especially saturated fats

56. According to the food pyramid, milk primarily supplies which nutrients?
    ① Vitamin C and calcium
    ② Calcium and protein
    ③ Iron and calcium
    ④ B-complex vitamins and protein

57. A variety of diets have been used over the years to deal with gastrointestinal disorders. Which statement best describes current thinking concerning diet and peptic ulcer disease?
    ① Eat what you like but avoid foods that are especially irritating
    ② Milk and milk products should be the foundation of peptic ulcer diets
    ③ Food and drink containing caffeine, chocolate, and alcohol can be taken in unrestricted amounts
    ④ Physicians are strongly encouraging compliance with the bland diet for conditions such as peptic ulcer

58. Which of the following statements about diabetes mellitus and diet are correct?
    ① The best kinds of carbohydrates to include are refined, simple carbohydrates
    ② The use of any alcoholic beverage is absolutely prohibited
    ③ The food choices available are extremely limited
    ④ Include high-fiber foods in menu planning

59. Which of the following statements is true?
    ① Blood cholesterol levels of 250 to 300 mg/dl are considered ideal
    ② Of the factors an individual can control, diet has the greatest effect on blood cholesterol levels
    ③ A high ratio of low-density lipoprotein (LDL) to high-density lipoprotein (HDL) is considered desirable
    ④ Lowering blood cholesterol levels requires both medication and dietary adjustments

60. The Food Guide Pyramid recently introduced by the U.S. Department of Agriculture:
    ① Places fruits and vegetables as the foundation of a healthy diet
    ② Graphically illustrates the approximate proportions of various foods needed for a healthy diet
    ③ Places meat, poultry, fish, dry beans, and nuts as the foundation of a healthy diet
    ④ Does not address placing fats, oils, and sweets in the diet

ANSWERS AND RATIONALES

1. Knowledge, planning, health (a)
   ❶ A low-fat diet is recommended to avoid aggravating gallbladder disease. These items are all acceptable on a low-fat diet.
   ② Ice cream would not be allowed on a low-fat diet.
   ③ All these are high-fat foods.
   ④ Avocado and chocolate milk are not allowed on a low-fat diet.

2. Knowledge, planning, health (b)
   ❶ Sugars should be eaten in moderation with an emphasis on complex carbohydrates.
   ②,③,④ These are all recommendations.

3. Comprehension, implementation, health (a)
   ❷ Recommended portions of vegetables are 3 to 5.
   ① Dairy products are adequate.
   ③ Sweets are not excessive.
   ④ Saturated fats are not excessive.

4. Comprehension, planning, physiologic (b)
   ❷ Fat-soluble vitamins are carried by fats. In a low-fat diet fat-soluble vitamins (such as vitamin A) may be deficient.
   ① Good sources of vitamin C, a water-soluble vitamin.
   ③ Good sources of potassium, a mineral.
   ④ Good sources of iron, a mineral.

5. Comprehension, implementation, physiologic (b)
   ❷ This food contains the lowest level of sodium.
   ① Corned beef is very high in sodium.
   ③ Lobster and canned peaches are high in sodium.
   ④ Macaroni and cheese is high in sodium.

6. Comprehension, assessment, physiologic (b)
   ❹ Protein is often restricted with renal patients, particularly with elevated BUN levels.
   ① Vegetables supply a variety of nutrients, however, they supply little protein.
   ② Alcoholics often need protein supplements to counteract poor eating habits.
   ③ Grapefruit supplies fiber and vitamin C, but not protein.

7. Application, assessment, health (b)
   ❸ Rumbling stomach indicates return of bowel sounds, which means peristalsis has started; hence, oral feedings can resume.
   ① Hunger does not necessarily mean bowel sounds have returned.
   ② Distention could indicate lack of peristalsis.
   ④ Although she may be able to tolerate food, this does not indicate return of peristalsis.

8. Comprehension, application, health (b)
   ❷ These foods are complementary proteins and inexpensive ways of supplying essential amino acids.
   ① Pasta does supply vitamins and energy and is healthy for the diet. It does not answer the question about protein.
   ③ This may be true for people in this society, but it does not give her any helpful information.
   ④ It is healthy for them to eat vegetables; however, it does not answer the question.

9. Comprehension, planning, physiologic (b)
   ❹ Contains foods liquid at room or body temperature, also many milk-based foods.
   ① Cottage cheese is on a soft diet.

② Pureed sweet potatoes and ground beef would be on a soft diet.
③ Bananas and baked squash would also be on a soft diet.

10. Knowledge, assessment, physiologic (a)
    ❶ Recurrent constipation can indicate a problem with nutrition.
    ② It is normal to feel fatigue after exertion, particularly if exercise is not done on a regular basis.
    ③ This is a normal pattern for many individuals.
    ④ This is normal for healthy mucous membranes.

11. Comprehension, planning, physiologic (b)
    ❹ The tomato sauce, mashed potatoes, and strawberries are all good sources of vitamin C—the vitamin especially needed for tissue healing.
    ① No good source of vitamin C. Peaches are a source of vitamin A.
    ② Although mashed potatoes supply vitamin C, there are other, better choices. Carrots are a source of vitamin A.
    ③ Squash is a source of vitamin A but none of these foods is a good source of vitamin C.

12. Knowledge, implementation, physiologic (b)
    ❸ This procedure is indicated when the remainder of the GI tract is functioning.
    ① Positive bowel sounds indicate that oral feedings can be given.
    ② You must have a functioning GI tract to use enteral feedings.
    ④ This is a drastic move for a patient refusing to eat. Patient's rights become involved. There are many other noninvasive measures that can be used to encourage intake.

13. Knowledge, implementation, health (b)
    ❹ Practices such as storing vitamin C foods cut up rather than whole, storing unwrapped, and overcooking in large amounts of water will significantly decrease the amount of vitamin C in a substance.
    ① Vitamin C is a water-soluble vitamin that needs to be replenished each day.
    ② Current research indicates vitamin C has a minor effect on reducing the number and severity of cold symptoms.
    ③ Symptoms of vitamin A deficiency, not vitamin C.

14. Comprehension, implementation, health (b)
    ❹ Food habits are established early and are difficult to change. Incorporating favorite foods will enhance compliance.
    ① This is closing communication and may or may not enhance compliance.
    ② This understanding may exist but it does not encourage compliance.
    ③ This attack may have been mild but behaviors should be changed to help prevent a more serious one.

15. Knowledge, implementation, health (a)
    ❸ Most processed foods have sodium added.
    ① Canned vegetables generally have sodium added.
    ② Portions of meat should be monitored because it is high in sodium; however, it is only part of the answer.
    ④ Checking with the physician is always a good idea; however, there are helpful instructions that a nurse can provide.

16. Comprehension, evaluation, physiologic (b)
- ❸ About 60% of total calories of the diet should come from carbohydrates. Of this, 40% should come from complex forms such as pastas and whole grains. They break down more slowly than simple sugars, thus providing a steadier blood level.
- ① About 15% of carbohydrates come from simple sugars such as those found in fruit or milk.
- ② Artificial sweeteners can be used in moderation, but only as part of a balanced diet.
- ④ Teenagers find support with peers and it is important that they spend time with them. Healthy choices can be made at most fast-food restaurants.

17. Knowledge, application, safe environment (a)
- ❶ Popcorn can cause a choking hazard for small children.
- ② Apples are permitted for toddlers.
- ③ Chocolate cake may not be nutritious; unless there is concern about calories it is not a hazard.
- ④ Toddlers should receive whole milk to help promote growth and energy metabolism.

18. Comprehension, application, physiologic (b)
- ❸ Patients should always check with their pediatrician. Cereals, often containing iron supplements, are generally the first foods given, followed by fruits and vegetables. New food should be introduced at 5- to 6-day intervals to detect the possibility of allergic reactions.
- ① Breast milk, with supplements of fluoride and iron being introduced at 4 to 6 months respectively, is recommended. Solid foods are introduced gradually at 5 to 6 months once the need of the infant to suck begins to diminish.
- ② Patients should always check with their pediatrician. It is true that they may have different feelings; however it is in within the realm of nursing practice for the nurse to give patients basic nutritional information.
- ④ Cereals are generally the first foods given.

19. Knowledge, implementation, physiologic (b)
- ❸ TPN is used long term in cases of major surgery, when a patient is unable to obtain sufficient oral nourishment.
- ① TPN does not utilize oral route. Nasogastric tubes are used for short term use (approximately 4 to 6 weeks).
- ② TPN does not utilize the gastrointestinal route.
- ④ PPN (peripheral parenteral nutrition) is short term (approximately 10 days) and placed in a peripheral vein.

20. Application, implementation, health (b)
- ❸ Malnutrition contributes to a compromised immune system. This is one way to have control over his health.
- ① This answer closes communication. How does the nurse know he will ever be ready to talk?
- ② Written material is appropriate after a discussion as a reinforcement.
- ④ The nurse has no way of knowing whether this is true or not.

21. Application, evaluation, health (b)
- ❶ Decreasing fat intake and watching portion size will help to control weight. Weight management is a current recommendation for many coronary conditions.
- ② Cholesterol is supplied in the diet as well as manufactured by the body. It has specific functions in the body.
- ③ Yes, cholesterol has specific functions in the body, but beyond infancy it does not have to be supplied in the diet.

- ④ A negative statement that does not indicate he really understands why exercise is an important part of a changing lifestyle.

22. Application, implementation, physiologic (b)
- ❸ Current medications are very effective in decreasing acid secretions. A well-balanced diet provides nutrients for healing.
- ① A bland diet is no longer considered effective in healing ulcers.
- ② Dairy products provide only transitional relief and contain an undesirable fat content.
- ④ It is better to eat 3 full meals. Any food intake produces acid.

23. Knowledge, implementation, physiologic (b)
- ❶ A high-fiber diet is recommended for diverticulosis because it helps prevent the development of high pressure segments and increases the volume and weight of fecal material in the colon.
- ② Bland diets are sometimes recommended following gastric surgery or in peptic ulcer disease.
- ③ Low-fiber diets may be ordered in diverticulitis (inflammatory stage), ulcerative colitis, or before and after bowel surgery.
- ④ Low-fat diets may be used in gallbladder disease, cardiovascular disease, or obesity.

24. Knowledge, application, physiologic (b)
- ❸ These are symptoms most typical of a deficiency of C and B_{12}. The aging process may increase the need for these nutrients because of impaired absorption and decreased intake.
- ① These are fat soluble and therefore stored in the liver.
- ②,④ The symptoms are not typical of these vitamin deficiencies.

25. Knowledge, implementation, physiologic (b)
- ❸ It is recommended that smokers increase their Vitamin C by approximately 100 mg/day.
- ① Vitamin A is fat soluble and can be toxic in megadoses.
- ② Vitamin K is synthesized by the body.
- ④ Vitamin B has not been shown to be deficient in smokers.

26. Knowledge, planning, physiologic (a)
- ❶ All three are high in potassium.
- ② Good sources of vitamin D but not potassium.
- ③ Good sources of vitamin C but not potassium.
- ④ Good sources of calcium and phosphorus but not potassium.

27. Knowledge, planning, health (b)
- ❹ Table salt contains a great amount of sodium. Substituting other flavorings for salt can make it easier to cut down on the amount of salt used.
- ① Canned and processed meats are high in salt.
- ② Dairy products contain much salt.
- ③ Fresh fruits and vegetables are low in salt and can be used freely on a sodium-restricted diet.

28. Application, implementation, health (b)
- ❶ Fats should be included because they perform specific functions, including providing a feeling of fullness and carrying fat-soluble vitamins A, D, E, and K.
- ② The U.S. dietary guidelines advocate the reduction of total fat intake to no more than 30% of caloric intake.
- ③ This is true, however, it causes alarm and does not give information to promote a healthy choice.

④ Protein does build new cells and carbohydrates supply energy; this does not make this nutrient-restricted diet a healthy diet.

29. Knowledge, implementation, physiologic (a)
❸ A healthy weight-loss diet should be balanced and include exercise.
① This is true but it does not completely answer the question.
② This is false. A variety of nutrients are needed for a healthy diet.
④ This is true, however, it does not answer the question.

30. Knowledge, planning, health (a)
❷ Lactose intolerance refers to the inability to digest milk sugar (lactose) because of a deficiency of the enzyme lactose.
① Contains no milk, so would not interfere with digestion.
③ Contains no lactose, such as in milk products.
④ Contains no lactose.

31. Knowledge, assessment, health (a)
❶ Many nutrients are lost in the cooking process.
② There is no correlation between a meal's price and its nutritive value.
③ Grading of canned goods is related to appearance rather than nutritive value.
④ Refined products have many of the nutrients removed, whereas those that are fortified have had additional nutrients added.

32. Comprehension, implementation, physiologic (b)
❸ Irregular eating habits and age are two factors (among others) that identify potential risk factors.
① This is only 4 pounds above the 25 to 35 pounds recommended for a normal weight woman.
② This is normal; caused by increasing pressure of the uterus on the diaphragm.
④ Anemia in pregnancy is often caused by increased blood volume. True anemia should be diagnosed by blood work and treated by a physician.

33. Application, implementation, health (b)
❷ For nonendurance events plain water prevents dehydration. Minerals are obtained in the diet.
① Minerals can be replaced in the diet.
③ Athletes involved in endurance events may possibly need a 10% sugar solution to replace water and carbohydrates.
④ Vitamins do not provide energy.

34. Knowledge, assessment, physiologic (a)
❷ NIDDM occurs mostly in adults, especially those who are overweight.
① Insulin-dependent diabetes (IDDM) occurs mostly in children.
③ Weight loss over a safe period of time is often an effective control for NIDDM.
④ NIDDM occurs more frequently in overweight individuals.

35. Knowledge, implementation, physiologic (b)
❹ The primary purpose of protein is tissue building. Carbohydrates spare protein from energy use to permit them to be used in tissue building.
① Vitamins are supplied in the food and often in supplements as well. They permit the more efficient use of energy; they do not, however, supply energy.
② Proteins supply nitrogen.

③ This is true; however, it does not completely answer the question.

36. Comprehension, assessment, health (b)
❸ Meat and dairy products are the main source of protein in our diets.
① Green, leafy vegetables and dried fruits can be good sources of iron.
② Bread and cereal group can supply many B complex vitamins.
④ Many fruits and vegetables can be good sources of vitamins A, D, C, and K.

37. Knowledge, assessment, health (a)
❹ Metabolism slows down in the older person; therefore, fewer calories are needed.
① Frequently there is less tolerance to fat and it is harder to digest.
② Vitamin and mineral intake should be maintained, and perhaps increased, to account for decreased absorption.
③ Fluid intake should be increased to help eliminate waste products.

38. Comprehension, evaluation, physiologic (b)
❸ Cardiac arrhythmias are a serious consequence of potassium deficiency. Hypokalemia is frequently associated with diuretic therapy.
① Indicates a deficiency of riboflavin.
② Deficiency of vitamin C.
④ Deficiency of B complex vitamins or niacin.

39. Knowledge, planning, health (b)
❶ Mineral oil is indigestible and, if taken with meals, carries fat-soluble vitamins with it as it leaves the body.
② Because it is indigestible, mineral oil doesn't add calories; but it can't be considered a good idea to use it routinely because of its action on fat-soluble vitamins and as a laxative.
③ Not irritating but not a good idea.
④ Mineral oil adds no calories because it isn't digested.

40. Comprehension, implementation, physiologic (a)
❹ Foods included in a bland diet are mild flavored and nonirritating. They reduce peristalsis and excessive flow of gastric juices.
① Roast beef, tomatoes, and coffee are not allowed on a bland diet; they are too irritating to the digestive tract.
② Fried foods and carbonated beverages are not allowed on a bland diet.
③ Iced beverages and raw vegetables are not allowed on a bland diet.

41. Knowledge, planning, health (c)
❷ Honey contains botulism spores, which could be a problem for very young babies (older children and adults are not affected by the spores).
① Current advice from the American Academy of Pediatrics suggests not beginning solid food until 3 months of age.
③ It is better not to get the baby used to the taste of additives, such as sugar and salt, that have no significant nutritional value.
④ Most allergies to eggs are caused by the white, not the yolk.

42. Knowledge, planning, health (b)
   ❹ Of the choices provided, rice cereal causes the fewest allergic reactions in children.
   ① Eggs, especially the egg white, cause many cases of food allergies.
   ② Cow's milk is known to cause allergic reactions in certain children.
   ③ Wheat, oats, and barley cereals cause more allergic reactions than does rice cereal.

43. Knowledge, planning, health (a)
   ❶ Eating high-carbohydrate foods such as dry toast or crackers on awakening is a common suggestion for alleviating morning sickness.
   ② Fluids should be ingested between meals.
   ③ High-fat foods are a common cause of nausea and should be avoided.
   ④ High-carbohydrate foods may help alleviate the nausea.

44. Knowledge, planning, physiologic (a)
   ❹ Dried fruits are excellent alternative sources of iron.
   ① Good sources of vitamin A, not iron.
   ② Milk and other dairy products contain very little iron.
   ③ Refined cereals have had much of the valuable nutrients removed.

45. Comprehension, planning, physiologic (b)
   ❸ Iron absorption is enhanced when given with vitamin C. Citrus juices are excellent sources of vitamin C.
   ① Milk and dairy products contain no vitamin C.
   ② Fish liver oils contain vitamins A and D, not C.
   ④ Green, leafy vegetables contain vitamins A, E, and K, not C.

46. Knowledge, assessment, health (a)
   ❷ The exchange system is based on the fact that each food within an exchange is equivalent in nutrients to every other one. Therefore substituting one food for another within an exchange does not significantly alter the diet.
   ① One advantage of using the exchange system is that specialized foods are not needed.
   ③ Food exchanges are important to space nutrient ingestion over the entire day so the body is able to metabolize each.
   ④ The recommended number of exchanges is usually set up by a dietician, but substitution is easily done by the diabetic patient.

47. Application, planning, physiologic (a)
   ❷ All fruits and fruit juices are on the fruit exchange and so can be substituted for blackberries.
   ① Milk is on the milk exchange.
   ③ Cheese is on the meat exchange (protein foods).
   ④ Pecans are on the fat exchange.

48. Application, implementation, physiologic (b)
   ❹ An egg, because it is protein, is on the meat exchange, the biscuit on the bread exchange, and the 2 teaspoons of butter are two fat exchanges.
   ① No milk, one bread, and two fat exchanges.
   ② No milk or fruit exchange and two fats.
   ③ No vegetable exchange and two fats (1 teaspoon = one exchange).

49. Comprehension, evaluation, health (a)
   ❷ Oranges and orange juice are readily digestible and absorbed carbohydrate.
   ① Crackers are a starchy carbohydrate and take longer to be digested and absorbed.
   ③ Bread and butter (starch and fat) both take longer to be absorbed.
   ④ Cereal is also a starch and takes longer to be absorbed.

50. Application, planning, physiologic (b)
   ❶ Low protein provided by this diet limits end products of protein metabolism—an important consideration in kidney disease.
   ② Steak and milk provide more protein than is desirable for this patient.
   ③ Hamburger and milk provide protein not desirable in this case.
   ④ Liver, cottage cheese, eggs, and cream provide a high-protein diet.

51. Knowledge, planning, physiologic (a)
   ❸ Clear liquids, nonresidue, nonirritating, and non–gas forming.
   ① Cream-based soups are considered full liquids.
   ② Sherbet is a full liquid.
   ④ Orange juice is a full liquid.

52. Knowledge, planning, physiologic (a)
   ❶ A diet low in residue to avoid irritating the colon, but high in vitamins and proteins to replace nutrients that are frequently lost in ulcerative colitis and provide for tissue repair.
   ② High residue may further irritate the already irritated colon.
   ③ Patients with colitis frequently need increased amounts of calories.
   ④ No reason for low-sodium or low-carbohydrate diet.

53. Knowledge, implementation, physiologic (b)
   ❹ Soft diets are easier to digest, thereby reducing the workload of the heart.
   ① Unless the patient is overweight, no specific reason to reduce calories.
   ② Not the primary reason for the soft diet in this situation.
   ③ Decreasing irritation to the digestive tract would be a consideration in certain gastrointestinal disorders, not cardiovascular.

54. Application, planning, physiologic (b)
   ❷ A high-fiber diet provides the bulk that stimulates peristalsis, thereby decreasing constipation.
   ① Very little residue is provided by this diet.
   ③ All foods on this diet provide very little residue.
   ④ Again, very little residue the way these foods are prepared.

55. Knowledge, assessment, health (b)
   ❹ Fats, especially saturated fats, are prime contributors to high blood cholesterol levels and atherosclerotic heart disease.
   ① Total calories need to be reduced only if the individual is overweight.
   ② Carbohydrates should constitute approximately 50% to 60% of total caloric intake.
   ③ Polyunsaturated fats should replace saturated fats in dietary considerations.

56. Knowledge, assessment, health (a)
   ❷ Milk and milk products are excellent sources of calcium and protein.
   ① Milk and milk products are poor sources of vitamin C.
   ③ Milk is a poor source of iron.
   ④ Milk is a poor source of B complex vitamins.

57. Knowledge, assessment, health (b)

❶ Currently, medical experts think that the severe restrictions of the past are not warranted and that a diet of omitting only what irritates is healthier.

② Milk increases the secretion of gastric acid more than it buffers it.

③ Caffeine, chocolate, and alcohol are strong stimulants of gastric acid.

④ Use of the bland diet has decreased because there is no evidence that such a restrictive diet helps the healing process.

58. Knowledge, planning, health (a)

❹ Including high-fiber foods in menu planning lowers blood glucose and blood cholesterol levels.

① The best carbohydrates are unrefined, high-fiber, complex carbohydrates.

② Although it should be taken with food and in limited amounts, a moderate amount of alcohol (1 to 2 oz once or twice a week) can be consumed.

③ The exchange list system of menu planning allows a wide variety of food choices.

59. Knowledge, planning, health (a)

❷ The two primary sources of cholesterol are the diet and that which is synthesized by the body. Diet is the primary controllable factor.

① The recommendation is that blood cholesterol levels be maintained at below 200 mg/dl.

③ LDL is considered to be "bad cholesterol" and should be lowered in relation to HDL.

④ Dietary treatment is the primary treatment for high blood cholesterol. Medications are added only if dietary measures fail to bring cholesterol levels down to targeted levels.

60. Knowledge, assessment, environment (c)

❷ The pyramidal shape graphically places those foods to be eaten the most (breads, cereals, and pasta) at the broad base, followed upward by lesser foods to the tip, which illustrates that fats, oils, and sweets are to be eaten sparingly.

① Breads, cereals, and pasta are at the base, followed by fruits and vegetables.

③ Only 2 to 3 servings of meats, poultry, fish, and eggs are needed as compared with 6 to 11 servings of cereal and pasta.

④ Fats, oils, and sweets are at the top of the pyramid, indicating that they are to be eaten sparingly.

Chapter 5 Medical-Surgical Nursing

This chapter presents the nursing assessment of medical-surgical patients and is grouped according to the body system affected. Following the nursing process, frequent patient problems and recommended nursing care are identified and discussed. A selected group of major diagnoses, medical management, and nursing care plans is included. Although assessment of each system's functioning and problems is isolated, the student must remember that total patient assessment is necessary each time a patient is given care. The chapter begins with a brief overview of anatomy and physiology before moving on to the anatomy and physiology of the individual body systems, which precede the respective medical diagnoses. Nursing assessment, care and responsibility for the patient before and after surgery, diagnostic testing, and nursing care procedures are discussed. Medications, the specific nursing responsibilities they entail, and their adverse effects are addressed in Chapter 3, Pharmacology.

ANATOMY AND PHYSIOLOGY: AN OVERVIEW

A. Anatomy: the study of the structure of the body, its many parts, and their relationship to one another
B. Physiology: the study of how the body and its many parts function
C. Homeostasis: a state of constancy or equilibrium within the body
D. Anatomic terminology
  1. Anatomic position: the body is erect, with arms at sides and palms turned forward
  2. Anterior: toward the front of the body
  3. Posterior: toward the back of the body
  4. Cranial: near the head
  5. Superior: toward the head
  6. Inferior: toward the lower aspect
  7. Medial: toward the midline
  8. Lateral: toward the side
  9. Proximal: nearest the origin of a structure
  10. Distal: farthest from the origin of a structure
E. Body cavities
  1. Dorsal: pertaining to the back; has two subdivisions that are continuous with each other
    a. Cranial: the space inside the skull; contains the brain
    b. Spinal: extends from the cranial cavity nearly to the end of the vertebral column; contains the spinal cord
  2. Ventral: pertaining to the front; contains structures of the chest and abdomen; has two subdivisions
    a. Thoracic: chest cavity; contains the heart, lungs and large blood vessels; separated from the lower cavity by the diaphragm
    b. Abdominopelvic: one large cavity with no separation
      (1) Abdominal: upper portion; contains stomach, liver, gallbladder, pancreas, spleen, kidneys, and most of the intestines
      (2) Pelvic: lower portion; contains urinary bladder, lower part of intestines and internal reproductive organs

Structural Units

CELL

A. Definition: the basic unit of structure and function of all living things; made of protoplasm (meaning "original substance"), which is composed of carbon, oxygen, hydrogen, sulfur, nitrogen, and phosphorus; vary in size and shape
B. Structures and functions
  1. Structural parts
    a. Cytoplasmic membrane: keeps cell whole and intact; allows certain substances to pass through and prevents others from entering
    b. Cytoplasm: area where most cellular activity occurs; the working and storage area
    c. Nucleus: the control center; directs cell activity and is necessary for reproduction; the site of the genetic material DNA
  2. Characteristics of cells
    a. Irritability: responds to stimuli
    b. Growth and reproduction: gets larger in size and continues species
    c. Metabolism: chemical reaction consisting of:
      (1) Anabolism: forming new substances to build new cell material
      (2) Catabolism: breaking down of substances into simpler substances and disposing of waste
    d. Contractability: the ability to shorten
    e. Conductivity: ability to transfer an electrical charge
  3. Functions
    a. Movement of substances through cell membranes
      (1) Diffusion: movement of particles and water molecules through a fluid or membrane; dissolved particles become evenly distributed throughout fluid
      (2) Osmosis: movement of water and particles through a semipermeable membrane
      (3) Filtration: movement of water and particles through a membrane because of a greater pushing force on one side of the membrane
    b. Reproduction mitosis: process of cell division; distributes identical chromosomes (DNA molecules) to each cell formed; enables cells to reproduce their own kind

TISSUES

A. Definition: groups of similar cells having like functions
B. Classifications and functions
  1. Epithelial: cells are packed close together; contain no blood vessels; three main types
    a. Simple squamous: single layer of cells that substances can pass through; function is absorption; lines air sacs of lungs, lines blood vessels, and covers membranes that line body cavity
    b. Stratified squamous: several layers of closely packed cells; protect the body against invasion of microorganisms; outer layer of skin, epidermis
    c. Simple columnar: single layer of cells; lines the stomach, intestines, and respiratory tract; specializes in secreting mucus and in absorption
  2. Connective: cells are separated by intercellular material; located in all parts of the body; various types include areolar, adipose, bone, and cartilage; function is to support and protect.
  3. Muscle: three types of muscle tissue
    a. Skeletal or striated (voluntary): cells have striations; attach to bones; contractions are controlled voluntarily; cause movement
    b. Cardiac or striated (involuntary): cells have cross striations; contractions cannot be controlled; compose heart muscle; cause movement
    c. Visceral or nonstriated (smooth involuntary): cells appear smooth; help form walls of blood vessels and intestines; contractions cannot be controlled; cause movement
  4. Nerve: composed of cells called neurons; all neurons receive and conduct electrochemical impulses; important in control of the entire body

MEMBRANES

A. Definition: thin, soft sheets of tissue that cover, line, lubricate, and anchor body parts
B. Classification and functions
  1. Epithelial: lubricate and protect the body against infection; two types
    a. Mucous: line body cavities that open to the exterior (mouth, nose, intestinal tract, and urinary tract);

secrete mucus, which protects against bacterial invasion

   b. Serous: line cavities that do not open to the exterior; cover the lungs, stomach, and heart; secrete thin fluid that prevents friction

  2. Connective: cover bone or hold body parts in place

   a. Skeletal: cover bones and cartilage; support the bony structure

   b. Synovial: line joint cavities and secrete synovial fluid, which lubricates

   c. Fascial or fibrous: hold organs in place; superficial, connects the skin to underlying structures; deep, supports the internal organs (the viscera)

ORGANS

Structures composed of several tissues grouped together; they perform a more complex function than a single tissue; their composition and structure depend on their function

SYSTEMS

A. Definition: groups of organs that contribute to the function of the whole; they perform a more complex function than a single organ; no system can function independently of another system

B. Body systems and functions
  1. Integumentary (skin): covers and protects the body
  2. Musculoskeletal: supports and allows movement; body's framework
  3. Circulatory: transports food, water, oxygen, and waste
  4. Digestive: processes food and eliminates waste
  5. Respiratory: supplies oxygen and eliminates carbon dioxide
  6. Urinary: excretes waste
  7. Nervous: controls and coordinates body activities
  8. Endocrine: regulates body activities
  9. Reproductive: reproduction

THE MUSCULOSKELETAL SYSTEM
Anatomy and Physiology
Skeletal System (Fig. 5-1)

A. Functions
  1. Support: forms framework for body structures and provides shape
  2. Protection: protects the internal organs
  3. Movement: serves as levers that are activated by the contraction of an attached muscle
  4. Mineral storage: stores calcium and minerals used by the body when needed
  5. Produces blood cells: forms erythrocytes and thrombocytes and red marrow of bone

B. Bone composition
  1. Bone composed of 33% organic material and 67% inorganic mineral salts
  2. Collagen: organic part derived from a protein; fibrous material with a jellylike substance between the fibers; gives bone flexibility
  3. Inorganic substance consists of large amount of mineral salts, calcium phosphate, calcium carbonate, calcium fluoride, magnesium phosphate, sodium oxide, and sodium chloride; these minerals give bone its hardness and durability

C. Classification of bones

  1. Long bone: consists of diaphysis, epiphysis, and medullary cavity (e.g., femur)
  2. Short bone: contains more spongy bone than compact; generally cube shaped (e.g., wrist bone)
  3. Flat bone: thin and flat; has two thin layers of compact bone with a spongy bone between them; red blood cells are manufactured here (e.g., sternum)
  4. Irregular: do not fall into preceding categories; are not symmetrical (e.g., vertebrae)

D. Structure of long bones
  1. Similar to other bones in the body as to structure, development, and function
  2. Longer than wide; have a shaft with heads at both ends; bones of extremities are long bones
  3. Diaphysis or shaft: hollow cylinder of hard compact bone; contains medullary canal, which is filled with yellow bone marrow; in the adult it is primarily a storage area for adipose fat
  4. Epiphysis: the ends of the diaphysis composed of spongy bone covered by a thin layer of compact bone; contains red marrow where some red blood cells are manufactured during childhood and adolescence; erythropoietic activity in the adult mainly occurs in flat bones and vertebrae
  5. Periosteum: strong fibrous membrane that covers the bone; contains blood vessels, lymph vessels, nerves, and bone cells necessary for growth, repair, and nutrition
  6. Epiphyseal disk (flat plate of hyaline cartilage): allows for lengthwise growth of long bones; at puberty when growth stops, it calcifies and becomes the epiphyseal line
  7. Haversian canals: run lengthwise through bone matrix, carrying blood vessels and nerves to all areas of the bone; nourish the osteocytes or bone cell

E. Processes: bony prominences that serve as landmarks
  1. Acromion: highest point of the shoulder
  2. Olecranon: the upper end of the ulna, forms the point of the elbow
  3. Iliac crest: curved rim along the upper border of the ilium
  4. Ischial spine: lies at the back of the pelvic outlet
  5. Acetabulum: the deep socket in the hip bone
  6. Greater trochanter: the large protuberance located at the top of the shaft of the femur

F. Factors that affect bone growth and maintenance
  1. Heredity: each person has a genetic potential for height with genes inherited from both parents
  2. Nutrition: nutrients such as calcium, phosphorus, and proteins are raw materials of which bones are made of; without nutrients bones cannot grow properly
  3. Hormones: produced by endocrine glands; help regulate cell division, protein synthesis, calcium metabolism, and energy production
  4. Exercise: bearing weight, such as walking; without exercise bones become thin and fragile

G. Joints: point where bones meet; classification is determined by extent of movement
  1. Synarthroses: fibrous connective tissue holds joining bones close together; no movement (e.g., sutures in skull)
  2. Amphiarthroses: slight movement (e.g., joints between the vertebrae)
  3. Diarthroses: free movement; all have a joint capsule, a joint cavity, and a layer of cartilage

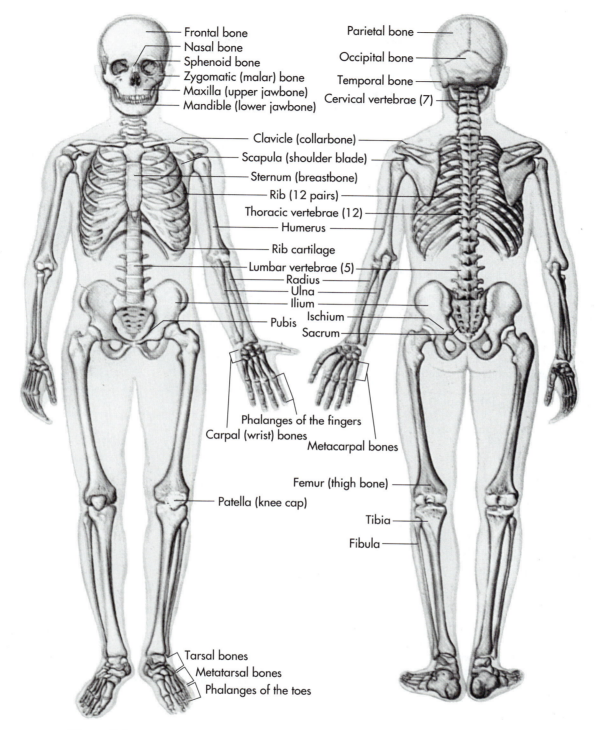

Frontal bone
Nasal bone
Sphenoid bone
Zygomatic (malar) bone
Maxilla (upper jawbone)
Mandible (lower jawbone)

Parietal bone
Occipital bone
Temporal bone
Cervical vertebrae (7)

Clavicle (collarbone)
Scapula (shoulder blade)
Sternum (breastbone)
Rib (12 pairs)
Thoracic vertebrae (12)
Humerus
Rib cartilage
Lumbar vertebrae (5)
Radius
Ulna
Ilium
Ischium
Pubis
Sacrum

Phalanges of the fingers
Carpal (wrist) bones
Metacarpal bones

Femur (thigh bone)

Patella (knee cap)

Tibia
Fibula

Tarsal bones
Metatarsal bones
Phalanges of the toes

Figure 5-1.   **The skeletal system.** (From Milliken ME, Campbell G: *Essential competencies for patient care,* St Louis, 1985, Mosby.)

a. Ball-and-socket joint: ball-shaped head of one bone fits into a concave socket of another bone (e.g., hip joint)
b. Hinge joint: allows movement in only two directions, flexion and extension (e.g., knee)
c. Pivot joint: small projection of one bone pivots in an arch of another bone (e.g., vertebrae of the neck)

d. Saddle joint: exists only between the metacarpal bone and a carpal bone of the wrist (e.g., thumb and wrist)
e. Gliding joint: bone surfaces slide over one another (e.g., wrist/ankle)
H. Ligaments: connective tissue bands that hold bones together
I. Tendons: connective tissue bands that attach bones to muscles
J. Bursa: a sac or cavity filled with fluid that reduces friction

Muscular System (Fig. 5-2)

A. Functions
1. Produces movement by contraction (Table 5-1)
2. Maintains posture
3. Produces heat and energy

B. Structure and types
1. Striated: skeletal, voluntary muscle; attached to bones and accounts for body movement; controlled consciously
2. Smooth: visceral, nonstriated, involuntary muscle; found in the walls of internal organs and blood vessels; works automatically
3. Cardiac: found only in the heart; striated, branched, and involuntary

C. Characteristics
1. Excitability: capacity to respond to stimulus
2. Contractility: ability to shorten and tighten
3. Extensibility: ability to stretch
4. Elasticity: ability to regain original size and shape
5. Tonicity: ability to maintain steady contraction

D. Contraction and movement
1. Muscles move bones by pulling on them; as muscle contracts, it pulls insertion bone toward its original bone
   a. Origin: attached to fixed structure of bone
   b. Insertion: attached to movable part
2. Several muscles contract at the same time to produce movement
   a. Prime mover: mainly responsible for producing movement
   b. Synergists: aid the prime mover in producing movement
3. To contract, muscle must first be stimulated by nerve impulses
   a. Subminimal stimulus: does not cause contraction
   b. Minimal stimulus: does cause contraction
   c. Maximal stimulus: causes all muscle fibers in muscle to contract
   d. Supramaximal stimulus: strength of stimulus is above maximal; no effect on strength of contraction
4. Types of contraction
   a. Isometric: increases the tension without causing movement
   b. Isotonic: produces movement
   c. Tonic: does not produce movement but increases firmness of muscles that maintain posture
   d. Twitch: a quick, jerky contraction
   e. Tetanic (tetanus): sustained contraction
5. Types of movement
   a. Flexion: makes angle at joint smaller
   b. Extension: makes angle at joint larger
   c. Abduction: moves part away from midline
   d. Adduction: moves part toward midline

MUSCULOSKELETAL CONDITIONS/DISORDERS

Musculoskeletal disorders may be acute or chronic. Acute problems are usually related to simple injuries. Chronic disorders may be more distressing to the patient because of loss of mobility and changes in self-image. The nurse needs to possess good skills in observation, positioning the patient safely, and use and care of equipment. The nurse is probably the most important health care provider in preventive care associated with complications of immobility.

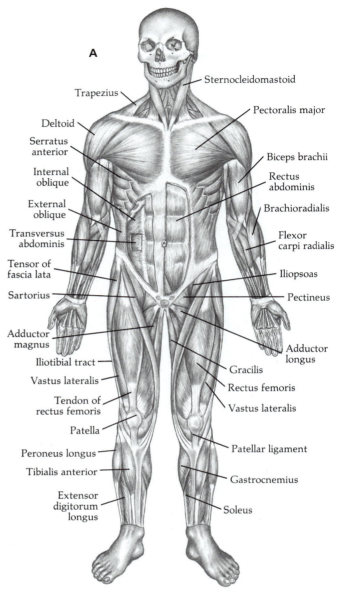

Figure 5-2.   Skeletal muscles of body. A, Anterior view. (From Thompson J, McFarland GK, Hirsch JE et al: *Mosby's clinical nursing,* ed 3, St Louis, 1993, Mosby.)

Nursing Assessment

A. Nursing observation (objective data)
1. General appearance
   a. Age
   b. Weight loss or weight gain
   c. Height changes: loss
   d. Abnormal gait
   e. Absence of extremity
   f. Deformity
   g. Malalignment
   h. Use of assistive devices
   i. Spinal curvature
2. Respirations
   a. Rate
   b. Depth
   c. Character; any difficulty

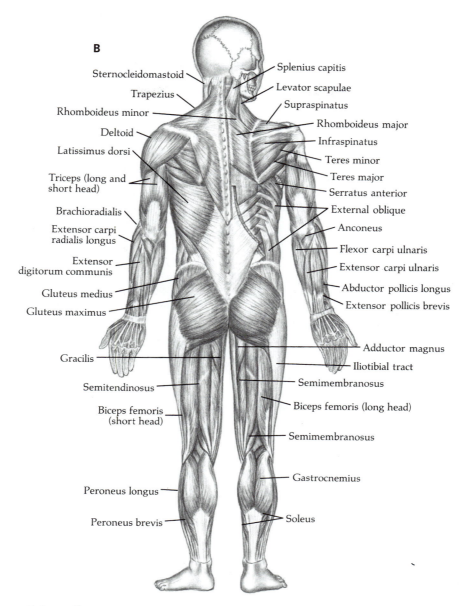

B

Sternocleidomastoid
Trapezius
Rhomboideus minor
Deltoid
Latissimus dorsi
Triceps (long and short head)
Brachioradialis
Extensor carpi radialis longus
Extensor digitorum communis
Gluteus medius
Gluteus maximus
Gracilis
Semitendinosus
Biceps femoris (short head)
Peroneus longus
Peroneus brevis

Splenius capitis
Levator scapulae
Supraspinatus
Rhomboideus major
Infraspinatus
Teres minor
Teres major
Serratus anterior
External oblique
Anconeus
Flexor carpi ulnaris
Extensor carpi ulnaris
Abductor pollicis longus
Extensor pollicis brevis
Adductor magnus
Iliotibial tract
Semimembranosus
Biceps femoris (long head)
Semimembranosus
Gastrocnemius
Soleus

Figure 5-2. cont'd.   Skeletal muscles of body. B, Posterior view. (From Thompson JM, McFarland GK, Hirsch JE et al: *Mosby's clinical nursing,* ed 3, St Louis, 1993, Mosby.)

Table 5-1	The Skeletal Muscles	
Muscle	**Location**	**Function**
Sternocleidomastoid	Neck	Flexion and rotation of head
Trapezius	Upper back	Helps hold head erect; also assists in moving the head sideways
Latissimus dorsi	Lower back	Extension and adduction of upper arm
Pectoralis major	Chest	Flexion and adduction of upper arm
Deltoid	Shoulder	Abduction of upper arm
Biceps brachii	Anterior upper arm	Flexion of arm and forearm
Triceps brachii	Posterior upper arm	Extension of arm and forearm
Gluteus maximus	Fleshy part of hips and buttocks	Extension of thigh
Gluteus medius	Lateral part of hips and buttocks	Abduction of thigh when limb is extended
Hamstring group	Posterior thigh	Flexion of lower leg and extension of thigh
Quadriceps femoris	Anterior thigh	Flexion of thigh and extension of lower leg
Gastrocnemius	Calf of leg	Helps in extension of foot and flexion of leg

3. Pulse
  a. Presence of: check above and below injured/casted part
  b. Rate, quality, character
4. Neurovascular status
  a. Assessment of skin color and temperature
  b. Pulses, presence of
  c. Intact sensation (noting numbness)
  d. Motor function
  e. Sensation and capillary refill
5. Motor function
  a. Compare affected and unaffected sides
  b. Limited ability or loss of ability to move body part
  c. Diminished muscle strength to passive resistance
  d. Limited range of motion (ROM)
  e. Degree of ability to perform activities of daily living (ADLs)
6. Pain and swelling
  a. Location, character, frequency duration, alleviating/aggravating factors
  b. Bony enlargements or soft tissue swelling
B. Patient description (subjective data)
  1. Pain
    a. Patient's account of location, character, frequency, duration, onset
  2. Stamina
    a. Weakness, fatigue
    b. Changes in ability to perform activities of daily living
  3. Report of recent injury
    a. Description
    b. Evaluation/treatment
  4. Motor function
    a. Pain with movement
    b. Limited movement/difficult gait
  5. General
    a. Maintenance of weight
    b. Changes in appetite
    c. Tolerance of activities of daily living

Diagnostic Tests/Methods

A. Serum laboratory studies
  1. Complete blood count (CBC): an aid in determining anemia or the presence of infection
  2. Erythrocyte sedimentation rate (ESR): elevation is evidenced during inflammatory processes
  3. Rheumatoid factor: a protein found in the blood of most persons afflicted with rheumatoid arthritis
  4. Uric acid: high concentration is found in persons who have gout
  5. Lupus erythematosus (LE) cell
    a. A cell identified in persons with lupus
    b. Normally there are no LE cells in the blood
B. Procedures
  1. Roentgenogram (x-ray): a film to determine the presence of a deformity, fracture, or tumor of the skeletal system
  2. Aspiration: withdrawal of fluid from a joint to obtain a specimen for diagnostic purposes
  3. Bone biopsy: removal and examination of bone tissue
  4. Myelogram: x-ray examination of the spinal cord after injection with radiopaque dye

5. Bone scan: isotope imaging of the skeleton
6. Computerized tomography (CT): use of roentgen rays to provide accurate images of thin cross sections of the body
7. Magnetic resonance imaging (MRI): aid for the diagnosis of musculoskeletal conditions through the clear differentiation of various types of tissue, such as bones, fat, and muscle
8. Arthroscopy: endoscopic examination that allows for direct visualization of a joint
9. Electromyography (EMG): used to evaluate nerve conduction in skeletal muscle
10. Positron emission tomography (PET): using an isotope, scans the brain for evaluation of structure function
C. Nursing intervention for myelogram
  1. After procedure, have patient remain flat in bed 12 to 24 hours before allowing him or her to resume usual activities
  2. Encourage fluids to 2000 to 3000 ml every 24 hours
  3. Observe for alterations in normal motor and sensory states
  4. Observe for nausea and vomiting

Frequent Patient Problems and Nursing Care

A. Disturbance in self-concept; body image related to immobility
  1. Provide atmosphere of acceptance
  2. Express empathy, warmth, and friendliness
  3. Encourage acceptance of self-limitations
  4. Encourage self-performance
B. Impairment of skin integrity; potential breakdown related to immobility/assistive devices
  1. Change the patient's position frequently
  2. Keep the skin clean, dry, and lubricated
  3. Massage bony prominences
  4. Provide sheepskin or polyurethane foam padding
C. Potential for injury: joint contracture related to incorrect body alignment
  1. Place hands, feet, and knees in the natural position of function
  2. Provide devices to protect against poor alignment of body part
  3. Assist in performance of active and passive ROM exercises
  4. Provide trapeze over the patient's bed
  5. Avoid knee gatch position/pillow under knee
D. Potential respiratory secretion congestion related to ineffective airway clearance
  1. Change the patient's position frequently
  2. Encourage coughing and deep breathing
  3. Observe for coughing, fever, and green-yellow sputum
E. Potential thrombus and emboli related to impaired physical mobility/edema
  1. Encourage patient to move lower extremities
  2. Encourage adequate hydration
  3. Avoid use of knee gatch/pillow under knee
  4. To avoid release of emboli, never rub legs
  5. Use of elastic stockings
  6. Daily calf measurements
F. Bone pain related to bone fracture or disease
  1. Inspect and palpate the painful site looking for inflammation, edema, bruising, tenderness, and skin warmth

2. Support the affected body part
3. Apply warm, moist compress to affected body part where prescribed
4. Give prescribed analgesic
5. Evaluate effectiveness of pain relief measures

G. Potential limited ROM related to cast or traction confinement, joint pain, stiffness, or inflammation
   1. Explain the reason for and intended effect of ROM exercises
   2. Maintain body alignment
   3. Provide total exercising of muscles and joints except if severe pain or inflammation is present; contraindicated if recent surgery was performed on or near the joint

H. Alteration in comfort: pain related to cast
   1. Massage the area around the cast, except for leg casts
   2. Pad rough edges
   3. Elevate extremity
   4. Inspect the skin for irritation
   5. Observe for cyanosis of the extremity in a cast
   6. Observe for complaints of numbness and tingling of extremity
   7. Observe cast for indentations

I. Self-care deficits (feeding, bathing, and hygiene) related to impaired physical mobility
   1. Assist with ADLs
   2. Provide self-care aids/devices
   3. Teach self-care activities

Major Medical Diagnoses

RHEUMATOID ARTHRITIS

A. Definition: a chronic, systemic disease in which inflammatory changes occur throughout the body's connective tissue destroying joints internally; joints most involved are hands, wrists, elbows, knees, and ankles

B. Pathology: cause is unknown; related theories include autoimmune, microorganisms, viruses, and genetic predisposition

C. Signs and symptoms
   1. Subjective
      a. Sore, stiff, swollen joint(s)
      b. Fatigue
      c. Weakness
      d. Malaise
      e. Loss of appetite
   2. Objective
      a. Low-grade fever
      b. Weakened grip
      c. Anemia
      d. Weight loss
      e. Subcutaneous nodes
      f. Enlarged lymph nodes
      g. Joint deformity
      h. Muscle atrophy
      i. Limited ROM
      j. Edema and tenderness of joint
      k. Extraarticular symptoms: lung, heart, blood vessels, muscle, eye, and skin

D. Diagnostic tests/methods
   1. Elevated ESR
   2. Slightly elevated white blood cell (WBC) count
   3. Presence of serum rheumatoid factors
   4. Synovial fluid aspiration
   5. X-ray film reveals joint deformity
   6. Low hemoglobin and hematocrit

E. Treatment
   1. Antiinflammatory agents, analgesics, corticosteroids, gold salts, and immunosuppressive drugs
   2. Heat applications such as paraffin dip, hot packs, and warm tub baths or showers for analgesia or muscle relaxation
   3. Surgical intervention to prevent deformities or remove damaged joints
   4. Physical therapy to maintain optimal function

F. Nursing intervention
   1. Provide undisturbed periods of rest
   2. Use firm mattress, foot boards, splints, and sandbags to maintain proper body alignment
   3. Encourage self-performance activities such as combing hair, feeding self, and brushing teeth
   4. Provide ROM exercises within limits of pain tolerance

OSTEOARTHRITIS

A. Definition: a local joint disorder affecting weight-bearing joints; results in disintegration of the cartilage covering the ends of bones

B. Pathology: cause is unknown; predisposing factors include aging, joint trauma, and obesity

C. Signs and symptoms
   1. Subjective
      a. Pain after exercise; relieved by rest
      b. Morning stiffness
      c. Muscle spasms
      d. Reduced strength
   2. Objective
      a. Limited ROM
      b. Crepitant joint
      c. Prominent bony enlargement

D. Diagnostic tests: x-ray studies reveal joint abnormalities

E. Treatment
   1. Weight reduction to relieve strain
   2. Heat and massage for aching and stiffness
   3. Physical therapy to maintain optimum level of functioning
   4. Drugs to relieve symptoms
      a. Analgesics
      b. Antiinflammatory agents
      c. Steroids
   5. Surgical intervention to prevent deformity, relieve inflammation, delay progression, or replace affected joint

F. Nursing intervention
   1. Encourage patient to express feelings concerning disorder
   2. Provide moist heat, massage, and prescribed exercise, if ordered, to relax muscle and relieve stiffness or discomfort

GOUTY ARTHRITIS (GOUT)

A. Definition: a disorder in which excessive amounts of uric acid are retained in the blood

B. Pathology
   1. Cause is related to a disorder of purine metabolism
   2. Uric acid crystals are deposited in the joints and cartilage and form lumps (tophi)

3. Deposits cause local irritation and an inflammatory response
4. Men older than 30 years of age are most commonly affected

C. Signs and symptoms
1. Subjective
    a. Acute pain, swelling, and inflammation of great toe (most affected joint)
    b. Headache
    c. Malaise
    d. Anorexia
    e. Pruritus (local)
2. Objective
    a. Skin over joint is swollen, warm, and red
    b. Limited ROM
    c. Tophi located in cartilage of ears, hands, and feet

D. Diagnostic tests/methods
1. Elevated serum uric acid level
2. Elevated ESR and WBC count

E. Treatment
1. Dietary restriction of foods high in purines
2. Uricosuric drugs to increase uric acid excretion
3. Allopurinol to inhibit uric acid formation
4. Colchicine to reduce pain and relieve swelling
5. Alkaline ash diet to increase urinary pH
6. Weight loss

F. Nursing intervention
1. Instruct patient to avoid foods high in purine content: liver, kidney, sweetbreads, sardines, and brains
2. Encourage physical activity to promote optimal muscular and skeletal function
3. Place bed cradle to prevent pain of part by linen pressure
4. Encourage fluid intake of 2000 to 3000 ml daily to avoid renal calculi unless contraindicated
5. Instruct patient to limit alcohol intake, which may precipitate an acute attack
6. Instruct patient to avoid salicylates because of antagonistic actions of uricosuric drugs

SYSTEMIC LUPUS ERYTHEMATOSUS (SLE)

A. Definition: a chronic multisystem inflammatory disorder involving the connective tissues, such as the muscles, kidneys, heart, and serous membranes; may affect the skin, lungs, and nervous system

B. Pathology
1. Cause is unknown; is believed to be an autoimmune disorder
2. Inflammation produces fibroid deposits and structural changes in connective tissue of organs and blood vessels
3. Results in problems with mobility, oxygenation, and elimination

C. Signs and symptoms
1. Subjective
    a. Abdominal, joint, and muscle pain
    b. Weakness; fatigue
    c. Depression
2. Objective
    a. Low-grade fever
    b. Weight loss
    c. Butterfly skin rash over bridge of nose and cheeks, which increases with exposure to the sun
    d. Anemia
    e. Alopecia

D. Diagnostic tests
1. Positive LE test
2. Elevated ESR
3. Increased gamma globulin levels
4. Positive antinuclear antibody titer
5. High anti-DNA test

E. Treatment
1. Corticosteroids, analgesics, and medications for anemia
2. Avoidance of exposure to sunlight

F. Nursing intervention
1. Provide emotional support to patient and family in coping with poor prognosis
2. Encourage alternative activity and planned rest periods
3. Instruct to avoid persons with infections, undue exposure to sunlight, and emotional stress, which can cause exacerbations
4. Encourage intake of foods high in iron content: liver, shellfish, leafy vegetables, and enriched breads and cereals

SCLERODERMA (PROGRESSIVE SYSTEMIC SCLEROSIS)

A. Definition: fiberlike changes in the connective tissue throughout the body caused by collagen deposits and subsequent fibrosis

B. Pathology
1. An insidious, chronic, progressive disorder usually beginning in the skin
2. Skin becomes thick and hard; fingers and toes become fixed in a position
3. Other disorders that occur are difficulty in swallowing, impaired gastrointestinal (GI) mobility, cardiac and renal problems, and osteoporosis

C. Signs and symptoms
1. Subjective
    a. Sweating of hands and feet
    b. Stiffness of hands
    c. Muscle weakness
    d. Joint pain
    e. Dysphagia
2. Objective
    a. Increased pigmentation or dyspigmentation
    b. Dilated capillaries of lips, fingers, face, and tongue

D. Diagnostic tests/methods
1. Positive LE cell test
2. False-positive syphilis test

E. Treatment
1. Skin care to prevent formation of decubiti
2. Physical therapy
3. Analgesics for joint pain
4. Corticosteroids

F. Nursing intervention
1. Provide emotional support to patient and family in promoting physical and psychologic needs
2. Encourage moderate exercise to promote muscular and joint function
3. Force fluids
4. Advise to avoid cold temperatures; use gloves to remove items from freezer
5. Plan rest periods

6. Provide assistive devices to help with activities of daily living (eating, grooming)

POLYARTERITIS NODOSA

A. Definition: a collagen disease that results in inflammation and necrosis in the walls of small- to medium-sized arteries
B. Pathology
   1. Impairment of artery supply alters organ systems
   2. Most involved structures are muscles, kidneys, liver, and GI tract
C. Signs and symptoms
   1. Subjective
      a. Prolonged fever
      b. Malaise
      c. Weakness
      d. Weight loss
   2. Objective
      a. Palpable nodules along arterial walls
      b. Subcutaneous nodules
      c. Hematuria
D. Diagnostic tests/methods
   1. Positive rheumatoid factor
   2. Elevated ESR
E. Treatment: corticosteroids
F. Nursing intervention
   1. Provide emotional support to patient and family in dealing with poor prognosis
   2. Provide comfort measures for relief of symptomatic pain
   3. Encourage balanced food intake for weight loss
   4. Encourage moderate exercise, when able, to maintain muscle tone and slow development of disability

OSTEOMYELITIS

A. Definition: bone inflammation caused by direct or indirect invasion of an organism
B. Pathology: bacteria enter bloodstream through an open fracture, open wound, or by secondary invasion from blood-borne infection from a distant site such as bone or infected tonsils
C. Signs and symptoms
   1. Subjective
      a. Tenderness over the bones
      b. Painful movement; limited mobility
      c. Malaise
   2. Objective
      a. Fever
      b. Chills
      c. Heat, swelling, and redness of the skin over the bone
      d. Signs of sepsis
      e. Wound drainage
D. Diagnostic tests/methods
   1. Positive blood cultures
   2. Elevated ESR
   3. Elevated WBC count
   4. X-ray film may not reveal abnormalities for 5 to 10 days from onset
E. Treatment
   1. Antibiotic therapy
   2. Drainage from abscess with continuous irrigation of wound
   3. Surgical removal of necrotic bone

F. Nursing intervention
   1. Use strict aseptic technique when changing dressings
   2. Keep affected limb in proper alignment with pillows and sandbags
   3. Maintain drainage and secretion precautions for disposal of dressings
   4. Provide a high-calorie, high-protein diet and adequate hydration
   5. Provide undisturbed rest periods
   6. Move affected body part gently, because of severe pain

OSTEOPOROSIS

A. Definition: metabolic bone disorder in which bone mass is decreased
B. Pathology
   1. Common in postmenopausal women
   2. May be result of deficit of estrogen and androgens, prolonged immobilization, insufficient calcium intake or absorption, or endocrine disorder
   3. Sites usually affected are vertebrae, pelvis, and femur
C. Signs and symptoms
   1. Subjective: backache; worsens with sitting, standing, coughing, and sneezing
   2. Objective
      a. Kyphosis
      b. Loss of height
      c. Pathologic fractures
D. Diagnostic test: x-ray film reveals bone demineralization and compression of vertebrae
E. Treatment
   1. Physical activity and exercise to prevent disuse atrophy
   2. Estrogen replacement to provide calcium balance
   3. Diet high in protein and calcium
   4. Vitamin D supplements
   5. Support of spine with brace or corset
F. Nursing intervention
   1. Encourage use of walker or cane to stabilize balance when ambulating
   2. Encourage fluid intake of 2000 to 3000 ml daily, unless contraindicated, to avoid formation of renal calculi
   3. Give instruction on those foods high in protein and calcium content
   4. Emphasize need to follow prescribed daily activity and exercise
   5. If confined to bed, give passive and active ROM exercises
   6. Teach safety measures to protect from fractures

OSTEOGENIC SARCOMA

A. Definition: a tumor located in the bone composed of cells derived from connective tissue
B. Pathology
   1. Highly malignant tumor metastasizing through the lymph nodes to the lungs
   2. Affects children, adolescents, and young adults
   3. Usually occurs in shaft of long bones, especially affecting the knee
C. Signs and symptoms
   1. Subjective: pain
   2. Objective:
      a. Restricted ROM
      b. Swelling

c. Weight loss

d. Anemia

D. Diagnostic tests/methods

    1. X-ray examination to reveal lesion in the extremity and chest; CT scan

    2. Biopsy examination to evaluate cells

    3. Frozen section for rapid diagnosis of possible malignant lesion

E. Treatment

    1. Chemotherapeutic agents to reduce and retard growth

    2. Radiation therapy to destroy malignant tissue

    3. Amputation of affected limb or resection of tumor

F. Nursing intervention

    1. Provide emotional support to patient and family to reduce fear and anxiety

    2. Provide diet high in protein and caloric content

    3. If patient undergoes amputation procedure, follow special nursing actions (refer to amputations)

    4. If patient is receiving radiotherapy

       a. Provide noninfectious environment

       b. Avoid ointments, lotions, powders, and washing of port (treated) areas

       c. Do not remove markings on skin

       d. Observe site for redness, swelling, itching, and drying

OSTEOMALACIA

A. Definition: a disorder in which widespread softening and demineralization of bones occur

B. Pathology

    1. Possible causes

       a. Vitamin D deficiency resulting from poor dietary intake of vitamin D

       b. Body's inability to absorb or use vitamin D

       c. Lack of ultraviolet rays

    2. The effect of parathyroid hormone on bone resorption and calcium absorption is decreased

    3. Most affected bones are spine, pelvis, and lower extremities

C. Signs and symptoms

    1. Subjective

       a. Rheumatic-type pain

       b. Weakness

    2. Objective

       a. Waddling gait

       b. Spontaneous fractures

       c. Bone deformities

D. Diagnostic tests/methods

    1. Reduced calcium and phosphorus serum levels

    2. X-ray examination reveals fracturelike lines of affected bones

E. Treatment

    1. Therapeutic doses of vitamin D

    2. High dietary intake of calcium and phosphorus

F. Nursing intervention

    1. Change patient's position gradually

    2. Teach good body mechanics

    3. Encourage intake of foods high in calcium: meat, shellfish, and dark green, leafy vegetables

    4. Emphasize need to maintain weight in normal range

    5. Instruct on avoidance of heavy lifting

    6. Safety measures to prevent fractures

OSTEITIS DEFORMANS (PAGET'S DISEASE OF BONE)

A. Definition: an inflammatory condition in which certain bones become soft, thick, and deformed

B. Pathology

    1. Cause is unknown: occurs mainly in men in middle age or older

    2. Disease disturbs new bone tissue with bones becoming enlarged and coarse in texture

C. Signs and symptoms

    1. Subjective

       a. Bone pain; worsens at night

       b. Tenderness on pressure of the bones

       c. Back pain

       d. Headache from enlarged skull

       e. Deafness or blindness caused by pressure from overgrowth of bone

    2. Objective

       a. Pathologic fractures

       b. Decrease in height

       c. Bowing of femur and tibia

       d. Enlarged skull

D. Diagnostic tests/methods

    1. Skeletal x-ray film reveals bone enlargement and denseness

    2. Elevated serum alkaline phosphate value

    3. Urinary excretion of hydroxyproline is increased

E. Treatment

    1. Androgen therapy for men; estrogen therapy for women to reverse hypercalciuria, if present

    2. Salicylates for pain

F. Nursing intervention

    1. Observe for stress fractures

    2. Emphasize need for maintenance of normal weight

    3. If fracture occurs and patient becomes immobilized

       a. Limit calcium intake to avoid renal calculi

       b. Provide high fluid intake to avoid hypercalcemia

    4. Safety measures to prevent fractures

HERNIATED NUCLEUS PULPOSUS (SLIPPED DISK OR RUPTURE OF INTERVERTEBRAL DISK)

A. Definition: protrusion of the nucleus pulposus, which compresses the nerve roots of the spinal cord

B. Pathology

    1. Site usually affected is between L4 and L5, L5 and sacrum, C5 and C6, or C6 and C7

    2. Causes may be straining of the spine in an unnatural position, degenerative changes, heavy lifting when bending from the waist, and accidents

C. Signs and symptoms

    1. Subjective

       a. Cervical disk

          (1) Stiff neck

          (2) Shoulder pain descending down the arm into the hand

          (3) Numbness of arm and hand

       b. Lumbosacral disk: low-back pain radiating down the posterior thigh

    2. Objective

       a. Cervical disk

          (1) Sensory disturbances of the hand

          (2) Atropy of biceps and triceps

       b. Lumbosacral disk

(1) Difficulty in ambulating
(2) Lasègue's sign: pain in back and leg while raising heel with knee straight
(3) Numbness of leg and foot
(4) Foot drop

D. Diagnostic tests/methods
1. X-ray examination to reveal narrowing disk space
2. Myelogram to localize site
3. Electromyography
4. CT scan of the spine
5. MRI of spine

E. Treatment
1. Cervical traction (cervical disk); traction to lower extremities (lumbosacral disk)
2. Bed rest, heat application, and analgesics
3. Surgical intervention
   a. Laminectomy: removal of a portion of the vertebra and excision of the ruptured portion of the nucleus pulposus
   b. Spinal fusion: permanent binding of the vertebrae
   c. Chemonucleolysis: dissolving of the affected disk through the injection of chymopapain

F. Nursing intervention
1. Encourage patient to verbalize feelings related to immobility, fears, and future impairment
2. Observations for traction
   a. Check that it is hanging free and has not fallen or become caught in bed grooves
   b. Observe for frayed cords and loosened knots
3. Give back care to promote circulation and relax muscles
4. Maintain proper body alignment
5. Provide diet high in fiber with adequate hydration to avoid constipation and straining
6. Instruct patient on principles of body mechanics
7. If patient has myelogram procedure
   a. Position flat for period prescribed by physician
   b. Encourage adequate hydration
8. If patient undergoes surgical intervention, follow general postoperative nursing actions
   a. Observe for leakage of cerebrospinal fluid on surgical dressing; reinforce dressing until inspected by physician
   b. Change position by log rolling to prevent motion of spinal column
   c. Provide straight-backed chair for patient to sit in; feet must be on floor
   d. Discharge instructions include
      (1) Avoid heavy lifting and climbing stairs
      (2) Avoid riding in car
      (3) Avoid forward flexion of head (cervical laminectomy)

FRACTURES

A. Definition: a break in the continuity of bone that may be accompanied by injury of surrounding soft tissue, producing swelling and discoloration

B. Pathology
1. Most fractures are a result of trauma; pathologic fractures result from disorders such as osteoporosis, malnutrition, bone tumors, and Cushing's syndrome
2. Types of fractures
   a. Closed (simple): skin is intact over the site
   b. Open (compound): break in skin is present over the fracture site; the ends of the bone may or may not be visible
   c. Complete: fracture line extends completely through the bone
   d. Incomplete (partial): fracture line extends partially through the bone; one side breaks while the opposite side bends
   e. Comminuted: more than one fracture with bone fragments either crushed or splintered into several pieces
   f. Greenstick: splintering of one side of a bone (most often seen in children because of soft bone structure)
   g. Impacted: one bone fragment is driven into another bone fragment

C. Signs and symptoms
1. Subjective
   a. Pain on movement of body part
   b. Tenderness
   c. Loss of function
   d. Muscle spasms
2. Objective
   a. Deformity
   b. Edema
   c. Bruising
   d. Crepitus

D. Diagnostic test: x-ray examination to confirm location and direction of fracture line

E. Treatment
1. Reduction of the fracture consists of pulling the broken bone ends to correct alignment and regain continuity; usually a cast is applied or the part may be placed in a traction device
   a. Closed reduction: manual manipulation to bring ends into contact
   b. Open reduction: surgical intervention to cleanse the area and attach devices to hold the bones in position
2. Cast application to immobilize, support, and protect the part during the healing process
3. Traction to apply a pulling force in two directions to realign the bones
   a. Skin traction is temporarily applied: light weights that are attached to the skin with strips of adhesive tape
      (1) Buck's extension: exerts a straight pull on the limb; used for fractures of upper and lower leg, hip dislocation, and pelvic injuries
      (2) Bryant's traction: vertical extension of lower extremities, hip flexed 90 degrees, knees extended, and buttocks clear of the bed (see Fig. 8-15, p. 394) for reduction of femur or hip dislocation in very young children
      (3) Russell traction: a sling is placed behind the knee to create an upward pull of the knee, and at the same time a horizontal force is exerted on the tibia and fibula; used for fractures of femurs
   b. Skeletal traction provides continuous reduction by the attachment of a device to the bone
      (1) Kirschner wires or Steinmann pins are surgically inserted through the skin and bone; a traction bow or stirrup is attached to the wire or pin to exert a longitudinal pull and control rotation

(2) Crutchfield tongs are inserted into parietal areas of the skull to obtain hyperextension; used for spinal fractures

(3) Halo traction-halo loop for alignment of cervical area; loop is attached to a halo vest or cast

F. Nursing intervention
1. Provide emergency nursing care of fractures (refer to Chapter 10)
2. Provide nursing care for the patient with a cast
   a. Observe for neurovascular impairment of limb: color, temperature, pulse, sensation, and motor function
   b. Elevate extremity in cast on pillow
   c. Promote drying of cast by exposing it to air
   d. Inspect for skin irritation under edges of cast: apply lotion, pad edges, and apply tape to edge of cast
   e. If drainage is present on the cast, measure and note
   f. Observe for possible infection: increased temperature, foul odor from cast, edema, and "hot spots" over the cast
   g. Observe for complications
      (1) Pulmonary emboli: if emboli lodges in the lungs, patient may experience dyspnea, anxiety, restlessness, chest pain, cough, hemoptysis, and increase in temperature
      (2) Fat emboli: similar to pulmonary emboli, except the emboli is a fat globule, probably arising from central area of the fractured bone
      (3) Compartment syndrome occurs when circulation to the muscles is compromised; look for changes in neurocirculatory status
   h. Educate patient on home cast care
3. Provide nursing care for the patient in traction
   a. Inspect and maintain ropes, knots, and pulleys; taut rope rides easily over pulleys; knots should not slip and should be unobstructed
   b. Inspect and maintain weights: hang freely, off the floor and free of bedding
   c. Observations for skin traction
      (1) Inspect skin condition at distal ends of bandages (wrist and heel) for possible skin breakdown
      (2) Ensure that tapes do not encircle a limb, are applied smoothly, and are applied on skin that is free of irritation
      (3) Assess neurovascular status: color, pulses, warmth, and sensation
   d. Observations for skeletal traction
      (1) Inspect insertion points daily for signs and symptoms of infection
      (2) Provide dressing change or wound care aseptically to prevent infection
      (3) Inspect pins, wires, and skeletal apparatus for sharp ends that may catch on bed linen
      (4) Assess neurovascular status
   e. Examine and give skin care to all pressure points on which the patient rests
   f. Provide foot support to prevent foot drop, especially for patients with Russell traction or Buck's extension
   g. Observe for thrombophlebitis, especially for the patient with Russell traction because of pressure to the popliteal space

h. Encourage diet high in protein and vitamins to promote healing
i. Encourage 2000 to 3000 ml fluid intake daily to prevent complications such as constipation, renal calculi, and urinary tract infections
j. Encourage patient to perform ROM and isometric exercises
k. Maintain proper position and good alignment

FRACTURED HIP
A. Definition: fracture of the hip joint
B. Pathology
   1. Site of fracture
      a. Inside the joint (intracapsular or neck of the femur)
      b. Outside the joint (extracapsular or base of the neck of the femur)
   2. Elderly women experience high incidence because of osteoporosis
C. Signs and symptoms
   1. Subjective: pain
   2. Objective
      a. Leg appears shorter than nonaffected extremity
      b. Foot points upward and outward on affected side (external rotation)
      c. Edema
      d. Discoloration
D. Diagnostic test: x-ray study confirms discontinuity of the bone
E. Treatment
   1. Russell traction or Buck's extension: before open reduction to prevent muscle spasms if surgery is not contraindicated
   2. Closed reduction with application of hip spica cast if the fracture occurred in the intertrochanteric site
   3. Open reduction and implantation of a prosthesis to replace head and neck of femur or fixation device to secure fragments of the fracture
      a. Austin Moore prosthesis
      b. Thompson prosthesis
      c. Neufeld nail and screws
      d. Smith-Petersen nail
      e. Ziekel nail
F. Nursing intervention
   1. Provide nursing care of the patient in traction as outlined previously in section on Fractures
   2. Be aware of coexisting problems such as diabetes or cardiac, vascular, or neurologic disorders
   3. Considerations for the geriatric patient
      a. Complications of immobility
      b. Reduced tolerance to drugs
      c. Delayed healing because of nutritional problems related to the elderly
   4. Keep side rail up and provide trapeze to facilitate movement
   5. Encourage patient to participate in activities of daily living: eating, bathing, and combing hair
   6. Provide postoperative care
      a. Inspect dressings and linen for drainage and bleeding
      b. Provide trochanter roll to prevent external rotation of legs
      c. Provide and maintain proper alignment; adduction, external rotation, or acute flexion of the hip can dislocate hip before it is healed

d. Encourage quadriceps-setting exercises

e. Assist the patient to learn to use walker, ambulating with a nonweight-bearing technique

ARTHROPLASTY

A. Definition: replacement of a joint, which may be necessary to restore function, relieve pain, and correct deformity

B. Pathology: arthritic changes damage the joint, resulting in impaired mobility, pain, and deformity; hip, knee, fingers, elbow, and shoulder are commonly affected

C. Signs and symptoms
1. Subjective
   a. Pain
   b. Limited ROM
   c. Limited weight-bearing ability
2. Objective
   a. Limited ROM
   b. Edema and skin character changes around affected joint

D. Diagnostic tests/methods
1. X-ray studies confirm joint changes and damage
2. Arthroscopy provides direct visualization and inspection of joint changes

E. Treatment: a prosthetic device used to replace the articulating joint surfaces (hip, knee, shoulder, elbow, and fingers)

F. Nursing intervention
1. Proper positioning postoperatively (e.g., if hip is replaced, maintain affected leg in abduction)
2. Wound care: monitor drains, note blood loss, and monitor dressing status
3. Monitor continuous passive ROM machine, if used for knee replacement
4. Assist with prescribed activity and encourage prescribed exercise
5. Monitor pain; provide pain control
6. Assess neuromuscular function
7. Monitor skin integrity

AMPUTATION

A. Definition surgical removal of part or all of an extremity

B. Pathology
1. Majority of amputations result from blood vessel disorders causing inadequate oxygen supply to the tissue
2. Other indications for amputation are gas gangrene, malignant tumors, septic wounds, severe trauma, and burns
3. Usually a skin flap is constructed for prosthetic equipment

C. Signs and symptoms
1. Subjective
   a. Gas gangrene and septic wounds: pain
   b. Peripheral vascular diseases
      (1) Pain
      (2) Tingling
2. Objective
   a. Gas gangrene and septic wounds
      (1) Fever
      (2) Edema
      (3) Foul odor
      (4) Bronze or blackened wound

      (5) Necrosis
   b. Peripheral vascular diseases
      (1) Edema
      (2) Pallor
      (3) Shiny, hairless skin
      (4) Hyperpigmentation
      (5) Ulcer formation
   c. Arterial diseases
      (1) Pallor
      (2) Cyanosis
      (3) Diminished pulses
      (4) Pain on pressure

D. Diagnostic tests/methods
1. Oscillometry
2. Arteriography
3. Skin temperature studies
4. X-ray examination
5. Doppler flow studies

E. Treatment
1. Psychologic preparation
2. Rehabilitation preparation
3. Nutritional status buildup
4. Prosthetic device

F. Nursing intervention
1. Provide preoperative care
   a. Encourage expression of feelings by providing honesty concerning loss of limb
   b. Explain to the patient the possibility of experiencing pain in the amputated limb (called *phantom limb pain*)
   c. Explain to the patient that he or she will undergo a program of exercises that includes strengthening of upper extremities, transferring from bed to chair, and ambulating with a walker or crutches
2. Provide postoperative care
   a. Provide routine postoperative care
   b. Monitor for bleeding and have a large tourniquet available to apply around the residual limb in the event of hemorrhage
   c. Apply elastic (Ace) bandages in a crisscross or figure-8 pattern only
   d. Elevate the residual limb 8 to 12 hours on a pillow; remove after 12 hours to prevent hip contracture; place in prone position 1 hour out of every 4 hours to prevent hip contractures
   e. Prevent outward rotation by placing trochanter roll along the outer side of the residual limb
   f. Instruct the patient not to hang the residual limb over the edge of the bed, wheelchair, chair, or handrail of his or her crutches to avoid residual limb contracture
   g. When conditioning of the residual limb is ordered, begin by having the patient push the residual limb against a pillow and progress to pushing against a firmer surface
   h. Teach the patient to massage the residual limb to soften the scar and improve vascularity
   i. Use TENS (transcutaneous electrical nerve stimulator) for relief of phantom limb pain
   j. Encourage progressive ambulation and physical therapy

RESPIRATORY SYSTEM
Anatomy and Physiology

A. Respiration: the taking in of oxygen, its use in the tissues, and the giving off of carbon dioxide; has two stages
   1. External: exchange of oxygen and carbon dioxide between body and outside environment; consists of inhalation and exhalation

2. Internal: exchange of carbon dioxide and oxygen between the cells and the interstitial fluid surrounding the cells

B. Organs (Figs. 5-3, 5-4, 5-5, 5-6)
   1. Nose:
     a. Divides into two cavities separated by nasal septum
     b. Ciliated mucosa lines the cavities and traps inhaled foreign particles

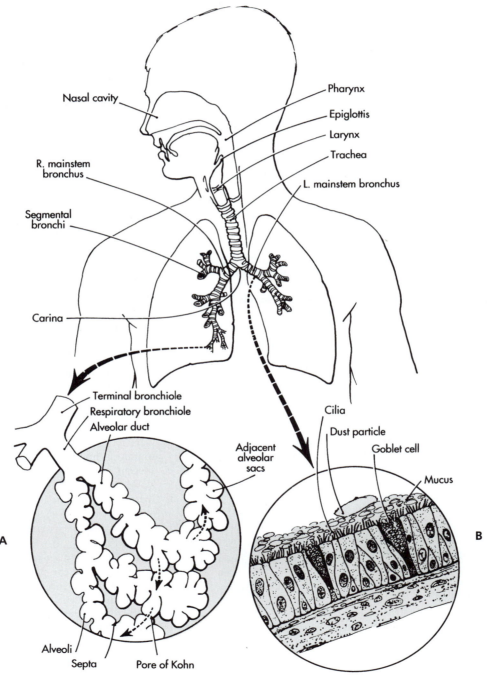

Figure 5-3. **Structures of the respiratory tract. A,** Pulmonary functional unit, **B,** Ciliated mucous membrane. (From Hoeman SP: *Rehabilitation nursing: process and application,* ed 2, St Louis, 1996, Mosby.)

c. Filters, warms, and moistens air
d. Serves as organ of smell
   (1) Receptors located in olfactory epithelium of upper part of nasal cavity
   (2) Stimulates appetite and flow of digestive juices
   (3) Senses of smell and taste work together to give flavor to food
e. Paranasal sinuses: lighten skull, act as resonance chamber in speech
2. Pharynx: passageway for food and air; divided into three parts
   a. Nasopharynx (behind nose): contains adenoids; eustachian tube, which drains the middle ear, opens into the nasopharynx
   b. Oropharynx (mouth): contains tonsils, which are lymphatic tissue
   c. Laryngopharynx: opens into larynx toward front and into esophagus toward back
3. Larynx (voice box)
   a. Formed by nine cartilages in boxlike formation
   b. Thyroid cartilage forms the Adam's apple
c. Epiglottis: flap of elastic cartilage that closes off the larynx when swallowing food
d. Produces sound; vocal cords vibrate with expelled air
e. Passageway for air to the trachea
4. Trachea (windpipe): tube reinforced by C-shaped rings; open ends of rings face posteriorly toward the esophagus and allow esophagus to expand when swallowing food; solid portion keeps the trachea open for the passage of air
5. Bronchi
   a. Formed by the division of the trachea into two branches; distribute air to the lungs' interior; called bronchial tree
   b. Right main bronchus is larger and more vertical; aspiration is more common by this route
   c. Bronchi divide into smaller branches called bronchioles
   d. Bronchioles divide into smaller tubes and terminate in the alveoli
   e. Alveoli: microscopic air sacs that resemble bunches of grapes; composed of a single, thin layer of squamous epithelium; external surface surrounded with

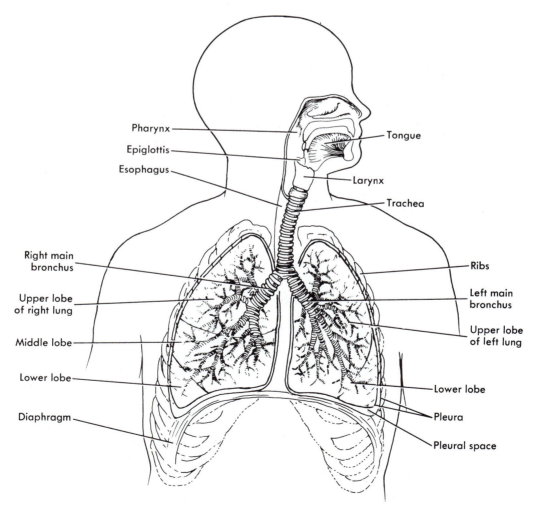

Figure 5-4. **Anatomy of the thorax and lungs.** (From Long et al: *Medical-surgical nursing: a nursing process approach*, ed 3, St Louis, 1993, Mosby.)

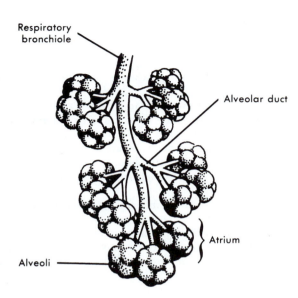

Figure 5-5. **Respiratory unit.** (From Long et al: *Medical-surgical nursing: a nursing process approach*, ed 3, St Louis, 1993, Mosby.)

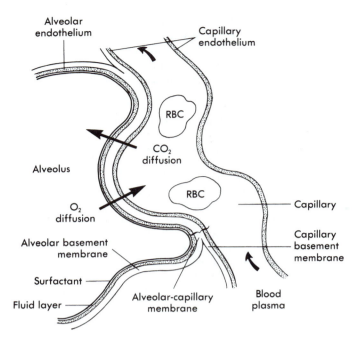

Figure 5-6. **Alveolar-capillary membrane.** (From Long et al: *Medical-surgical nursing, a nursing process approach*, ed 3, St Louis, 1993, Mosby.)

spider webbed pulmonary capillaries; here the gas exchanges occur, oxygen passes from the alveoli into the capillary blood, and carbon dioxide leaves the blood to enter the alveoli
6. Lungs
   a. Cone shaped; upper part is the apex; broad lower part is the base; base is concave and rests on diaphragm
   b. Tissue is porous and spongy
   c. Pleura: thin, moist, slippery membrane covering lungs; prevents friction during breathing movement
C. Physiology
   1. Two phases of breathing: inspiration and expiration
   2. Respiration controlled by respiratory center in medulla oblongata
   3. Carbon dioxide stimulates respiration
   4. Muscles of respiration
      a. Diaphragm: dome shaped; separates thoracic and abdominal cavities; contracts and relaxes
      b. Intercostals: between the ribs; elevate the ribs and enlarge the thorax during inspiration
   5. Mechanism of inspiration
      a. Contraction of diaphragm causes thorax to expand
      b. The lungs cling to the thoracic wall as a result of the attachment of the pleural membranes
      c. Intrathoracic pressure decreases
      d. The volume within the lungs (intrapulmonary) increases, and gases in the lungs spread out to fill the space
      e. Result is a decrease in gas pressure, and a partial vacuum sucks air into the lungs; air continues to move into the lungs until intrapulmonic pressure equals atmospheric pressure
   6. Mechanism of expiration

   a. Respiratory muscles relax and thorax decreases in size
   b. Intrathoracic and intrapulmonary volumes decrease
   c. As volume decreases, gases are forced closer together, and intrapulmonary pressure rises higher than atmospheric pressure
   d. Gases flow out of lungs and equalize pressure inside and outside the lung
   7. Volumes of air exchanges
      a. Total lung capacity (TLC): total volume of air present in the lungs after maximum inspiration
      b. Vital capacity (VC): volume of air that can be expelled after maximum inspiration
      c. Tidal volume (TV): volume of air exhaled after normal inspiration
      d. Residual volume (RV): amount of air remaining in lung after maximum expiration

Respiratory Conditions/Disorders

All cells of the body depend on adequate oxygenation and removal of carbon dioxide for health. The respiratory system is dependent on central nervous system regulation and on the cardiovascular system for blood supply. Respiratory distress or dysfunction may be secondary to disease in another system. Many pulmonary diseases are chronic. Therefore it is essential that the nurse make a complete respiratory assessment of all patients and include this in nursing care planning, even when the primary diagnosis is unrelated to the respiratory system.

The following are terms used to describe respirations:

bradypnea   slow respirations
Cheyne-Stokes   periods of apnea alternating with rapid respirations
DOE   dyspnea on exertion

dyspnea   difficulty breathing; may be subjective or objective

Kussmaul breathing   fast, deep, and labored respirations

orthopnea   difficulty breathing in a supine position; relieved by sitting up

paroxysmal nocturnal dyspnea   transient episodes of acute dyspnea that occur a few hours after falling asleep

SOB   short of breath

tachypnea   rapid respirations

wheeze   sound as air moves out through bronchi and bronchioles that have been narrowed by spasm, swelling, and secretions

Nursing Assessment

A. Nursing observations (objective data)
  1. Respirations
     a. Rate
     b. Depth
     c. Characteristics (wheezing); any difficulty breathing
  2. Oxygen deprivation (note any)
     a. Restlessness
     b. Yawning
     c. Anxiety
     d. Drowsiness
     e. Confusion
     f. Disorientation
  3. Cough
     a. Frequency
     b. Relationship to activity and precipitating factors
     c. Production of sputum
     d. Describe completely (e.g., dry, productive, nonproductive, hoarse, barking, moist, or hacking)
  4. Lung sounds (adventitious)
     a. Crackles
     b. Wheezes
     c. Friction rub
  5. Sputum (note the following)
     a. Consistency (e.g., thick, tenacious, watery, or frothy)
     b. Amount (e.g., scant, moderate, or copious)
     c. Color (e.g., white, yellow, pink, rust, blood tinged, or green)
     d. Odor
  6. Skin color
     a. Pallor, ashen, or ruddy
     b. Cyanosis (bluish discoloration): observe lips, nail beds, and mucous membranes
  7. Skin
     a. Temperature
     b. Diaphoresis
  8. Vital signs
     a. Pulse: note rate, quality and characteristics
     b. Blood pressure
     c. Temperature (rectal; tympanic)
     d. Pulse oximetry
  9. Nasal discharge
  10. Voice: huskiness
B. Patient description (subjective data)
  1. Cough
  2. Pain
  3. Difficulty breathing
  4. Fatigue or weakness
  5. Sputum

C. Patient history
  1. Use of extra pillows needed to sleep
  2. Respiratory illness or difficulty
  3. Injuries
  4. Use of medications or respiratory aids
  5. Smoking
  6. Seasonal exacerbations

Diagnostic Tests/Methods

A. Chest x-ray examination: a picture of lung tissue from different angles; based on a knowledge of normal anatomy and usual changes in disease, diagnosis of many conditions can be made (e.g., tumors, pneumonia); there is no preparation and no special care or observations after x-ray examination
B. Bronchoscopy
  1. Direct inspection of the trachea and bronchi through a scope passed via the nose or mouth; with this procedure specimens are obtained for biopsy and culture; foreign bodies can be removed (e.g., fish bones)
  2. Nursing responsibilities: provide general preparation as that for a surgical procedure (see Chapter 2); after procedure monitor vital signs, provide oral hygiene, and observe for cough and blood-streaked sputum; do not allow patient to eat or drink until gag reflex returns
C. Bronchogram
  1. Visualization of bronchial tree through x-ray examination after introducing radiopaque dye; patient is given sedative and antispasmodic
  2. Nursing responsibilities: provide postural drainage to aid in removal of dye; encourage deep breathing and coughing; do not allow patient to eat or drink until gag reflex returns
D. CT scan: produces clear, anatomic images of the chest cavity
E. Ultrasound: image of area is created by high-frequency sound; used for specific data relative to lung capacities
F. MRI: image created by magnetic resonance, a noninvasive procedure
G. Thoracentesis
  1. Needle aspiration of fluid from pleural cavity (space); local anesthesia is used
  2. Nursing responsibilities: maintain proper positioning; support and reassure patient during the procedure; monitor vital signs during and after the procedure
H. CBC: WCB count changes from normal values may indicate infection
I. Arterial blood gases
  1. Measurement of the partial pressure of oxygen and carbon dioxide in the blood; arterial puncture is performed
  2. Nursing care: once the blood sample is obtained, apply constant pressure to the site for 5 minutes; apply pressure dressing; inspect site frequently for hematoma and pain; distally for skin temperature, color
J. Culture and sensitivity
  1. Throat or nasopharynx
  2. Sputum
     a. Identifies organisms and specific medication to which patient will respond
     b. Nursing responsibilities: obtain before starting antibiotics; first sputum in the morning usually has the most organisms
K. Sputum analysis

1. Acid-fast bacillus (AFB): determines presence of mycobacterium tuberculosis
2. Cytology: assists in the diagnosis of lung carcinoma

L. Pulmonary function tests: determine extent of respiratory difficulty and evaluate function of respiratory system; measure vital capacity, tidal volume, and total lung capacity; no special preparation or nursing care after testing

M. Lung scan-Positron emission tomography (PET): radioisotopes are inhaled or administered intravenously; a scanning device records the pattern of radioactivity; used in diagnosing vascular diseases (e.g., pulmonary embolism); no special preparation or nursing care

N. Biopsy examination
   1. Removal of a small amount of tissue to identify disease; biopsy may be of a lymph node to determine if the disease has spread into the lymphatic system
   2. Nursing care: provide general preoperative and postoperative care (see Chapter 2)

Frequent Patient Problems and Nursing Care

A. Activity intolerance related to fatigue and weakness: body cells' demand for oxygen is not met; the patient tires easily and becomes short of breath
   1. Protect from exertion; provide care; space activities appropriately
   2. Plan care to include rest periods
   3. Leave bed in low position
   4. Leave call bell and all personal belongings within easy reach
   5. Provide oxygen with humidity as ordered
   6. Limit conversation

B. Risk for injury related to dizziness: caused by diminished oxygen to the brain cells
   1. Provide all care as in preceding list
   2. Maintain safety; use side rails
   3. Make neurologic assessment every 4 hours (q4h)

C. Altered oral mucous membrane related to mouth breathing
   1. Encourage fluids if allowed
   2. Provide oral hygiene q2h
   3. Lubricate lips with nonpetroleum base product

D. Altered breathing pattern related to orthopnea
   1. Place a pillow longitudinally under back
   2. Provide table with pillow for headrest in extreme difficulty
   3. Use footboard to prevent slipping down in bed
   4. Semi- to high-Fowler's position

E. Ineffective airway clearance; impaired gas exchange related to dyspnea and coughing
   1. Oxygen therapy: maintain safety of equipment and proper care and observations
   2. Organize care and work efficiently to conserve patient's energy
   3. Plan rest periods
   4. Position in semi- to high-Fowler's position; use two pillows
   5. Provide soft diet and small, frequent feedings
   6. Avoid gas-forming foods
   7. Prevent constipation and straining
   8. Use rectal thermometer; take tympanic temperature
   9. Make accurate observations about cough and sputum
   10. Obtain specimens as needed
   11. Provide tissues and bag for disposal in easy reach
   12. Provide sputum cup if needed
   13. Change position q2h
   14. Encourage deep breathing
   15. Encourage fluids q2h
   16. Provide oral hygiene q2h
   17. Provide postural drainage if ordered (see Chapter 2)
   18. Give expectorants as ordered (see Chapters 2 and 3)

F. Anxiety related to dyspnea, fatigue, and weakness
   1. Maintain quiet environment
   2. Remain calm
   3. Explain everything slowly and carefully
   4. Provide physical and mental rest
   5. Answer call lights promptly
   6. Provide frequent contacts
   7. Offer realistic encouragements
   8. Provide restful diversion (e.g., music)
   9. Encourage patients to express feelings and concerns

G. Alteration in nutrition, less than body requirements, related to dry mouth from mouth breathing, foul taste and odor from sputum, and fatigue; may affect desire for food
   1. Make mealtime pleasant
   2. Provide oral hygiene before each meal
   3. Remove used tissues and sputum cups
   4. Request food preferences
   5. Give small, frequent, attractively served meals

Major Medical Diagnoses

SINUSITIS

A. Definition: inflammation of one or more of the sinuses of the frontal, ethmoid, sphenoid, or maxillary bones; secretions become infected; is acute but becomes chronic if not treated or leads to complications: septicemia, meningitis, brain abscess

B. Cause: results from the spread of organisms from the nose or trapped secretions interfering with drainage (e.g., nasal polyps or edema from allergy)

C. Signs and symptoms
   1. Pain and headache
   2. Nasal secretions, possibly purulent and blood tinged
   3. Elevation of temperature; mild leukopenia

D. Diagnostic tests/methods
   1. Patient history and physical assessment
   2. X-ray examination

E. Treatment
   1. Irrigation and inhalation of steam
   2. Antibiotics and decongestants (see Chapter 3)
   3. Surgery (e.g., Caldwell-Luc [infected maxillary sinus is removed through an incision under the upper lip] or ethmoidectomy)

F. Nursing intervention
   1. Administer nonnarcotic analgesics or nasal constrictors (see Chapter 3)
   2. Provide moist steam
   3. Provide hot wet pack
   4. Give general preoperative and postoperative care (see Chapter 2); note specific orders for care or observations

EPISTAXIS (NOSEBLEED)

A. Definition: bleeding from the nose

B. Cause: may be spontaneous, related to direct trauma, or a result of a systemic diseases (e.g., hypertension or blood dyscrasias); may be caused by local irritation from chronic infections or low-humidity environment

C. Sign: bleeding; shock if profuse
D. Diagnostic tests/methods: patient history and physical examination; platelet, HCT, HBG if profuse
E. Treatment (only if bleeding cannot be stopped)
  1. Nasal packing
  2. Cauterization of site with 10% silver nitrate stick
  3. Epinephrine spray
  4. Treatment of systemic disease
  5. Hemostatic agents
F. Nursing intervention
  1. Maintain patent airway (direct patient to breathe through mouth); have suction available
  2. Control bleeding: pinch nose firmly with fingers on soft part of nose; position in high-Fowler's with head forward
  3. Instruct patient to expectorate blood (swallowing will cause vomiting)
  4. Apply ice or cold compresses to nasal area to constrict blood vessels
  5. Monitor vital signs
  6. Avoid hot liquids
  7. Provide oral hygiene
  8. Reassure patient and family

DEVIATED SEPTUM
A. Definition: airway obstruction caused by deflection of bone and cartilage in the nasal septum
B. Causes
  1. Trauma
  2. Congenital
C. Diagnostic test/methods
  1. Patient history
  2. Physical assessment
  3. X-ray examination
D. Treatment: surgery-submucous resection (SMR), performed through the mucous membrane within the nares; bone and cartilage are removed
E. Nursing intervention
  1. Provide general preoperative and postoperative care (see Chapter 2)
  2. Before surgery inform patient that nasal packing will be in place 24 to 48 hours; nasal breathing will not be possible; there will be a temporary loss of smell; sneezing must be avoided; and there will be pain, discoloration, and swelling around the eyes
  3. Maintain airway; place patient on side or in semi-Fowler's position; monitor respirations
  4. Provide oral hygiene every 1 to 2 hours
  5. Provide ice compresses; note bleeding on dressing; inspect back of throat for trickle of blood
  6. Use rectal thermometer
  7. Provide liquid diet when tolerated; encourage fluids; prevent constipation
  8. Discourage forceful coughing

POLYPS
A. Definition: grapelike swellings of tissue; nasal polyps obstruct breathing and block sinus drainage (see sinusitis)
B. Treatment: surgical removal

LARYNGITIS
A. Definition: an inflammation and swelling of the mucous membrane lining of the larynx
B. Cause: local irritation (e.g., smoking, spread of infection from elsewhere in the upper respiratory tract, or abuse of vocal cords)
C. Signs and symptoms
  1. Hoarseness
  2. Pain
  3. Loss of voice
  4. Cough
D. Diagnostic tests/methods
  1. Physical assessment
  2. Patient history
  3. Indirect laryngoscopy
E. Treatment and nursing intervention
  1. Rest voice; provide alternate means of communication
  2. Removal of cause
  3. Provide moist steam inhalations
  4. Administer astringent or antiseptic spray (see Chapter 3)

CARCINOMA OF THE LARYNX
A. Description: squamous cell carcinoma grows, spreads, and metastasizes; the rate of growth is determined by location of the lesion in the larynx
B. Causes: related to heavy smoking, chronic laryngitis and vocal abuse, and alcohol consumption
C. Signs and symptoms
  1. Hoarseness
  2. Signs of metastasis: pain, lump in throat, difficulty swallowing, dyspnea, and enlarged, painful lymph nodes
  3. Anxiety (i.e., concerning surgery; confirmation of diagnosis; disfigurement)
D. Diagnostic tests/methods
  1. Patient history
  2. Visual examination (laryngoscopy)
  3. Biopsy examination
  4. Laryngeal tomography
E. Treatment: Surgery
  1. Removal of larynx (laryngectomy) (partial or complete)
  2. Radical neck dissection: wide excision including lymph nodes, epiglottis, thyroid cartilage, and muscle tissue; a permanent tracheostomy is performed
  3. Radiotherapy with surgery
F. Nursing intervention
  1. Provide general preoperative and postoperative care (see Chapter 2)
  2. Immediate postoperative care
    a. Maintain patent airway; patient may have a permanent tracheostomy (see nursing care and suctioning of a patient with a tracheostomy-Chapter 2); there will be a shorter tube (laryngectomy tube); place patient in semi-Fowler's position; frequent mouth care
    b. Observe dressing qh; connect wound drains to suction as ordered; prevent movement of head
  3. Continued postoperative care
    a. Provide method of communication (e.g., magic slate), leave call bell close to hand, and answer promptly in person
    b. Assist and be supportive as alternate methods of speech are learned (e.g., esophageal speech or use of mechanical voice box)
    c. Provide high-calorie, high-protein diet (may require tube feedings at first)

d. Arrange for a visit from someone who has had a similar operation and satisfactory rehabilitation

PNEUMONIA

A. Description: an inflammation of the lungs or part of the lung (e.g.; left lower lobe [LLL] pneumonia); secretions fill the alveolar sacs, which is a good medium for bacterial growth; the inflammation spreads to adjacent sacs; spaces of the lung consolidate with thick exudate; irritation may cause bleeding, and sputum has the characteristic rusty color; exchange of air is difficult and, in advanced conditions, not possible

B. Causes: bacterial infections and viruses are spread by respiratory secretions (droplets); chemical irritation; fungi and other organisms; aspirations; patients with poor health and low natural resistance to infection are more susceptible (e.g., the elderly, those with chronic illness, and immunocompromised individuals should consider receiving pneumovax vaccine as a preventative measure)

C. Signs and symptoms
   1. Dyspnea, short of breath, pain on inspiration, shallow breathing, signs of air hunger, orthopnea, and oxygen deprivation
   2. Marked elevation in temperature
   3. Cough: painful and dry at first, then productive with copious amounts of thick sputum (color according to organism)

D. Diagnostic tests/methods
   1. Patient history
   2. Physical assessment with auscultation of chest
   3. Chest x-ray examination
   4. Sputum culture and sensitivity
   5. CBC

E. Treatment
   1. Specific and broad-spectrum antibiotics (see Chapter 3)
   2. Antipyretics, analgesics (codeine), expectorants, and bronchodilators (see Chapter 3)
   3. Intravenous (IV) fluids; encourage oral fluids
   4. Oxygen with humidity; incentive spirometer

F. Nursing intervention
   1. Provide optimum rest: provide care; help patient conserve energy; schedule rest periods; limit conversation; keep personal items and call bell within easy reach; alleviate anxiety
   2. Maintain oxygen with humidity
   3. Isolate as indicated, especially patients with oral and nasal secretions; provide for proper disposal (see Isolation Technique, Chapter 2)
   4. Liquefy secretions: force fluids (3000 ml daily or more); observe and document production of sputum; suction as necessary
   5. Provide oral hygiene q2h
   6. Monitor vital signs q4h; use rectal thermometer; monitor lung sounds
   7. Assist with loosening of secretions: have patient turn, cough, and deep breathe q2h (splint chest if painful); observe and document cough; may need aerosol treatment
   8. Maintain adequate nutrition: provide liquid-to-soft diet high in protein and calories
   9. Maintain IV fluids and medication schedule to ensure continued blood levels
   10. Position for comfort (high-Fowler's or lying on affected side)

PLEURISY

A. Description: inflammation of the pleural membranes (local or diffuse); may or may not have fluid exudate; when fluid is present, the condition is pleural effusion, when purulent, the condition is empyema

B. Cause: infections (e.g., pneumonia, lung abcess, trauma, fungus, tuberculosis, lung cancer, congestive heart failure, or ascites)

C. Signs and symptoms
   1. Sharp pain on inspiration (referred to shoulder, abdomen, or affected side)
   2. Dyspnea and cough
   3. Anxiety
   4. Elevation of temperature
   5. Decreased breath sounds
   6. Pleural rub

D. Diagnostic tests/methods
   1. Chest x-ray examination
   2. Patient history
   3. Physical assessment including auscultation of chest
   4. Examination of pleural fluid obtained via thoracentesis and laboratory analysis

E. Treatment (according to cause)
   1. Analgesics and antibiotics
   2. Drainage of fluid: thoracentesis, then chest tubes to underwater seal drainage with suction
   3. Oxygen if dyspnea is severe; alleviate pain by turning patient to affected side

F. Nursing intervention: see plan for patient with chest tubes (the box to the right); provide diet high in protein, calories, minerals, and vitamins; alleviate anxiety

PNEUMOTHORAX/HEMOTHORAX

A. Description
   1. Pneumothorax: air in pleural space allowing for partial or complete collapse of the lung
   2. Hemothorax: blood in pleural space

B. Causes
   1. May be spontaneous
   2. Trauma (e.g., knife wound or fractured rib that punctures lung)
   3. Postoperative (e.g., where the thoracic cavity has been entered)
   4. Diagnostic (e.g., CVP line, thoracentesis, pleural biopsy)

C. Signs and symptoms
   1. Sudden, sharp chest pain (when spontaneous)
   2. Anxiety: diaphoresis, rapid pulse, and rapid respirations
   3. Vertigo
   4. Decreased blood pressure
   5. Decreased breath sounds
   6. Dyspnea

D. Diagnostic tests/methods
   1. Patient history and physical assessment
   2. Chest x-ray examination

E. Treatment
   1. Closure of wound with airtight dressing
   2. Aspiration of fluids and air; water-seal drainage
   3. Analgesics
   4. Thoracentesis

F. Nursing intervention
   1. Provide nursing care and observations as necessary for primary diagnosis

Patient with Chest Tubes

Description

Drainage tubes are inserted between ribs into the pleural cavity to allow for drainage of secretions, blood, or air; the tube(s) is attached to an underwater seal system to allow for expansion of the lung and to prevent air from entering the pleural cavity; the drainage system may or may not be attached to suction

Indications

Chest surgery
Stab wounds of the chest
Pleural effusion
Spontaneous pneumothorax

Nursing intervention

Do complete assessment of the respiratory system q2h; place patient in semi-Fowler's position; provide oxygen with humidity

Prevent complications of immobility: have patient turn, deep breathe, and cough q2h; encourage patient to ambulate as ordered and as condition allows; splint chest to cough

Encourage fluids to liquefy secretions; provide tissues and bag for proper disposal; provide sputum cup

Provide oral hygiene q2h

Anticipate pain, medicate as needed, observe respirations 30 minutes after administration of sedative or analgesic

Observe underwater seal system qh
    Drainage color and amount
    Rise and fall of water in bottle (or suction) going to patient
    Bubbling (if connected to suction)

Alleviate anxiety

Pace activities to allow for periods of rest

---

2. Place patient in high-Fowler's position
3. Monitor vital signs
4. Administer oxygen
5. Provide nursing care for a patient with chest tubes as described in the box above
6. Provide instructions on tube/dressing care if discharged with chest tube in place

INFLUENZA

A. Description: acute disease that may occur as an epidemic; recovery is usually complete; no permanent immunity results; complications and death may occur in patients with chronic or debilitating conditions, especially cardiac or pulmonary
B. Cause: virus
C. Signs and symptoms
    1. Headache, chest pain, nuchal rigidity, and muscle ache
    2. Elevated temperature
    3. Coughing, sneezing, dry throat, nasal discharge, and herpetic lesions

    4. Gastrointestinal symptoms; nausea, vomiting, and anorexia
    5. Weakness
D. Diagnostic tests/methods: patient history and physical assessment
E. Treatment
    1. Prevention with vaccines; influenza vaccine recommended on a yearly basis
    2. Symptomatic
F. Nursing intervention
    1. Provide rest, assist with care; provide quiet environment and dim lighting
    2. Encourage fluids
    3. Relieve symptoms: provide antipyretics, analgesics

PULMONARY TUBERCULOSIS

A. Description: a chronic, progressive infection; alveoli are inflamed, and small nodules are produced called primary tubercles; the tubercle bacillus is at the center of the nodule (these become fibrosed); the area becomes calcified and can be identified on x-ray film; the person who has been infected harbors the bacillus for life; it is dormant unless it becomes active during physical or emotional stress
B. Cause: *Mycobacterium tuberculosis,* Koch's bacillus, an acid-fast bacillus (AFB) spread by droplets from an infected person
C. Signs and symptoms
    1. Malaise; patient is easily fatigued
    2. Chest pain, cough, and hemoptysis (coughing up blood from the respiratory tract)
    3. Elevation of temperature and night sweats
    4. Anorexia and weight loss
    5. Anxiety (i.e., fear of chronic disease, fear of public rejection)
D. Diagnostic tests/methods
    1. Patient history and physical assessment
    2. Chest x-ray examination
    3. Sputum specimen for AFB; aspiration of gastric fluid for AFB if unable to obtain specimen
    4. Tuberculin skin testing (e.g., tine or Mantoux test)
E. Treatment
    1. Antituberculin drugs for 18 to 24 months (see Chapter 3)
    2. Rest (physical and emotional)
    3. Diet high in carbohydrates, proteins, and vitamins (especially B_6)
    4. Surgical resection of affected lung tissue or involved lobe (only when necessary)
F. Nursing intervention
    1. Provide rest; assist with or provide care; plan rest periods; limit conversation; leave personal items in easy reach
    2. Prevent transmission: ensure proper isolation (AFB; tuberculosis); provide tissues and bag for disposal; encourage proper use of tissues; insist on patient covering mouth and nose when coughing or sneezing; provide mask for patient if necessary; room must be equipped with special means of ventilation
    3. Provide frequent, small meals and nutritious snacks; mouth care after meals
    4. Avoid chills; keep skin dry and clean; protect from drafts, especially at night
    5. Allay fears of patient and family about transmission: encourage proper adherence to drug maintenance;

explain how organism is carried, transmitted, and destroyed (nurse must be aware that a tuberculin test is recommended for all contacts with a person with tuberculosis [TB];) a positive test result does not mean the disease has manifested but indicates that the organism has entered the body and that the body has produced antibodies at some point; explain need for multiple, long-term drug therapy

CHRONIC OBSTRUCTIVE PULMONARY DISEASE
Chronic obstructive pulmonary disease (COPD) includes chronic and frequently progressive pulmonary disorders that affect expiratory air flow; asthma, chronic bronchitis, and pulmonary emphysema may occur independently or together.

ASTHMA
A. Description: spasms of the bronchial muscle occur; edema and swelling of the mucosa produce thick secretions; air flow is obstructed; air enters and is trapped; a characteristic wheeze accompanies attempts to exhale through narrowed bronchi; breathing is labored; coughing is attempted, but patient fails to expectorate satisfactory amounts; patient experiences great anxiety; the attacks last 30 to 60 minutes, often with normal breathing between attacks; if attack is difficult to control, and is resistant to all forms of treatment, it is called *status asthmaticus*
B. Causes
   1. Recurrent respiratory infection
   2. Allergic reaction
   3. Physical or emotional stress may provoke attack in a person with asthma
C. Signs and symptoms
   1. Shortness of breath, expiratory wheeze, labored respirations, diaphoresis, use of accessory muscles, and flaring nostrils
   2. Thick, tenacious sputum (after acute attack)
   3. Anxiety or feeling of suffocation, dyspnea
D. Diagnostic tests/methods: patient history and physical examination, ABGs, allergy testing, pulmonary function
E. Treatment
   1. Removal of cause (source of allergy) or desensitization
   2. Low-flow, humidified oxygen
   3. Bronchodilators, mast cell inhibitors, corticosteroids, or sedatives (see Chapter 3)
F. Nursing intervention
   1. Reduce anxiety: provide time to listen; do not leave patient alone during attack
   2. Remove cause: keep environment free from dust and other allergens
   3. Provide continuous humidity as ordered
   4. Encourage fluids; maintain IV as ordered
   5. Position for maximum comfort and breathing: have patient sit in high-Fowler's position with arms supported by over-bed table
   6. Prevent secondary infections: avoid staff and visitors with upper respiratory infections
   7. Teach abdominal breathing
   8. Do not allow smoking; refer patient for help in quitting
   9. Avoid exposure to cold, wet weather
   10. Instruct on preventive treatment for exertional asthma

CHRONIC BRONCHITIS
A. Description: chronic, progressive infection accompanied by hypersecretion of mucus by the bronchioles; without treatment and prevention of acute attacks, the alveolar sacs and capillaries will extend and destruct
B. Causes
   1. Asthma
   2. Acute respiratory tract infections (e.g., pneumonia, influenza, smoking, and air pollution contribute to incidence)
   3. Familial tendency
C. Signs and symptoms
   1. Problems related to acute infection
   2. Cough, productive with thick, white sputum; sputum is blood tinged as disease progresses (cough is greatest on arising)
D. Diagnostic tests/methods
   1. Patient history
   2. Pulmonary testing to rule out other disease (e.g., tuberculosis or malignancy)
E. Treatment
   1. Prevent irritation of bronchial mucosa: encourage patient to discontinue smoking and change aggravating conditions in occupation or home environment
   2. Prevent upper respiratory tract infection: maintain optimum health, adequate rest, and high-protein, high-vitamin diet
   3. Provide bronchodilators, antibiotics, corticosteroids, and influenza vaccine during epidemics (see Chapter 3)
F. Nursing intervention
   1. Provide care to relieve patient problems (see discussion on frequent patient problems and nursing care outlined earlier in this chapter)
   2. Loosen, liquefy, and remove secretions: provide postural drainage and chest percussion as ordered; encourage fluids
   3. Involve patient and family in care and care planning
   4. Do not allow smoking; refer patient for help in quitting

EMPHYSEMA
A. Description: a chronic, progressive condition in which the alveolar sacs distend, rupture, and destroy the capillary beds; the alveoli lose elasticity, inspired air is trapped; inspiration is difficult and expiration is prolonged; the lung tissue becomes fibrotic; exchange of gases is not possible; anxiety increases; signs of oxygen deprivation are evident
B. Cause (see discussion on bronchitis)
C. Signs and symptoms
   1. Dyspnea on exertion (later, dyspnea on slightest exertion and orthopnea); inspiration is difficult; expiration is prolonged, accompanied by wheeze
   2. Chronic cough; productive, purulent sputum in copious amounts
   3. Difficulty talking: speaks in short, jerky sentences
   4. Cerebral anoxia: is drowsy and confused; may become unconscious and go into coma
   5. Barrel chest
   6. Anorexia, weight loss, and weakness
D. Diagnostic tests/methods
   1. Patient history and physical examination
   2. Chest x-ray examination

3. Pulmonary function tests
4. Arterial blood gases; CBC
5. Sputum analysis
E. Treatment (see discussion on bronchitis)
F. Nursing intervention
1. Loosen, liquefy, and remove secretions: provide postural drainage and chest percussion as ordered; encourage fluids; administer expectorants as needed
2. Promote respiratory function: breathing exercises and coughing
3. Administer oxygen; oxygen is administered in low concentrations only (1 to 2 L); oxygen can be dangerous when the carbon dioxide level of the blood is high; the respiratory center of the brain becomes accustomed to the low blood oxygen level; if oxygen increases, respiratory rate will slow significantly
4. Prevent and control infections: administer antibiotics; avoid contact with people with upper respiratory tract infections; avoid smoking
5. Provide rest: limit exertion of any type; provide care; minimize conversation; assist with all movements (e.g., turning and getting into chair)
6. Include family in care and care plan; be understanding that this condition is chronic
7. Teach pursed-lip breathing; abdominal breathing
8. Encourage small, frequent meals

CANCER OF THE LUNG
A. Description: primary or secondary (from metastasis [e.g., from prostate]) malignant tumor; bronchogenic carcinoma is the most common primary tumor; is usually without symptoms until late stages when metastasis has occurred to brain, spinal cord, or esophagus; treatment is difficult in late stages and usually is symptomatic; prognosis is poor unless detected and treated early
B. Cause: strongly related to smoking, air pollution, and chemical irritants
C. Signs and symptoms (occur in late stages)
1. Productive cough with blood-streaked sputum
2. Dyspnea and chest pain
3. Fatigue, anorexia, and weight loss
D. Diagnostic tests/methods
1. CT scan; MRI
2. Examination of sputum for cells (cytology)
3. Bronchial biopsy examination
E. Treatment
1. Surgery: procedure depends on size and location of tumor (lobectomy, pneumonectomy, or laparoscopic thoracotomy)
2. Radiation
3. Chemotherapy
4. Photodynamic therapy with laser
F. Nursing intervention
1. Provide nursing care for symptoms (see discussion on frequent patient problems and nursing care earlier in chapter)
2. Provide preoperative and postoperative nursing care (see Chapter 2)
a. Maintain patent airway; administer oxygen; have patient turn, cough, and deep breathe q2h; a patient with a pneumonectomy must not cough; do not

turn on operative side until physician orders (prevent mediastinal shift)
b. Provide special care for a patient with chest tubes (rarely used, but still a possibility)

THE CARDIOVASCULAR, PERIPHERAL, AND HEMATOLOGIC SYSTEMS
Anatomy and Physiology of the Circulatory System
A. Functions
1. Major function: transports oxygen, carbon dioxide, cell wastes, nutrients, enzymes, and antibodies throughout the body
2. Secondary function: contributes to the body's metabolic functions and maintenance of homeostasis
B. Heart (Fig. 5-7)
1. Hollow, cone-shaped muscular organ the size of a man's fist; functions as pump
2. Positioned in thoracic cavity between the sternum and thoracic vertebrae
3. Apex extends slightly to the left and rests on the diaphragm, approximately at the level of the fifth rib; a stethoscope should be placed at the apex to count an apical pulse
4. Layers
a. Pericardium: outer covering; consists of two layers of serous membrane that is lubricated and prevents friction when the heart beats
b. Myocardium: dense fibrous connective tissue; the wall of the heart
c. Endocardium: a thin, serous lining that helps the blood flow smoothly through the heart; lines the heart chamber
5. Chambers
a. Atria: upper chambers: primarily receiving chambers; not important in the pumping action of the heart
(1) Right atrium: receives deoxygenated blood from the superior and inferior vena cava
(2) Left atrium: receives oxygenated blood from the lungs by way of the four pulmonary veins
b. Ventricles: lower chambers; the dispensing chambers; have the major responsibility of forcing blood out into large arteries
(1) Right ventricle: receives blood from right atrium and pumps blood to lungs by way of the pulmonary artery
(2) Left ventricle: does the major work of the heart; has the thickest wall; pumps blood to all parts of the body by way of the aorta
(3) Interventricular or interatrial septum: divides the heart longitudinally
6. Valves: permit flow of blood in only one direction
a. Tricuspid: allows blood to flow from right atrium into right ventricle
b. Pulmonary semilunar: allows blood to flow out of right ventricle into pulmonary artery

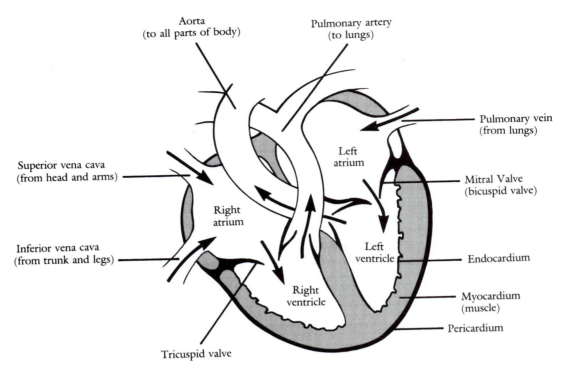

Figure 5-7. **Structures of the heart.** (From Sorrentino SA: *Mosby's textbook for nursing assistants,* ed 4, St Louis, 1995, Mosby.)

c. Mitral or bicuspid: allows blood to flow from left atrium to left ventricle

d. Aortic semilunar: allows blood to flow out of left ventricle into aorta

7. Physiology
   a. Cardiac cycle: refers to one complete heartbeat, consisting of contraction or systole and relaxation or diastole of the atria and ventricles
   b. Auscultatory sounds: heard through a stethoscope; the first sound, systolic, is longer and louder because of the closure of the cuspid valves; the second sound, diastole, is shorter and softer because of the closure of the semilunar valves
   c. Conduction system
      (1) Functions: initiates heartbeat; conducts electrical impulses around heart; coordinates heartbeat
      (2) Components
         (a) Sinoatrial (SA) node: the pacemaker of the heart, sets and regulates the beat by sending electrical impulses to the atria and the AV node
         (b) Atrioventricular (AV) node: receives impulses from SA node; transmits electrical impulses by way of bundle of His to the ventricles
         (c) Bundle of His: fibers that begin at AV node and follow the interventricular septum; divides into Purkinje's fibers
         (d) Purkinje's fibers: conducting fibers; stimulate the ventricles to contract
   d. Heart rates: controlled by internal and external factors

      (1) Bradycardia: slower than normal rate, less than 60 beats/min
      (2) Tachycardia: faster than normal rate, more than 100 beats/min
      (3) Extrasystole: premature beat
      (4) Sinus arrhythmia: a deviation from the normal pattern of the heartbeat resulting from changes in the rate and depth of breathing or other benign causes

C. Blood vessels
   1. Arteries: elastic, muscular-conducting tubes; carry blood away from the heart and to the capillaries; all arteries (except pulmonary) carry oxygenated blood
      a. Aorta: the largest artery, from which all other arteries branch out and become smaller and smaller
      b. Arterioles: extremely small arteries; branch into the capillaries
   2. Veins: thin-walled tubes that have one-way valves to prevent backflow of blood; transport blood back to the heart; all veins (except pulmonary) carry deoxygenated blood
      a. Venae cavae: largest veins; enter the right atrium
         (1) Superior vena cava: returns blood from the head, arms, and thoracic region
         (2) Inferior vena cava: returns blood from body regions below the diaphragm
      b. Venules: extremely small veins; collect blood from the capillaries
   3. Capillaries: microscopic vessels; carry blood from arterioles to venules; exchange of nutrients and waste products occurs in capillaries
D. Types of circulation

1. Systemic: blood flows from the left ventricle into the aorta, through the body, and back to the right atrium; provides oxygen-rich, nutrient-laden blood to body organs
2. Pulmonary: blood flows from the right ventricle into the pulmonary artery, to the lungs, and then back to the left atrium through the pulmonary vein; its function is to carry blood to the lungs for gas exchange and return it to the heart
3. Portal: detour of venous blood from stomach, pancreas, intestines, and spleen through the liver, where it is processed, and returned by way of the inferior vena cava; excess glucose is removed and stored in the liver as glycogen; poisonous substances are removed and detoxified

E. Blood
  1. Functions
    a. Transports oxygen and carbon dioxide to and from lungs
    b. Transports nutrients, hormones, and waste products
    c. Helps maintain acid-base balance, electrolyte balance, and fluid balance
    d. Carries substances that help fight infection
    e. Acts to maintain homeostasis
  2. Composition
    a. Plasma: liquid, straw-colored portion of blood
      (1) Approximately 90% water
      (2) Contains blood proteins (fibrinogen, prothrombin, albumin, gamma globulin)
      (3) Contains mineral salts (electrolytes), hormones, nutrients, oxygen, carbon dioxide, and waste products (urea, lactic acid, and uric acid)
    b. Formed elements
      (1) Erythrocytes: red blood cells (RBCs)
        (a) Contain hemoglobin, which carries oxygen to cells and carbon dioxide from cells
        (b) Originate in red bone marrow
        (c) Life span is 100 to 120 days
        (d) Destroyed by the spleen, liver, and bone marrow
        (e) Normal range: male, 4.5 to 6.2 million per cubic millimeter; female, 4 to 5.5 million per cubic millimeter
      (2) Leukocytes: white blood cells (WBCs)
        (a) Principal function is to fight infection
        (b) Able to multiply rapidly
        (c) Classified according to whether they contain visible granules in their cytoplasm
          ■ Granulocytes: include neutrophils, eosinophils, and basophils
          ■ Agranulocytes: include lymphocytes and monocytes
        (d) Formation is in red bone marrow and by lymphatic tissue in lymph nodes, thymus, and spleen
        (e) Normal range: 5000 to 10,000 per cubic millimeter
      (3) Thrombocytes: platelets
        (a) Aid in clotting process
        (b) Originate in bone marrow
        (c) Normal range: 200,000 to 400,000 per cubic millimeter
  3. Blood types

    a. Every person belongs to one of the four groups: type A, type B, type AB, or type O; and is classified as either Rh positive or Rh negative
    b. Type A blood: A antigens in RBCs, anti-B antibodies in plasma
    c. Type B Blood: type B antigens in RBCs, anti-A antibodies in plasma
    d. Type AB blood: has type A and type B antigens in RBCs; no anti-A or anti-B antibodies in plasma; type AB called universal recipient
    e. Type O blood; no type A or type B antigens in RBCs; both anti-A and anti-B antibodies in plasma; type O is called universal donor blood
    f. Rh-positive blood: Rh-factor antigen in RBCs
    g. Rh-negative blood: no Rh factor in RBCs; no anti-Rh antibodies in plasma
    h. Harmful effects can result from a blood transfusion if donor's RBCs become agglutinated by antibodies in the recipient's plasma

F. Lymphatic system: represents an accessory route for return of fluid from interstitial spaces to cardiovascular system; consists of lymphatic vessels, lymph nodes or glands, and spleen
  1. Lymph: transparent fluid in surrounding spaces between tissue cells; made of water and end products of cell metabolism; referred to as intercellular or interstitial fluid
  2. Function of system
    a. Lymphatic vessels: return fluid and proteins to blood
    b. Lymph nodes: filter injurious particles such as microorganisms and cancer cells
    c. Tonsils: filter and remove bacteria or pathogens entering the throat
    d. Thymus: most active during early life; relates immune reaction through puberty; atrophies at adulthood
  3. Spleen: consists of lymphoid tissue
    a. Forms lymphocytes and monocytes
    b. Destroys old RBCs
    c. Stores blood until needed and then releases it into circulation

G. Immunity: the body's defense system against diseases and substances interpreted as nonself; mediated by T- and B-lymphocytes of the circulatory system; the functions of lymphocytes in immunity by cell type are
  1. T-lymphocytes: originate from stem cells in thymus; responsible for cellular immunity (a slow response) to an antigen; act against most bacteria, viruses, tumor cells, and foreign organs or grafts; clone into types of regulatory cells-helper and suppressors
    a. Helper T-cells: interact directly with B-cells by stimulating activity of B-cells on killer T-cells
    b. Killer T-cells: directly attack virus-infected cells, promote lysis
    c. Suppressor T-cells: terminate normal immune response
  2. B-lymphocytes: originate mainly in fetal liver and lymphoid tissue during first few months of life; responsible for humoral immunity (a rapid response) to an antigen
    a. Clone antibody producing plasma cells
    b. Protect against toxin
  3. Naturally acquired immunity

a. Active: acquired through contact with disease
b. Passive: acquired from antibodies obtained through placenta and mother's milk
4. Artificially acquired immunity
a. Active: immunization with vaccines
b. Passive: administration of immune serum

CARDIOVASCULAR CONDITIONS/DISORDERS

Diseases related to the cardiovascular system are the leading cause of death in the United States. Cardiovascular health problems occur across the age continuum. To reduce death and disability, three major objectives include early detection of the disease, appropriate treatment to control the disease progression, and reduction of predisposing factors by promoting screening, education, and patient care of cardiovascular health.

Nursing Assessment

A. Nursing observations
  1. Vital signs
    a. Temperature
    b. Pulse: character, rate, rhythm, and any irregularities
    c. Respiration: character, rate; note abnormalities
  2. General appearance
    a. Note skin temperature, character, and color (jaundice, cyanosis, pallor); note clamminess
    b. Distended neck veins
    c. Dyspnea on exertion
    d. Limited or reduced ability to perform activities of daily living
    e. Clubbing of fingers
    f. Presence of edema; pedal or sacral (if supine)
  3. Heart sounds
    a. Note bruits in carotids
    b. Abnormal heart sounds/dysrhythmias
    c. Precordial movements/thrills
B. Patient description (subjective data)
  1. Chest pain
    a. Onset, location, frequency, duration, radiation,
    b. Alleviating/aggravating factors
    c. Chest pain may occur during periods of physical and emotional stress (emotions, eating, exercise, environment); pain may radiate to arm or jaw, or may occur at rest
  2. Easily fatigued
    a. Can no longer perform usual activities without frequent rest periods
    b. Intolerance of exercise/exertion
  3. Palpitations
  4. Dizziness/fatigue feeling, especially when arising or standing
  5. Cough
    a. Frothy or blood tinged (hemoptysis)
    b. Nocturnal cough
  6. Family history of heart disease and hypertension
  7. Dyspnea on exertion

Diagnostic Tests/Methods

A. Electrocardiogram (ECG)
  1. A tracing of the electrical activity of the heart
  2. A tool used to identify abnormal cardiac rhythms (dysrhythmias) and coronary atherosclerotic heart disease
  3. Reassure the patient that the ECG is recording the electrical impulses of the heart and is not delivering any electrical impulses to the body
B. Stress test
  1. A procedure designed to detect cardiac ischemia that develops during exercise or exertion
  2. A heart tracing (ECG) is recorded and monitored while a patient performs an activity such as stair climbing, pedaling a stationary bicycle, or walking on a treadmill
C. Blood tests
  1. Complete blood count (CBC): analyzes components of the blood
    a. Low hemoglobin and hematocrit indicate anemia
    b. Elevated WBC count indicates inflammation/infection
  2. Erythrocyte sedimentation rate (ESR): may indicate inflammation
  3. Blood urea nitrogen (BUN) and creatinine: to detect the effects of heart disease on the kidneys
  4. Serum enzymes and isoenzymes (serum glutamic oxaloacetic transaminase [SGOT], creatine phosphokinase [CPK], and lactate dehydrogenase [LDH]): will elevate in a myocardial infarction
  5. Serum lipids: elevated blood lipids have been associated with coronary disease
  6. Blood cultures: if bacterial endocarditis is suspected
  7. Coagulation studies: useful in monitoring anticoagulant therapy
  8. Serum electrolytes: detect imbalances in sodium, potassium, and calcium
  9. Arterial blood gases: monitor oxygenation and acid-base balance
D. Urinalysis: to determine the effects of heart disease on the kidney
E. Holter monitoring
  1. Portable monitor designed and equipped to record the patient's heartbeat during a 24-hour period; a written record of the patient's activity is kept simultaneously; helpful in determining dysrhythmias
  2. Assist the patient in the recording of activity
F. Coronary angiography
  1. A roentgenogram of the coronary circulation facilitated by the introduction of contrast medium into the artery to outline the vessel and determine the extent of the disease process
  2. After the study the patient must be observed for bleeding from the puncture site and have a cardiovascular status check of the involved area (pulses and skin temperature)
G. Chest x-ray examination: a standard chest roentgenogram is used to determine heart size and shape
H. Echocardiography (ultrasound cardiography)
  1. Echoes from sound waves are used to study the movements and dimensions of cardiac structures; determines abnormalities
  2. Information derived includes size of cardiac structures
I. Radionuclide studies
  1. Tracing material is injected intravenously, and the radioactivity concentration over a body part is recorded
  2. Size, shape, and filling of the heart chambers can be recorded; heart damage as well as cardiac circulation can also be evaluated

J. Cardiac catheterization
    1. A cardiac catheter is introduced through a vein or artery and is advanced through the system; pressures of the heart chambers and pulmonary arteries are recorded and blood is analyzed; a contrast dye can be injected for visualization of certain structures to detect defects
    2. Patient may feel a warm flushing sensation on injection of the dye; some patients experience chest pain
    3. Patient observations after examination: monitor bleeding at the insertion site, check pulses and skin warmth in the involved area, and check heart rate and rhythm
K. Oscillometry: a noninvasive test that measures the amplitude of pulsations over an artery

Frequent Patient Problems and Nursing Care

A. Pain related to decreased cardiac output; overactivity
    1. Evaluate and record onset, duration, and intensity
    2. Note any associated symptoms (nausea, vomiting, dyspnea, etc.)
    3. Monitor vital signs and record
    4. Give vasodilators as prescribed; monitor for effectiveness and observe for side effects
    5. If pain is unrelieved in 15 minutes by drugs or rest, notify physician
    6. Reinforce patient teaching regarding diet, drugs, planned exercise, and stress management
    7. Record reactions to treatment and nursing care
B. Ineffective breathing pattern related to dyspnea
    1. Monitor vital signs and record
    2. Note character and rate of respirations
    3. Elevate the head of the bed at least 30 degrees
    4. Help patient assume an orthopneic position when necessary
    5. Auscultate chest and note the presence of abnormal lung and heart sounds
    6. Monitor oxygen therapy
    7. Monitor intake and output
    8. Record reactions to treatment and nursing care
    9. Give diuretics, cardiotonics, and bronchodilators as prescribed and monitor for side effects
    10. Note color, character, and amount of sputum
C. Decreased cardiac output related to dysrhythmias
    1. Monitor vital signs and record
    2. Note and report any changes in the vital signs
    3. Auscultate chest, noting any abnormal heart sounds and report abnormalities
    4. Give antidysrhythmic drugs as prescribed and monitor for side effects
    5. Monitor for and report any associated symptoms
D. Impaired tissue perfusion related to edema
    1. Note and record location and degree
    2. Elevate legs
    3. Change positions when in bed
    4. Note degree of pitting
    5. Note "weeping" of skin areas
    6. Monitor for skin breakdown
    7. Give prescribed diuretics and cardiotonics
    8. Note the presence of tenderness in the upper quadrant of the abdomen
    9. Note the presence of ascites
    10. Note daily weight
    11. Record intake and output
    12. Limit fluid intake as prescribed
    13. Reinforce teaching for reduction of dependent edema
E. Fatigue/activity intolerance related to reduced cardiac reserve
    1. Encourage progressive ambulation
    2. Encourage progressive resuming of activities of daily living
    3. Provide for planned activity and rest periods
    4. Monitor for signs of fatigue
    5. Stop activity at the first sign of intolerance
    6. ROM exercises
    7. Provide prescribed diet
    8. Reinforce patient instruction of planned exercise
F. Alteration in tissue perfusion related to decreased cardiac output
    1. Observe for presence of postural hypotension
    2. Assist patient to dangle legs over the side of the bed before standing
    3. Instruct patient to get up slowly
    4. Assess patient's pulse when standing
G. Fluid volume excess related to decreased cardiac output
    1. Note daily weight; report weight changes
    2. Record intake and output
    3. Monitor serum electrolytes
    4. Limit fluids as prescribed
    5. Provide salt-restricted diet if ordered
    6. Give diuretic medication as prescribed
    7. Reinforce instructions regarding diet, drugs, and weight control
H. Alteration in tissue perfusion related to hypertension
    1. Monitor vital signs and report changes
    2. Provide sodium-restricted diet as prescribed
    3. Provide cholesterol-controlled diet if prescribed and monitor for side effects
    5. Instruct in the avoidance of risk factors (smoking, stress, and obesity)
    6. Reinforce teaching in the areas of diet, weight control, avoidance of risk factors, and home monitoring of blood pressure

Major Medical Diagnoses

ARTERIOSCLEROSIS-ATHEROSCLEROSIS

A. Definition
    1. Arteriosclerosis: a process in which the arterial walls harden, thicken, and lose their elasticity, resulting in restricted blood flow
    2. Atherosclerosis: one form of arteriosclerosis; fatty plaques form on the intima (inner layer) of the arteries
B. Pathology
    1. The underlying mechanism is the formation of fatty plaque deposits in the arteries
    2. The plaque increases in size and ultimately obstructs blood flow to vital areas
C. Arteriosclerosis is associated with the following health problems
    1. Coronary artery disease
    2. Angina pectoris
    3. Myocardial infarction
    4. Hypertension
    5. Peripheral vascular disease
    6. Cerebrovascular accidents (strokes)

D. Signs and symptoms vary, depending on the arteries affected by the sclerosing process
   1. Extremity involvement
      a. Cramping pain (intermittent claudication)
      b. Numbness and tingling
      c. Reduced circulation causing ulceration or pain
      d. Outward changes: skin pallor, cool skin, reduced or absent pulses, loss of leg hair, and skin ulceration
   2. Coronary involvement
      a. Chest pain
      b. Dyspnea
      c. Palpitations
      d. Fainting (syncope)
      e. Fatigue
E. Diagnostic tests/methods
   1. Patient history and physical examination
   2. Arteriograms
   3. ECG
   4. Oscillometry
F. Treatment
   1. Dietary restriction of fat and cholesterol
   2. Vasodilating drugs
   3. Cholesterol-lowering drugs
   4. Elimination or reduction of risk factors
      a. Smoking
      b. Obesity
      c. Stress
      d. Lack of exercise
   5. Weight management
   6. Planned exercise
   7. Prevention of pressure in extremities
   8. Use of special devices such as bed cradles
   9. Bypass surgery or removal of plaques may be considered
G. Nursing intervention
   1. Assess and document signs and symptoms
   2. Protect the extremity from trauma
   3. Monitor protective devices (bed cradles, pads, etc.)
   4. Provide skin care to ulcerated areas or areas affected by reduced circulation
   5. Monitor pulses and skin character of involved extremities
   6. Report changes in the involved extremities
      a. Absence of pulse
      b. Cyanosis
      c. Increased pain
      d. Temperature change (coldness)
   7. Monitor for signs and symptoms of infection in ulcerated areas
   8. Provide slow, progressive physical activity as prescribed
   9. Give prescribed diet
   10. Administer prescribed drugs
   11. Relieve pain from ischemia
   12. Avoid cold and provide adequate warmth to prevent vasoconstriction
   13. Avoid clothing that impairs circulation
   14. Educate patient and family regarding avoidance of risk factors, dietary management, medication, and activity

ANGINA PECTORIS
A. Definition: episodes of acute chest pain resulting from insufficient oxygenation of myocardial tissue, caused by decreased blood flow to the area

   1. Episodes occur most frequently during periods of physical or emotional exertion
      a. Exercise
      b. Eating a heavy meal
      c. Environmental temperature extremes
   2. Episodes seldom last more than 15 minutes
B. Causes
   1. The major cause is atherosclerosis
   2. Narrowed coronary arteries obstruct blood flow; thus oxygen carried by the blood cannot sufficiently meet tissue demands, particularly during periods of exertion
C. Signs and symptoms
   1. Substernal chest pain, usually brought on by exertion
   2. Radiation of pain to the jaw or an extremity
   3. Dyspnea
   4. Anxiety or feeling of impending doom
   5. Tachycardia
   6. Diaphoresis
   7. Sensation of heaviness, choking, or suffocation
   8. Indigestion
D. Diagnostic tests/methods
   1. Patient history and physical examination
   2. ECG
   3. Holter monitoring
   4. Coronary angiography
   5. Stress testing
   6. Chest x-ray examination
   7. Serum lipid and enzyme values
E. Treatment
   1. Relief of chest pain through the use of vasodilating drugs (e.g., nitrates, beta blockers, calcium channel blockers), sedatives, and analgesics
   2. Dietary restriction of fat and cholesterol
   3. Planned exercise
   4. Weight management
   5. Stress management
   6. If conservative measures are unsuccessful, coronary bypass surgery or an angioplasty may be considered
F. Nursing intervention
   1. Assess and document signs and symptoms and reactions to treatment
   2. Administer vasodilating medication and monitor for side effects
   3. Instruct patient to inform the nursing staff at the onset of an anginal attack
   4. Provide emotional support and assurance
   5. Provide prompt relief of pain
   6. Monitor vital signs, particularly during an attack
   7. Educate patient and family regarding diet, activity, drug therapy, and avoidance of risk factors

HYPERTENSION (HIGH BLOOD PRESSURE)
A. Definition: characterized by persistent elevation of blood pressure in which the systolic pressure is above 140 mm Hg and the diastolic pressure is above 90 mm Hg
   1. Primary hypertension (essential): a persistent elevation of blood pressure without an apparent cause
      a. Actual cause is unknown
      b. Primarily, small blood vessels are affected; peripheral resistance increases; and blood pressure rises
      c. Constricted blood vessels eventually cause damage to organs that rely on a blood supply from these vessels

2. Secondary hypertension: a persistent elevation of blood pressure associated with another disease state
   a. Renal disease
   b. Toxemia
   c. Adrenal dysfunction
   d. Atherosclerosis
   e. Coarctation of the aorta
B. Predisposing factors
   1. Smoking
   2. Obesity
   3. Heavy salt and cholesterol intake
   4. Heredity
   5. Aggressive, hyperactive personality
   6. Age: develops between 30 and 50 years of age
   7. Sex: primarily men over 35 years of age and women over 45 years of age
   8. Race: blacks have twice the incidence of whites
   9. Birth control pills and estrogens
C. The heart brain, kidney, and eyes can be damaged if the hypertensive state continues without correction
D. Signs and symptoms may be insidious and vague; a person can have the disorder and not know it
   1. Tinnitus
   2. Light-headedness
   3. Blurred vision
   4. Irritability
   5. Fatigue
   6. Tachycardia and palpitations
   7. Occipital, morning headaches
   8. Nosebleeds (epistaxis)
   9. Dyspnea on exertion
E. Diagnostic tests/methods
   1. Patient history and physical examination
   2. Series of resting blood pressure readings
   3. Routine urinalysis, BUN, and serum creatinine to screen for renal involvement
   4. Serum electrolytes to screen for adrenal involvement
   5. Blood sugar levels to screen for endocrine involvement
   6. Lipid profile
   7. Chest x-ray examination
   8. ECG
   9. Holter monitoring
   10. Funduscopic eye examination
F. Treatment
   1. Lowering blood pressure through the use of antihypertensive drugs
   2. Sodium-restricted diet
   3. Cholesterol-controlled diet
   4. Weight management
   5. Stress management
   6. Reduction or elimination of smoking
   7. Planned exercise
G. Nursing intervention
   1. Assess and document signs and symptoms and reactions to treatments
   2. Administer prescribed medication
   3. Observe for and report drug-related side effects
   4. Monitor weight every day (qd) to evaluate initial diuretic therapy
   5. Monitor intake and output to evaluate initial diuretic therapy

6. Monitor vital signs, particularly blood pressure, under the same conditions qd
7. Provide planned activity and rest periods
8. Provide prescribed diet
   a. Calorie controlled
   b. Sodium restricted
   c. Cholesterol controlled
9. Educate patient and family
   a. Drug therapy and side effects
   b. Dietary restrictions; weight management
   c. Elimination of risk factors, such as smoking
   d. Activity
   e. Blood pressure monitoring
   f. Need for participation in and compliance with the prescribed regimen

MYOCARDIAL INFARCTION (HEART ATTACK)

A. Definition: the obstruction of a coronary artery or one of its branches
   1. The obstruction results in the death of the myocardial tissue supplied by that vessel
   2. The myocardial tissue dies because of oxygen deprivation (Fig. 5-8)
   3. The heart's ability to regain or maintain its function depends on the location and size of the area of infarction
B. A myocardial infarction can occur whenever a coronary artery or branch of the artery becomes occluded by a thrombus, emboli, or the atherosclerotic process
C. Signs and symptoms
   1. "Crushing" chest pain lasting longer than 15 minutes and unrelieved by rest or drugs
   2. Shortness of breath
   3. Nausea and vomiting

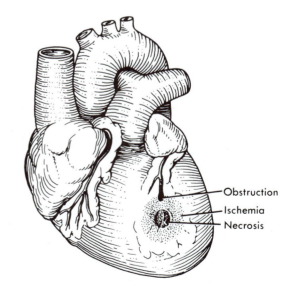

Figure 5-8. Myocardial infarction: areas of ischemia and necrosis. (From Billings DM, Stokes LG: *Medical-surgical nursing: common health problems of adults and children across the life span*, St Louis, 1986, Mosby.)

4. Tachycardia
5. Diaphoresis and pallor
6. Temperature rise after 48 hours
7. Elevation of the cardiac enzymes
8. Dysrhythmias
9. Anxiety
D. Diagnostic tests/methods
   1. Patient history and physical examination
   2. ECG
   3. Cardiac enzyme studies (SGOT, LDH, CPK-MB)
   4. Chest x-ray examination
E. Treatment
   1. Analgesic drugs to relieve pain
   2. Oxygen to relieve respiratory distress
   3. Vasopressor drugs to prevent circulatory collapse (cardiogenic shock)
   4. Cardiac monitoring to detect dysrhythmias
   5. Hemodynamic monitoring: internal monitoring of the blood pressure and pulmonary artery pressure
   6. Bed rest with progressive activity to allow the damaged myocardium to heal
   7. Intravenous (IV) fluids to provide for IV drug administration
   8. Cardiopulmonary resuscitation in the event of cardiac standstill (arrest)
   9. Pacemaker insertion
   10. Anticoagulant therapy
   11. Thrombolytic therapy to dissolve blood clot and restore blood flow
   12. Nitrates
F. Nursing intervention
   1. Provide pain relief
   2. Provide ongoing assessment and documentation of symptoms and reactions to treatment
   3. Administer and monitor oxygen
   4. Record vital signs qh during the acute period
   5. Record intake and output qh during the acute period
   6. Provide bed rest during the acute period and progressive activity as prescribed
      a. Apply antiembolism stockings
      b. Allow patient out of bed to use bedside commode (less taxing to the cardiovascular system)
      c. Monitor pulse during periods of activity
   7. Avoid activities that produce straining (Valsalva's maneuver) to avoid taxing the cardiovascular system
      a. Administer stool softeners as prescribed
      b. Caution patient against straining when attempting a bowel movement
   8. Provide diet as prescribed
      a. May start out on liquids and then progress
      b. Sodium and cholesterol may be restricted
      c. Caffeine may be restricted
   9. Give prescribed antidysrhythmics and monitor for side effects
   10. Give prescribed cardiotonics and diuretics and monitor for side effects
   11. Monitor for complications
      a. Cardiogenic shock: circulatory collapse caused by decreased cardiac output; the vital organs are not being perfused
         (1) Monitor vital signs every 15 minutes
         (2) Record intake and output qh

         (3) Report changes in rate, rhythm, and conductivity
         (4) Observe and report signs and symptoms of restlessness, diaphoresis, pallor, low blood pressure, and tachycardia
         (5) Administer and monitor prescribed vasopressors and antidysrhythmics
         (6) Administer oxygen as prescribed
         (7) Provide cardiac and hemodynamic monitoring (hemodynamic monitoring refers to the internal monitoring of blood pressure and pulmonary artery pressure)
      b. Pulmonary edema: left ventricle failure (pumping mechanism) caused by strain on a diseased heart; cardiac output (the amount of blood pumped out by the heart to the body per minute) is reduced, resulting in lung congestion
         (1) Observe and report symptoms of anxiety, dyspnea, orthopnea, frothy, pink-tinged sputum, rales, decreased urine output, and dependent edema
         (2) Record vital signs every 15 minutes
         (3) Record intake and output qh
         (4) Place bed in high-Fowler's position
         (5) Administer cardiotonics and diuretics as prescribed and monitor for side effects
         (6) Administer and monitor oxygen therapy
         (7) Be prepared to administer analgesics to allay anxiety and reduce respiratory rate
         (8) Provide emotional support to patient and family

CONGESTIVE HEART FAILURE
A. Definition: failure of the pumping mechanism of the heart resulting in an insufficient blood supply to meet the body's needs
B. Causes
   1. The underlying mechanism in congestive heart failure (CHF) involves the failure of the pumping mechanism of the heart to respond to the metabolic changes of the body
   2. The end result is a heart that cannot supply a sufficient amount of blood in relation to the body's needs and to the amount of blood returning to the heart (venous return); pressure builds up in the vascular beds on the affected side of the heart
C. CHF is described in terms of left-sided or right-sided failure, depending on which side is affected
D. Signs and symptoms are divided into left-sided failure and right-sided failure, although both sides may be affected
   1. Left-sided failure leads to pulmonary congestion
      a. Dyspnea
      b. Orthopnea
      c. Nonproductive cough that worsens at night
      d. As severity of failure increases, frothy, blood-tinged sputum is noted
      e. Anxiety and restlessness
      f. Fatigue
   2. Right-sided failure may follow left-sided failure and results in systemic venous congestion
      a. Weight gain caused by fluid accumulation in the tissues
      b. Dependent edema in the form of ankle edema or sacral edema

c. Ascites caused by the collection of fluid in the abdominal cavity; ascites may also hinder respiration

d. Fatigue

e. Gastrointestinal symptoms such as nausea, vomiting, and anorexia

f. Decreased urine output

E. Diagnostic test/methods

1. Patient history and physical examination including the findings of edema, abnormal heart sounds, and the presence of rales with dyspnea (orthopnea)

2. Chest x-ray examination

3. ECG

4. Arterial blood gas studies

5. Liver function studies

6. Renal function studies

F. Treatment

1. Drug therapy: digitalization, diuretics, and sedatives

2. Recording of weight qd

3. Monitoring intake and output

4. Oxygen therapy

5. Hemodynamic monitoring

6. Restricting fluids

7. Restricting dietary sodium

8. Bed rest with progressive activity

9. Elevate the head of the bed on blocks

10. Monitor vital signs

G. Nursing intervention

1. Provide ongoing assessment and documentation of signs, symptoms, and reactions to treatment

2. Monitor oxygen therapy

3. Record vital signs every 15 minutes to 2 hours during the acute phase

4. Record intake and output qh during the acute phase

5. Weigh patient qd

6. Administer and monitor prescribed cardiotonics, diuretics, and sedatives; observe for side effects

7. Determine the amount of activity that produces the least discomfort to the patient

8. Monitor for dependent edema

a. Ankle edema when sitting upright

b. Sacral edema when in supine position

9. Raise the head of the bed as prescribed

10. Observe for complications of bed rest

a. Have patient turn, cough, and take deep breaths

b. Apply antiembolism stockings

11. Provide emotional support to the patient and family

12. Provide a diet low in sodium if prescribed

13. Educate the patient and family concerning dietary management, drug therapy, and activity

14. Restrict fluids as ordered

VALVULAR CONDITIONS

A. Valvular dysfunction results in either stenosis or insufficiency of the heart valves

1. Valvular stenosis results from cardiac infections; the valve leaflets (cusps) become fibrotic and thicken and may even fuse together, thus hindering blood flow

2. Valvular insufficiency occurs in much the same way as valvular stenosis; after repeated infections the valve leaflets (cusps) become inflamed and scarred and no longer close completely; the incomplete closure allows blood to leak from the left ventricle into the left atrium during systole

B. Blood flow through the heart is altered, resulting in decreased cardiac output, systemic and pulmonary congestion, and dilation of the heart chambers

C. Causes

1. Rheumatic heart disease is the primary cause of valvular dysfunction

2. Other causes include syphilis, bacterial endocarditis, and congenital malformations

D. Signs and symptoms

1. Mitral stenosis

a. Dyspnea on exertion

b. Orthopnea

c. Pink-tinged sputum

d. Fatigue

e. Palpitations

f. Heart murmur

2. Mitral insufficiency

a. Fatigue

b. Dyspnea or exertion

c. Heart murmur

d. Orthopnea

e. Pulmonary congestion

3. Aortic stenosis

a. Fatigue

b. Angina

c. Syncope

d. Heart murmur

e. Congestive heart failure

4. Aortic insufficiency

a. Palpitations

b. Dyspnea

c. Fatigue

d. Orthopnea

e. Anginal pain occurring even at rest

E. Diagnostic tests/methods

1. Patient history and physical examination; a murmur is a common finding of the examination

2. ECG

3. Chest x-ray examination: to determine heart size

4. Cardiac catheterization: may reveal pressure changes

5. Echocardiogram: provides information concerning structure and function of valves

6. Laboratory studies

F. Treatment

1. Mitral stenosis

a. Antibiotics administered prophylactically to prevent recurrences of causative agents

b. Drug therapy: diuretics, cardiotonics, and antidysrhythmics

c. Restricted sodium diet

d. Planned activity and avoidance of symptom-producing activity

e. Surgical correction of the defect

(1) Mitral commissurotomy: the fused valve leaflets are separated, and the mitral opening may be dilated

(2) Valve replacement: diseased valve is replaced with a prosthetic valve

2. Mitral insufficiency

a. Planned exercise and avoidance of symptom-producing activity

b. Sodium-restricted diet

c. Drug therapy; diuretics, cardiotonics, antidysrhythmics, and vasodilators
d. Surgical correction
   (1) Valvuloplasty: repair of the existing valve
   (2) Valve replacement
3. Aortic stenosis
   a. Prevention of infective endocarditis
   b. Treatment of symptoms
   c. Drug therapy: diuretics, nitrates, and cardiotonics
   d. Sodium-restricted diet
   e. Valve replacement
G. Nursing intervention
   1. Assess and document signs and symptoms and reaction to treatments
   2. Administer prescribed medication and observe patient for side effects
   3. Provide a calm, quiet environment
   4. Allow patient and family to verbalize their anxieties and fears
   5. Monitor vital signs and report changes
   6. Weigh the patient qd
   7. Provide the prescribed diet
      a. Nutritionally well balanced
      b. Sodium restricted to prevent fluid retention
   8. Progressive activity as prescribed
      a. Consider the patient's limitations
      b. Provide rest periods
   9. Monitor intake and output if diuretics are used
   10. Educate patient and family concerning diet, drugs, activity, and need for compliance
   11. Vocational counseling may be needed if the patient has a demanding job

INFLAMMATORY DISORDERS OF THE HEART
A. Definition: diseases resulting from acute or chronic inflammation of the lining of the heart and valves caused by bacteria or viruses, trauma, or other factors
   1. Pericarditis: an inflammation of the pericardium
      a. The result is a loss of elasticity or fluid accumulation within the pericardial sac
      b. Heart failure and cardiac tamponade may result
   2. Myocarditis: an inflammation of the myocardium
      a. The result is impairment of contractility
      b. Myocardial ischemia and necrosis may result
   3. Endocarditis: an inflammation of the inner lining of the heart and valves associated with a streptococcal infection
   4. Rheumatic heart disease
      a. Usually associated with rheumatic fever
      b. Rheumatic fever is an inflammatory process that can affect all the layers of the heart
      c. Cardiac impairment results from swelling and scarring of valve leaflets, leading to valvular changes (mitral insufficiency, aortic insufficiency, and pericarditis)
B. Signs and symptoms
   1. Chest pain
   2. Dyspnea
   3. Chills and intermittent fever
   4. Weakness and fatigue
   5. Diaphoresis
   6. Anorexia
   7. Dysrhythmias

8. Elevated cardiac enzymes
9. Friction rubs (auscultatory sound created by the rubbing together of two serous surfaces)
10. Presence of Aschoff bodies (collection of cells and leukocytes in the interstitial layers of the heart)
11. New heart murmur or an abnormal heart sound
12. Existing streptococcal infection
13. Cardiac enlargement
14. Joint involvement
C. Diagnostic tests/methods
   1. Patient history and physical examination
      a. History of recent infections
      b. History of heart disease
   2. ECG
   3. Chest x-ray examination
   4. Cardiac enzyme studies
   5. Blood cultures
   6. Echocardiogram: to assess valvular disease and vegetation (growth of scar tissue)
   7. Laboratory studies: CBC, electrolytes, ESR
   8. Radionuclide studies: to assess heart structure and heart damage
D. Treatment
   1. Identification and elimination of the infecting agent
   2. Drug therapy: antibiotics, cardiotonics, antiinflammatory agents, analgesics, and corticosteroids
   3. Blood cultures
   4. Oxygen
   5. Rest and planned activity
   6. Well-balanced diet
   7. Prevention of exposure to other infectious agents
E. Nursing intervention
   1. Assess and document signs and symptoms and reactions to treatment
   2. Maintain a calm, quiet environment
   3. Administer prescribed drugs and monitor for side effects
   4. Evaluate the patient's understanding of the disease process and the need for compliance
   5. Alleviate pain
   6. Allay patient's and family's fears and anxieties
   7. Monitor vital signs and report changes
   8. Observe for signs and symptoms of complications (tachycardia, dyspnea, and orthopnea)
   9. Educate patient concerning the illness, diet, drugs, activity, avoidance of infections, dental care, vocational counseling, and compliance to the regimen

Peripheral Vascular Conditions

Peripheral vascular disease refers to vascular disorders exclusive of those affecting the heart. The underlying factor in peripheral vascular disease is the arteriosclerotic process. Blood flow is slowed because of vessels that are narrowed or obstructed. The lack of normal blood flow causes tissue changes (see Arteriosclerosis under Assessment of the cardiovascular system). Vascular disease related to the lower extremities is discussed in this section.

Nursing Assessment

A. Nursing observation
   1. Skin of the lower extremities
      a. Redness (hyperemia) of the leg when in a dependent position
      b. Cold or blue feet

c. Varicose veins
d. Sparse hair distribution
e. Lesions or stasis ulcers
f. Edema
g. Dermatitis or brown pigmentation of the skin
2. Delayed capillary filling
3. Diminished or absent pulses
   a. Rigidity (hardness) of the vessels
   b. Palpable vibration of the vessels (thrill)
4. Assess major arteries for bruits (an auscultatory sound taking the form of a buzzing or humming sound)
5. Differences in leg circumference
6. Thickening of nail beds

B. Patient description (subjective data)
1. Leg cramps
2. Aching calves
3. Leg numbness
4. Leg pain occurring during exercise (claudication)
5. Loss of sensation in the leg(s)
6. Past or present history
   a. Alcohol excess
   b. Diabetes mellitus
   c. Hypertension
   d. Thrombophlebitis

Diagnostic Tests/Methods

A. Chest x-ray examination for abnormalities
B. Oscillometry: a noninvasive test that measures the amplitude of pulsations over an artery
C. Doppler ultrasonography: a device that emits sound waves that can be used to measure the amount of blood flow through a vessel
D. Arteriography: Used to determine the location and extent of the disease process
E. Venography: radiographic study used to determine the location and size of a blood clot, vessel distention, and development of collateral circulation
F. Trendelenburg test
1. Used to determine valvular competency
2. The leg is elevated to 90 degrees, and a tourniquet is placed around the thigh
3. The patient stands, and the vein-filling pattern is observed
4. Normally the veins fill slowly from below in 20 to 30 seconds; the rate of filling should not greatly accelerate when the tourniquet is removed
G. Lung scan
1. Used to assess the presence of pulmonary embolism and lung damage
2. An intravenous, radiographic isotope is injected into the patient
3. Pulmonary circulation is assessed with a scanning device
4. The patient also inhales a radioactive gas and is scanned to determine lung distribution of this gas
H. Arterial blood gas analysis: used to assess the adequacy of ventilation
I. X-ray examination of the abdomen: may show evidence of an aneurysm
J. Blood tests
1. CBC: for routine evaluation
2. ESR: used to determine the presence of an inflammatory process
3. Coagulation studies (platelet count, bleeding time, prothrombin time [PT], and partial thromboplastin time [PTT]): used to determine the existence of blood disorders

Frequent Patient Problems and Nursing Care

A. Pain related to intermittent claudication
1. Evaluate and record onset, duration, and intensity
2. Provide rest during the episode
3. Determine the amount of exercise the patient can tolerate before claudication occurs
4. Assess for and report claudication occurring without activity
5. Educate the patient to avoid exposure to cold and maintain warmth
B. Fluid volume excess as evidenced by edema of the lower extremities/decreased cardiac output
1. Note and record location and degree
2. Instruct patient to avoid activity that places the legs in a dependent position for prolonged periods
3. Instruct patient to avoid wearing constricting clothing around the legs
4. Monitor for skin breakdown
5. Elevate legs
C. Impaired skin integrity related to stasis ulcers
1. Note location and character of ulceration
2. Maintain bed rest with leg elevation
3. Perform prescribed wound care
4. Instruct patient to avoid trauma to the legs
5. Instruct patient in proper skin care measures
6. Reinforce patient teaching in the area of drugs, diet, activity, and skin care

Major Medical Diagnoses
ARTERIOSCLEROSIS OBLITERANS
A. Definition: a chronic arteriooclusive disease
1. Progresses slowly and insidiously
2. The medial and intimal layers of arteries become inflamed and thrombosed
3. There is loss of vessel elasticity, and plaques obstruct blood flow
4. Vessels primarily affected are the femoral and carotid arteries
B. Causes
1. Associated with atherosclerotic process
2. Predisposing factors include hypertension, smoking, hyperlipidemia, obesity, and a positive family history
C. Signs and symptoms
1. Intermittent claudication
2. Pain in the legs at rest
3. Impotence
4. Paresthesia
5. Pallor or blanching on elevation of leg
6. Hyperemia (redness) or dusky appearance of the leg(s) when dependent
7. Loss of hair on extremities
8. Absent or diminished pulses
D. Diagnostic tests/methods
1. Patient history and physical examination
2. Oscillometry
3. Doppler ultrasonography

4. Arteriography
5. Laboratory studies
E. Treatments
  1. Protection of extremity from injury
  2. Prevention and control of infection
  3. Drug therapy: vasodilators, analgesics, and antibiotics
  4. Weight-reduction diet if patient is obese
  5. Bed rest
  6. Avoidance of smoking
  7. Surgical management: endarterectomy (removing the obstructing plaque) or a bypass graft
F. Nursing intervention
  1. Assist the patient in obtaining body warmth and warmth to the extremity
    a. Warm room
    b. Warm bath
    c. Warm clothes such as socks
  2. Avoid applying direct heat to the affected part
  3. Protect the affected part from trauma and pressure
    a. Use bed cradle
    b. Assess skin lesions and monitor for signs of infection
    c. Caution patient against wearing anything that constricts
  4. Give prescribed drugs and monitor for side effects
  5. Assess the affected part qd
    a. Assess skin color, temperature, and circulation
    b. Monitor for pain
  6. Provide emotional support
  7. Educate the patient and family regarding
    a. Hygiene and avoidance of infection
    b. Rest and planned exercise
    c. Protection from injury
    d. Diet
    e. Drugs
    f. Improvement of circulation

BUERGER'S DISEASE (THROMBOANGIITIS OBLITERANS)

A. Definition: an inflammatory process primarily affecting arteries that causes occlusion, thrombosis, and ultimately ischemia
  1. Medium-sized distal arteries of the legs are primarily affected
  2. Veins can also be affected
B. Causes
  1. Exact cause is unknown
  2. Associated with smoking
  3. Men in the 25- to 40-year age group who smoke are at risk
  4. Familial tendency
C. Signs and symptoms
  1. Coldness of the extremities
  2. Diminished or absent pulses
  3. Numbness and tingling
  4. Cramping pain (intermittent claudication)
  5. Pain at rest, not associated with activity
  6. Skin ulceration
  7. Aggravation of symptoms by exposure to cold environment
  8. Change in appearance of extremities
  9. Muscle atrophy
  10. Slow-healing cuts
  11. Gangrene
  12. Sensitivity to cold

D. Diagnostic tests/methods
  1. Patient history and physical examination
  2. Oscillometry
  3. Doppler ultrasonography
  4. Arteriography
  5. Laboratory studies
  6. ECG
  7. Chest x-ray examination
E. Treatment
  1. Restricting smoking
  2. Drug therapy: vasodilating drugs, analgesics, and anti-coagulants
  3. Moderate exercise
  4. Avoidance and treatment of infection
  5. Protection from trauma
  6. Sympathectomy (disruption of nerve impulses to a particular area)
  7. Nerve blocks (use of drug injections to block nerve impulses)
  8. Amputation, as a last resort
F. Nursing intervention
  1. Support the patient in his effort to stop smoking
  2. Give prescribed vasodilators, analgesics, and anti-coagulants; monitor for side effects
  3. Document location and character of pain
  4. Assist the patient in maintaining warmth
  5. Educate the patient and family concerning drug therapy, activity, and avoidance of smoking, exposure to cold, constricting clothing, and trauma

RAYNAUD'S DISEASE

A. Definition: a peripheral vascular disease affecting digital arteries
  1. Disease occurs primarily in women
  2. Exposure to environmental cold, emotional stress, or tobacco use produces spasms of the arteries
  3. Hands and arms are usually affected
B. Cause
  1. Exact cause is unknown
  2. Associated with collagen diseases in women
C. Contributing factors
  1. Pressure to the fingertips such as that encountered by typists and pianists
  2. Use of hand-held vibrating equipment on a regular basis
D. Signs and symptoms
  1. Numbness and tingling
  2. Blanching of digits and cyanosis
  3. Hyperemia
  4. Coldness
  5. Dryness and atrophy of the nails
  6. Pain
  7. Punctate (small hole) lesions of the fingertips
  8. Eventual gangrene of the fingertips
E. Diagnostic tests/methods
  1. Patient history and physical examination
  2. Doppler ultrasonography
  3. Arteriography
  4. ECG
  5. Chest x-ray examination
F. Treatment
  1. Drug therapy with vasodilators
  2. Sympathectomy: in advanced cases

3. Elimination of smoking
4. Avoidance of stressful situations
5. Avoidance of exposure to cold

G. Nursing intervention
1. Document location and characteristics of pain
2. Observe affected areas qd
3. Administer prescribed vasodilators and analgesics; monitor for side effects
4. Instruct patient to avoid activities that precipitate spasms
5. Instruct patient to avoid exposing the hands to the cold without proper protection
6. Support patient's effort to give up smoking
7. Offer emotional support and allay anxiety
8. Educate patient and family concerning drug therapy, avoidance of cold, protection from trauma/infection, and prevention of spasms

ANEURYSMS

A. Definition: the enlargement or ballooning of an artery, usually caused by trauma, congenital weakness, arteriosclerosis, or infection; aorta is most frequently affected artery
B. Causes
1. Causes are varied, but the prime culprit is arteriosclerosis; plaque formation causes degenerative changes leading to loss of vessel elasticity, weakness, and dilation
2. Syphilis
3. Infections
4. Congenital disorder
5. Trauma
6. Risk factors: obesity, smoking, hypertension, stress, high blood cholesterol levels
C. Signs and symptoms
1. Abdominal
a. Increased blood pressure
b. Visible or palpable pulsating mass
c. Pain or tenderness in the abdominal area
2. Thoracic
a. Dyspnea
b. Dysphagia
c. Hoarseness or cough
d. Severe chest pain
3. Ruptured aneurysm
a. Anxiety
b. Restlessness
c. Pain
d. Diminished pulses
e. Hypotension and shock
D. Diagnostic tests/methods
1. Patient history and physical examination
2. Chest x-ray examination
3. Abdominal x-ray examination
4. Ultrasonography
5. Angiography/arteriography
6. Routine ECG
7. Laboratory studies
E. Treatment
1. Conservative measures
a. Drug therapy: antihypertensives, pain relievers, and negative inotropic agents
b. Correct hydration and electrolyte imbalances
c. Decreased activity

2. Surgical repair
a. Resection and replacement with a prosthesis of Teflon or Dacron
b. Resection and replacement with a graft
F. Nursing intervention
1. Provide immediate postoperative care
a. Assess vital signs and peripheral pulses every 15 minutes; then decrease the frequency as ordered
b. Record intake and output qh
c. Compare extremities for warmth and color
d. Administer IV fluids at prescribed rate
e. Relieve pain with prescribed analgesic
f. Monitor oxygen therapy
g. Give prescribed prophylactic antibiotics as ordered
h. Assess level of consciousness every 1 to 2 hours
i. Auscultate lung sounds and bowel sounds at least q4h
j. Monitor for dysrhythmias
k. Have patient turn, cough, and deep breathe at least q2h
2. Other postoperative considerations
a. Provide antiembolism stockings
b. Provide emotional support and allay anxiety
c. Encourage early ambulation as prescribed
d. Instruct patient to observe for changes in the extremities such as color and warmth
e. Instruct patient on assessments of peripheral pulses

PHLEBITIS AND THROMBOPHLEBITIS

A. Definition: inflammatory disorders of the veins
1. Phlebitis: inflammation of a vein
2. Thrombophlebitis: inflammation of a vein with clot formation
B. Causes
1. The inflammation and clot formation are associated with venous stasis, vessel damage, and enhanced blood coagulability
2. Situations that produce venous stasis include immobility, prolonged periods of standing, wearing confining clothing, and increased abdominal pressure
C. Signs and symptoms
1. Redness and pain along vein path
2. Elevation of temperature
3. Swelling
4. Positive Homans' sign (pain on dorsiflexion of the foot)
5. Area is sensitive to the touch
D. Diagnostic tests/methods
1. Patient history and physical examination
2. Doppler ultrasonography
3. Venography
4. Laboratory studies: CBC, ESR, and coagulation studies
5. Lung scan to rule out pulmonary embolism
E. Treatment
1. Bed rest
2. Anticoagulant therapy
3. Thrombolytic therapy
4. Vasodilators
5. Warm, moist packs to the affected leg (some physicians prefer ice packs to the area)
6. Antiembolism stockings
7. Elevation of affected extremity
8. Surgical intervention is required in only a small percentage of patients

F. Nursing intervention
1. Assess and document signs and symptoms
2. Administer analgesics as ordered and monitor for side effects
3. Elevate leg as ordered; avoid the use of a knee gatch or pillow under the affected knee; avoid crossing legs
4. Apply warm, moist heat as ordered
5. Assess thigh and calf measurements qd
6. Monitor vital signs q4h
7. Maintain bed rest as ordered
8. Apply antiembolism stockings on unaffected leg
9. Avoid massaging calf of affected leg
10. Avoid constrictive clothing
11. Monitor anticoagulant therapy
12. Monitor for bleeding tendencies
    a. Bleeding gums
    b. Epistaxis
    c. Bruising easily
    d. Melena
    e. Petechiae
13. Monitor hemoglobin and hematocrit levels
14. Educate patient and family concerning drug therapy, avoiding activities that aggravate the existing state, and monitoring for signs and symptoms of complications
15. Monitor patient for complications such as an embolism

EMBOLISM

A. Definition: a blood clot circulating in the blood
B. Causes
1. The clot may be a fragment of an arteriosclerotic plaque, or it may have originated in the heart
2. If large, an embolism may lodge in a vessel bifurcation and obstruct the flow of blood to vital organs or tissues
3. Most emboli arise from deep vein thrombi; the embolus travels in the bloodstream until it lodges in a narrowed area, usually the lungs
C. Signs and symptoms: depend on the area involved
1. Pain at the site
2. Shock
3. Areas supplied by the involved vessel evidence pallor, coldness, numbness, tingling, and cyanosis
4. Sudden onset of dyspnea
5. Cough and hemoptysis
6. Chest pain
7. Tachycardia
8. Tachypnea
D. Diagnostic tests/methods
1. Patient history and physical examination
2. Lung scan
3. Chest x-ray examination
4. Arterial blood gases
E. Treatment
1. Oxygen therapy
2. IV fluids
3. IV anticoagulants
4. Analgesics
5. Thrombolytic agents
F. Nursing intervention
1. Assess and document signs and symptoms and reactions to treatments
2. Monitor vital signs
3. Monitor arterial blood gas reports

4. Administer prescribed analgesic and monitor for side effects
5. Administer anticoagulants as prescribed and monitor for bleeding tendencies
6. Monitor oxygen therapy
7. Give ROM exercises
8. Provide antiembolism stockings
9. Educate patient and family concerning drug therapy, monitoring for bleeding tendencies, and restriction of activities

VARICOSE VEINS

A. Definition: dilated, tortuous leg veins resulting from blood back-flow caused by incomplete valve closure; this leads to congestion and further enlargement
B. Causes
1. Basic cause of varicosities is unknown
2. Predisposing factors: heredity, pregnancy, obesity, and aging
C. Signs and symptoms
1. Leg fatigue and aching
2. Leg cramping and pain
3. Heaviness in the legs
4. Dilated veins
5. Ankle edema
D. Diagnostic tests/methods
1. Patient history and physical examination
2. Venography
3. Trendelenburg test
E. Treatment
1. Rest with elevation of legs
2. Exercise
3. Support stockings
4. Avoid prolonged standing, sitting, and crossing the legs
5. Weight management
6. Surgical vein stripping/ligation; vein sclerosing
7. Laser
F. Nursing intervention
1. After surgery check legs for color, movement, temperature, and sensation
2. Provide leg exercises as prescribed
3. Reinforce the importance of weight management
4. Instruct the patient to avoid prolonged sitting and standing
5. Avoid constrictive clothing

Hematologic Conditions

Disorders of hemopoiesis refer to problems of the blood-forming tissues. These include the blood cells, bone marrow, spleen, and lymph system. This discussion includes descriptions of the anemias, leukemia, and acquired immunodeficiency syndrome.

Nursing Assessment

A. Nursing observations
1. Pulse
   a. Character, rate, rhythm
   b. Note tachycardia or periods of palpitations
2. Respirations
   a. Character, rate, rhythm
   b. Tachypnea
   c. Dyspnea on exertion
   d. Shortness of breath (SOB)

3. Blood pressure: Hypotension, perhaps orthostatic
4. Temperature: Unexplained occurrences of elevation, sometimes accompanied by chills and sweating
5. Skin
   a. Color: pallor, cyanosis
   b. Pruritus
   c. Bruising
   d. Slow to heal cuts
   e. Bleeding from nose or mouth
6. Oral mucousal changes
   a. Mouth ulcerations
   b. Bleeding gums
   c. Smooth tongue
7. Motor
   a. Incoordination
   b. Loss of usual stamina
   c. Changes in ability to perform activities
   d. Intolerance to exertion (climbing stairs, usual housework, walking)
B. Patient description (subjective)
   1. Changes in ability to perform activities of daily living
   2. Self-reported increase in weakness and fatigue
   3. Dyspnea on exertion
   4. Changes in appetite
      a. Weight loss
      b. Anorexia
      c. Nausea and vomiting
   5. Skin
      a. Easily bruises
      b. Bleeding from gums, nose
   6. Mood changes: irritable
   7. Progressive symptoms
      a. Onset of headaches
      b. Onset of fatigue
      c. Numbness, tingling, burning feet
      d. Intermittent swollen, tender lymph nodes

Diagnostic Tests/Methods

A. Red blood cell (RBC) count
   1. The blood study is used in routine screenings and provides information about the hematologic system
   2. Circulating RBC counts elevate in conditions such as anemia and hypoxia
B. Erythrocyte indexes (mean cell volume, mean cell hemoglobin concentration, and mean cell hemoglobin)
   1. Aid in describing the anemias
   2. Provide a relationship between the number, size, and hemoglobin content of the RBCs
C. Hemoglobin and hematocrit levels
   1. Provide an index to the severity of the anemia
   2. Hematocrit refers to the number of packed RBCs found in 100 ml of blood
   3. Hemoglobin is the oxygen-carrying component of the RBC and is more reliable in determining the severity of the anemia
D. Reticulocyte count
   1. Provides information concerning the cause of the anemia
   2. Indicates whether the anemia is a result of diminished production or excessive loss or destruction of RBCs
E. Sedimentation rate
   1. Not specific to anemias

2. Elevated ESR suggests the presence of an underlying disease process; therefore further workup may be indicated
F. Serum iron
   1. Helpful in classifying the anemia
   2. Useful in differentiating an acute from a chronic disorder
G. Total iron-binding capacity (TIBC): helpful in classifying the anemia and differentiating between an acute and a chronic disorder
H. Serum bilirubin
   1. Useful in evaluating the degree of RBC hemolysis
   2. Bilirubin is formed from the hemoglobin of destroyed RBCs
   3. Elevations may indicate the increased destruction of RBCs caused by a particular disease process
I. Schilling test
   1. Used in classifying anemias, particularly a vitamin B_{12} disorder
   2. Helps differentiate between an intrinsic factor deficiency and an intestinal absorption disorder
   3. Patient preparation
      a. The patient may be instructed to take nothing by mouth (NPO) before the test
      b. Oral radioactive vitamin B_{12} is administered
      c. Nonradioactive parenteral dose is given 2 hours later
      d. Urine collection follows
      e. A third of the vitamin appears in the urine; little or no radioactivity in the urine suggests a gastrointestinal malabsorption problem
      f. Procedure may be repeated with the addition of intrinsic factor to the oral vitamin B_{12}
      g. Nonabsorption of B_{12} without intrinsic factor but absorption with the intrinsic factor is suggestive of pernicious anemia
   4. Nursing intervention
      a. Explain the basic procedure to the patient
      b. Maintain NPO
      c. Collect the urine at the specified time
J. Vitamin B_{12} level
   1. Used to help classify the anemias
   2. Provides an index for determining the adequacy of B_{12} levels and the need for further evaluation
   3. Vitamin B_{12} is important for normal hematopoiesis
K. Serum folate level
   1. Folic acid is another important factor in hematopoiesis
   2. Useful in classifying the anemias
L. Gastric analysis
   1. Nasogastric tube is inserted and then histamine is injected to stimulate gastric secretions
   2. Gastric contents are aspirated and analyzed
   3. Achlorhydria (absence of hydrochloric acid) is a feature of pernicious anemia
M. Sickle cell preparation
   1. The reaction of the blood specimen in hypoxia is observed
   2. Sickling of cells in hypoxia suggests sickle cell trait or sickle cell anemia
N. Hemoglobin electrophoresis
   1. An electric field separates the specimen into the various types of hemoglobin present
   2. Hemoglobins S and A suggest sickle cell anemia or trait
   3. Hemoglobin F suggests thalassemia

O. Bone marrow biopsy
1. Bone marrow aspiration provides information about blood cell production
2. Test may be used in patients suspected of having leukemia, aplastic anemia, and other hematologic disorders
3. Sample of marrow may be obtained from the sternum, iliac crest, vertebrae, or vertebral body
4. Procedure
    a. The skin over the designated area is prepared and anesthetized
    b. The needle is inserted into the center of the bone, and a small amount of marrow is aspirated
5. Nursing intervention
    a. Allay patient's anxiety before examination
    b. Assist with the marrow as instructed
    c. Place patient in a comfortable position after the procedure
    d. Monitor pain status (soreness remains for several days)
    e. Monitor puncture site for bleeding

P. WBC count and differential
1. Determines the total number of leukocytes
2. The differential helps analyze each type of WBC and determine if the amount present is in proper proportion
3. Aids in the diagnosing of infection and blood disorders such as leukemia

Q. Platelet count
1. Evaluates adequacy of platelet levels
2. If platelet levels drop below a certain level, spontaneous hemorrhage is possible

R. Serum for HIV: determines the presence of the HIV antibodies

S. Lymphangiography: radiologic examination used to detect lymph node involvement

Frequent Patient Problems and Nursing Care

A. Activity intolerance related to weakness and fatigue
1. Provide planned activity and rest periods
2. Monitor for signs of fatigue
3. Reinforce patient teaching of planned activity and exercise
4. Assist patient with activities of daily living
5. Assess vital signs as ordered

B. Potential alteration in tissue perfusion related to hypotension
1. Observe for evidence of postural hypotension
2. Assist patient to dangle legs over the side of the bed before standing
3. Instruct patient to get up slowly
4. Assess patient's pulse when standing

C. Ineffective breathing pattern related to dyspnea on exertion
1. Note the degree or kind of activity that causes dyspnea
2. Note character and rate of respirations during the episodes
3. Instruct the patient to stop the activity and relax when dyspnea is experienced
4. Assist the patient in planning activities so that dyspnea will not occur
5. Reinforce patient teaching regarding planned exercise and rest periods

D. Impaired swallowing caused by ulcerations of the mouth and tongue
1. Assess the ulcerated areas qd
2. Provide mouth care with a soft-bristle brush or cotton swab
3. Offer soothing mouthwashes every 2 to 4 hours
4. Instruct the patient to avoid ingesting food or drink that may aggravate the ulcers

E. Fluid volume deficit related to hemorrhage
1. Assess for signs of bleeding
    a. Tarry stools
    b. Hematuria
    c. Bleeding gums
    d. Bleeding tendency
    e. Petechiae
    f. Epistaxis
2. Protect from trauma and injury
3. Avoid parenteral injections
4. Have patient use soft-bristle brush for mouth care
5. Monitor vital signs at least q4h
6. Monitor hemoglobin and hematocrit values
7. Encourage intake of fluids and the prescribed diet

F. High risk for infection related to interference with the immune system
1. Prevent exposure to others with infection
2. Monitor for signs and symptoms of infection
3. Give prescribed drugs and monitor for side effects
4. Place in protective isolation if ordered

Major Medical Diagnoses
ANEMIA CAUSED BY DECREASED RBC PRODUCTION

A. Normally there is a balance between RBC production and RBC destruction; however, alterations do occur that significantly affect RBC production
1. Iron deficiency anemia
    a. Results from insufficient dietary intake of iron, which is needed for the formation of hemoglobin and RBCs
    b. Other causes: malabsorption, blood loss, and hemolysis
2. Pernicious anemia
    a. Caused by a lack of intrinsic factor in the GI tract
    b. Intrinsic factor is needed for the absorption of vitamin B_{12}
    c. Anemia usually results from a loss of the mucosal surface of the GI tract, which secretes intrinsic factor
    d. Patients undergoing total gastrectomies and small bowel resections are at risk
3. Folic acid deficiency anemia
    a. Folic acid is required in the synthesis of DNA, which in turn is necessary for the production of RBCs
    b. Common causes: poor diet (lacking in green, leafy vegetables, citrus fruits, liver, grains, and dried beans), malabsorption, and drugs that interfere with the absorption of folic acid
4. Thalassemia
    a. Unlike the other three anemias, thalassemia is a genetic disorder resulting in abnormal hemoglobin synthesis
    b. The main problem is an inadequate production of normal hemoglobin; hemolysis is a secondary problem
    c. People of Mediterranean ancestry are at risk

d. Mild forms of this anemia (thalassemia minor) may be asymptomatic

e. Patients with a more severe hemolytic form (thalassemia major) may experience hepatomegaly, splenomegaly, jaundice, and bone marrow hypertrophy

B. Signs and symptoms
  1. Skin changes
     a. Pallor
     b. Jaundice
     c. Pruritus
     d. Dermatitis
  2. Eye and visual disturbances
     a. Blurred vision
     b. Scleral icterus
  3. Mouth
     a. Glossitis
     b. Smooth tongue
     c. Ulcerations of the mucosa
  4. Cardiovascular
     a. Tachycardia
     b. Murmurs
     c. Angina
     d. Congestive heart failure (CHF)
     e. Hypotension
  5. Respiratory
     a. Tachypnea
     b. Dyspnea on exertion
     c. Orthopnea
  6. Neurologic
     a. Dizziness
     b. Headaches
     c. Irritability
     d. Depression
     e. Incoordination
     f. Impaired thought processes
  7. Gastrointestinal (GI)
     a. Nausea and vomiting
     b. Anorexia
     c. Hepatomegaly
     d. Splenomegaly
  8. General
     a. Weight loss
     b. Weakness and fatigue
     c. Bone pain
     d. Numbness, tingling, and burning of the feet
C. Diagnostic tests/methods
  1. Patient history and physical examination
  2. Routine chest x-ray examination
  3. Routine ECG
  4. Schilling test
  5. Gastric analysis
  6. CBC/red blood cell indexes
  7. Bone marrow aspiration or biopsy
  8. Serum iron level
D. Treatment
  1. Iron therapy
  2. Increase dietary iron intake
  3. Vitamin B_{12} replacement (pernicious anemia)
  4. Folic acid replacement
  5. Use of hematinics
  6. Blood transfusions (thalassemia)

E. Nursing intervention
  1. Assess and document signs and symptoms and reactions to treatments
  2. Provide planned activity alternated with rest periods
  3. Assist patient with activities of daily living to avoid fatigue
  4. Monitor supplemental oxygen therapy in use
  5. Administer prescribed drugs and monitor for side effects
  6. Monitor blood transfusions
  7. Provide oral hygiene, particularly if mouth ulcers are present
  8. Provide the prescribed diet
  9. Instruct patient to get up from bed or chair slowly to avoid dizziness
  10. Instruct patient on avoiding and preventing exposure to infection
  11. Support patient and allay anxiety
  12. Educate patient and family concerning drugs, diet therapy, and planned activity

ANEMIA CAUSED BY RBC DESTRUCTION

A. Definition: a process in which RBCs are being destroyed faster than they are produced
B. Known causes of RBC destruction
  1. Snake venom
  2. Infections
  3. Drugs or chemicals
  4. Heavy metals or organic compounds
  5. Antigen antibody reaction
  6. Splenic dysfunction
  7. Congenital causes
     a. Thalassemia: a group of hereditary hemolytic anemias characterized by a defect or defects in one or more of the hemoglobin polypeptide chains
     b. Sickle cell anemia: see Chapter 8, Pediatric Nursing
     c. Spherocytosis: A hemolytic anemia characterized by spherocytes (small, globular erythrocytes without the characteristic central pallor) in the blood; the abnormal cells are destroyed by the spleen
     d. Glucose-6-phosphate dehydrogenase (G6PD) deficiency: a hemolytic disorder brought on by stressors such as infection, certain drugs, acidosis, and toxic substances; individuals with this genetic disorder are relatively symptom free until they experience the stressor that initiates the hemolytic process
C. Signs and symptoms
  1. Anemia
  2. Jaundice
  3. Splenomegaly
  4. Hepatomegaly
  5. Weakness and fatigue
  6. Skin pallor
  7. Anorexia
  8. Weight loss
  9. Dyspnea
  10. Tachycardia
  11. Tachypnea
  12. Hypotension
  13. Cholelithiasis (gallstones): caused by excessive bilirubin
D. Diagnostic tests/methods
  1. Patient history and physical examination

2. Laboratory studies
3. Routine chest x-ray examination
4. Routine ECG
5. Bone marrow biopsy
6. Renal studies to monitor kidney status

E. Treatment
1. Identify the causative agent
2. Blood or blood product replacement
3. Supportive care
4. Genetic counseling
5. Splenectomy to halt the destruction of abnormal RBCs by the spleen
6. Maintain renal function
7. Maintain fluid and electrolyte balance

F. Nursing intervention
1. Assess and document signs and symptoms and reactions to treatment
2. Monitor vital signs as ordered and report abnormalities
3. Allay fears and anxieties
4. Provide planned exercise and rest periods
5. Caution patient to get up slowly form the bed or chair to avoid postural hypotension
6. Assist patient with activities of daily living
7. Monitor intake and output
8. Monitor laboratory studies
9. Encourage intake of fluids
10. Provide prescribed diet
11. Administer prescribed drugs and monitor for side effects
12. Educate patient and family concerning drugs, diet, activity, and compliance to the prescribed regimen

APLASTIC ANEMIA (HYPOPLASTIC)

A. Definition: a failure of the bone marrow to produce adequate amounts of erythrocytes, leukocytes, and platelets

B. Exact cause is unclear (idiopathic)
1. May be congenital
2. Related to radiation exposure
3. Results from a disorder that suppresses bone marrow (cancer)
4. Exposure to toxic substances may be a contributing factor

C. Signs and symptoms
1. General symptoms of anemia; refer to the preceding outlines in this section
2. Susceptibility to infection
3. Fever
4. Bleeding tendencies

D. Diagnostic tests/methods
1. Patient history and physical examination
2. Laboratory studies, particularly WBC count and platelet count; a reduced WBC count predisposes patient to infection; a low platelet count predisposes patient to a bleeding disorder
3. Bone marrow biopsy examination to evaluate blood cell production
4. Routine chest x-ray examination
5. Routine ECG

E. Treatment
1. Identify the causative agent
2. Supportive care

3. Administration of blood or blood products
4. Hydration with IV fluids
5. Protect from injury and infections
6. Prevent hemorrhage
7. Splenectomy
8. Bone marrow transplant

F. Nursing intervention
1. Assess and document signs and symptoms and reactions to treatment
2. Monitor vital signs at least q4h
3. Monitor for and report signs of bleeding
4. Give prescribed medication and monitor for side effects
5. Avoiding fatiguing the patient; provide planned exercise and rest periods
6. Prevent injury and exposure to infection
7. Neutropenic precautions may be necessary
8. Monitor supplemental oxygen if ordered
9. Provide and encourage the prescribed diet
10. Allay fears and anxiety
11. Provide oral hygiene, avoiding aggravation of bleeding gums
12. Provide skin care using protective devices and frequent repositioning
13. Educate patient and family concerning drug therapy, diet, planned activity, avoidance of injury and infection, monitoring for bleeding tendencies, and compliance with the regimen

LEUKEMIA

A. Definition: a disorder of the hematopoietic system characterized by an overproduction of immature WBCs
1. As the disease progresses, fewer normal WBCs are produced
2. The abnormal cells continue to multiply and eventually infiltrate and damage the bone marrow, spleen, lymph nodes, and other organs

B. Classification of leukemias
1. Two major categories are acute and chronic
   a. Acute leukemia has a rapid onset; cells in this phase are young, undifferentiated, and immature
   b. Chronic leukemia has a gradual onset; cells are mature and differentiated
2. Further classification: identifying the type of WBC involved
   a. Acute granulocytic leukemia: the myeloblasts proliferate; myeloblasts are the precursors of granulocytes
   b. Acute lymphoblastic leukemia: immature lymphocytes proliferate in the bone marrow
   c. Chronic granulocytic leukemia: excessive neoplastic granulocytes are found in the bone marrow
   d. Chronic lymphocytic leukemia: characterized by inactive, mature appearing lymphocytes

C. Leukemia is considered a neoplastic process; cause is unknown

D. Predisposing factors
1. Familial tendency
2. Viral origin
3. Exposure to chemicals
4. Exposure to radiation

E. Once leukemia is diagnosed, the aim of therapy is to prolong survival by attaining a state of remission

1. Management of acute leukemia aggressive
2. Management of chronic leukemia aims to control the disorder and maintain remission
3. All forms of leukemia are fatal if untreated

F. Signs and symptoms
1. General symptoms of anemia
2. Decreased resistance to infection
3. Fever
4. Bleeding tendencies
5. Enlarged lymph nodes
6. Splenomegaly
7. Hepatomegaly
8. Elevated WBC count
9. Low platelet count and low hemoglobin and hematocrit levels
10. Poor appetite
11. Mouth ulcers
12. Diarrhea

G. Diagnostic test/methods
1. Patient history and physical examination
2. Laboratory studies to evaluate peripheral blood
3. Bone marrow biopsy
4. Routine chest x-ray examination
5. Routine ECG
6. Lymph node biopsy examination

H. Treatment
1. Drug therapy: chemotherapeutic agents, analgesics, sedatives, and antibiotics
2. Radiation therapy (prophylactic measure)
3. Bone marrow transplants are still under investigation
4. Hydration with IV fluids
5. Replacement of blood and blood products
6. Monitoring renal status
7. Protection against infection (neutropenic precautions if needed)
8. Prevention of hemorrhage

I. Nursing intervention
1. Assess and document signs and symptoms and reactions to treatment
2. Prevent patient from being exposed to infection
   a. Screen visitors
   b. Monitor WBC counts
   c. Good hand washing
3. Avoid fatigue
   a. Provide planned exercises and rest periods
   b. Assist patient with activities of daily living
4. Monitor for bleeding tendencies
5. Administer blood or blood components as ordered and monitor for side effects
6. Monitor intake and output
7. Encourage intake of fluids
   a. Keep fluids at the bedside
   b. Provide patient with favorite fluids
8. Administer prescribed medication as ordered and monitor for side effects
   a. Analgesics and sedatives
   b. Antiemetics
9. Monitor IV fluids
   a. Monitor the IV site for infiltration
   b. Monitor rate
10. Allay anxieties and fears

11. Monitor vital signs at least q4h and report abnormalities (an elevated temperature may be the only sign of infection in an immunocompromised patient)
12. Monitor supplemental oxygen if ordered
13. Provide and encourage the prescribed diet
14. Provide oral hygiene, which avoids aggravation of bleeding and drying of the mouth; carefully monitor oral status
15. Provide skin care to include the use of protective devices and frequent repositioning
16. Educate patient and family concerning drug therapy, diet, activity, monitoring for bleeding tendencies, avoidance of injury and infection, and compliance with the regimen

ACQUIRED IMMUNODEFICIENCY SYNDROME (AIDS)

A. Definition: a viral disorder that disrupts the balance of T-lymphocytes and ultimately destroys them, rendering the body incapable of defending itself against infection; course is progressive and fatal

B. Cause: infection with HIV (human immunodeficiency virus)
1. The virus is spread by sexual contact; sharing of infected needles; and infected blood and blood products
2. Infected mothers can pass the virus to the unborn baby during the gestational period, the birth process, or breast feeding
3. The virus may also enter the body when contaminated blood or body fluids come in contact with broken skin surfaces

C. Signs and symptoms (vary with each patient; may harbor the virus, but be asymptomatic for months and/or years)
1. Swollen lymph glands
2. Recurrent fever; night sweats
3. Weight loss; diminished appetite
4. Chronic diarrhea
5. Fatigue
6. White patches or lesions in the mouth
7. Presence of opportunistic infections such as *Pneumocystis carinii* (pneumonia) and Kaposi's sarcoma (purplish skin lesions)
8. Dry cough; shortness of breath
9. Centers for Disease Control clinical categories (Table 5-2)
   a. Category A: categories B and C have not occurred; asymptomatic HIV infection; persistent, generalized lymphadenopathy; acute HIV infection
   b. Category B: category C has not occurred; presence of conditions commonly associated with HIV
   c. Category C: once in this category, person remains in this category; all clinical conditions listed as associated with advanced HIV disease or AIDS
10. Symptoms may occur as early as 2 to 6 weeks after exposure, or individual may be asymptomatic for months or years. Seroconversion (when the bloodwork changes from a "negative" to a "positive" for HIV antibodies) may not occur for 8 to 12 weeks or longer. Retesting is advisable 6 months after exposure, then at 1 year. Further testing is left up to the health care provider.

D. Diagnostic tests/methods
1. Patient history and physical examination
2. Serum for HIV antibodies

| Table 5-2 | 1993 Revised Classification System for HIV Infection and Expanded AIDS Surveillance Case Definition for Adolescents and Adults |

	Clinical Categories*		
CD4 Cell Categories	(A) Asymptomatic or PGL	(B) Symptomatic, Not (A) or (C) Conditions	(C) AIDS-Indicator Conditions
> 500/mm³	A1	B1	C1
200-499/mm³	A2	B2	C2
< 200/mm³ AIDS-indicator cell count	A3	B3	C3

Centers for Disease Control and Prevention: Impact of the expanded AIDS surveillance case definition on AIDS case reporting–US first quarter, 1993, *MMWR* 42(16):308-310, 1993a.

*Description of Clinical Categories
A: One or more of the conditions listed below with documented HIV infection. Conditions listed in categories B and C must not have occurred.
   –Asymptomatic HIV infection
   –Persistent generalized lymphadenopathy (PGL)
   –Acute (primary) HIV infection with accompanying illness or history of acute infection
B: Symptomatic conditions that meet at least one of the following criteria: (a) the conditions are attributed to HIV infection and/or are indicative of a defect in cell-mediated immunity; or (b) the conditions are considered by physicians to have a clinical course or management that is complicated by HIV infection. Examples of conditions in clinical category B include, but are not limited to:
   –bacterial endocarditis, meningitis, pneumonia, or sepsis
   –candidiasis, vulvovaginal that is persistent (greater than one month duration) or poorly responsive to therapy
   –candidiasis, oropharyngeal (thrush)
   –cervical dysplasia, severe; or carcinoma
   –constitutional symptoms, such as fever (38.4° C) or diarrhea lasting more than one month
   –hairy leukoplakia, oral
   –herpes zoster (shingles), involving at least two distinct episodes or more than one dermatome
   –idiopathic thrombocytopenic purpura
   –listeriosis
   –*Mycobacterium tuberculosis*, pulmonary
   –nocardiosis
   –pelvic inflammatory disease
   –peripheral neuropathy
C: Any condition listed in the 1993 surveillance case definition for AIDS. The conditions in clinical category C are strongly associated with severe immunodeficiency, occur frequently in HIV-infected individuals, and cause serious morbidity or mortality.
Adapted from Harkness and Dincher: *Medical surgical nursing: total patient care*, ed 9, St Louis, 1996, Mosby.

3. Presence of opportunistic infections
   a. *Pneumocystis carinii* pneumonia
   b. Kaposi's sarcoma
4. Bronchial biopsy (tests for presence of opportunistic infections)
5. Lumbar puncture (tests for neurological evidence of infections)
6. CT scan
7. Enzyme-linked immunosorbent assay (ELISA); detects antibodies for HIV; false positives may occur
8. Western blot test: used to confirm the results of a positive ELISA test; detects HIV antibodies
9. CD-4 cell counts: if less than 200 there is an increased risk for opportunistic infections (see Table 5-2)
E. Treatment
   1. Treatment is instituted according to the symptoms
   2. Protect the patient from opportunistic infections
   3. Zidovudine (AZT, Retrovir)
   4. Didanosine

5. Zalcitabine
6. Nutritional support
7. Treatment of opportunistic infections
F. Nursing care
   1. Assess and document signs and symptoms and reactions to treatment
   2. Monitor vital signs
   3. Monitor arterial blood gas, CBC, and platelet count
   4. Administer prescribed medication and monitor for side effects
   5. Employ blood and body fluid precautions (Note: this should be followed when caring for all patients)
      a. Wear protective clothing (gloves, masks, goggles, gowns, etc.) as needed for the procedure
      b. Wash hands thoroughly
      c. Label specimens accordingly
      d. Dispose of contaminated articles properly
   6. Plan activity followed by rest periods
   7. Encourage physical independence

8. Monitor oxygen therapy
9. Monitor pain status and provide analgesia and comfort measures
10. Support patient and allay anxiety
11. Educate the patient and family concerning mode of spread, protective measures, and home care

LYMPHOMA

A. Definition: a group of malignancies originating in the stem cell of the bone marrow
B. Causes: unknown, possibly linked to viruses, genetics, environmental exposures, and possibly autoimmune links
C. Two main types
  1. Hodgkin's disease
  2. Non-Hodgkin's lymphoma
D. Signs and symptoms
  1. Swollen, painless lymph nodes
  2. Fever, chills
  3. Weight loss
  4. Night sweats
  5. Fatigue
  6. Loss of usual stamina; changes in ability to perform ADLs
E. Diagnostic test/methods
  1. History and physical exam
  2. Complete blood count/red blood cell indices
  3. Blood chemistry: alkaline phosphatase, gamma globulin
  4. Serum protein electrophoresis
  5. Urine electrophoresis
  6. Lymph node biopsy
  7. Bone marrow biopsy
F. Treatment
  1. Staging laparotomy with splenectomy (to improve response to chemotherapy)
  2. Chemotherapy
  3. Radiation therapy
G. Nursing care
  1. Assess and document signs and symptoms and reactions to treatment
  2. Monitor vital signs
  3. Monitor lab studies
  4. Prevention of infection and recognition of early signs
  5. Planned activity; rest periods
  6. Monitor oxygen therapy if ordered
  7. Monitor pain status and provide comfort measures
  8. Give support and allay anxiety
  9. Maintain hydration

THE GASTROINTESTINAL SYSTEM
Anatomy and Physiology

A. Organs (Fig.5-9)
  1. Mouth (buccal cavity)
    a. Receives food; aids in digestion; aids in speaking
    b. Consists of hard and soft palate, teeth, tongue, and salivary glands
      (1) Teeth
        (a) Deciduous: baby teeth
        (b) Permanent: appear at approximately 6 years of age
        (c) Incisors: cut food
        (d) Canines: tear food
        (e) Molar: grind food
      (2) Salivary glands, parotid, submandibular, submaxillary; manufacture saliva, which contains ptyalin to begin the chemical breakdown of food
      (3) Tongue: also organ of taste
        (a) Receptors (taste buds, located in tongue): stimulated only if substance is in solution
        (b) Four kinds: sweet (tip of tongue); sour (side of tongue); salty (tip of tongue); bitter (back part of tongue)
        (c) Stimulates appetite and flow of digestive juices
    c. Functions
      (1) Ingestion of food
      (2) Mastication of food
      (3) Lubrication of food
      (4) Digestion of starch with salivary amylase
  2. Pharynx: transports food
  3. Esophagus: muscular tube; conducts food from pharynx to stomach
  4. Stomach:
    a. J-shaped pouch; varies in size depending on contents; stores food and changes it into chyme
    b. Three divisions
      (1) Fundus: upper portion; the cardiac sphincter between the esophagus and fundus; controls the entrance of food
      (2) Body: the largest, central portion
      (3) Pylorus: lower portion above the small intestine; the pyloric sphincter controls the passage of food into the duodenum
    c. Glands: secrete gastric juices and enzymes (including hydrochloric acid): the chemical breakdown of protein begins in the stomach
      (1) Pepsin: begins digestion of protein
      (2) Lipase: acts on emulsified fat
      (3) Renin: acts on casein (a protein) in milk
      (4) Gastrin (hormone): related to the control of gastric secretions; not an enzyme
      (5) Hydrochloric acid: makes stomach content acid and activates enzymes
    d. Chyme: the semiliquid contents of the stomach, consisting of partially digested food and gastric enzymes
    e. Functions
      (1) Storage of food
      (2) Breakdown of food by churning
      (3) Liquefying of food with hydrochloric acid
      (4) Digestion of protein with enzyme, pepsin
  5. Small intestine: extends from the pyloric sphincter to the ileocecal valve, which prevents backflow of material and regulates forward flow
    a. Size: approximately 20 ft (600 cm) long and 1 inch (2.5 cm) in diameter
    b. Three major divisions
      (1) Duodenum: approximately 10 inches (25 cm) long; curves around head of the pancreas; pancreatic and common bile duct enter below pyloric sphincter
      (2) Jejunum: approximately 8 ft (240 cm) long
      (3) Ileum: approximately 12 ft (360 cm) long; terminal part
    c. Functions

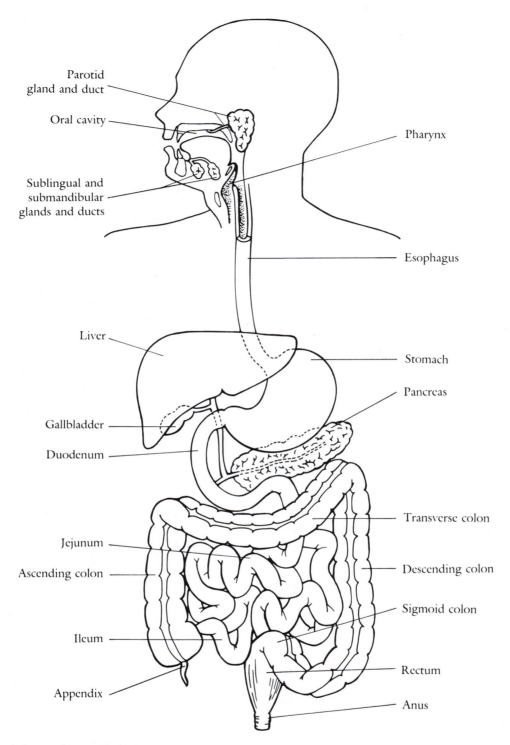

Parotid
gland and duct

Oral cavity

Sublingual and
submandibular
glands and ducts

Pharynx

Esophagus

Liver

Stomach

Pancreas

Gallbladder

Duodenum

Transverse colon

Jejunum

Ascending colon

Descending colon

Sigmoid colon

Ileum

Rectum

Appendix

Anus

Figure 5-9.   **Digestive system.** (From Sorrentino SA: *Mosby's textbook for nursing assistants*, ed 4,
St Louis, 1995, Mosby.)

(1) Digestion of food
(2) Absorption of food
d. Intestinal glands, pancreas, liver, and gallbladder
secrete digestive enzymes that complete the chemical
breakdown of food
(1) Bile (formed in the liver and stored in the gallbladder): not an enzyme; emulsifies fat

(2) Trypsin (pancreas): digests proteins into amino
acids
(3) Amylase (pancreas): digests starches into sugars
(4) Lipase (pancreas): digests fat into simplest
forms (fatty acids and glycerol)
(5) Erepsin (intestine): digests proteins into amino
acids

(6) Lactose, maltose, sucrose (secretions of the small intestine): digest sugar into simplest forms (glucose, fructose, galactose)

6. Large intestine
   a. Size: approximately 5 to 6 ft (150 to 180 cm) long and 2½ inches (6 cm) in diameter
   b. Divisions
      (1) Cecum: a blind pouch approximately 3 inches (7.5 cm) long; appendix attaches to distal end; located in right lower quadrant
      (2) Colon: ascending, continues up right side; transverse, extends across to the left; descending, descends on left side of pelvis
      (3) Sigmoid: S-shaped portion; extends to rectum
      (4) Rectum: approximately 8 inches (20 cm) long
      (5) Anus: terminal opening: guarded by internal and external sphincters
   c. Functions
      (1) Reabsorption of fluids
      (2) Temporary storage of fecal matter; defecation

B. Accessory organs (see Fig. 5-9)
   1. Liver: largest organ in body; lies below diaphragm in upper right quadrant of abdominal cavity
      a. Metabolizes carbohydrates, fats, and proteins
      b. Detoxifies harmful substances
      c. Produces and stores heparin and fibrinogen
      d. Stores glycogen and vitamins A, B, B_{12}, and K
      e. Manufactures bile; hepatic duct drains bile into gallbladder
   2. Gallbladder: small sac embedded in the interior surface of the liver
      a. Concentrates and stores bile
      b. Releases bile through the common bile duct into the duodenum when fat enters the small intestine
   3. Pancreas: long, triangular gland; lies behind the stomach; produces enzymes that break down food particles; secretes enzymes into the duodenum; has two functions
      a. Exocrine gland; secretes digestive enzymes that neutralize chyme
      b. Endocrine gland: islets of Langerhans; secretes insulin for utilization of glucose; secretes glucagons to regulate blood sugar level

C. Functions
   1. Digestion: two processes
      a. Mechanical: chewing, swallowing, and peristalsis of food; ends with elimination
      b. Chemical: breakdown of food into simpler compounds by the action of enzymes on food
   2. Absorption
      a. Occurs in small intestine
      b. Most water absorbed in large intestine
   3. Metabolism: the sum of all body functions to convert simple compounds into living tissue
      a. Catabolism: process in which substances are broken down into simpler substances, resulting in the release of heat and energy
      b. Anabolism: the building phase in which simpler substances are combined to form more complex substances (conversion of food into living tissues)
      c. Basal metabolism: the amount of energy (calories) used by the body when at rest

Gastrointestinal Disorders/Conditions

The GI system provides a means by which food and fluids enter the body and are converted into elements that help maintain the human organism. It is important to note that other systems of the body influence this system. The endocrine system, central nervous system, and autonomic nervous system all serve as regulators to the GI system.

Nursing Assessment

A. Nursing observations (objective data)
   1. Vital signs
   2. Skin character/color
      a. Gingivitis
      b. Stomatitis
      c. Jaundice
   3. Hematemesis: emesis is like coffee grounds in appearance, signifying digested blood
   4. Stool changes
      a. Melena (tarry stool)
      b. Clay-colored (lack of bile pigment)
      c. Frothy, foamy, foul-smelling (seen in pancreatitis)
      d. Constipation
      e. Diarrhea
      f. Changes in size and/or shape (may indicate colon lesion)
   5. Urine color: dark urine (tea-colored)
   6. Hemorrhoids
   7. Abdominal distention
   8. Edema

B. Patient description (subjective data)
   1. General
      a. History of GI-related problems
      b. Family history of GI-related problems
   2. Weight
      a. Loss or gain
      b. Appetite changes: increase or decrease
   3. Dietary/eating changes
      a. Presence of nausea/vomiting
      b. Difficulty chewing
      c. Dysphagia
      d. Occurrence of indigestion or dyspepsia
      e. Intolerance to certain foods
      f. Presence of pain: relationship to meals/eating
   4. Changes in bowel habit
      a. Diarrhea
      b. Constipation
      c. Alternating diarrhea and constipation
      d. Gas formation
   5. Easily bruised

Diagnostic Tests/Methods

A. Patient history and physical examination
B. Examination of stool
   1. Examination of stool for occult (hidden) blood
   2. Fecal analysis: analysis of stool for mucus, pus, blood, parasites, and fat content
   3. Nursing intervention
      a. Instruct the patient in the proper collection of the specimen
      b. Take the specimen to the laboratory promptly
C. Radiographic examination
   1. Upper GI series

a. Patient ingests contrast medium (barium)

b. Movement of the medium through the esophagus and into the stomach is observed by fluoroscopy; x-ray films are also taken

  (1) Aids in identification of esophageal and stomach pathology

  (2) Nursing intervention

    (a) Explain procedures to the patient

    (b) Patient is usually NPO before the examination

    (c) Enemas or cathartics may be given before and after the examination

    (d) Allay patient's anxiety

2. Lower GI series (barium enema)

a. The filling of the colon with barium is observed by fluoroscopy; x-ray films of the colon are also taken

b. Aids in the detection of abnormalities or defects in the colon such as lesions, polyps, tumors, and diverticula

c. Nursing intervention

  (1) Explain procedures to the patient

  (2) Patient is usually NPO before the examination

  (3) Enemas or cathartics may be given before and after the examination

  (4) Allay patient's anxiety

3. Gallbladder series (oral cholecystography)

a. Patient is given an oral radiographic dye to ingest the evening before the examination

b. The gallbladder is visualized to detect gallstones and obstruction of the biliary tract

c. Nursing intervention

  (1) Explain procedures to the patient

  (2) Administer the radiographic dye as prescribed

  (3) Maintain NPO after the dye is given

  (4) Allay patient's anxiety

4. Cholangiography

a. Aids in the visualization of the biliary duct system

b. Three methods

  (1) Intravenous cholangiography (IVC): a radiographic dye is administered intravenously, and x-ray films are taken

  (2) Percutaneous transhepatic cholangiography: under fluoroscopy a cannula is inserted into the liver and bile duct; a radiographic dye is injected into the duct, and filling is observed

  (3) Operative or T-tube cholangiography: contrast medium is instilled into the common bile duct, cystic duct, or gallbladder using a fine needle or catheter during surgery or via an existing T-tube postoperatively

c. Nursing intervention

  (1) Explain procedures to the patient

  (2) Maintain NPO as ordered

  (3) Monitor the patient for bleeding or bile leakage if the percutaneous approach was used

5. Barium swallow: barium contrast study used to detect esophageal abnormalities

D. Endoscopy

1. Endoscopy of the upper GI tract (esophagoscopy, gastroscopy, gastroduodenoscopy, esophagogastroduodenoscopy)

a. Visualization of the esophagus, stomach, or duodenum with a lighted scope

b. Useful in detecting inflammation, ulceration, tumors, and other lesions

c. Nursing intervention

  (1) Explain procedures to the patient

  (2) Obtain signed consent

  (3) Maintain NPO as ordered

  (4) Administer preoperative medication as ordered

  (5) After the examination, maintain NPO until the gag reflex returns

2. Colonoscopy/sigmoidoscopy

a. Visualization of the internal structures of the colon with a fiberoptic scope

b. Lesions, tumors, and polyps may be visualized, and a biopsy may be performed

c. Nursing intervention

  (1) Explain procedures to the patient

  (2) Prepare patient with enemas and cathartics as ordered

  (3) After the examination, observe for rectal bleeding and signs of perforation (malaise, distention, and tenesmus)

E. Ultrasonography

1. Noninvasive test that uses echoes from sound waves to visualize deep structures of the body

2. No special preparation is needed

3. Useful in detecting masses, fluid accumulation, cysts, tumors, etc.

F. Scans (liver and pancreas)

1. Assessment of size, shape, and position of the organ

2. Radionuclide is injected intravenously, and a scanning device picks up the radioactive emissions, which are recorded on paper

3. Nursing intervention

a. No preparation is required for liver scanning

b. Fasting and dietary preparation may be ordered for pancreatic scanning

c. Explain procedures to the patient

d. Allay patient's anxiety

G. Computerized tomography (CT scan)

1. Noninvasive, radiologic imaging technique that takes exposures of the body or body part at different depths

2. No special preparation is necessary

H. Liver biopsy

1. Invasive procedure in which a needle is inserted into the liver through a small incision in the skin and a sample of liver tissue is obtained

2. The incision is usually made on the right side, at the sixth, seventh, eighth, or ninth intercostal space

3. Nursing intervention

a. Obtain signed consent

b. Explain procedure to the patient

c. Take baseline vital signs

d. Provide assistance during the procedure

e. After the procedure monitor the vital signs every 15 minutes to 1 hour; carry out prescription for bed rest (position flat or on the right side), assess the site and monitor for complications

I. Laboratory studies

1. Serum amylase

a. Measures the secretion of amylase by the pancreas

b. Useful in diagnosing pancreatitis

2. Serum lipase

a. Measures the secretion of lipase by the pancreas
b. Useful in diagnosing pancreatitis
3. Serum bilirubin and spot urine amylase: indicates the liver's ability to conjugate and excrete bilirubin
4. Coagulation studies (PT and PTT): useful in analyzing hemostatic functions
5. Liver enzyme studies (SGOT, serum glutamic-pyruvic transaminase [SGPT], and LDH): elevations usually indicate liver damage
6. Hepatitis-associated antigen (HAA): presence suggests hepatitis
7. Ammonia levels: elevated in advanced liver disease
8. Urine amylase: elevated amylase levels indicate pancreatic dysfunction

J. Gastric analysis
1. Gastric contents are analyzed primarily for hydrochloric acid content
2. Acidity (pH), volume, and cytology may also be determined

K. D-xylose tolerance test
1. This study evaluates absorption
2. Xylose in water is given orally
3. A urine collection of several hours follows; the amount of D-xylose in the urine is measured
4. Abnormal amounts of D-xylose in the urine indicate a malabsorption problem
5. Nursing intervention
   a. Explain procedure to the patient
   b. Maintain NPO before the examination
   c. Give patient instructions on collecting the urine

Frequent Patient Problems and Nursing Care

A. Pain related to stomatitis
1. Give soft, bland foods
2. Encourage intake of fluids that do not aggravate the condition
3. Encourage the use of soothing mouth rinses
4. Administer topical medication as prescribed

B. Impaired swallowing related to gingivitis
1. Give mouth irrigations as prescribed
2. Offer soft, bland foods and liquids
3. Instruct the patient in the benefit of good oral hygiene and professional dental cleaning

C. Potential fluid volume deficit related to nausea and vomiting
1. Observe character and quantity of emesis
2. Observe for associated symptoms
3. Observe for precipitating factors
4. Administer antiemetics as prescribed
5. Offer ice chips
6. Maintain cool environment
7. Apply a cool compress to the neck and forehead for comfort
8. Offer sips of clear liquids such as 7-Up
9. Reduce environmental stimuli such as noise, unpleasant odors, and unpleasant sights
10. Encourage rest and deep breathing
11. Serve patient's favorite foods
12. Limit food servings
13. Provide mouth care after episodes of emesis

D. Impaired swallowing related to dysphagia
1. Provide patient with favorite foods arranged attractively
2. Provide soft, bland foods that can easily be chewed
3. Provide small, frequent feedings
4. Avoid irritating food and fluid
5. Monitor intake
6. Administration topical medication as ordered

E. Alteration in nutrition, less than body requirements, related to anorexia
1. Assess status of the anorexia
2. Monitor intake of food and fluid
3. Determine patient's food likes and dislikes
4. Prepare patient for meals
   a. Relieve pain
   b. Provide mouth care
   c. Assist patient to a comfortable position
   d. Use patient screen for privacy
   e. Remove unpleasant stimuli from patient's view
5. Prepare food tray
   a. Serve food at the proper temperature
   b. Make the tray attractive
   c. Serve appropriate quantities (large quantities may reduce the appetite)

F. Potential fluid volume deficit related to diarrhea
1. Document character, consistency, number, and appearance of stools
2. Assess for associated symptoms
3. Monitor intake and output
4. Administer antidiarrheals as prescribed and monitor for side effects
5. Avoid milk and milk products
6. Increase fluid intake to at least 3000 ml daily
7. Monitor vital signs at least q4h
8. Identify symptoms of electrolyte imbalance
9. Monitor laboratory reports for electrolyte values

G. Constipation related to decreased peristalsis/activity
1. Administer enemas, stool softeners, and cathartics as ordered
2. Encourage fluids to at least 3000 ml daily
3. Provide hot drinks to stimulate peristalsis
4. Encourage a diet high in fiber
5. Check for an impaction
6. Encourage exercises
7. Instruct patient concerning proper diet, increased fluid intake, exercise, and avoidance of laxative abuse

Major Medical Diagnoses

ESOPHAGITIS
A. Definition: an inflammation of the esophagus; more common in middle age
B. Causes
1. Inflammation of the esophagus may be brought on by irritants (food and tobacco), bacteria, or trauma (also see hiatal hernia)
2. Fungal: *Candida*
3. Reflux esophagitis: an incompetent lower esophageal sphincter allows a reflux of gastric contents into the esophagus
4. Malignancy
5. Prolonged nasogastric intubation
6. Repeated vomiting
C. Signs and symptoms
1. Heartburn (epigastric distress)
2. Pain with eructation or regurgitations

3. Dysphagia
4. Pain associated with ingestion of citrus liquids, alcohol, or hot or cold fluid
5. Symptoms aggravated by recumbency
6. Bleeding

D. Diagnostic tests/methods
   1. Patient history and physical examination
   2. Barium swallow
   3. Esophagoscopy and biopsy
   4. Routine chest x-ray examination

E. Treatments
   1. Avoid food and fluids that aggravate the symptoms
   2. Administer antacids, analgesics, and sedatives
   3. Elevate head of bed on shock blocks
   4. Maintain bland diet
   5. Surgery may be necessary if conservative measures fail
      a. Fundoplication: plication (making tucks) in the fundus of the stomach around the lower end of the esophagus
      b. Vagotomy and pyloroplasty: interruption of the impulses carried by the vagus nerve to reduce gastric secretions; the pylorus is also surgically manipulated to provide a larger conduit between the stomach and the duodenum

F. Nursing intervention
   1. Assess signs and symptoms and reactions to treatments
   2. Provide small, frequent feedings of bland, low-roughage foods
   3. Discourage intake of food close to bedtime
   4. Administer medication as prescribed and monitor for side effects
   5. Place in semi-Fowler's position

ESOPHAGEAL VARICES

A. Definition: dilated vessels that occur at the lower end of the esophagus

B. Causes
   1. Dilation of these vessels is usually a complication arising from cirrhosis of the liver
   2. Veins in the lower esophagus become distended as a result of increased portal pressure; the varices may rupture, causing hemorrhage and subsequent shock

C. Signs and symptoms
   1. Usually no signs and symptoms appear until the varices become ulcerated
   2. Hematemesis and coffee-ground emesis
   3. Melena
   4. Tachycardia
   5. Hypotension
   6. Low hemoglobin and hematocrit levels

D. Diagnostic tests/methods
   1. Patient history and physical examination: history of alcoholism may exist
   2. Fiberoptic endoscopy
   3. Laboratory studies: hemoglobin, hematocrit, and liver function studies
   4. Angiography
   5. Barium swallow
   6. CT scan
   7. Ultrasound

E. Treatment
   1. Blood and blood product replacement

2. Control of bleeding through ice water lavages, insertion of Sengstaken-Blakemore tube, and vitamin K therapy
3. Laboratory studies to monitor bleeding status and effectiveness of treatments
4. Hydration with IV fluids
5. Monitor intake and output
6. Surgery if needed to control bleeding
7. Injection of the bleeding varices with a sclerosing agent to control the bleeding

F. Nursing intervention
   1. Provide ongoing assessment of signs and symptoms and reactions to treatment
   2. Monitor vital signs at least q4h and monitor vital signs every half hour if bleeding is occurring
   3. Record intake and output qh if varices are bleeding
   4. Monitor fluids: assess the site and monitor flow rate
   5. Give prescribed medication as ordered and monitor for side effects
   6. Allay patient's anxieties and fears
   7. Assess all emesis and stool for the presence of blood
   8. Monitor laboratory studies and inform physician of incoming laboratory test values
   9. Keep head of bed elevated
   10. Monitor the Sengstaken-Blakemore tube if in use; keep scissors taped to the head of the bed in case of emergency
   11. Note the character of respirations

HIATAL HERNIA

A. Definition: a protrusion of the proximal area of the stomach through a weakened area of the diaphragm into the thoracic cavity (Fig. 5-10)

B. Causes
   1. Congenital weakness
   2. Increased abdominal pressure
   3. Trauma
   4. Relaxation of the musculature
   5. Gastric reflux may flow into the esophagus, causing inflammation and ulceration

C. Signs and symptoms
   1. Heartburn (pyrosis)
   2. Sternal pain after a heavy meal
   3. Regurgitation
   4. Feeling of fullness
   5. Dysphagia
   6. Dyspnea

D. Diagnosis tests/methods
   1. Patient history and physical examination
   2. Upper GI series (barium swallow)
   3. Esophagoscopy
   4. Routine chest x-ray examination

E. Treatment
   1. Conservative
      a. Elevation of the head of the bed on shock blocks
      b. Bland diet with frequent small feedings
      c. Avoidance of caffeine, alcohol, and chocolate
      d. Drug therapy with anticholinergics and antacids
      e. Weight management
      f. Avoidance of activities that increase intraabdominal pressure
   2. When conservative measures fail, surgery is indicated: fundoplication—"wrapping" the upper part of the stomach around the esophageal sphincter to prevent reflux

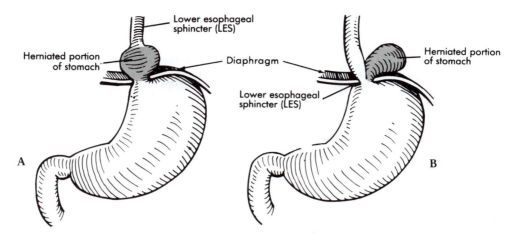

Figure 5-10. **Hiatal hernia. A**, Sliding hernia. **B**, Paraesophageal hernia. (From Phipps et al: *Medical-surgical nursing: concepts and clinical practice,* ed 5, St Louis, 1995, Mosby.)

a. Nasogastric tube
b. IV therapy
c. Drug therapy with analgesics and antiemetics
d. Monitor vital signs
e. Monitor intake and output

F. Nursing intervention
1. Assess and document signs and symptoms and reactions to treatments
2. Administer prescribed drugs and monitor for side effects
3. Monitor vital signs at least every shift and more often if surgery was performed
4. Monitor intake and output if surgery was performed
5. Provide the prescribed diet
6. Inform the physician if gastric reflux is reported by the patient after surgery
7. Educate patient and family concerning drug therapy, diet, activities to avoid, and the need for compliance

GASTRITIS

A. Definition: an inflammation in the mucosal lining of the stomach; the condition may be acute or chronic
B. Gastritis may be caused by bacteria, drugs, or toxins that cause the lining of the stomach to become inflamed and edematous
C. Signs and symptoms
1. Nausea and vomiting
2. Anorexia
3. Epigastric tenderness
4. Feeling of fullness
5. Cramping
6. Diarrhea
7. Fever
D. Diagnostic tests/methods
1. Patient history and physical examination
2. Identification of a causative agent
3. Laboratory studies
4. Stool culture
5. Endoscopy with biopsy

6. Gastric analysis
E. Treatment
1. Supportive care
2. Bed rest
3. NPO if nausea or vomiting is severe
4. Hydration with IV fluids
5. In severe cases a nasogastric tube is inserted
6. Drug therapy: antiemetics, antacids, and H_2 receptor antagonists
7. Progressive diet when acute symptoms subside
8. Restriction of smoking
F. Nursing intervention
1. Assess and document signs and symptoms and reactions to treatments
2. Monitor vital signs at least q4h
3. Monitor intake and output
4. Provide the prescribed diet
5. Administer medication as prescribed and monitor for side effects
6. Note amount and character of emesis and diarrhea
7. Monitor IV fluids
8. Educate patient and family concerning drug therapy, diet, activities, and any restrictions

CANCER OF THE STOMACH

A. Cancer can develop anywhere in the stomach
B. Causes
1. Exact cause is unknown
2. Familial tendency is suspected
3. Predisposing conditions: chronic gastric ulcers and gastritis
C. Signs and symptoms
1. Loss of appetite; early satiety
2. Weight loss
3. Weakness and fatigue
4. Pain
5. Melena
6. Anemia
7. Hematemesis

8. Dizziness
9. Indigestion or dysphagia
10. Constipation
D. Diagnostic tests/methods
1. Patient history and physical examination
2. Laboratory studies
3. Stool analysis
4. Gastric analysis
5. Barium studies
6. Gastroscopy
E. Treatment
1. Preoperative therapy
a. Correct nutritional deficiencies
b. Treat anemias
c. Blood replacement
d. Gastric decompression with a nasogastric tube
2. Surgery: removal of the cancerous lesion or tumor along with a margin of normal tissue
3. Radiation therapy and chemotherapy may be used if the patient is not expected to undergo surgery
a. Combination therapy has a better response rate
b. Single-agent therapy has proved to be of little value
F. Nursing intervention
1. Preoperative care
a. Support the patient and family
b. Assess and document signs and symptoms and reactions to treatments
c. Provide and encourage the prescribed diet
d. Monitor vital signs at least q8h
e. Monitor blood and fluid replacement therapy
f. Provide preoperative teaching
2. Postoperative care (immediate)
a. Have patient turn, cough, and breathe deeply
b. Monitor nasogastric suctioning and tube patency
c. Monitor vital signs as ordered
d. Record intake and output
e. Administer prescribed medication and monitor for side effects
f. Assess dressing
g. Assess for bowel sounds
h. Encourage early ambulation and ROM exercises to prevent thrombosis
i. Provide antiembolism stockings
j. Relieve pain with drugs and supportive measures
3. Postoperative period
a. Provide six to eight small feedings
b. Weigh patient qd while in hospital to monitor weight loss
c. Reduce fluids taken with meals if not tolerated
d. Educate patient and family concerning drug therapy, dietary restrictions, activity, wound care, and compliance with the regimen

PEPTIC ULCERS
A. Definition: ulcerations in the mucosal lining of the distal esophagus, stomach, or small intestine (duodenum or jejunum); duodenal ulcers are more common than gastric ulcers, and men are more prone to ulcers than women
B. Cause: exact cause is unknown; recurrent or refractory ulcers linked with *Helicobacter pylori* infections
C. Predisposing factors
1. Stress

2. Smoking
3. Heavy caffeine ingestion
4. Ingestion of certain drugs (ASA, steroids, NSAIDs)
5. Infection of the mucosa by *H. pylori*
D. Signs and symptoms
1. Loss of appetite
2. Weight loss or gain
3. Pain (gnawing, burning)
4. Melena
5. Anemia
6. Hematemesis; coffee-ground emesis
7. Occasional nausea or vomiting
8. Dark, tarry stools
E. Diagnostic tests/methods
1. Patient history and physical examination
2. Gastroscopy and duodenoscopy
3. Barium studies
4. Gastric analysis
5. Laboratory studies
F. Treatment
1. Conservative
a. Rest
b. Drug therapy: antacids, anticholinergics, histamine receptor antagonists, sedatives, and analgesics
c. Elimination of smoking and caffeine
d. Reduction of stress
e. Bland diet with small, frequent feedings
f. In acute situations the patient may be NPO and have nasogastric tube inserted
2. Surgical intervention
a. Closure if perforation has occurred
b. Pyloroplasty and vagotomy if the gastric outlet is obstructed
c. Total or partial resection of the stomach to remove the ulcerated area(s)
G. Nursing intervention
1. Conduct ongoing assessment of signs and symptoms and reactions to treatments
2. Monitor vital signs at least q4h
3. Administer the prescribed medication and monitor for side effects
4. Provide the prescribed diet
5. Provide physical and emotional rest
6. Monitor for signs and symptoms of complications (perforation, hemorrhage, and obstruction)
7. Instruct patient regarding elimination of smoking, avoidance of certain foods, and reduction of stress
8. Educate patient and family concerning drug therapy, diet and dietary restrictions, avoidance of stress, and the need for compliance with the prescribed regimen

OBSTRUCTION
A. Definition: a mechanical or neurologic abnormality inhibiting the normal flow of gastric or intestinal contents
B. Obstructions may result from scar tissue formation, cancer, or strangulated hernias; all are mechanical barriers to the normal flow of gastric or intestinal contents
C. A neurologic obstruction, in the form of a paralytic ileus, causes interference with innervation, thus hindering normal peristaltic activity
D. Signs and symptoms
1. Abnormal pain and distention

2. Projectile vomiting
3. Nausea
4. Possible absence of bowel sounds or increase in bowel sounds
5. Cramping
6. Abdomen may be tense (distended)
7. Obstipation (chronic constipation)

E. Diagnostic tests/methods
1. Patient history and physical examination
2. Flat plate of the abdomen
3. Laboratory studies

F. Treatment
1. Surgery is the treatment for mechanical obstructions
2. Gastric or intestinal decompression to decrease nausea and vomiting
3. Hydration with IV therapy
4. Prophylactic antibiotics
5. Monitor intake and output
6. Supportive care

G. Nursing intervention
1. Assess and document signs and symptoms and reactions to treatments
2. Monitor vital signs at least q4h
3. Record intake and output
4. Monitor the decompression tube and assess quantity and character of drainage
5. Provide mouth care while patient is intubated
6. Administer prescribed medication and monitor for side effects
7. Maintain NPO
8. Monitor the states of distention and hydration
9. Provide routine postoperative care if patient undergoes surgery

CROHN'S DISEASE (REGIONAL ENTERITIS)

A. Definition: an inflammatory disease affecting primarily the small bowel and also possibly the large bowel; the intestinal lining ulcerates, and scar tissue forms; bowel becomes thick and narrow
B. Cause is unknown; stricture, obstruction, and perforation can occur as a result of this disorder; malabsorption of fluid and nutrients is also associated with this disorder
C. Signs and symptoms (aggravated by illness/stress)
1. Abdominal pain and cramping
2. Diarrhea
3. Weight loss
4. Fever
5. Anemia
6. Weakness and fatigue
7. Anorexia
8. Abdominal tenderness
D. Diagnostic tests/methods
1. Patient history and physical examination
2. Laboratory studies: CBC, electrolytes, clotting studies
3. Stool examination
4. Endoscopy
5. Proctosigmoidoscopy and biopsy examination
6. Barium studies
E. Treatment
1. Drug therapy: sedatives, antidiarrheals, antibiotics, steroids, hematinics, anticholinergics, and analgesics
2. Hydration with IV therapy

3. Correct nutritional deficiencies
4. Provide symptomatic relief
5. In severe cases the patient may be NPO, have a naso-gastric tube, and require blood transfusions
6. High-calorie, high-protein, low-residue diet
7. Surgery is indicated if there is fistula formation, bleeding, perforation, or obstruction

F. Nursing intervention
1. Assess and document signs and symptoms and reactions to treatments
2. Monitor vital signs q4h
3. Record intake and output
4. Provide and encourage the prescribed diet
5. Assist with activities of daily living
6. Monitor the number, amount, and character of stools
7. Monitor hydration status
8. Assess for abdominal distention
9. Maintain skin integrity and monitor for anal excoriation
10. Provide support to the patient
11. Administer prescribed medication and monitor for side effects
12. Educate patient and family concerning drug therapy, dietary restrictions, and compliance; ostomy care if applicable

ULCERATIVE COLITIS

A. Definition: an inflammatory disorder of the large bowel; the inflammatory process begins in the distal segments of the colon and ascends
1. The mucosa ulcerates, bleeds, and becomes edematous and thickens
2. Perforations and abscesses can occur
3. The colon eventually loses its elasticity, and its absorptive ability is reduced
B. Cause is unknown, although it has been associated with stress, autoimmune factors, and food allergies
C. Signs and symptoms
1. Abdominal cramping pain with diarrhea
2. Nausea
3. Dehydration
4. Cachexia
5. Weight loss
6. Anorexia
7. Bloody diarrhea
8. Anemia
D. Diagnostic tests/methods
1. Patient history and physical examination
2. Laboratory studies reveal anemia and electrolyte imbalance: CBC, electrolytes
3. Stool examination
4. Proctosigmoidoscopy
5. Barium studies
E. Treatment
1. Drug therapy: sedatives, antidiarrheals, antibiotics, steroids, hematinics, anticholinergics, and analgesics
2. Correction of malnutrition
3. Hydration with IV therapy
4. Colectomy with ileostomy if other medical treatment fails
5. Provide symptomatic relief
6. Monitor weight
7. Monitor intake and output

8. Parenteral hyperalimentation may be necessary
9. Psychotherapy
F. Nursing intervention
   1. Assess and document signs and symptoms and reactions to treatments
   2. Provide emotional as well as physical rest
   3. Monitor number, amount, and characteristics of stools
   4. Provide skin care measures to avoid anal excoriation
   5. Monitor intake and output
   6. Monitor vital signs q4h
   7. Weigh patient qd
   8. Increase intake of fluids
   9. Provide the prescribed diet
   10. Administer prescribed medication and monitor for side effects
   11. Assess bowel sounds q4h
   12. Assist with activities of daily living
   13. Provide emotional support
   14. Educate patient and family concerning drug therapy, dietary restrictions, avoidance of stress, and compliance with the prescribed regimen

DIVERTICULOSIS/DIVERTICULITIS

A. Definition: *diverticulum*—an outpouching of the mucosa of the colon
   1. Diverticulosis: the existence of diverticula in the large intestine
   2. Diverticulitis: an inflammation of the diverticulum
B. Cause of diverticulosis is unknown; theories include a congenital weakness of the colon, colon distention, constipation, and inadequate dietary fiber
C. Signs and symptoms
   1. Abdominal cramps
   2. Lower-quadrant tenderness
   3. Constipation or constipation alternating with diarrhea
   4. Fever
   5. Occult bleeding
   6. Elevated WBC count
D. Diagnostic tests/methods
   1. Patient history and physical examination
   2. Laboratory studies
   3. Stool examination for occult blood
   4. Sigmoidoscopy
   5. Colonoscopy
   6. Barium studies
E. Treatment
   1. High-residue diet
   2. Drug therapy: bulk laxatives, antibiotics, stool softeners, and anticholinergics
   3. In more severe cases the patient may be NPO and require IV therapy
   4. Surgery: colon resection for obstruction and hemorrhage
F. Nursing intervention
   1. Assess and document signs and symptoms and reactions to treatments
   2. Provide increased roughage in the diet
   3. Increase intake of fluids
   4. Administer prescribed medication and monitor for side effects
   5. Instruct patient to avoid activity that increases intraabdominal pressure (straining at stool, lifting, bending, and wearing restrictive clothing)

   6. Educate patient and family concerning drug therapy, dietary restrictions, and avoidance of constipation and activity that increases intraabdominal pressure

COLON/RECTAL CANCER AND POLYPS

A. Definition: the cancerous process can invade the large intestine; cancer of the colon and rectum may take the form of well-defined tumor or cancerous polyp: a polyp is a pouch-like structure projecting from the wall of the bowel; polyps may be cancerous or benign
B. Cause of colon cancer is unknown; persons with colon polyps, lesions, diverticula, or ulcerative colitis are monitored closely for malignant changes in the bowel
C. Signs and symptoms
   1. Changes in bowel pattern
   2. Rectal bleeding
   3. Changes in the shape of stool
   4. Weakness and fatigue
   5. Weight loss
   6. Rectal pain
   7. Abdominal pain
   8. Anemia
D. Diagnostic tests/methods
   1. Patient history and physical examination
   2. Laboratory studies
   3. Barium studies
   4. Proctosigmoidoscopic examination
E. Treatment
   1. Surgical resection of the affected area/creation of a colostomy if necessary
   2. Chemotherapy
   3. Radiation therapy
   4. Supportive therapy
F. Nursing intervention (also see nursing care plan for cancer of the stomach)
   1. Assess and document signs and symptoms and reactions to treatments
   2. Monitor vital signs at least q4h and more often during the postoperative periods
   3. Record intake and output
   4. Monitor dressings and wound drainage
   5. Relieve pain
   6. Administer prescribed medication and monitor for side effects
   7. Provide psychologic support
   8. Monitor colostomy site
   9. Monitor perineal area if drain or packing has been inserted
   10. Assist patient with sitz baths if ordered
   11. Assist patient with activities of daily living as needed
   12. Monitor hydration status
   13. Encourage increased fluid intake
   14. Educate patient and family concerning drug therapy, diet, activities, colostomy care, and adaptation to everyday activity

HEMORRHOIDS

A. Definition: varicosities or dilated vessels in the rectal and anal area
B. Cause: hemorrhoids result from increased abdominal pressure such as that during pregnancy and from prolonged periods of sitting and standing; constipation and obesity are also predisposing factors

C. Signs and symptoms vary from no symptoms at all to pain, itching, and bleeding
D. Diagnostic tests/methods
   1. Patient history and physical examination
   2. Digital examination
   3. Proctoscopy
E. Treatment
   1. Symptomatic relief in mild cases
      a. Topical medication to shrink the mucous membrane
      b. Stool softeners and laxatives to keep stool soft and avoid straining
      c. Sitz baths to relieve pain
      d. High-fiber diet to keep stools soft
   2. Rubber-band ligation of internal hemorrhoids: the constriction impairs circulation; the tissues become necrotic and slough off
   3. Hemorrhoidectomy: the surgical excision of hemorrhoids
      a. Removal may be by clamp, excision, or cautery
      b. Postoperative treatments are similar to those identified previously for symptomatic relief
F. Nursing intervention
   1. Assess and document signs and symptoms and reactions to treatments
   2. Alleviate pain with analgesics, positioning, and sitz baths
   3. Administer prescribed medication and monitor for side effects
   4. Monitor vital signs at least q4h
   5. Monitor dressings for drainage
   6. Monitor voiding after surgery
   7. Assist with gradual return to activity
   8. Encourage increased fluid intake
   9. Provide patient with rationale for avoiding constipation and prolonged sitting and standing
   10. Educate patient and family concerning drug therapy, high-fiber diet, activity, and avoidance of constipation

CHOLELITHIASIS/CHOLECYSTITIS

A. Definition:
   1. Cholelithiasis: the presence of gallstones in the gallbladder or biliary tree
   2. Cholecystitis: an inflammation of the gallbladder usually associated with the presence of gallstones
B. Cause
   1. Cholelithiasis is believed to be precipitated by chemical changes in bile
      a. Bile stasis, infections of the gallbladder, and metabolic changes can precipitate stone formation
      b. Stones may lodge in the biliary tree, causing obstruction and biliary colic (Fig. 5-11)
   2. Cholecystitis: may be brought on by cholelithiasis or the presence of an organism in the gallbladder
C. Signs and symptoms
   1. Indigestion after a meal high in fat
   2. Nausea and vomiting
   3. Flatulence
   4. Belching
   5. Right upper-quadrant pain radiating to the back or shoulder
   6. Fever
   7. Jaundice
   8. Clay-colored stools

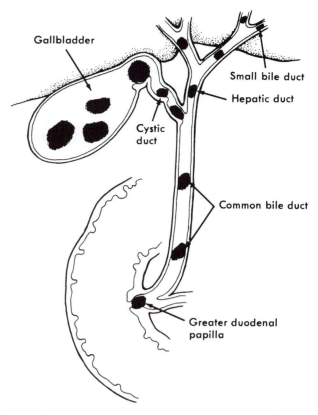

Figure 5-11. Common sites of gallstones. (From Phipps et al: *Medical-surgical nursing: concepts and clinical practice,* ed 5, St Louis, 1995, Mosby.)

   9. Dark-colored urine
   10. Elevated WBC count
D. Diagnostic tests/methods
   1. Patient history and physical examination
   2. Laboratory studies
   3. Oral cholecystography
   4. IV cholangiography
   5. Ultrasound of gallbladder
E. Treatment
   1. Hydration with IV fluids
   2. Drug therapy: analgesics, antibiotics, and antispasmodics
   3. Drug therapy to dissolve stones has been effective in certain patients
   4. Low-fat diet
   5. Lithotripsy (use of shock waves to disintegrate gallstones) has been attempted in patients having few stones
   6. Surgical removal of the gallbladder (cholecystectomy) or gallstones (cholecystostomy)
   7. Laparoscopic choleceptectomy (removal through an endoscope inserted through the abdominal wall)
F. Nursing intervention
   1. Assess and document signs and symptoms and reactions to treatments
   2. Administer prescribed medication and monitor for side effects
   3. Alleviate pain and promote comfort

4. Monitor IV therapy
5. Provide the prescribed diet
6. Monitor the state of hydration
7. Assess vital signs at least q4h
8. Provide postoperative care: monitor dressing, nasogastric tube, and T tube (tube is inserted into the common bile duct during surgery if the common bile duct is explored) (Fig. 5-12)
9. Educate patient and family concerning drug therapy, dietary restrictions, and wound care if surgery was performed

HEPATITIS
A. Definition: inflammation of the liver
B. Causes
  1. Drugs or chemicals (toxic hepatitis)
  2. Viral origin (hepatitis A [HAV] and B [HBV])
  3. Multiple blood transfusions (hepatitis non-A or non-B)
C. The most common forms of HAV and HBV
  1. HAV: infectious hepatitis
    a. Transmitted by the fecal-oral route
    b. Incubation period is approximately 2 to 7 weeks
    c. May be spread by contaminated food, water, milk, and shellfish
  2. HBV: serum hepatitis
    a. Associated with contaminated needles and syringes
    b. Transmitted through blood or blood products and pricking of the skin with contaminated equipment
    c. May also be spread through feces, urine, saliva, and semen
    d. Patients are prone to exacerbations and complications (cirrhosis) from the disease
    e. Incubation period is approximately 6 to 26 weeks
    f. Immunization available: given to newborn, then again at 2 and 6 months of age
  3. Hepatitis C (HCV; formerly known as non-HAV and non-HBV) and hepatitis E
    a. Name given to forms of hepatitis caused by a virus genetically different from hepatitis A or B
    b. Associated with blood transfusions, particularly from paid donors; previous IV drug use
    c. No specific antigen is associated with the form
    d. Similar to hepatitis B in characteristics but course is insidious in the beginning
    e. HCV now tested on all blood donors
D. Signs and symptoms: (early symptoms of HAV may be more severe)
  1. Fever and chills
  2. Headache
  3. Respiratory symptoms
  4. Anorexia
  5. Nausea and vomiting
  6. Liver tenderness
  7. Jaundice and itching
  8. Elevated liver enzymes
  9. Elevated prothrombin time (PT) values
  10. Elevated bilirubin levels
  11. Presence of HAV in feces and serum
  12. Presence of the hepatitis surface antigen HB_sAg
  13. Clay-colored stools and dark-colored urine
E. Diagnostic tests/methods
  1. Patient history and physical examination

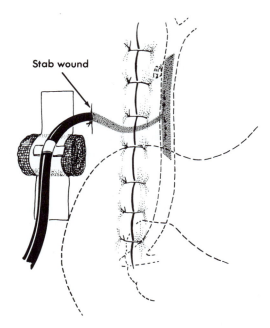

Stab wound

Figure 5-12. Section of T-tube emerging from stab wound may be placed over roll of gauze anchored to skin with adhesive tape to prevent its lumen from being occluded by pressure. (From Phipps et al: *Medical-surgical nursing: concepts and clinical practice*, ed 5, St Louis, 1995, Mosby.)

  2. Laboratory studies: hepatitis-associated antigen (HAA); liver profile
  3. Stool examination
  4. Urinary bilirubin and urobilinogen
  5. Liver biopsy
F. Treatment
  1. Monitor liver function studies
  2. Bed rest with bathroom privileges
  3. High-calorie, high-carbohydrate, high-protein, moderate-fat diet
  4. Topical lotions to alleviate dry, itchy skin
  5. Hydration with IV therapy
  6. Administration of vitamin K preparations
  7. Monitor for bleeding tendencies and progression of the illness
  8. Blood and body fluid precautions
  9. Passive immunity
G. Nursing intervention
  1. Assess and document signs and symptoms and reactions to treatments
  2. Monitor skin, stool, and urine color
  3. Promote balanced activity and rest periods
  4. Maintain blood and body fluid precautions
  5. Monitor IV therapy
  6. Assess intake and output
  7. Monitor vital signs at least q4h
  8. Provide and encourage the prescribed diet
  9. Support the patient and family
  10. Administer prescribed medication and monitor for side effects
  11. Monitor for bleeding tendencies

12. Educate patient and family concerning drug therapy, the prescribed diet, activity level, and monitoring for complications

CIRRHOSIS

A. Definition: cell degeneration occurring in the liver wherever scar tissue replaces normally functioning tissue
B. Cirrhosis is a complication of alcoholism, hepatitis, biliary disease, and certain metabolic disorders
C. Whatever the cause of the liver destruction, the course of cirrhosis is the same
   1. Liver parenchyma dies and regenerates, and fibrous tissue (scarring) occurs
   2. This alteration in structure progresses in the liver, causing problems in hepatic blood flow and normal liver function; in time the liver fails
D. Major complications of cirrhosis
   1. Portal hypertension: hypertension resulting from the obstruction of normal blood flow through the portal system; the obstruction is caused by changes in the liver from the cirrhotic process
   2. Esophageal varices (refer to Esophageal varices at the beginning of this section)
   3. Ascites: the accumulation of fluid in the peritoneal or abdominal cavity, which is a later symptom in cirrhosis
   4. Hepatic coma (encephalopathy): a condition of advanced liver disease; blood enters the general circulation without being properly detoxified by the liver
E. Signs and symptoms
   1. Headache
   2. Nausea and vomiting
   3. Weight loss
   4. Anorexia
   5. Jaundice
   6. Abdominal pain
   7. Fatigue and weakness
   8. Liver enlargement and fibrosis
   9. Bleeding disorders caused by disruption in the manufacture of vitamin K-dependent factors
   10. Edema
   11. Telangiectasis (blood vessels develop a spiderlike appearance)
   12. Ascites
   13. Esophageal varices
   14. Hepatic coma
F. Diagnostic tests/methods
   1. Patient history and physical examination
   2. Laboratory studies to assess liver function
   3. Liver scan
   4. Liver biopsy
G. Treatment
   1. Rest with activity as tolerated
   2. Nutritious diet with protein level determined by liver functioning
   3. If ascites is present, restrict fluid and sodium, monitor weight, and monitor intake and output
   4. Monitor for complications such as ascites, esophageal varices, and hepatic coma
   5. Drug therapy to reduce ammonia levels, prevent bleeding, reduce edema, and provide comfort
H. Nursing intervention
   1. Assess and document signs and symptoms and reactions to treatments

2. Administer prescribed medication and monitor for side effects
3. Provide and encourage the prescribed diet
4. Promote comfort
5. Monitor vital signs at least q4h and report abnormalities
6. Monitor status of ascites
   a. Record weight
   b. Assess measurements of extremities and abnormal girth
   c. Monitor intake and output
7. Provide planned exercise and rest periods
8. Assist patient with activities of daily living
9. Monitor skin status and take measures to prevent skin breakdown
10. Protect against infection
11. Provide diversional activity
12. Offer emotional support
13. Provide ongoing assessment for evidence of hepatic encephalopathy
   a. Monitor for symptoms of lethargy, confusion, twitching, tremors, sweetish breath odor, fever, and increasing somnolence
   b. Eliminate dietary protein
   c. Administer prescribed drugs and enemas to reduce ammonia levels
   d. Monitor IV fluids
   e. Give narcotics and sedatives cautiously
14. Also see Care of patient with esophageal varices at the beginning of this section
15. Educate patient and family concerning home-bound care

PANCREATITIS

A. Definition: an acute or chronic inflammation of the pancreas
B. Pancreatitis is associated with biliary disease, infections, drug toxicity, nutritional deficiencies, and ingestion of alcohol
C. The digestive enzymes of the pancreas are released into the pancreatic tissue, causing inflammation
   1. As the condition progresses, ischemia, duct obstruction, and necrosis may occur
   2. Bleeding occurs if tissue necrosis affects vessels
   3. Pancreatic abscesses may occur if bacteria invade the necrotic tissue
   4. In chronic pancreatitis the tissue becomes fibrotic and normal function is compromised
D. Signs and symptoms
   1. Acute pancreatitis
      a. Epigastric pain that radiates to the back
      b. Eating tends to aggravate pain
      c. Patient may assume a side-lying position with knees bent for comfort
      d. Nausea and vomiting
      e. Low-grade fever
      f. Hypotension
      g. Tachycardia
      h. Jaundice
      i. Elevated WBC count
      j. Shock: if there is blood vessel or tissue erosion
   2. Chronic pancreatitis
      a. Abdominal pain
      b. Weight loss
      c. Steatorrhea (foul-smelling, foamy stool)
      d. Diabetes mellitus if beta function is affected

E. Diagnostic tests/methods
 1. Patient history and physical examination
 2. Laboratory tests, particularly electrolytes, amylase, lipase, and liver enzymes
 3. Pancreatic scan and sonography
 4. Visualization of the pancreatic duct (endoscopy)
 5. X-ray studies
F. Treatment
 1. Control of pain
 2. Hydration with IV fluids
 3. Correction of any bleeding
 4. Nasogastric tube and NPO to reduce pancreatic secretions
 5. Drug therapy: analgesics, antibiotics, steroids, vitamins, and pancreatic extracts
 6. Diet that does not stimulate pancreatic secretions
 7. Control of blood glucose levels if beta cells are affected
G. Nursing intervention
 1. Assess and document signs and symptoms and reactions to treatments
 2. Administer prescribed medication and monitor for side effects
 3. Provide the prescribed diet
 4. Explain dietary restrictions to patient
 5. Monitor vital signs at least q4h
 6. Monitor IV therapy
 7. Promote comfort and relieve pain
 8. Provide emotional support
 9. Assess intake and output
 10. Relieve nausea and vomiting if present
 11. Note color, character, and amount of urine and stool
 12. Monitor jaundice if present
 13. Monitor the nasogastric tube and secretions
 14. Educate patient and family concerning drug therapy, diet and dietary restrictions, avoidance of alcohol, monitoring steatorrhea, blood glucose monitoring (glucometer), and compliance with the regimen

CANCER OF THE PANCREAS

A. Cancer of the pancreas can affect any portion of the pancreas, including the beta cells; metastasis readily occurs to adjacent structures
B. Cancerous tissue impairs normal pancreatic function, primarily by causing obstruction and hindering the flow of pancreatic secretions
C. Signs and symptoms
 1. Early symptoms may be vague
  a. Nausea and vomiting
  b. Anorexia
  c. Weight loss
  d. Weakness and fatigue
 2. Later symptoms
  a. Pain
  b. Jaundice
  c. Diabetes mellitus
D. Diagnostic tests/methods
 1. Patient history and physical examination
 2. Laboratory studies
 3. Pancreatic scan and sonography
 4. X-ray studies
 5. Visualization of the pancreatic duct
E. Treatment
 1. Supportive therapy

 2. Surgical excision: Whipple's procedure may be performed removing the head of the pancreas, lower portion of the common bile duct, distal portion of the stomach, and the duodenum
 3. Palliative surgery: to restore bile and pancreatic output
 4. Chemotherapy
F. Nursing intervention: see Cancer of the stomach, p. 194

APPENDICITIS

A. Definition: inflammation of the appendix
B. Signs and symptoms
 1. Right lower-quadrant pain
 2. Nausea and vomiting
 3. Anorexia
 4. Fever
 5. Elevated WBC count
C. Diagnostic tests/methods
 1. Patient history and physical examination
 2. Laboratory tests, particularly a WBC count
D. Treatment
 1. Supportive therapy
 2. Immediate surgical removal (appendectomy)
E. Nursing intervention
 1. Assess and document signs and symptoms and reactions to treatments
 2. Monitor IV fluids
 3. Provide comfort measures such as an ice pack to the abdomen and analgesia
 4. Administer prescribed drugs and monitor for side effects
 5. Monitor vital signs as ordered
 6. Encourage progressive ambulation after surgery
 7. Monitor the dressing and operative site after surgery
 8. Educate patient and family concerning drug therapy, activity restrictions, and care of the operative site

PERITONITIS

A. Definition: infection and subsequent inflammation of the peritoneal membrane by trauma or bacterial invasion
B. The inflammation may be localized or widespread and may affect the organs of the abdominal cavity; adhesions, abscesses, and obstructions may occur
C. Signs and symptoms
 1. Nausea and vomiting
 2. Abdominal pain
 3. Abdominal rigidity and distention
 4. Fever
 5. Paralytic ileus
 6. Fluid and electrolyte imbalance
 7. Elevated WBC count
 8. Constipation; diarrhea
D. Diagnostic tests/methods
 1. Patient history and physical examination
 2. Laboratory tests including a WBC count, electrolytes, and blood cultures
E. Treatment
 1. Identification of the causative agent
 2. Intestinal decompression
 3. Hydration with IV therapy
 4. Pain control
 5. Drug therapy: analgesics and antibiotics
 6. Monitoring vital signs

7. Monitoring intake and output
8. Controlling the spread of infection

F. Nursing intervention
1. Assess and document signs and symptoms and reactions to treatment
2. Assess vital signs every 1 to 2 hours during the acute period
3. Monitor intake and output
4. Administer prescribed medication and monitor for side effects
5. Provide comfort and relief of pain
6. Assess bowel sounds
7. Maintain NPO during the acute period
8. Maintain nasogastric tube and monitor output during the acute period
9. Support patient and allay anxieties
10. Place patient in semi-Fowler's position
11. Have patient turn, cough, and deep breathe at least q2h

HERNIAS

A. Definition: a protrusion of an organ or structure through the wall of the containing cavity
B. Hernias may occur around the umbilical area, inguinal area, diaphragm, femoral ring, and at the site of an incision
C. Hernias are categorized as
1. Reducible: can be returned to its normal position
2. Irreducible: cannot be returned to the normal position
3. Incarcerated: obstruction of intestinal flow
4. Strangulated: blood supply is cut off (occluded)—surgical emergency
D. Causes
1. Congenital weakness in the containing wall
2. Weakness in containing wall is related to straining and the aging process
3. Trauma
4. Increased intraabdominal pressure (obesity or pregnancy)
E. Signs and symptoms
1. Protrusion of a structure without symptoms
2. Appearance of a protrusion when straining or lifting
3. In certain instances there may be pain
4. If the intestine is obstructed, there may be distention, pain, nausea, and vomiting
F. Diagnostic methods: patient history and physical examination
G. Treatment
1. Surgery is the treatment of choice
a. Herniorrhaphy: surgical repair of the hernia
b. Hernioplasty: the surgical reinforcement of the weakened area
2. Use of a truss (a support worn over the hernia to keep it in place)
H. Nursing intervention
1. Assess and document signs and symptoms and reactions to treatments
2. Assess vital signs every shift before surgery
3. Report any symptoms of coughing, sneezing, or upper respiratory tract infection noted before surgery because this will weaken the surgical repair
4. Apply ice packs as ordered to control pain and swelling
5. Monitor voidings following inguinal hernia repair
6. Educate patient and family concerning care of the operative site, activity restrictions, and avoidance of constipation

THE NEUROLOGIC SYSTEM
Anatomy and Physiology

The nervous system acts as a coordinated unit both structurally and functionally

A. Functions
1. Regulates system
2. Controls communication among body parts
3. Coordinates activities of body system
B. Divisions
1. Central nervous system (CNS): brain and spinal cord; interprets incoming sensory information and sends out instruction based on past experiences
2. Peripheral nervous system (PNS): cranial and spinal nerves extending out from brain and spinal cord; carry impulses to and from brain and spinal cord
3. Autonomic nervous system: functional classification of the PNS; regulates involuntary activities
4. Somatic nervous system: functional classification of the PNS; allows conscious or voluntary control of skeletal muscles
C. Structure and physiology
1. Neurons or nerve cells: respond to a stimulus, connect it into a nerve impulse (irritability), and transmit the impulse to neurons, muscle, or glands (conductivity), consists of three main parts
a. Cell body: contains nucleus and one or more fibers or processes extending from cell body
b. Dendrites: conduct impulses toward cell body; neuron has many dendrites
c. Axons: conduct impulses away from cell body; neuron has one axon
2. Types of neurons
a. Motor (efferent): conduct impulses from CNS to muscle and glands
b. Sensory (afferent): conduct impulses toward CNS
c. Connecting (interneuron): conduct impulses from sensory to motor neurons
3. Synapse: chemical transmission of impulses from axon to dendrites
4. Myelin sheath: protects and insulates the axon fibers; increases the rate of transmission of nerve impulses
5. Neurilemma: sheath covering the myelin; found in PNS; function is regeneration of nerve fiber
6. Neuroglia: connective or supporting tissue, important in reaction of nervous system to injury or infection
7. Ganglia: clusters of nerve cells outside CNS
8. White matter: bundles of myelinated nerve fibers; conducts impulses along fibers
9. Gray matter: clusters of neuron cell bodies; fibers not covered with myelin; distributes impulses across selected synapses
D. Central nervous system
1. Brain (Fig. 5-13)
a. Cerebrum: largest part of brain; outer layer called cerebral cortex; cortex composed of dendrites and cell bodies; controls mental processes; highest level of functioning (Table 5-3)
b. Cerebellum: controls muscle tone coordination and maintains equilibrium
c. Diencephalon: consists of two major structures located between cerebrum and midbrain

Table 5-3	Specific Functions of Cerebral Cortexes
Frontal cortex	Conceptualization Abstraction Judgment formation Motor ability Ability to write words Higher level centers for autonomic functions
Parietal cortex	Highest integrative and coordinating center for perception and interpretation of sensory information Ability to recognize body parts Left versus right Motor movement
Temporal cortex	Memory storage Auditory integration Hearing
Occipital cortex	Visual center Understanding of written material

From Long et al: *Medical surgical nursing: a nursing process approach*, St Louis, 1993, Mosby.

    (1) Hypothalamus: regulates the autonomic nervous system; controls blood pressure; helps maintain normal body temperature and appetite; controls water balance and sleep

    (2) Thalamus acts as a relay station for incoming and outgoing nerve impulses; produces emotions of pleasantness and unpleasantness associated with sensations

  d. Brainstem: connects the cerebrum with the spinal cord

    (1) Midbrain: relay center for eye and ear reflexes

    (2) Pons: connecting link between cerebellum and rest of nervous system

    (3) Medulla oblongata: contains center for respiration, heart rate, and vasomotor activity

2. Spinal cord

  a. Inner column composed of gray matter, shaped like an H, made up of dendrites and cell bodies; outer part composed of white matter, made up of bundles of axons called tracts

  b. Function: sensory tract conducts impulses to brain; motor tract conducts impulses from brain; center for all spinal cord reflexes

3. Protection for CNS

  a. Bone: vertebrae surround cord; skull surrounds brain

  b. Meninges: three connective tissue membranes that cover brain and spinal cord

    (1) Dura mater: white fibrous tissue; outer layer

    (2) Arachnoid: delicate membrane, middle layer; contains subarachnoid fluid

    (3) Pia mater: inner layer, contains blood vessels

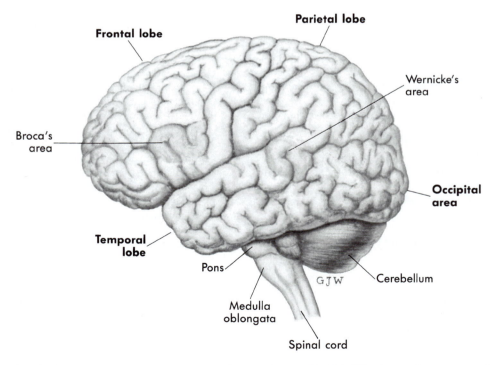

Figure 5-13. **Lateral view of the brain.** (From Howman SP: *Rehabilitation nursing: process and application*, ed 2, St Louis, 1996, Mosby.)

c. Spaces
  (1) Epidural between dura mater and the vertebrae
  (2) Subdural space: between dura mater and arachnoid
  (3) Subarachnoid space: between arachnoid and pia mater, contains cerebrospinal fluid
  d. Cerebrospinal fluid: acts as a shock absorber; aids in exchange of nutrients and waste materials
E. Peripheral nervous system
  1. Carries voluntary and involuntary impulses
  2. Cranial nerves (Table 5-4)
  3. Spinal nerves: 31 pairs; conduct impulses necessary for sensation and voluntary movement; each group named for the corresponding part of the spinal column
F. Autonomic nervous system
  1. Part of PNS; controls smooth muscle, cardiac muscle, and glands
  2. Two divisions
    a. Sympathetic: "fight or flight" response; increases heart rate and blood pressure; dilates pupils
    b. Parasympathetic: dominates control under normal conditions; maintains homeostasis

Neurologic Conditions

Pathology of the central nervous system (CNS) arises from injuries, new growths, vascular insufficiency, infections, and as complications secondary to other diseases. Patient problems are related to interference with normal functioning of the affected tissue.

The following terms are used in describing the patient with a neurologic impairment.

anesthesia   complete loss of sensation
aphasia   loss of ability to use language
auditory/receptive aphasia   loss of ability to understand
expressive aphasia   loss of ability to use spoken or written word
ataxia   uncoordinated movements
coma   state of profound unconsciousness
convulsion   involuntary contractions and relaxation of muscle
delirium   mental state characterized by restlessness and disorientation
diplopia   double vision
dyskinesia   difficulty in voluntary movement
flaccid   without tone—limp
neuralgia   intermittent, intense pain along the course of a nerve
neuritis   inflammation of a nerve or nerves
nuchal rigidity   stiff neck
nystagmus   involuntary, rapid movements of the eyeball
papilledema   swelling of optic nerve head
paresthesia   abnormal sensation without obvious cause, with numbness and tingling
spastic   convulsive muscular contraction
stupor   state of impaired consciousness with brief response only to vigorous and repeated stimulation
tic   spasmodic, involuntary twitching of a muscle
vertigo   dizziness

Nursing Assessment

A. Nursing observations
  1. Mental status: drowsiness or lethargy, ability to follow commands
  2. Level of consciousness (LOC): ability to be aroused in response to verbal and physical stimuli; ranges from awake and alert to "coma"; Glasgow Coma Scale (Table 5-5) is the usual guide for assessing and describing the degree of conscious impairment, based on three determinants:

Table 5-4	Cranial Nerves		
Cranial nerves	**Conducts impulses**		**Function**
I Olfactory	From nose to brain		Sense of smell
II Optic	From eye to brain		Vision
III Oculomotor	From brain to eye and eye muscles		Contraction of upper eyelid; maintain position of eyelid; pupillary reflexes
IV Trochlear	From brain to external eye muscles		Eye movements
V Trigeminal	From skin and mucous membranes of head and teeth to chewing muscles		Sensations of head and teeth; muscles of chewing
VI Abducens	From brain to external eye muscles		Eye movements
VII Facial	From taste buds of the tongue and facial muscles to muscles of facial expression		Taste; facial expression
VIII Acoustic	From organ of Corti to brain		Hearing
Vestibular branch	From semicircular canals to brain		Balance
IX Glossopharyngeal	From pharynx and posterior to third of tongue to brain; also from brain to throat muscles and salivary glands		Sensations of tastes, sensations of pharynx; swallowing; secretion of saliva
X Vagus	From throat and organs in thoracic and abdominal cavities to brain; to muscles of throat and abdominal cavities		Important in swallowing, speaking, peristalsis, and production of gastric juices
XI Accessory	From brain to shoulder and neck muscles		Rotation of head and raising shoulders
XII Hypoglossal	From brain to muscles of tongue		Movement of tongue

Table 5-5	Glasgow Coma Scale	
	Stimuli	**Score**
Eyes open	Spontaneously	4
	To speech	3
	To pain	2
	None	1
Best verbal response	Oriented	5
	Confused	4
	Inappropriate words	3
	Incomprehensible	2
	None	1
Best motor response	Obeys commands	5
	Localizes to pain	4
	Flexes to pain	3
	Extends arm to pain	2
	None	1

From Long et al: *Medical surgical nursing: a nursing process approach*, ed 3, St Louis, 1993, Mosby.

a. Eye opening
b. Motor response
c. Verbal response
3. Orientation
   a. Time: knows month or year
   b. Place: has general knowledge of where patient is (e.g., hospital)
   c. Person: knows own name; able to name relative or friend
4. Behavior: is it appropriate for the situation
5. Emotional response: is it appropriate for the situation
6. Memory: capability for early and recent recall
7. Speech: presence of aphasia, appropriate speech, words distinct or slurred
8. Vital signs: temperature, pulse, respirations, and blood pressure
9. Ability to follow simple directions
10. Eyes
    a. Pupillary reaction to light: the pupils are periodically assessed with a flashlight to evaluate and compare size, configuration, and reaction. Differences between both eyes and from previous assessments are compared for similarities and differences
    b. Movement of lids and pupils
11. Motor function: coordination, gait, balance, posture, strength, and functioning
12. Bladder and bowel control
13. Ears for drainage (may indicate CSF leak)
14. Facial expression for symmetry
15. Sensation for
    a. Pain
    b. Light touch, pressure
    c. Smell
16. Rancho Los Amigos Scale: A scale of cognitive functioning that was developed to aid in assessment and treatment after traumatic brain injury (TBI)

a. No response; patient is completely unresponsive to any stimuli
b. Generalized response; reacts inconsistently and non-purposefully to stimuli
c. Localized response; reacts specifically yet inconsistently to stimuli
d. Confused-agitated; in agitated state yet has decreased ability to process information
e. Confused-inappropriate; appears alert, able to respond to simple commands fairly consistently
f. Confused-appropriate; has goal-directed behaviors, needs cues
g. Automatic-appropriate; oriented, does daily routine, has shallow recall of actions
h. Purpose-appropriate; aware and oriented, able to recall and integrate past and recent events
B. Patient description (subjective data)
   1. History of head injury, loss of consciousness, vertigo, weakness, headache, sleep problems, paralysis, seizures, or diplopia
   2. Complains of pain, numbness, problems with elimination, memory loss, difficulty concentrating, drowsiness, or visual problems
   3. Medications taken
C. History from family
   1. Medical
   2. Activities of daily living (ADLs)
   3. Behavior

Diagnostic Tests/Methods

A. Computerized tomography (CT; CAT scan): computer analysis of tissues as x-rays pass through them; has replaced many of the usual tests; no special preparation or care after test
B. Lumbar puncture (spinal tap)
   1. Description: under local anesthesia a puncture is made at the junction of the third and fourth lumbar vertebrae to obtain a specimen of cerebrospinal fluid; cerebrospinal fluid pressure can be measured; this procedure is also used to inject medications (e.g., spinal anesthesia) and in diagnostic x-ray examination to inject air or dye (e.g., myelogram)
   2. Nursing intervention
      a. Monitor vital signs
      b. Keep patient supine 4 to 8 hours
      c. Observe for headache and nuchal rigidity
      d. Monitor site for leakage
C. Cerebral angiography
   1. Description: intraarterial injection of radiopaque dye to obtain an x-ray film of cerebrovascular circulation
   2. Nursing intervention after procedure
      a. Related to dye: observe for allergic reaction: urticaria, decreased urinary output, respiratory distress, and difficulty swallowing; have tracheostomy set available
      b. Related to injection site
         (1) Provide ice pack and bed rest
         (2) Monitor vital signs
         (3) Observe for pain, tenderness, bleeding, temperature, color
D. Electroencephalography (EEG)
   1. Description: electrodes are placed on unshaven scalp with tiny needles and electrode jelly

2. Nursing intervention
   a. Anticipate patient's fears about electrocution; do not give stimulants/depressants before test
   b. No smoking or caffeinated beverages; patient needs to eat a full meal before the test; fasting may cause hypoglycemia and alter brain waves
   c. Stress need for restful sleep before test; sleep deprivation may cause abnormal brain waves
   c. Wash hair and scalp after procedure to remove jelly
   d. Patient may resume all previous activities
E. Brain scan
   1. Description: after an IV injection of a radioisotope, abnormal brain tissue will absorb more rapidly than normal tissue; this can be detected with a Geiger counter to diagnose brain tumors
   2. Nursing intervention
      a. No observations
      b. Patient may resume all previous activities
F. Magnetic resonance imaging (MRI)
   1. Description: MRI uses a combination of radio waves and a strong magnetic field to view soft tissue (does not use x-rays or dyes); produces a computerized picture that depicts soft tissues in high-contrast color
   2. Nursing intervention
      a. Before the procedure, instruct the patient to remain perfectly still in the narrow cylinder-shaped machine
      b. Inform the patient that there will be no pain or discomfort, but there is no room for movement during the MRI
      c. No specific care or observations are necessary after the procedure
G. Myelography (MEG)
   1. Description: injection of a radiopaque dye into the subarachnoid space via a lumbar puncture; performed to locate lesions of the spinal column or ruptured vertebral disk
   2. Types of agents used: Metrizamide and Pantopaque; if Metrizamide is used the patient should not take phenothiazines, tricyclic antidepressants, CNS stimulants, or amphetamines for 24 to 48 hours before test; after the procedure is completed, Pantopaque dye is removed; leaving it in would cause meningeal irritation; Metrizamide is water soluble and does not need to be removed
   3. After procedure with Pantopaque, the patient lies flat in bed for 6 to 8 hours; after procedure with Metrizamide patient's head must be elevated 30 to 50 degrees for 6 to 8 hours; fluids are encouraged; common side effects include nausea, vomiting, and possibly seizures; check with physician when medications withheld prior to test may be given; with both types of agents observe site for leakage of CSF; strength and sensation in lower extremities should be assessed; encourage fluids; maintain bedrest; monitor vital signs; observe for headache, pain, and dizziness
H. Positron emission tomography (PET scan)
   1. The patient inhales or is injected with a radioactive substance
   2. The computer can diagnose and determine level of functioning of an organ
   3. Exposure to radiation is minimal and no special care is indicated
I. Skull x-ray examination: no preparation; no nursing care or observations indicated afterward

Frequent Patient Problems and Nursing Care

A. Impaired physical mobility related to progression of primary disease
   1. Give specific care and assessment as required
   2. Perform neurologic assessment every 2 to 4 hours
   3. Initiate all nursing care measures to prevent complications of immobility
   4. Use of assistive devices
B. Risk for injury/infection related to "fixed eyes" (no blinking)
   1. Protect with eye shields
   2. If needed remove dried exudate with warm saline solution and mineral oil
   3. Close eyes
   4. Inspect for inflammation
C. Ineffective breathing pattern related to neuromuscular impairment
   1. Maintain patent airway, suction as needed, and elevate head 20 to 30 degrees
   2. Have tracheostomy set available
   3. Provide oxygen with humidity
   4. Monitor vital signs q2h
   5. Provide oral hygiene q2h
   6. Lubricate lips
D. Risk for alteration in body temperature related to neuromuscular impairment
   1. Assess rectal temperature q2h
   2. Use external heating and cooling, (e.g., hypo-hyperthermia machine)
E. Risk for aspiration related to neuromuscular impairment
   1. Maintain NPO
   2. Position patient on side; turn q2h
   3. Provide nasogastric tube feedings
   4. Monitor IV fluids
F. Risk for injury related to restlessness, involuntary motions, or seizures
   1. Maintain safety (e.g., padded side rails, bed in low position)
   2. Follow precautions, care, and observations for a patient with seizures (see Convulsive Disorders, p. 207)
G. Altered patterns of urinary elimination related to neuromuscular impairment
   1. Oliguria (urinary retention)
      a. Provide indwelling catheter care
      b. Monitor intake and output qh
   2. Incontinence
      a. Wash, dry, and inspect skin as needed
      b. Implement measures to prevent decubitus ulcers
      c. Implement bladder training
H. Bowel incontinence/constipation related to neuromuscular impairment
   1. Incontinence
      a. Wash, dry, and inspect skin as needed
      b. Implement measures to prevent decubitus ulcers
      c. Implement bowel training
   2. Constipation
      a. Record bowel movements
      b. Provide stool softeners, laxatives, and enemas as ordered
      c. Check for impaction; disimpact as needed
      d. Encourage fluids as tolerated

e. Encourage activity as tolerated
f. Increase fiber in the diet

I. Fear/anxiety related to pain; complications; surgery; possible disfigurement, disability, or dependency; fatal prognosis
1. Explain everything (actions) carefully
2. Encourage patient to express feelings
3. Report to health team
4. Involve family/significant others in care

J. Other possible patient problems include
1. Self care deficit: perform own ADLs related to sensory-motor impairments
2. Altered nutrition: less than body requirements related to dysphagia and fatigue
3. Grieving related to actual/perceived loss and/or uncertain future
4. Impaired swallowing related to chewing difficulties, muscle paralysis
5. Activity intolerance related to fatigue and difficulty in performing ADLs
6. Fatigue related to weakness, spasticity, fear of injury, and stressors
7. Risk for social isolation related to spasticity, change in body image
8. Risk for injury related to visual field, motor, or perception deficits
9. Altered family processes related to physiologic deficits, role disturbances, uncertain future
10. Sensory-perceptual alterations specifically related to hypoxia secondary to trauma, progression of disease process
11. Impaired communication related to dysarthria and/or aphasia secondary to physiological changes
12. Risk for fluid volume deficit related to vomiting secondary to increased intracranial pressure (IICP)

SPECIAL SITUATIONS
A. The patient in coma
1. Unconscious state in which the patient is unresponsive to verbal or painful stimuli; this occurs with many primary diseases; the patient depends on the nurse for maintenance of all basic human needs, nourishment, bathing, elimination, respiration, prevention of complications, and assessment and provision of care for problems (A to J in the preceding outline)
2. Nursing intervention
a. Include family in nursing care and care planning as much as possible
b. Note level of consciousness (LOC) (see Nursing assessment of the neurologic patient, p. 203) every 15 minutes if LOC decreases; assess every 1, 2, or 4 hours as LOC improves
c. Demonstrate respect in patient's presence
d. Provide a quiet, restful environment
e. Speak to patient; use proper name; introduce self, and explain all care before starting
f. Provide privacy

B. The patient with paralysis
1. Paraplegia: paralysis of the lower extremities from sudden injury (e.g., automobile accident) or progressive degenerative disease (e.g., multiple sclerosis) to the spinal cord; there may be no motion or sensory function or reflexes; there may be uncontrollable muscle

spasms; perspiration ceases and then becomes profuse; there is a loss of bladder and bowel control; sexual dysfunction, anxiety, fear, depression, anger, and embarrassment are major patient problems; patient may be totally dependent
2. Quadriplegia (tetraplegia): paralysis of all four extremities from sudden injury (e.g., diving accident) or progressive degenerative disease (e.g., amyotrophic lateral sclerosis [ALS]); symptoms and patient problems include those encountered with paraplegia, as well as autonomic dysreflexia
3. Nursing intervention
a. Take measures to prevent complications of immobility
b. Provide bowel and bladder training
c. Prevent deformity: maintain joint mobility and correct alignment
d. Encourage fluid intake
e. Provide high-protein diet
f. Encourage independence according to ability
g. Communicate and work closely with the physiatrist, physical therapist, occupational therapist, and other members of the rehabilitation team
h. Include family in nursing care and planning

Major Medical Diagnoses
INCREASED INTRACRANIAL PRESSURE (IICP)
A. Description: fluid accumulation or a lesion takes up space in the cranial cavity, producing IICP; the brain is gradually compressed, or life-sustaining functions cease; may be sudden or progress slowly
B. Causes: tumors, hematoma, edema from trauma, and abscesses from infections
C. Signs and symptoms: related to primary diagnosis
1. Headache, restlessness, and anxiety
2. Vomiting: recurrent, projectile, and not related to nausea or meals
3. Change in pupil response to light
4. Seizures
5. Respiratory difficulty: irregular, Cheyne-Stokes, or Kussmaul breathing
6. Blood pressure elevates, with wide pulse pressure
7. Pulse increases at first then slows to 40 to 60 beats/min, regular and strong
8. Altered LOC: becomes lethargic, speech slows, becomes confused, and shows decreased level of response
9. Visual disturbances: diplopia and blurred vision
10. Progressive weakness or paralysis
11. Loss of consciousness, coma, and death
D. Diagnostic tests/methods: neurologic assessment by physician and nurse
E. Treatment: depends on cause
1. Surgical intervention (craniotomy)
2. Steroids, anticonvulsants, mannitol, dexamethasone (Decadron), or urea to decrease edema
F. Nursing intervention
1. Elevate head to semi-Fowler's position; never place in Trendelenburg position
2. Monitor vital signs every 15 minutes
3. Prevent aspiration; place patient on side
4. Maintain airway; O_2 therapy as necessary
5. Observe pupillary response (usually unequal and may not react to light)

6. Report any change in LOC immediately
7. Provide special care and observation when a patient has a seizure
8. Provide care and safety for an unconscious patient
9. Monitor IV fluids closely to prevent overhydration

CONVULSIVE DISORDERS

A. Description: frequently a convulsion or seizure is not a disease but a symptom of a neurologic disorder; epilepsy is a disease characterized by a disposition for seizures; the following are types of seizures
   1. Generalized or grand mal: there may be a premonition or sign (aura); the individual cries out, loses consciousness, and enters a tonic phase (the body is rigid, and the jaw is clenched); then there is a clonic phase, with jerking movements of muscles, cessation of respirations, and fecal and urinary incontinence; lasts 1 to 2 minutes followed by a short period of unresponsiveness
   2. Partial or petit mal: loss of consciousness that lasts 5 to 30 seconds, during which time normal activities may or may not cease; there may be amnesia concerning this time
   3. Jacksonian (motor): a focal seizure that may be limited to jerky movements of one extremity; may precede a grand mal seizure
B. International Classification of Epileptic Seizures (see box in column 2).
C. Causes:
   1. May be secondary to another condition: cerebrovascular accident (CVA), head injury, brain tumor, markedly elevated temperature, toxins, or electrolyte imbalance
   2. Epilepsy may have no known cause; onset usually is in childhood, before 30 years of age
D. Patient problems
   1. Related to primary disease
   2. Fear of injury
   3. Anxiety related to a chronic, lifelong disease
   4. Embarrassment
   5. Fear of public rejection
   6. Side effects of drug therapy
E. Diagnostic tests/methods
   1. Specific tests to identify lesions
   2. EEG, CT scan, MRI, and brain mapping
F. Treatment
   1. Treat and remove cause, if known
   2. Anticonvulsant drugs (see Chapter 3)
   3. Surgery-stereotactic (electrical stimulation to locate and resect [destroy] epileptogenic focus)
G. Nursing intervention
   1. Provide accurate observation and documentation including: aura, time of onset, whether seizure is generalized or focal, specific parts of body involved, progression of seizure; duration of seizure, eye movement, loss of consciousness, loss of bowel and bladder control, condition after seizure, memory loss, weakness, and any injury caused by seizure
   2. Encourage patient to wear medical identification tag
   3. Have suction available
   4. Secure airway for easy accessibility
   5. During generalized (grand mal) seizure
      a. Insert airway between teeth before seizure (do not force)
      b. Maintain airway

International Classification of Epileptic Seizures

Partial (focal) seizures (consciousness may not be impaired): With motor symptoms, with special sensory symptoms, with autonomic symptoms, with psychic symptoms. May become complex partial seizures. May evolve to generalized seizures

Generalized seizures (involve the entire brain; consciousness is lost): May last from several seconds to minutes. Types: absence seizures, myoclonic seizures, clonic seizures, tonic seizures, tonic-clonic seizures, atonic seizures

Unclassified seizures: unable to classify because of incomplete/inadequate data

---

   c. Prevent head injury
   d. Place patient on side if possible
   e. Protect extremities from injury by guiding movements
   f. Do not restrain
   g. Loosen clothing
   h. Remove pillows
   i. Maintain safety until fully conscious

TRANSIENT ISCHEMIC ATTACKS (TIAs)

Altered cerebral tissue perfusion related to a temporary neurologic disturbance
A. Manifested by sudden loss of motor or sensory function
B. Lasts for a few minutes to a few hours
C. Caused by a temporarily diminished blood supply to an area of the brain
D. Patient is at high risk for developing a stroke
E. Medical management is indicated (control of hypertension, low-sodium diet, possible anticoagulant therapy, stop smoking)
F. Nursing care would include close observation and assessment; specific care based on treatment

CEREBROVASCULAR ACCIDENT (CVA) (STROKE)

A. Description: decreased blood supply to a part of the brain caused by rupture, occlusion, or stenosis of the blood vessels; onset may be sudden or gradual; symptoms and patient problems depend on location and size of area of brain with reduced or absent blood supply (left CVA results in right-sided involvement often associated with speech problems; right CVA results in left-sided involvement often associated with safety/judgment problems)
B. Causes: increased incidence with aging
   1. Atherosclerosis
   2. Embolism
   3. Thrombosis
   4. Hemorrhage from a ruptured cerebral aneurysm
   5. Hypertension
C. Signs and symptoms
   1. Altered level of consciousness
   2. Change in mental status: decreased attention span, decreased ability to think and reason, difficulty following simple directions

3. Communication: motor or sensory aphasia, difficulty reading, writing, speaking, or understanding
4. Bowel or bladder dysfunction: retention, impaction, or incontinence
5. Seizures
6. Limited motor function: paralysis, dysphagia, weakness, hemiplegia, loss of function, or contractures
7. Loss of sensation/perception
8. Headaches and syncope
9. Loss of temperature regulation and elevated temperature, pulse, and blood pressure
10. Absent gag reflex (aspiration)
11. Unusual emotional responses: depression, anxiety, anger, verbal outbursts, and crying; emotional lability
12. Problems related to immobility (see Chapter 2)

D. Diagnostic tests/methods
1. Physical assessment and patient or family history
2. EEG, CT scan, lumbar puncture, cerebral angiography, or carotid ultrasonography

E. Treatment
1. Remove cause, prevent complications, and maintain function; rehabilitation to restore function
2. Provide antihypertensives, anticoagulants, and stool softeners (see Chapter 3)
3. Surgical removal of clot, repair of aneurysm, carotid endarterectomy or balloon angioplasty

F. Nursing intervention
1. Maintain bed rest; provide complete care; use turning sheet, foot board, firm mattress, pillows; and trochanter rolls to maintain proper body alignment; anticipate needs and leave things within reach (e.g., call bell)
2. Reposition patient q2h; provide passive and active ROM exercises; place patient in chair as soon as allowed; use flotation mattress or sheepskin
3. Provide bath, inspect, and provide nursing measures to prevent decubitus ulcers
4. Provide oxygen with humidity; have patient cough and take deep breaths q2h if possible; maintain airway; suction as needed; prevent aspiration; keep head turned to side; place in semi-Fowler's position
5. Ensure adequate nutrition and fluid and electrolyte balance; provide nasogastric/gastrostomy tube feeding; maintain IV fluids; provide soft diet when tolerated; use total parenteral nutrition (TPN); aspiration precautions
6. Establish means of communication: call bell, pad and pencil, and nonverbal gestures; use simple commands; speak slowly, explain all care; provide speech therapy
7. Be nonjudgmental about personality changes; encourage family participation; provide diversional activities; praise accomplishments realistically
8. Assess LOC; maintain safety in environment; use side rails; restrain only as necessary
9. Observe for IICP
10. Monitor vital signs q4h
11. Ensure elimination; check bowel sounds; monitor bowel movements; monitor intake and output; provide indwelling catheter care; then conduct bowel and bladder training
12. Provide care, safety, and precautions for a patient with seizures
13. Provide support for family
14. Schedule physical and occupational therapy as soon as possible
15. Provide nursing measures to prevent complications of immobility (see Chapter 2)
16. Encourage self-care

BRAIN TUMOR
A. Description: a benign or malignant growth that grows and exerts pressure on vital centers of the brain, depressing function and causing increased pressure
B. Cause: unknown
C. Signs and symptoms: individual, depending on location and size
1. Personality changes, fear, and anxiety
2. Headaches, dizziness, and visual disturbance (e.g., double vision)
3. Seizures
4. Pituitary dysfunction
5. Signs of IICP
6. Local paresthesia or anesthesia
7. Aphasia
8. Problems with coordination

D. Diagnostic tests/methods
1. Patient history and physical examination
2. Neurologic assessment including EEG, CT scan, angiography, and MRI

E. Treatment: surgical removal if possible (craniotomy), frequently combined with radiotherapy and chemotherapy

F. Nursing intervention
1. Perform timely neurologic assessment and documentation
2. Provide safety and assist with care as needed
3. Be nonjudgmental about personality changes; encourage the patient to express feelings
4. Provide postoperative care
    a. Anticipate and provide care as needed to maintain airway
    b. Provide safety and observation during a seizure
    c. Regulate body temperature
    d. Position on unoperated side
    e. Elevate head only under medical order
    f. Inspect dressing every 30 minutes for hemorrhage or drainage (leakage of cerebrospinal fluid)
    g. Make neurologic assessment qh until patient is stable and then q4h; observe for IICP
    h. Provide care for the patient in coma as indicated earlier in this section

HEAD INJURIES
A. Description: trauma to scalp, skull, or brain; a fracture to the skull may result, either a simple break in the bone or bone fragmentation that penetrates the brain tissue; can also cause hemorrhage, concussion, or contusion
1. Cerebral concussion: injury to the head; patient may be dazed or unconscious for a few minutes; some functions (e.g., memory) may be impaired for as long as several weeks
2. Cerebral contusion: head injury causing bruising of brain tissue; person experiences stupor, confusion, or loss of consciousness; if severe, may go into coma
3. Cerebral laceration: a break in continuity of brain tissue
B. Cause: blow to the head (e.g., from a fall or automobile accident

C. Signs and symptoms: individual, according to location and extent of blow
1. Nausea and vomiting
2. Lethargy: increasing loss of consciousness to impending coma
3. Disorientation
4. Drainage of cerebrospinal fluid from ear or nose (Battle's sign)
5. Convulsions
6. Problems related to IICP

D. Diagnostic tests/methods
1. Patient history and physical/neurologic assessment
2. X-ray examination
3. Angiography, Doppler studies
4. CT scan, MRI
5. PET

E. Treatment
1. Anticonvulsions, corticosteroids, mannitol—if cerebral edema
2. Maintenance of fluid balance
3. Surgery

F. Nursing intervention
1. Provide care as discussed for a patient with IICP (see previous outline)
2. Neurologic assessment qh
3. Maintain airway
4. Give care as required for the unconscious patient if necessary
5. Take precautions for a patient with seizures
6. Observe for serous or bloody discharge from ears/nose

MULTIPLE SCLEROSIS

A. Description: a chronic, progressive disease of the brain and spinal cord; lesions cause degeneration of the myelin sheath and interfere with conduction of motor nerve impulses; there are periods of remissions and exacerbations; onset occurs in young adults; it has an unpredictable progression

B. Cause: unknown, exacerbates with stress

C. Signs and symptoms vary with individual
1. Ataxia
2. Paresthesia
3. Weakness and loss of muscle tone
4. Loss of sense of position
5. Vertigo
6. Blurred vision, diplopia, nystagmus, patchy blindness that may progress to total blindness
7. Inappropriate emotions: euphoria/apathy/depression
8. Dysphagia
9. Slurred speech
10. Bladder and bowel dysfunction: incontinence or retention
11. Sexual dysfunction: impotence, diminished sensation
12. Spasticity as disease progresses

D. Diagnostic tests/methods
1. Patient history and physical/neurologic assessment
2. CT Scan
3. MRI
4. Examination of cerebrospinal fluid (CSF)

E. Treatment: symptomatic—corticosteroids during acute exacerbations

F. Nursing intervention
1. Provide care to prevent complications of immobility (see Chapter 2)

2. Encourage patient to maintain independence
3. Encourage patient to participate in care plan
4. Encourage high-caloric, high-vitamin, high-protein diet; provide nutrition that can be swallowed easily
5. Provide bowel and bladder training (may have indwelling catheter)
6. Provide diversional activities
7. Provide safety
8. Allow time for patients to express concerns about disabilities and dependencies: be supportive
9. Avoid precipitating factors that cause exacerbations (fatigue, cold, heat, infections, stress)
10. Patient/family education

PARKINSON'S DISEASE

A. Definition: a progressive, degenerative disease causing destruction of nerve cells in the basal ganglia of the brain caused by a deficiency of dopamine; limbs become rigid, fingers have characteristic pill-rolling movement, and head has to-and-fro movement; the patient has a bent position and walks in short, shuffling steps; facial expression becomes blank with wide eyes and infrequent blinking (Parkinson's mask); intelligence is not affected

B. Cause: unknown

C. Signs and symptoms
1. Tremor
2. Voluntary movement is slow and difficult; coordination is poor (ataxia)
3. Impaired chewing and eating; excessive salivation and drooling
4. Speech is slow and patient is soft spoken; written communication is difficult
5. Excessive sweating
6. Emotional changes: depression, paranoia, and eventually confusion
7. Dependency

D. Diagnostic tests/methods
1. Patient history and physical assessment
2. Neurologic assessment

E. Treatment: many patients respond to drug therapy, and the disease is controlled with medication for the remainder of their lives; others have no response, and the disease progresses to a state of invalidism and immobility (usually treated with a combination of drugs) (see Chapter 3); surgeries—stereotaxic, fetal dopamine transplant, adrenal medullary transplant

F. Nursing intervention
1. Encourage patient to maintain independence as much as possible in hygiene and dressing; include patient in planning all aspects of care as much as possible
2. Encourage participation in previous work and social and diversional activities (avoid social withdrawal)
3. Help patient avoid embarrassment while eating; use straws, wipe drooling saliva, use bib, and keep clothing clean; use utensils with large handles for easy grip
4. Recommend a soft diet or one of a consistency the patient is able to chew
5. Provide diversion (activity therapy)
6. Encourage daily exercises as tolerated, especially walking; take safety measures
7. Encourage patient to avoid fatigue
8. Help patient to avoid frustration; emphasize capabilities rather than limitations

9. Reinforce speech, physical, and occupational therapy treatment protocols
10. Administer stool softeners to avoid constipation
11. Provide bowel and bladder training
12. Be patient when patient is slow or clumsy
13. Establish a means of communication
14. Enhance cognitive skills (reorient frequently)
15. Prevent pneumonia; force fluids; turn patient when in bed and encourage patient to be out of bed as much as possible
16. Provide mouth care q4h
17. Encourage family participation in all aspects of rehabilitation

AMYOTROPHIC LATERAL SCLEROSIS (ALS)
A. Definition: also known as Lou Gehrig's disease, ALS is a degenerative disease that affects the upper or lower motor neurons of the brain, the spinal cord, or both
B. Cause: unknown; a genetic link or a slow-moving viral infection is suspect
C. Signs and symptoms
   1. Fatigue, weight loss
   2. Difficulty doing fine motor tasks (buttoning a shirt)
   3. Progressive muscle weakness; muscle wasting; atrophy
   4. Dysphagia (difficulty swallowing)
   5. Dysarthria (difficult speech)
   6. Tongue fasciculation (twitching)
   7. Jaw clonus (involuntary tightening/relaxing of muscles)
   8. Spasticity of flexor muscles
   9. Respiratory difficulty
   10. Involvement of upper/lower extremities; one side of body affected more than other (late in disease process)
   11. No sensory loss; patient remains alert
   12. Death usually occurs 5 to 10 years from onset; caused by respiratory or bulbar paralysis
D. Diagnostic tests/methods: no specific test is available to diagnose ALS; an electromyography (EMG) may be done initially to rule out other neuromuscular diseases
E. Treatment: symptomatic relief as disease progresses; surgery may be necessary to insert a gastrostomy tube during the latter stages of the disease
F. Nursing intervention
   1. Provide care to prevent complications of immobility
   2. Promote adequate nutrition; implement safety measures
   3. Provide adequate rest periods; avoid hot baths or traveling in hot weather
   4. Provide alternative means of communication
   5. Prevent bowel and bladder problems with adequate diet; medications to prevent urinary tract infections/constipation; bowel and bladder training programs may be necessary
   6. Promote skin integrity
   7. Assist in maintaining activities of daily living
   8. Assist in maintaining a clear airway; encourage use of a tucked chin position when eating or drinking; use of a suction machine; ventilator may be used for respiratory assist during latter stages of disease
   9. Patient/family education
   10. Facilitate coping/adjustment; be supportive and allow patient and family to express their concerns; refer to local support group

Spinal Cord Impairment
The vertebral column houses the spinal cord. A small cartilage disk acts as a cushion between the vertebrae. All sensory and motor nerves to the neck, trunk, and extremities branch out from the spinal cord. The degree of disability and patient problems is related to the part of the body controlled by the injured or diseased nerves.

HERNIATED INTERVERTEBRAL DISK (SEE MUSCULOSKELETAL CONDITIONS)

SPINAL CORD LESION
A. Description: a growth compressing the spinal cord; may be benign or malignant; interferes with nerve function
B. Cause: unknown
C. Signs and symptoms: individual, according to area involved
D. Diagnostic tests/methods
   1. Patient history
   2. Myelography
   3. Neurologic assessment
E. Treatment: Surgical removal
F. Nursing intervention: See Care of a patient with a laminectomy, p. 155

SPINAL CORD INJURIES
A. Description: trauma to spinal cord may cause complete or partial severing of the spinal cord; if severing is complete, there is permanent paralysis of body parts below site of injury; when there is partial damage, edema may cause a temporary paralysis
B. Cause: accident (e.g., automobile, shooting, or diving)
C. Signs and symptoms: individual, according to level of spinal cord involved (signs of spinal shock)
   1. Respiratory distress
   2. Paralysis
D. Diagnostic tests/methods: physical examination
E. Treatment
   1. Immobilization: Crutchfield tongs, halo traction, back brace, or body cast
   2. Surgery, corticosteroids, mannitol
F. Nursing intervention
   1. See Care of a patient with paralysis, p. 206; observe for complications of spinal shock
   2. Maintain airway and respiratory function
   3. See Emergency care of a patient with a spinal cord injury, p. 444 (Chapter 10)

THE ENDOCRINE SYSTEM
Anatomy and Physiology
A. Classification and secretions
   1. Exocrine glands: have ducts (tubes); secretions carried to an external or internal surface of the body by ducts (e.g., lacrimal gland)
   2. Endocrine glands: ductless; secretions by glands (hormones) carried to body tissue by blood and lymph
B. Endocrine glands and hormones (Fig. 5-14 and Table 5-6)
   1. Pituitary: located at base of the brain in a saddle-like depression of the sphenoid bone at the base of brain; called the master gland, approximately the size of a grape; composed of two parts

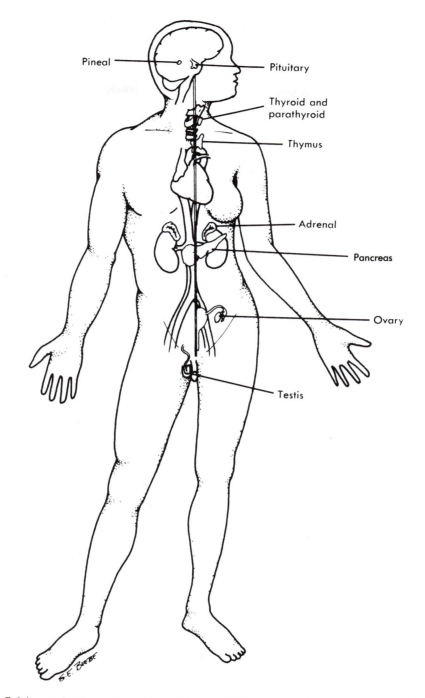

Figure 5-14. Endocrine system. (From Phipps et al: *Medical surgical nursing: concepts and clinical practice,* ed 5, St Louis, 1995, Mosby.)

a. Anterior lobe: secretes many hormones
b. Posterior lobe: secretes two hormones
2. Thyroid: located in the neck inferior to the Adam's apple; easily palpated; the largest of the endocrine glands; consists of two lobes joined by a narrow band (isthmus)
3. Parathyroid (four glands): located on posterior surface of the thyroid; regulates calcium level in the blood
4. Adrenal
    a. Two small glands; curve over the top of the kidneys
    b. Each gland has two separate parts: inner area (medulla) and outer area (cortex); produces different hormones

c. Medulla: mimics the action of the sympathetic nervous system
d. Cortex: outer part of the adrenals: produces three major groups of steroid hormones
5. Gonads (sex glands)
    a. Ovaries in female: located in pelvic cavity; produce ova and two hormones, estrogen and progesterone; do not function until puberty
    b. Testes in male: suspended in a sac called the scrotum outside the pelvic cavity; produce sperm and sex hormone, testosterone

Table 5-6	Endocrine Glands, Hormones, and Actions
Endocrine glands and hormones	**Actions of hormones**
Anterior pituitary	
Corticotropin (adrenocorticotropic hormone [ACTH])	Stimulates the adrenal cortex to produce and secrete glucocorticoid hormones
Somatotropic hormone (STH)	Stimulates growth of body cells
Thyroid-stimulating hormone (TSH)	Stimulates the thyroid gland to produce and release thyroid hormone

Gonadotropic hormones (GTH)
    Luteinizing hormone (LH)
    Follicle-stimulating hormone (FSH)
    Lactogenic hormone (prolactin)
	Affect growth, maturity, and function of primary and secondary sex organs

Posterior pituitary	
Antidiuretic hormone (ADH)	Promotes sodium and water retention in the kidney; increases blood pressure
Oxytocin	Initiates and maintains labor; influences the breasts to release milk
Thyroid	
Thyroxine	Regulates the metabolic rate of all body cells
Pancreas	
Insulin	Promotes glucose use by the cell and decreases blood sugar level
Glucagon	Promotes glucose release from the liver and increases blood sugar level
Adrenal cortex	
Glucocorticoids (includes cortisol and cortisone)	Assist the body to respond to stress; concerned with carbohydrate, fat, and protein metabolism; reduces inflammation
Mineralocorticoids (includes aldosterone)	Promote sodium and water retention in the kidney and potassium excretion
Sex hormones (androgens, estrogen, and progesterone)	Mainly affect development of secondary sex characteristics
Adrenal medulla	
Epinephrine (adrenaline) and norepinephrine (noradrenaline)	Constrict blood vessels and channel the blood to vital internal organs to prepare the body for emergency situations
Ovaries	
Estrogen	Promotes development of female sex characteristics, growth of female sex organs, and development of the uterine wall for implantation of the fertilized ovum; regulates menstruation
Progesterone	Prepares the uterine wall for implantation of the fertilized ovum; maintains the placenta and pregnancy; regulates menstruation
Testes	
Androgens (includes testosterone)	Stimulates development of the secondary male sex characteristics; essential for normal functioning of male sex organs

6. Islets of Langerhans: located within the pancreas; consist of alpha and beta cells
   a. Alpha cells: produce glucagon
   b. Beta cells: secrete hormone insulin
7. Pineal: lies just above midbrain; secretes melatonin, which inhibits gonadotropic hormone (GTH) secretion; exact function in man unclear

C. Functions: regulators of body functions
   1. Growth and development
   2. Reproduction
   3. Metabolism
   4. Fluid and electrolyte balance

Conditions/Disorders

The endocrine system is composed of numerous glands and hormones. These hormones are chemical messengers for other target glands or cells. A disturbance in one of the secreting glands may affect the regulation of another gland; therefore the patient may experience multiple problems and have varying needs. Some of the hormonal disturbances may affect patient appearance, personality, and stamina. Part of the nursing intervention is aimed at providing support and education for the patient and the family. Some patients must undergo lifelong hormonal therapy as the result of the endocrine disorder that affects them.

Nursing Assessment

A. Nursing observations
  1. General appearance
  2. Vital signs
  3. Weight
  4. Skin
     a. Color
        (1) Pallor
        (2) Flushed
        (3) Yellow pigmentation
        (4) Bronze pigmentation
        (5) Purple striae over obese areas
     b. Temperature
     c. Dry
     d. Moist
     e. Excess diaphoresis
     f. Poor wound healing
  5. Hair
     a. Dry
     b. Brittle
     c. Thin
  6. Nails
     a. Dry
     b. Thin
     c. Thick
  7. Musculoskeletal
     a. Muscle mass distribution
     b. Fat distribution
     c. Change in height
     d. Changes in body proportions: enlarged ears, nose, jaws, hands, and feet
     e. Diminished muscle strength
  8. Central nervous system
     a. Personality changes
     b. Alterations in consciousness
        (1) Listlessness
        (2) Slowed cognitive ability
        (3) Stupor
        (4) Seizures
        (5) Confusion
        (6) Coma
     c. Slowed, hoarse speech
     d. Reflexes
        (1) Trousseau's sign
        (2) Chvostek's sign
  9. Eyes
     a. Periorbital edema
     b. Protruding eyeball (exophthalmos)
     c. Drooping eyelids (ptosis)
  10. Gastrointestinal system
     a. Anorexia
     b. Polyphagia
     c. Polydipsia
     d. Constipation
     e. Diarrhea
     f. Nausea and vomiting
  11. Cardiovascular system
     a. Hypertension
     b. Hypotension
     c. Tachycardia
     d. Bradycardia
  12. Respiratory system
     a. Tachypnea
     b. Acetone breath
     c. Kussmaul-Kien respirations
  13. Renal system
     a. Polyuria
     b. Oliguria
  14. Reproductive system
     a. Menstrual disturbances
     b. Libido disturbances
     c. Galactorrhea (excess mammary gland secretion in females)
     d. Gynecomastia (increased breast tissue in males)
B. Patient description (subjective data)
  1. Pain
     a. Headache
     b. Skeletal pain
     c. Back pain
     d. Muscle spasms
  2. Appetite
     a. Anorexia
     b. Polyphagia
  3. Weakness
  4. Numbness
  5. Tingling
  6. Mood swings
  7. Nausea
  8. Intolerance to heat or cold
  9. Polydipsia
  10. Polyuria, nocturia, and dysuria
  11. Decreased libido and impotence
  12. Frequent infections

Diagnostic Tests/Methods

A. Serum laboratory studies
  1. Protein-bound iodine (PBI)
     a. The thyroid hormone, thyroxine, contains iodine that binds itself to blood proteins; therefore, the function of the thyroid gland is evaluated by measuring the amount of this iodine
     b. Factors that may alter test findings
        (1) Ingestion of drugs or administration of dyes containing iodine
        (2) Mercurial diuretics or estrogen
        (3) Pregnancy
  2. Iodine 131 uptake (radioactive iodine thyroid uptake)
     a. Measures the amount of radioactive iodine that has concentrated in the thyroid gland after ingestion of the iodine preparation
     b. Test findings may be altered by recent ingestion of iodides or use of radiographic dyes
     c. A normal thyroid gland removes 15% to 50% of iodine from the bloodstream
  3. Basal metabolic rate (BMR): measures the amount of oxygen consumed by the body while the patient is in a state of complete mental and physical rest
  4. T_3 (triiodothyronine): measures thyroid function indirectly by evaluating whether radioactive triiodothyronine binds to a serum specimen
  5. T_4 (thyroxine): measures the amount of thyroxine in the circulation
  6. Thyroid-stimulating hormone (TSH) radioimmunoassay: indicator of thyroid-stimulating hormone production based on pituitary function; measures TSH levels

7. Fasting blood sugar (FBS)
   a. Measures the amount of glucose in the bloodstream during a fasting period
   b. No food is permitted for 12 hours before the test
   c. Normal value: 80 to 120 mg/dl
8. Postprandial blood sugar
   a. Evaluates the patient's ability to dispose of blood glucose after a meal
   b. Normal value: 80 to 120 mg/dl serum
9. Glucose tolerance test (GTT)
   a. Determines patient response to a measured dose of glucose
   b. Normal value: blood glucose climbs to a peak of 140 mg/dl serum in the first hour and returns to normal by the second or third hour
10. Serum potassium
    a. Measures the amount of K in the bloodstream
    b. Normal range: 3.5 to 5.0 mEq/L
11. Serum sodium
    a. Measures the amount of Na in the bloodstream
    b. Normal range: 135 to 145 mEq/L
12. Total serum calcium
    a. Measures the amount of Ca in the bloodstream
    b. Normal range: 4.8 to 5.2 mEq/L (9 to 11 mg/dl)
13. Serum ketones: determines the amount of ketones produced by the metabolism of fat
14. Blood pH
    a. Measures the acid-base status of the blood
    b. Normal arterial blood findings: pH 7.35 to 7.45
    c. Normal venous blood findings: pH 7.31 to 7.41
15. Serum phosphorus: measures the amount of serum phosphorus in the bloodstream
16. Adrenocorticotropic hormone (ACTH) stimulating test (or glucocorticoid-stimulating test)
    a. Evaluates the changes in adrenocortical function produced by the administration of ACTH
    b. ACTH is administered intramuscularly (IM) or intravenously (IV)
    c. For the IM methods a blood specimen is obtained 1 hour after the administration of ACTH
    d. For the IV method a 24-hour urine specimen is collected and analyzed
17. Cortisone suppression test: used to differentiate between Cushing's syndrome and Cushing's disease
18. Plasma cortisol
    a. Hormonal study of the adrenal cortex
    b. Low levels are seen in Addison's disease
    c. Elevated levels indicate Cushing's syndrome
19. Plasma cortisol response to ACTH
    a. Hormonal study of the adrenal cortex
    b. Patient's blood specimen is drawn in a fasting state and examined for plasma cortisol levels
    c. Next ACTH is administered IM, and a second blood sample is withdrawn
    d. A rise in the plasma cortisol level in the second specimen is normal
20. Urine 17-ketogenic steroids
    a. Measures adrenocortical function
    b. Urine specimen is collected for a 24-hour period and should be kept cold
B. Urine laboratory studies
   1. Twenty-four–hour quantitative sugar specimen

a. An evaluation of the patient's glucose loss over a 24-hour period
b. Normally the urine is free of sugar
c. Nursing implications
   (1) Have the patient void and discard the specimen at the beginning of the 24-hour period
   (2) Save all urine voided in a container provided by the laboratory
   (3) At the end of the 24 hours, have the patient void again and save the specimen in the container
2. Urine pH
   a. Measures the acid-base balance of the urine
   b. Normal range: pH 4.8 to 7.5
3. Quantitative urinary calcium: measures the amount of Ca in a 24-hour urine specimen after a period of Ca deprivation
4. Vanillylmandelic acid (VMA) test
   a. Determines the amount of urinary excretion of the end product of catecholamine metabolism
   b. Factors that may alter test findings
      (1) Ingestion of coffee, tea, chocolate, bananas, vanilla-containing food, or aspirin
      (2) Stress
C. Scans
   1. Thyroid scan: radionucleotide study of the thyroid to determine function
   2. CT scan: used to visualize cross sections of tissue

Frequent Patient Problems and Nursing Care

A. Self-esteem disturbance related to body image
   1. Observe the patient for loss of appetite, insomnia, disinterest in self, and unwillingness to discuss alteration in body image
   2. Encourage patient to express feelings
   3. Encourage communication with significant other
B. Altered nutrition, less than body requirements, related to noncompliance with therapeutic diet
   1. Observe the patient for diet intolerance such as refusal to eat, complaints of foods, and eating of foods that are contraindicated
   2. Explain to the patient and family the reason for and intended effect of therapeutic diet and necessity of maintaining it until discontinued by physician
   3. Instruct the patient and family on prescribed food selection
C. Knowledge deficit related to prescribed medication
   1. Explain to the patient and family the dosage and method of administering prescribed drugs
   2. Provide information about the purpose of the drug and potential side effects
   3. Describe symptoms that should be reported to the physician
   4. Explain where therapeutic supplies may be obtained
   5. Evaluate the patient's response to teaching
D. High risk for injury related to toxic effects of iodine preparations. Discontinue iodides if evidence of the following exists
   1. Swelling of buccal mucosa
   2. Excessive salivation
   3. Swelling of neck glands
   4. Skin eruptions

E. High risk for injury related to hypoglycemia
1. Observe for complaints of headache, nervousness, hunger, dizziness, pallor, and sweating (diaphoresis)
2. Assess vital signs
3. Give quick-acting carbohydrate
   a. Orange juice
   b. Coca-Cola
   c. Granulated sugar
   d. Crackers
   e. Hard candy
4. If patient is unconscious: give instant glucose (buccally); glucagon (SC); IV glucose
5. Have laboratory withdraw serum specimen for glucose assessment
6. Assess reason for reaction after situation has been controlled
   a. Length of time since last meal
   b. Correct amount of food eaten or meal omitted
   c. Correct dosage of insulin
   d. Kinds of activities or situation before reaction
F. High risk for injury (seizures) related to hypocalcemia
1. Observe for complaints of numbness, tingling, cramping, or spastic movements of extremities
2. Emergency treatment requires administration of IV calcium
3. Prevent airway obstruction
   a. Keep airway (seizure stick) at bedside
   b. Provide suction machine at bedside
   c. Provide tracheostomy set at bedside
4. Prevent injury by putting padding along side rails, easing patient to floor, or removing constrictive clothes
5. Monitor and record vital signs
6. Note frequency, time, level of consciousness, and length of seizure

Major Medical Diagnoses

HYPERPITUITARISM
A. Definition: overproduction of growth hormone by the anterior pituitary gland
B. Pathology
1. Increased activity of the gland usually results from a secreting pituitary tumor
2. Two major disorders arise from hypersecretion
   a. Gigantism: develops in children; hypersecretion before the growth plate closes, results in bone and tissue growth
   b. Acromegaly: a disorder in adults caused by hypersecretion after closure of the epiphyses of the long bones
C. Signs and symptoms
1. Subjective
   a. Headache
   b. Visual disturbances
   c. Weakness
2. Objective
   a. Coarse facial features: enlarged ears, nose, lips, tongue, and jaws
   b. Broad hands, fingers, and feet
   c. Palpable, enlarged visceral organs
   d. Disturbances in carbohydrate metabolism, menstruation, and libido
   e. Gynecomastia in the male; galactorrhea in the female

f. Symmetrical bone overgrowth (gigantism)
g. Increased heights; 8 to 9 ft (gigantism)
D. Diagnostic tests/methods
1. X-ray studies of jaws, sinuses, hands, and feet
2. Changes in physical appearance
3. CT scan to identify tumor
4. Cerebral arteriography to identify tumor
5. Growth hormone assay
E. Treatment
1. Surgical intervention: hypophysectomy (excision of the pituitary gland); excision of tumor with laser
2. Irradiation of the pituitary gland
3. Medication to treat symptoms related to other hormonal disturbances as a result of hypersecretion
F. Nursing intervention
1. Assist the patient to accept altered body image emphasizing person's value as an individual
2. Explain the basis for altered sexual functioning
3. Emphasize need for lifelong medical follow-up
4. If the patient has undergone hypophysectomy
   a. Follow nursing care as for the patient who has undergone intracranial surgery
   b. Observe for potential postoperative complications
      (1) Adrenal insufficiency
      (2) Hypothyroidism
      (3) Diabetes insipidus

HYPOPITUITARISM (SIMMONDS' DISEASE)
A. Definition: total absence of all pituitary secretions
B. Pathology: occurs after destruction of the pituitary gland by surgery, infection, injury, hemorrhage, or tumor
C. Signs and symptoms
1. Subjective
   a. Lethargy
   b. Loss of muscle strength
   c. Weakness
   d. Menstrual irregularities
2. Objective
   a. Emaciation
   b. Pallor
   c. Dry, yellow skin
   d. Diminished axillary and pubic hair
   e. Decreased muscle size
   f. Increased susceptibility to infection
D. Diagnostic tests/methods
1. T_3 and T_4
2. Urine 17-ketogenic steroids
E. Treatment
1. Replacement hormones
2. Surgical ablation if tumor is present in pituitary gland
F. Nursing intervention
1. Emphasize need for lifelong medical follow-up
2. Teach the patient self-administration of drug: purpose, proper dosage, and potential side effects
3. Follow nursing care as for the patient who has undergone intracranial surgery

HYPERTHYROIDISM (GRAVES' DISEASE AND THYROTOXICOSIS)
A. Definition: overactivity of the thyroid gland with hypersecretion of T_4
B. Pathology

1. Metabolic rate is increased, resulting in a high amount of energy and oxygen expenditure
2. May be caused by decreased production of thyroid-stimulating hormone (TSH) by malfunctioning pituitary gland; which results in high T_4 serum concentration
3. May be attributed to enlarged thyroid gland caused by decreased iodine intake
C. Signs and symptoms
   1. Subjective
      a. Polyphagia
      b. Hyperexcitability/personality changes
      c. Heat intolerance
      d. Insomnia
      e. Amenorrhea
      f. Diarrhea/constipation
      g. Increased appetite
      h. Fatigue/weakness
   2. Objective
      a. Weight loss
      b. Exophthalmos
      c. Excessive sweating
      d. Increased pulse rate
      e. Fine hand tremors
      f. Warm, flushed skin
      g. Elevated blood pressure
      h. Bruit over thyroid
D. Diagnostic tests: increased laboratory values of T_3, T_4, ^{131}I uptake, PBI, and BMR confirm hyperthyroidism; thyroid scan
E. Treatment
   1. Medication to inhibit T_4 production
   2. Radioactive iodine to destroy thyroid gland cells to decrease T_4 secretion
   3. Drugs to control tachycardia and hyperexcitability
   4. Subtotal or total thyroidectomy
F. Nursing intervention
   1. Teach the patient and family signs and symptoms of hypothyroidism when patient is receiving thyroid-inhibiting drugs
      a. Increased body weight
      b. Sensitivity to cold
      c. Fatigue
      d. Dry skin, hair, and nails
      e. Slow, hoarse speech
      f. Constipation
   2. Encourage adequate nutrition for increased energy expenditure
      a. High-calorie, high-vitamin, and high-carbohydrate intake
      b. Between-meal snacks
      c. Increased fluid intake
      d. Avoidance of caffeine
   3. Plan undisturbed rest periods to restore energy: provide cool, quiet, nonstressful environment
   4. Advise the patient to elevate the head of bed while recumbent to improve eye drainage
   5. If the patient has undergone surgery
      a. Place patient on back in a low-Fowler's or semi-Fowler's position to avoid strain on sutures
      b. Observe dressing for hemorrhage or constriction of the throat; examine back of neck for pooling of blood

c. Keep tracheostomy set at bedside in event of respiratory obstruction caused by hemorrhage, edema of glottis, laryngeal nerve damage, or tetany
d. Encourage patient to cough and expectorate secretions from throat and bronchi
e. Observe for signs of thyroid storm (may occur as a result of gland manipulation during surgery): fever, tachycardia, and restlessness
f. Observe for signs of tetany (may occur if parathyroids are accidentally removed); numbness and tingling around mouth, carpopedal spasms, convulsions

HYPOTHYROIDISM

A. Definition: absence or decreased production of T_4 by the thyroid gland
B. Pathology
   1. The disorder causes a depression of metabolic activity, resulting in physical and mental sluggishness
   2. There are three classifications of hypothyroidism
      a. Cretinism: total absence of T_4 from birth
      b. Hypothyroidism without myxedema: mild thyroid failure in older children and adults
      c. Hypothyroidism with myxedema: a severe form of gland failure in adults
C. Signs and symptoms
   1. Subjective
      a. Lethargy
      b. Fatigues easily
      c. Cold intolerance
      d. Constipation
   2. Objective
      a. Increased body weight with loss of appetite
      b. Coarse facial features
      c. Slow, hoarse speech
      d. Dry skin, hair, and nails
      e. Bradycardia
      f. Impaired memory
      g. Slowed thought process
      h. Personality changes
D. Diagnostic tests: decreased laboratory values of T_3, T_4, ^{131}I uptake, PBI, and BMR confirm hypothyroidism; thyroid scan
E. Treatment: thyroid-replacement drugs
F. Nursing intervention
   1. Educate the patient on self-administration of drug: purpose, proper dosage, and potential side effects
   2. Emphasize need for lifelong medical follow-up
   3. Teach the patient and family signs and symptoms of hyperthyroidism when receiving thyroid-replacement drugs: chest pain, tachycardia, nervousness, headache, excessive sweating, heat intolerance, and weight loss
   4. Encourage decreased caloric intake to avoid weight gain
   5. Encourage application of emollients to soothe dry skin

HYPERPARATHYROIDISM

A. Definition: oversecretion of parathormone by the parathyroid gland(s)
B. Pathology
   1. Results in calcium loss from the bones and an increased secretion of calcium and phosphorus by the kidneys
   2. Usually the result of a parathyroid tumor

C. Signs and symptoms
  1. Subjective
    a. Fatigue
    b. Thirst; poor appetite
    c. Nausea
    d. Back pain
    e. Skeletal pain
    f. Pain on weight bearing
    g. Constipation
    h. Visual disturbances
  2. Objective
    a. Pathologic features
    b. Vomiting
    c. Kidney stones composed of calcium phosphate
D. Diagnostic tests
  1. Quantitative urinary calcium
  2. Total serum calcium
  3. Serum phosphorus
  4. X-ray film to reveal skeletal changes
E. Treatment: surgical resection of parathyroid gland
F. Nursing intervention
  1. Observe for postoperative conditions (refer to postoperative nursing interventions under diseases of the thyroid gland: hyperthyroidism)
  2. Observe for tetany: tingling of hands and feet, facial muscle spasms, and muscle twitching
  3. Protect from accidents: position carefully, keep bed low, keep side rails up, and assist to ambulate
  4. Explain rationale for low-calcium, low-phosphorus diet
  5. Encourage adequate hydration and dietary fiber to avoid constipation

HYPOPARATHYROIDISM

A. Definition: undersecretion of parathormone by the parathyroid glands
B. Pathology
  1. Insufficiency of parathormone causes a decrease of the serum calcium level and slows bone resorption
  2. Serum phosphorus value rises
  3. Increased neuromuscular irritability results in tetany
C. Signs and symptoms
  1. Subjective
    a. Lethargy
    b. Painful muscle spasms
    c. Tingling of hands and feet
    d. Visual disturbances
  2. Objective
    a. Dry skin, hair, and nails
    b. Respiratory distress caused by laryngeal spasms
    c. Convulsions
D. Diagnostic tests/methods
  1. Quantitative urinary calcium
  2. Total serum calcium
  3. Positive Trousseau's sign (spasms of fingers and hands after application of blood pressure cuff to arm)
  4. Presence of Chvostek's sign (hyperactivity of facial muscle in response to tapping near the angle of the jaw)
  5. X-ray studies reveal increased bone density
E. Treatment
  1. Calcium replacement in chronic cases
  2. Calcium gluconate IV for emergency treatment
  3. Diet high in calcium and low in phosphorus

  4. Vitamin D preparation
F. Nursing intervention
  1. Keep endotracheal tube and tracheostomy set at bedside at all times when caring for patients with acute tetany
  2. Promote rest with a quiet, calm, and low-lit environment
  3. Explain need for diet high in calcium but low in phosphorus: avoid milk, cheese, and egg yolks
  4. Emphasize importance of lifelong medical follow-up; serum calcium level should be assessed at least three times a year

DIABETES MELLITUS

A. Definition: insufficiency or absence of insulin production by pancreatic islets, creating a disturbance in carbohydrate metabolism as well as a deficiency in protein and fat conversion
B. Pathology
  1. Develops when there is a persistent deficiency of insulin
  2. May be caused by trauma, infection, or tumor of the pancreas or increased insulin requirements attributable to obesity, pregnancy, infection, or stress
  3. Those at risk: women over 40 years of age and individuals who are obese or who have a familial tendency to diabetes
  4. Two classifications
    a. Type I: insulin dependent diabetes mellitus (IDDM) (formerly juvenile diabetes): rapid onset with no production of insulin; affects children and adolescents; is controlled with insulin
    b. Type II: noninsulin-dependent diabetes mellitus (NIDDM) (formerly adult onset): gradual onset; may be controlled by diet, oral hypoglycemic drugs, or insulin injection
  5. Lack of insulin disrupts transportation of glucose into cells, and cells become energy exhausted; cells must use proteins and fats as a compensatory mechanism
  6. Blood sugar level becomes elevated because of lack of insulin in the cells
  7. Cellular dehydration occurs because blood sugar pulls water from the cells into the bloodstream
  8. Glucose builds up in urine, creating osmotic pull; kidneys cannot reabsorb water
C. Signs and symptoms
  1. Subjective
    a. Polyuria and nocturia
    b. Polydipsia
    c. Polyphasia
    d. Weakness
    e. Blurred vision
  2. Objective
    a. Hyperglycemia
    b. Glycosuria
    c. Polyuria
    d. Ketosis
    e. Weight loss
    f. Retarded wound healing
D. Diagnostic tests/methods
  1. Presence of polyuria, polydipsia, and polyphagia
  2. Family and medical history
  3. Laboratory studies: FBS, postprandial blood sugar, GTT, and glycosylated hemoglobin
  4. Twenty-four hour urine quantitative sugar specimen

E. Treatment
   1. Drug therapy for hyperglycemia; refer to Chapter 3, Pharmacology, for indicated nursing actions
   2. Therapeutic diet with controlled calories to correct and avoid obesity
      a. American Diabetes Association (ADA) food exchange list widely prescribed by physicians (see Appendix G)
      b. Identifies calorie intake of protein (15% to 20%), carbohydrates (50% to 60%), fats (no more than 30%)
F. Nursing intervention
   1. Assist patient in adjusting to condition: allow verbalization of feelings, offer reassurance, and give support at patient's own pace
   2. Emphasize need to comply with diet and eat meals at prescribed times
   3. Instruct the patient and family on signs of impending hypoglycemia: diaphoresis, pale, cold, and clammy skin, nervousness, hunger, mental confusion; give orange juice, sugar, or hard candy
   4. Encourage prompt treatment of minor injuries or irritation to skin
   5. Emphasize importance of continued medical follow-up, regular vision examinations, and foot care
   6. Patient teaching should include
      a. Self-blood glucose level monitoring
      b. Self-injection of insulin: selection of equipment, sites of injection, rationale for rotation, accurate withdrawal of insulin, injection technique, and peak action time of insulin
      c. How to use food substitution
      d. Instructions on foot care: hygiene, proper trimming of toenails, proper fit of shoes and stockings, and treatment of minor abrasions
      e. Relationship between exercise and blood glucose
   7. Instruction to patient and family on signs and symptoms of impending ketoacidosis: hot, dry, flushed skin, polydipsia, fruity odor of breath, nausea, and abdominal pain
   8. Administration of insulin by way of pump
      a. Method of needle insertion and filling of syringe
      b. Instruction on site rotation and needle change q48h
      c. Remove pump and cover needle and tubing for bathing

DIABETIC COMA (KETOACIDOSIS)

A. Definition: excess glucose and acid (ketones) in the bloodstream
B. Pathology
   1. A response to insufficient insulin levels
   2. Fats are mobilized for energy; fatty acids are rejected by muscles, resulting in buildup of acids in the bloodstream
   3. Body's buffer system becomes exhausted
C. Signs and symptoms
   1. Subjective
      a. Weakness
      b. Polydipsia
      c. Abdominal pain
      d. Nausea
      e. Headache
      f. Polyphagia
   2. Objective
      a. Hot, dry, flushed skin

   b. Listlessness and drowsiness
   c. Kussmaul's respirations
   d. Sweet or acetone breath
   e. Hypotension
   f. Confusion
   g. Polyuria
   h. Nausea/vomiting
   i. Coma
D. Diagnostic tests
   1. Elevated serum glucose level
   2. Elevated serum and urinary ketones
   3. Lowered blood pH
E. Treatment
   1. Insulin replacement
   2. Correct electrolyte and pH imbalance
   3. Fluid replacement
F. Nursing intervention
   1. Give insulin as ordered; have another person check to prevent error
   2. Monitor and record vital signs and intake and output
   3. Test for glucose and acetone levels; record on diabetic flow sheet
   4. Position patient with head of bed elevated 30 degrees
   5. Maintain patent airway
   6. Give oral care q4h and when required (prn); keep lips and mouth moist
   7. Assess level of consciousness
   8. Observe patient for signs of hypoglycemia: pale, cool, clammy skin, lethargy, and hypotension
   9. Instruct patient and family on factors and signs of impending ketoacidosis
   10. Explain importance of balance among diet, exercise, and insulin
   11. Before discharge provide diabetic alert band or chain

HYPERGLYCEMIC HYPEROSMOLAR NONKETOTIC COMA (HHNC)

A. Definition: similar to ketoacidosis, but occurs in noninsulin-dependent diabetes (NIDDM); ketosis does not develop
B. Pathology: high serum glucose levels increase osmotic pressure; this leads to polyuria, and dehydration occurs at the cellular level
C. Signs and symptoms
   1. Subjective
      a. Polyuria
      b. Polydipsia
      c. Drowsiness
      d. Confusion
   2. Objective
      a. Dry, hot skin
      b. Flushed skin
      c. Hyperglycemia
      d. Glycosuria
      e. Hypotension
D. Diagnostic tests (see Ketoacidosis)
E. Treatment (see Ketoacidosis)
F. Nursing intervention (see Ketoacidosis)

HYPOGLYCEMIA (INSULIN SHOCK)

A. Definition: abnormally low level of glucose in the bloodstream
B. Pathology

1. Accelerated glucose is removed from the serum
2. May be caused by overproduction or overdosage of insulin
3. Omission of a meal or too little food eaten by a patient receiving insulin
4. Too much exercise without extra food; rapid onset
C. Signs and symptoms
   1. Subjective
      a. Hunger
      b. Weakness
      c. Visual disturbances
      d. Tingling lips and tongue
      e. Nervousness
   2. Objective
      a. Pale, moist skin
      b. Tremors
      c. Tachycardia
      d. Hypotension
      e. Muscle weakness
      f. Disorientation
      g. Coma
D. Diagnostic test: lowered serum glucose level
E. Treatment
   1. Sweetened fluids or sugar given orally; oral glucose preparations
   2. Glucagon subcutaneously or IM
   3. Glucose IV
F. Nursing intervention
   1. Give medications as ordered
   2. Monitor and record vital signs and intake and output
   3. Patient teaching should include
      a. Always carry and ingest quick-acting carbohydrate when initial signs appear; fruit juices, sweetened sodas, granulated sugar, or hard candy
      b. Prevent medication error by having another person check dosage
      c. Record each administration of medication to avoid duplication
      d. Always wear medical identification tag
      e. Remember to eat a regular meal after raising glucose level to prevent a rebound effect

DIABETES INSIPIDUS

A. Definition: water metabolism disorder related to hyposecretion of antidiuretic hormone (ADH) by the posterior pituitary lobe
B. Pathology
   1. Renal tubules are unable to reabsorb water, resulting in elimination of large amounts of water
   2. Hyposecretion may occur in conjunction with lung cancer, head injuries, pituitary tumor, myxedema, or encephalitis
   3. Other causes may result from malfunctioning, surgical removal, or atrophy of the pituitary gland
C. Signs and symptoms
   1. Subjective
      a. Polydipsia
      b. Polyuria
   2. Objective
      a. Signs of dehydration (loss of skin turgor, dry skin and mucous membranes, and cracked lips)
      b. Low specific gravity (sp gr) (1.001 to 1.006)

c. Increased fluid intake (5 to 40 L/24 hr)
d. Increased urine output (5 to 25 L/24 hr)
e. Electrolyte imbalance
D. Diagnostic method: restriction of fluid intake to observe changes in urine volume and concentration
E. Treatment: vasopressin replacement
F. Nursing intervention
   1. Monitor and record intake and output
   2. Monitor specific gravity
   3. Weigh patient daily

PRIMARY HYPERALDOSTERONISM (CONN'S SYNDROME)

A. Definition: hypersecretion of aldosterone by the adrenal cortex
B. Pathology
   1. Usually caused by a tumor(s), which results in renal retention of sodium and excretion of potassium
   2. Leads to inability of kidneys to concentrate urine (acidify)
C. Signs and symptoms
   1. Subjective
      a. Headache
      b. Polyuria and polydipsia
      c. Paresthesia
   2. Objective
      a. Hypertension with postural hypotension
      b. Signs of kidney damage: flank pain, chills, fever, and increased frequency of voiding
      c. Low specific gravity
D. Diagnostic tests
   1. Low serum potassium level
   2. Elevated serum sodium value
   3. Elevated urinary aldosterone level
   4. Increased urine pH
   5. X-ray study reveals cardiac hypertrophy caused by chronic hypertension
E. Treatment: surgical removal of adrenal tumor
F. Nursing intervention
   1. Monitor and record blood pressure, specific gravity, and intake and output
   2. Identify and explain diet high in potassium and low in sodium
   3. Provide fluids to meet excessive thirst
   4. If the patient has undergone adrenalectomy
      a. Protect the patient from exposure to infections
      b. Follow general postoperative nursing actions
   5. Once patient is convalescent, teach the patient self-administration of drugs: purpose, proper dosage, and potential side effects
   6. Before discharge obtain medical identification tag

CUSHING'S SYNDROME

A. Definition: hyperactivity of the adrenal cortex
B. Pathology
   1. Excessive cortisol is secreted
   2. Disorder results from abnormal growth of cortices or tumor to one of the glands
   3. May occur because of pituitary gland dysfunction, causing excessive production of adrenocorticotropic hormone (ACTH)
C. Signs and symptoms
   1. Subjective
      a. Weakness

b. Bruises easily
c. Amenorrhea
d. Decreased libido
e. Changes in secondary sex characteristics
2. Objective
a. Fat deposits to face, back of neck, and abdomen
b. Decreased muscle mass on limbs
c. Unusual growth of body hair
d. Purple striae over obese areas
e. Impaired wound healing
f. Hypertension
g. Mood lability
D. Diagnostic tests
1. Increased plasma cortisol levels
2. ACTH stimulating test
3. Cortisone suppression test
E. Treatment
1. Drugs to inhibit cortisol production
2. Bilateral adrenalectomy
3. Resection of pituitary gland
4. Potassium supplements
5. Diet with sodium restriction
F. Nursing intervention
1. Assist patient in adjusting to altered body image
2. Place in noninfectious environment
3. Maintain diet low in calories, carbohydrates, and sodium and high in potassium
4. Weigh patient daily
5. Monitor glucose and acetone levels
6. Follow general postoperative nursing actions if patient undergoes adrenalectomy
7. Once the patient is convalescent, instruct on self-administration of replacement hormones and drugs: proper dosage, purpose, and potential side effects

ADDISON'S DISEASE
A. Definition: hypofunction of adrenal cortex
B. Pathology
1. As a result of dysfunction, adrenal cortex shrinks and atrophies
2. Disorder usually originates within itself or may result from destruction of the adrenal cortex
3. Results in disturbances of sodium and potassium
C. Signs and symptoms
1. Subjective
a. Weakness and fatigue
b. Anorexia and nausea
c. Depression
d. Diarrhea
e. Abdominal pain
2. Objective
a. Weight loss
b. Hypotension
c. Hypoglycemia
d. Bronze or tan skin pigmentation
e. Susceptibility to infection
f. Dysrhythmias
D. Diagnostic tests
1. Eight-hour IV ACTH test
2. Plasma cortisol response to ACTH
3. Low serum sodium level
4. High serum potassium level

E. Treatment
1. Replacement of adrenal cortex hormones
2. Restoration of sodium and potassium balance
3. Diet high in sodium and low in potassium, with adequate fluids
F. Nursing intervention
1. Monitor and record vital signs and intake and output
2. Weigh patient daily
3. Observe for sodium imbalance: increased body weight, pitting edema, puffy eyelids, coughing, and diaphoresis
4. Observe for potassium imbalance: lethargy, flaccid muscles, anorexia, hypotension, and dysrhythmias
5. Provide small, frequent feedings
6. Observe for hypoglycemia: weakness, clammy skin, tremors, and mental confusion
7. Before discharge obtain medical identification tag
8. Emphasize need for compliance to diet and medication regimen
9. Observe for addisonian crisis (causes: stress, surgery, trauma, infection, withdrawal of medication): hypotension, asthenia, abdominal pain, confusion, shock, and vascular collapse
10. Teach patient to avoid infections and stressful situations

PHEOCHROMOCYTOMA
A. Definition: hyperactivity of the adrenal medulla
B. Pathology: caused by tumor in adrenal medulla, resulting in increased secretion of epinephrine and norepinephrine
C. Signs and symptoms
1. Subjective
a. Headache
b. Visual disturbances
c. Nervousness
d. Heat intolerance
2. Objective
a. Hypertension (blood pressure may be as high as 220/140)
b. Orthostatic hypotension
c. Tachycardia
d. Hyperglycemia
e. Blanching of skin
f. Weight loss
g. Dysrhythmias
h. Diaphoresis
D. Diagnostic tests
1. Chemical and pharmacologic drug tests to differentiate from hypertension or hyperthyroidism
2. X-ray studies to reveal adrenal medullary tumor
3. Twenty-four hour urine collection for vanillylmandelic acid (VMA) and metanephrines
4. Arteriography
5. CT scan
6. Intravenous pyelogram
E. Treatment
1. Surgical excision of tumor
2. Drugs to control hypertension and dysrhythmias
F. Nursing intervention
1. Monitor blood pressure q4h and record
2. Plan undisturbed rest periods: cool, quiet, nonstressful environment
3. Encourage adequate hydration: record intake and output

4. If patient undergoes adrenalectomy, follow general postoperative nursing actions: observe for adrenal crisis—falling blood pressure, tachycardia, elevated temperature, restlessness, convulsions, and coma
5. Patient teaching should include
   a. Self-administration of medications: purpose, proper dosage, and potential side effects
   b. Signs of impending adrenal crisis
   c. Avoidance of exposure to infection; report symptoms of infections to physician
   d. Avoidance of stressful situations
   e. Emphasize need for adequate rest and good nutrition
6. Provide medical identification tag

THE RENAL (URINARY) SYSTEM
Anatomy and Physiology
A. Organs (Figs. 5-15 and 5-16)
  1. Kidneys: bean shaped and reddish brown lie against posterior abdominal wall; right kidney is slightly lower than the left
    a. External structure
      (1) Hilus: concave notch; blood vessels, nerves, lymphatic vessels, and ureters enter the kidneys at this point
      (2) Renal capsule; protective fibrous tissue surrounding kidneys
    b. Internal structure
      (1) Cortex: outer portion; the greater portion of the nephron is located here
      (2) Medulla: inner portion; consists of 12 cone-shaped structures (pyramids); tip of pyramid points toward renal pelvis and drains waste and excess water into pelvis
      (3) Pelvis: funnel shaped; forms upper end of ureter and receives waste and water
    c. Nephron: basic unit of function; microscopic structure composed of capillaries; approximately 1 million per kidney; control the processes of filtration, reabsorption, and secretion (Fig. 5-17)
      (1) Glomerulus: filtering unit; process of urine formation begins
      (2) Renal tubules: reabsorption occurs in the proximal convoluted tubules, through Henle's loops, and the distal convoluted tubules; then the collecting tubules pass the final urine product into the pelvis
  2. Ureters: two long, narrow tubes; transport urine from kidney to bladder by peristalsis
  3. Bladder: elastic, muscular organ, capable of expansion; stores urine; assists in voiding (micturition: the release of urine or voiding)
  4. Urethra: narrow, short tube from bladder to exterior; exterior opening called the meatus

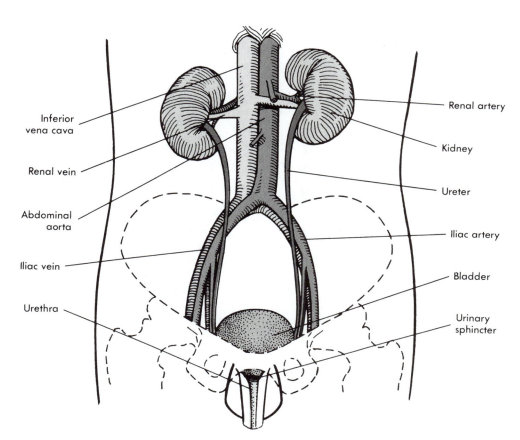

Figure 5-15. **Organs and other structures of urinary system.** (From Phipps et al: *Medical-surgical nursing: concepts and clinical practice*, ed 5, St Louis, 1995, Mosby.)

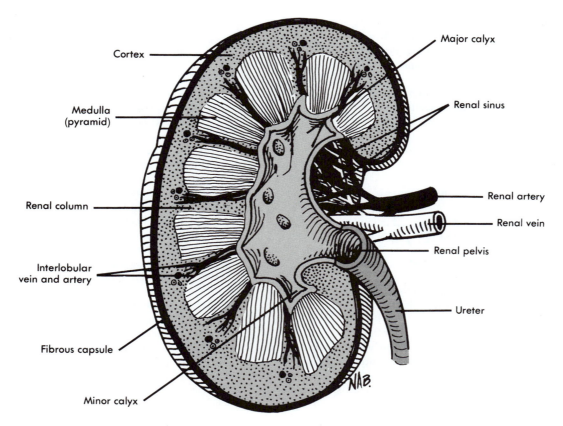

Figure 5-16.   Frontal section of kidney. (From Phipps et al: *Medical-surgical nursing: concepts and clinical practice,* ed 5, St Louis, 1995, Mosby.)

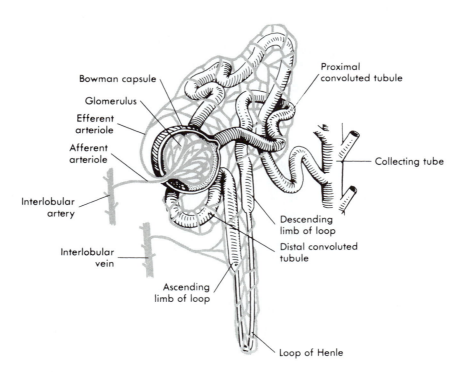

Figure 5-17.   Nephron. (From Phipps et al: *Medical-surgical nursing: concepts and clinical practice,* ed 5, St Louis, 1995, Mosby.)

a. Female: approximately 1¼ to 2 inches (3 to 5 cm) long; transports urine

b. Male: approximately 8 inches (20 cm) long; transports urine and is a passageway for semen

B. Functions

1. Excretion: nitrogen-containing waste (urea, uric acid, and creatinine) is excreted; normal daily output is 1200 to 1500 ml

2. Maintenance of water balance: absorbs more or less water depending on intake; normally, intake is approximately equal to output

3. Regulates acid balance; reabsorbs or actively secretes excess acids and bases produced by cell metabolism

C. Urine composition

1. Clear, yellowish, slightly aromatic, and slightly acid

2. Contains 95% water and 5% solids, which includes urea, uric acid, creatinine, ammonia, sodium, and potassium; specific gravity (sp gr) indicates amount of the dissolved solids; normal range: 1.05 to 1.03 sp gr

3. Abnormal substances: glucose, blood protein, RBC, bile, and bacteria

Conditions of the Renal (Urinary) System

The urinary system regulates the composition and volume of the blood. It excretes metabolic wastes and fluids and maintains fluid and electrolyte balance and acid-base balance. Malfunction of this system has generalized effects on the body's normal physiology. Frequently patients are older and have chronic medical problems (e.g., cardiac); these must be considered when nursing care is planned (e.g., many diagnoses and procedures require additional fluids as a natural irrigation; increased fluids might be contraindicated in the patient with a cardiac condition). Problems of the male reproductive system are discussed in this section.

The following terms are used to describe urine output:

anuria   absence of urine output

bacteriuria   bacteria in the urine

dribbling   voiding without stream, in small amounts, frequently or constantly

dysuria   painful or difficult urination

enuresis   involuntary voiding while asleep

frequency   voiding often and in small amounts

hematuria   blood in the urine

hesitancy   cannot immediately empty full bladder when the desire is present

incontinence   partial or complete inability to control urine output

micturition   voiding, urination

nocturia   awakening to void

overflow incontinence   leakage of urine in small amounts while bladder remains full and distended

polyuria   excessive production and excretion of urine

residual urine   urine remaining in the bladder after voiding

retention   inability to excrete urine from bladder

urgency   an intense stimulus to void (may cause incontinence)

voiding   micturition, elimination of urine

Nursing Assessment

A. Nursing observations

1. Observe bladder for distention: lower abdominal area will be rigid, tense, swollen, and sensitive to the touch

2. Assess urine: amount, color, odor, opacity (clear or cloudy), presence of sediment, mucus, or clots

3. Check catheter (if indwelling) for drainage and meatus for irritation or secretions

4. Check genitals (scrotum, labia, and anal area) for irritation, rashes, and lesions

5. Monitor fluid and electrolyte balance

6. Check eyes, extremities, presacral area, and scrotum for edema

7. Monitor vital signs: note elevation of temperature and blood pressure

8. Note problems related to aging (i.e., urgency, stress incontinence)

B. Patient description (subjective data)

1. Change in voiding habits

2. Problems with elimination

3. Urethral discharge

4. Burning on voiding

5. Pain: suprapubic or flank

C. Obtain patient history regarding

1. Normal urinary and bowel elimination habits

2. Medical problems with the urinary system (e.g., stones or sexually transmitted diseases [STDs])

3. Medical problems with other body systems (i.e., cardiac); trauma

4. Medications

5. Diet

6. Food or medication allergies

7. Decreased urinary stream

8. Pain or spasms: what precipitated this and what relieved it

9. Discharge

10. Edema

Diagnostic Tests/Methods

A. Blood studies

1. Blood urea nitrogen (BUN): normal level 10 to 20 mg/dl; urea is an end product of protein metabolism and is excreted by the kidneys in urine; an increase indicates impaired renal function

2. Creatinine: normal level 0.5-1.3 mg/dl; elevation indicates decreased renal function

3. Acid and alkaline phosphatase: normal value varies with laboratory; increase may indicate metastasis to bone or liver from the kidney; nurse must assess for bone fracture or liver pathology

4. Albumin: globulin ratio is usually 2:1; a change indicates damage to nephron and loss of albumin in the urine; patient retains fluid and has edema

B. Urine studies

1. Routine urine: a single voided specimen to observe and compare to known normal specimens; results give information about renal function and systemic health

2. Specific gravity (sp gr): normal value 1.010 to 1.030; change indicates dehydration or inadequate kidney function; a single voided specimen is required

3. Urine culture and sensitivity (see Chapter 2)

4. Phenolsulfonphthalein test (PSP): after an IV injection of PSP dye, urine specimens are collected to measure amounts excreted; delay in excretion indicates renal disease; nurse collects specimens as directed by laboratory

5. Creatine: 24-hour urine collection to measure creatinine excreted; oral fluids are encouraged (see Chapter 2: Collecting a 24-hour specimen, p. 19)

C. X-ray procedures
   1. Kidneys, ureter, bladder (KUB): an abdominal x-ray study that gives baseline information about size, shape, and placement of organs; flatus and stones are visualized; no preparation or care after procedure is required
   2. Intravenous pyelogram (IVP): an IV injection of a radiopaque dye that is rapidly excreted by the kidney; this tests renal function, and the x-ray films outline renal pelvis, ureters, bladder, and urethra; nursing responsibilities: keep NPO before procedure; after procedure observe for allergic reaction to dye; note voiding
   3. Retrograde pyelogram: visualization of upper genitourinary (GU) tract by injecting radiopaque dye through ureteral catheters to locate obstruction (e.g., stone or tumor); nursing implications: preparation is the same as for preoperative preparation (see Chapter 2); after procedure monitor vital signs, anticipate pain, and administer analgesics, note voiding, and observe urine
   4. Cystoscopy: a direct visualization of the bladder and urethral orifices; a cystoscope is inserted through the urethra into the bladder; the bladder is distended with sterile solution; stones, tumors, and polyps can be diagnosed; urine can be observed entering the bladder from each ureter to evaluate renal function; instruments may be passed through the cystoscope to crush stones, take biopsy specimens, or pass catheters into ureters; nursing responsibilities: provide general preoperative and postoperative care (see Chapter 2); after procedure determine what was done during procedure; assess urinary function; observe urine; provide care and observation of a patient with indwelling catheter (see Chapter 2)

Frequent Patient Problems and Nursing Care

A. Incontinence (types: urge, total, stress, reflex, and functional) related to catheter use, infection, tissue damage, immobility
   1. Minimize embarrassment; provide privacy
   2. Wash, dry, and inspect skin and take measures to prevent decubitus ulcers (pressure sores)
   3. Provide bladder training

B. Impaired skin integrity related to retention of metabolic wastes and resulting toxicity (uremia)
   1. Urea is excreted through the skin, causing odor and pruritus: provide frequent and thorough skin care; wash and pat dry
   2. Confusion and disorientation; may progress to state of unconsciousness and coma; provide all care; maintain safety (see earlier discussion of comas under The Neurologic System)
   3. Nausea and vomiting: provide mouth care q2h
   4. Renal failure: see Nursing care for patient with chronic renal failure, p. 227

C. Pain related to bladder spasms: bladder spasms caused by catheter irritation are intermittent in the suprapubic area, radiating to the urethra
   1. Assess type, location, and severity of pain
   2. Check catheter for obstruction; irrigate as ordered

3. Administer medication as ordered (Antispasmodics, see Chapter 3)
4. Reassure patient that spasms are not abnormal

D. Fluid volume deficit related to dehydration
   1. Use hydration methods (encourage fluids)
   2. Monitor intake and output

E. Risk for infection/injury (hematuria) related to surgery and/or pathogens
   1. Monitor signs and symptoms; vital signs
   2. Administer medication as ordered
   3. Note characteristics or urine at each voiding
   4. Encourage fluids if not contraindicated
   5. Report and document clots noted in urine
   6. Maintain patency and gravity drainage of catheters
   7. Assess for signs of anemia (weakness and fatigue)
   8. Provide nursing care and safety as indicated
   9. Reassure patient that blood-tinged urine is not unusual after instrumentation or surgery

F. Urinary retention related to surgery
   1. Take nursing measures to assist patient with voiding (see Chapter 2)
   2. Monitor intake and output
   3. Encourage fluids if not contraindicated

G. Anxiety related to sexual dysfunction, impending surgery, and/or possible change in body image and/or function
   1. Provide time to listen to patient express feelings
   2. Explain all care and procedures; reassure often
   3. Be honest; provide privacy; avoid embarrassing situations
   4. Praise patient's progress toward discharge goals

H. Potential fluid excess
   1. Assess deep skin (i.e., sacral, feet)
   2. Monitor lung sounds

Major Medical Diagnoses

CYSTITIS
A. Definition: inflammation of the bladder mucosa; is difficult to cure; recurs and may be chronic
B. Pathology: is usually a bacterial infection
   1. May be secondary to infection elsewhere in urinary system (e.g., urethritis)
   2. Contamination during catheterization or instrumentation
   3. An obstruction causing urinary stasis in the bladder (e.g., enlarged prostate or urethral stricture)
C. Signs and symptoms
   1. Burning, dysuria, urgency, frequency, nocturia, hematuria, and pyuria
   2. Low-back pain and bladder spasms
   3. Elevation of temperature
D. Diagnostic tests/methods
   1. Patient history and assessment
   2. Urine culture, IVP, voiding cystoureterogram
E. Treatment: systemic medications, urinary antiseptics, antibiotics, sulfonamides, and antispasmodics (see Chapter 3)
F. Nursing intervention
   1. Encourage fluids: 3000 ml daily over that of dietary intake unless contraindicated
   2. Provide and supervise proper perineal care
   3. Provide diet that acidifies urine (e.g., cranberry juice)
   4. Monitor temperature and administer antipyretics as ordered
   5. Provide sitz baths
   6. Teach preventive measures (i.e., compliance with treatment, follow-up care)

URETHRITIS

A. Definition: inflammation of the urethra; may develop scar tissue and stricture, causing obstruction, cystitis, and nephritis
B. Pathology
  1. Prostatitis; injury during instrumentation or catheterization
  2. Gonococcus infection; chlamydial infection
C. Signs and symptoms
  1. Urgency
  2. Frequency
  3. Dysuria
  4. Burning on urination
  5. Purulent discharge
D. Diagnostic tests/methods
  1. Patient history and physical examination
  2. Culture of discharge
E. Treatment
  1. Antibiotics
  2. Dilatation for stricture
F. Nursing intervention
  1. Sitz baths
  2. Isolation as indicated
  3. Demonstrate and supervise thorough hand washing
  4. Care of Foley catheter

PYELONEPHRITIS

A. Definition: infection of the kidney; may be acute or become chronic; kidney becomes edematous, mucosa is inflamed, and multiple abscesses may form; the kidney will become fibrotic, and uremia may develop
B. Pathology
  1. Ascending infection from an infection lower in the GU tract
  2. Staphylococcal or streptococcal infection carried in the blood
C. Signs and symptoms
  1. Markedly elevated temperature (102° to 105° F); shaking, chills
  2. Nausea and vomiting
  3. Dysuria, burning, frequency, pyuria, and hematuria
  4. Flank pain and tenderness in kidney
  5. Increased WBC count
D. Diagnostic tests/methods
  1. Urine culture and sensitivity
  2. Patient history and physical examination
  3. IVP
E. Treatment: urinary antiseptics and specific antibiotics (see Chapter 3); follow-up care for at least 1 year
F. Nursing intervention
  1. Prevent dehydration: encourage fluids and maintain IV therapy
  2. Provide rest and conserve energy
  3. Prevent chill; keep skin dry and clean
  4. Provide mouth care q2h
  5. Provide soft diet
  6. Provide and assist with pericare; demonstrate proper technique and hand washing
  7. Anticipate pain: administer analgesics and local heat
  8. Administer antiemetic as needed
  9. Control temperature: administer antipyretics and sponge baths as ordered

CALCULI (LITHIASIS)

A. Definition: formation of stones in the urinary tract caused by deposits of crystalline substance that normally remain in solution and are excreted in the urine; may be found in the kidney, ureters, or bladder; vary in size from renal calculi that can be as large as an orange or as small as grains of sand; can obstruct urine flow, causing chronic infection, backflow, hydronephrosis, and gradual destruction of kidney; many small stones pass spontaneously
B. Cause
  1. Infection
  2. Urinary stasis
  3. Dehydration and concentration of urine
  4. Metabolic diseases (e.g., gout, hyperparathyroidism)
  5. Immobility (see Dangers of immobility, Chapter 2)
  6. Familial tendency
  7. Elevated uric acid
  8. Excessive calcium intake
C. Signs and symptoms
  1. Pain (can be extreme) radiates down flank to pubic area
  2. Frequency and urgency
  3. Hematuria and pyuria
  4. Diaphoresis, nausea, vomiting, and pallor (related to pain)
D. Diagnostic tests/methods: x-ray studies—KUB, IVP; urine studies—ultrasonography, cystoscopy, serial blood calcium and phosphorus levels
E. Treatment: depends on location—stones are removed; normal urine production and elimination are restored; recurrence is prevented
  1. Cystoscopy and crushing of stones (lithotripsy)
  2. Dislodging ureteral stone by passing ureteral catheter; laser lithotripsy
  3. Surgery to remove ureteral or kidney stone
    a. Pyelolithotomy: removal of stones from renal pelvis
    b. Nephrolithotomy: incision through kidney and removal of stone
    c. Ureterolithotomy: removal of ureteral calculus
    d. Transcutaneous shock wave lithotripsy: ultrasonic waves used to disintegrate renal calculi
F. Nursing intervention
  1. Provide general preoperative and postoperative nursing care (see Chapter 2)
  2. Supervise and explain diet restrictions as ordered according to type of stone
  3. Provide analgesics as ordered
  4. Observe, describe, and strain all urine
  5. Maintain gravity drainage: never clamp ureteral or nephrostomy catheters
  6. Observe patency of catheters: usually never irrigate renal or ureteral catheters
  7. Record output from each catheter separately; immediately report scanty output from one tube
  8. Encourage fluids (but keep NPO if there is nausea, vomiting, or abdominal distention)
  9. Strain urine

HYDRONEPHROSIS

A. Definition: an accumulation of fluid in the renal pelvis; there is distention of the renal tubules, calyces, and pelvis; renal tissues are destroyed from pressure; leads to uremia (azotemia)

B. Pathology
   1. Congenital defective drainage; blockage from stones or scar tisues
   2. Reflux (backup) from obstructed bladder neck in benign prostatic hypertrophy
C. Signs and symptoms
   1. Related to cause
   2. Infection
   3. Flank tenderness and pain
D. Diagnostic tests/methods
   1. Patient history and physical examination
   2. Blood serum tests (urea/creatinine)
   3. IVP, ultrasonography
E. Treatment
   1. Remove cause
   2. Provide for adequate urinary drainage (e.g., bladder catheter or nephrostomy tube)
   3. Antibiotics
F. Nursing intervention
   1. Provide rest
   2. Provide medication and care as needed for symptoms (e.g., elevation of temperature or pain)
   3. Assess for and provide care as indicated for patient with uremia

BLADDER TUMORS

A. Definition: benign or malignant lesions that ulcerate into the mucous membrane; bladder capacity is decreased; benign tumors tend to recur and become malignant
B. Pathology
   1. Related to cigarette smoking and exposure to dyes (environmental-nitrates, benzene, rubber, petroleum)
   2. Chronic bladder irritation (e.g., stones or infection)
   3. Related to aging
C. Signs and symptoms
   1. Painless, gross hematuria
   2. Anemia
   3. Signs of bladder infection: dysuria, frequency, urgency, and chills
D. Diagnostic tests/methods
   1. Patient history and physical examination
   2. X-ray studies: IVP, KUB, and retrograde pyelogram
   3. Cystoscopy and biopsy examination
   4. Renoscan, ultrasonography, CT, MRI
E. Treatment
   1. Removal of the tumor through cystoscopy if benign
   2. Surgery
      a. Partial cystectomy
      b. Cystectomy: total removal of the bladder and provision for urinary diversion
      c. Radiation, intravesicular, external
      d. Chemotherapy, intravesicular
      e. Fulguration (coagulation)
      f. Experimental therapy (photodynamic therapy—use of photosensitivity agent and laser destruction of tumor cells)
      g. Interferon (Roferon-A)
F. Nursing intervention: give according to method of treatment (see specific sections)
   1. Be supportive of patient concerns expressed
   2. General pre- and postoperative care (see Chapter 2)

URINARY DIVERSION

A. Definition: surgical intervention to allow for urinary elimination; the bladder is removed; the procedure is permanent
   1. Ileal conduit (ileal passageway): a small segment of ilium is separated from the intestine and the distal end is brought out of the abdomen to form a stoma; the ureters are implanted into this ileal pouch; urine flows continuously from the renal pelvis through the ureters into the ileal pouch and into a collecting bag
   2. Ureterointestinal implant: the ureters are anastomosed into the sigmoid colon or rectum; urine is mixed with feces, and evacuation is controlled from the anal sphincter
   3. Cutaneous ureterostomies: the ureters are implanted on the abdomen, forming one or two stomas that drain urine continuously into drainage bags
   4. Continent ileal urinary reservoir (Koch pouch): the ureters are anastomosed to an isolated segment of ileum, which has a one-way valve; urine is drained by periodic insertion of a catheter
   5. Nephrostomy (may be long-term): tubes are inserted in the pelvis of each kidney, brought through the skin, and connected to a closed drainage system
B. Indication: cancer of the bladder
C. Patient problems (depends on procedure)
   1. Susceptibility to infection
   2. Anxiety or depression about diagnosis and change in body image
   3. Inability to control elimination
   4. Embarrassment
   5. Odor if urine leaks onto skin; risk for impaired skin integrity
D. Nursing intervention (varies with procedures)
   1. Provide general preoperative and postoperative care (see Chapter 2)
   2. Provide time to listen to patient fears and anxieties
   3. Assess fluid and electrolyte imbalance
   4. Maintain integrity of the skin: clean, inspect, and change drainage bag as needed
   5. Monitor temperature
   6. Monitor urine output from each catheter/tube; maintain separate output records for each; if nephrostomy tubes-contact physician if tube fails to drain urine, if urine is grossly bloody, or if patient complains of sudden severe flank pain
   7. Stoma care (see Ileostomy, colostomy); may need to have stoma dilated in postoperative period
   8. Monitor fluid and electrolyte balance
   9. Prevent infection: maintain asepsis; encourage fluids; patient must know when to seek medical attention for pain or elevation of temperature
   10. Do not give patient laxatives or enemas (rectal implant)
   11. Arrange a visit from a person who has undergone a similar procedure (with permission of physician and patient)
   12. Elimination of odor in drainage bags; use weak solution of vinegar

KIDNEY TUMOR

A. Definition: most tumors of the kidney are malignant; no early symptoms are presented
B. Cause: unknown
C. Signs and symptoms (only in late stages)

1. Hematuria with no pain
2. Low-grade temperature
3. Weight loss
4. Anemia
5. Symptoms related to metastasis (e.g., bone pain)

D. Diagnostic tests/methods
   1. Renal arteriogram: IVP and KUB
   2. Renal biopsy examination
E. Treatment
   1. Surgery: radical nephrectomy
   2. Radiation
   3. Chemotherapy
F. Nursing intervention
   1. Provide nursing care for individual symptoms
   2. Provide general nursing care: before and after surgery, during radiation, and for a patient receiving chemotherapy (see specific discussions)

ACUTE RENAL FAILURE (RENAL SHUTDOWN)

A. Definition: sudden damage to the kidneys causing cessation of function and retention of toxins, fluids, and end products of metabolism; patient may recover, or disease may become chronic or be fatal
B. Causes: blood transfusion reaction, shock, toxins, burns, renal ischemia, nephrotoxins, trauma, or reaction to chemotherapy
C. Signs and symptoms
   1. Lethargy, headache, and drowsiness; convulsion; may go into coma
   2. Nausea, vomiting, and diarrhea
   3. Sudden oliguria or anuria
   4. Increased bleeding time
   5. Electrolyte imbalance
   6. Abnormal BUN and creatinine levels
   7. Paresthesia
D. Diagnostic tests/methods
   1. Patient history and physical examination
   2. Blood serum tests, especially potassium
   3. Renal scar
   4. Nephrotomography
   5. Retrograde pyelogram
   6. Ultrasonography, CT, MRI
   7. Urinalysis
E. Treatment
   1. Removal of cause
   2. Peritoneal dialysis
   3. Hemodialysis
F. Nursing intervention
   1. Provide nursing observations and care as indicated for primary problem
   2. Provide care and observations as indicated for patient with chronic renal failure (see following outline)
   3. Provide nursing care as indicated for patient receiving peritoneal dialysis (see later outline)
   4. Provide nursing care as indicated for patient receiving hemodialysis (see later outline)
   5. Offer emotional support

CHRONIC RENAL FAILURE (END-STAGE RENAL DISEASE)

A. Definition: progressive kidney damage; the nephron deteriorates; the kidneys stop functioning; this is the final stage of many chronic diseases (e.g., hypertension)

B. Causes
   1. Glomerulonephritis, pyelonephritis, polycystic kidney, or urinary tract obstruction, diabetes
   2. Essential hypertension
   3. Lupus erythematosus
   4. Toxic agents
   5. Vascular disorders
C. Signs and symptoms (Fig. 5-18)
   1. Malaise
   2. Nausea and vomiting
   3. Anemia
   4. Oliguria
   5. Hyperkalemia
   6. Twitching (from low serum calcium and increased phosphorus levels); pathologic fracture
   7. Hypertension (from fluid retention)
   8. Very susceptible to infection: delayed wound healing and ulcers in the mouth
   9. Bleeding tendency
   10. Uremic frost: urea is excreted in perspiration onto the skin, and small crystals can be seen; this causes severe pruritus
   11. Headaches and visual disturbances, disorientation, convulsions, coma, and death
D. Diagnostic tests/methods
   1. Patient history and physical examination
   2. Serum blood tests
   3. Kidney function tests; BUN; creatinine level
   4. X-ray studies
   5. Renal arteriograms
   6. Nephrotomograms
   7. Kidney biopsy
E. Treatment
   1. Remove (treat) cause
   2. Hemodialysis
   3. Peritoneal dialysis
   4. Kidney transplant
F. Nursing intervention
   1. Monitor fluid balance: weigh patient daily; record intake and output
   2. Maintain asepsis: provide catheter care, prevent infections, and encourage frequent hand washing; do not expose patient to staff or visitors with upper respiratory tract infections
   3. Conserve energy: provide care, maintain rest periods
   4. Provide safety: place side rails up (see earlier discussion on Care of patient in coma, p. 206)
   5. Relieve pruritus: wash patient frequently with tepid water; do not use soap; handle skin gently; use skin lotion; cut nails; apply calamine lotion
   6. Assist with administration of transfusion
   7. Provide oral hygiene every 1 to 2 hours; use cotton swabs and antiseptic mouthwash; apply mineral oil to lips
   8. Provide soft, high-carbohydrate, low-potassium, low-sodium, low-protein diet in small feedings
   9. Restrict fluids as ordered
   10. Anticipate cardiac arrest: monitor vital signs
   11. Assess LOC: orient as necessary
   12. Provide nursing care and precautions as indicated for a patient with seizures (see discussion of Convulsive disorders)

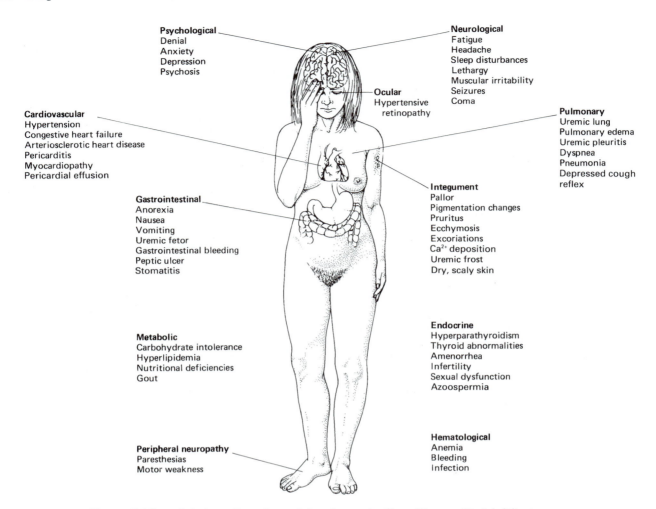

Psychological
Denial
Anxiety
Depression
Psychosis

Neurological
Fatigue
Headache
Sleep disturbances
Lethargy
Muscular irritability
Seizures
Coma

Ocular
Hypertensive
retinopathy

Cardiovascular
Hypertension
Congestive heart failure
Arteriosclerotic heart disease
Pericarditis
Myocardiopathy
Pericardial effusion

Pulmonary
Uremic lung
Pulmonary edema
Uremic pleuritis
Dyspnea
Pneumonia
Depressed cough
reflex

Integument
Pallor
Pigmentation changes
Pruritus
Ecchymosis
Excoriations
Ca^{2+} deposition
Uremic frost
Dry, scaly skin

Gastrointestinal
Anorexia
Nausea
Vomiting
Uremic fetor
Gastrointestinal bleeding
Peptic ulcer
Stomatitis

Metabolic
Carbohydrate intolerance
Hyperlipidemia
Nutritional deficiencies
Gout

Endocrine
Hyperparathyroidism
Thyroid abnormalities
Amenorrhea
Infertility
Sexual dysfunction
Azoospermia

Peripheral neuropathy
Paresthesias
Motor weakness

Hematological
Anemia
Bleeding
Infection

Figure 5-18.   **Clinical manifestations of chronic uremia.** (From Hoeman SP: *Rehabilitation nursing: process and application,* ed 2, St Louis, 1996, Mosby.)

13. Provide nursing measures to prevent dangers of immobility (see Chapter 2)
14. Anticipate and prevent bleeding
    a. Observe stool, urine, sputum, and vomitus
    b. Monitor vital signs, lab valves
    c. Use soft swab for mouth care
    d. Avoid injections if possible
15. Reinforce instructions for kind of drug therapy (i.e., erythropoietin, iron, minerals, antihypertensives, phosphate binders, and ion-exchange resins)

PERITONEAL DIALYSIS (FIG. 5-19)
A. Description: toxins, end-products of metabolism, and fluids are removed from the blood through the peritoneal membrane; a catheter is passed into the peritoneal cavity; dialyzing fluid, which is similar to plasma, is instilled by gravity into the abdominal cavity, and the catheter is clamped; toxins and electrolytes, which are in greater concentration in the blood vessels of the peritoneal membrane, pass into the dialyzing fluid; after 1 hour the catheter is unclamped, and the fluid drains out by gravity

B. Patient problems
    1. Risk for infection related to dialysis procedure
    2. Self-care deficit related to discomfort and immobility
C. Nursing intervention
    1. Record baseline vital signs; complete assessment; carefully measure fluid instilled/drained
    2. Maintain surgical asepsis; prevent peritonitis
    3. Assist patient with self-care activities
    4. Observe for complications (hypotension, pain, respiratory distress, hypovolemia, peritonitis, atelectasis)

HEMODIALYSIS
A. Description: blood leaves the patient through an arterial cannula and travels through coils placed in a solution; dialysis takes place, and the detoxified blood returns to the patient's venous circulation; a surgically created arteriovenous fistula (connection) is necessary for repeated dialysis

B. Patient problems
    1. Self-esteem disturbance related to threatened self-image
    2. Powerlessness related to dependency on machine

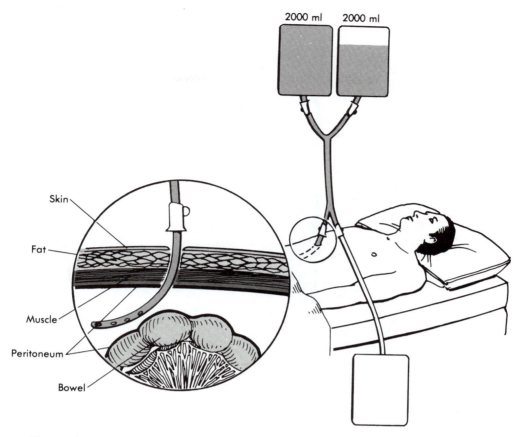

Figure 5-19.   **Patient receiving peritoneal dialysis.** Dialysis fluid is being infused into the peritoneal cavity. (From Phipps et al: *Medical-surgical nursing: concepts and clinical practice*, ed 5, St Louis, 1995, Mosby.)

3. Risk for infection related to the hemodialysis procedure
4. Anxiety related to lifelong, life-threatening disease
C. Nursing intervention
1. Maintain surgical asepsis
2. Assess bruit patency
3. Provide emotional support; alleviate anxiety
4. Provide patient teaching

KIDNEY TRANSPLANT
A. Removal of the diseased kidney and transplantation of a normal kidney is sometimes performed for patients with advanced renal failure; restores normal function; less expensive than dialysis after first year
B. Patient problems
1. Risk for infection related to altered immune system secondary to medications
2. Anxiety related to possibility of organ rejection

MALE REPRODUCTIVE SYSTEM
Anatomy and Physiology (Fig. 5-20)
A. External genitals
1. Scrotum: skin-covered pouch; lies outside of pelvic cavity; contains testes, epididymis, and lower part of vas

deferens; lower body temperature here is necessary for reproduction
2. Penis: erectile tissue; organ of coitus (sexual intercourse); serves as passageway for urine and semen
B. Testes: small oval glands in scrotum; produce spermatozoa; secrete testosterone
C. Ducts
1. Seminiferous tubules: formation of sperm
2. Epididymis: narrow, tightly coiled tubes; provides temporary storage space for immature sperm
3. Vas deferens: continuation of the epididymis; lies near surface of scrotum; called the spermatic cord
4. Ejaculatory: pass through prostate; ejaculate semen into urethra
D. Accessory glands
1. Seminal vesicles: located on each side of the prostate; empty secretion into the prostatic ampulla
2. Prostate: encircles the upper area of the urethra; secretes alkaline fluid; increases sperm motility
3. Cowper's gland: located below prostate; produces an alkaline secretion that is primarily a lubricant during sexual intercourse
E. Semen: alkaline fluid (pH 7.5); the major bulk (60%) is secreted by the seminal vesicles; the remaining 40% is secreted by other accessory organs

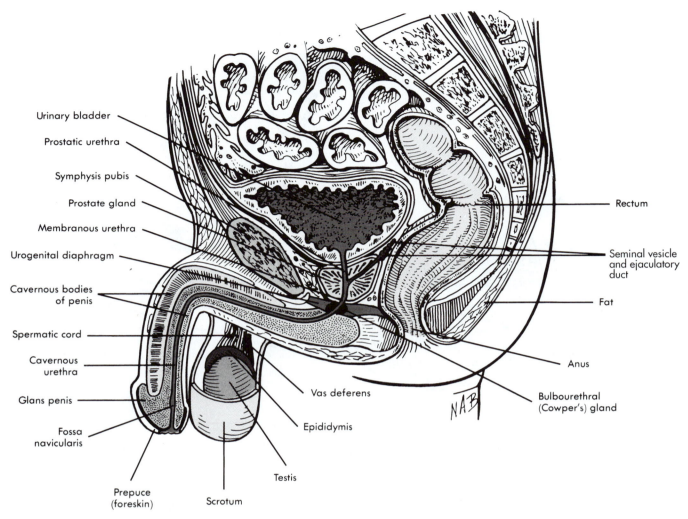

Figure 5-20. **Male organs of reproduction.** (Adapted from Long et al: *Medical-surgical nursing: nursing process approach*, ed 3, St Louis, 1993, Mosby.)

Labels on figure:
Urinary bladder
Prostatic urethra
Symphysis pubis
Prostate gland
Membranous urethra
Urogenital diaphragm
Cavernous bodies of penis
Spermatic cord
Cavernous urethra
Glans penis
Fossa navicularis
Prepuce (foreskin)
Scrotum
Testis
Epididymis
Vas deferens
Rectum
Seminal vesicle and ejaculatory duct
Fat
Anus
Bulbourethral (Cowper's) gland

F. Function
1. Reproduction
2. Production of testosterone

Conditions/Disorders of the Male Genitourinary System

BENIGN PROSTATIC HYPERTROPHY (BPH)

A. Description: the prostate gland slowly enlarges (hypertrophies) and extends upward into the bladder; outflow of urine is obstructed; the urinary stream is smaller, and voiding is difficult; a pouch is formed in the bladder as the gland continues to enlarge; stasis of urine occurs; obstruction causes gradual dilation of ureters and kidneys; may cause hydronephrosis; when obstruction is complete, there is acute urinary retention

B. Cause: unknown; increased incidence with age, usually over 50 years of age; related to smoking

C. Signs and symptoms
1. Dysuria, frequency, nocturia, urgency, retention, burning on urination, and decreased force of stream
2. Urinary tract infection
3. Acute urinary retention

D. Diagnostic tests/methods
1. Patient history and assessment; palpation through rectal examination
2. IVP, cystoscopy, and retrograde pyelography
3. Urine culture
4. BUN
5. Serum creatinine
6. Transrectal ultrasonography

E. Treatment
1. Immediate
a. Bladder drainage with indwelling catheter
b. Decompression
c. Antibiotics as indicated
d. Suprapubic cystotomy and insertion of catheter for long-term drainage
2. Surgery: type depends on patient's age and size of enlargement (open approaches)
a. Transurethral resection of the prostate (TURP): an

instrument is passed through the urethra to the prostate; under direct visualization, small pieces of the obstructing gland are removed with electric wire; the bleeding points are cauterized; there is no incision; bleeding is a common postoperative problem

    b. Suprapubic (transvesical) prostatectomy: a low incision is made over the bladder; the bladder is opened, and the prostatic tissue is removed through an incision into the urethral mucosa; two drainage tubes are inserted (a cystotomy tube and a Foley catheter); these are connected to a continuous bladder irrigation setup

    c. Retropubic prostatectomy: a low abdominal incision is made; the bladder is not entered

    d. Perineal prostatectomy: the gland is removed through an incision in the perineum; the entire gland and capsule are removed

    e. Bilateral vasectomy may be performed with a prostatectomy to reduce risk of epididymitis

  3. Other treatment methods

    a. Finasteride (Proscar), an androgen hormone inhibitor, can be used to decrease symptoms, may arrest prostate enlargement

    b. Transcystoscopic urethroplasty: balloon dilatation of prostatic urethra

    c. TUIP: transurethral incision at bladder neck

    d. Short-term effects treatment involving microwaves

F. Nursing intervention

  1. On admission, complete assessment related to

    a. Aging

    b. Possible infection

    c. Anxiety

    d. Medical problems associated with aging: diabetes, cardiovascular, hearing, sight, and gastrointestinal

  2. Encourage fluids if not contraindicated; monitor intake and output

  3. Maintain gravity drainage of indwelling catheter

  4. Provide general preoperative and postoperative care (see Chapter 2)

  5. Provide specific postoperative care; depends on the procedure performed

    a. Maintain gravity drainage of indwelling catheter

    b. Keep irrigation flowing (note clots); maintain a closed, continuous irrigation; ensure drainage not obstructed

    c. Maintain asepsis; change dressing when wet (may need physician's order); there may be fecal incontinence if a perineal prostatectomy was performed

    d. Monitor vital signs; hematuria is expected; report frank bleeding or clots

    e. Use oral thermometer (no rectal treatments)

    f. Encourage patient to avoid straining; encourage fluids; provide stool softeners

    g. Observe for bladder spasms; note if catheter is draining freely; irrigate by syringe as ordered; administer antispasmodics

    h. Administer analgesic as needed for postoperative pain

    i. Monitor intake and output; record all drainage tubes separately

    j. Sitz bath for pain and inflammation if perineal prostatectomy

    k. Provide care instructions if patient is discharged with indwelling catheter

CANCER OF THE PROSTATE

A. Definition: a malignant tumor; it has no symptoms until it has become large or metastasized

B. Cause: unknown; increased incidence with age (all men older than 40 years should have rectal examinations yearly)

C. Signs and symptoms

  1. Early tumor has no symptoms

  2. Frequency, nocturia, dysuria, and urinary retention

  3. Back pain

  4. Symptoms from metastasis

D. Diagnostic tests/methods

  1. Rectal examination

  2. Biopsy examination (needle or a pin)

  3. Acid phosphatase

  4. Transrectal ultrasonography

  5. Prostate-specific antigen level (PSA)

  6. Serum alkaline phosphatase level (elevated in bone metastasis)

  7. Bone scan to assess metastasis

  8. Pelvic or spinal radiographs

  9. MRI, CT

E. Treatment surgery

  1. Radical perineal prostatectomy (removal of prostate, capsule, and seminal vesicles)

  2. Bilateral orchiectomy (removal of both testicles)

  3. TURP

  4. Estrogen therapy

  5. Agonists of luteinizing hormone—releasing hormone

  6. Radiation (external, interstitial, spot)

F. Nursing intervention

  1. See nursing intervention for a patient with BPH

  2. Be supportive as concerns are expressed about a malignancy and feminization from estrogens; answer questions; refer problems to physician

  3. Pain control for terminally ill patient; may consider hospice care

HYDROCELE

A. Definition: a cystic mass filled with fluid that forms around the testicle

B. Causes

  1. Infection

  2. Trauma

C. Signs and symptoms

  1. Swelling of testicle

  2. Discomfort in sitting and walking

D. Diagnostic tests/methods: assessment

E. Treatment

  1. Aspiration (usually only in children)

  2. Injection of a sclerosing solution

  3. Surgical removal of the sac (hydrocelectomy)

F. Nursing intervention

  1. Provide usual preoperative and postoperative care (see Chapter 2)

  2. Scrotal support (elevation) may be necessary during postoperative period

  3. Be supportive to concerns expressed by patient

CANCER OF THE TESTES

A. Definition: an uncommon malignancy; usually no systemic symptoms are present until metastasis occurs; can be diagnosed early only by examination and finding a hard,

nontender mass (testicular self-examination should be done monthly); age of incidence is usually in early 30s
B. Treatment
1. Surgery: orchiectomy
2. Radiotherapy
3. Chemotherapy
4. Possibly radical: lymph node dissection
C. Nursing intervention: related to treatment selected

FEMALE REPRODUCTIVE SYSTEM
Anatomy and Physiology

A. External genitals
1. Vulva
   a. Labia majora: two long folds of skin on each side of the vaginal orifice outside of the labia minora
   b. Labia minora: two flat, thin, delicate folds of skin that are highly sensitive to manipulation and trauma; enclose the region called the vestibule, which contains the clitoris, the urethral orifice, and the vaginal orifice
   c. Clitoris: very sensitive erectile tissue; becomes swollen with blood during sexual excitement
   d. Vaginal orifice: opening into vagina; hymen, fold of mucosa, partially closes orifice and generally is ruptured during first sexual intercourse
   e. Bartholin's glands: located on each side of vaginal orifice; secrete lubrication fluid
2. Perineum: between vaginal orifice and anus; forms pelvic floor
B. Internal organs (Fig. 5-21)
1. Ovaries: main sex glands
   a. Located on either side in pelvic cavity
   b. Produce ova, which form in the graafian follicles
   c. Graafian follicle produces estrogen
   d. Rupture of a follicle releases an ovum (ovulation)
   e. Ruptured follicles become glandular mass called corpus luteum
   f. Corpus luteum secretes estrogen, but mainly progesterone
2. Fallopian tubes
   a. Extend from point near ovaries to uterus; no direct connection between ovaries and tubes
   b. Fimbriae: fingerlike extensions on tubes; pick up ova and transport into fallopian tubes
   c. Fertilization occurs in outer one third of the fallopian tubes

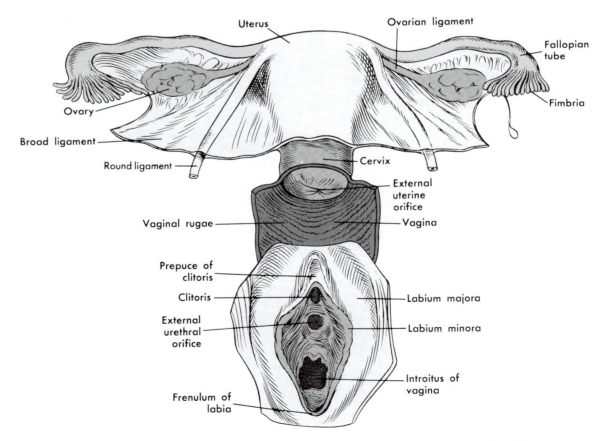

Figure 5-21.   **Female internal organs of reproduction.** Major ligaments are shown. (From Phipps et al: *Medical-surgical nursing: concepts and clinical practice*, ed 5, St Louis, 1995, Mosby.)

3. Uterus
  a. Upper portion rests on upper surface of bladder; the lower portion is embedded in pelvic floor between the bladder and the rectum
  b. Pear-shaped, hollow organ that expands tremendously to accommodate a fetus
  c. Divisions
    (1) Body: upper main part
    (2) Fundus: bulging upper surface of the body
    (3) Cervix: neck of the uterus
  d. Endometrium: uterine lining; sloughs off during menstruation
  e. Functions
    (1) Menstruation
    (2) Pregnancy
    (3) Labor
4. Vagina
  a. Located between rectum and urethra
  b. Structure: wrinkled mucous membrane (rugae); capable of great distention
  c. Functions
    (1) Lower part of birth canal
    (2) Receives semen from male
    (3) Passageway for menstrual flow
C. Breasts (mammary glands)
  1. Located over pectoral muscles
  2. Size depends on adipose tissue rather than glandular tissue
  3. Consists of lobes, lobules, and milk-secreting cells (acini)
  4. Ducts lead to the opening called the nipple
  5. Areola: pigmented area surrounding the nipple
D. Function
  1. Reproduction
  2. Production of estrogen and progesterone
E. Menstrual cycle (Fig. 5-22)
  1. Phases: regulated primarily by the hormonal control of pituitary gland, ovaries, and uterus
    a. One ovum discharged each month from an ovary; ripens in the graafian follicle; follicle-stimulating hormone (FSH) from anterior lobe of pituitary stimulates the formation of the follicle
    b. Estrogen produced by the follicle builds up the endometrium in expectation of a fertilized ovum
    c. Ovum is discharged into the fallopian tube by luteinizing hormone (LH) from the anterior lobe pituitary; follicle is converted into the corpus luteum
    d. Postovulation: corpus luteum secretes progesterone and estrogen for final preparation of the endometrium
    e. Premenstrual: the gradual drop in progesterone and estrogen leads to menses
  2. Length of cycle: usually 28 days; highly variable; ovulation occurs midway
  3. Menopause (climacteric) the gradual cessation of menstrual cycle; the ability to bear children ends; occurs at approximately 45 years of age
    a. Ovaries lose their ability to respond to hormones
    b. Decrease in levels of estrogen and progesterone
      (1) Failure to ovulate
      (2) Monthly flow is less, is irregular, and gradually ceases
      (3) Reproductive organs atrophy

Conditions/Disorders of the Female Reproductive System

Childbearing is the major physiologic function of the female reproductive system. Disorders of this system are distressing to the patient because of interference with sexuality, conception, and self-image. The nurse plays an important role by clearly providing information to the concerned patient.

Nursing Assessment

A. Nursing observations (objective data)
  1. General appearance
  2. Vital signs
  3. Weight
  4. Breasts
    a. Contour
    b. Skin dimpling
    c. Nodules
      (1) Size
      (2) Consistency
      (3) Mobile or fixed
    d. Nipples
      (1) Asymmetry
      (2) Retraction
      (3) Rash
      (4) Ulceration
      (5) Discharge
  5. External genitalia
    a. Irritation
    b. Redness
    c. Excoriation
    d. Bulge
  6. Introitus
    a. Irritation
    b. Redness
    c. Excoriation
    d. Nodules
  7. Discharge
    a. Color
    b. Malodorous
    c. Consistency
B. Patient description (subjective data)
  1. Lower abdominal pain and cramping
  2. Backache
  3. Stress incontinence
  4. Urinary frequency and urgency
  5. Urine or fecal material draining from vaginal tract
  6. Breasts
    a. Tenderness
    b. Burning
    c. Swelling
    d. Pain
    e. Nipples
      (1) Tenderness
      (2) Burning
  7. External genitalia
    a. Itching
    b. Burning
  8. Introitus
    a. Burning
    b. Itching
    c. Tenderness
    d. Dyspareunia (painful intercourse)

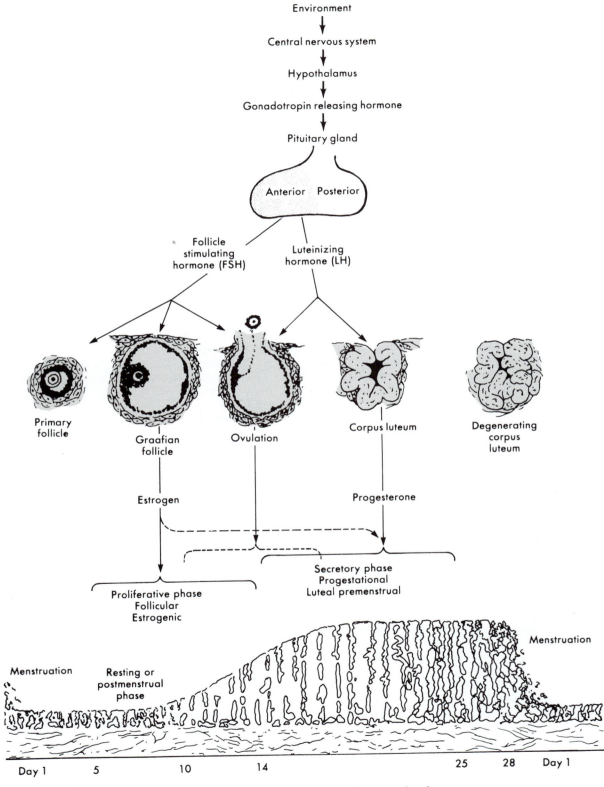

Figure 5-22. Hormonal control of menstrual cycle.

9. Menstrual cycle
   a. Duration of cycles
   b. Number of days between cycles
   c. Associated symptoms
      (1) Pain
      (2) Headache
      (3) Irritability
      (4) Depression
      (5) Insomnia

Diagnostic Tests/Methods

A. Serum laboratory studies
   1. Luteinizing hormone (LH)
      a. Stimulates progesterone secretion
      b. Diminished levels may relate to prolonged, heavy menses
      c. Elevated levels may result in short, scanty menses
   2. Follicle-stimulating hormone (FSH)
      a. Stimulates estrogen secretion
      b. Diminished levels may relate to bleeding between cycles
      c. Elevated levels may result in excessive uterine bleeding
   3. Thyroid function tests
      a. Used to rule out menstrual abnormality secondary to thyroid dysfunction
      b. Diminished thyroid hormone secretion may result in bleeding between cycles, irregular menses, or absence of menstrual flow
   4. Adrenal function tests
      a. Used to rule out menstrual abnormality secondary to adrenal dysfunction
      b. Elevated or decreased production of adrenal cortex hormone secretion may result in amenorrhea
B. Procedures
   1. Pelvic examination: to inspect and assess the external genitalia, perineal and anal areas, introitus, vaginal tract, and cervix
      a. Have patient empty bladder
      b. Place patient in the lithotomy position
      c. Flex and abduct patient's thighs
      d. Place patient's feet in stirrups
      e. Extend patient's buttocks slightly beyond the edge of the examining table
   2. Laparoscopy: visualization of the pelvic structures with a lighted laparoscope inserted through the abdominal wall
   3. Culdoscopy: visualization of the ovaries, fallopian tubes, and uterus with a lighted instrument inserted through the vaginal tract
      a. After procedure, position patient on abdomen to expel air
      b. Monitor for vaginal bleeding
      c. Instruct patient to abstain from intercourse, douching, and use of tampons until advised by physician
   4. Colposcopy: visualization of the cervix with an instrument that magnifies tissue
   5. Papanicolaou smear test (Pap smear): a sample of cervical scrapings is obtained for study under a microscope for evidence of malignant cell changes
      a. Follow nursing actions as in a pelvic examination
      b. Write patient's name on the frost side of the slide, handling edges only
      c. Smear the specimen on a glass slide
      d. Place a drop of a fixative, dry, and send to laboratory

   e. Reinforce importance of Pap smears as recommended by the American Cancer Society
   6. Cervical biopsy examination: removal of tissue to examine for presence of malignancy
      a. After procedure, advise patient to rest and avoid strenuous activity for 24 hours
      b. Leave packing in place until physician permits removal (usually 12 to 24 hours)
      c. Monitor for vaginal bleeding
      d. Instruct patient to abstain from intercourse, douching, and use of tampons until advised by physician
      e. Explain that there will be a malodorous discharge that may last 3 weeks; daily bath should help control this
   7. Conization
      a. Removal of cone-shaped tissue of the cervix for analysis of cancerous cells
      b. Indicated for removal of diseased cervical tissue
      c. Nursing intervention
         (1) Maintain packing 12 to 24 hours
         (2) Monitor for bleeding
         (3) Instruct patient to abstain from intercourse, douching, and use of tampons until advised by physician
   8. Schiller's test
      a. Application of a dye to the cervix to aid in detecting cancerous cells
      b. Normal vaginal cells will stain a deep brown
      c. Abnormal cells with not absorb the dye
      d. Nursing intervention: recommend to patient that a perineal pad be used to protect clothes from stain
   9. Ultrasonography
      a. A sound frequency that reflects an image of the pelvic structures
      b. An aid in confirming ovarian and uterine tumors
   10. Culture and sensitivity
      a. The culture of a specimen of exudate suspected of infection
      b. The sensitivity of an antibiotic to the microorganism
   11. Dilatation and curettage (D & C)
      a. A diagnostic and therapeutic procedure
      b. The cervix is dilated to scrape the lining of the uterine cavity with a curet
      c. Nursing intervention
         (1) After procedure, provide sterile perineal pads and record amount of drainage
         (2) Encourage voiding to prevent urinary retention
         (3) Instruct patient to abstain from intercourse, douching, and use of tampons until advised by physician
   12. Mammography: an x-ray examination of the breasts to detect tumors
   13. Thermography: infrared photography used to detect breast tumors
   14. Xerography: an x-ray examination of the breasts and skin that provides good definition of the tissue
   15. CT; MRI

Frequent Patient Problems and Nursing Care

A. Anxiety related to modesty
   1. Keep the patient's body covered at all times
   2. Provide privacy

3. Speak with the patient during the examination or procedure

B. Knowledge deficit related to understanding of menstruation
1. Provide factual information related to the process of menstruation
2. Describe abnormalities associated with menstruation
3. Describe emotional changes associated with menstruation
4. Teach menstrual hygiene
   a. Change perineal pad or tampon every 3 to 4 hours
   b. Remove napkin front to back
   c. Alternate sanitary napkins and tampons qd to prevent toxic shock syndrome or back flow of menstruation

C. Knowledge deficit related to menstrual abnormalities: explain which menstrual symptoms are considered abnormal
1. Flow occurring more frequently than every 21 days
2. Flow occurring less frequently than every 35 days
3. Duration of less than 3 days
4. Duration of more than 7 days
5. Use of 12 or more perineal pads per 24 hours

D. Pain related to menstruation
1. Assess location, duration, onset, and quality of pain
2. Apply heating pad to the abdomen
3. Provide warm liquids of patient's choice
4. Provide massage to lumbar area
5. Provide pain relief medication as ordered by physician

E. Knowledge deficit related to breast self-examination (BSE)
1. Recommend that breasts be examined 7 days after onset of menstruation every month (Fig. 5-23)
2. Instruct patient on technique of breast self-examination
   a. Inspect breasts in front of mirror with arms at sides
   b. Observe breasts with arms raised above the head
   c. With hands on hips, lean forward and contract chest muscles
3. Lying supine, palpate each breast with flat part of fingers and continue in a circular movement to nipple
4. Observations of the breasts
   a. Size
   b. Symmetry

How to do BSE

1. Lie down and put a pillow under your right shoulder. Place your right arm behind your head.
2. Use the finger pads of the three middle fingers on your left hand to feel for lumps or thickening. Your finger pads are the top third of each finger.

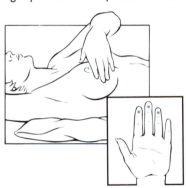

3. Press hard enough to know how your breast feels. If you're not sure how hard to press, ask your health care provider. Or try to copy the way your health care provider uses the finger pads during a breast exam. Learn what your breast feels like most of the time. A firm ridge in the lower curve of each breast is normal.

4. Move around the breast in a set way. You can choose either the circle (A), the up and down line (B), or the wedge (C). Do it the same way every time. It will help you to make sure that you've gone over the entire breast area and to remember how your breast feels each month.

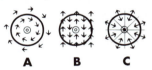

A   **B**   **C**

5. Now examine your left breast using right hand finger pads.
*   You might want to check your breasts while standing in front of a mirror right after you do your BSE each month. You might also want to do an extra BSE while you're in the shower. Your soapy hands will glide over the wet skin making it easy to check how your breasts feel.*

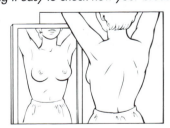

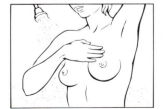

Figure 5-23.   Breast self-examination. (Courtesy of American Cancer Society from: Harkness and Dincher: *Medical-surgical nursing: total patient care,* ed 9, St Louis, 1996, Mosby.)

c. Skin texture

d. Color

e. Nipple position

f. Nipple discharge

F. Knowledge deficit related to menopause

1. Describe accompanying symptoms associated with menopause

   a. Irregular menses

   b. Hot flashes

   c. Night sweats

   d. Insomnia

   e. Depression

   f. Anxiety

2. Onset is usually after age 40 years

3. Explain that menopause does not interfere with sexuality

4. Recommend use of lubricant before intercourse

5. Recommend use of contraception for 6 months after the last menstrual period

Major Medical Diagnoses

MENSTRUAL ABNORMALITIES

DYSMENORRHEA

A. Definition: intense pain at the time of menses

B. Cause: uterine spasms cause cramping of the lower abdomen

C. Signs and symptoms

1. Subjective

   a. Headache, backache

   b. Abdominal pain

   c. Chills

   d. Nausea

2. Objective

   a. Fever

   b. Vomiting

D. Diagnostic method: pelvic examination to rule out other physical disorders

E. Treatment

1. Analgesics, such as nonsteroidal antiinflammatory agents

2. Local application of heat

3. Pelvic exercises

4. D & C

F. Nursing intervention

1. Instruct patient on avoidance of fatigue and overexertion during menstrual period

2. Instruct patient on ingestion of warm beverages before onset of pain to prevent attack

PREMENSTRUAL TENSION SYNDROME (PMS)

A. Definition: a number of symptoms occurring a few days before menstruation

B. Cause: cause is unclear; may be related to fluid retention combined with emotional tension; usually disappears with onset of menstruation

C. Signs and symptoms

1. Subjective

   a. Breast tenderness

   b. Headache

   c. Nausea

   d. Depression

   e. Insomnia

   f. Irritability

   g. Fatigue

2. Objective: weight gain 2 to 10 days before onset of menstruation

D. Diagnostic method: assessment of specific symptoms and psychologic health

E. Treatment

1. Diuretics

2. Mild sodium restriction

3. Mild tranquilizers

4. Well-balanced diet

5. Exercise

F. Nursing intervention

1. Assist patient in working out a diet with decreased sodium content

2. Instruct patient to decrease consumption of coffee, alcohol, and nicotine during latter half of menstrual cycle

AMENORRHEA

A. Definition: absence of menstrual periods

B. Causes

1. Diabetes

2. Debilitating illness

3. Malnutrition

4. Obesity

5. Extreme anxiety

6. Anemia

7. Oral contraceptives

8. Chronic nephritis

9. Tumors of the endocrine glands

C. Signs and symptoms

1. Subjective: anxiety

2. Objective

   a. Absence of menses by age 17 years (primary amenorrhea)

   b. Failure of a menstrual period (secondary amenorrhea)

D. Diagnostic tests/methods

1. Pelvic examination

2. LH level

3. FSH level

4. Thyroid function test

5. Adrenal function test

E. Treatment: according to cause

F. Nursing intervention

1. Encourage patient to follow prescribed orders to ensure success of therapeutic plan

2. Provide clear explanations related to cause of disorder to decrease anxiety

MENORRHAGIA (HYPERMENORRHEA)

A. Definition: excessive menstrual flow (amount or duration)

B. Causes

1. Uterine tumors

2. Pelvic inflammatory disease

3. Endocrine disturbances

C. Signs and symptoms

1. Subjective

   a. Feeling of pelvic heaviness

   b. Fatigue

2. Objective

   a. Profuse menstrual bleeding with clots

   b. Pale, tired appearance

D. Diagnostic tests/methods

1. Pelvic examination

2. LH level
3. FSH level
4. Thyroid function test
5. Adrenal function test
6. RBC count
E. Treatment
   1. According to cause
   2. D & C
F. Nursing intervention
   1. Encourage intake of foods high in iron content
   2. Encourage planned rest periods
   3. Instruct the patient to count number of pads used during an abnormal period
   4. Weigh each pad before and after use to estimate blood loss

METRORRHAGIA

A. Definition: bleeding between menstrual intervals
B. Pathology
   1. Causes are similar to those of menorrhagia
   2. Break-through bleeding may occur with use of contraceptive pills
   3. May be early symptom of cervical cancer
C. Signs and symptoms
   1. Subjective
     a. Feeling of pelvic heaviness
     b. Fatigue
   2. Objective
     a. Spotting or bleeding between menstrual periods
     b. Tired appearance
D. Diagnostic tests/methods
   1. Pelvic examination
   2. LH level
   3. FSH level
   4. Thyroid function test
   5. Adrenal function test
   6. RBC count
   7. Pap smear
E. Treatment: according to cause
F. Nursing intervention
   1. Instruct the patient on how to keep accurate records of bleeding episodes
   2. Encourage continued medical follow-up because of possible cervical changes associated with cancer

VAGINITIS

A. Definition: inflammation of the vaginal mucosa
B. Pathology
   1. Invasion of virulent organisms permitted by changes in normal flora; pH becomes alkaline
   2. Causes:
     a. Trichomoniasis: parasitic organism
     b. *Candida albicans* (moniliasis): fungal organism
     c. Atrophic (senile): occurs in postmenopausal women because of atrophy of vaginal mucosa
     d. Bacterial: invasion by staphylococci, streptococci, *Escherichia coli, Chlamydia,* or *Gardnerella vaginalis*
     e. Foreign body
     f. Allergens or irritants
C. Signs and symptoms
   1. Trichomoniasis: thick, white or yellow, frothy, malodorous discharge causing itching, burning, and excoriation of vulva

   2. Monilial: thick or watery, white or yellow, curdlike discharge; mucosa becomes reddened
   3. Atrophic: blood-flecked discharge with burning and itching of the vagina and dyspareunia
   4. Bacterial: profuse, yellow mucoid discharge with irritation to vulva and urethra; fishy or foul odor
   5. Foreign body: blood-tinged serosanguineous or purulent discharge; foul odor; may be thin or thick
   6. Allergens/irritants: increase in usual secretions, itching, burning, rash
D. Diagnostic tests/methods: culture and sensitivity; pelvic exam
E. Treatment
   1. Trichomoniasis: metronidazole (Flagyl), floraquin tablets administered vaginally, and carbarsone suppositories administered rectally; sitz baths to relieve itching
   2. Candidiasis: nystatin (Mycostatin) or gliconazole (Monistat) creme daily for 14 days; sitz baths to relieve itching
   3. Atrophic: antibiotics and estrogen therapy
   4. Bacterial: antibiotics and sulfonamide creams
   5. Foreign body: removal of object; use of antibiotics
   6. Allergens or irritants: removal of cause; use of topical steroid ointment if necessary
F. Nursing intervention
   1. Reassure patient during vaginal examination to decrease anxiety
   2. Instruct patient on perineal hygiene: cleansing front to back
   3. In the event of trichomoniasis, instruct patient to abstain from intercourse or have partner wear a condom, because this infection can be transmitted
   4. Advise patient to use perineal pads because of increased discharge
   5. Teach patient importance of compliance with treatment

UTERINE CANCER (ENDOMETRIUM)

A. Definition: new growth of abnormal cells in the uterine lining
B. Pathology
   1. Spreads to cervix, fallopian tubes, ovaries, bladder, and rectum
   2. Associated factors are women over 50 years of age, obesity, diabetes, and hypertension
   3. Prognosis is good if identified in early stages
C. Signs and symptoms
   1. Subjective
     a. Postmenopausal bleeding
     b. Bleeding between cycles
     c. Bleeding after intercourse
     d. Watery vaginal discharge
   2. Objective
     a. Uterine enlargement
     b. Suspicious Pap test results
D. Diagnostic tests/methods
   1. D & C
   2. Tissue biopsy examination
E. Treatment
   1. Surgical intervention
     a. Panhysterectomy (removal of uterus and cervix)
     b. Oophorectomy (removal of ovaries)
     c. Salpingectomy (removal of fallopian tubes)

2. Chemotherapy
3. Radiation
F. Nursing intervention: refer to section on Cancer of the cervix, p. 241

UTERINE FIBROID TUMORS
A. Definition: a benign tumor located in the uterus
B. Pathology
   1. Develops slowly, symptoms occur only in relation to size, location, and number of tumors present
   2. Occurs in 25% of women over 35 years of age
C. Signs and symptoms
   1. Subjective
      a. Menstrual disturbances
      b. Backache
      c. Frequent urination
      d. Constipation
   2. Objective; uterine enlargement
D. Diagnostic tests/methods
   1. Pelvic examination
   2. Laparoscopy
E. Treatment
   1. Excision of the myoma is indicated for small tumors
   2. Hysterectomy (removal of uterus) with preservation of ovaries is indicated for large tumors
F. Nursing intervention
   1. Explain to patient that tumors may decrease in size after menopause
   2. Encourage patient to verbalize concerns
   3. If patient undergoes myomectomy, follow general postoperative nursing measures related to abdominal surgery
   4. If the patient undergoes a hysterectomy, follow nursing interventions covered under Cancer of the cervix, p.241

ENDOMETRIOSIS
A. Definition: tissue resembling the endometrial membrane grows in another location in the pelvic cavity
B. Pathology
   1. During menstrual period, endometrial cells are stimulated by ovarian hormone
   2. Bleeding into surrounding tissue occurs, causing inflammation
   3. Condition may result in adhesions, fusion of pelvic organs, bladder dysfunction, stricture of bowel, or sterility
C. Signs and symptoms: symptoms usually appear in women over 30 years of age
   1. Subjective
      a. Discomfort of pelvic area before menses, becoming worse during menstrual flow, and diminishing as flow ceases
      b. Dyspareunia
      c. Fatigue
   2. Objective: infertility
D. Diagnostic tests/methods
   1. Laparoscopy
   2. Culdoscopy
E. Treatment
   1. Hormonal therapy to suppress ovulation
   2. Surgical intervention: hysterectomy, oophorectomy, or salpingectomy

F. Nursing intervention
   1. Provide emotional support
   2. If patient is young, advise not to delay family because of risk of sterility
   3. Explain that hormonal drug may cause pseudopregnancy and irregular bleeding
   4. If patient is middle aged, advise her that menopause may stop progression of condition
   5. Follow general postoperative nursing actions if the patient undergoes surgical procedure
      a. Observe for vaginal hemorrhage, malodorous vaginal discharge, or vaginal discharge other than serosanguineous discharge
      b. Observe for urine retention, burning, frequency, or urgency to void
      c. Listen for renewed bowel sounds
   6. Patient teaching on discharge
      a. Heavy lifting, prolonged standing, walking, and sitting are contraindicated
      b. Sexual intercourse should be avoided until approved by physician

PELVIC INFLAMMATORY DISEASE (PID)
A. Definition: inflammation of the pelvic cavity
B. Pathology
   1. Pathogenic organisms are introduced into the cervix
   2. PID may be confined to one or more structures: fallopian tubes, ovaries, pelvic peritoneum, pelvic veins, or pelvic tissue
   3. May result in adhesions, strictures, or sterility
   4. Most common causative organism: gonococcus
   5. Also caused by staphylococci or streptococci
C. Signs and symptoms
   1. Subjective
      a. Abdominal pain
      b. Pelvic pain
      c. Low-back pain
      d. Nausea
   2. Objective
      a. Malodorous, purulent discharge
      b. Fever
      c. Vomiting
D. Diagnostic tests/method: culture and sensitivity test and CBC; pelvic exam; laparoscopy
E. Treatment
   1. Antibiotic therapy
   2. Analgesics
F. Nursing intervention
   1. Provide nonjudgmental, accepting attitude
   2. Place patient in semi-Fowler's position to provide dependent pelvic drainage
   3. Apply heat to abdominal area if ordered to improve circulation and provide comfort
   4. Patient teaching should include
      a. Take shower instead of tub bath
      b. Perineal hygiene: wipe from front to back
      c. How to recognize if sexual partner is infected with gonococcus: discharge from penis of whitish fluid with painful urination (not all males are symptomatic)
      d. Importance of routine physical examinations, because gonococcal infection is asymptomatic in females
      e. Reinforce "safe sex" guidelines

VAGINAL FISTULA

A. Definition: tubelike opening between two internal organs
B. Pathology
  1. Causes include radiation therapy, gynecologic surgery, or traumatic childbirth
  2. Results in impaired blood supply and sloughing of tissue, leading to abnormal opening
  3. Four types affect female reproductive organs
    a. Ureterovaginal: between ureter and vagina; urine leaks into vagina
    b. Vesicovaginal: between bladder and vagina; urine leaks into vagina
    c. Urethrovaginal: between urethra and vagina; urine leaks into vagina
    d. Rectovaginal: between rectum and vagina; flatus and fecal matter leak into vagina
C. Signs and symptoms
  1. Subjective
    a. Leakage of urine, flatus, and fecal matter
    b. Pain in affected area
  2. Objective
    a. Excoriation
    b. Malodor
D. Diagnostic methods
  1. Symptoms and physical examination
  2. Patient history of radiation therapy
  3. Intravenous pyelogram (IVP)
  4. Cystoscopy
E. Treatment
  1. Small fistula may heal spontaneously
  2. Surgical excision
  3. Temporary colostomy for rectovaginal fistula
F. Nursing intervention
  1. Provide psychologic support: offer reassurance and acceptance
  2. Encourage patient to verbalize feelings; express empathy
  3. Observe vaginal discharge and record
  4. Change perineal pad q4h and prn
  5. Instruct on perineal hygiene
  6. Provide sitz bath and irrigation solutions for hygiene if ordered
  7. Follow general postoperative nursing actions if patient undergoes surgery
    a. Observe Foley catheter for drainage at all times
    b. Caution patient not to strain when having a bowel movement

PROLAPSED UTERUS

A. Definition: downward displacement of the uterus through the vaginal orifice
B. Pathology
  1. A result of weakened supporting muscles and ligaments of the pelvis
  2. Causes include childbirth injuries, repeated pregnancies with short intervals between, menopausal atrophy, and congenital weakness
C. Signs and symptoms
  1. Subjective
    a. Pain in lower abdomen
    b. Feeling of pressure within pelvis
    c. Stress incontinence
    d. Dyspareunia
    e. Backache
  2. Objective
    a. Urinary stasis
    b. Elongated cervix
D. Diagnostic methods
  1. Signs and symptoms
  2. Pelvic examination
E. Treatment
  1. Placement of a pessary in the vagina to support uterus
  2. Surgical suspension of the uterus
  3. Hysterectomy if condition is postmenopausal
F. Nursing intervention
  1. Approach unhurriedly, demonstrate calmness, and encourage expression of feelings to decrease anxiety
  2. Explain all procedures
  3. Follow general postoperative nursing actions
    a. Chart number of perineal pads used during 8-hour period
    b. Observe for hemorrhage
    c. Observe for vaginal discharge other than serosanguineous fluid
    d. Listen for renewed bowel sounds
    e. Observe for urinary retention and pelvic congestion

CYSTOCELE AND RECTOCELE

A. Definition
  1. Cystocele: abnormal protrusion of the bladder against the vaginal wall
  2. Rectocele: abnormal protrusion of part of the rectum against the vaginal wall
B. Pathology
  1. Result of weakened supporting muscles and ligaments of the pelvis
  2. Causes include childbirth injuries, repeated pregnancies with short intervals between, menopausal atrophy, and congenital weakness
C. Signs and symptoms
  1. Subjective
    a. Pelvic pressure; backache
    b. Stress incontinence and dysuria (cystocele)
    c. Constipation or incontinence of feces and flatus (rectocele)
  2. Objective
    a. Residual urine after voiding (cystocele)
    b. Hemorrhoids (rectocele)
D. Diagnostic methods
  1. Signs and symptoms
  2. Pelvic examination
E. Treatment
  1. Anterior colporrhaphy to adjust cystocele
  2. Posterior colporrhaphy to adjust rectocele
F. Nursing intervention
  1. Administer catheter care twice a day (bid) and prn
  2. Splint abdomen when coughing
  3. Place in low-Fowler's position or flat in bed to avoid pressure on suture line
  4. Explain to patient that she should respond to bowel stimuli to avoid suture strain
  5. After each bowel movement, clean perineum with warm water and soap; pat dry anterior to posterior
  6. Apply heat lamp, anesthetic spray, or ice packs if ordered to relieve discomfort
  7. Patient teaching includes:

a. Heavy lifting and prolonged standing, walking, and sitting are contraindicated

b. Sexual intercourse should be avoided until approved by physician

c. Pelvic exercises

OVARIAN TUMORS

A. Definition: a mass of tissue growing on the ovary; is usually asymptomatic until large enough to cause pressure

B. Pathology: two classifications
   1. Ovarian cyst: a benign condition but may transform to a malignancy; may be small, containing clear fluid, or may be filled with a thick yellow fluid; size varies
   2. Malignant tumors: a cancerous growth found on the ovary; can be the primary site of the cancer or secondary site caused by metastasis from the GI tract, breast, pancreas, or kidneys

C. Signs and symptoms
   1. Subjective
      a. Pelvic pain
      b. Menstrual disturbances
      c. Abdominal distention
      d. Constipation
      e. Dyspareunia
   2. Objective: palpable mass

D. Diagnostic tests/methods
   1. Culdoscopy
   2. Ultrasonography
   3. Biopsy examination

E. Treatment
   1. Cyst may be observed for regression in size
   2. Oophorectomy (removal of ovaries)
   3. Removal of all reproductive organs
   4. Estrogen replacement therapy
   5. X-ray therapy and chemotherapy
   6. Radiation therapy

F. Nursing intervention
   1. If patient undergoes oophorectomy, follow general postoperative nursing care related to abdominal surgery
   2. If the patient undergoes surgery for removal of all abdominal reproductive organs, follow nursing intervention covered below under cancer of the cervix
   3. Assist the patient in dealing with changes of body image

CANCER OF THE CERVIX

A. Definition: new growth of abnormal cells in the neck of the uterus

B. Pathology
   1. Early stage is confined to epithelial cervical layer
   2. Will continue to invade surrounding area such as bladder and rectum
   3. Metastasizes to lungs, bones, and liver

C. Signs and symptoms
   1. Subjective
      a. Asymptomatic in early stage
      b. Menstrual disturbances
      c. Postmenopausal bleeding
      d. Bleeding after intercourse
      e. Watery discharge
   2. Suspicious Pap test result

D. Diagnostic tests/methods
   1. Pap smear
   2. Cervical biopsy examination
   3. Colposcopy
   4. Schiller's test
   5. Conization

E. Treatment
   1. Panhysterectomy (excision of uterus and cervix)
   2. Radiation in advanced case
   3. Chemotherapy

F. Nursing intervention
   1. Reassure patient and family that adjustment to illness can be slow
   2. Acknowledge that patient must adapt to illness according to her age, developmental stage, and past life experiences
   3. If patient is to receive internal radium implant
      a. Provide isolation
      b. Instruct patient to maintain supine or side-lying position
      c. Explain to patient and visitors that the amount of time spent with patient will be limited to avoid overexposure to radiation
      d. Provide high-protein, low-residue diet to avoid straining of bowels, which may dislodge implant
      e. Maintain high fluid intake: 2000 to 3000 ml daily
      f. Insert Foley catheter to prevent bladder distention
      g. Administer antiemetics as ordered
   4. If the patient undergoes surgery, follow general postoperative nursing actions
      a. Observe for vaginal hemorrhage, malodorous vaginal discharge, or any vaginal discharge other than serosanguineous discharge
      b. Observe for urinary retention
      c. Change perineal pads every 3 to 4 hours and prn
      d. Listen for renewed bowel sounds

BARTHOLIN CYSTS

A. Definition: a tumorlike capsule formed of retained secretions

B. Pathology
   1. May develop as a consequence of an earlier bacterial infection of these structures
   2. Formation of these cysts results from obstruction in the outlet of these glands

C. Signs and symptoms
   1. Subjective
      a. Pain on walking
      b. Dyspareunia
   2. Objective: mobile nodule

D. Diagnostic methods
   1. Pelvic examination
   2. Palpable nodule

E. Treatment
   1. Incision and drainage
   2. Antiseptic wound packing

F. Nursing intervention
   1. Reassure the patient that normal function of the gland will be regained after the procedure
   2. After surgery provide a sterile perineal pad q4h and prn
   3. Provide sterile wound care as ordered
   4. Instruct on perineal hygiene
   5. Provide sitz baths for increased circulation and comfort
   6. On patient's discharge from the hospital explain that the surgical wound is susceptible to bacterial infection until healing has taken place

FIBROCYSTIC BREAST DISEASE

A. Definition: fiberlike tumors of the breast tissue with cyst formation
B. Pathology
  1. Cause is unknown; possible hormonal imbalance
  2. Condition occurs during reproductive years and disappears with menopause
  3. A benign condition affecting 25% of women over 30 years of age
C. Signs and symptoms
  1. Subjective: breast tenderness and pain
  2. Objective: small, round, smooth nodules
D. Diagnostic tests/methods
  1. Mammography
  2. Thermomastography
  3. Xerography
E. Treatment: Conservative
  1. Aspiration
  2. Biopsy examination to rule out malignancy
F. Nursing intervention
  1. Explain importance of monthly breast self-examination
  2. Encourage patient to seek medical evaluation if nodule forms because cystic disease may interfere with early diagnosis of breast malignancy

CANCER OF THE BREAST

A. Definition: small, painless, fixed lump most frequently located in the upper, outer portion of the breast
B. Pathology
  1. Risk factors increase with age
  2. Influenced by heredity
  3. Sites of metastasis: lymph nodes, lungs, liver, bone, brain
  4. Other risk factors
    a. Obesity
    b. Diet high in fat and protein
    c. Nulliparity
    d. Parity after age 35
    e. Menarche before 11 years of age
    f. Menopause after 55 years of age
    g. History of cancer in one breast
C. Signs and symptoms
  1. Subjective: nontender nodule
  2. Objective:
    a. Enlarged axillary nodes
    b. Nipple retraction or elevation
    c. Skin dimpling
    d. Nipple discharge
D. Diagnostic tests/methods
  1. Mammography
  2. Thermography
  3. Xerography
  4. Breast biopsy examination
E. Treatment
  1. Lumpectomy: removal of the lump and partial breast tissue; indicated for early detection
  2. Mastectomy
    a. Simple mastectomy: removal of breast
    b. Modified radical mastectomy: removal of breast, pectoralis minor, and some of adjacent lymph nodes (the pectoralis major is preserved)

c. Radical mastectomy: removal of the breast, pectoral muscles, pectoral fascia, and nodes
  3. Oophorectomy, adrenalectomy, or hypophysectomy to remove source of estrogen and those hormones that stimulate the breast tissue
  4. Radiation therapy to destroy malignant tissue
  5. Chemotherapeutic agents to shrink, retard, and destroy cancer growth
  6. Corticosteroids, androgens, and antiestrogens to alter cancer that is dependent on hormonal environment
F. Nursing intervention
  1. Provide atmosphere of acceptance, frequent patient contact, and encouragement in illness adjustment
  2. Introduce a person who has successfully undergone the same experience: arrange contact from Reach to Recovery representative
  3. Encourage grooming activities such as hair, nails, teeth, and skin
  4. Arrange attractive environment
  5. If the patient is receiving radiation or chemotherapy, explain and assist her with potential side effects
    a. Nausea and vomiting
    b. Anorexia
    c. Diarrhea
    d. Stomatitis
    d. Malaise
    f. Itching
    g. Hair loss (alopecia)
  6. If the patient has undergone surgical intervention, follow postoperative nursing actions
    a. Elevate affected arm above level of right atrium to prevent edema
    b. Drawing blood or administering parenteral fluids or taking blood pressure on affected arm is contraindicated
    c. Monitor dressing for hemorrhage; observe back for pooling of blood
    d. Empty Hemovac and measure drainage q8h
    e. Assess circulatory status of affected limb
    f. Measure upper arm and forearm, bid, to monitor edema
    g. Encourage exercises of the affected arm when approved by physician; avoid abduction
      (1) Brushing hair
      (2) Squeezing ball
      (3) Feeding self
  7. Patient teaching on discharge
    a. Exercise to tolerance
    b. Sleep with arm elevated
    c. Elevate arm several times daily
    d. Avoid injections, vaccinations, and taking of blood pressure in affected arm
    e. Never allow blood to be drawn from or IV started in affected arm

PAGET'S DISEASE OF THE BREAST

A. Definition: cancer of the nipple
B. Pathology
  1. Rare occurrence affecting women over 40 years of age
  2. Spreads from nipple to areola to part of the breasts; ulcerates

C. Signs and symptoms
  1. Subjective
    a. Itching
    b. Swelling
  2. Objective
    a. Blistering
    b. Discharge
    c. Nipple retraction
D. Diagnostic method: biopsy examination
E. Treatment: mastectomy
F. Nursing intervention: refer to nursing intervention as previously outlined under Cancer of the breast, p. 242

SEXUALLY TRANSMITTED INFECTIOUS DISEASES (STDS)
SYPHILIS

A. Description: caused by a spirochete, *Treponema pallidum;* appears in three stages; transmitted through sexual contact or warm blood
  1. Primary stage: after an incubation period of 10 to 60 days (usually 3 weeks), during which there are no symptoms, an ulcer or chancre appears at the site of entry; it contains many organisms and is highly infectious; there may be minor local discomfort or mild generalized symptoms (e.g., headache or lymph node enlargement); without treatment it heals in 3 to 5 weeks
  2. Secondary stage: 3 weeks later it appears as a mild rash on skin (usually palms of hands and soles of feet) and as papules on mucous membranes; all lesions contain organisms and are highly contagious; symptoms may be mild or generalized (e.g., bone pain, sore throat, hair loss in patches, or lymph node changes); lasts a few weeks and becomes dormant if not treated; patient is infectious for about 1 year
  3. Third or latent stage: 10 to 30 years later the spirochetes, which have been deposited in tissues and organs are in lesions (gummas); these destroy the tissue; common sites are the CNS, eyes, and the aorta
B. Signs and symptoms: relate to organ involved (e.g., aortic aneurysm)
C. Diagnostic tests/methods
  1. Primary stage: microscopic examination of smear
  2. Second and third stages: blood serum tests (e.g., VDRL and Wassermann)
D. Treatment: penicillin or tetracycline (patient and partner)

GONORRHEA

A. Definition: a highly communicable disease; there is inflammation of the urethra and spread to other organs of the genital tract; incubation period is 3 to 4 days
B. Cause: *Neisseria gonorrhoeae,* transmitted by sexual contact
C. Signs and symptoms
  1. Female patients may have no early symptoms or purulent vaginal discharge, dysuria, or urgency; untreated, it may spread to other organs in the pelvic cavity (see discussion of Pelvic imflammatory disease [PID], p. 239)
  2. Male patients have purulent urethral discharge and burning on urination; may develop urethral stricture; epididymitis, prostatitis
D. Diagnostic tests/methods

  1. Patient history and physical examination
  2. Smear or culture
E. Treatment: penicillin or tetracycline; ceftriaxone (a cephalosporin) for penicillinase-resistant strains

HERPES GENITALIS

A. Description: fluid-filled vesicles on genitalia form crusts, causing generalized symptoms such as elevated temperature; pain; may have no symptoms; there are recurrent episodes; problems arise in pregnancy; is believed to predispose to cervical cancer
B. Cause: herpesvirus hominis type 2 HSV
C. Treatment: symptomatic; topical or oral antiviral agents (acyclovir [Zovirax]); no cure
D. Recommend use of barrier forms of contraception

CHLAMYDIA TRACHOMATIS

A. Definition: most common STD in the United States; causes symptoms similar to gonorrheal infections
B. Cause: *Chlamydia trachomatis*
C. Signs and symptoms
  1. Males: urethritis, dysuria, frequency, watery mucoid discharge; complications include epididymitis, prostatitis, infertility
  2. Females: often asymptomatic; mucopurulent cervicitis, dysuria, frequency, local soreness; complications include salpingitis, PID, ectopic pregnancy, and infertility
D. Diagnostic tests/methods: urogenital smear analysis for enzyme or antibody
E. Treatment: antibiotic therapy (doxycycline, tetracycline, erythromycin)

CONDYLOMATA ACUMINATA

A. Definition: also referred to as genital/venereal warts; often seen with other STDs such as gonorrhea and trichomoniasis; highly contagious
B. Cause: human papilloma virus (HPV)
C. Signs and symptoms: initially single, small papillary growths that grow into large cauliflower-like masses, profuse foul-smelling vaginal discharge, bleeding; may progress to genital and cervical dysplasia, cancer
D. Diagnostic tests/methods: inspection of urinary meatus, vulva, labia, vagina, cervix, penis, scrotum, anus, perineum; culture and biopsy
E. Treatment
  1. Cryotherapy with liquid nitrogen or cryoprobe
  2. Laser therapy
  3. Acid treatments
  4. Surgery
  5. Chemotherapy (5FU)

TRICHOMONIASIS/CANDIDIASIS

A. Definition: very common STD; symptoms frequently seen only in women
B. Cause: *Trichomonas vaginalis* and *Candida albicans,* respectively
C. Signs and symptoms: itching; discharge
D. Diagnostic tests/methods: culture and inspection of affected tissues
E. Treatment: antifungals; antiprotozoal drugs (metronidazole [Flagyl])

INTEGUMENTARY SYSTEM
Anatomy and Physiology

A. Structure of skin: (Fig. 5-24) includes epithelial, connective, and nerve tissue; consists of sweat and oil glands; is soft and has elasticity
1. Epidermis: outermost layer; cells are flat and tough; no blood supply
   a. Cells undergo constant cellular change by mitosis
   b. Contains pigment (melanin); amount of pigment varies among races and individuals
2. Dermis: "true skin"; the inner layer, composed of living cells
   a. Connective tissue framework
   b. Contains blood vessels, nerves, hair roots, and oil and sweat glands
   c. The ridges and grooves form the pattern for fingerprints, unique to each individual
   d. Nerve endings provide sensation (touch)
      (1) Receptors: small, round bodies (tactile corpuscles)
      (2) Located in dermis; numerous in tips of fingers, toes, and tongue
      (3) Allows perception of heat, cold, and pain
3. Subcutaneous tissue: lies under dermis
   a. Contains fat cells, which give the skin its smooth appearance
   b. Serves as a shock absorber and insulates deeper tissues
4. Glands
   a. Sebaceous (oil glands)
      (1) Excrete oily substance (sebum)
      (2) Keep skin soft and moist
   b. Sudorifeous (sweat glands)
      (1) Secrete perspiration
      (2) Part of the body's heating and regulating equipment
5. Appendages
   a. Hair: covers the skin except on the palms of the hands and the soles of the feet; composed of dead keratinized cells
      (1) Shaft: the hair above the skin
      (2) Follicle: a tiny sac from which the hair root grows
   b. Nails: tightly packed cells of scaly epidermis
      (1) Roots are living cells; visible ends are dead cells
      (2) They protect the tips of the fingers and toes
      (3) The pink coloring comes from the blood supply in the nail bed
B. Functions
   1. Protection: protects deeper tissues from pathogenic organisms and harmful chemicals
   2. Excretion: limited to water and urea; only a small amount of waste products are eliminated
   3. Regulation: helps regulate body temperature and fluid content
   4. Sensory: contains millions of nerve endings that provide sensory reception to pressure, touch, pain, and temperature
   5. Vitamin D production—effect of sunlight
C. Effects of aging: skin, hair, nails (Table 5-7)

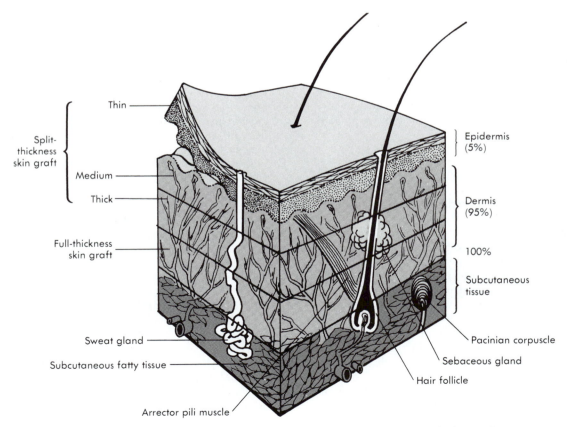

Figure 5-24. **Structures of the skin and skin layers.** (From Long et al: *Medical-surgical nursing: a nursing process approach,* ed 3, St Louis, 1993, Mosby.)

Table 5-7	Changes from Aging in Skin, Hair, and Nails	
Parameters	**Observable changes**	**Cause**
Skin		
Color	Paleness in white skin	Decreased vascularity of dermis; loss of melanocytes
	Brown spots (senile lentigines)	Hyperpigmentation
	Purple patches (senile purpura)	Blood leaking from poorly supported, fragile capillaries
Moisture	Dry skin, decreased perspiration	Decreased sebaceous and sweat gland activity
Elasticity, turgor	Decreased elasticity	Loss of collagen and elastic fibers
	Loose folds and wrinkles	
	Decreased turgor	
Texture	Some rough areas	Environmental effects over time and decreased moisture
	Thinner, more transparent skin	Thinning of epidermis from decreased vascularity of dermis; loss of underlying tissue
Hair		
Color	Grayness	Decreased number of melanocytes in hair
Consistency	Thinner on head and body	Decreased density and rate of hair growth
	Coarser in nose of men	Increased density of nasal hair
Distribution	Loss of hair on head and body	Decreased rate of hair growth; decreased hormones; decreased peripheral circulation
	Increased hair on face of women	Higher androgen-to-estrogen ratio
Nails	More brittle	Slowing of nail growth; decreased peripheral circulation
	Longitudinal ridges	
	Thickening and yellowing of toenails	

From Long et al: *Medical surgical nursing: a nursing process approach*, ed 3, St Louis, 1993, Mosby.

Conditions/Disorders of the Integumentary System

The skin is the body's barrier and protection from the environment. It prevents loss of body fluids and protects tissues and organs from external injury and organisms. Temperature regulation, sensation, and excretion of small amounts of water and sodium chloride are functions of the skin. Maximum health and healing of the skin are maintained by proper nutrition, hydration, electrolyte balance, exercise, and rest. Problems arise from systemic allergies (e.g., food and medication, exposure to external irritants such as chemicals, plants, and cosmetics, exposure to sun, parasites, microorganisms, injury, and new growths).

The following terms are used to describe skin lesions:

atheroma fatty patch or thickening on skin

bleb blister filled with fluid

bulla large blister filled with fluid, as occurs with burns

comedo blackhead or acne

cyst sac or capsule containing fluid or semisolid material (e.g., sebaceous cyst of scalp)

erythema red area (e.g., sunburn)

excoriation abrasion of the outer layer of skin (e.g., friction trauma)

exudate fluid, usually containing pus, bacteria, and dead cells (e.g., fluid from infected wound)

fissure groove, crack, or slit as occurs with ulceration

furuncle painful erythematous raised lesion (e.g., boil)

hive solid, raised, and itchy area (wheal), usually the result of allergy

macule small, flat discolored area (e.g., freckle)

maculopapular multiple lesions consisting of both macules and papules (e.g., early chickenpox)

mole flat or raised pigmented growth (e.g., birthmark)

nevus congenital raised, pigmented growth (e.g., birthmark or mole)

nodule small, solid mass (e.g., swollen lymph node)

papule small, red, raised elevation (e.g., measles)

petechia red pinpoint hemorrhage; seen in some blood diseases

pustule small elevation on the skin containing purulent fluid (e.g., acne)

ulcer depression (e.g., open lesion on skin)

urticaria hives (e.g., blood transfusion reaction)

vesicle small sac containing serous or sanguineous fluid (e.g., pimple)

wheal raised lesion, usually accompanied by itching (e.g., mosquito bite)

Nursing Assessment

A. Nursing observations
   1. Skin
      a. Color: any deviation from normal, (e.g., pallor, cyanosis, jaundice, or blanching)
      b. Turgor: evaluate hydration and elasticity
      c. Lesions and rashes: size, location, color, drainage, and crusts
      d. Skin temperature for inconsistency: areas cool or warm to the touch

e. Cleanliness and hygiene
f. Odor
g. Pressure areas for existing or potential decubitus ulcers
2. Hair and scalp
a. Unusual distribution or absence of scalp and body hair; lesions
b. Texture: smooth or coarse
c. Parasites: scalp and pubic
3. Nails
a. Cleanliness
b. Brittleness
c. Length
B. Patient description (subjective data)
1. History to include onset, changes, and presence of itching, pain, or burning
2. Factors that make condition worse/better
3. Allergies
4. Recent changes in environment and diet
5. Medications taken
6. Concerns about appearance, change in body image, and disfigurement
7. Changes in activities or life-style caused by disease

Frequent Patient Problems and Nursing Care

A. Body image disturbance related to disfigurement
1. Show acceptance by being nonjudgmental
2. Plan time to allow patient to express feelings
B. Pain related to pruritus (itching)
1. Administer antipruritics and antihistamines (see Chapter 3)
2. Keep nails short
3. Use cotton bedding and clothing; avoid rough fabrics
4. Encourage use of cotton gloves when sleeping
5. Bathe with tepid water; use minimal soap; pat dry using no friction
6. Give oil, medicated, or starch baths
C. Risk for infection/injury related to open lesions
1. Use aseptic technique in cleaning
2. Maintain isolation only if patient is infectious
3. Use dressings only when necessary and apply loosely with gauze and nonallergenic tape
D. Impaired skin integrity related to seborrhea: oily scalp with shedding of greasy scales
1. Give frequent shampoos
2. Use medicated shampoos; rinse thoroughly

Major Medical Diagnoses

CONTACT DERMATITIS

A. Definition: an inflammatory response of the skin with redness, edema, thickening of the skin, and frequent scaling; there may be vesicles and papules
B. Cause: an allergic reaction or unusual sensitivity when a substance comes in direct contact with the skin (e.g., poison ivy, soaps, cleaning agents, and fabrics)
C. Symptoms: pruritus; erythema
D. Diagnostic test/methods
1. Allergy testing
2. Patient history and assessment
E. Treatment
1. Systemic medication: antihistamines, antipruritics, and corticosteroids (see Chapter 3)

2. Topical medication: corticosteroids (see Chapter 3)
3. Remove cause
F. Nursing intervention
1. Prevent scratching
2. Give tepid baths
3. Cut nails
4. Administer prn medications as soon as possible

PSORIASIS

A. Definition: a chronic condition in which there are patches of inflammation that are red and covered with silvery scales that shed; these usually occur on elbows, knees, lower back, and scalp; they may cover the entire body
B. Cause: unknown, may be a family tendency, symptoms increase during stress and high anxiety; other related factors are alcoholism, trauma, and infection
C. Signs and symptoms
1. Pruritus, mild to severe
2. Depression related to appearance
D. Diagnostic methods: patient history and physical appearance
E. Treatment (individual)
1. Topical medication: coal tars and corticosteroids (see Chapter 3)
2. Systemic medication: corticosteroids and methotrexate (in severe cases) (see Chapter 3)
3. Exposure to ultraviolet light; photochemotherapy
4. Anxiolytics
5. Antimetabolites
F. Nursing intervention
1. During bath gently remove scales with cloth or brush
2. Occlusive dressing may be wrapped in plastic

HERPES SIMPLEX (COLD SORE/FEVER BLISTER) TYPE I (HSV-I)

A. Definition: a group of blisters on a reddened base usually on or near mouth or genitalia
B. Cause: a viral infection precipitated by an upper respiratory tract infection or elevation of temperature from systemic infection; frequently related to emotional upset, menstrual cycle, or general immunosuppression
C. Signs and symptoms
1. Pain and local discomfort
2. Distress about appearance
D. Diagnostic methods: physical assessment; viral isolation by tissue culture
E. Treatment: lasts about 1 week; antiviral agents (acyclovir) administered topically or systemically
F. Nursing intervention: none indicated

HERPES ZOSTER (SHINGLES)

A. Definition: crops of vesicles and erythema following sensory nerves on face and trunk; higher incidence in the elderly
B. Cause: varicella zoster virus (chickenpox)
C. Signs and symptoms
1. Severe pain
2. Elevation of temperature
3. Malaise
4. Anorexia
5. Pruritus
D. Diagnostic methods: physical examination; vesicles follow sensory nerve paths
E. Treatment: no specific treatment (symptomatic only); analgesics may be used for pain; usually subsides in 3 weeks

(pain may last for months); antivirals, corticosteroids, antibiotics (capsaicin [Zostrix])
F. Nursing intervention
1. Keep patient in isolation while vesicles are present
2. Apply topical lotions to lesions for itching
3. Give baths or compresses for cooling and soothing
4. Prevent scratching and secondary infection
5. Anticipate pain: medicate as needed
6. Provide small, frequent, well-balanced meals
G. Varicella vaccine (Varivax)

NEOPLASMS
A. Definition: any new and abnormal growth; may be of varied size and location
B. Cause
1. Benign: unknown
2. Malignant: related to exposure to the sun and chemical and physical irritants, such as pipe smoking
C. Signs and symptoms: anxiety: related to diagnosis and change in physical appearance
D. Diagnostic test: biopsy examination: high cure rate with early detection
E. Treatment: see Table 5-8
F. Nursing intervention
1. Assess all patients for skin lesions
2. Discuss with patient the importance of reporting any changes in moles
3. Give general preoperative and postoperative care (see Chapter 2)
4. Provide general care for patient receiving radiotherapy (see Chapter 2)
5. Give general care for patient receiving chemotherapy (see Chapter 3)
G. Classification of common skin tumors (Table 5-8)

BURNS
A. Definition: a wound in which the skin layers and underlying tissue is destroyed
B. Causes
1. Heat—dry or moist (e.g., fire)
2. Chemical (e.g., acids)
3. Electrical (e.g., lightning or electrical wires)
4. Radiation (e.g., sun)
5. Mechanical (e.g., friction from rope)
C. Signs and symptoms: depend on depth (Table 5-9) and area involved
1. Infection: there is destruction of the body's first line of defense and time postburn (hypovolemic and diuretic stage)
2. Loss of body tissue (protein)
3. Loss of fluid and electrolytes (edema)
4. Pain
5. Respiratory distress
6. Immobilization
7. Disfigurement
8. Impending shock
D. Diagnostic methods: physical assessment
E. Treatment
1. Respiratory evaluation, maintenance of airway, and possible tracheostomy; edema of lung tissue from smoke inhalation may cause increased secretions
2. Replacement of fluids and electrolytes with IV solutions: plasma, blood, dextran, and electrolytes
3. Emergency wound care: removal of foreign material; avoidance of contamination
4. Prevention of infection: tetanus immune globlin and antibiotics
5. Analgesics for pain (see Chapter 3)

Table 5-8 Classification of Common Tumors of the Skin

Classification	Description	Treatment
Benign	Nevus, brown or black mole	Observe for changes: remove only if irritated or changes are observed
Premalignant or potentially malignant	Senile keratosis: brownish scaly spots on face and hands of aging persons	Surgical removal or topical medication or cryosurgery
	Leukoplakia: shiny white patches on mucous membranes of mouth and female genitalia	Removal of irritating teeth; oral hygiene. For genitalia: surgical excision; biopsy
	Moles (nevi) that bleed, grow, or are irritated or crusted	May become malignant and are surgically removed
	Black, smooth moles	
Malignant	Squamous cell carcinoma: begin as a warty growth and grow and become ulcerated; found on exposed surfaces of the body (tongue and lip)	Early surgical removal
	Basal cell carcinoma: a slow-growing tumor; results from exposure to the sun	Chemosurgery, electrosurgery, or surgical removal
	Malignant melanoma: black tumor that metastasized	Widespread excision

Table 5-9	**Description of Burns**		
Classification	**Depth**	**Description**	**Possible cause**
Superficial or shallow partial thickness	Epidermis	Red and dry; painful; may have edema; no scarring	Sunburn
Deep partial thickness	Epidermis and some dermis	Mottled, pink to red blisters; painful; leave scar	Hot oil
Full thickness partial	Epidermis, dermis, and subcutaneous tissue	Black or bright red eschar forms leathery covering; leaves scar; may have no pain	Fire
Full thickness deep	All of the above plus subcutaneous fat, fascia, muscle, and bone (nerve endings, hair follicles, and sweat glands are destroyed)	Black; there is no pain	Fire

6. Prevention of shock: plasma expanders; keep patient warm; monitor vital signs, urine output
7. Wound treatment method
   a. Open method exposure; wound heals by epithelialization of eschar; this method requires reverse isolation; eschar must be removed by debridement (cutting away), whirlpool baths, and escharotomy (incision into eschar)
   b. Topical medications (see Chapter 3)
   c. Grafts: to minimize infection and fluid loss; may be temporary because they are frequently rejected; this method allows for growth of new tissue underneath the protection of the graft
      (1) Autograft: transplantation of skin from patient's own body; care must also be given to donor site; can also grow skin in test tube, then do graft procedure
      (2) Homograft (allograft): transplantation of tissue from living human
      (3) Heterograft: transplantation from animal (pig or cow—xenograft)
      (4) Synthetic material used in grafting
   d. Cosmetic surgery may be performed during recovery phase
F. Nursing intervention
   1. Anticipate and prevent respiratory distress; maintain airway, monitor breathing qh then q4h (see Chapter 2); keep tracheostomy equipment available
   2. Maintain fluid balance: monitor IV fluids; monitor urine output qh through indwelling catheter; monitor sp gr qh; weigh patient qd
   3. Anticipate infection: maintain asepsis and reverse isolation; administer antibiotics; monitor temperature q2h; keep patient warm
   4. Anticipate pain: give frequent sedation as ordered, especially before dressing change (administered intravenously during early phase of treatment)
   5. Prevent dangers of immobilization (see Chapter 2); provide proper alignment to prevent deformities (may be uncomfortable or painful); prevent skin surfaces from touching; use turning frames and cradles

6. To enhance tissue repair, diet must be high in calories (6000 calories qd) and high in protein; tube feeding or total parenteral nutrition may be necessary
7. Anticipate shock: assess level of consciousness and mental status; monitor pulse rate and blood pressure
8. Anticipate Curling's ulcer (stress ulcer): at the end of the first week assess for gastrointestinal distress or bleeding
9. Be aware of anxiety: provide diversional activities; allow time for patient to verbalize feelings; encourage contact with family; involve patient as much as possible with planning and self-care; administer tranquilizers and sedation as necessary

SENSORY SYSTEMS
VISUAL SYSTEM
Anatomy and Physiology (Figs. 5-25, 5-26)
A. Lies in a protective bony orbit in the skull
B. Eyebrows, eyelids, and lashes also protect the eye
C. Sphere consists of three layers of tissue
   1. Sclera: thick, white fibrous tissue (white of eye); a transparent section over the front of the eyeball, the cornea, permits light rays to enter
   2. Choroid: the middle vascular area: brings oxygen and nutrients to the eye: choroid extends to ciliary body (two smooth muscle structures), which helps control shape of the lens; the front is a pigmented section (iris), which gives the eye color; in the center of the iris lies the pupil, the "window of the eye" (allows light to pass to lens and retina)
   3. Retina: inner layer; physiology of vision takes place; contains receptors of optic nerve; neurons are shaped like rods and cones; cones permit perception of color, rods permit perception of light and shade
D. Chambers
   1. Anterior: contains aqueous humor, maintains slight forward curve in cornea
   2. Posterior: contains vitreous humor: maintains spherical shape of eyeball

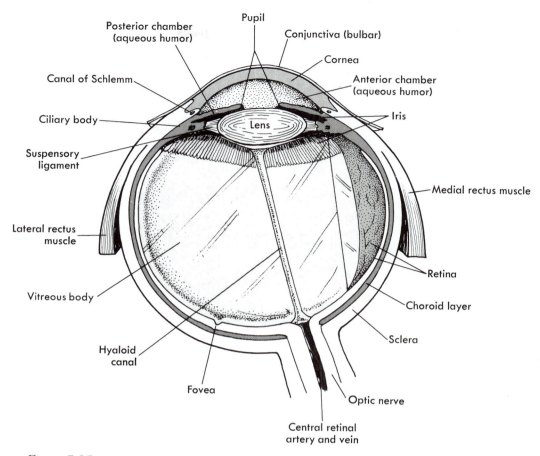

Figure 5-25. **Horizontal section through left eyeball.** (From Phipps et al: *Medical-surgical nursing: concepts and clinical practice,* ed 5, St Louis, 1995, Mosby.)

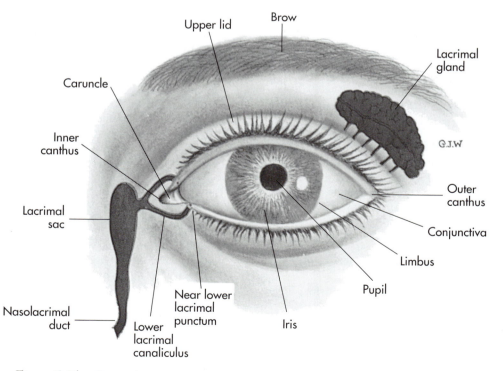

Figure 5-26. **External eye structures** (From Long et al: *Medical-surgical nursing: a nursing process approach,* ed 3, St Louis, 1993, Mosby.)

E. Conjunctiva: mucous membrane that covers eyeball and eyelid; keeps eyeball moist
F. Lens: transparent structure behind iris; focuses light rays on retina
G. Lacrimal apparatus: gland located in upper, outer part of eye; produces tears to lubricate and cleanse; nasolacrimal duct is located in nasal corner, tears drain into nose
H. Normal intraocular pressure: 10 to 21 torr (mm Hg)

Conditions/Disorders of the Eye

Sight is the most important sense to most people. Visual acuity is dependent on general good health, CNS regulation of movement and conduction, and condition of the structures of the eye. Changes in vision are frequently indicative of systemic disease; routine examination of the eye can provide information about diseases in other systems. The nurse must assess the eyes of each patient under his or her care. Although the incidence of blindness and visual impairment increases with age, problems are seen in patients of all ages.

Nursing Assessment

A. Nursing observations
  1. Glasses, contact lenses, or false eyes
  2. Tearing, discharge (clear or purulent), and color of sclera (white, yellow, or pink)
  3. Accuracy and range of vision
  4. Edema of eyelids; crusting; blinking, rubbing; redness
  5. Clouded appearance over pupil; protrusion or bulging of eye(s); pupil response to light
  6. Squinting or drooping (ptosis) of lid
  7. Symmetry
B. Patient description (subjective data)
  1. Double vision (diplopia), decreased or absent vision in one or both eyes, or blurred or clouded vision
  2. Sensitivity to light (photophobia), spots, halos around lights, flashes of light, or problems seeing in the dark
  3. Eye fatigue, itching, pain, tearing, burning, or headache
C. Note patient history of
  1. Stumbling
  2. Trauma of face or eyes
  3. Contact lenses or eye medication
  4. Changes in vision and any related circumstances
  5. Any systemic medications taken

Diagnostic Tests/Methods

A. Ophthalmoscope: assessment of the interior of eye
B. Tonometer: measurement of intraocular pressure; increased pressure may indicate early glaucoma; recommended every 3 years for individuals between 35 and 40 years of age and on a yearly basis for individuals over 40
C. Fields of vision: testing to measure sight on one or both sides (peripheral vision); perimetry
D. Refraction: measurement of light refraction and lenses required for visual acuity
E. Slit lamp: examination of intraocular structures with a high-intensity light beam (corneal abrasions, iritis)
F. Snellen chart: assessment of visual acuity
G. Retinal angiography: retinal vessels

Eye Care Professionals

A. Ophthalmologist (also called *oculist*): a medical doctor who specializes in diagnosis, treatment, and surgery of the eyes, including the prescribing of glasses
B. Optometrist: educated and licensed to test for refractive problems; may prescribe and fit glasses; may, within limits, diagnose disease, prescribe medication, or treat eye diseases (laws vary among states)
C. Optician: fills prescription for corrective lenses as prescribed by physician; fits glasses properly

Frequent Patient Problems and Nursing Care

A. Anxiety/fear related to concerns about loss of vision, altered lifestyles, ability to function, employment, plans for the future, and altered body image: allow time for the patient to express feelings
B. Risk for infection related to drainage
  1. Clean as necessary with normal saline solution
  2. Gently apply compresses to loosen if necessary
  3. Use aseptic technique; wipe from inner canthus to outer canthus
  4. If drainage is purulent, dispose of properly
C. Risk for injury related to need for corrective lenses
  1. Glasses must be kept clean and in a protective case
  2. Contact lenses are kept in a case with *R* and *L* to designate which eye the lens fits; obtain directions for soaking from patient
  3. If patient is dependent on lenses, obtain permission for patient to wear glasses or lenses when going for diagnostic tests
D. Risk for injury related to photophobia
  1. Keep room dim and evenly lighted
  2. Keep blinds adjusted to avoid glare

Major Medical Diagnoses

LOW VISION
A. Definition: low vision refers to defects that cannot be corrected with lenses
B. Cause: disease of the eye itself, in the visual pathways to the brain, or in the receptors in the brain
C. Signs and symptoms: vision may be blurred and images distorted; vision may be clear only at close range; shades of color may not be distinguishable

TOTAL OR LEGAL BLINDNESS
A. Definition: legal blindness is the ability to see at no more than 20 feet (6 m) what normally should be seen at a distance of 200 feet (60 m)(20/200); this may also refer to severe restrictions in peripheral fields of vision (after corrective lenses are used)
B. Pathology
  1. Degeneration, glaucoma, detached retina, or diabetic retinopathy
  2. Trauma or laceration
  3. Inflammation or optic neuritis
  4. Vascular or hypertensive retinopathy
  5. Neoplasms of the brain or eye
  6. Cataract
C. Patient problems
  1. Inability to care for self (dependency)
  2. Frustration
  3. Occupational hazards
  4. Boredom
D. Nursing intervention
  1. Allow as much independence as possible; help make use of existing vision; encourage use of any visual aids

recommended by physician (e.g., special lenses, large-type books, and cane); provide reading material in braille for the patient who has learned this method
2. Do not touch patient without talking; always address patient by name; introduce yourself; and tell patient when you are leaving the room
3. Explain all care and treatments; encourage patient to participate in planning care
4. At mealtime, indicate position of utensils and placement of food on dish by comparing it to numbers on a clock (e.g., "the potato is at 3 o'clock")
5. Orient patient to room and entire unit; point out hazards and obstacles (doors and windows); explain location of furniture, bathroom, call bell, and telephone; keep things in the same place
6. Leave bedside table, call bell, and personal items in close reach
7. Maintain safety; keep unit uncluttered, floor clean and dry, bed in low position, and side rail(s) up as necessary; tell patient position of bed and side rails
8. Guide the ambulatory patient by placing patient's arm on yours while walking slowly
9. Provide diversion: radio and books on tapes; be aware of local agencies in your community; many libraries have braille books or tapes available

REFRACTIVE DISORDERS
A. Definition: inability of the refractory media to converge light rays and focus on retina
  1. Myopia (nearsightedness): the eyeball is too long; light rays focus at a point before reaching the retina
  2. Hyperopia (farsightedness): the eyeball is shorter than normal; light rays focus beyond the retina
  3. Presbyopia: a gradual loss of elasticity of the lens; there is decreased ability to focus on near objects
  4. Astigmatism: unequal curve in the shape of the cornea or lens; vision is distorted
B. Cause: unknown; may be inherited
C. Symptoms: diminished or blurred vision
D. Diagnostic tests/methods
  1. Patient history
  2. Refraction
E. Treatment: corrective lenses (glasses or contact lenses); keratorefractive surgery
F. Nursing intervention
  1. Encourage proper care of lenses
  2. Encourage follow-up checkups as indicated

CONJUNCTIVITIS
A. Definition: infection or inflammation of the conjunctiva
B. Causes: bacteria, usually *Staphylococcus,* allergens, chemical reactions, and chlamydial or viral infections
C. Patient problems
  1. Very contagious (especially in young children)
  2. Purulent drainage and itching
  3. Photophobia
  4. Tearing
D. Diagnostic method: physical assessment; culture and sensitivity of conjunctival scrapings
E. Treatment: ophthalmic antibiotics (see Chapter 3)
F. Nursing intervention
  1. Prevent transmission to others: encourage frequent hand washing

2. Provide warm compresses; cleanse eyelids; remove crusts before administering ophthalmic medications
  a. Discourage rubbing of eyes
  b. Isolate personal items (towels, washcloths, and pillowcases)

CATARACT
A. Definition: the crystalline lens becomes clouded and opaque (not transparent)
B. Causes
  1. Trauma
  2. Congenital
  3. Related to diabetes
  4. High incidence in the elderly (senile cataracts)
  5. Heredity
  6. Infections
  7. Longtime exposure to the sun; ultraviolet rays
C. Signs and symptoms
  1. Loss of vision
  2. Progressive blurring
  3. Haziness with eventual complete loss of sight
D. Diagnostic tests/methods
  1. Examination with ophthalmoscope
  2. Patient history
  3. Ultrasonography
E. Treatment: surgical removal of opaque lens, usually on an outpatient basis; after surgery, corrective lenses are necessary (glasses, contact lenses, or surgical implantation of an artificial lens [IOL])
F. Nursing intervention
  1. Give general preoperative care (see Chapter 2)
  2. Provide nursing care as for the patient with low vision
  3. Postoperative management depends on surgical procedure; be careful to adhere to physician's order; general principles: have patient avoid coughing, bending, or rapid head movements; provide bed rest for a specified time (usually 2 hours); keep patient flat or in low-Fowler's position; have patient deep breathe (avoid coughing); be sure patient avoids straining (give stool softener); help patient avoid vomiting (an antiemetic will be ordered; administer as needed); observe dressing; report pain or bleeding; position patient with unoperated side down

GLAUCOMA
A. Definition: intraocular pressure increases because of a disturbance in the circulation of aqueous humor; there is an imbalance between production and drainage as the angle of drainage closes
  1. Acute (closed-angle) glaucoma: dramatic onset of symptoms; immediate treatment is required, usually surgery
  2. Chronic (open-angle) glaucoma: symptoms progress slowly and are frequently ignored; if disease is not detected early, it may lead to permanent loss of vision
B. Pathology
  1. Familial tendency
  2. Related to age; incidence increases over 40 years of age
  3. Secondary to injuries and infections
C. Signs and symptoms
  1. Loss of peripheral vision (tunnel vision), halos around lights, and permanent loss of vision (a leading cause of blindness)

2. Pain, malaise, nausea, and vomiting
3. Pupils fixed and dilated
4. Reduced visual acuity at night

D. Diagnostic tests/methods
   1. History of symptoms
   2. Measurement of visual fields
   3. Measurement of intraocular pressure
   4. Gonioscopy: measures angle of the anterior chamber

E. Treatment
   1. Miotics to decrease intraocular pressure (see Chapter 3)
   2. Surgery: iridectomy (an incision through the cornea to remove part of the iris to allow for drainage); laser trabeculoplasty (relieves excess intraocular pressure); trabeculectomy (new opening made to bypass obstruction and facilitate flow of aqueous humor)
   3. Continued medical supervision

F. Nursing intervention
   1. Encourage patient to wear medical identification tag
   2. Administer eye medications on schedule
   3. Inform the patient to avoid drugs with atropine; discourage straining and lifting
   4. Give preoperative and postoperative care according to that for a patient with a cataract; pay careful attention to specifics in physician's orders

DETACHED RETINA

A. Definition: the sensory layer of the retina pulls away from the pigmented layer, vitreous humor may leak into the space occupying the position the retina normally assumes

B. Cause: usually unknown and spontaneous; may be related to sudden blow to the head or follow eye surgery (e.g., removal of cataract)

C. Signs and symptoms
   1. Loss of vision in affected area (may be complete loss)
   2. Painless
   3. Visual disturbance (blurring)
   4. Spots and flashes of light

D. Diagnostic tests/methods
   1. Patient history and physical assessment
   2. Retinal examination with ophthalmoscope
   3. Ultrasonography
   4. Slit lamp

E. Treatment: depends on area of detachment
   1. Bed rest
   2. Prevention of extension of detachment
   3. Mydriatics
   4. Surgical intervention: laser photocoagulation; cryopexy; diathermy; scleral buckling; pneumatic retinopexy, and vitrectomy

F. Nursing intervention
   1. Provide individual care according to location of detachment; physician's orders will be specific
   2. Maintain absolute rest; restrict activity; patch eye to limit eye movement; may use eye shield; patient position based on location of retinal detachment
   3. Prepare patient for postoperative care: inform patient that both eyes may be patched and he or she may be unable to see
   4. Postoperative care: position patient exactly as ordered; maintain eye patch(es); have patient deep breathe and avoid coughing; administer medication for pain; provide care as needed for a person with limited sight

G. Patient problems
   1. Anxiety related to possibility of permanent vision loss
   2. Self-care deficit related to imposed activity restrictions
   3. Pain related to surgical correction and unusual positioning

AUDITORY SYSTEM
Anatomy and Physiology (Figs. 5-27, 5-28)

A. External ear (pinna or auricle): outer, visible portion, shaped like a funnel; gathers sound and sends it into the auditory canal, which is lined with tiny hairs and secretes cerumen, a waxy substance; canal extends to the eardrum, also called the tympanic membrane

B. Middle ear: small, flattened space; contains three small bones called ossicles: malleus (hammer), incus (anvil), and stapes (stirrup); bones are mobile and vibrate; conduct sound waves; the eustachian tube extends into nasopharynx and equalizes the pressure in the middle ear to that of atmospheric pressure

C. Internal ear (labyrinth): vestibule; cochlea, snail-shaped bony tube, contains organ of Corti (organ of hearing); semicircular canals are the receptors for equilibrium and head movements

D. Function
   1. Transmission of sound waves; result is hearing
   2. Maintenance of equilibrium

Conditions of the Ear

Hearing problems are not as obvious initially during assessment as are many other problems. Hearing loss may be misinterpreted. Many people associate hearing aids with dependency or disfigurement or signs of aging and refuse to wear them. Yet the sense of hearing contributes to well-being and safety. This assessment (hearing) must be made for each patient cared for.

Nursing Assessment

A. Nursing observations
   1. Difficulty hearing or understanding verbal communication
   2. Not responding to loud or sudden noises
   3. Use of hearing aid, lip reading, or sign language
   4. Drainage, dried secretion, or deformities of the ear

B. Patient description (subjective data)
   1. Earache or headache
   2. Difficulty hearing (or lack of hearing) in one or both ears
   3. Itching, drainage, pressure or full feeling
   4. Ringing, buzzing, popping, or echoes
   5. Vertigo
   6. Medications taken

C. Note history of
   1. Ear infections
   2. Ear surgery
   3. Head injury
   4. Medication taken

Diagnostic Tests/Methods

A. Audiometry: a hearing test to determine ability to discriminate sounds, voices, and degrees of loudness and pitch

B. Otoscopy: visual examination of the ear canal and tympanic membrane

C. Weber's test: a tuning fork is struck and placed midline on the patient's forehead; the patient is asked where the sound

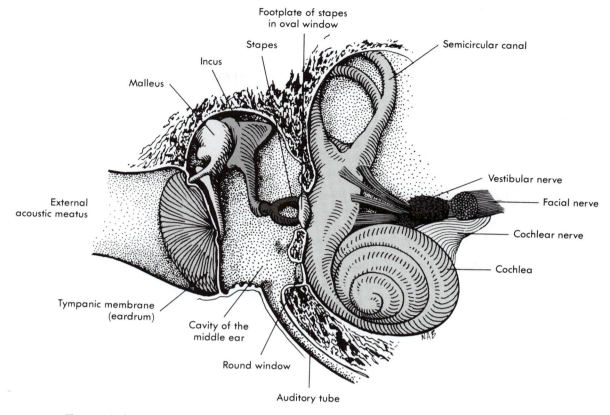

Footplate of stapes
in oval window

Stapes

Incus

Malleus

Semicircular canal

External
acoustic meatus

Vestibular nerve

Facial nerve

Cochlear nerve

Cochlea

Tympanic membrane
(eardrum)

Cavity of the
middle ear

Round window

Auditory tube

Figure 5-27. **Structures of the ear.** (From Long et al: *Medical-surgical nursing: a nursing process approach,* ed 3, St Louis, 1993, Mosby.)

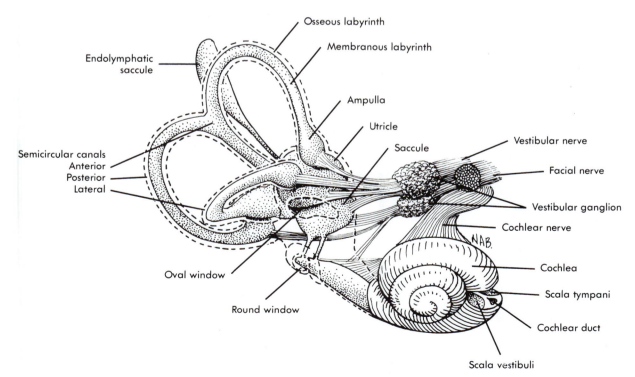

Osseous labyrinth

Membranous labyrinth

Endolymphatic
saccule

Ampulla

Utricle

Saccule

Vestibular nerve

Semicircular canals
Anterior
Posterior
Lateral

Facial nerve

Vestibular ganglion

Cochlear nerve

Cochlea

Oval window

Scala tympani

Round window

Cochlear duct

Scala vestibuli

Figure 5-28. **Structures of the inner ear.** (From Long et al: *Medical-surgical nursing: a nursing process approach,* ed 3, St Louis, 1993, Mosby.)

is heard; in this test of conduction, sounds should be heard equally well in each ear

D. Rinne test: the tuning fork is struck and placed on the mastoid process of the skull behind the ear; the fork is removed, and the patient indicates when the sound can no longer be heard; the still vibrating fork is then placed near the external ear canal; normally the sound will be heard longer through air conduction than through bone

E. Caloric stimulation test (CST): tests vestibular reflexes of the inner ear that control balance

F. Electronystagmography: monitors eye movements; done with CST

The Patient with Impaired Hearing

A. Definition
   1. Conductive hearing loss occurs when injury or disease interferes with the conduction of sound waves to the inner ear (e.g., cerumen in canal)
   2. Sensory hearing loss occurs when there is malfunction of the inner ear, auditory nerve, or auditory center in the brain (e.g., toxic effect to eighth cranial nerve from drugs [aspirin])
B. Patient problems
   1. Inability to communicate
   2. Inability to hear hazards in the environment (e.g., automobiles)
   3. Frustration, anxiety, anger, and insecurity
   4. Misinterpretation of communication
C. Treatment: according to cause (cochlear implants, stapedectomy); frequently none
D. Nursing intervention
   1. Find out if a hearing aid can be fitted
      a. Encourage patient to wear it
      b. Test batteries for function
      c. Make sure hearing aid is turned on
      d. Protect hearing aid from breakage; ask patient or family about usual care and storage
   2. Attract patient's attention before speaking
   3. Do not touch patient until he or she is aware that you are in the room
   4. Speak face to face; articulate clearly but not too slowly; move close to patient; avoid covering mouth with hand
   5. Provide alternate methods of communication
      a. Find out if patient lip-reads or uses sign language
      b. Provide magic slate or pad and pencil
   6. Nursing intervention after surgery
      a. Give general preoperative and postoperative care (see Chapter 2)
      b. Report drainage immediately
      c. Observe for facial nerve injury: inability to close eyes or pucker lips
      d. Anticipate vertigo: provide safety
      e. Be sure patient avoids blowing nose
      f. Note specific instructions from physician for positioning, activity, and diet

Major Medical Diagnoses

MÉNIÈRE'S SYNDROME

A. Definition: a chronic disease with sudden attacks of vertigo and tinnitus (ringing in the ear) with progressive hearing loss; attacks last a few minutes to a few weeks; usually occurs in women over 50 years of age

B. Cause: unknown; related to fluid in cochlea—either increased production or decreased absorption
C. Signs and symptoms
   1. Vertigo
   2. Nausea and vomiting
   3. Ringing in the ears and hearing loss
D. Diagnostic tests/methods: patient history; physical examination; neurologic assessment; CST; radiography; electronystagmography
E. Treatment
   1. Diuretics, low sodium diet, vasodilators, antihistamines, and antiemetics
   2. Surgery: endolymphatic shunt (reduces pressure and controls vertigo); destruction of the labyrinth as a last resort
F. Nursing intervention
   1. Bed rest; position of comfort
   2. Maintain quiet and safety
   3. Low-sodium diet
   4. Provide specific nursing care as that for patient with limited hearing (see above)
   5. Provide general preoperative and postoperative care (see Chapter 2)
   6. Provide nursing care for patient after ear surgery

MASTOIDITIS

A. Definition: infection of the mastoid process; may be acute or chronic; not common because of antibiotics
B. Cause: extension of middle ear infection that was inadequately treated
C. Signs and symptoms
   1. Elevation of temperature
   2. Headache, ear pain, and tenderness over mastoid process
   3. Drainage from ear
D. Treatment
   1. Antibiotics
   2. Surgery
      a. Simple mastoidectomy: removal of infected cells
      b. Radical mastoidectomy: more extensive excision resulting in some degree of hearing loss
E. Nursing intervention
   1. See above for Care of patient with impaired hearing
   2. Provide general preoperative and postoperative care (see Chapter 2)
   3. Provide nursing care for patient after ear surgery (see previous outline)

OTOSCLEROSIS

A. Definition: a progressive formation of new bone tissue around the stapes preventing transmission of vibrations to the inner ear
B. Cause: unknown
C. Signs and symptoms
   1. Loss of hearing
   2. Ringing or buzzing (tinnitus)
D. Treatment
   1. Hearing aid
   2. Surgery; stapedectomy (removal of diseased bone and replacement with prosthetic implant)
E. Nursing intervention
   1. Provide general care for patient who is hearing impaired (see previous outline)

2. Give general preoperative and postoperative care (see Chapter 2)
3. Follow specific orders from physician
4. Provide general nursing care for patient after ear surgery (see previous outline)

SUGGESTED READING

Applegate E: *The anatomy and physiology learning system: textbook,* Philadelphia, 1995, WB Saunders.

Burke SR: *Human anatomy and physiology in health and disease,* Albany, New York, 1992, Delmar.

Cole G: *Fundamental nursing concepts and skills,* ed 2, St Louis, 1996, Mosby.

Dirksen et al: *Clinical companion to medical surgical nursing,* St Louis, 1996, Mosby.

Elkin et al: *Nursing interventions and clinical skills,* St Louis, 1996, Mosby.

Harkness G, Dincher JR: *Medical surgical nursing: total patient care,* ed 9, St Louis, 1996, Mosby.

Harkness G, Dincher JR: *Workbook to accompany total patient care: foundations and practice of adult health nursing,* ed 9, St Louis, 1996, Mosby.

Hoeman SP: *Rehabilitation nursing: process and application,* ed 2, St Louis, 1995, Mosby.

Hole JW Jr: *Essentials of human anatomy and physiology,* ed 4, Dubuque, Iowa, 1992, WC Brown.

Long et al: *Medical-surgical nursing: a nursing process approach,* ed 3, 1993, Mosby.

Marieb E: *Human anatomy and physiology,* Menlo Park, Calif, 1996, Benjamin Cummings.

Memmler et al: *Structure and function of the human body,* ed 6, Philadelphia, 1996, Lippincott.

Mosby's medical, nursing and allied health dictionary, ed 4, St Louis, 1994, Mosby.

Perry AG, Potter PA: *Basic nursing: theory and practice,* ed 3, St Louis, 1995, Mosby.

Phipps et al: *Medical-surgical nursing: concepts and clinical practice,* ed 5, St Louis, 1995, Mosby.

Physicians' desk reference, Montreal, NJ, Medical Economics (published annually).

Scanlon V, Sanders T: *Essentials of anatomy and physiology,* ed 2, 1995, FA Davis.

Scherer JC: *Introductory medical-surgical nursing,* ed 6, Philadelphia, 1995, JB Lippincott.

Smeltzer SC, Bare BG: *Brunner's textbook of medical-surgical nursing,* ed 8, Philadelphia, 1996, JB Lippincott.

Tate P, Seeley RR: *Understanding the human body,* St Louis, 1994, Mosby.

Thibodeau GA: *Structure and function of the body,* ed 9, St Louis, 1992, Mosby.

Thompson et al: *Mosby's clinical nursing,* ed 3, St Louis, 1993, Mosby.

Tucker et al: *Patient care standards: nursing process, diagnosis and outcome,* ed 5, St Louis, 1996, Mosby.

REVIEW QUESTIONS

Answers and rationales begin on p. 274.

1. Formed elements in the blood that aid in blood clotting are called:
   ① Antibodies
   ② Leukocytes
   ③ Erythrocytes
   ④ Platelets

2. The body's continual response to changes in the external and internal environment is called:
   ① Homeostasis
   ② Diffusion
   ③ Osmosis
   ④ Filtration

3. The ability of a cell to reproduce is called:
   ① Osmosis
   ② Crenation
   ③ Lyse
   ④ Mitosis

4. The immunity that occurs when a person is given a substance containing antibodies or antitoxins is called:
   ① Active
   ② Autoimmune
   ③ Passive
   ④ Permanent

5. The part of the cell necessary for reproduction is the:
   ① Cytoplasm
   ② Nucleus
   ③ Protoplasm
   ④ Cytoplasmic membrane

6. The hormone that regulates the metabolic rate of body cells is:
   ① Oxytocin
   ② Aldosterone
   ③ Thyroxin
   ④ Cortisone

7. The ovaries produce the hormones:
   ① Estrogen and testosterone
   ② Progesterone and testosterone
   ③ Estrogen and progesterone
   ④ Progesterone and prolactin

8. A greater amount of body heat is lost when surface blood vessels:
   ① Contract
   ② Dilate
   ③ Increase the production of sweat
   ④ Help the skeletal muscles relax

9. The pigmented area surrounding the nipple is the:
   ① Areola
   ② Bartholin's gland
   ③ Cowper's gland
   ④ Urochrome

10. The hormone produced by the testes is:
    ① Progesterone
    ② Estrogen
    ③ Testosterone
    ④ Aldosterone

11. Connective tissue that attaches muscles to bones is called:
    ① Tendons
    ② Ligaments
    ③ Cartilage
    ④ Osseous

12. The lymphatic system is a collection of vessels and tissues that:
    ① Destroys enzymes
    ② Manufactures erythrocytes
    ③ Localizes infections and filters foreign cells
    ④ Filters and aids in blood clotting

13. A patient with a low hemoglobin level would be deficient in which of the following essential minerals:
    ① Copper
    ② Magnesium
    ③ Calcium
    ④ Iron

14. Bile is important in the digestive process because it:
    ① Dissolves meat fibers and makes them easier to digest
    ② Breaks down fat globules so they can be more easily digested
    ③ Digests simple fats and sugars
    ④ Changes complex sugars to glucose

15. The tissue that forms a protective covering for the body and lines the intestinal and respiratory tract is called:
    ① Periosteum
    ② Pericardium
    ③ Epithelial
    ④ Connective

16. Regurgitation of food is prevented by the:
    ① Cardiac sphincter
    ② Rugae
    ③ Chyme
    ④ Pyloric sphincter

17. Nutrients that the body uses are absorbed primarily in the:
    ① Liver
    ② Stomach
    ③ Small intestine
    ④ Large intestine

18. Muscles whose functions are to close off body openings are:
    ① Abductors
    ② Sphincters
    ③ Extensors
    ④ Flexors

19. Tears drain into the nose through the:
    ① Ciliary body
    ② Lacrimal gland
    ③ Eustachian tube
    ④ Nasolacrimal duct

20. The first eight deciduous teeth to appear through the gums of a baby are:
    ① Eye teeth
    ② Molars
    ③ Incisors
    ④ Canines

21. Respiration and heart rate are controlled by the:
    ① Cerebellum
    ② Cerebrum
    ③ Medulla
    ④ Pons

22. The main function of the large intestine is to:
    ① Absorb digested food
    ② Absorb water from waste material
    ③ Produce digestive enzymes
    ④ Secrete digestive enzymes

23. The movement that propels food down the digestive tract is called:
① Pylorospasm
② Rugae
③ Mastication
④ Peristalsis

24. The end product of protein metabolism is:
① Amino acids
② Ptyalin
③ Hydrochloric acid
④ Glucose

25. The completion of digestion occurs in the:
① Large intestine
② Stomach
③ Small intestine
④ Sigmoid

26. The function of the liver includes the following *except:*
① Production of digestive enzymes
② Detoxification of harmful substances
③ Manufacture of bile
④ Production of heparin and fibrinogen

27. To function adequately, the thyroid gland must have a sufficient supply of:
① Calcium
② Phosphorus
③ Iron
④ Iodine

28. The exchange of nutrients and waste products occurs in the:
① Capillaries
② Veins
③ Arterioles
④ Venules

29. The chamber of the heart that receives venous blood from body tissues is:
① Right atrium
② Left atrium
③ Right ventricle
④ Left ventricle

30. The hormone released by the medulla at times of an emergency is called:
① Insulin
② Aldosterone
③ Epinephrine
④ Testosterone

31. The reabsorption of water from the kidney tubules is promoted by:
① Oxytocin
② Calcitonin
③ Antidiuretic hormone (ADH)
④ Prolactin (PRL)

32. The exchange of oxygen and carbon dioxide in the lungs occurs in the:
① Bronchi
② Alveoli
③ Bronchioles
④ Venules

33. The pacemaker of the heart is the:
① AV node
② Bundle of His
③ Purkinje fibers
④ SA node

34. All arteries carry oxygenated blood with the exception of the:
① Pulmonary
② Aorta
③ Coronary
④ Carotid

35. Immunity occurring in the early months of an infant's life results from the functioning of which gland?
① Thyroid
② Thymus
③ Pineal
④ Pituitary

36. The large, rounded portion at the upper and lateral portion of the femur most often involved in hip fractures is the:
① Acetabulum
② Acromion
③ Greater trochanter
④ Olecranon process

37. The major function of the periosteum is to:
① Produce RBCs
② Produce yellow bone marrow
③ Provide a structure for blood, lymph, and nerves
④ Provide storage for adipose fat

38. The muscular structure that forms the floor of the pelvis is the:
① Peritoneum
② Perineum
③ Mons pubis
④ Rectus abdominis

39. Assessment of a patient's integumentary system includes checking:
① Blood pressure and pulse
② Blood sugar levels
③ Rashes, bruises, and decubitus
④ Rashes, bruises, and blood sugar levels

40. Observing that a teenager has many blackheads, you know one cause would be blockage of the:
① Ceruminous gland
② Lacrimal gland
③ Sebaceous gland
④ Sudoriferous gland

41. Normal urine has the following characteristics *except:*
① Clear, amber liquid
② Nitrogenous waste products
③ Slightly aromatic
④ High specific gravity

42. Grooves and ridges that make up fingerprints are located in the:
① Elastic skin tissue
② Subcutaneous layer of tissue
③ Upper surface of the dermis
④ Upper surface of the epidermis

43. The hormone that regulates blood composition and blood volume by acting on the kidney is:
① Antidiuretic (ADH)
② Aldosterone
③ Parathormone
④ Oxytocin

44. Muscles obtain energy from:
① Glycogen and acetylcholine
② Carbohydrates and lactic acid
③ Oxygen and acetylcholine
④ Oxygen and glycogen

45. An injury to the left motor area of the cerebrum would cause paralysis of:
    ① The right side of the body
    ② The left side of the body
    ③ Both arms and legs
    ④ Both arms

46. The large, flat, dome-shaped muscle that assists in breathing is the:
    ① Latissimus dorsi
    ② Sternocleidomastoid
    ③ Diaphragm
    ④ Gastrocnemius

47. The part of the nervous system that directs the digestion of food and the circulation of blood is the:
    ① Sensory
    ② Interneurons
    ③ Sympathetic
    ④ Parasympathetic

48. Regulation of body temperature is a function of the:
    ① Medulla
    ② Hypothalamus
    ③ Cerebral cortex
    ④ Cerebellum

49. The organ of hearing is the:
    ① Tympanic membrane
    ② Organ of Corti
    ③ Semicircular canal
    ④ Malleus

50. The equalizing of pressure in the middle ear with atmospheric pressure is the function of the:
    ① Eustachian tube
    ② Labyrinth
    ③ Oval window
    ④ Ossicles

51. Electrolyte balance is maintained chiefly by the action of the:
    ① Bladder
    ② Kidney
    ③ Islets of Langerhans
    ④ Gonads

52. Insulin is produced in the:
    ① Pineal gland
    ② Duodenum
    ③ Islets of Langerhans
    ④ Liver

53. Which statement best describes the T-cells in the immunity response?
    ① Responsible for humoral immunity
    ② Act against bacteria, viruses, tumor cells, and foreign organs
    ③ Clone into helpers and suppressors
    ④ Clone antibody-producing plasma cells

54. The primary function of the fluid within the eyeball is to:
    ① Dilate the pupil
    ② Produce tears
    ③ Regulate the thickness of the lens
    ④ Give and maintain shape of the eyeball

55. When caring for a patient in skin traction it is important for the nurse to:
    ① Encourage diet high in carbohydrates and vitamins
    ② Limit fluid intake to 1000 ml/day
    ③ Limit patient's activities to maintain effectiveness of traction
    ④ Assess circulatory status

56. If a patient's problem was related to blockage of the bile duct by a stone, the nurse could anticipate the stool to appear:
    ① Tarry
    ② Very watery
    ③ Clay colored
    ④ Full of mucus

57. A patient with diabetes is being managed on a split dose of 70/30 isophane insulin suspension (NPH insulin) at 7:30 AM and 4:30 PM. At 2:30 PM one afternoon, the patient calls the nurses' station stating that she is not feeling well. On assessment, the nurse notes her skin is cool and clammy, her hands are shaking, and she appears very apprehensive. The glucometer blood sugar is 45 mg/dl. The most appropriate nursing intervention for the patient's current symptoms is to provide:
    ① Four ounces of fruit juice
    ② Twelve ounces of diet drink
    ③ A large candy bar
    ④ A cube of sugar

58. A patient diagnosed with Type I (juvenile onset) diabetes mellitus is receiving Humulin R by sliding scale. Glucometer readings show a blood sugar of 250 mg/dl. Based on this finding the patient will receive 6 units of Humulin R. Following subcutaneous administration, the nurse should monitor for symptoms of hypoglycemia at the peak time of insulin, which occurs _____ hours after the injection:
    ① 2 to 3
    ② 4 to 6
    ③ 7 to 8
    ④ 9 to 10

59. In a patient recovering from orthopedic surgery or a patient with a fracture, the complication of osteomyelitis might be signaled through which of the following symptoms?
    ① Numbness and delayed capillary refill
    ② Edema, pain, and drainage
    ③ Chest pain and dyspnea
    ④ Paresthesia and bluish skin discoloration

60. A 64-year-old patient has undergone a craniotomy for removal of a meningioma. Which of the following questions would be the most appropriate in assessing a possible complication of this patient's surgery?
    ① "Have you noticed any salty or sweet-tasting drainage coming from your incision?"
    ② "Do you have any headache when you turn to your left side?"
    ③ Are you hungry or thirsty yet?"
    ④ Do you feel that you need to sleep more?"

61. The nurse is caring for a patient with AIDS. He/she must suction the patient's tracheostomy. Which of the following personal protective equipment should be worn by the nurse?
    ① Mask and gloves
    ② Mask and gown
    ③ Gloves and gown
    ④ Mask with eyeshield and gloves

62. The primary concern of the nurse caring for a patient who has an immune deficiency is:
    ① Protection of the patient from infection
    ② To encourage participation in group activities to build the immune system
    ③ To instruct the patient to wear a face mask
    ④ To implement contact isolation precautions

63. A patient with muscular dystrophy has been assigned to your unit. Which of the following observations would be characteristic of this disease?
   ① Pillrolling
   ② Waddling gait
   ③ Shuffling gait
   ④ Tardive dyskinesia

64. A 65-year-old active male who has been complaining of difficulty dressing, weight loss, fatigue, and progressive muscle weakness is diagnosed with amyotropic lateral sclerosis (ALS). When planning care for a patient with ALS, a priority nursing intervention would include:
   ① Increased periods of exercise
   ② Alternative means of communication
   ③ Clear airway maintenance
   ④ Facilitating coping/adjustment to diagnosis

65. A 79-year-old female patient who states that she has "always been healthy" is being treated for a urinary tract infection. The nurse observes that she uses her diaphragm during inspiration and plans to teach her to "purse" lip breathe, based on the understanding that:
   ① Older persons need to consciously think about taking deep breaths.
   ② The older one becomes, the more likely one will develop COPD.
   ③ Age-related changes of loss of elastic recoil of the lungs occur.
   ④ Older people lose the use of their intercostal muscles.

66. In severe cases of degenerative joint disease, a treatment that would facilitate pain reduction and improve joint function is:
   ① Arthrodesis
   ② Laparoscopy
   ③ Arthroscopy
   ④ Arthroplasty

67. A nurse caring for a patient with amyotrophic lateral sclerosis (ALS) must continually assess for signs and symptoms of disease progression. Which of the following signs and symptoms would indicate disease progression?
   ① Aphasia, flexor muscle spasticity, and jaw clonus
   ② Flexor muscle spasticity, dysarthria, and respiratory difficulty
   ③ Dysphagia, dysarthria, and spasticity of flexor muscles
   ④ Sensory loss, jaw clonus, and dysarthria

68. An aim of disease management for an overweight patient with a painful weight-bearing joint is control of symptoms. To help control joint strain, the nurse should teach the patient about the importance of:
   ① Exercising the involved joint
   ② Taking medication at the first sign of pain
   ③ Applying intermittent heat application
   ④ Weight reduction and maintenance

69. Large weight-bearing joints are frequently involved in osteoarthritis. Common characteristics of involved joints include:
   ① Tenderness and crepitus
   ② Bilateral inflammation and immobility
   ③ Pain resulting from destruction of supportive structures
   ④ Fluid within the joint along with inflammatory tissue changes

70. A 60-year-old with a history of osteoarthritis is overweight and leads a sedentary life-style. Lately, his left hip has been particularly painful especially when weight bearing. During the initial assessment of this patient, an important piece of information for the nurse to obtain in planning his care is:
   ① Use of alcohol and tobacco
   ② Hobbies and interests
   ③ Use of a cane, walker, or crutches
   ④ Food likes and dislikes

71. Should an insulin-dependent patient lose consciousness during a hypoglycemic reaction, before food or drink can be administered by mouth, a suitable alternative for the nurse to consider would include:
   ① Administering intravenous (IV) insulin
   ② Sitting the patient up and placing small amounts of a beverage in her mouth
   ③ Placing crushed crackers in the patient's mouth and making her swallow
   ④ Placing prepared glucose concentrate between the cheek and the gum and allowing it to absorb

72. A patient has been diagnosed with acromegaly. The nurse is aware that this condition is caused by an overproduction of:
   ① Prolactin
   ② Cortisol
   ③ Thyroid hormone
   ④ Growth homone

73. The nursing assistant asks the nurse about the turning schedule for a patient who had a right pneumonectomy yesterday. The nurse explains that the patient should be turned every hour from:
   ① Back to left side to right side
   ② Back to left side to back
   ③ Left side to right side to left side
   ④ Back to right side to back

74. A patient diagnosed with right-sided CHF, who is receiving oxygen, questions why the nurse is placing "a clothespin" on her finger. The nurse explains that it is a pulse oximetry machine that will help determine how much:
   ① "Energy she is using"
   ② "Oxygen to give her"
   ③ "Of her heart medication she needs"
   ④ "Her heart is beating"

75. A patient is admitted to the hospital with cirrhosis of the liver related to alcohol abuse and malnutrition. He is jaundiced, has ascites, and has recently experienced dyspnea. When planning care for this patient the nurse is aware that the ascites is primarily caused by which of the following situations?
   ① Increased production of albumin
   ② Portal hypertension
   ③ Increased production of ammonia
   ④ Blockage of the common bile duct

76. A nurse is assisting a physician with a thoracentesis. Upon completion of the procedure, the physician applied a dressing over the puncture site. A student asks the nurse the type of dressing and why it was needed. The nurse's most appropriate response is:
   ① "A clean dressing is used to prevent the patient from infecting the puncture site"
   ② "The physician has his special way of doing things. A bandaid would do"
   ③ "A sterile occlusive dressing is done because of the needle placement"
   ④ "A wet-to-dry dressing is used in case there is any leakage"

77. A patient had a right lower lobectomy at 10 AM. It is now 2 PM. The nurse knows that the best turning schedule for the patient is:
① Right side to back to left side to right side
② Left side to back to left side to back
③ Back to left semiprone to back
④ Back to right semiprone to back

78. A patient with cholelithiasis is experiencing right upper quadrant pain after eating a meal that was high in fat and asks the nurse for an explanation of how his diet can precipitate pain. The most appropriate response by the nurse would be:
① "There is an inadequate absorption of both fat and soluble vitamins"
② "Foods high in fat are harder to digest"
③ "Obstructed bile flow limits the amount of bile available to emulsify fat"
④ "The ducts from the liver and pancreas become obstructed"

79. The nurse is caring for a patient who has had a subtotal thyroidectomy. The nurse is aware that accidental removal of the parathyroid glands could occur and will monitor the patient for
① Seizures
② Tetany
③ Loss of the gag reflex
④ Renal shutdown

80. The patient with a hiatal hernia and reflux syndrome is having discomfort lying in a supine position and is having trouble sleeping. An appropriate intervention by the nurse would be:
① Suggesting that the head of the bed be raised on cinder blocks
② Removing high-acid food from the diet
③ Recommending a glass of milk and a sandwich just before going to bed
④ Suggesting a hot cup of coffee or cocoa before retiring for the night

81. The nurse is to prepare a patient for a proctoscopic exam that is to be performed in the treatment room of the nursing unit. For this procedure, the nurse will position the patient in which position?
① Sims'
② Supine
③ Prone
④ Dorsal recumbent

82. When reviewing patient histories, which of the following patients would the nurse consider to be at greater risk of developing an oral form of cancer?
① Two-year history of smoking
② Poor dental hygiene
③ Frequent bouts of tonsilitis
④ Alcohol abuse

83. The nurse is teaching a patient newly diagnosed with diabetes about reducing the risk of hypoglycemia. Teaching will include all of the following *except:*
① Space meals no farther than four hours apart
② Engage in moderate, planned daily exercise
③ Take your diabetes medicine by noon each day
④ Carry a form of rapid-acting sugar with you at all times

84. When instructing a female patient about antibiotic therapy, the nurse should alert the patient about a disorder that can occur from a disturbance in the normal vaginal flora, particularly during or after antibiotic therapy. The condition is commonly known as:
① Tetany
② Candidiasis
③ Graves' disease
④ Herpes zoster

85. In planning the nursing care of a patient with Addison's disease, a priority of nursing care is:
① Permitting all activity as desired by the patient
② Providing diversional activities
③ Protecting the patient from stress and exertion
④ Planning a well-balanced diet and nourishing snacks

86. A patient with Addison's disease is being regulated with medication. The nurse knows that the goal of therapy is aimed primarily at:
① Reducing the white blood cell count
② Maintaining the red blood cell count level
③ Restoring electrolyte balance
④ Increasing bone marrow functioning

87. A patient awakens and states that she is having difficulty breathing. The nurse can provide relief to the patient by *first:*
① Remaining calm
② Elevating the head of the bed
③ Suctioning her
④ Medicating for pain

88. A patient who recently returned to the unit after a bronchoscopy starts to wheeze and appears frightened. The nurse's most appropriate response to the patient's obvious concern is:
① "Wheezing frequently occurs after this type of test"
② "This is a sign that the local anesthetic is wearing off"
③ "This means that your gag reflex is returning"
④ "I will notify your physician that this is occurring"

89. A neighbor comes to your house after striking her right arm against the mailbox out by her icy walkway. She cannot drive herself to the hospital, and asks you for assistance. As you are talking with your neighbor, you also note that the right lower arm is angulated, but the skin is intact. First-aid measures would include
① Call 911
② Splint the affected area
③ Wrap the area in a warm compress
④ Keep the affected area below the level of the heart

90. Following a lobectomy a patient has difficulty doing deep breathing and productive coughing exercises. The use of an incentive spirometer hasn't helped the situation. Nursing notes indicate the patient's cough is weak and dry and that he tires easily. The most appropriate plan of action the nurse should consider is to:
① Encourage the patient to drink 8 to 10 glasses of water a day
② Ask the physician for PRN throat lozenges and cough demulcent orders
③ Report to the physician and ask if aerosol treatments may help
④ Increase the room temperature to 70° F and humidity to 70%

91. A patient's sputum has suddenly become pink and frothy. The nurse has gathered the following data during her assessment. Which of the data is *significant* and needs to be reported and documented?
    ① Decreased appetite
    ② Respirations 16, regular, easy
    ③ Complaints of dull headache
    ④ Coughing when supine

92. Management of hypertension is very important because of the effects that hypertension has on other organs. Organs most frequently affected by the hypertensive state include:
    ① Liver, lung, and stomach
    ② Heart, brain, and kidney
    ③ Liver, stomach, and colon
    ④ Brain, blood, and bladder

93. A patient is scheduled for a pulmonary angiogram and wants to know what will happen. The nurse explains that:
    ① She will receive a local anesthetic and a tube will be inserted through her nose
    ② She will be placed in a big hollow tube and must remain completely still
    ③ She will wear a clip on her nose and breathe into a machine
    ④ A dye will be injected through an IV and an x-ray will be taken

94. A 69-year-old patient wants to know why she must have a chest x-ray now, since the physician just performed a thoracentesis on her 15 minutes ago. The nurse's most appropriate response to the patient's concern is:
    ① "This test is a double check to see that the physician removed all the fluid"
    ② "This test should have been done before the procedure, but the physician wouldn't wait"
    ③ "The chest x-ray is routinely done after this type of procedure to make sure everything is all right"
    ④ "The chest x-ray is done to make sure the physician didn't nick your lung"

95. A patient is scheduled for a CAT scan of the thorax using contrast medium. The nurse is preparing the patient as per standard procedure for this type of diagnostic test. Which of the actions by the nurse indicates proper protocol is being followed?
    ① Restricting fluids to 1000 cc 4 hours before the test
    ② Placing the patient on NPO status for at least 4 hours before the test
    ③ Allowing the patient to have her usual meal
    ④ Telling the patient she will be on bedrest for 4 hours after the test

96. A 45-year-old patient experienced an acute episode of sharp chest pain, breathing difficulty, and change in breath sounds. She is scheduled for a ventilation/perfusion lung scan. When explaining the reason for the procedure to staff the nurse explains that it:
    ① Was scheduled because the patient may have had a pulmonary embolus
    ② Was ordered to rule out acute myocardial infarction
    ③ Measures vital lung capacity to rule out a pulmonary tumor
    ④ Involves a contrast dye injected IV to check circulation of blood flow through the heart

97. A 33-year-old patient, scheduled for a thoracentesis to instill medication, wants to know where the needle will be placed. The nurse shows her by placing her hand:
    ① Below the patient's diaphragm
    ② Between the patient's second and third rib
    ③ Between the patient's fifth and sixth rib
    ④ Between the patient's eighth and ninth rib

98. The physician has ordered oxygen at 6L per nasal cannula for his patient. While the nurse is preparing the necessary equipment, the patient asks about the bottle of water and cannister, stating she didn't have all that stuff the last time she needed oxygen. The nurse's most appropriate response would be which of the following?
    ① "Apparently they had different equipment when you were here last"
    ② "Based on the ordered rate, humidification is necessary to keep your nose from becoming too dry"
    ③ "Most patients feel more comfortable when the oxygen is humidified"
    ④ "Humidity decreases the fire hazard of using oxygen"

99. Hepatic coma is a complication associated with cirrhosis. When caring for a patient with the disease, it is important the nurse is aware that measures to prevent hepatic coma include which of the following?
    ① Eliminate carbohydrates from the diet
    ② Eliminate protein from the diet
    ③ Give soapy enemas
    ④ Perform iced saline lavages

100. The nurse is caring for a patient in diabetes ketoacidosis. In the acute phase of this condition, the nurse will expect to administer what type of insulin?
    ① Regular
    ② Lente
    ③ NPH
    ④ Glucotrol

101. Glucose is primarily used as _____ by a cell.
    ① A protein source
    ② An energy source
    ③ Repair material
    ④ Protoplasm

102. A common cause of diabetic ketoacidosis is:
    ① Stress
    ② Infection
    ③ Excess insulin
    ④ Insufficient calories in the diet

103. The nurse is aware that mitral stenosis and mitral insufficiency have similar symptoms. A symptom common to both is:
    ① Syncope
    ② Angina
    ③ Murmur
    ④ Constipation

104. The nurse is monitoring a patient on bed rest for symptoms of fluid retention and dependent edema. The nurse knows that a good area to assess for the presence of edema is the:
    ① Hands
    ② Knees
    ③ Feet
    ④ Sacrum

105. Uncontrolled hypertension over time can affect the heart, brain, kidney, and eyes. The patient wants the nurse to tell him the name of the recommended annual eye exam he is to have. The best response by the nurse would be to explain the examination called a:
    ① Vision screen
    ② Tonometer test
    ③ Fundoscopic exam
    ④ Visual fields exam

106. A patient with a CVA, who has paresis of her left side and weighs 90 kg, is incontinent of urine and perspires heavily. The nurse instructs the nursing assistant to:
    ① Pull the patient up in bed at least once a shift
    ② Keep the patient off the affected side when positioning the patient
    ③ Get help to move and reposition the patient
    ④ Lower the temperature in the room

107. Because of pneumonia, a dark-skinned patient has spent most of the day in bed. Which of the following might cause the nurse the most concern during skin assessment rounds?
    ① A productive cough when she moves
    ② A dark, almost purple area over her right scapula
    ③ Complaints of feeling cool
    ④ Complaints of feeling "stiff"

108. The nurse notes that the edges of her patient's incisional area are not healing properly. The patient had a thoracotomy a week ago and has not been eating well. Which of the following actions would be most appropriate for the nurse to pursue?
    ① Sit down and help the patient with menu selection
    ② Encourage the patient to exercise more
    ③ Ask the physician for an antidepressant order
    ④ Offer mouth care before each meal

109. A patient who has had frequent bouts of pneumonia spends most of her time in bed, insisting that the head of her bed remain at 90 degrees. Because she has reddened areas on her coccyx, the nurse teaches her that:
    ① She needs to stay off her back for the next 24 hours
    ② The head of the bed should be kept at 15 to 30 degrees
    ③ She keeps getting pneumonia because of the moisture that forms on her skin
    ④ Her buttocks hurt because the skin over the bones is dying

110. A patient complained of dizziness immediately after receiving eardrops. This may indicate that:
    ① The eardrops were administered too quickly
    ② The auditory canal is occluded
    ③ The ear drops were very warm
    ④ He is having an allergic reaction

111. Symptoms of hypertension are vague and subtle. In assessing hypertensive patients, the nurse may observe symptoms of:
    ① Increased urination, fatigue, and blurred vision
    ② Nausea, vomiting, and nosebleeds
    ③ Chest pain, shortness of breath, and nervousness
    ④ Blurred vision, irritability, and occipital headaches

112. Your patient with multiple sclerosis requires intermittent catheterizations and is apprehensive. When she asks why this is necessary, the nurse's best response is:
    ① "You need to discuss this with your physician"

② "It will empty your bladder completely at certain times each day"
③ "It guarantees that you will not be incontinent"
④ "It relieves any pressure on your bowels so you will not become constipated"

113. A patient who has been receiving high doses of oxygen is suspected of developing oxygen toxicity. Besides observing for hallucinations and confusion, which of the following should be assessed for?
    ① Halos around lights
    ② Loss of peripheral vision
    ③ Increased shallow respirations
    ④ Uncontrolled muscular twitching

114. A patient diagnosed with chronic renal failure is becoming more confused. Because all previous laboratory test results were within normal range, which of the following would be of concern to the nurse and should be reported?
    ① Potassium of 5.5 mEq/L
    ② Glucose of 90mg/100ml
    ③ Platelet count of 150,000/mm^3
    ④ Leukocyte count of 5,500/mm^3

115. A patient refuses to cough and deep breathe or to use the incentive spirometer. Besides assessing respirations and laboratory results, which of the following data would indicate beginning respiratory acidosis?
    ① Warm, flushed skin
    ② Numbness of fingers
    ③ Peripheral cyanosis
    ④ Facial twitching

116. In the acute phase of treatment for a myocardial infarction, supplemental oxygen is administered to a patient. The main goal of oxygen therapy is to:
    ① Increase oxygen supply to myocardial tissue
    ② Prevent ventricular fibrillation
    ③ Decrease anxiety and restlessness
    ④ Prevent shock

117. A patient who had a CVA three years ago has been admitted with blisters and tiny open areas on her buttocks. No drainage is present at this time. The most appropriate dressing for the nurse to use for this patient is:
    ① Hydrophilic
    ② Steri-strips
    ③ Hydrophobic
    ④ Wet-to-dry

118. A patient was recently admitted because of a motor vehicle accident. Which of the following observations would cause the nurse to monitor intake and output closely?
    ① Capillary refill less than 3 seconds
    ② Elastic skin turgor
    ③ Crackles in lower lobes
    ④ Amber aromatic urine

119. During routine AM rounds, the nurse notes that a patient with chronic pulmonary disease is more forgetful today. The nurse also notes an unusual odor on the patient's breath while assessing lung sounds. It is essential that the nurse evaluate the patient within the hour because the patient:
    ① May need to be oriented to her environment more today
    ② May be developing a respiratory infection
    ③ May need more encouragement to eat today
    ④ Is at risk for developing acidosis

120. After a patient has joint arthroplasty, the nurse is vigilant in monitoring for complications. In the immediate postoperative phase, which of the following assessments must be reported immediately?
① Nausea
② Neurocirculatory compromise
③ Infiltration of intravenous fluids
④ Inability to cough productively

121. A patient being treated for kidney failure complains of nausea, diarrhea, and postural dizziness. Her pulse is rapid, thready, and regular. The most appropriate action by the nurse would be to:
① Monitor her output hourly
② Assess her level of consciousness twice/shift
③ Make her NPO until the diarrhea clears
④ Notify the RN or physician of these complaints

122. The nurse is caring for the periostomal area of a patient who had a urinary diversion 2 weeks ago. Which of the following actions is most appropriate?
① Cleansing the area with soap and water and patting dry
② Applying baby oil to the area and stoma
③ Moistening the stoma and area with aloe lotion
④ Massaging the area 3 to 4 times a day

123. Your patient with multiple sclerosis has a neurogenic bladder. When evaluating the patient's response to medical therapy, which of the following medications would you expect to be therapeutic for this bladder problem?
① Oxybutynin chloride (Ditropan)
② Bethanechol (Urecholine)
③ Propantheline bromide (Pro-Banthine)
④ Trimethoprim sulfamethoxazole (Bactrim, Septra)

124. To best prepare the patient for a cystoscopy where no x-rays will be taken, the nurse:
① Administers enemas until clear
② Shaves the pubic area
③ Inserts an indwelling catheter
④ Encourages fluid intake

125. A patient returns to the unit following a TURP with a continuous bladder irrigation and is complaining of bladder spasms. Which of the following interventions can the nurse implement to help relieve this problem?
① Increase the flow rate of the irrigating solution
② Raise the collecting drainage bag to the level of the bladder
③ Encourage relaxation techniques to avoid straining to pass urine
④ Elevate the scrotum on towels

126. During a patient's annual physical an enlarged boggy prostate is noted by the physician. Based on this information, which of the following data is most important?
① Hesitancy, change in urine stream
② Color and odor of urine
③ Constipation and smoking history
④ Type and amount of fluids taken daily

127. A patient diagnosed with hyperthyroidism and exhibiting signs of exophthalmus has been complaining of dry eyes. Which of the following physician's orders would the nurse expect to implement to meet the patient's comfort needs?
① Artificial tears
② Mydriatic eye drops
③ Antibiotic ointment
④ Prone position for sleep and rest

128. In a patient with myasthenia gravis, which of the following drugs would the nurse question if they were ordered?
① Neostigmine (Prostigmin)
② Neomycin (Mycifradin)
③ Prednisone (Deltasone)
④ Pyridostigmine (Mestinon)

129. A patient with a ureterostomy is to adhere to an acid ash diet. Which of these menu selections should the nurse question?
① Cereal with cranberries, bowl of prunes
② Fish, buttered noodles, peanuts for dessert
③ Chicken with rice, cheese slices
④ Steak, creamed vegetables, glass of milk

130. When a patient returns from dialysis she is diaphoretic, restless, vomiting, and has tachycardia. Which of the following actions by the nurse is most appropriate *initially*?
① Apply a cool washcloth to the patient's forehead and monitor vital signs
② Encourage frequent sips of water and elevate foot of bed
③ Lower the head of the bed, elevate the foot of the bed, turn the patient on her side
④ Decrease the temperature in the room and turn the patient on her side

131. When assessing a patient's range of motion, the nurse notices that the patient has trouble extending his right arm out from his side. Moving a body part away from the midline is called:
① Abduction
② Adduction
③ Flexion
④ Pronation

132. The patient is frail and evidences muscle atrophy in both upper and lower extremities. A good choice for the nurse to consider for an intramuscular injection would be:
① Gluteus medius
② Deltoid
③ Gastrocnemius
④ Sartorius

133. The nurse is aware that the cause of Cushing's syndrome is most commonly an overproduction of which hormone?
① Growth hormone
② Thyroid hormone
③ Cortisol
④ Epinephrine

134. A 4-day postoperative patient is most uncomfortable because of abdominal distention. The nurse prepares the patient for ambulation by splinting the abdominal wound based on the understanding that:
① Sustained stress disrupts wound layers and tissue repair
② This allows for deeper respirations and coughing
③ Persons with abdominal distention hesitate to move
④ An abdominal binder would restrict her movements

135. The patient with hypertension is upset that he is having to undergo treatment and states, "I don't feel bad. Why is the doctor making such a fuss?" The best reply by the nurse is:
① "I can see that you are angry; we can talk later when you are in a better mood."
② "Why are you acting this way? We are all trying to help you!"
③ "I'll tell the doctor that you are questioning his care!"
④ "There may be no symptoms with hypertension, but organ damage can occur if this problem continues without correction."

136. The nurse is assessing a patient for evidence of a hypoglycemic reaction. Which assessments indicate this reaction?
    ① Polyuria, dysuria, and fever
    ② Glycosuria, hematuria, and tachypnea
    ③ Pale, clammy skin and confusion
    ④ Ketonuria, fruity odor to the breath, and hot/dry skin

137. A patient is typed and crossed-matched for blood he may receive in surgery. He is found to be of the type that is considered the "universal donor." The nurse knows that his blood type is:
    ① A
    ② B
    ③ AB
    ④ O

138. A patient who is a diabetic twisted her ankle, fell, and sustained a skin abrasion. She asks the nurse to apply an ice wrap to her ankle. The nurse hesitates based on the understanding that:
    ① The open area will become infected
    ② Diabetics have a greater potential for injury related to cold
    ③ She first will need to get an x-ray of the ankle
    ④ Rebound swelling may occur when the ice is removed

139. A 76-year-old stroke patient continues to complain of numbness and discomfort in her right knee. The most appropriate nursing intervention to ensure her comfort is to:
    ① Administer the PRN heat wrap ordered for joint stiffness
    ② Administer the PRN medication ordered for temperature over 101° F
    ③ Secure an order for an ice wrap to the right knee
    ④ Visit with the patient and reposition her

140. A patient with a chest wound was transferred to the subacute unit and is complaining of increased pain at the wound site, which is covered with a dry 4 × 4 dressing. Based on the information given by the patient, the nurse knows this may mean that:
    ① The pain medication is no longer effective
    ② An infection is developing
    ③ The dressing is too tight
    ④ The dressing needs to be changed

141. A 70-year-old patient, who is 3 days postpneumonectomy, develops an infection of the surgical site. When securing supplies for the wet-to-dry dressing changes, the nurse orders Montgomery straps, based on the understanding that these:
    ① Are more cost effective
    ② Are less likely to cause additional infection
    ③ Will cause less trauma to the skin
    ④ Will decrease the need for frequent dressing changes

142. A patient who had chest surgery has a taped, windowed, sterile dressing covering the surgical site. A nursing goal is to maintain skin integrity of the surrounding tissues. To meet this goal, when removing the dressing the nurse needs to:
    ① Explain each step of the procedure
    ② Soak the old dressing with normal saline before attempting removal
    ③ Apply sterile gloves, loosen all tape first and lift up, bringing the edges toward her
    ④ Loosen tape by pulling toward the incision and, using the thumb, gently pull skin away from tape

143. A dark-skinned patient is at high risk for a pressure ulcer. You assess her pressure points for blanching. The color that describes blanching in patients with dark skin is:
    ① Pale, like someone who is anemic
    ② Grayish, like ashes in a fireplace
    ③ Hyperemic, like the color of a plum
    ④ Pinkish, like circles of red blush makeup

144. When assessing his patient who is in kidney failure, the physician suspects electrolyte imbalance based on her symptoms. Which of the following are signs of electrolyte imbalance and should be reported to the physician?
    ① Nausea, vomiting, increased depth of respirations
    ② Anxiety, abdominal cramps, irregular heartbeat
    ③ Crackles, nausea, excessive thirst
    ④ Dry lips, loss of weight, dark amber urine

145. A 36-year-old patient being treated with chemotherapy for lung cancer has just received a rapid infusion of 3 units of whole blood and is complaining of numbness in his fingertips, lips, and tongue. While taking his blood pressure, the nurse noted a twitching of the patient's wrist and fingers which she promptly reported to the team leader based on the knowledge that:
    ① These are signs that the cancer has spread
    ② The signs are adverse effects of chemotherapy
    ③ These are signs of hypocalcemia
    ④ The signs indicate respiratory distress

146. A middle-aged male who has cancer of the lung started receiving TPN yesterday. The patient's wife asks you to explain what the TPN feeding is doing for her husband. The best response would be:
    ① "These feedings are the safest type of feeding for debilitated persons."
    ② "These feedings contain all the essential nutrients that can't be given through small veins."
    ③ "These tube feedings place the necessary nutrients directly into the stomach."
    ④ "These feedings make eating unnecessary. This keeps your husband from tiring so easily."

147. A paracentesis may be performed to reduce the discomfort related to ascites. What nursing actions would the nurse anticipate in assisting with the procedure?
    ① Place patient in right lateral position to facilitate drainage
    ② Record amount and color of fluid removed
    ③ Prepare the area by cleansing with warm, soapy water and drape with sterile towels
    ④ Assist with the application of a simple sterile dressing after the procedure

148. Nursing observations of a patient with severe liver dysfunction with accompanying jaundice would include which of the following?
    ① Dark stools, yellow sclera, and dark urine
    ② Clay-colored stools, yellow sclera, and blood-tinged urine
    ③ Clay-colored stools, pruritus, and dark urine
    ④ Dark stools, pruritus, and amber urine

149. A patient who is very weak secondary to her lung cancer requires frequent suctioning of her nasopharynx. Based on the standards of care, you check the suction machine and adjust the pressure setting to:
    ① 50 to 95 mm Hg
    ② 95 to 110 mm Hg

③ 110 to 115 mm Hg
④ 135 to 150 mm Hg

150. A patient who has a thoracotomy tube in his left thorax is apprehensive and afraid to move. The tube is attached to water-seal chest drainage. The appropriate teaching for this patient is to:
① Comb his hair with his left arm every 4 to 6 hours.
② Avoid any sudden movements or turning.
③ Apply lotion around the tube after his bath.
④ Keep the side rails up while in bed.

151. The water seal chamber of the patient's chest drainage set-up has stopped fluctuating. The suction control is working properly. The chest tube has been in place for 2 days. The most appropriate action for the nurse to do first is to:
① Notify the physician or RN of this development
② Ask the patient to bear down and perform a Valsalva maneuver
③ Check the tubing for dependent loops
④ Add reinforcing tape around the tube insertion site

152. The nurse is instructing the patient on how to prevent most upper airway infections. She/he should stress frequent good hand washing and encourage the patient to:
① Maintain proper dental hygiene
② Stay in air conditioning as much as possible
③ Use more disposable Kleenex
④ Take megadoses of vitamin C daily

153. During a care conference, the RN asks you if the nursing diagnosis of ineffective clearance related to bronchial secretions is still appropriate for the patient. You can best evaluate this by:
① Taking the patient's temperature
② Checking the rate and strength of the patient's pulse
③ Counting the patient's respirations for 1 full minute
④ Listening for clear breath sounds

154. The position the majority of patients with respiratory tract infections find to be the most comfortable is:
① Low Fowler's
② High Fowler's
③ Left lateral
④ Semiprone

155. A patient with influenza has ineffective airway clearance related to bronchial secretions. To assist the patient in bringing up bronchial secretions, the nurse should plan to:
① Monitor intake and output
② Limit visitors
③ Increase room humidity to 60%
④ Encourage liberal fluid intake of 2000 cc/day

156. The patient's left thoracotomy tube is connected to water-seal drainage. When the patient is sitting in a chair, the nurse should make sure that the tube and drainage system remain:
① Connected on the bed frame
② Even with the level of the patient's heart
③ On a towel sitting on the floor
④ Below her chest

157. The patient has severe pharyngitis and has developed an elevated temperature, chills, and a skin rash. A sputum specimen for culture and sensitivity has been ordered. The nurse reports the skin rash based on the understanding that:

① Medicated creams need to be ordered
② Antibiotics need to be started
③ The patient may be developing scarlet fever
④ The rash may be very painful

158. The patient who had a right lower lobectomy 5 days ago is being discharged. The instructions the patient is given should include:
① Avoiding soft or low chairs
② Avoiding lifting items over 5 pounds until the incision is healed
③ Taking sponge baths until his follow-up physician appointment
④ Staying indoors until outdoor activities are approved by the physician

159. Your patient begins to complain of pruritus and you notice that she has been scratching and has excoriated areas. Your plan is to make her comfortable and her skin pliable. This can best be achieved by:
① Cutting her fingernails to the top of her fingertips
② Keeping the environment cool and at 40% humidity
③ Checking to see what medication she is receiving
④ Administering a PRN nonsteroidal antiinflammatory drug (NSAID)

160. Damage to the laryngeal nerve may occur following a thyroidectomy. The nurse observes for symptoms of:
① Hoarseness
② Frothy sputum
③ Positive Chvostek's sign
④ Choking sensation

161. Following a thyroidectomy, the accidental removal of the parathyroid glands would precipitate the symptoms of tetany. Nursing observations for evidence of tetany would include:
① Unrelenting headache and blurred vision
② Hypertension and somnolence
③ Painful muscle spasms of the hands and face
④ Blood-tinged urine and frequency

162. A patient diagnosed with hyperthyroidism is extremely nervous and anxious. The nurse notes she comes from a large, close-knit family, which is constantly hovering over her. An important aspect for the nurse to consider when planning this patient's care would include:
① Maintaining a calm, relaxed environment
② Encouraging visitors to help stimulate patient interactions
③ Placing her in a semiprivate room or ward to foster interaction and release tension
④ Providing for frequent interactions between the patient and the staff

163. A patient who is being evaluated for congestive heart failure is scheduled for an x-ray and asks why a chest x-ray is necessary for his cardiac workup. The best reply by the nurse is:
① "Ask your doctor to explain this to you."
② "You can ask to speak to the radiologist once you are in x-ray."
③ "This study will outline the vessels of your heart and and show the degree of heart disease."
④ "This study will be useful in determining the size of your heart."

164. A 73-year-old black male with a history of hypertension and arteriosclerosis was admitted from the nursing home for observation. The nursing home attendant reported noticing that the patient had become more withdrawn, had trouble using his right hand, and that the right side of his mouth sagged. The nurse would be alert for progressive signs of:
① Angina
② Hypertension
③ Myocardial infarction
④ Cerebrovascular accident

165. A patient undergoing a gastrectomy may develop which of the following problems postoperatively?
① Diabetes mellitus
② Esophageal reflux
③ Pernicious anemia
④ *Helicobacter pylori* infection

166. The nurse is aware that a sound measure for preventing hepatitis B is:
① Testing blood donors
② Adding bleach to the water
③ Avoiding blood donations
④ Avoiding consumption of all shellfish

167. A young patient with a diagnosis of Crohn's disease has had a recent ileostomy. The patient asks the nurse what sports he should avoid when returning to school. The best response by the nurse is:
① Swimming
② Track
③ Football
④ Shot put

168. A patient who develops peritonitis should be evaluated for fever and:
① Reduced urine output
② Abdominal muscular rigidity
③ Increased bowel motility
④ Nervousness

169. When planning to teach a newly diagnosed patient with Type I diabetes mellitus, it is essential that the nurse is aware that cardinal symptoms of diabetes mellitus include:
① Headache, hypertension, and hyperglycemia
② Polyuria, polydipsia, and polyphagia
③ Lethargy, slowed mental processes, and hypotension
④ Clammy skin, tremors, and polyuria

170. Thirty percent of all patients with cirrhosis develop esophageal varices. Early management is directed toward treatment of bleeding. Because of this, it is essential the nurse be knowledgeable of treatment strategies for these patients, which include:
① Gastric lavage with room–temperature saline solution
② Use of Sengstaken-Blakemore tube and iced saline lavages
③ Administration of vasodilators, antibiotics, and antacids
④ Administration of platelets and refrigerated blood

171. A patient has longstanding stasis dermatitis of the legs. The nurse's main concern is to:
① Maintain intact skin on her legs
② Administer antiinflammatory drugs as ordered
③ Wear gloves when applying ointments to her legs
④ Keep her from bathing with soap

172. You are assigned to do the meds and treatments on a patient who received a skin graft 5 days ago. Which of the following orders for the donor site on the left thigh would you question?
① Wet-to-dry dressing changes every 6 hours
② Out of bed ad lib
③ Give analgesics as necessary for discomfort
④ Apply bed cradle to the foot of the bed

173. When warm compresses are applied to your patient's eyes, she has an allergic reaction. The most appropriate nursing action would be to:
① Wear sterile gloves and use sterile technique
② Wear clean gloves and use clean technique
③ Tape compresses in place
④ Warm the solution in a microwave

174. The nurse is to administer an antibiotic eye ointment to a patient with a bacterial infection of his right eye. The nurse would:
① Place an eye pad on the eye after administering the ointment
② Wear gloves to administer the ointment
③ Place the ointment on the eyeball
④ Use the unit's stock supply of ointment

175. The patient returning home after a right cataract extraction with an intraocular lens implant needs to be instructed to:
① Sleep on his left side
② Restrict fluid intake to 1000 cc/day
③ Shower and shampoo every other day
④ Avoid watching television

176. You are to administer eye medications for a group of 6 patients, all of whom have glaucoma. You know it is vital that these medications be given as ordered. This is based on the understanding that:
① Giving medications on time is part of your job
② These medications keep the pupil constricted to permit better aqueous humor drainage
③ Glaucoma is a leading cause of blindness
④ The patient will experience severe eye pain if a dose is late

177. A patient, who has noticed that she tends to bump into objects, is being tested for glaucoma. The nurse explains to her that with glaucoma:
① Circulation to the brain is decreased
② Blindness is an eventual result
③ Her sense of balance is disturbed
④ A decrease in peripheral vision is a first symptom

178. Your patient, who has been treated for glaucoma for 4 months, recently had a CVA. As you are caring for her in the rehabilitation unit, she questions you about difficulty seeing after she receives her eyedrops. You explain that:
① The blurred vision after receiving the drops will decrease with prolonged use
② Bright lights are to be avoided
③ The room should be dark right after the eyedrops are inserted
④ Smoking while receiving these drops is contraindicated

179. You just learned that your patient is suspected of having a retinal detachment. The patient is presently in bed and it is important that you:
① Explain and show that her call light is within easy reach

② Tell her that she will receive antiemetics to prevent insomnia

③ Remind her that she will remain on bed rest for 3 to 4 weeks

④ Assure her that she will receive eye drops for the ocular pain

180. A 5-year-old patient has an upper respiratory infection. When teaching him how to blow his nose, the nurse tells him to:
   ① Blow with both nostrils open
   ② Blow one side of his nose at a time
   ③ Keep his mouth open when blowing one side at a time
   ④ Shut his eyes while blowing hard

181. A patient, who is being treated with furosemide (Lasix) for her CHF, has begun to experience tinnitus. The nurse tells her that:
   ① The sounds she hears are normal
   ② This is caused by nerve deafness
   ③ She will not be able to drive
   ④ This may be related to her new medication

182. A postoperative measure following a hemorrhoidectomy that the nurse will anticipate is:
   ① Use of a fecal tube to reduce gas pain
   ② Changing occlusive rectal dressings
   ③ Encouraging warm showers
   ④ Administering laxatives and stool softeners

183. The nurse is assessing a nursing home resident who has just been admitted from the ER to the orthopedic unit. The diagnosis is a "probable right femoral neck fracture." The patient is to be placed in traction. Before the application of the traction, the nurse observes the affected femur and finds it to be in what position?
   ① Supination and internal rotation
   ② Pronation and internal rotation
   ③ Leg lengthening and lateral rotation
   ④ Leg shortening and external rotation

184. A patient is diagnosed with Cushing's syndrome. Overproduction of hormones may place the patient at risk of developing which one of the following?
   ① Hyperglycemia
   ② Hyperkalemia
   ③ Hypocalcemia
   ④ Hypoinsulinemia

185. An important nursing assessment of a client in hypovolemic shock is:
   ① Checking urine output
   ② Monitoring bowel movements
   ③ Assessing pedal pulses
   ④ Checking for the presence of jugular venous distention

186. The patient has lymphoma and is undergoing chemotherapy. Periodically, the physician orders a complete blood count (CBC). The nurse is aware that the lab work is to monitor for:
   ① Thalassemia
   ② Bone marrow depression
   ③ Cancer in remission
   ④ Increasing platelet counts

187. Which of the following diets would be best for a patient with hyperthyroidism?
   ① Low-purine, high-fat, 1000-calorie diet
   ② High-protein, high-calorie, high-carbohydrate diet with snacks

③ Clear liquids in the form of 6 small feedings
④ 2-gram low-sodium diet with an evening snack

188. A 27 year old entered the clinic with symptoms of nervousness, racing heart, and weight loss. Thyroid function studies were performed and a diagnosis of hyperthyroidism was made. The nurse is aware that other symptoms of hyperthyroidism include:
   ① Dry skin, intolerance to cold, and slowed responses
   ② Urinary frequency, blurred vision, frequent infections
   ③ Increased sweating, hand tremor, and excitability
   ④ Constipation, depression, and brittle hair

189. If a hypertensive patient's management includes a diuretic, an important aspect of patient education would include:
   ① Drinking at least a quart of liquids a day
   ② Refraining from caffeine and caffeine-containing products
   ③ Maintaining a high-potassium diet
   ④ Avoiding spicy and high-fat, high-cholesterol foods

190. A patient has been diagnosed with primary hypertension. Which one of the following medications is designed to lower blood pressure?
   ① Cimetidine (Tagamet)
   ② Ibuprofen (Motrin)
   ③ Digoxin (Lanoxin)
   ④ Hydrochlorothiazide (HydroDIURIL)

191. The nurse needs to obtain a sterile urine specimen for culture and sensitivity. The best way to obtain this specimen in a patient with an indwelling Foley catheter is to:
   ① Disconnect the catheter from the drainage tubing and let the urine drip into the sterile bottle
   ② Use a needle and syringe to withdraw urine from the tubing port and inject the specimen into the sterile bottle
   ③ Place a towel under the bag and open the drainage valve at the bottom of the drainage bag
   ④ Remove the old Foley, using a straight catheter, and recatheterize

192. The patient's wife is concerned because her husband, who suffered a CVA 3 days ago, laughs and cries inappropriately. The nurse's best reply is:
   ① "This is a normal healing sign for someone who has had a CVA."
   ② "I ignore him when he starts acting like that."
   ③ "He has what is called 'emotional lability.' This may occur after a stroke."
   ④ "Men your husband's age like to tease us by acting this way."

193. A head trauma patient has impaired speech but seems to understand what is said to him. The nurse needs to include which of the following in his plan of care?
   ① Keep the room dimly lighted
   ② Allow extra time for communication
   ③ Avoid the use of gestures
   ④ Keep voice level, soft, and low

194. A patient who had a CVA 2 weeks ago, has dysphagia. Based on these data the nurse tells the aide to:
   ① Keep the patient in bed
   ② Speak loudly when talking
   ③ Allow extra time for him to answer her
   ④ Make sure he swallows his food

195. The patient requires nasopharyngeal suctioning. The nurse places the suction catheter into sterile solution. The underlying principle for this action is to:
① Maintain sterile technique
② Prevent tissue trauma
③ Check patency of the tube
④ Check the suction's pressure

196. The nurse performing nasopharyngeal suctioning applies suction for a maximum of 10 seconds at a time. The underlying principle for this action is that it:
① Maintains catheter tube patency
② Prevents contamination of the catheter
③ Allows patient to breathe normally
④ Prevents improper tube placement

197. The nurse observes that her patient, age 60, has stress incontinence each time she coughs or gets out of bed. The nurse understands that:
① Hormonal changes place older women at risk for stress incontinence
② Her patient is not emptying her bladder completely
③ The nerves controlling the bladder are affected
④ Her patient's bladder is displaced in her pelvic cavity

198. A patient who grows her own fruits and vegetables is concerned that her urine, which is red in color, indicates that she is bleeding. The most appropriate response from the nurse is:
① "You must increase your milk intake to about 8 to 10 glasses a day."
② "This is nothing to be concerned about. Let me know if it is still happening next week"
③ "Tell me, do you feel any pain or pass flatus when you urinate?"
④ "Tell me, what types of vegetables and fruits have you been eating?"

199. A 25 year old sustained an injury to his spinal cord at the C5 level. Based on a spinal cord injury at this level, the nurse would most likely expect the patient to have loss of:
① His emotions
② Movement of all extremities
③ His sexual desires
④ Speaking ability

200. In a patient with chronic bronchitis, which of the following early signs of hypoxemia should the nurse watch for?
① Dyspnea, hypotension, bradycardia
② Bradycardia, wheezing, confusion
③ Capillary refill >3 seconds, SOB, confusion
④ Restlessness, tachycardia, yawning

201. A patient is being transferred to the unit where he is to be observed following a 2-day stay in coronary care for a possible myocardial infarction. He is receiving several medications and is complaining of a headache. Which of the following medications commonly causes the side effect of headache?
① Lanoxin
② Tylenol
③ Nitroglycerin
④ Potassium chloride

202. A 36-year-old female has been experiencing intermittent episodes of mild chest pain and shortness of breath, particularly with exertion but also at rest. So far the cardiac work-up of lab studies and EKG are negative. The physician wants to see if the symptoms are aggravated or precipitated by activity. The nurse will anticipate counseling the patient in the use of
① A glucometer
② Urine collection
③ A Doppler flow study
④ A Holter monitor

203. Treatment of mild hypertension usually involves control by use of conservative measures. A factor that a hypertensive patient is unable to control is
① Smoking
② Obesity
③ Lack of exercise
④ Genetic predisposition

204. After a 4-day stay in the coronary care unit, a patient is transferred to an intermediate care unit. Because he has been on extended bed rest, the nursing care plan includes monitoring for thrombophlebitis. The nurse is aware that symptoms of thrombophlebitis include:
① Numbness and tingling of an extremity
② Coldness and paleness of the involved area
③ Absence of pulses and reduced sensation
④ Pain and red streaking along the vein path

205. A patient with a diagnosis of myocardial infarction has been admitted to the coronary care unit. The nurse assesses the patient's breath sounds and hears fine crackles in the lower lung bases. This symptom may indicate:
① Dysrhythmias
② Pneumonia
③ An extension of the myocardial infarction
④ Lung congestion from heart failure

206. When ambulating a patient with right hemiparesis, you should stand on the patient's:
① Right side and hold one arm on the gait belt on the patient's waist
② Left side and hold one arm around the patient's waist
③ Right side and 12 inches behind the patient
④ Left side and hold the patient's right hand

207. Your patient is very anxious about going home, and you need to give her discharge teaching. You must remember that her
① Anxiety is hidden anger at being discharged too soon
② Feelings are based on fear of the unknown
③ Concerns are self-centered
④ Anxiety may interfere with her ability to understand or remember the instructions

208. A patient has chronic respiratory disease and is newly-diagnosed with Alzheimer's disease. In planning his care, the nurse should prioritize his care as:
① Safety, physiological assessment, comfort
② Psychological care, personal integrity, comfort
③ Safety, pain relief, cueing
④ Physiological assessment, reorientation, cueing

209. A patient has started receiving bronchodilators (Theophylline). When checking for toxic and side effects, the nurse should observe for:
① Hypotension, abdominal cramping, diarrhea
② Urticaria, nausea and vomiting, dehydration
③ Restlessness, tachycardia, insomnia
④ Anorexia, blurred vision, cramps

210. Your patient has had emphysema for 3 years and has dyspnea even at rest. Which of the following observations is characteristic of the disease?

① Dry, hacking cough
② Elevated body temperature
③ Use of accessory muscles of respiration
④ Hemoptysis

211. A patient with bilateral hearing aids complains of ear pressure and is subsequently diagnosed with right ear otitis media. The nurse instructs the aide in his care, which includes:
① Turning the hearing aids' sensitivity levels higher
② Wiping off the right hearing aid with an alcohol sponge after removal
③ Making sure the patient receives his ear drops before putting in his hearing aid
④ Leaving the right hearing aid out of the patient's ear

212. A patient is to receive 1000 cc of 5% dextrose in water plus 40 mEq KCL in 12 hours. In checking the flow rate, how many ccs should the patient receive per hour?
① 42 cc/hr
② 83 cc/hr
③ 100 cc/hr
④ 125 cc/hr

213. A patient is at risk for a pulmonary embolism secondary to deep vein thrombosis. Which expected outcome is appropriate for the patient?
① No pain with respiratory effort
② Participates in ADL
③ Maintains stable weight
④ Demonstrates effective coughing techniques

214. The nurse is determining an asthmatic patient's achievement of the goals for the nursing diagnosis: Activity intolerance related to imbalance between oxygen supply and demand. Which of the following expected outcomes is appropriate?
① No evidence of anxiety
② Demonstrated knowledge of disease process
③ Able to perform ADL
④ Clear breath sounds

215. A patient scored 5 on the Rancho Los Amigos Scale, meaning that she is confused-inappropriate. The nurse expects this patient to:
① React inconsistently and nonpurposefully to stimuli
② Appear alert and be able to respond to simple commands fairly consistently
③ Show goal-directed behavior but depend on external input for direction
④ Be in a heightened state of activity with decreased ability to process information

216. Following a myocardial infarction a patient receives the anticoagulant Coumadin. The nurse is aware that monitoring is of extreme importance for which of the following adverse effects?
① Blurred vision
② Vomiting
③ Epistaxis
④ Back pain

217. A patient is being evaluated because of complaints of cervical neck pain. As part of the evaluation, the intent is to rule out the possibility of a ruptured disc. Which of the following is a common symptom of cervical disc involvement?
① Stiff neck
② Difficulty walking

③ Numbness of the lower extremities
④ Atrophy of the gastrocnemius muscle group

218. Which of the following interventions will the nurse anticipate implementing for a patient with a diagnosis of a myocardial infarction?
① Adjusting the bed to Trendelenburg's position
② Maintaining prescription of complete bed rest for at least 5 days
③ Providing clear, room-temperature liquids throughout hospitalization
④ Administering a stool softener to prevent straining with bowel movements

219. A concern for a patient having experienced a recent myocardial infarction is the development of cardiogenic shock. Signs of cardiogenic shock include:
① Hot, dry skin, rapid respirations, and mental confusion
② Bounding pulses, clammy skin, and fever
③ Hypotension, weak pulses, and clammy skin
④ Hypertension, shallow respirations, and chest pain

220. Building construction is going on next to your unit. You are concerned about the noise level and plan to encourage your patients to:
① Keep their TVs off so as not to add to the noise
② Wear temporary ear protectors during the hours construction is going on
③ Request a transfer to another unit
④ Practice distraction techniques during the construction hours

221. A diabetic patient is being treated for pneumonia. She received 22 units of regular insulin at 6:30 AM and was unable to eat her breakfast. The nurse needs to observe for:
① Increased urine output
② Polydipsia
③ Somnolence
④ Diaphoresis

222. The nurse is determining how well a patient with tuberculosis has achieved the goals for the nursing diagnosis: Ineffective breathing pattern related to sputum production. Which of the following expected outcomes is appropriate?
① Stable weight
② Clear breathing sounds
③ Negative sputum culture
④ Verbalizes need for Isoniazid (INH)

223. A patient has Ménière's disease and is taking medication for the vertigo. You are with the patient during a severe attack. Which of the following helps reduce the vertigo?
① Encourage the patient to move slowly to a chair
② Take an additional dose of meclizine (Antivert)
③ Increase fluid intake to 2000 cc/day
④ Darken the room

224. A patient suffers from presbycusis. Based on your understanding of this condition, which of the following best states nursing concerns for the patient?
① At risk for alteration in comfort (physical)
② At risk for injury: falls
③ At risk for alteration in family roles
④ At risk for increasing alteration in sensory perception, auditory

225. A patient fell in the bathroom, hitting her head on the commode. In monitoring her vital signs, which of the following blood pressures would indicate that the patient is experiencing an increase in intracranial pressure?
    ① Systolic decreasing, diastolic decreasing
    ② Systolic decreasing, diastolic increasing
    ③ Systolic increasing, diastolic decreasing
    ④ Systolic increasing, diastolic increasing

226. Your patient, who wears a hearing aid in her left ear, has sensory perceptual alteration: Auditory, related to decreased hearing secondary to cerumen buildup. The most appropriate plan is to:
    ① Encourage chewing motions and daily washing of the ears
    ② Encourage periodic ear washing in the clinic
    ③ Encourage increasing fluid intake to 2000 cc/day
    ④ Encourage cleaning the hearing aid with hydrogen peroxide

227. The nurse is watching for any early, untoward effects in a patient who just had a lumbar puncture done. The nurse should be assessing for:
    ① Delayed capillary refill of the lower extremities
    ② Complaints of headache
    ③ Difficulty with bladder control
    ④ Change in blood pressure

228. You are evaluating your patient's ability to demonstrate correct technique in doing an ear irrigation. The pinna in an adult is pulled:
    ① Up, back, and out
    ② Up, forward, and in
    ③ Down, back, and in
    ④ Down, forward, and in

229. You are presenting a class on hearing difficulties of the elderly to the aides. Behavioral clues indicating difficulty in hearing and the need for evaluation by an otolaryngologist include:
    ① Complaining of ringing in the ears
    ② Avoiding face-to-face contact
    ③ Changing body positions frequently
    ④ Speaking while others are talking

230. In a patient who has a stage 2 decubitus ulcer and pneumonia, the nurse makes the following observations. Which one is the priority?
    ① Temperature of 99.6° F (37.5° C)
    ② Facial flushing
    ③ Tachypnea
    ④ Productive cough

231. In distinguishing between a sprain and a fracture, the nurse would be more suspicious of a fracture if which of the following signs were present on assessment?
    ① Edema
    ② Deformity
    ③ Limited movement
    ④ Tenderness to palpation of the area

232. An adult patient is placed in Buck's extension traction to the left leg. The nurse is aware that this type of traction can be useful in which of the following injuries?
    ① Neck sprains
    ② Spinal fractures
    ③ Shoulder dislocations
    ④ Lower extremity and hip fractures

233. There are several complications associated with Russell's traction. The nurse will monitor the patient for which one of the following?
    ① Drainage at the cast site
    ② Signs of compartment syndrome
    ③ Pressure under the popliteal space
    ④ Evidence of undue skin pressure from under the boot

234. Which one of the following special precautions will the nurse incorporate into the plan of care for an 82-year-old patient who has undergone an open reduction and internal fixation of the hip?
    ① Monitor for nutritional problems
    ② Maintain proper extremity alignment
    ③ Keep the side rails in an elevated position
    ④ Frequent inspection of linen and dressings for drainage

235. In planning preoperative care for a patient about to undergo a below-the-knee amputation, the nurse may focus on postoperative care by explaining
    ① Elements of the exercise program
    ② Postoperative measures to control pain
    ③ Turning, coughing, and deep breathing maneuvers
    ④ Visiting hours immediately after the surgery

236. A 42-year-old male fractured his right tibia and fibula and arrives on the unit following an open reduction and application of a long plaster cast. Two hours after arriving on the unit, the patient complains of severe pain in his right leg. The best nursing action would be to:
    ① Administer the oral pain medication as ordered
    ② Turn the patient, rub his back, and straighten the linen
    ③ Evaluate the neurocirculatory status of the affected leg
    ④ Check the right leg to make sure that it is elevated and externally rotated

237. Your patient is being instructed on postlumbar puncture care. She is apprehensive about getting "sick with a terrible headache like her neighbor did when she had that test done." Your most appropriate response is:
    ① "Moving about after the test is the best way to prevent a headache."
    ② "You will need to remain flat on your stomach after the test. This will prevent the headache."
    ③ "You will be able to drink fluids after the test. That, as well as lying flat, helps most people."
    ④ "With all the advances in medicine, these types of headaches are not common anymore."

238. In a patient with emphysema, the priority nursing diagnosis is: Alteration in nutritional status related to fatigue secondary to work of breathing. In planning to instruct the patient, which of the following instructions refers to the nursing diagnosis?
    ① Eat several small meals each day
    ② Keep the oxygen between 1 and 2 L/min
    ③ Increase fluid intake to 8 glasses/day
    ④ Increase hours of sleep throughout the day

239. You noticed that your patient has new areas of ecchymosis. Based on your understanding that some skin lesions may result from toxic, metabolic, or allergic reactions to drugs, which of these newly-ordered drugs would you suspect?
    ① Mafenide acetate (Sulfamylon)
    ② Warfarin (Coumadin)
    ③ Penicillin G (Bicillin)
    ④ Salicylates (Trilisate)

240. The nurse on the previous shift charted that the patient was drowsy. Which of the following behaviors would support this description of the patient's level of consciousness?
    ① Responds appropriately when aroused
    ② Absence of response even to painful stimuli
    ③ Incomplete arousal to painful stimuli
    ④ Response to verbal command is inconsistent, vague
241. A patient is being observed for increased intracranial pressure. Which classification of drugs, besides anticonvulsants and corticosteroids, would you expect to be ordered?
    ① Narcotic analgesics
    ② Antiemetics
    ③ Osmotic diuretics
    ④ Antibiotics
242. The nurse is distributing health literature on prostate cancer. Which of the following blood tests is recommended by the American Cancer Society as a screening test for this type of cancer?
    ① CEA (carcinogenic embryonic antigen)
    ② PSA (prostate-specific antigen)
    ③ DRE (digital rectal exam)
    ④ ELISA (enzyme-linked immunoabsorbent assay)
243. In a head trauma patient being treated for increased intracranial pressure, which of the following would be *least likely* to cause complications?
    ① Isometric exercises
    ② Aerobic exercises
    ③ Passive range of motion exercises
    ④ High Fowler's position
244. Your patient has just returned to his room after undergoing a myelogram using Pantopaque (iodine-based) dye. What position is most therapeutic for this patient?
    ① Up ad lib
    ② Supine for at least 6 to 8 hours
    ③ Head of bed elevated 15 degrees
    ④ Head of bed elevated 60 degrees
245. In teaching your patient who experiences migraine headaches, which of these behaviors indicates that the patient teaching has been successful?
    ① The patient states that she needs to exercise daily
    ② The patient states that she will wear sunglasses when outdoors
    ③ The patient states that she will take an aspirin daily to prevent the headache
    ④ The patient identifies the factors that trigger her headaches
246. You are teaching a health class to adolescent men about the testicular self-exam and testicular cancer. Which of the following would you stress as a warning sign that needs to be reported to a physician?
    ① A tight prepuce that cannot be retracted
    ② Urinary urgency and frequency
    ③ A dull ache in the lower abdomen
    ④ Pain upon urination
247. The nurse is aware of the circulatory pathway through the heart. In congestive heart failure, symptoms of dyspnea, pedal edema, and increased abdominal girth most likely signal a problem with which part of the heart?
    ① Mitral valve
    ② Aortic valve
    ③ Right ventricle
    ④ Left ventricle

248. A diabetic patient has developed an elevated temperature, cough, and congested breath sounds. The physician orders a complete blood count (CBC) "stat." When the results are received, the nurse will focus on what part of the CBC to help guide her care of the patient?
    ① White blood cells
    ② Hemoglobin and hematocrit
    ③ Red blood cell indices
    ④ Platelet count and morphology
249. The nurse is assessing a patient who is in a long-leg cast. The nurse is aware that this patient had an abraded area of the involved leg, and has been in this cast for 7 days now. A very warm spot is noted in a particular area of the cast. The nurse knows that a hot spot could indicate:
    ① That the cast is too tight
    ② Swelling under the cast
    ③ Inflammation under the cast
    ④ A foreign body under the cast
250. A hypertensive patient has been started on a medication that can cause orthostatic hypotension. The nurse can explain to the patient that this side effect can be minimized by:
    ① Wearing antiembolic stockings
    ② Limiting the sodium in the diet
    ③ Resting after each meal
    ④ Sitting on the edge of the bed momentarily before arising
251. A patient reports that his anginal pain increases with exertion. The nurse is aware that angina pectoris indicates:
    ① Problems with the mitral valve
    ② Insufficient blood supply to the heart muscle
    ③ A myocardial infarction
    ④ A thrombosed cerebral artery
252. A patient's injuries sustained in a car accident have resulted in cerebral edema. Which of the following is the most appropriate position for this patient?
    ① Supine
    ② Prone
    ③ Low- to mid-Fowler's
    ④ Mid- to high-Fowler's
253. In a patient receiving continuous bladder irrigations following a transurethral prostatectomy, the nurse assesses that the catheter may be blocked. The most appropriate instruction the nurse should give the patient is to:
    ① Try to void around the catheter
    ② Deep breathe, cough, and remain perfectly still until the doctor arrives
    ③ Notify the nurse if he notices a change in the color of the drainage in the bag
    ④ Increase fluid intake to 4000 cc/day
254. A patient has returned from having a myelogram using Metrizamide (water-based) dye. Which of the following postprocedure actions is most appropriate?
    ① Encourage fluids
    ② Secure a bedside commode
    ③ Spray the room with a room deodorizer
    ④ Administer all drugs withheld before the procedure

255. A patient, diagnosed with a seizure disorder, is being treated with phenytoin (Dilantin) and valproic acid (Depakene). Which of the following statements should the nurse consider the priority teaching need for this patient?
    ① Must use good oral hygiene
    ② Must increase intake of green, leafy vegetables
    ③ Must carry a padded tongue blade at all times
    ④ Must sleep 6 to 8 hours each night

256. In a patient with cerebral edema, which of the following nursing plans is most appropriate?
    ① Administer stool softeners as ordered
    ② Encourage a full glass of water with each medication
    ③ Keep the room dark and quiet
    ④ Medicate for pain before ambulation

257. Patients with sensory dysfunction, such as persons with paraplegia, have many teaching needs. Which one of the following is a high-priority teaching need?
    ① Importance of doing own weight shifts for 5 minutes qh
    ② Importance of decreasing calcium intake
    ③ Importance of avoiding cold or very hot foods
    ④ Importance of adequate fluid intake of 2000 cc/day

258. The patient has been maintaining an acid ash diet and has been instructed to avoid certain medications and foods. Which of the following may the patient have?
    ① Salt substitutes
    ② Antacids
    ③ Sulfa drugs
    ④ NutraSweet

259. The patient has chronic renal failure. You are evaluating his knowledge of the dietary restrictions. Which of the following statements by the patient reflects changes to keep within the dietary restrictions?
    ① "I never did eat much meat."
    ② "I eat a lot of bread and potatoes."
    ③ "I'd better watch how many pickles and olives I eat."
    ④ "Bananas give me gas, so I avoid them."

260. Your patient just underwent a cystoscopy. Immediately following this procedure, which of the following nursing actions is most appropriate?
    ① Taking vital signs
    ② Administering the PRN narcotic ordered for pain
    ③ Applying cool towels to the lower abdomen
    ④ Assisting the patient off the table to the wheelchair

261. Your patient has had a cutaneous ureterostomy performed and has catheters (stents) inserted through the ureters to drain the renal pelvis. One of your main concerns is:
    ① Preventing contamination of the stents with stool
    ② Testing urine for protein, blood, and glucose
    ③ Maintaining patency of the stents
    ④ Irrigating the stents

262. Your patient has Parkinson's disease and takes the following medications: amantadine (Symmetrel) and trihexyphenidyl hcl (Artane). In evaluating the effectiveness of these medications, which of the following therapeutic responses would you expect?
    ① Decreased salivation, less tremor of head/hands at rest
    ② Expressions of depression and thoughts of suicide
    ③ Normal vital signs, propulsive gait
    ④ Less visual blurring and mental confusion

263. A concern of the nurse who is caring for an HIV-positive patient is to provide education. The nurse should explain how the patient can prevent:
    ① AIDS
    ② Pneumonia
    ③ Hypotension
    ④ Opportunistic infections

264. The nurse is aware that oral hypoglycemic agents may be used for patients with diabetes mellitus who have:
    ① Obesity
    ② Liver disease
    ③ Type I (juvenile onset) diabetes
    ④ Some insulin production

265. A patient is admitted to the unit in diabetic ketoacidosis. The most common cause of ketoacidosis is:
    ① Stress
    ② Infection
    ③ Too much insulin
    ④ Not enough food

266. What type of insulin would the nurse expect to give to a patient in diabetic ketoacidosis?
    ① NPH
    ② Lente
    ③ Ultra-Lente
    ④ Regular

267. A 76-year-old patient with severe arthritis is taking large doses of an antiinflammatory medication that has a side effect of gastric irritation. Patient teaching should include instructions to:
    ① Avoid driving
    ② Take with food
    ③ Discontinue if CNS effects develop
    ④ Take on an empty stomach to enhance absorption

268. When assessing and planning care for any patient it is essential that the nurse be knowledgeable about the disease process. When preparing for a new patient with the diagnosis of rheumatoid arthritis, the nurse should be aware that the disease is a:
    ① Local joint disease
    ② Self-limited illness
    ③ Disease of striated muscles
    ④ Chronic and systemic disease

269. Rheumatoid arthritis can be managed with rest, exercise, and medication. The nurse must be aware that first-line pharmacologic management includes use of:
    ① Narcotic analgesics
    ② Muscle relaxants
    ③ Antiinflammatory agents
    ④ Calcium channel-blocking agents

270. In the patient who has a cystostomy drain in place following a suprapubic prostatectomy, the nurse should:
    ① Assess the perineal dressing for drainage
    ② Take vital signs more frequently
    ③ Catheterize the patient if he complains of bladder fullness
    ④ Assess the abdominal dressing and change PRN

271. In the patient suspected of having benign prostatic hypertrophy, the common, most frequent, and disturbing signs to assess for are:
    ① Dysuria, nocturia
    ② Hematuria, groin discomfort
    ③ Flank pain, chills
    ④ Bladder stones, malaise

272. The patient with a cervical spinal injury exhibits spasticity of the extremities. Which of the following types of

medications will assist in decreasing the spasticity for the patient?

① Muscle relaxants such as baclofen (Lioresal)
② Vasodilators such as terazosin hcl (Hydrin)
③ Narcotic analgesics such as morphine sulfate (Roxanol)
④ NSAIDs such as tolmetin sodium (Tolectin)

273. The patient with an arteriovenous fistula and graft in the left forearm receives hemodialysis 3 times a week. The nurse should plan to:

① Keep the patient on bed rest
② Irrigate the fistula every 4 hours
③ Take the blood pressure on the right arm
④ Monitor I and O hourly

274. In a patient with the nursing diagnosis of Knowledge deficit related to TURP, the expected outcome is that the patient will describe activity restrictions. Which of the following teaching points is most appropriate?

① Avoid straining at stool for 4 to 6 weeks by using stool softeners as necessary
② Do Kegel perineal exercises every 4 to 6 hours for the next 2 weeks
③ Report any dribbling that occurs in the next 2 weeks
④ Monitor appearance of urine and report if urine becomes persistently bright red

275. During the fifth day in coronary care, a patient with a diagnosis of myocardial infarction develops dyspnea, has blood-tinged, frothy sputum, and becomes very anxious. These symptoms may indicate:

① Pulmonary edema
② Emphysema
③ Pulmonary embolism
④ Chronic obstructive pulmonary disease

ANSWERS AND RATIONALES

1. Knowledge (a)
   ④ Platelets stick together and form a plug that seals the wound. They release chemicals that eventually result in formation of clot.
   ① Antibodies are produced in response to a specific antigen.
   ② Leukocytes are WBCs, which destroy pathogens.
   ③ Erythrocytes are RBCs, which carry oxygen from lungs to tissues.

2. Knowledge (a)
   ① The body is constantly stabilizing and equalizing its environment to prevent any sudden or severe change.
   ② Diffusion is the process of dissolved particles being distributed evenly throughout a fluid.
   ③ Osmosis is the movement of water through a permeable membrane.
   ④ Filtration is the movement of water and solutes through a membrane because of a greater pushing force on one side of the membrane.

3. Knowledge (a)
   ④ The DNA molecules in the nucleus of a cell duplicate themselves, and the cell divides, forming two cells.
   ① Osmosis is the movement of water through a permeable membrane.
   ② Crenation is the shrinking of red cells placed in a hypertonic salt solution.
   ③ Lysis is the swelling of red cells placed in a hypotonic salt solution.

4. Knowledge (a)
   ③ In acquiring passive immunity the body of the recipient plays no active part in response to an antigen.
   ① In active immunity the resistance to a disease results from the development of antibodies within the body.
   ② Autoimmune immunity occurs by the body's producing antibodies to its own tissue.
   ④ Newborn babies receive a short-term immunity as a result of the antibodies of their mother.

5. Knowledge (a)
   ② The functional unit is suspended near the center of the cell and has the property of division.
   ① Cytoplasm is the portion of the protoplasm of a cell outside the nucleus.
   ③ Protoplasm is a thick, viscous substance that exists only in cells.
   ④ The cytoplasmic membrane encloses the cytoplasm.

6. Knowledge (a)
   ③ Produced by the thyroid gland, thyroxin controls the rate at which glucose is burned and converts it to heat and energy.
   ① Oxytocin initiates and maintains labor.
   ② Aldosterone promotes sodium and water retention in the kidney.
   ④ Cortisone assists the body to respond to stress and reduces inflammation.

7. Knowledge (a)
   ③ Estrogen and progesterone promote development of the female sex characteristics and sex organs and regulate menstruation for the purpose of reproduction.
   ①,② Testosterone is produced in the testes.
   ④ Prolactin is produced in the pituitary gland.

8. Comprehension (b)
   ② Dilation of the blood vessels brings more blood to the surface so that heat can be dissipated.
   ① Contraction slows the amount of blood in the veins and serves to protect the skin and deeper tissue from excess heat loss.
   ③ The production of sweat is increased by dilation of blood vessels but is not the primary cause of loss of body heat.
   ④ An increase in blood supply constricts muscles rather than relaxing them.

9. Knowledge (a)
   ① The area is located slightly below the center of each breast and contains slightly raised areas (glands of Montgomery).
   ② Bartholin's glands lie on each side of the vaginal outlet.
   ③ Cowper's glands are located on either side of the urethra and just below the prostate gland in the male.
   ④ Urochrome gives urine its color.

10. Knowledge (a)
    ③ The male sex glands produce the hormone that regulates male sex characteristics.
    ① Progesterone is produced by the ovaries.
    ② Estrogen is produced by the ovaries.
    ④ Aldosterone is produced by the adrenal cortex.

11. Knowledge (a)
    ① The connective tissue is made of dense fibrous tissue in the shape of a cord and has great strength.
    ② Ligaments attach bones to bones.
    ③ Cartilage makes a slick surface for rotation and absorbs shock.
    ④ Osseous is commonly called bony tissue.

12. Knowledge (b)
    ③ The lymphatic system drains excess fluids through a series of filters, lymph nodes, where bacteria and foreign bodies are trapped and destroyed.
    ① The lymphatic system destroys bacteria.
    ② Erythrocytes are manufactured primarily in long bones.
    ④ Clotting of blood is aided by platelets.

13. Comprehension (c)
    ④ Iron is an essential mineral in the formation of hemoglobin.
    ① Copper assists in the use of iron.
    ② Magnesium is essential in general metabolism.
    ③ Calcium is essential in bone and tooth formation.

14. Knowledge (b)
    ② Fat globules must be broken down into very small particles (emulsified) to be digested. Bile is the enzyme that emulsifies fat.
    ① Bile does not act on the protein that is part of meat fiber. Pepsin and hydrochloric acid break down protein.
    ③ Bile does not assist in the breakdown of sugar, only fats.
    ④ The liver cells convert complex sugar, glycogen, to glucose.

15. Comprehension (a)
    ③ Epithelial tissue has many forms—flat and irregular, square, long and narrow—that are arranged in single or many layers to form a protective covering and lining.
    ① Periosteum is a connective tissue covering the bone.
    ② Pericardium is a fibrous sac lined with serous membrane that surrounds the heart.
    ④ Connective tissue supports and connects other tissues and parts of the body.

16. Comprehension (a)
    ❶ The cardiac sphincter separates the esophagus from the stomach region close to the heart.
    ② Rugae are the folds in the stomach lining.
    ③ Chyme is a semiliquid mixture of gastric juices and food.
    ④ The pyloric sphincter is located between the distal end of the stomach and the proximal end of the small intestine and determines how long food stays in the stomach.

17. Comprehension (a)
    ❸ The small intestine secretes enzymes that digest proteins and carbohydrates, and most of the digestive process, absorption, occurs in the small intestine.
    ① The liver has many functions, such as storing glucose and manufacturing bile.
    ② The stomach serves as a storage pouch and a digestive organ.
    ④ The large intestine stores and eliminates waste and reabsorbs water.

18. Knowledge (a)
    ❷ Circular muscles contract when stimulated, closing an opening.
    ① Adduction is movement toward the body.
    ③ Extensors cause the angle of the joint to become larger.
    ④ Flexors cause the angle of the joint to become smaller.

19. Knowledge (a)
    ❹ A small opening into the nose at the inner corner of the eye allows the fluid to drain through.
    ① The ciliary body is a smooth muscle structure to which the lens is attached.
    ② The lacrimal gland releases tears into the anterior surface of the eyeball.
    ③ The eustachian tube connects the middle ear chambers with the throat.

20. Knowledge (a)
    ❸ Incisors are the four top and bottom front teeth.
    ① Eye teeth, or canines, appear later in the baby.
    ② Molars are the last to appear, usually by 2 to 2 1/2 years.
    ④ Canines are another name for eye teeth and appear after the incisors.

21. Knowledge (a)
    ❸ Many gray matter areas that form the cranial nerves are located in the medulla and are involved in the control of vital activities.
    ① The cerebellum controls muscle tone, coordination, and equilibrium.
    ② The cerebrum controls the highest level of functioning, sensation, memory, reasoning, and intelligence.
    ④ The pons carries messages between the cerebrum and the medulla.

22. Knowledge (a)
    ❷ As peristalsis moves content along, water is absorbed through the walls into the circulation, and the remaining cellulose passes on to the rectum.
    ① Absorption of food occurs in the small intestine.
    ③ Enzymes are produced in the mouth, stomach, pancreas, and small intestine.
    ④ Enzymes are secreted from the mouth, stomach, pancreas, and small intestine.

23. Knowledge (a)
    ❹ The progressive, wavelike movement that occurs involuntarily forces food forward.

    ① Pylorospasm is a spasm of the pyloric sphincter.
    ② Rugae are large folds of mucous membrane.
    ③ Mastication is chewing.

24. Comprehension (b)
    ❶ Gastric and intestinal enzymes gradually break down the protein molecule into its separate amino acids.
    ② Ptyalin is an enzyme found in saliva.
    ③ Hydrochloric acid is an enzyme found in the stomach.
    ④ Glucose is the breakdown product of carbohydrates.

25. Knowledge (a)
    ❸ The process of digestion is accelerated, and, as the food moves through the loops of the intestine, it is digested and absorbed by the villi into the blood and lymph capillaries.
    ① The large intestine absorbs water after digestion is completed.
    ② The process of digestion continues in the stomach.
    ④ Sigmoid is a part of the large intestine.

26. Comprehension (b)
    ❶ Bile is produced in the liver but is not an enzyme.
    ②,③,④ Is a function of the liver.

27. Comprehension (b)
    ❹ Iodine is an element that aids in the formation of thyroxin, which is a hormone produced in the thyroid.
    ① Calcium aids in the formation of bones and teeth.
    ② Phosphorus aids in the calcification of bones and teeth.
    ③ Iron is essential in the formation of hemoglobin.

28. Comprehension (a)
    ❶ Capillaries connect arterioles with venules and function as exchange vessels.
    ② Veins transport the blood back to the heart.
    ③ Arterioles carry blood to capillaries.
    ④ Venules carry blood from capillaries to veins.

29. Comprehension (a)
    ❶ Deoxygenated blood returns from body tissues through the superior and inferior vena cava into the right atrium.
    ② Left atrium receives oxygenated blood.
    ③ Right ventricle receives deoxygenated blood from the right atrium.
    ④ Left ventricle receives oxygenated blood from the left atrium.

30. Knowledge (a)
    ❸ Epinephrine is a hormone manufactured in the adrenal medulla and increases blood pressure and heart rate.
    ① Insulin is manufactured in the pancreas and decreases blood sugar levels.
    ② Aldosterone is produced in the adrenal cortex and aids in regulating electrolytes and water balance.
    ④ Testosterone is produced by the testes and stimulates growth and development of sex organs.

31. Comprehension (c)
    ❸ Antidiuretic hormone (ADH) produced in the posterior pituitary promotes reabsorption.
    ① Oxytocin produced in the posterior pituitary causes uterine muscles to contract.
    ② Calcitonin is produced in the thyroid and assists in decreasing calcium level in blood.
    ④ Prolactin is produced in the anterior pituitary and promotes growth of all body tissues.

32. Comprehension (a)
    ❷ The diffusion of gas occurs across the thin, squamous epithelium lining of the alveoli.
    ① The bronchi carry air to the right and left lung.
    ③ Bronchioles are the smallest branches of the bronchi.
    ④ Venules collect blood from capillaries.

33. Knowledge (a)
    ❹ SA node, located in the right atrium, starts each heart beat.
    ① AV node receives the impulse from SA node.
    ② Bundle of His receives the impulse from AV node.
    ③ Purkinje fibers receive impulses from bundle of His, resulting in the contraction of the ventricles.

34. Comprehension (a)
    ❶ The pulmonary artery carries deoxygenated blood from the heart.
    ② Aorta carries oxygenated blood from the heart.
    ③ Coronary artery carries oxygenated blood to the heart.
    ④ Carotid artery carries oxygenated blood to the brain.

35. Comprehension (a)
    ❷ T-cells are lymphocytes that are produced by the thymus and produce an immunity.
    ① The thyroid influences cell metabolism.
    ③ The pineal secretes melatonin, which may regulate sexual development.
    ④ The pituitary produces many hormones that affect growth and development, protects the body in stressful situations, promotes reabsorption of water, etc.

36. Comprehension (b)
    ❸ The greater trochanter is the ball-like head, which articulates with the hip bone.
    ① Acetabulum is the deep socket in the hip bone.
    ② Acromion is the highest point of the shoulder.
    ④ Olecranon process is the upper end of the elbow; forms point of elbow.

37. Comprehension (a)
    ❸ Periosteum is a strong fibrous membrane that covers the bone and provides growth, nutrition, and repair.
    ① Red blood cells are formed in red marrow of bone.
    ② Yellow bone marrow is a fatty material found inside the long bone.
    ④ Adipose tissue is stored in the diaphysis or shaft.

38. Comprehension (a)
    ❷ Perineum is the external region between vulva and anus in a female or between scrotum and anus in the male and forms the pelvic floor.
    ① Peritoneum lines the abdominal cavity and folds over abdominal organs.
    ③ Mons pubis is the fatty rounded area overlying the pubic symphysis.
    ④ Rectus abdominis is an abdominal muscle.

39. Comprehension (b)
    ❸ The integumentary system includes the skin and appendages. Rashes, bruises, and decubitus are noted on the skin.
    ① Blood pressure and pulse are considered part of the respiratory and cardiovascular system.
    ② Blood sugar levels would be an assessment of the endocrine system, pancreas.
    ④ Although rashes and bruises are considered in assessment of the integumentary system, blood sugar levels are assessed with the endocrine system.

40. Comprehension (b)
    ❸ Sebaceous glands produce an oily secretion for lubrication. Blackheads are a mixture of dirt and sebum and collect at the openings of the sebaceous glands.
    ① Ceruminous glands or wax glands are in the ear.
    ② Lacrimal glands produce tears, which keep the conjunctiva of the eye moist.
    ④ Sudoriferous glands are sweat glands that regulate body temperature.

41. Comprehension (b)
    ❹ Normal urine has a low specific gravity.
    ① Urine is a clear, amber liquid.
    ② Urine is composed of nitrogenous waste products.
    ③ Urine is slightly aromatic.

42. Comprehension (b)
    ❸ The upper surfaces of the dermis have raised and depressed areas that are unique to each individual and thus a means of identification.
    ① Elastic connective tissue is found in the subcutaneous layer.
    ② The subcutaneous layer is below the dermis.
    ④ Upper surface of the epidermis consists of the outermost cells that are constantly lost to wear and tear.

43. Comprehension (c)
    ❷ Aldosterone is released by the adrenal cortex in response to decreased blood volume, decreased blood sodium ions, or increased potassium ions.
    ① ADH prevents excess water loss in the urine.
    ③ Parathormone regulates calcium-ion homeostasis of the blood.
    ④ Oxytocin stimulates uterine muscles during birth.

44. Knowledge (b)
    ❹ Oxygen prevents the accumulation of lactic acid, which can cause muscle fatigue, and glycogen, which is a source of food.
    ① Acetylcholine is important in the transmission of nerve impulses and synapses.
    ② Lactic acid is a waste product and causes muscle fatigue.
    ③ Acetylcholine is important in the transmission of nerve impulses and synapses.

45. Comprehension (b)
    ❶ The left motor control center in the brain controls the right side of the body because of the crossing of the nerve tracts within the brain.
    ② The left side of the body is controlled by the right side of the brain.
    ③ Only one side of the body is affected if an injury is to only one side of the brain.
    ④ Only one arm would be affected, depending on which side of the brain was injured.

46. Comprehension (a)
    ❸ The diaphragm separates the abdomen from the thoracic cavity. It contracts with inspiration and relaxes with expiration.
    ① The latissimus dorsi is located in the middle lower back.
    ② The sternocleidomastoid is located alongside the neck.
    ④ The gastrocnemius is located in the calf of the leg.

47. Comprehension (c)
    ❹ The parasympathetic division of the autonomic nervous system maintains homeostasis by regulating digestion and circulation.

① Sensory neurons carry impulses toward the CNS.
② Interneurons (connecting) conduct impulses from the sensory neurons to the motor neurons.
③ The sympathetic nervous system controls the "fight or flight" response.

48. Comprehension (a)
❷ The hypothalamus is an important autonomic nervous system center and controls body temperature.
① Medulla controls heart rate, blood pressure, breathing, and swallowing.
③ Cerebral cortex is the outer layer of the cerebrum.
④ Cerebellum controls muscle tone and coordination and coordinates action of the voluntary muscles.

49. Comprehension (b)
❷ The snail-like cochlea is the organ of Corti and contains hearing receptors.
① Tympanic membrane is the eardrum.
③ Semicircular canal controls equilibrium.
④ Malleus is part of the middle ear.

50. Comprehension (c)
❶ The eustachian tube connects the middle ear with the throat; swallowing or yawning equalizes the pressure, which allows the eardrum to vibrate easily.
② The labyrinth is the internal ear.
③ Sound waves are passed through the oval window to the internal ear.
④ Ossicles are the three tiny bones in the middle ear.

51. Comprehension (c)
❷ When water intake is excessive, the kidneys excrete generous amounts of urine; if water intake is lost, they produce less urine; the process is regulated by hormones.
① The bladder is the reservoir for urine.
③ Islets of Langerhans produce insulin.
④ Gonads are the sex glands.

52. Comprehension (a)
❸ The islets of Langerhans are located in the pancreas and produce insulin.
① Pineal gland is found in the brain and atrophies at an early age.
② Insulin is released into the duodenum, a division of the small intestine.
④ The liver produces bile.

53. Comprehension (b)
❷ Primary function is to act against most bacteria, viruses, tumor cells, and foreign organs.
① B-cells are responsible for humeral immunity.
③ T-cells do clone into helpers and suppressors to carry out primary function, but statement 2 is most explicit.
④ B-cells clone antibody-producing plasma cells.

54. Knowledge (b)
❹ The aqueous humor, a watery fluid that fills most of the eyeball, maintains the slight forward curve of the cornea.
① Dilation of the pupil is regulated by the involuntary iris muscle.
② The lacrimal gland produces tears.
③ The thickness of the lens is regulated by the contraction of the ciliary body.

55. Knowledge, assessment, physiologic (b)
❹ This is important—skin color, warmth, sensation, and pulses should be checked frequently.

① Diet should be high in protein and vitamins to promote healing.
② Fluid intake should be increased to 2000 to 3000 cc/day to prevent such complications as constipation, renal calculi, and urinary tract infections.
③ Isometric and ROM exercises are encouraged.

56. Comprehension, assessment, physiologic (a)
❸ With blockage by a stone, little or no bile passes into the small intestines. Bile gives stool its classic color.
① May indicate upper GI bleeding or a normal change if the patient is on iron therapy.
②, ④ Not characteristic of a gallbladder dysfunction.

57. Comprehension, implementation, physiologic (b)
❶ Should raise blood glucose level.
② Diet drinks will not help in raising the blood glucose level.
③ May raise glucose to a higher level than required.
④ Insufficient amount to raise glucose level; will take several sugar cubes.

58. Comprehension, implementation, physiologic (a)
❶ Most fast-acting insulins peak in 2 to 4 hours following administration.
②,③,④ Not standard peak times for fast-acting insulins.

59. Comprehension, assessment, physiologic (b)
❷ Classic symptoms.
① Symptoms of neurocirculatory impairment.
③ May indicate embolism.
④ Symptoms of neurologic impairment.

60. Application, assessment, physiologic (c)
❶ Salty or sweet-tasting drainage from the operative area may indicate cerebral spinal fluid is leaking.
② Headache is frequent after craniotomy, usually caused by stretching or irritation of nerves of the scalp during the operation. Position shouldn't affect headache unless the left is the operative side.
③ Neither hunger nor temporary anorexia would indicate a possible complication. You would anticipate thirst postoperatively.
④ The patient has had general anesthesia so sleepiness is expected but level of consciousness changes are critical.

61. Application, implementation, environment (b)
❹ A mask with an eyeshield and gloves are need to protect the caregiver's hands and eyes from direct contact or spraying of infected secretions.
① A plain mask will not offer adequate protection against spraying of secretions.
② A plain mask will not offer adequate protection against spraying of secretions. Gloves are also needed to prevent direct contact exposure.
③ A mask is required to protect the eyes from accidental spraying of secretions from tracheostomy.

62. Comprehension, implementation, environment (c)
❶ The immunocompromised individual is unable to resist foreign agents and is susceptible to overwhelming infection.
② The immune deficient patient is encouraged not to be around groups of people, as this increases the risk of infection.
③ The nursing staff wears face masks to prevent spread of microorganisms to the patient.
④ Protective isolation precautions are implemented.

63. Comprehension, assessment, physiologic (b)
    ❷ The pelvis of a patient with muscular dystrophy widens, causing a waddling gait.
    ① Pillrolling is a common behavior associated with Parkinson's disease.
    ③ A shuffling gait is a common behavior also associated with Parkinson's disease.
    ④ Tardive dyskinesia is an irreversible condition of involuntary muscle movements seen in patients taking antipsychotic medications.

64. Application, planning, psychosocial (b)
    ❹ A patient newly diagnosed with ALS needs support from family and health care professionals. Of all the responses, this is a priority at this time.
    ① Periods of exercise are necessary, but they would not be increased. Adequate periods of rest are a necessity for this patient.
    ②,③ Unrelated to situation at this time; a priority during later stages of the disease.

65. Comprehension, planning, physiologic(a).
    ❸ It is true that it takes longer to inspire or expire air because of age-related physiologic changes.
    ① This is not a proven fact for the elderly.
    ② This is not a proven correlation.
    ④ It is true that there may be stiffness of the chest wall.

66. Comprehension, implementation, physiologic (a)
    ❹ For severe disease, accompanied by pain and loss of ROM, reconstruction of one or both articulating joint surfaces may be needed.
    ① Stabilizes joint by restricting ROM.
    ② Not performed on joints.
    ③ Diagnostic aid used to visualize the inside of a joint.

67. Comprehension, assessment, physiologic (b)
    ❸ These are signs rested during later stages of the disease; others include jaw clonus and respiratory difficulty.
    ① Aphasia is not a symptom noted in ALS; the patient can speak, but has difficulty doing so.
    ② Flexor muscles become spastic, not flaccid.
    ④ There is no sensory loss experienced with ALS; the patient remains alert.

68. Comprehension, implementation, environment (a)
    ❹ Obesity increases strain on weight-bearing joints; reduction of weight minimizes some of the presenting symptoms.
    ① Does not reduce joint strain, but maintains existing range of motion.
    ② Does not control strain in joints.
    ③ Provides comfort in strained joints.

69. Knowledge, assessment, physiologic (b)
    ❶ Classic finding.
    ②,③,④ More common in rheumatoid arthritis.

70. Comprehension, planning, environment (a)
    ❸ Current use of assistive devices is important in planning care and for safety considerations.
    ① Excessive use of alcohol is a consideration in any patient; tobacco use does not play a role in priority planning in this case.
    ② Significant for planning of diversional activity if hospitalization is prolonged.
    ④ May be significant if patient is not eating properly.

71. Application, implementation, physiologic (c)
    ❹ Commercial glucose concentrates can be absorbed between the buccal mucosa and gum; when patient fully awakens, give a fast-acting carbohydrate by mouth.
    ① Insulin lowers glucose levels; patient's blood glucose level needs to be elevated in hypoglycemia.
    ②,③ These actions will place patient at risk of aspiration; should not attempt getting patient to swallow unless she is fully conscious.

72. Knowledge, planning, physiologic (a)
    ❹ An increase in growth hormone after the epiphyseal plates close leads to acromegaly.
    ① Prolactin is not associated with acromegaly.
    ② Cortisol is made by the adrenal cortex; an overproduction causes Cushing's syndrome.
    ③ Overproduction of thyroid hormone is referred to as hyperthyroidism.

73. Application, implementation, environment (b)
    ❹ Allows the fluid left in the space to consolidate and lessens the possibility of mediastinal shift.
    ①,②,③ Inappropriate. Increases risk of mediastinal shift when placed on unaffected side.

74. Comprehension, implementation, physiologic (a)
    ❷ Monitors arterial oxygen saturation and can be used to regulate oxygen rate.
    ① The machine does not measure metabolic rate.
    ③ This is the physician's responsibility.
    ④ The machine does not measure heart rate.

75. Comprehension, planning, physiologic (b)
    ❷ Increased hydrostatic pressure in the portal system causes fluid to collect in the peritoneal space.
    ① Decreased albumin level is associated with ascites.
    ③ Ammonia levels may be elevated but do not cause cirrhosis.
    ④ Does not cause ascites.

76. Comprehension, implementation, environment (b)
    ❸ This is standard practice.
    ① A clean dressing is not a sterile dressing.
    ② This is not correct, is inappropriate, and is degrading to the physician.
    ④ Not a sterile dressing, which is standard practice.

77. Application, implementation, physiologic (b)
    ❶ A patient with a lobectomy may be turned to either side.
    ②,③,④ Does not allow for full expansion and drainage of all remaining lobes.

78. Application, implementation, physiologic (b)
    ❸ Bile is needed to emulsify fat. When fat requires bile for emulsification, the gallbladder contracts in an effort to release the bile to be used in this process. A diseased gallbladder that must contract causes a sensation of pain.
    ① Although a portion of this statement is true, this does not explain the mechanism by which pain is produced.
    ② Foods high in fat require bile released by the gallbladder to aid in the emulsification process.
    ④ It is possible that the duct leading from the liver to the gallbladder may become blocked, but it is less likely to involve the pancreas in most acute presentations.

79. Comprehension, evaluation, physiologic (a)
    ❷ Accidental removal of the parathyroid glands can lead to tetany, because the glands secrete a hormone that regulates calcium balance.

① A seizure is possible in tetany, but is not one of the initial symptoms.

③,④ Not associated with accidental parathyroid removal.

80. Comprehension, implementation, physiologic (a)
    ❶ Elevating the head of the bed will reduce the chance of reflux into the esophagus.
    ② This suggestion will not reduce bedtime discomfort.
    ③ This will only increase symptoms. Eating is recommended 3 hours before bedtime.
    ④ Will only increase symptoms.

81. Knowledge, implementation, environment (a)
    ❶ This is an appropriate position to start out this exam.
    ② This position does not provide good access to the rectal area.
    ③ Not the preferred position for good access to the rectum.
    ④ Does not provide good access to the rectal area.

82. Comprehension, assessment, physiologic (b)
    ❹ Alcohol is an irritant that can predispose the patient who is abusing alcohol to cancer.
    ① Although smoking is a risk factor, it is more a risk for lung cancer.
    ②,③ Not usually a risk factor.

83. Comprehension, planning, environment (a)
    ❸ Medication is taken first thing in the morning before breakfast.
    ① Meals spaced farther apart place patient at risk of hypoglycemia.
    ② Planned daily exercise is encouraged.
    ④ Hypoglycemia can be countered with the ingestion of a rapid-acting sugar.

84. Knowledge, implementation, environment (a)
    ❷ Yeast overgrowth is a side effect of antibiotic therapy.
    ① A condition caused by low levels of serum calcium.
    ③ A thyroid condition in which there is overproduction of thyroid hormone.
    ④ A viral infection. Herpes type II can invade the genital area, but is associated with antibiotic use.

85. Comprehension, planning, physiologic (b)
    ❸ Stress and exertion can overtax the patient and increase the risk of an addisonian crisis.
    ① Activity has to be planned and moderated.
    ② Diversional activity does not take priority over #3.
    ④ Again, this is part of the care of most patients, but the priority is reducing the risk of an addisonian crisis.

86. Comprehension, planning, physiologic (a)
    ❸ Addison's disease is a failure to produce the needed hormones by the adrenal cortex (glucocorticoids and mineralocorticoids) that help regulate electrolyte balance.
    ①,②,④ Addison's disease does not involve blood cell deveopment or bone marrow function; see response in #3

87. Application, implementation, environment (b)
    ❷ Raising the head of the bed may relieve the dyspnea if it is paroxysmal nocturnal dyspnea.
    ① Is helpful but doesn't physically relieve the underlying cause.
    ③ Is not necessary based on information given. Also, suctioning may cause trauma to mucous membranes.
    ④ Not appropriate. In addition, some pain medication may depress respirations.

88. Application, implementation, physiologic (b)
    ❹ May indicate bronchospasm and laryngospasms.
    ① Not usual; may indicate complications.
    ② Wheezing is abnormal; not a usual indication that anesthesia is wearing off.
    ③ Return of a gag reflex does not include wheezing.

89. Application, implementation, physiologic (a)
    ❷ Splinting protects the fracture, immobilizes the arm, and may prevent worsening of the situation.
    ① Use 911 only in true emergencies.
    ③ Warmth may actually cause an increase in edema and does not immobilize the fracture.
    ④ Elevate the affected extremity.

90. Application, planning, physiologic (b)
    ❸ If mucus is too thick for the patient to expectorate, aerosol treatments would help.
    ① Is appropriate but may not be as effective or act as quickly as #3.
    ② These actions would relieve the throat irritation but not assist in making his cough productive.
    ④ Inappropriate. The high humidity may make breathing more difficult.

91. Application, implementation, physiologic (b)
    ❹ May be associated with left-sided heart failure.
    ① May be caused by a variety of factors.
    ② VS should be documented although easy, regular respirations are normal.
    ③ This may have a variety of causes.

92. Knowledge, assessment, physiologic (a)
    ❷ Commonly affected by hypertension.
    ① Not associated with complications related to hypertension.
    ③ See rationale for #1.
    ④ Brain may be affected, but the blood and bladder are not associated with hypertensive complications.

93. Knowledge, implementation, physiologic (a)
    ❹ Correct definition.
    ① Definition of a bronchoscopy.
    ② Definition of an MRI.
    ③ Definition of spirometry.

94. Comprehension, implementation, environment (c)
    ❸ Necessary to assess for a pneumothorax.
    ① Also possible to note with chest x-ray, but not the primary reason.
    ② Inappropriate and unethical relative to the physician.
    ④ True, but stated in a way that would alarm the patient.

95. Application, implementation, physiologic (a)
    ❷ This is correct based on the use of the contrast medium (dye).
    ①,③ Not proper procedure; patient should be NPO.
    ④ This is not necessary; patient's activity has nothing to do with standard protocol for this test under normal circumstances.

96. Comprehension, assessment, physiologic (b)
    ❶ Used to determine areas of lung being ventilated, but not perfused, because of an obstruction or clot in the pulmonary circulation.
    ② Inappropriate test for this medical diagnosis (acute myocardial infarction).
    ③ Inappropriate test for this medical diagnosis (pulmonary tumor).
    ④ Definition of a cardiac catheterization.

97. Knowledge, implementation, physiologic (a)
    ❹ This is the most common location, less likely to puncture the lung.
    ① More appropriate for a paracentesis.
    ②,③ Improper placement.

98. Application, implementation, psychosocial (b)
    ❷ When flow rate is more than 4L/min humidification is necessary.
    ① Not really responsive to patient's concern.
    ③ True, however, is incomplete in rationale.
    ④ Humidity does not increase safety factors when oxygen is in use; also, such a statement may be cause for patient concern.

99. Comprehension, implementation, physiologic (a)
    ❷ Conversion of protein produces ammonia; ammonia affects the brain tissue.
    ① Carbohydrates are tolerated by a diseased liver.
    ③ Cation-exchange enemas remove toxic wastes.
    ④ Will not decrease ammonia levels.

100. Knowledge, implementation, physiologic (a)
    ❶ Regular insulin is fast acting and is used in the acute phase.
    ②,③ These are intermediate-acting insulins and do not act rapidly to lower blood sugar. They are not first choices.
    ④ This is an oral agent and is not used in the acute phase of DKA.

101. Knowledge (a)
    ❷ Glucose provides energy for fat and muscle cells.
    ① Glucose is sugar, not protein.
    ③ Glucose is an energy source.
    ④ Is not protoplasm.

102. Knowledge, assessment, physiologic (a)
    ❷ Infection can cause fluctuations to occur in blood sugar, usually in the form of elevations.
    ① Stress has been associated with aggravating blood sugar, but not in causing DKA in and of itself.
    ③ Excess insulin is associated with lowering blood glucose (hypoglycemia).
    ④ Also associated with hypoglycemia.

103. Comprehension, assessment, physiologic (a)
    ❸ Changes in the heart valve commonly manifest as murmurs.
    ① Syncope is not a usual symptom in these forms of valvular disease.
    ② Though chest pain is a symptom associated with the heart, it is not common to all valvular disease.
    ④ Unrelated to valvular disease.

104. Comprehension, assessment, physiologic (a)
    ❹ In a bedridden patient, dependent edema will pool at the sacrum.
    ①,② See #4.
    ③ In an ambulatory patient, dependent edema will be evidenced in the feet.

105. Comprehension, implementation, psychosocial (b)
    ❸ The fundoscopic exam is useful in examining the retina of the eye for changes that are suggestive of those accompanying hypertension.
    ① Merely tests visual acuity.
    ② Evaluates pressure within the eye and is useful in monitoring glaucoma.
    ④ Evaluates peripheral vision and is useful in monitoring glaucoma and in evaluating neurological problems.

106. Application, planning, environment (a)
    ❸ The incontinence, perspiration, and weight put her at risk for a pressure ulcer.
    ① Not appropriate; would also require assistance; shearing forces can cause breakdown.
    ② She could be positioned on her left side with appropriate support.
    ④ Inappropriate; may predispose to complications.

107. Application, assessment, physiologic (b)
    ❷ In dark-skinned persons skin under pressure appears darker than surrounding skin and may even take on a purplish hue.
    ① May mean she is able to bring up mucus on her own.
    ③ May be normal for the patient; age is unknown.
    ④ Patient may have secondary diagnosis of arthritis; age is unknown; remaining in bed in one position can also contribute to this type of complaint.

108. Application, planning, environment (b)
    ❶ Wound healing is limited by poor protein, vitamin, and caloric intake.
    ② Appropriate action, but not for this patient at this time.
    ③ Inappropriate. Nothing indicates that the decreased appetite is caused by depression; nurses do not diagnose.
    ④ All patients should be given this opportunity; not the most appropriate response.

109. Application, implementation, environment (b)
    ❷ Keeping the head of the bed below 30 degrees will reduce shearing of the skin.
    ① A turning schedule that is adhered to will be more effective.
    ③ Incorrect information is being given.
    ④ Inappropriately stated; also nerve endings may be compromised and pain may not be present.

110. Comprehension, assessment, safe environment (a)
    ❸ Eardrops should be warmed to body temperature (no more than 38° C). Vertigo may result from high or low temperatures.
    ① Although eardrops should be slowly instilled and allowed to flow into the canal, the rate most likely did not cause the vertigo.
    ② Occluded canal may cause vertigo. However, his vertigo occurred immediately following administration of the eardrops.
    ④ Most unlikely, although possible if being given for the first time. Not the best response.

111. Knowledge, assessment, physiologic (a)
    ❹ Common manifestations.
    ① Increased urination is not commonly associated with hypertension.
    ② Nausea and vomiting are not common manifestations.
    ③ Not common manifestations.

112. Comprehension, implementation, health (a)
    ❷ Intermittent catheterization is a part of a bladder retraining program. The objective is to periodically empty the bladder to decrease infections and incontinence.
    ① Inappropriate. Doesn't answer the patient's concern.
    ③ Inappropriate. The patient may be incontinent between catheterizations.
    ④ Inappropriate. Not a purpose of intermittent catheterization.

113. Knowledge, assessment, environment (a)
    ❸ Changes indicating decreased vital capacity or respiratory distress are signs of oxygen toxicity.
    ① Is a sign of Digoxin toxicity.
    ② Is a sign of glaucoma.
    ④ Is a sign of alkalosis or electrolyte imbalance.

114. Application, implementation, physiologic (a)
    ❶ At high end of normal range, failing kidneys cause abnormal buildup of electrolytes such as Na, Cl, K.
    ②,③,④ These are normal results.

115. Knowledge, assessment, physiologic (a)
    ❶ Is a sign of respiratory acidosis.
    ② Is a sign of respiratory alkalosis, metabolic alkalosis.
    ③ Is a sign of tissue hypoxia.
    ④ Is a sign of hypocalcemia.

116. Comprehension, planning, physiologic (a)
    ❶ A goal of therapy to restore oxygen to a damaged myocardium.
    ② A goal of overall management.
    ③ High anxiety levels may increase oxygen demand.
    ④ Oxygen does not prevent shock.

117. Application, implementation, environment (a)
    ❸ Are nonabsorbent, waterproof. Purpose is to protect the ulcer from contamination.
    ① Are absorbent. Purpose is to draw excessive drainage away from ulcer site.
    ② Purpose is to keep skin edges approximated.
    ④ Purpose is to debride or promote drainage.

118. Application, evaluation, physiologic (a)
    ❸ May indicate overhydration.
    ① Normal capillary refill time.
    ② Normal skin turgor.
    ④ Normal color and odor of urine.

119. Application, planning, environment (b)
    ❹ Persons with pulmonary disease are at risk for acidosis, secondary to CO_2 retention.
    ① Does not warrant checking within the next hour.
    ②,③ Not enough data to support this assumption.

120. Application, assessment, physiologic (b)
    ❷ Changes in the neurologic or circulatory status of the involved extremity indicate a complication.
    ① Is not associated with serious sequelae.
    ③,④ Not a postoperative complication.

121. Application, planning, environment (a)
    ❹ These are signs of hyponatremia.
    ① Inappropriate to monitor hourly.
    ② May be appropriate for continued assessment of the patient.
    ③ Inappropriate without communicating with RN or physician.

122. Application, implementation, physiologic (a)
    ❶ Maintains cleanliness. Is preventive skin care for maintaining integrity of skin.
    ②,③ Moisture provides growth medium for fungal infections. Oils and creams may be irritating to the skin.
    ④ Inappropriate; unnecessary action.

123. Knowledge, evaluation, physiologic (b)
    ❶ Acts by exerting a direct antispasmodic effect on smooth muscle such as the bladder.
    ② Cholinergic drugs helpful with atonic bladder.
    ③ Used for complaints of urinary frequency and urgency.
    ④ Is an antiinfective.

124. Application, implementation, physiologic (a)
    ❹ This ensures a continuous flow of urine in case specimens are needed, and aids in preventing multiplication of bacteria that may be introduced during the procedure.
    ① Bowel prep required if x-rays are taken. Enemas till clear may be unsafe depending on the number/amount administered.
    ② Unnecessary for this procedure.
    ③ Inappropriate; see rationale for correct response.

125. Comprehension, implementation, physiologic (a)
    ❸ The catheter produces the sensation of fullness. Attempting to strain to pass urine around the catheter causes the bladder muscles to contract, resulting in a painful bladder spasm.
    ① Is not an independent nursing action. May add to patient discomfort.
    ② Unsafe practice. May cause fluid backflow and introduce bacteria into the bladder.
    ④ Inappropriate; elevation of the scrotum will not decrease bladder spasms.

126. Comprehension, assessment, physiologic (a)
    ❶ These are the early symptoms.
    ② Is related and may indicate a UTI. General.
    ③,④ Part of any health history. General.

127. Comprehension, implementation, physiologic (b)
    ❶ Keeps the eyes (cornea) from drying out.
    ② Dilate eyes; do not lubricate.
    ③ Do not lubricate eyes.
    ④ Increases risk of corneal abrasion and eye problems.

128. Application, implementation, physiologic (b)
    ❷ Potentiates muscle weakness because of effect on myoneural junction.
    ① Blocks the action of cholinesterase at the myoneural junction and allows acetylcholine to act. Is therapeutic.
    ③ Corticosteroids are sometimes used as an adjunct therapy. Is therapeutic.
    ④ Blocks the action of cholinesterase at the myoneural junction and allows acetylcholine to act. Is therapeutic.

129. Application, planning, physiologic (b)
    ❹ Is an alkaline ash diet.
    ①,②,③ Appropriate as an acid ash diet.

130. Application, implementation, physiologic (a)
    ❸ The patient is displaying signs of hypovolemia. Initial measures would be those for shock. Turning on side helps prevent aspiration.
    ① Important to monitor vital signs; application of a cool cloth is a later measure.
    ② Sips of water are inappropriate if patient is going into shock.
    ④ Decreasing the room temperature is not relative to situation; turning on side helps to prevent aspiration.

131. Knowledge, assessment, physiologic (a)
    ❶ Abduction moves part away from midline.
    ② Adduction moves part toward midline.
    ③ Flexion makes angle at a joint smaller.
    ④ Pronation rotates a part to face downward.

132. Comprehension, planning, environment (a)
    ❶ Gluteus medius is a deep muscle located in the upper outer-quadrant of the hip and buttocks.
    ② Deltoid is a shallow muscle located in the upper arm and the patient is said to have muscle wasting.
    ③ Located in the posterior lower leg.
    ④ Sartorius winds down the thigh, ileum to the tibia.

133. Knowledge, assessment, physiologic (a)
    ❸ An overproduction of adrenal cortex hormones is associated with Cushing's syndrome.
    ① Overproduction of this hormone leads to acromegaly or giantism.
    ② Overproduction leads to hyperthyroidism.
    ④ Epinephrine is an adrenal medulla catecholamine.

134. Comprehension, implementation, environment (b)
    ❶ Additional stress placed on the tissues by movement and/or coughing may disrupt the healing tissues.
    ② This is true; however, the question asked why you would do this when getting her out of bed.
    ③ May be true; however, not the best choice.
    ④ It shouldn't if applied properly.

135. Comprehension, implementation, psychosocial (a)
    ❹ Acknowledge the patient's feelings and state the simple facts.
    ① The feeling tone is acknowledged, but the patient is not allowed the time for further verbalization.
    ② Statements should not start out with "why."
    ③ This will place the patient on the defensive and discourage further expression of feelings.

136. Comprehension, assessment, physiologic (a)
    ❸ Low blood sugar (hypoglycemic) symptoms.
    ①,② Not associated with hypoglycemia.
    ④ Symptoms of ketoacidosis.

137. Knowledge, assessment, physiologic (a)
    ❹ This type has no A or B antigens and can receive blood that is A, B, or O, provided the Rh factor is also compatible.
    ①,②,③ Can only receive blood that is compatible.

138. Comprehension, implementation, environment (c)
    ❷ Is true. The other circulatory and sensory changes that may occur with diabetes should also be considered.
    ① This is an abrasion and if cared for properly should not become infected.
    ③ Not enough data given.
    ④ Rebound swelling should not occur if the time of the cold application is no longer than 20 to 30 minutes.

139. Application, implementation, psychosocial (b)
    ❹ This is the least restrictive and intrusive. Visiting allows the nurse to assess the patient, provides the patient with distraction, and promotes her self-esteem. Repositioning would relieve strain.
    ①,③ Inappropriate. The older adult has a greater sensitivity to heat. CVA victims who have some neurosensory impairment may not be able to determine when complications of heat/cold applications occur.
    ② Giving this medication the way the order is written would violate the principles of medication administration.

140. Comprehension, evaluation, physiologic (b)
    ❷ Severe or increased pain in a wound may indicate that an infection or hematoma may be developing.
    ① Not likely after 6 days.
    ③ Is unlikely; a 4 × 4 is not used as a compression or pressure dressing.
    ④ Inspection of site is necessary; however, a soiled dressing is not always associated with pain.

141. Application, implementation, physiologic (b)
    ❸ Skin of older adults is fragile and may not tolerate adhesive tape. Frequent tape applications should be avoided.

① Although this is true, 3 explains the physiologic rationale for use of Montgomery straps, which is priority over cost.
    ② Inappropriate response; increase in infection would not be caused by the method used to secure the dressing.
    ④ The frequency of dressing changes is based on physician orders and/or the amount of drainage. The straps secure the dressing in place.

142. Application, implementation, physiologic (a)
    ❹ This provides countertraction and will minimize trauma of tissues. This should decrease patient discomfort.
    ① Should be done; however, this was not the principle asked for.
    ② Soaking is not necessary. Moistening may be indicated if the dressing adheres to the site or resistance is felt during removal.
    ③ Clean gloves are appropriate for removing dressing. Bringing the edges toward her would expose any drainage present.

143. Knowledge, assessment, physiologic (a)
    ❷ Is true. In dark-skinned persons, pressure areas appear darker. With blanching, these areas appear gray.
    ① Is descriptive in light-skinned persons.
    ③ Is a sign of pressure, not blanching.
    ④ May be a sign of pressure.

144. Application, assessment, physiologic (a)
    ❷ All are signs of hyperkalemia.
    ① These are vague, generalized signs and symptoms.
    ③ Are signs of fluid imbalance.
    ④ Are signs of fluid deficit.

145. Comprehension, implementation, environment, (a)
    ❸ Rapid administration of blood containing citrate predisposes the patient to hypocalcemia.
    ① Numbness is a symptom that can result from a variety of causes unrelated to metastatic carcinoma.
    ② Adverse signs of chemotherapy include nausea, vomiting, hair loss, and myelosuppression.
    ④ Signs of adult respiratory distress syndrome include shortness of breath, rapid breathing, tachycardia, and elevated blood pressure.

146. Comprehension, implementation, psychosocial (a)
    ❷ Does contain water, protein, carbohydrates, fats, electrolytes, vitamins, and trace elements. The subclavian vein or another large vein is used because of the high osmolarity of the nutrients.
    ① Septicemia is a possible complication.
    ③ Nutrients enter the circulatory system.
    ④ Inappropriate. Persons may take food orally while receiving TPN.

147. Knowledge, implementation, physiologic (a)
    ❷ Usually 1000 to 1500 ml is removed or enough to relieve symptoms; larger amounts place the patient at risk of developing hypovolemic shock; color is an indicator of infection and bleeding.
    ① High-Fowler's is the preferred position.
    ③ The abdomen is always prepared aseptically.
    ④ A sterile pressure dressing is applied to prevent leakage.

148. Knowledge, assessment, physiologic (a)
    ❸ Damaged parenchymal cells are unable to metabolize bilirubin, which gives the stool its normal color; bilirubin in the circulation causes jaundice, pruritus, and dark urine.

① Stools are clay colored because of the liver's inability to metabolize bilirubin.

② Urine is dark in liver dysfunction.

④ Stools are clay colored, and urine is dark.

149. Application, implementation, environment (a)

❸ Appropriate setting for adults.

① Appropriate setting for infants.

② Appropriate setting for children.

④ Inappropriate, unsafe; too much pressure exerted on mucous membranes.

150. Application, implementation, health (c)

❶ Encourages use of the arm and shoulder on the affected side. Movement of the affected side may increase confidence and decrease apprehension. Encourages joint mobility.

② Inappropriate; discourages normal ADL and ROM and may increase apprehension.

③ Inappropriate; a Vaseline occlusive dressing should be in place.

④ Raising side rails may make him feel more secure or may be a type of restraint.

151. Application, evaluation, environment (a)

❸ This would stop the tidaling.

① A complete assessment of the patient and the equipment should be performed first.

② Inappropriate; would not help pinpoint the reason tidaling has ceased.

④ Inappropriate to do at insertion site. A Vaseline occlusive dressing is at this location. Reinforcing all connecting sites may be helpful if a leak was present.

152. Knowledge, planning, health (a)

❶ Maintains healthy oral mucous membranes and decreases the risk of organisms entering the bloodstream.

② May be unrealistic.

③ Increased cost of using disposables is a factor. Proper disposal of used Kleenex would need to be taught.

④ Increased cost to patient. Not proven to be effective and may be dangerous practice.

153. Application, evaluation, physiologic (a)

❹ This would indicate that secretions have not accumulated.

① Would indicate an infection and/or dehydration.

② Inappropriate for this nursing diagnosis.

③ This would give the opportunity to assess the effort of breathing.

154. Knowledge, evaluation, physiologic (a)

❶ Provides for better drainage of secretions.

② Causes more postnasal drip. Not as comfortable because of frequent swallowing.

③,④ Secretions may pool. Patent airway may be occluded by this position.

155. Comprehension, planning, physiologic (a)

❹ Would help liquify secretions.

① Monitoring would give one factor of the patients' hydration status.

② Does not relate to the nursing diagnosis.

③ Humidity would be too high, adding to the effort of breathing. Sometimes increasing room humidity can aid in liquifying mucus that is thick and difficult to expectorate.

156. Application, planning, physiologic (a)

❹ To allow gravity drainage and prevent fluid backup.

① Inappropriate; may interfere with gravity drainage or cause fluid backup, depending on the height of the bed frame.

② Inappropriate. Is unsafe at this level.

③ The towel would not add to or maintain a patent safe drainage system.

157. Comprehension, implementation, physiologic (a)

❸ Persons with pharyngitis caused by streptococci may develop the complication of scarlet fever.

① Inappropriate. Nothing is ordered until the proper testing is completed. Reporting is necessary to obtain proper testing.

② Penicillin or antibiotics are the treatment of choice for streptococcal pharyngitis. Antibiotics should not be started until the specimen for C&S has been obtained.

④ Unusual, unless infected by scratching.

158. Application, implementation, physiologic (a)

❷ Lifting heavier items puts unnecessary stress on the healing site.

① May sit on these chairs. Should scoot to edge of seat and push up, using legs and arms together to rise up.

③ May shower/bathe. Site may be covered with a piece of Saran or plastic wrap.

④ Unnecessary restriction.

159. Knowledge, planning, physiologic (b)

❷ Cool temperatures cause vasoconstriction, and a comfortable room humidity prevents skin dryness.

① This would decrease the likelihood of skin excoriation.

③ True that pruritus may be a result of a drug reaction; however, this would not immediately add to the patient's comfort.

④ Administering medications that may not be needed is inappropriate.

160. Comprehension, assessment, physiologic (a)

❶ Increasing hoarseness will occur.

② Does not occur with laryngeal nerve damage.

③ Indicates tetany.

④ May indicate hemorrhage.

161. Comprehension, assessment, physiologic (b)

❸ Classic symptoms of carpopedal spasm and facial twitch.

①,②,④ Not classic symptoms of tetany.

162. Comprehension, planning, psychosocial (a)

❶ Calm environment is important; these patients are usually in a hyperexcitable state.

② Visitors may need to be limited to avoid overtaxing the patient's energies.

③ Private room ensures better control over the environment.

④ Provide a supportive environment; do not overtax the patient.

163. Comprehension, implementation, psychosocial (a)

❹ Chest x-ray can reveal an enlarged heart and help augment other diagnostic testing to rule in or rule out CHF.

①,② A simple explanation of the test is within the purview of nursing. Any questions requiring extensive explanations or indicating that the patient is truly not understanding his status should be left to the patient's physician(s).

③ A chest x-ray does not outline vessels in a way that would confirm the degree or extent of the disease process. That would require angiography.

164. Application, assessment, physiologic (a)
    ❹ Muscle weakness and personality changes herald the possibility of neurological problems.
    ① Chest pain on exertion is a common symptom.
    ② May have no symptoms at all, or symptoms of headache, fatigue, irritability.
    ③ Neurological signs are not as common as prodromal symptoms of an MI.

165. Comprehension, assessment, physiologic (b)
    ❸ Following this procedure there may be a loss of sufficient intrinsic factor
    ① Diabetes is a pancreatic problem resulting from insufficient amounts of insulin.
    ② Reflux refers to the backward flow of gastric contents through an incompetent sphincter, allowing gastric juices to flow into the esophagus.
    ④ *H. pylori* may be found in the gastric mucosa and is suspected of causing peptic ulcers that will recur, unless the *H. pylori* is eradicated.

166. Knowledge, implementation, environment (a)
    ❶ Protection of the blood supply is a sound way to prevent hepatitis B, hepatitis C, and HIV.
    ② May reduce the risk of ingestion of some pathogens.
    ③ One cannot get a bloodborne disease by merely donating blood.
    ④ The environment that the product is grown in as well as the preparation and cooking process are all factors. Shellfish are associated with hepatitis A.

167. Application, implementation, environment (a)
    ❸ Contact sports that carry the risk of blunt blows to the abdomen are usually avoided and discouraged.
    ①,②,④ Noncontact sports carry a reduced risk of injury.

168. Comprehension, assessment, physiologic (a)
    ❷ A common assessment finding in peritonitis.
    ① May occur as a late symptom, if the infection is not brought under control.
    ③ Frequent stooling or diarrhea is not a herald symptom.
    ④ This symptom is common in several conditions, including hypoglycemia.

169. Knowledge, planning, physiologic (a)
    ❷ Cardinal symptoms.
    ① Hypertension is not a common symptom; some patients with high ketone levels have reported headaches.
    ③,④ Not cardinal symptoms.

170. Comprehension, implementation, physiologic (a)
    ❷ The tube is a triple-lumen tube with an esophageal balloon to control bleeding of varices; one lumen is for lavage and one is for suction.
    ① Iced saline solution is used.
    ③ Vasodilators do not control bleeding.
    ④ Platelets need not be replaced; refrigerated blood lacks prothrombin and coagulation factors needed for clotting.

171. Application, planning, physiologic (a)
    ❶ Intact skin is the body's major defense.
    ② Stasis dermatitis is caused by decreased circulation.
    ③ Medications are not a treatment of choice.
    ④ Soap will further compound any dryness that may be present. #1 is the better choice.

172. Application, implementation, environment (b)
    ❶ May cause infection. Area usually kept dry.
    ② Activity does not need to be restricted.
    ③ Is appropriate treatment. Maintain patient comfort.
    ④ Is appropriate treatment. Allows more air circulation.

173. Application, planning, environment (a)
    ❷ Clean technique may be used for allergic reaction.
    ① Sterile technique required if an infection or ulceration is present.
    ③ Inappropriate. No pressure should be exerted on the eyeball.
    ④ No solution should ever be warmed in a microwave. It is unpredictable. Temperature of compresses should not exceed 49° C (120° F).

174. Knowledge, planning, environment (a)
    ❷ Gloves should be worn.
    ① Eye pads are contraindicated in general eye infections because they enhance bacterial growth.
    ③ Ointment should be placed in the conjunctiva.
    ④ All patients should have their own tubes of ointment to prevent cross-infection.

175. Knowledge, planning, physiologic (a)
    ❶ To prevent pressure on the suture line of the operated eye.
    ② Restricting fluids is inappropriate.
    ③ Should avoid showers and shampooing as soap may irritate the eye.
    ④ TV is okay. Reading is to be avoided. Back-and-forth eye motion may loosen stitches.

176. Comprehension, planning, physiologic (a)
    ❷ This is the physiologic action of the pharmacologic therapy.
    ① This is true of any medication.
    ③ This is true, but not the appropriate rationale.
    ④ This may occur after multiple consecutive missed doses.

177. Comprehension, implementation, physiologic (a)
    ❹ This is the only true statement.
    ① Is not directly related to glaucoma.
    ② Blindness is not always a result if glaucoma is diagnosed and treated.
    ③ Is not directly related to glaucoma.

178. Comprehension, implementation, environment (b)
    ❶ This is true.
    ② Bright lights are usually not harmful.
    ③ Darkness is not necessary.
    ④ This is not based on a physiologic reason.

179. Knowledge, implementation, environment (b)
    ❶ Safety precaution.
    ② This may be given if nausea and/or vomiting were present.
    ③ Bed rest is only for the preoperative period and 3 to 5 days postoperatively.
    ④ Retinal detachment produces anxiety and fear but usually not pain.

180. Application, implementation, physiologic (b)
    ❶ Prevents excessive pressure.
    ② Excessive pressure from nose blowing can force infected secretions up the eustachian tube into the middle ear.
    ③ Keeping mouth open is not necessary. Should blow with the nostrils open.
    ④ Excessive pressure from nose blowing can force infected secretions up the eustachian tube into the middle ear.

181. Knowledge, implementation, physiologic (b)
    ❹ Some diuretics and antibiotics are ototoxic, causing tinnitus and dizziness.
    ① Untrue.
    ② Some patients may experience tinnitus.
    ③ This would be an extreme result.
182. Comprehension, planning, physiologic (a)
    ❹ A comfort measure to reduce irritation and promote healing.
    ① Gas formation is not a common problem in this procedure.
    ② Seldom used. Packing and loose dressings to collect drainage may still be used.
    ③ Sitz baths are more soothing.
183. Comprehension, assessment, physiologic (c)
    ❹ The involved leg may be shorter because of the pull of the muscles nearest the fracture site, and the leg rotates outward (external).
    ①,② Supination and pronation are terms associated with the upper extremities.
    ③ There is usually a shortening, not a lengthening; and the foot of the affected side is externally rotated.
184. Knowledge, assessment, physiologic (a)
    ❶ An overproduction of hormones is associated with increasing blood sugar.
    ② Hypokalemia may occur.
    ③ Usually associated with precipitating tetany.
    ④ An underproduction of insulin is associated with a pancreatic problem.
185. Comprehension, assessment, physiologic (a)
    ❶ Hypovolemia may affect kidney perfusion. Kidney status is measured by output.
    ② BMs are not traditionally red flags for hypovolemia.
    ③ Pedal pulses can be affected by conditions other than hypovolemia.
    ④ Distention is associated with fluid overload or heart failure.
186. Comprehension, assessment, physiologic (a)
    ❷ Chemotherapy can cause bone marrow depression. A lowering of the white blood cell count can place the patient at risk of infection.
    ① Not associated with lymphoma treated by chemotherapy.
    ③ The CBC may augment other studies but does not directly indicate a disease in remission.
    ④ Platelet counts usually decrease rather than increase with chemotherapy.
187. Application, planning, physiologic (b)
    ❷ Diet should supply calories, protein, and carbohydrates caused by the increased metabolic demands imposed by the disease.
    ① Calories are insufficient; restriction of purine is not necessary.
    ③ Will not meet the metabolic demands of the body.
    ④ Sodium restrictions are not usually indicated.
188. Knowledge, assessment, physiologic (a)
    ❸ Classic symptoms of hyperthyroidism.
    ① Typical of hypothyroidism.
    ② Not a classic symptom of thyroid dysfunction.
    ④ Typical of hypothyroidism.

189. Comprehension, implementation, health (a)
    ❸ Many diuretics cause excretion of both sodium and potassium; it is important to maintain adequate potassium levels for proper heart function.
    ①,②,④ Not an aspect of teaching in diuretic therapy.
190. Knowledge, planning, physiologic (a)
    ❹ Diuretic.
    ① Suppresses gastric acid secretion.
    ② Antiinflammatory.
    ③ Cardiotonic.
191. Application, implementation, environment (a)
    ❷ Maintains an intact drainage system. Less likely that urine specimen will become contaminated.
    ① Disrupts the patency of the system. Increases likelihood of contamination and a urinary tract infection.
    ③ Urine collecting in the drainage bag likely to have organisms present, thereby giving inaccurate test results.
    ④ Unnecessary actions. Increases risk to patient of acquiring trauma and/or infection.
192. Comprehension, implementation, psychosocial (a)
    ❸ Is an emotional change that is common after a CVA. Emotional lability may or may not be appropriate to the situation.
    ① Is common but normal.
    ② Inappropriate. Encourages negative behavior modification technique. The patient has emotional lability.
    ④ Inappropriate. The patient is not acting this way on purpose.
193. Application, implementation, physiologic (a)
    ❷ Communication takes longer when speech is impaired.
    ① Inappropriate. May be a safety hazard.
    ③ Gestures may be appropriate and supplement the intended message. Would be inappropriate if patient is hallucinating or misinterprets.
    ④ Inappropriate. May add to communication misinterpretation.
194. Comprehension, assessment, physiologic (a)
    ❹ Dysphagia means difficulty swallowing. He may need to double-swallow between bites.
    ① Inappropriate. Unnecessary restriction.
    ② Not necessary. No indication that patient is hearing impaired.
    ③ Is a good practice for any person who has had a CVA. However, not specific to this question.
195. Comprehension, implementation, physiologic (a)
    ❷ Lubrication would allow easier insertion.
    ① This is a sterile technique, but not the underlying principle.
    ③ This is a result. It is not the underlying principle.
    ④ May be a result, but is not the underlying principle.
196. Comprehension, implementation, physiologic (a)
    ❸ This is true. It also allows rest for the patient and minimizes tissue trauma.
    ① Inappropriate principle; action will not maintain patency unless done continuously.
    ② Inappropriate principle; action will not prevent contamination of the catheter.
    ④ Inappropriate principle; action will not prevent improper tube placement.

197. Knowledge, planning, physiologic (a)
❶ This is true. Weakened pelvic muscles may also be a cause.
② Inappropriate assumption; this is called "residual" and is not usually a factor in stress inconvenience.
③ Inappropriate assumption; muscles and nerves are usually involved, not nerves alone.
④ Inappropriate assumption; this may be true but other symptoms would be evident, such as back pain.

198. Comprehension, evaluation, psychosocial (a)
❹ Seeks more data and demonstrates attentive listening. Beets, blackberries, rhubarb, and some medications may turn the urine red or orange.
① Milk increase is not necessary. Liquids should normally be around 2000 cc/day. This response gives a quick fix.
② False reassurance. This is belittling patient's concern.
③ Does show nurse is listening. Nurse is seeking more data. However, response #4 is individualized and therefore a better choice.

199. Comprehension, knowledge, physiologic (a)
❷ Injuries above C5 cause quadriplegia.
① Emotions remain intact. However, grief and mourning reactions and depression frequently occur.
③ Desire remains. However, may be affected by emotional reactions to the trauma and its effects.
④ Speaking ability remains intact.

200. Comprehension, assessment, physiologic (b)
❹ These are early signs reflecting heart's attempt to compensate through tachycardia. Yawning is body's way to take deep breaths to increase oxygen to brain.
① Are signs of prolonged or severe oxygen deprivation.
② Wheezing usually not present. Bradycardia and confusion are later signs.
③ All are later signs of severe hypoxemia.

201. Comprehension, evaluation, physiologic (b)
❸ Nitrates have a vasodilating effect and are often the cause of headaches, at least initially.
① Not a common side effect.
② Commonly taken for headache discomfort.
④ Usually used to counter side effects of hypokalemia.

202. Comprehension, planning, environment (a)
❹ The monitor will record a tracing of the heart during various activities and is compared with activities that the patient is documenting as well.
① Evaluates capillary blood sugar levels.
② Urines are used to evaluate various conditions, but not heart activity during exertion.
③ Evaluates blood flow.

203. Comprehension, planning, physiologic (a)
❹ Genetic factors that predispose a person to hypertension cannot be controlled by the patient.
① Can be controlled by smoking cessation.
② Can be controlled by diet and exercise programs.
③ An exercise program can be started.

204. Knowledge, assessment, physiologic (a)
❹ Classic symptoms of thrombophlebitis.
① More of a neurologic manifestation.
②,③ Symptoms are arterial in nature.

205. Comprehension, assessment, physiologic (c)
❹ As the heart fails, circulating blood backs up into the pulmonary tree; a sign of congestion is rales (crackles) in lung bases.

①,②,③ Not associated with manifestation of pulmonary congestion related to heart failure.

206. Application, implementation, environment (a)
❶ Should stand on the affected side and support with gait belt. Gait belt provides stability, provides greater control in assisting patient without putting undue pressure on patient's body and/or nurse.
② Inappropriate. Does not provide patient with a base of support.
③ Not a safe practice. Patient may hesitate or tip backward.
④ Inappropriate. A patient with right-sided weakness requires the nurse to stand on the right side. Reaching over to hold the patient's right hand may change patient's center of gravity and tip her forward. Awkward body mechanics for the nurse.

207. Comprehension, planning, psychosocial (a)
❹ Patient's anxiety and concerns need to be addressed first. This allows her to express any fears and questions. Teaching will be heard once patient's concerns are answered.
① Unknown if true. This is an assumption.
② May be true. However, it is an assumption until patient is given opportunity to express her concerns.
③ Inappropriate assumption.

208. Comprehension, planning, environment (b)
❶ Safety should come first. In this patient's case, use Maslow's hierarchy of needs.
② Safety should be first priority.
③ Response #1 is better choice. Situation did not indicate pain was present. Assessment of respiratory function would be more appropriate and more individualized.
④ Safety should be first priority.

209. Knowledge, assessment, physiologic (a)
❸ Toxic levels (lab value of theophylline >20 ug/ml) accompanied by these signs. May also have palpitations or develop seizures.
①,②,④ Not typical side effects of theophylline-bronchodilators.

210. Knowledge, assessment, physiologic (a)
❸ Characteristic barrel-shaped chest, loss of elasticity, and narrowed bronchioles increase work effort to move air. The patient compensates by using accessory muscles.
① Coughs with copious amount of mucopurulent sputum.
② Not common.
④ Not usually present.

211. Application, evaluation, health (b)
❹ Hearing aids should not be worn during an ear infection. Leaving the hearing aid out allows for drainage and observation of the site and prevents complications.
① Would only distort the sound more. It is unsafe.
② May damage the ear mold.
③ Hearing aids should not be worn during an ear infection.

212. Knowledge, implementation, environment (a)
❷ 1000/12 hr 83.3 = 83 cc/hr.
①,③,④ Incorrect math calculation.

213. Comprehension, evaluation, physiologic (b)
❶ Persons with a pulmonary embolism experience pain related to ischemia caused by obstruction of small pulmonary arterial branches, process in lung, described as pleuritic chest pain.

② Relates to activity intolerance or interest in doing own self-care. May be an indication of lessened anxiety.

③ Appetite, weight, nutritional status not a usual problem for patients with a pulmonary embolism.

④ Related to an ineffective airway clearance problem.

214. Comprehension, evaluation, psychosocial (a)
❸ Being able to do own ADL indicates activity tolerance is increased.
① Anxiety is most likely related to being unable to breathe.
② Related to a knowledge deficit diagnosis.
④ Related to the physiologic effects.

215. Comprehension, assessment, psychosocial (b)
❷ Correct description.
① Describes Level II = Generalized response.
③ Describes Level VI = Confused-appropriate.
④ Describes Level IV = Confused-agitated.

216. Comprehension, evaluation, physiologic (a)
❸ Bleeding is a serious side effect of anticoagulant therapy. Nursing measures focus on monitoring for signs of ease in bleeding or active bleeding.
① A common side effect of many medications.
② A common side effect of many medications. Hematemesis would be a serious side effect.
④ Not a common side effect of this class of medications; and is not suggestive of bleeding.

217. Comprehension, assessment, physiologic (a)
❶ Neck pain, decreased neck mobility caused by pain, and upper extremity motor /sensory changes are common symptoms.
②,③ May be symptoms in lumbar involvement.
④ Muscle atrophy of this group is not a finding when the cervical region is involved.

218. Comprehension, planning, physiologic (b)
❹ Reduces risk of constipation and straining, which may put a strain on damaged myocardium.
① Not a standard of care in MI.
② Prolonged bed rest is no longer advocated.
③ Not a standard of care in MI.

219. Comprehension, assessment, physiologic (a)
❸ Not classic symptoms of this type of shock.
①,②,④ Classic symptoms of cardiogenic shock.

220. Comprehension, planning, health (a)
❷ OSHA (Occupational Safety and Health Administration) says that unprotected exposure to noise levels of 90 db (decibels) over an 8-hour day is considered excessive, and must be avoided. Ear plugs/ protectors can reduce noise reaching the middle ear by 10 db to 30 db.
① Does not address the need to reduce the number of decibels of the original noise.
③ A possible action. However, may be unrealistic for all patients to move.
④ Inappropriate. Does not decrease number of decibels reaching the middle ear.

221. Comprehension, assessment, physiologic (a)
❹ Diaphoresis is a symptom of hypoglycemia which may result when taking insulin without eating, or from a sudden increase in activity, or body demands such as illness, surgery, or stress.
①,② Is a symptom of hyperglycemia.
③ Is a late sign of either hypoglycemia or hyperglycemia. Nurse needs to be aware of earlier signs.

222. Comprehension, evaluation, psychosocial (b)
❷ Indicates that sputum has been expectorated from the lungs.
① Relates to decreased appetite and altered nutrition.
③ Demonstrates effectiveness of therapy.
④ Relates to a knowledge deficit nursing diagnosis.

223. Application, implementation, environment (a)
❶ To prevent falling and to decrease vertigo sensation, person has to be still and avoid all head movements that aggravate the spinning sensation.
② Would only be appropriate if a PRN had been ordered.
③ Normal hydration is 2000 cc/day. At times a diuretic may be prescribed to help decrease fluid volume of endolymph.
④ May increase sensation of vertigo. Bright, glaring lights should be avoided.

224. Comprehension, planning, health (a)
❹ Presbycusis is the term used to describe hearing loss associated with aging.
① Inappropriate; hearing loss does not usually affect physical comfort.
② Is possible if unaware of environmental sounds. However, it is not a common cause.
③ Inappropriate; hearing loss does not usually affect family roles.

225. Comprehension, evaluation, physiologic (b)
❸ Widening pulse pressure is a sign of increased ICP.
①,②,④ Is not a sign of widening pulse pressure.

226. Knowledge, planning, health (b)
❶ Chewing and daily ear hygiene aids in the removal of cerumen.
② May be necessary. However, subjects patient to a procedure that could be prevented through health-promoting habits.
③ Allows for hydration, but not directly related to cerumen buildup.
④ May damage the hearing aid.

227. Comprehension, assessment, physiologic (a)
❷ Some patients experience a spinal headache after removal of CSF.
① Capillary refill would assess oxygenation of tissues. Should not be directly related to this procedure.
③ Inappropriate. Bladder control affected by many factors. Should not be directly affected by this practice.
④ Inappropriate. Blood pressure affected by many factors. Should not be directly affected by this procedure.

228. Knowledge, evaluation, health (a)
❶ Allows for maximum straightening of the auditory canal.
②,③,④ May occlude auditory canal.

229. Application, assessment, health (a)
❶ May indicate a problem in inner ear.
② Frequently watch face to lip read.
③ May be true if position changes were to lean forward to hear better.
④ This behavior may result from a variety of factors that are not hearing related.

230. Application, implementation, physiologic (a)
    ❸ Airway, breathing, and circulation is the first priority. Rapid respirations that are shallow and irregular need immediate action.
    ① Need to know patient's previous temperature.
    ② May indicate many things. Need further data. It is not a priority.
    ④ May indicate therapy is effective. Need further data. It is not a priority.

231. Comprehension, assessment, physiologic (a)
    ❶ Both sprains and fractures may evidence edema.
    ② Angulation deformities, shortening of a limb are suggestive of a break in bone continuity.
    ③ Both types of injuries may evidence limited movement.
    ④ Both types of injuries may evidence tenderness. Contused soft tissue structures are tender/painful, thus limiting mobility as well.

232. Knowledge, planning, physiologic (a)
    ❹ Commonly used to reduce femoral fractures.
    ①,②,③ Buck's is not designed for use in these fractures/injuries.

233. Comprehension, evaluation, physiologic (a)
    ❸ Russell's usually uses a sling device whereby the upper area of the sling may slide under the knee (popliteal space) and compromise circulation.
    ① There is no cast in this type of traction.
    ② There is no encircling device in this type of traction.
    ④ A boot device is not common in this type of traction, but skin pressure is a problem; see response #3.

234. Comprehension, planning, physiologic (a)
    ❶ Delayed wound healing because of nutritional problems is common in the elderly.
    ②,③,④ Intervention is appropriate regardless of patient's age.

235. Comprehension, planning, physiologic (a)
    ❶ Specifically focusing on rehabilitation and the elements involved and rationale should expedite recovery, by gaining the patient's cooperation.
    ②,③,④ All are elements of general preoperative teaching plans.

236. Application, implementation, physiologic (b)
    ❸ When pain is severe, evaluate the neurologic and circulatory status first; initial presentation of complications may be that of severe pain.
    ① Evaluate the patient's status first; then give ordered medication; be suspicious of pain unrelieved by medication.
    ② Provide supportive care.
    ④ Elevation reduces edema; leg rotation is not usually a standard measure.

237. Comprehension, implementation, psychosocial (a)
    ❸ Hydration and lying flat for 4 to 6 hours helps those individuals who may develop a spinal headache. This response addresses her concerns and gives a plan of action.
    ① This is not a proven fact. Some individuals will develop a headache.
    ② Staying prone versus supine does not give any additional benefit. May increase patient's apprehension, as she may be fearful of moving. This is not a comfortable position to maintain.
    ④ May belittle patient's concerns.

238. Comprehension, planning, health (b)
    ❶ Easier on the patient to eat small, frequent meals. A large meal is physiologically and emotionally overwhelming to a person with decreased appetite. COPD patients lose weight because of decreased appetite and work of breathing.
    ② Does not relate to nursing diagnosis.
    ③ Does help with hydration status and to keep secretions moist.
    ④ Unrealistic. As dyspnea progresses, patients are unable to sleep well because of the conscious effort to breathe. Pacing activities would decrease fatigue.

239. Application, assessment, physiologic (b)
    ❷ Also may cause purpura, petechiae.
    ① Usual adverse skin reaction is an erythematous rash.
    ③ Adverse skin reaction is rash or urticaria.
    ④ Adverse skin reaction is urticaria.

240. Knowledge, assessment, physiologic (a)
    ❶ Accurate. Other behaviors include sleepiness, very short attention span, able to respond verbally. Fends off painful stimuli with purposeful movement.
    ② Descriptive of deep coma state.
    ③,④ Descriptive of stuporous state.

241. Comprehension, implementation, physiologic (a)
    ❸ Also known as hyperosmolar drugs. Mannitol (Osmitrol) is an example. These agents draw water from the edematous brain.
    ① Should be used carefully; may mask LOC or cause respiratory depression.
    ② May be ordered if nausea is present.
    ④ May be ordered if open wound is caused by trauma.

242. Knowledge, assessment, health (a)
    ❷ Is recommended as an annual test for all men age 50 and older.
    ① Is a blood test used as a monitoring tool to evaluate a cancer patient's response to treatment or for recurrence of the disease.
    ③ Is a screening test for BPH or cancer of prostate. It is *not* a blood test. It is an exam recommended for all men over the age of 40.
    ④ One of the diagnostic tests for HIV.

243. Application, implementation, physiologic (a)
    ❸ Will not increase systemic blood pressure because they are not resistive.
    ①,② Unsafe. Causes sudden increase in blood pressure and intracranial pressure.
    ④ Unsafe. May cause flexion of hips and/or neck. Both of these positions may cause sudden increase in intracranial pressure.

244. Comprehension, implementation, physiologic (a)
    ❷ Is a heavy dye and the physician strives to remove all the dye to prevent irritation of the meninges. Lying flat may help to lessen chance of headache.
    ① Unsafe. Besides headache, must assess for strength and sensation of lower extremities first.
    ③,④ Inappropriate. Any dye remaining may rise.

245. Comprehension, evaluation, psychosocial (a)
    ❹ Is individualized. Discovery of triggering factors demonstrates understanding of disease process and preventative health habit.
    ① Not directly related. However, may relieve stress, which is frequently a trigger of headaches.

② There is no proof that sunlight triggers these types of headaches.

③ Acetylsalicylic acid (aspirin) is seldom effective for classic migraine. Taking it as a preventive may not be a healthful habit.

246. Knowledge, assessment, health (a)
❸ The ache may be in the groin. Other signs are a lump or enlargement of a testicle, heaviness or sudden collection of fluid in the scrotum, and/or enlargement or tenderness of the breasts.
① Describes phimosis.
②,④ Not a warning sign of testicular cancer.

247. Knowledge, assessment, physiologic (b)
❸ Right ventricle problems cause a pooling and backup of blood entering the heart from the systemic circulation.
①,②,④ The ventricles by design are for pumping. Most heart failure is left-sided. Left-sided failure can then lead to right-sided problems and associated symptoms.

248. Comprehension, planning, physiologic (b)
❶ Principal function of white blood cells is to fight infection, which is signaled by an elevation of the WBCs. Infection in a patient with diabetes can cause blood sugar fluctuations.
②,③,④ Though important to the overall informational process, these components of the blood count are not as useful as the WBC in this scenario.

249. Comprehension, assessment, physiologic (a)
❸ A hot spot is usually a sign of inflammation under the cast.
① Tightness of a cast is displayed in changes of the neurocirculatory symptoms.
② Swelling will cause tightness of the cast and affects the neurocirculatory status.
④ An object or foreign body beneath the cast, if large enough, may initially be evidenced by changes in neurocirculatory status.

250. Comprehension, implementation, physiologic (a)
❹ This gives the body a chance to adjust the circulation to the effects of gravity.
① Hose will not prevent hypotension.
② Limiting dietary sodium is used in the treatment of hypertension, but will not prevent hypotension.
③ Will not prevent hypotension.

251. Comprehension, assessment, physiologic (a)
❷ Anginal pain is caused by myocardial ischemia (insufficient blood and oxygen to the heart muscle).
① An incompetent valve is not a direct cause of angina.
③ No cell death occurs.
④ Angina is a cardiac problem, not a cerebral (brain) problem.

252. Application, implementation, physiologic (a)
❸ Promotes venous return.
①,② May increase intracranial pressure.
④ Causes flexion of hips and perhaps neck.

253. Application, implementation, physiologic (b)
❸ Clot may dislodge itself; bright red or darker color may indicate hemorrage.
① This would cause painful bladder spasms.
② May increase the patient's anxiety. The coughing may also increase the patient's discomfort.
④ May increase the patient's discomfort. He is already at risk for fluid and electrolyte imbalance because of absorption of the irrigation fluid.

254. Comprehension, implementation, physiologic (a)
❶ Aids in absorption of dye. Metrizamide dye is water-soluble and does not need to be removed.
② Not usually necessary.
③ Common side effects of this dye include nausea, vomiting, seizures with the peak time of risk 4 to 8 hours postprocedure.
④ Phenothiazines, tricyclic antidepressants, CNS stimulants, or amphetamines should not be taken 24 to 48 hours preprocedure or immediately postprocedure. These drugs lower seizure threshold.

255. Application, implementation, physiologic (a)
❶ Persons taking this anticonvulsant are especially prone to developing gingival hyperplasia.
② Inappropriate; not relative to the situation given; see #4.
③ Inappropriate; not a patient responsibility.
④ Adequate rest and diet are important. Choice #1 is individualized to situation and the better choice.

256. Application, planning, physiologic (a)
❶ Valsalva maneuver is avoided, as it will cause increased thoracic pressure, which indirectly causes increased intracranial pressure.
② Fluids are usually restricted until edema is resolved.
③ May ease discomfort if patient complains of headache and/or photosensitivity.
④ May be unsafe. Sensory perceptual alterations may be present. Ambulation may not be ordered until patient is alert, oriented, and has decreased cerebral edema. Certain classifications of pain medications may cause respiratory depression.

257. Application, planning, physiologic (a)
❶ Is at high risk for decubitus ulcer. Sensory loss prevents perception of pain and pressure, the warning signs of tissue injury. If able to, encourage patient involvement.
② Inappropriate; adequate calcium intake is essential for all individuals.
③ Inappropriate; not relative to situation.
④ Is not individualized to persons with sensory/motor loss.

258. Application, planning, physiologic (c)
❹ No known effect on urine acidity.
①,② Causes an alkaline urine
③ Sulfa drugs require an alkaline urine for maximum drug absorption.

259. Application, evaluation, physiologic (a)
❸ A diet high in carbohydrates and restricted in sodium, potassium, phosphorus, and protein.
①,②,④ Doesn't indicate a change in dietary habits.

260. Application, implementation, physiologic (b)
❹ Blood that drained from the legs while in the lithotomy position will flow back into vessels of the feet and legs as the person stands. Dizziness, fainting can occur from the sudden change in distribution.
① Although bleeding, perforation of bladder, and sepsis are complications of this procedure, the effect on VS would not be immediately evident.
② Not usually necessary.
③ Inappropriate; not relevant to situation.

261. Comprehension, implementation, physiologic (a)
   ❸ Hydronephrosis can occur rapidly if obstruction occurs.
   ① The stents are not near the rectum. Contamination with stool unlikely.
   ② Inappropriate; may be ordered but not related to situation.
   ④ Inappropriate; not irrigated, patency essential.

262. Application, evaluation, physiologic (a)
   ❶ Adjunctive treatment, both agents decrease extrapyramidal symptoms.
   ② The medications mentioned are not antidepressants.
   ③ VS not affected with Parkinson's; propulsive shuffling gait is a sign of muscular rigidity and loss of postural reflexes.
   ④ Not symptoms of Parkinson's.

263. Comprehension, implementation, physiologic (a)
   ❹ The patient may have a weakened immune system and should avoid the risk of infection.
   ① HIV-positive patients can develop AIDS, but there is no failsafe way to prevent it.
   ② A specific pneumonia is commonly seen in AIDS, but prevention goes beyond this one problem.
   ③ Hypotension is not a primary concern over prevention of infection.

264. Knowledge, implementation, physiologic (a)
   ❹ Oral agents are useful in treating diabetes when some beta cell function exists.
   ① Obesity is not a measurement for beta cell function.
   ② Most agents are cleared by the liver, but this fact is unrelated to the need for functioning beta cells.
   ③ Type I diabetes usually is associated with no beta cell function.

265. Comprehension, implementation, physiologic (a)
   ❷ Infection increases metabolism and increases the demand for insulin.
   ① Can affect glucose level, but is not a primary cause.
   ③ Not enough insulin is available for the bodys' needs.
   ④ Associated with hypoglycemia, not ketoacidosis.

266. Comprehension; implementation, physiologic (a)
   ❹ Regular insulin is rapid-acting.
   ①,② Is not rapid-acting insulin.
   ③ Is a long-acting insulin and would take too long to work.

267. Comprehension, implementation, health (a)
   ❷ Reduces gastric irritation.
   ① Does cause an appreciable change in mentation or awareness.
   ③ CNS effects are not commonly associated with this group of drugs.
   ④ Gastric irritation will occur on an empty stomach and may lead to nausea, vomiting.

268. Knowledge, planning, physiologic (a)
   ❹ Disorder tends to progress, and involvement of other systems is common with advancement of the disorder.
   ① This is more characteristic of osteoarthritis.

② Rheumatoid arthritis that appears in early childhood may run its course and dissipate in later years, but this is not true in the majority of cases.
   ③ Rheumatoid arthritis is a disease of joints as well as supportive structures.

269. Knowledge, assessment, environment (a)
   ❸ Reduce the inflammatory process.
   ①,② Not a first-line drug of choice.
   ④ Not classically used in management of rheumatoid arthritis.

270. Application, implementation, physiologic (a)
   ❹ The dressing is easily soaked with urine through the drain. Urine is irritating to the skin.
   ① No dressing present. Would be appropriate if patient had perineal resection.
   ② Inappropriate; vital signs would be done following usual procedure unless otherwise ordered.
   ③ Inappropriate. Most patients having a suprapubic prostatectomy also have a CBI for 24 to 48 hours. If no Foley catheter in place, would need physician's order.

271. Knowledge, assessment, physiologic (a)
   ❶ Awakening at night to void is most common. Pain on urination is sign of cystitis that most men find disturbing.
   ② Hematuria may result from blood vessels that have been overstretched. Groin pain not present in most men.
   ③ May result if UTI develops because of stasis of urine.
   ④ May develop. However, are not common signs.

272. Comprehension, implementation, physiologic (a)
   ❶ Decreases tone and involuntary movements and helps relieve anxiety and tension.
   ② Inappropriate; vasodilators will not decrease spasticity.
   ③ Inappropriate; narcotic analgesics are not given for spasticity.
   ④ Inappropriate; NSAIDs will not decrease tone.

273. Application, implementation, physiologic (a)
   ❸ Taking the BP in left arm may cause compression and/or occlude the fistula. Any compression, tight clothing, or carrying objects with arm bent is to be avoided.
   ① Unnecessary to do so; patients discharged with this in place.
   ② Inappropriate; not procedure.
   ④ Fluids may be restricted. Some patients may have urine output. Hourly monitoring is usually not appropriate.

274. Application, planning, physiologic (b)
   ❶ Straining may initiate bleeding.
   ②,③,④ Inappropriate for the expected outcome.

275. Analysis, assessment, physiologic (b)
   ❶ Common manifestation of heart failure.
   ②,③,④ Not associated with heart failure.

Chapter 6 Mental Health Nursing

The licensed practical/vocational nurse (LP/VN) requires a knowledge of mental health nursing principles in a variety of practice settings. Basic mental health concepts are useful in understanding the response to diseases and dysfunctions of both physical and social systems. Each person responds to disease and disorder in accordance with his or her own basic personality traits, past experiences, intelligence, and innate coping mechanisms. These concepts are explored and studied in mental health nursing.

Holism

A. Definition: a concept of health—holds that illness results from a complex interaction between the mind and body and the internal and external alterations that disturb the natural balance

B. Approaches to treatment: multifaceted approaches are used to treat disturbances, rather than simply relying on treatments aimed at specific symptoms; these approaches include the following dimensions
   1. Physical
   2. Psychologic
   3. Cultural
   4. Socioeconomic

Mental Health Continuum

A. Mental health and mental illness are seen as opposite poles on a continuum

B. The precise point at which an individual is deemed mentally ill is determined not only by the specific behavior exhibited but also by the context in which the behavior is seen

C. Some behaviors considered deviant in one setting are considered normal in another setting

D. Variations are based on the culture, the time or era, the specific personal characteristics of the individual, and many other variables

E. Behaviors of the mentally ill are exaggerations of normal human behaviors

Mental Health

A. Definition: an individual's ability to manage life's problems and to derive satisfaction from living throughout various life stages

B. Persons may experience times of greater or lesser satisfaction with life, and at times of lesser satisfaction may seek the assistance of a therapist

C. No clear set of characteristics specific to mental health can be identified
   1. All behavior is considered meaningful and may be interpreted as the individual's effort to adapt or cope with the environment
   2. At times some adaptations fail; others are continued long after the need for them has passed; still others may be directed to an undesired end

Mental Illness

A. Definition: a pattern of behavior that is disturbing to the individual or to the community in which the individual resides
   1. The person who is mentally ill acts in ways that seem unrelated to the current reality
   2. Relationships with family and friends are disturbed
   3. The person's ability to work and to contribute to his or her own welfare may be impaired
   4. The person often experiences subjective discomfort
   5. The person may exhibit symptoms such as hallucinations or delusions

B. Historical perspective of mental illness
   1. Early history
      a. Mentally ill persons were thought to be possessed by supernatural forces
      b. Mentally ill persons were ostracized from society or mistreated in other ways
      c. Mentally ill persons were regarded as messengers of the gods or as divinely possessed
      d. Attitudes did not change significantly until the modern era
   2. Classical era (Greco-Roman)
      a. Certain attitudes changed toward mental illness
      b. Early scientific interest led to various descriptive or classification systems
      c. The idea of divine possession was rejected in favor of the concept of humors
      d. Humors were thought to be basic internal fluids capable of controlling behavior
      e. The terms melancholia and hysteria are derived from these ancient beliefs
   3. The Middle Ages
      a. Return to the idea of divine possession and spiritual explanations of mental illness
      b. The mentally ill person was often mistreated by incarceration

---

Historic Highlights

Eighteenth century

Phillipe Pinel (1745-1826, France): freed mentally ill persons from chains

Benjamin Rush (1746-1813, United States): founded Pennsylvania Hospital; the father of American psychiatry

Nineteenth century

Florence Nightingale (1860, England): founder of modern nursing

Dorothea Dix (1802-1887, United States): promoted legislation to establish mental hospitals

Linda Richards (1873, United States): first psychiatric nurse

Daniel Tuke (1827-1895, England): founded York Retreat based on Quaker principles

Twentieth century

Clifford Beers (1876-1943, United States): wrote the book, *The Mind that Found Itself,* generating public concern for the treatment of mentally ill persons

Adolf Meyer (1866-1950, United States): Director of the Johns Hopkins Clinic; founder of the mental hygiene movement

Emil Kraepelin (1856-1926, Germany): classified mental disorders

Eugene Bleuler (1857-1939, Switzerland): coined the word *schizophrenia* and classified it into types

Sigmund Freud (1856-1939, Austria): developed psychoanalytic theory; revolutionized psychiatry

Carl Jung (1875-1961, Switzerland): developed a personality theory that included the concepts of introversion and extroversion

Karen Horney (1885-1952, United States): theorized that culture had a great influence on mental illness

4. Modern era: numerous reforms were instituted (see the box on p. 292)
5. Later modern developments include
   a. Discovery of tranquilizing drugs: late 1950s
   b. Community mental health: 1960s; still in use today; aim is to provide care of mentally ill persons in their own communities rather than in large institutions: a primary goal of the community mental health concept is to return patients to their homes as quickly as possible and to foster the development of support systems in the community
   c. Patients released from large hospitals: late 1970s; large numbers of mentally ill persons were released into communities where they often did not receive treatment either because they did not seek it out or because adequate types of services were not available; this process is called *deinstitutionalization*; some believe that there is an increase of "street people" as a result of the process

The Nursing Role

A. The nursing process
   1. Assessment: The licensed practical nurse collects subjective and objective data through observation, interview, and examination. Data obtained through:
      a. Health history
      b. Mental status exam
         (1) General appearance
         (2) Affect and mood
         (3) Intellect and sensorium
         (4) Thought processes
         (5) Insight
      c. Results of psychological testing
         (1) Intelligence testing
         (2) Personality testing
      d. Self assessment; e.g., stress scale; decision-making trees
      e. Physical examination
   2. Diagnosis: Nurses diagnose and treat human responses to illness; the nursing diagnosis is formulated by the Registered Professional Nurse; the licensed Practical Nurse contributes to this phase of the nursing process through collection of objective and subjective data; potential nursing diagnoses identify the problem and the etiology of the problem; actual nursing diagnoses identify the problem, etiology, and signs and symptoms; the NANDA listing is used; sample actual and potential nursing diagnoses used in mental health nursing include:
      a. Anxiety (Panic) related to family rejection; manifested by chest discomfort, palpitations, dizziness, diaphoresis, and trembling
      b. Impaired social interaction related to negative role modeling; manifested by verbalized and observed discomfort in social situations
      c. High risk for violence: self-directed; related to history of suicide attempts.
      d. High risk for trauma; related to muscular incoordination
      The psychiatric-mental health areas of concern for formulating nursing diagnoses appear in the box on this page.
   3. Planning: the plan of care is based on the nursing diagnosis; specific nursing interventions are devised to attain specifically stated goals; when possible, goals should be developed jointly with the patient and cooperation enlisted; goals may be short term or long term; all goals should be prioritized, emphasizing reduction or elimination of the identified problem; goals usually include the anticipated length of time for accomplishment and the standard for judging whether the goal has been met
   4. Implementation: the planned nursing actions that assist the patient to achieve the identified goal e.g., health teaching, activities of daily living, other prescribed treatments, and medications; this is an ongoing phase, and reactions to treatment are observed and documented so that the care plan may be modified periodically as goals are met
   5. Evaluation: Outcome achievement is identified as well as the factors that affected the goal being met, partially met, or not met; this is followed by deciding whether to continue, modify, or terminate the plan; following evaluation of goal achievement the entire nursing process and care plan are reviewed, modified, or updated to reflect new nursing diagnoses
B. Principles of mental health nursing
   1. Understand your inner needs, thoughts, and feelings and be aware of how these affect patients

---

Psychiatric—Mental Health Nursing's Phenomena of Concern

Actual or Potential Mental Health Problems of Clients Pertaining to:
- The maintenance of optimal health and well-being and the prevention of psychobiological illness
- Self-care limitations or impaired functioning related to mental and emotional distress
- Deficits in the functioning of significant biological, emotional, and cognitive systems
- Emotional stress or crisis components of illness, pain, and disability
- Self-concept changes, developmental issues, and life process changes
- Problems related to emotions such as anxiety, anger, sadness, loneliness, and grief
- Physical symptoms that occur along with altered psychological functioning
- Alterations in thinking, perceiving, symbolizing, communicating, and decision making
- Difficulties in relating to others
- Behaviors and mental states that indicate the patient is a danger to self or others or has a severe disability
- Interpersonal, systemic, sociocultural, spiritual, or environmental circumstances or events that affect the mental and emotional well-being of the individual, family, or community
- Symptom management, side effects/toxicities associated with psychopharmacological intervention and other aspects of the treatment regimen

From American Nurses' Association: *A statement on psychiatric mental health clinical nursing practice and standards of psychiatric mental health clinical nursing practice.* Washington, DC, 1994, The Association.

2. Be aware of your own resources and limitations so as to function effectively in mental health nursing
3. Respect the patient as a person; take time to listen to what is said
4. Be aware of the patient's dignity; show patience and understanding
5. Be nonjudgmental and nonthreatening; patients must be accepted as they are
6. Be honest
7. Reassure patients by being available and allaying fears
8. Explain routine, rules, and regulations when appropriate
9. Maintain a calm, hopeful attitude
10. Encourage reality testing and avoid entering into patient's unrealistic thinking
11. Emphasize strengths that the patient displays by acknowledging healthy behavior; offer warm understanding but do not encourage overdependency or intimacy
12. Remember that all staff members are role models and are often viewed as authority figures by patients
13. Help reduce anxiety by making as few demands as possible on patients
14. Explain what is happening to the patient in simple, understandable language
15. Remain objective but do not display aloofness or distance; maintain your awareness of the patient's humanity and dignity
16. Maintain a nurse/patient relationship that is always realistic and professional
17. Remember that there is a reason for all behavior
18. Note that behavior is changed through emotional experience rather than through rational means
19. Allow patients to exercise all of their basic human rights
20. Use the least restrictive method(s) of controlling behavior, such as communication
21. Respect the confidentiality of the patient

C. Communications in mental health nursing
   1. Communication: a complex activity consisting of a series of events, each interdependent on the other, which results in a negotiated understanding between two or more people in a given situation
      a. Communication is not merely the exchange of information
      b. Each message (input) generates an extremely complex reaction that eventually leads to a selective response (output), which in turn becomes a new input for the communicators
   2. Modes of communication
      a. The most apparent form is verbal (written or spoken language); spoken is the more important in mental health nursing
      b. Spoken communication is always accompanied by at least one of the following additional communication forms
         (1) Paralanguage: voice quality, tones, grunts, and other nonword vocalizations
         (2) Kinesis: facial expression, gestures, and eye and body movements
         (3) Proxemics: the spatial relationship between persons
         (4) Touch and messages to other sensory organs: aromas and cultural artifacts (jewelry, clothing, hairstyle)

   c. Effective communications are
      (1) Efficient: messages are simple, clear, and timed correctly
      (2) Appropriate: relevant to the situation
      (3) Flexible: open to alteration based on perceived response
      (4) Receptive: allow feedback (checking and correcting by either or both parties)
   3. Therapeutic communication (see box on p. 298)
   4. Blocks to communication (Table 6-1)

D. Nurse-patient relationship
   1. One-to-one relationship between a nurse and a patient
   2. Patient centered
   3. Goal directed
   4. Not for mutual satisfaction
   5. Focus is on modification of patient behavior, increasing patient's self-worth, and developing patient's coping strategies
   6. Therapeutic, not social, relationship
   7. Phases
      a. Preorientation: data collection about the patient; self-analysis of attitudes, biases, and perceptions by the nurse
      b. Orientation: 2 to 10 sessions; become acquainted; establish trust and rapport; establish parameters of the relationship; contract discussions; identify patient problems; build on patient's strengths
      c. Working: begins when the patient demonstrates responsibility to uphold terms of the contract; establish priorities and goals with patient; help patient achieve behavior change (e.g., discussion, role playing); focus on the present; reinforce the contract terms as necessary
      d. Termination: begins during orientation phase; purpose is to conclude the relationship; focus on patient growth, help patient with expression of feelings about relationship closure

E. Applications of mental health nursing
   1. Community mental health center
   2. Partial hospitalization setting: day or night hospitals
   3. Mental health clinic
   4. Liaison: use of mental health workers in general hospital setting
   5. Alcohol and drug-abuse facilities and clinics
   6. Inpatient units
   7. Crisis intervention
   8. Health maintenance organizations

Personality Development

A. Definition: a consistent set of behaviors peculiar to a specific individual; the sum of thoughts, feelings, physical characteristics, and sociocultural biases on which all behavior is built
B. Heredity
   1. Personality is influenced by inherited characteristics, both physical and psychologic
   2. Controversy exists over the extent of genetic influence on specific human behaviors
C. Environment
   1. The environment is a strong determining factor in the individual's development
   2. Environment includes the intrauterine environment as well as all the external factors that influence the individual after birth

Table 6-1 Ineffective Responses that Hinder Therapeutic Communication

Response	Discussion	Nontherapeutic response	Therapeutic response
Offering false reassurance	The nurse, in an effort to be supportive and to make the client's pain disappear, offers reassuring cliches. This response is not based on fact. It brushes aside the client's feelings and closes off communication. Often, it is due to the nurse's inability to listen to the client's negative emotions. No one can predict the outcome of a situation.	"Don't worry, everything will be OK." "Things will be better soon; you'll see."	"I know you have a lot going on right now. Let's make a list and begin to discuss them one at a time. Working toward solutions will assist you to get through this."
Not listening	The nurse is preoccupied with other work that needs to be done, is distracted by noise in the area, is thinking about personal problems.	"I'm sorry, what did you say?" "Could you start again? I was listening to the other nurse."	"That is interesting. Please elaborate." "I really hear what you are saying…it must be difficult."
Offering approval	It is most important how a client feels about what he or she said or did. The client ultimately must approve of his or her own actions.	"That's good." "I agree—I think you should have told him."	"What do you think about what you said to him?" "How do you feel about it?"
Minimizing problem	The nurse may use this when it is difficult to hear the enormity of a particular problem. This is used in an effort to try to make the client feel better. It cuts off communication.	"That's nothing compared to that other client's problem." "Everyone feels that way at times, it's not a big deal."	"That is a very difficult problem for you." "That sounds pretty important for you to deal with."
Offering advice	This response undermines clients' ability to solve their own problems. It serves to render them dependent and helpless. If the solution provided by the nurse does not work, the client may blame the outcome on the nurse. Clients do not take responsibility for developing outcomes. The nurse maintains control and at the same time devalues the client.	"I think you should…" "In my opinion, it would be wise to…" "Why don't you do…" "The best solution is…"	"What do *you* think you should do?" "There can be several alternatives—let's talk about some. However, the final decision must be yours. I will listen to your problem and help you see it clearly. We can develop a pros and cons list which may assist you in solving the problem."
Giving literal responses	The nurse feeds into a client's delusions of hallucinations, denies client the opportunity to see reality. This does not provide a healthy response toward growth.	C: "That TV is talking to me." N: "What is it saying to you?" C: "There is nuclear power coming through the air ducts." N: "I'll turn off the A/C for a while."	N: "The TV is on for everyone." N: "There is cool air blowing from the vents. It is the A/C system."

Continued

	Ineffective Responses that Hinder Therapeutic Communication—cont'd		
Table 6-1			
Response	**Discussion**	**Nontherapeutic response**	**Therapeutic response**
Changing the subject	The nurse changes the topic at a crucial time because the discussion is too uncomfortable. It negates what the client seems interested in discussing. Communication will remain superficial.	C: "My mother always puts me down." N: "That's interesting, but let's talk about…"	N: "Tell me about that."
Belittling	The nurse puts down client's expressed feelings to avoid having to deal with painful feelings.	C: "I don't want to live anymore now that my child is gone." N: "Anyone would be sad, but that's no reason to want to die."	N: "The death must be very difficult for you. Tell me a little more about how you are feeling."
Disagreeing	The nurse criticizes the client who is seeking support.	"I definitely do not agree with your view." "I really don't believe that."	"Let's talk about the way you see that." "It seems hard to believe. Please explain further."
Judging	The nurse's responses are filled with his or her own values and judgments. This demonstrates a lack of acceptance of the client's differences. It will provide a barrier to further disclosures.	"You are not married. Do you think having this baby will solve your problems?" "This is certainly not the Christian thing to do." "You are thinking about divorce when you have three children?"	"What will having this baby provide for you?" "What do you think about what you are attempting to do?" "Let's discuss this option," or "Let's discuss other options."
Excessive probing	Serves to control the nature of the client's responses. The nurse asks many questions of clients before they are ready to provide the information. This is self-protective to the nurse by avoiding the anxiety of uncomfortable silences. The client feels overwhelmed and may withdraw.	"Why do you do this?" "What do you think was the real cause?" "Do you always feel this way?" "Why do you think that way?"	"Tell me how this is upsetting you." "Tell me what you believe to be the cause." "Tell me how you feel when that happens." "Explain your thinking on this if you can."
Challenging	This stems from the nurse's belief that if clients are challenged regarding their unrealistic beliefs, they will be coerced into seeing reality. The client may feel threatened when challenged, holding onto the beliefs more strongly.	"You are not the Queen of England." "If your leg is missing, then how can you walk this hall?"	"You sound like you want to be important." "It seems to you like you are missing a leg. Tell me more about that."
Superficial comments	The nurse gives simple or meaningless responses to clients. It suggests a lack of understanding regarding the client as an individual. The interactions remain superficial, maintaining distance between nurse and client. Nothing of significance gets communicated.	"Great day, huh!" "You should be feeling good; you are being discharged today." "Keep the faith; your doctor should be coming anytime now."	"What kind of day are you having?" "How are you feeling about leaving the hospital today?" "You look worried. Your doctor called and said he would be here within the hour."

Table 6-1   Ineffective Responses that Hinder Therapeutic Communication—cont'd

Response	Discussion	Nontherapeutic response	Therapeutic response
Defending	The nurse may believe she or he must defend herself or himself, the staff, or the hospital. The nurse may not take the time to listen to the client's concerns. Efforts need to be made to explore the client's thoughts and feelings.	"Your doctor is a good doctor. He would never say that." "We have a very experienced staff here. They would not ever do that."	"What has you so upset about your doctor?" "Tell me what happened on the evening shift."
Self-focusing	The nurse focuses attention away from the client by thinking about sharing his or her own thoughts, feelings, problems. The focus is taken away from the client who is seeking help. The nurse is more interested in what to say next instead of actively listening to the client.	"That may have happened to you last year, but it happened to me twice this month, which hurt me a great deal and..." "Excuse me but could you say that again? I have a response to make, but I want to be sure of what you said."	"Tell me about your incident and how it might relate to your sadness now." "If I heard you accurately, you said..."
Criticism of others	The nurse puts down others.	C: "The staff members on the day shift let me smoke two cigarettes." N: "The day shift is always breaking the rules. On this shift, we follow the one cigarette policy." C: "My daughter is hateful to me." N: "She must be just awful to live with."	N: "The policy is one cigarette, which we must follow." N: "It sounds like you are having a rough time now with your daughter."
Premature interpretation	The nurse does not wait until the client fully expresses thoughts and feelings related to a particular problem. This rushes the client and disregards his or her input. The nurse may miss what the client wants to explain.	"I think this is what you really mean." "You may think that way consciously, but your unconscious believes..."	"What do you think this means?" "So you think..."

From Fortinash KM, Holoday-Worret PA: *Psychiatric-mental health nursing*, St Louis, 1996, Mosby.

Therapeutic Communication Techniques

Listening
Definition: An active process of receiving information and examining reaction to the messages received
Example: Maintaining eye contact and receptive non-verbal communication
Therapeutic value: Nonverbally communicates to the patient the nurse's interest and acceptance

Broad Openings
Definition: Encouraging the patient to select topics for discussion
Example: "What are you thinking about?"
Therapeutic value: Indicates acceptance by the nurse and the value of the patient's initiative

Restating
Definition: Repeating the main thought the patient expressed
Example: "You say that your mother left you when you were 5 years old."
Therapeutic value: Indicates that the nurse is listening and validates, reinforces, or calls attention to something important that has been said

Clarification
Definition: Attempting to put into words vague ideas or unclear thoughts of the patient to enhance the nurse's understanding or asking the patient to explain what he means
Example: "I'm not sure what you mean. Could you tell me about that again?"
Therapeutic value: Helps to clarify feelings, ideas, and perceptions of the patient and provide an explicit correlation between them and the patient's actions

Reflection
Definition: Directing back the patient's ideas, feelings, questions, and content
Example: "You're feeling tense and anxious and it's related to a conversation you had with your husband last night?"
Therapeutic value: Validates the nurse's understanding of what the patient is saying and signifies empathy, interest, and respect for the patient

Humor
Definition: The discharge of energy through the comic enjoyment of the imperfect
Example: "That gives a whole new meaning to the word *nervous*," said with shared kidding between the nurse and patient
Therapeutic value: Can promote insight by making conscious repressed material, resolving paradoxes, tempering aggression, and revealing new options, and is a socially acceptable form of sublimation

Informing
Definition: The skill of information giving

Example: "I think you need to know more about how your medication works."
Therapeutic value: Helpful in health teaching or patient education about relevant aspects of patient's well-being and self-care

Focusing
Definition: Questions or statements that help the patient expand on a topic of importance
Example: "I think that we should talk more about your relationship with your father."
Therapeutic value: Allows the patient to discuss central issues and keeps the communication process goal-directed

Sharing Perceptions
Definition: Asking the patient to verify the nurse's understanding of what the patient is thinking or feeling
Example: "You're smiling but I sense that you are really very angry with me."
Therapeutic value: Conveys the nurse's understanding to the patient and has the potential for clearing up confusing communication

Theme Identification
Definition: Underlying issues or problems experienced by the patient that emerge repeatedly during the course of the nurse-patient relationship
Example: "I've noticed that in all of the relationships that you have described, you've been hurt or rejected by the man. Do you think this is an underlying issue?"
Therapeutic value: Allows the nurse to best promote the patient's exploration and understanding of important problems

Silence
Definition: Lack of verbal communication for a therapeutic reason
Example: Sitting with a patient and nonverbally communicating interest and involvement
Therapeutic value: Allows the patient time to think and gain insights, slows the pace of the interaction and encourages the patient to initiate conversation, while conveying the nurse's support, understanding, and acceptance

Suggesting
Definition: Presentation of alternative ideas for the patient's consideration relative to problem solving
Example: "Have you thought about responding to your boss in a different way when he raises that issue with you? For example, you could ask him if a specific problem has occurred."
Therapeutic value: Increases the patient's perceived options or choices

Modified from Stuart GW, Sundeen AJ: *Principles and practice of psychiatric nursing*, ed 5, St Louis, 1995, Mosby.

D. Physical basis: personality develops normally if the necessary physical basis is present
   1. The brain is the major organ of thought and is necessary to development of personality
   2. Other influential factors include a normally functioning endocrine system, which strongly influences behavior
E. Major theorists (Table 6-2)
F. Elements of personality (Freud)
   1. Levels of consciousness
      a. The unconscious: always outside the awareness of the individual; influences actions in ways the individual may not understand; thought to include dreams
      b. The preconscious: usually outside awareness; available to conscious mind in special circumstances such as under hypnosis or during therapy
      c. The conscious: ordinary awareness
   2. Structures: some theorists refer to personality structures
      a. Freud: ego, id, superego
      b. Berne: child, adult, parent
   3. Functions: each structure is thought to perform specific functions (Freud)
      a. Id/child: basic, innate psychic energy; emotional
      b. Ego/adult: mediates between person's perception and objective reality; always rational
      c. Superego/parent: incorporates societal values; judgmental and critical
G. Development levels: various theorists describe levels of development
   1. Freud: oral, anal, phallic, latency, genital
   2. Erikson: basic trust vs. mistrust; autonomy vs. shame and doubt; initiative vs. guilt; industry vs. inferiority; identity vs. role diffusion; intimacy vs. isolation; generativity vs. stagnation; ego integrity vs. despair
H. Development of the self-concept
   1. Developed through experience with other people, e.g., parents, siblings, relatives, peers, teachers, and other adults
      a. Feelings of adequacy or inadequacy
      b. Feelings of acceptance or rejection
      c. Opportunities for identification
      d. Expectations of values, goals, and behaviors
   2. Self-concept consists of
      a. Body image: one's perception of one's body
      b. Self-ideal: one's idea of what is "good" behavior
      c. Self-esteem: personal judgment of one's own worth
      d. Role: one's perception of how one fits into the society
      e. Identity: the combination of all of the above into a unified whole

STRESS

Hans Selye (1956) defined stress as "wear and tear on the body." All people are continuously exposed to varieties of stress: physical, chemical, psychologic, and emotional. Almost any situation, pleasant or unpleasant, that requires change leads to some level of stress. Stress produces a clearly identifiable response called the general adaptation syndrome. It is associated with concomitant physical and chemical changes that commonly occur in the body.

Ego Defense Mechanisms

Ego defense mechanisms are basic psychologic tools that individuals use at various times to manage life's crises. They may also be referred to as ego defenses, defense mechanisms, or protective mechanisms. As such, they defend the ego or self from untoward anxiety, help resolve conflicts, and return the individual to a point of psychologic homeostasis or comfort. They are usually outside conscious awareness and are not considered pathologic in and of themselves. They should not be removed or challenged until the individual is ready and has adequate strength to tolerate the stressful situation. Common defenses are listed in Table 6-3.

Mental Disturbances and Resources

ANXIETY

A. Definition: a state of alertness or apprehension, tension or uneasiness; a major component of all mental disturbances. Anxiety is an internal state experienced by the individual when there is a perceived threat to the physical body or to the psychologic integrity of the person; it interferes with concentration, focusing attention on the perceived threat; in its mild form anxiety serves to alert the person to danger and to prepare the body to react to danger; in its severe form it is debilitating and may immobilize the person and interfere with activities; anxiety is usually described in degrees or levels
B. Process (Figure 6-1)
   1. Adaptive coping: the problem creating the anxiety is resolved
   2. Palliative coping: the problem creating the anxiety is not resolved but rather temporarily reduced; the problem returns at a later date
   3. Maladaptive coping: energy is channeled toward reducing the anxiety and no effort is made to solve the problem
   4. Dysfunctional coping: the problem is not solved and the anxiety not reduced
C. Levels
   1. Mild (+1)
   2. Moderate (+2)
   3. Severe (+3)
   4. Panic (+4)
D. Assessment (Table 6-4)
E. Interventions
   1. Remain with the highly anxious patient; leaving the patient alone increases anxiety
   2. Reduce environmental stimuli or move the patient to a quiet area; the patient's ability to handle stimuli is compromised
   3. Remain in control and calm; the patient fears losing control, and needs to feel secure
   4. Communicate with clear, simple, short sentences because the patient's ability to deal with complex, abstract statements is compromised

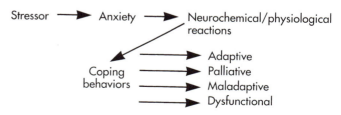

Figure 6-1. **Process of anxiety.** (From Keltner NL, Schwecke LH, Bostrom CE: *Psychiatric nursing*, ed 2, St Louis, 1995, Mosby.)

Table 6-2	A Comparison of the Development Stages Postulated by Freud, Sullivan, Erikson, and Piaget			
Freud	**Sullivan**	**Erikson**	**Piaget**

I) Oral stage (0-18 mo)
  a) The mouth is a source of satisfaction
  b) Two phases
    1) Passive
      Only interests are satisfying hunger and *sucking*
      Completely helpless, *security* is the greatest need
      Narcissistic and egocentric, operates on *pleasure principle*
      Omnipotent feelings are prevalent
    2) Active
      Biting is a mode of pleasure
      Continuous experimentation and associations
      Sensory discriminations.
      Differentiation between mental images and reality
      Differentiation of others and discovery of self
	I) Infancy (0-18 mo)
	  a) The mouth is a source of satisfaction
	  b) Mouth—takes in (sucking), cuts off (biting), and pushes out (spitting) objects introduced by others
	  c) Crying, babbling, and cooing are modes of communication used by the infant to call attention of adults to self
	  d) *Satisfaction response (pleasure principle).* Infant's biologic needs are met and a mutual feeling of comfort and fulfillment is experienced by mother and infant. (Mother gives and infant takes)
	  e) *Empathic observation.* Capacity to perceive feelings of others as his or her own immediate feelings in the situation
	  f) *Autistic invention.* State of symbolic activity in which the infant feels he or she is master of all he or she surveys
	  g) Experimentation, exploration, and manipulation are methods used to acquaint self with environment
		I) Oral-sensory stage (0-12 mo)
		  a) The mouth is a source of satisfaction and a means of dealing with anxiety-producing situations
		  b) Focus is on the development of the basic attitudes of *trust vs. mistrust*
		  c) Attitudes are formed through mother's reaction to infant needs
			I) Sensorimotor stage (0-12 mo)
			  a) Emphasis is on preverbal intellectual development
			  b) Learns relationships with external objects
			  c) Focus is on physical development with gradual increase in ability to think and use language

II) Anal stage (1½-3 yr)
  a) Primary activity is on learning muscular control association with urination and defecation (*toilet training period*)
  b) Exhibits more self-control; walks, talks, dresses, and undresses
  c) *Negativism*—assertion of independence
  d) Introduction of *reality principle*, ego development
	II) Childhood (1½-6 yr)
	  a) Begins with the capacity for communicating through speech and ends with a beginning need for association with peers
	  b) Uses language as a tool to communicate wishes and needs
	  c) Anus is power tool used to give or withhold a part of self to control significant people in his environment
		II Anal-muscular stage (1-3 yr)
		  a) Learns the extent to which the *environment* can be influenced by direct manipulation
		  b) Focuses on the development of the basic attitudes of *autonomy vs. shame and doubt*
		  c) Exerts self-control and willpower
			II) Preoperational stage (2-7 yr)
			  a) Learns to use symbols and language
			  b) Learns to imitate and play
			  c) Displays egocentricity
			  d) Engages in *animistic thinking*—endowment of objects with power and ability

Continued

Table 6-2	A Comparison of the Development Stages Postulated by Freud, Sullivan, Erikson, and Piaget—cont'd		
Freud	**Sullivan**	**Erikson**	**Piaget**
e) Superego begins to develop f) Engages in parallel play	d) Emergence and integration of *self-concept* and *reflected appraisal* of *significant persons* e) Awareness that postponing or delaying gratification of won wishes may bring satisfaction f) Begins to find limits in experimentation, exploration, and manipulation g) More aggressive h) Uses parallel play and curiosity to explore environment i) Uses exhibitionism and mastubatory activity to become acquainted with self and others j) Demonstrates a beginning ability to think abstractly		
III) Phallic stage (3-6 yr) a) *Libidinal energy* focus on the genitals b) Learns *sexual identity* c) *Superego* becomes internalized d) Sibling rivalry and manipulation of parents occurs e) Intellectual and motor facilities are refined f) Increased socialization and *associative play*		III) Genital-locomotor stage (3-6 yr) a) Learns the extent to which being *assertive* will influence the environment b) Focus is on the development of the *basic attitudes of initiative vs. guilt* c) Explores the world with senses, thoughts, and imagination d) Activities demonstrate direction and purpose e) Engages in first real social contacts through *cooperative play* f) Develops conscience	
IV) Latency (6-12 yr) a) *Quiet* stage in which sexual development lies dormant, emotional tension eases b) *Normal homosexual phase* For boys, gangs For girls, cliques c) Increased intellectual capacity d) Starts school	III) Juvenile stage (6-9 yr) a) Learns to form satisfactory relationship with peers b) *Peer norms* prevail over family norms c) Engages in *competition*, experimentation, exploration, and manipulation d) Able to cooperate and compromise	IV) Latency (6-12 yr) a) Learns to use energy to create, develop, and manipulate b) Focus is on the development of basic attitudes of *industry vs. inferiority* c) Able to initiate and complete tasks d) Understands rules and regulations	III) Concrete operations stage (7-11 yr) a) Deals with visible concrete objects and relationships b) Increased intellectual and conceptual development—uses logic and reasoning c) More socialized and rule conscious

Continued

Table 6-2	A Comparison of the Development Stages Postulated by Freud, Sullivan, Erikson, and Piaget—cont'd		
Freud	**Sullivan**	**Erikson**	**Piaget**

e) Identifies with teachers and peers
f) Weakening of home ties
g) Recognizes authority figures outside home, age of *hero worship*
	e) Demonstrates capacity to love
	f) Distinguishes fantasy from reality
	g) Exerts internal control over behavior
	
	IV) Preadolescence (9-12 yr)
	  a) Learns to relate to a friend of the same sex—*chum relationship*
	  b) Concerned with group success and derives satisfaction from group accomplishment
	  c) Shows signs of *rebellion*—restlessness, hostility, irritability
	  d) Assumes less responsibility for own actions
	  e) Moves from egocentricity to a more full social state
	  f) Uses experimentation, exploration, manipulation
	  g) Seeks *consensual validation* from peers
		e) Displays competence and productivity	

V) Genital stage (12 yr-early adulthood)
  a) Appearance of secondary sex characteristics, reawakening of sex drives
  b) Increased concern over physical appearance
  c) Strives toward independence
  d) Development of sexual maturity
  e) Identity crisis
  f) Identification of love object of opposite sex
  g) Intellectual maturity
  h) Plans future
	V) Early adolescence (12-14 yr)
	  a) Experiences physiologic changes
	  b) Uses rebellion to gain independence
	  c) Fantasizes, overidentifies with heroes
	  d) Discovers and begins relationships with opposite sex
	  e) Demonstrates heightened levels of anxiety in most interpersonal relationships
		V) Puberty and adolescence (12-18 yr)
		  a) Demonstrates an ability to integrate life experiences
		  b) Focus is on the development of the basic attitudes of *identity vs. role diffusion*
		  c) Seeks partner of the opposite sex
		  d) Begins to establish identity and place in society
			IV) Formal operations stage (11-15 yr)
			  a) Develops true abstract thought
			  b) Formulates hypothesis and applies logical tests
			  c) Conceptual independence

	VI) Late adolescence (14-21 yr)
	  a) Establishes an enduring intimate relationship with one member of the opposite sex
	  b) Self-concept becomes stabilized
		VI) Young adulthood (18-25 yr)
		  a) Primarily concerned with developing an intimate relationship with another adult	

Continued

Table 6-2	A Comparison of the Development Stages Postulated by Freud, Sullivan, Erikson, and Piaget—cont'd		
Freud	**Sullivan**	**Erikson**	**Piaget**
	c) Attains physical maturity d) Develops ability to use logic and abstract concepts VII) Adulthood (21 yr and older) 　a) Assumes responsibility relevant to station in life 　b) Maintains balance and involvement between self, family, and community 　c) Further develops creativity 　d) Reaffirms values in life	b) Focus is on the development of the basic attitudes of *intimacy and solidarity vs. isolation* VII) Adulthood (25-45 yr) 　a) Primarily concerned with establishing and maintaining a family 　b) Focus is on the development of the basic attitudes of *generativity vs. stagnation* 　c) Displays a marked degree of creativity 　d) Adjusts to circumstances of middle age 　e) Reevaluates life's accomplishments and goals VIII) Maturity (older than 45 yr) 　a) Acceptance of lifestyle as meaningful and fulfilling 　b) Focus is on the development of basic attitudes of *ego integrity vs. despair* 　c) Remains optimistic and continues to grow 　d) Adjusts to limitations 　e) Adjusts to retirement 　f) Adjusts to reorganized family patterns 　g) Adjusts to losses 　h) Accepts death with serenity	

Modified from Kreigh H, Perko J: *Psychiatric and mental health nursing: commitment to care and concern*, Reston, 1979, Reston Publishing.

| Table 6-3 | **Ego Defense Mechanisms** |

Defense mechanism	Example	Defense mechanism	Example
Compensation: Process by which a person makes up for a perceived deficiency by strongly emphasizing a feature that he regards as an asset.	A businessman perceives his small physical stature negatively. He tries to overcome this by being aggressive, forceful, and controlling in business dealings.	**Projection:** Attributing one's thoughts or impulses to another person. Through this process one can attribute intolerable wishes, emotional feelings, or motivations to another person.	A young woman who denies she has sexual feelings about a coworker accuses him without basis of being a "flirt" and says he is trying to seduce her.
Denial: Avoidance of disagreeable realities by ignoring or refusing to recognize them; probably simplest and most primitive of all defense mechanisms.	Mrs. P has just been told that her breast biopsy indicates a malignancy. When her husband visits her that evening, she tells him that no one has discussed the laboratory results with her.	**Rationalization:** Offering a socially acceptable or apparently logical explanation to justify or make acceptable otherwise unacceptable impulses, feelings, behaviors, and motives.	John fails an examination and complains that the lectures were not well organized or clearly presented.
Displacement: Shift of emotion from a person or object to another usually neutral or less dangerous person or object.	A 4-year-old boy is angry because he has just been punished by his mother for drawing on his bedroom walls. He begins to play "war" with his soldier toys and has them battle and fight with each other.	**Reaction formation:** Development of conscious attitudes and behavior patterns that are opposite to what one really feels or would like to do.	A married woman who feels attracted to one of her husband's friends treats him rudely.
Dissociation: The separation of any group of mental or behavioral processes from the rest of the person's consciousness or identity.	A man is brought to the emergency room by the police and is unable to explain who he is and where he lives or works.	**Regression:** Retreat in face of stress to behavior characteristic of any earlier level of development.	Four-year-old Nicole, who has been toilet trained for over a year, begins to wet her pants again when her new baby brother is brought home from the hospital.
Identification: Process by which a person tries to become like someone he admires by taking on thoughts, mannerisms, or tastes of that individual.	Sally, 15 years old, has her hair styled similarly to her young English teacher whom she admires.	**Repression:** Involuntary exclusion of a painful or conflictual thought, impulse, or memory from awareness. It is the primary ego defense, and other mechanisms tend to reinforce it.	Mr. R does not recall hitting his wife when she was pregnant.
Intellectualization: Excessive reasoning or logic is used to avoid experiencing disturbing feelings.	A woman avoids dealing with her anxiety in shopping malls by explaining that she is saving the frivolous waste of time and money by not going into them.	**Splitting:** Viewing people and situations as either all good or all bad. Failure to integrate the positive and negative qualities of oneself.	A friend tells you that you are the most wonderful person in the world one day, and how much she hates you the next day.
Introjection: Intense type of identification in which a person incorporates qualities or values of another person or group into his own ego structure. It is one of the earliest mechanisms of the child; important in formation of conscience.	Eight-year-old Jimmy tells his 3-year-old sister, "Don't scribble in your book of nursery rhymes. Just look at the pretty pictures," thus expressing his parents' values to his little sister.	**Sublimation:** Acceptance of a socially approved substitute goal for a drive whose normal channel of expression is blocked.	Ed has an impulsive and physically aggressive nature. He tries out for the football team and becomes a star tackle.
		Suppression: A process often listed as a defense mechanism but really a conscious counterpart of repression. It is intentional exclusion of material from consciousness. At times, it may lead to subsequent repression.	A young man at work finds he is thinking so much about his date that evening that it is interfering with his work. He decides to put it out of his mind until he leaves the office for the day.
Isolation: Splitting off of emotional components of a thought, which may be temporary or long term.	A second-year medical student dissects a cadaver for her anatomy course without being disturbed by thoughts of death.	**Undoing:** Act or communication that partially negates a previous one; primitive defense mechanism.	Larry makes a passionate declaration of love to Sue on a date. On their next meeting he treats her formally and distantly.

From Stuart GW, Sundeen SJ: *Principles and practice of psychiatric nursing*, ed 5, St Louis, 1995, Mosby.

Table 6-4	**Levels of Anxiety**		
Severity of anxiety	**Physical**	**Intellectual**	**Social and emotional**

Minimal (near 0)	Basal levels of:
	  Blood pressure
	  Pulse
	  Respiration rate
	  O_2 consumption
	Pupillary constriction
	Muscles relaxed
		Cognitive activity minimal
		Disregard for external environmental stimuli; no attempt to actively process information
		Focus typically on single, nonthreatening mental image
		States of altered consciousness
			No social interaction
			No attempt to deal with environmental stimuli
			Minimal emotional activity
			Feelings of indifference, invulnerability, and contentment prevail

Mild (+ 1)	Low-level sympathetic arousal Moderate to low skeletal muscle tension Body relaxed Voice calm, well-modulated	Perceptual field open; able to shift focus of attention readily Passively aware of external environment Self-referent thoughts positive; low concern for unexpected or negative outcomes	Behavior primarily automatic; habitual patterns and well-learned skills Positive feeling of security, confidence, and satisfaction dominate Solitary activities

Moderate (+ 2)	Sympathetic nervous system activation
	  ↑ Blood pressure
	  ↑ Pulse rate
	  ↑ Respiratory rate
	  Pupillary dilation
	  Sweat glands stimulated
	  Peripheral vascular constriction
	Increased muscular tension
	Heightened performance of well-learned skills
	Rate of speech increased, pitch heightened
	Increased alertness
		Narrowing of perception; attentional focus on specific internal or external stimuli
		Conscious effort in processing of information; optimal level for learning
		Self-referent thoughts ± mixed; some concern about personal ability or available resources necessary to solve problems; probability of positive outcomes increasingly uncertain
			Increased skill in learning and refining of skills; analyzing problematic situations; integrating cognitive and motor domains
			Feelings of challenge; drive to resolve problems or dilemmas
			Mixed sense of confidence/optimism with fear, lowered self-esteem, and potential inadequacy

Severe (+ 3)	Fight-flight response
	Stimulation of adrenal medulla
	  ↑ Catecholamines, accelerated heart rate, palpitations
	  ↑ Blood glucose
	  ↓ Blood flow to digestive system
	  ↑ Blood flow to skeletal muscles
	Muscles extremely tense
	Hyperventilation
	Physical actions increasingly agitated, pacing, wringing of hands, fidgeting, trembling
	May experience loss of appetite, nausea, "cold sweats"
	Rapid, high-pitched speech
	Facial expression:
	  poor eye contact, fleeting eye movements
		Perceptual capacity restricted; exclusive attention to singular stimuli (internal or external) or multifocal, fragmented processing of stimuli
		Problem solving inefficient, difficult
		Some threatening stimuli disregarded, minimized, denied
		Disorientation in terms of time and place
		Expected likelihood of negative consequences or outcomes high; estimates of personal self-efficacy low
			Flight behavior may be manifested by withdrawal, denial, depression, somatization
			Feelings of increasing threat, need to respond to situation are heightened
			Dissociating tendency; feelings are denied

Continued

Table 6-4	Levels of Anxiety—cont'd		
Severity of anxiety	**Physical**	**Intellectual**	**Social and emotional**
Panic (+ 4)	Continued physiologic arousal Actions disorganized, directionless; unable to execute simple motor tasks; fumbling, gross motor agitation, flailing May strike out verbally or physically; may attempt to withdraw from situation Eventual depletion of sympathetic neurotransmitters Blood redistributed throughout body Hypotension May feel dizzy, faint, or exhausted Appears pale, drawn, weary Facial expression: aghast, grimacing, eyes fixed Voice louder, higher pitched	Perception severely restricted, may be impervious to external stimuli Thoughts are random, distorted, disconnected, logical processing impaired Unable to solve problems; limited tolerance for processing novel stimuli (verbal, auditory, or visual) Preoccupied with thoughts of highly probable negative outcomes; conclusions may be drawn, negative consequences seen as inevitable	Emotionally drained, overwhelmed Reliance on earlier, more "primitive" coping behaviors: crying, shouting, curling up, rocking, freezing Feelings of impotence, helplessness, agony and desperation dominate; may be experienced as horror, dread, defenselessness; may be converted to anger, rage

From Keltner NL et al: *Psychiatric nursing: a psychotherapeutic management approach*, St Louis, 1991, Mosby.

5. Use of PRN medications may be necessary to decrease patient's anxiety to a manageable level: e.g., lorazepam (Ativan)
6. Encourage use of relaxation techniques
7. When appropriate, assist patient with recognizing early signs of anxiety and effective ways to prevent its escalation
8. Provide opportunities for discussion of the relationship of thoughts and verbalizations to anxiety
9. Implement seclusion and/or restraints if patient is a danger to self and/or others

PHOBIAS
A. Definition: irrational, continual fear of an activity, situation, object, or event
B. Types
   1. Agoraphobia (literal meaning, "fear of the marketplace") without panic attacks; fear of being away from a safe environment or person
   2. Social phobia: irrational fear of exposure to the scrutiny of others
   3. Simple phobia: a disabling fear of some specific object or situation, such as the fear of animals or of being in a high place
C. Assessment data
   1. Panic anxiety
   2. Anticipatory anxiety
   3. Recognition of phobia as irrational
   4. Uses defense mechanisms of displacement and repression
   5. Avoidance behaviors
   6. Interference with demands of daily activities

D. Interventions
   1. Acceptance of patient and his or her fears
   2. Encourage involvement in activities that do not increase anxiety
   3. Help patient recognize that his or her behavior is an attempt to cope with anxiety
   4. Use a calm, nonauthoritative approach
   5. Reassure patient that he or she will not be made to confront the phobia in treatment until ready to do so
   6. Systematic desensitization

OBSESSIVE COMPULSIVE DISORDER (OCD)
A. Definition: Obsessive thoughts (troublesome, persistent thoughts) and compulsions (ritualistic behaviors) that are repetitive
B. Assessment data
   1. Compulsive, ritualistic behavior
   2. Obsessive thoughts
   3. Alterations in normal functioning
   4. Fear of loss of control
   5. Feelings of guilt
   6. Suicidal thoughts/feelings
   7. Rumination (persistent meditation on thoughts)
   8. Insight impairment
   9. Feelings of worthlessness
   10. Decreased self-esteem
C. Interventions
   1. Allow patient time to perform rituals
   2. Ensure basic daily needs are met
   3. Redirect rumination positively

4. Do not, initially, call attention to or interfere with the compulsive act
5. Demonstrate concern for and interest in the patient
6. Encourage verbalization of concerns and feelings
7. As anxiety decreases and patient feels comfortable talking with staff, encourage the patient to talk about his or her behavior and thoughts
8. Encourage patient to try to reduce the frequency of compulsive behavior

F. Posttraumatic stress disorder: characteristic symptoms after a psychologically traumatic event; these include numbness of responses, frequently reliving the event, dreams, depression, and anxiety

PERCEPTION

A. Definition: awareness acquired through the five senses
B. Alterations: thought to be pathologies resulting from anxiety
    1. Illusion: misinterpretation of a sensory input
    2. Hallucination: a sensation without an external stimulus; may be
        a. Auditory: hearing nonexistent voices or sounds
        b. Olfactory: smelling nonexistent odors or aromas
        c. Visual: seeing nonexistent things, people, or animals
        d. Tactile: feeling somatic sensations
        e. Gustatory: experiencing flavors or tastes
    3. Delusion: a false belief, not based in fact, that cannot be changed by reasoning
        a. Delusions of grandeur: feelings of greatness
        b. Delusions of persecution: feelings of being mistreated
        c. Delusions of sin or guilt: feelings of deserving punishment
        d. Somatic delusions: feelings about the body or part of the body
        e. Ideas of reference: feeling that certain events or words have special meaning for self

THOUGHT DISORDERS

Schizophrenia is considered the psychiatric manifestation of thought disorder; this group of illnesses represents the largest number of mentally ill persons.

A. Types of schizophrenia
    1. Disorganized: includes frequent incoherence, non-systematized delusions, and inappropriate affect
    2. Catatonic: includes stupor, negativity, rigidity, excitement, and posturing
    3. Paranoid: includes persecutory delusions, grandiosity, delusional jealousy, and hallucinations
    4. Undifferentiated: does not fit criteria of other categories or combines them
    5. Residual: presence of residual symptoms (e.g., marked social isolation, inappropriate affect, odd beliefs) without delusions, hallucinations, or gross disorganization
B. Assessment data
    1. Delusions of being controlled
    2. Somatic delusions (grandiosity, religious, or nihilistic)
    3. Persecutory delusions accompanied by hallucinations
    4. Auditory hallucinations of a running commentary on behavior or thought
    5. Auditory hallucination on several occasions with content of more than one word

6. Incoherence, looseness of association, illogical thinking with a deterioration in function
7. Continuation of symptoms for 6 months or more, occurring before 45 years of age

C. Interventions
    1. Thought disorders
        a. Do not enter into patient's delusions; maintain your own view of reality without demeaning the patient's view of reality
        b. Do not argue about hallucinations: the patient views these as real
        c. Offer reassurance: most patients are experiencing pain from their symptoms
        d. Touch only with permission; the thought-disordered patient may have a distorted sense of his or her own person
        e. If you are afraid, be aware that the patient will sense this; be sure you have sufficient backup for your own safety and comfort
        f. Maintain patient safety

AFFECTIVE DISORDERS

Disturbances in feeling or affective disorders are classified as follows:

DEPRESSIVE DISORDERS

A. Major depression is the predominant mental illness in the United States and Canada with ranges from 7% to 12% in the male population and 26% to 30% in the female population
B. Assessment data
    1. Irritation
    2. Loss of interest in some or all usual activities
    3. Change in appetite: usually decreased
    4. Changes in weight: usually loss in weight
    5. Sleep disturbances: usually insomnia, but may be increased hours of sleep per day
    6. Withdrawal from family and friends
    7. Hopelessness and helplessness may become profound and may lead to delusions or fantasies of "ending it all"
    8. If left in this pattern, the patient eventually could justify how nonexistence may solve the problems
    9. The patient may start to dwell on death, and to devise a plan of self-destruction
    10. Self-destruction becomes the goal; this is suicidal ideation
C. See later sections on Suicide Prevention and Suicide Intervention

BIPOLAR DISORDERS

A. Category used when one or more manic episodes are noted whether or not a depressive episode is/has been experienced
B. Mania characterized by unstable mood, pressured speech, and increased motor activity

Intervention

A. Demonstrate sincere interest
B. Accept patient's feelings; anger may be directed to the nearest safe object: often the nurse
C. Allow patient to express feelings; for example, crying in a dignified environment

D. Encourage only the expression of feelings that you feel capable of handling; for example, do not encourage ventilation of feelings and then go on your lunch hour

E. If patient is overactive, limit setting or reduction of stimuli may be necessary

F. Avoid power struggles: use force only if necessary to protect patient or others in the environment

EATING DISORDERS

A. Obesity/compulsive overeating: consuming greater than required number of calories, which results in weight gain, usually considered more than 20% greater than the recommended weight for one's height

B. Anorexia nervosa: compulsive refusal to eat; person believes that he or she is overweight, regardless of his or her actual weight

C. Bulimia: an eating disorder characterized by episodes of binging and then purging; person may not appear overweight or underweight. Bulimia leads to other symptoms such as menstrual irregularities, gastric dilation, aspiration pneumonia, dental caries (caused by frequent vomiting), and esophagitis

See Anorexia nervosa and Bulimia in Pediatric Nursing, Chapter 8.

PERSONALITY DISORDERS

A. Paranoid personality: characterized by suspicion, rigidity, secretiveness, oversensitivity and alertness, distortions of reality, and the use of projection as a major defense mechanism

B. Borderline personality: at times moderately neurotic and at other times, overtly psychotic; extremely difficult to treat and often unstable after numerous treatment attempts
1. Assessment data
   a. Combined anger and depression
   b. Anhedonia (inability to experience pleasure)
   c. Social isolation
   d. Poor impulse control
   e. Dependency
   f. Substance abuse
   g. Sexual promiscuity
2. Interventions
   a. Be honest with patients
   b. These patients are often manipulative and attention seeking
   c. They tend to view people or situations as all good or all bad
   d. Patients need to begin developing meaningful relationships in which they can begin to trust
   e. Consistency is important; patients may split the staff to play one staff member against another

C. Codependency: meeting goals successfully by relying on another person for the answers. Characteristics of the codependent person include
1. Partners are dependent on each other to make a whole relationship
2. One of the partners in this relationship assumes a passive role
3. One or both may have low self-esteem
4. One or both may have low self-image
5. One or both may have an addictive disorder (alcohol, drugs, etc.)
6. They tend to be manipulative—there is a constant conflict either between them or within the family
7. They tend to operate in a series of delusions
8. Because of delusions, they tend to promote their version of any story as the absolute truth
9. They exhibit poor boundaries in relationships
10. They are somewhat to totally insensitive to others' emotions and feelings
11. If the codependency exists within family boundaries, it is highly likely that a dysfunctional family unit will emerge and the children will become a part of the codependency
12. Codependency may be intergenerational, and therefore cyclical

The treatment of codependent persons is designed by identifying the underlying emotions that are fostering the codependency

D. Substance abuse disorders: a pattern of pathologic use of substances that entails such things as need for daily use, loss of control, efforts to control use, overdoses, impairment of social functioning, family disruptions, legal problems, and so on; abuse is distinguished from dependency by tolerance of the substance (increasing use requires increasing doses to achieve the same effect) and the presence or absence of a withdrawal syndrome
1. Alcoholism
   a. Abuse is distinguished from recreational use by such features as daily drinking, frequent need for the chemical, blackouts, social impairment, and decreased ability to function, such as job loss, driving while intoxicated, arrests, and so forth
   b. Acute alcohol ingestion may result in a condition formerly known as delirium tremens (DTs), now known as acute alcohol withdrawal syndrome; key features are hallucinations, extreme agitation, and disorientation; treatment includes anxiolytics (benzodiazepines), anticonvulsants, and hydration
   c. Long-term use may lead to peripheral neuropathy, Wernicke's syndrome (confusion, ataxia, and abnormal eye movements), or Korsakoff's syndrome (alcoholic amnesia syndrome), which is manifested by memory loss and confabulation. These effects are largely caused by deficiency of thiamine and may be partially reversed by the provision of thiamine. Usually Korsakoff's syndrome is irreversible but may be arrested by thiamine replacement therapy and cessation of alcohol abuse
2. Barbiturate and sedative abuse (barbiturates, minor tranquilizers such as diazepam, benzodiazepines, etc.)
   a. Cross tolerant with alcohol
   b. May be used by "street addicts" when unable to obtain opiates
   c. Second most abused substance after alcohol in the United States
   d. Legally obtained drugs are often used by middle-class women who overuse tranquilizers
   e. Intoxication similar to alcohol
   f. There is a withdrawal syndrome similar to alcohol withdrawal
3. Opiates (heroin, morphine, etc.)
   a. Includes street addicts using IV heroin as well as "medical addicts" using various prescribed substances such as codeine

b. IV drug users are at a high risk for AIDS
c. Intoxication: pupil constriction, poor attention span, apathy, slurred speech, euphoria, and psychomotor retardation
d. There is a physical withdrawal syndrome
4. Cocaine
a. Stimulant
b. Increasing use among the middle class
c. Considered a social drug, many believe that it is not addictive
d. May be snorted or smoked as a "free-base" or as crack
e. Intoxication: poor judgment, poor impulse control, feeling of confidence, euphoria, talkative, rapid speech, pacing, elevated heart rate and blood pressure, dilated pupils, nausea, and sweating
f. May lead to hallucinations with prolonged use; severe depression occurs after the substance use is stopped, leading to strong psychologic craving
g. There does not appear to be a true withdrawal syndrome
5. Amphetamines
a. Abuse may begin in an effort to control weight
b. May be used IV by street addicts for a "rush"; may be combined with other drugs such as heroin or barbiturates
c. Intoxication: elevated heart rate and blood pressure, dilated pupils, chills, perspiration, nausea, and vomiting
6. Hallucinogens (LSD, mescaline, etc.)
a. Used much less than in the early 1970s
b. Use leads to altered perceptions and hallucinations; distorted perception of colors; illusions and delusions; unpredictable effects
c. Intoxication: perceptual changes; dilated pupils; increased pulse, sweating, anxiety, tremors; feelings of paranoia; and poor judgment
7. Cannabis (marijuana, hashish, etc.)
a. Widely used by various groups, usually smoked or eaten
b. Intoxication: increased pulse rate, bloodshot eyes, increased appetite, dry mouth, distorted perception of time, euphoria, and apathy
c. May precipitate panic attacks
8. Substance abuse interventions
a. Severe denial is a common defense mechanism
b. Keep the patient focused on the purpose of treatment
c. Manipulation may be used to obtain a substance for abuse
d. The nurse must remain nonjudgmental
e. These patients may require repeated attempts at treatment before they can conquer their addiction
f. Adequate diet, rest, and vitamin supplements are helpful
g. Long-term success is often achieved through a lifelong affiliation with abstinence programs such as Alcoholics Anonymous (AA) and Narcotics Anonymous (NA)
h. Alcoholism is usually treated in several steps, the first being detoxification. In detoxification, the alcoholic is withdrawn from the chemical through the use of a cross-tolerant substance, usually a benzodiazepine, which is administered for 3 to 5 days in decreasing doses. Frequently, alcoholics are referred to Alcoholics Anonymous
(1) Detoxification should occur in a controlled (monitored) setting because detoxification may become life threatening
(2) After the acute detoxification period of 3 to 5 days, intense counseling occurs
(3) The patient may find it beneficial to continue in a peer group setting on a regular full- or part-time schedule
(4) In some cases, additional treatment may be suggested in the form of halfway houses, which may offer up to 6 months to 1 year of treatment
i. Other forms of substance abuse are treated similarly, with combinations of detoxification, if needed, and supportive long-term treatment settings; opiate abusers may also be treated with methadone maintenance in attempts to prevent heroin use and allow the addict to return to more socially acceptable behavior patterns

PHYSICALLY BASED MENTAL DISORDERS
A. Organic brain syndrome may result from vascular disorders of the brain, brain infections, trauma, altered metabolism, poisoning, endocrine disorders, and deficiencies
1. Global involvement: confusion, delirium, and dementia
2. Selective involvement: may be limited to portions of the personality (e.g., amnesia, hallucinations, and psychosomatic disorders)
3. Functional impairment: has the features of psychosis (e.g. paranoia, depression, and mania)
4. Special needs of the elderly: special consideration is given to the role of declining physical attributes
a. There may be prejudices regarding the elderly
b. Most elderly persons do not suffer from senility
c. Apparent senility may be depression or other forms of illness (e.g., alcoholism)
d. The reaction to drugs of all types may be idiosyncratic among the elderly
e. Special techniques
(1) Life review
(2) Group work aimed at socialization such as remotivation
(3) Touch: many elderly are deprived of touch in the usual manner because of relational losses
Refer to Chapter 9, Nursing Care of the Older Adult
B. Mental retardation: subaverage intelligence; there are numerous causes including inherited defects in metabolism, genetic defects, birth injuries, and developmental anomalies
1. Mental retardation: classified as follows with interventions geared accordingly
a. Profoundly retarded: needs total nursing care in early stages; later may develop rudimentary ability to care for self; always requires some care
b. Severely retarded: may be able to care for self in protected environment; requires monitoring
c. Moderately retarded: usually capable of self-care but requires supervision when under stress
d. Mildly retarded: usually self-supporting; may require support of family or others when under stress

2. Special needs of children and adolescents: there are many similarities and some differences in the therapeutics for children and adolescents
   a. Services in hospitals are usually short and aimed at assessment and evaluation
   b. Most ongoing treatment is on an outpatient basis
   c. Treatment is action oriented, using such modalities as play therapy
   d. There are many issues of trust vs. mistrust
   e. There are issues of self-image, limit testing, and developmentally specific concerns
C. Other somatic manifestations of mental disturbance: several conditions have defined or suggested psychologic bases
   1. Ulcers
   2. Bowel disorders
   3. Cardiovascular disorders
   4. Asthma
   5. Allergies
   6. Eating disorders: anorexia, bulimia
   7. Headache
   8. Certain endocrine disorders

Death and Dying

Nursing intervention is aimed at ensuring the transition of the patient through each of the stages listed below. It is important to be aware of your own attitude about death and to ensure that you are meeting the patient's needs and not your own. Being nonjudgmental and allowing the expression of emotions by the patient are essential. Patient defenses are necessary in accepting his or her own death and should not be challenged. Elisabeth Kübler-Ross describes dying as a process that proceeds through the following stages

A. Shock and denial: the patient cannot actually accept or believe that he or she is going to die; may repress information, seek to escape the truth by seeking other opinions, and be unable to hear the real message
B. Anger and rage: a stage in which the patient becomes angry with the terrible truth of impending death; may be hypercritical of others, demanding, and resentful. Health care workers often bear the brunt of a patient's rage as they represent cure for others but not for him or her
C. Bargaining: in this stage, acceptance has begun, and the patient begins to bargain for more time or for some specific request; during this stage, wills may be finalized and legacies of various kinds bestowed. If possible, requests should be granted because they bring comfort to the dying person
D. Depression: after acceptance of the inevitable has begun, the person feels sad and alone. He or she may speak little, and cry often. Quiet acceptance is often the most helpful kind of intervention in this stage
E. Acceptance: once this occurs, the person is often seen as tranquil and at peace with himself. Again, the patient may speak little, since most of what he or she has to say to others has been said; although still sad, the patient has made his or her peace with death and has accepted the inevitable. This phase may last for months or longer

Grieving

George Engel (1964) defined grieving as a process of sequential steps similar to those in the dying process
A. Shock and disbelief: the person refuses to accept the loss, may feel stunned or numbed; similar to the first stage of dying

B. Developing awareness: the person may experience varying degrees of physical symptoms such as nausea, vomiting, and loss of appetite. Crying is common, anger may be felt and expressed toward the lost person for the act of desertion. Anger may be self-directed and recriminations made
C. Restitution (resolution): acceptance occurs and is aided by the culturally approved modes of grieving such as funerals and wearing black
D. The process of grieving may take more than 1 year; all stages must be experienced for grief to be successfully completed. If grieving is not successful, it may lead to one of the following
   1. Delayed reaction: a later reaction to the loss; delay is caused by repressing reality; it may result in more painful experiences than the normal immediate reaction
   2. Distorted reactions: may include the development of symptoms similar to the lost person's: medical illnesses, social isolation, agitated depression, increased use of alcohol or other drugs

Crisis Intervention

Generally, there are common components in all crisis situations. With this knowledge, strategies are developed to assist people through a crisis and minimize its detrimental effects.
A. Crisis: an event that disturbs the equilibrium of the individual or family
B. The disturbance leads to development of certain symptoms, most notably, anxiety and depression
C. These feelings continue until a need is felt to reduce or alleviate them
D. If the person or family has adequate coping mechanisms, the problem will be resolved and balance restored
E. Without coping mechanisms, anxiety and depression increase to intolerable levels
F. Interventions are aimed at providing short-term therapy to increase coping behaviors
G. Most crises are resolved within 6 to 8 weeks
H. Intervention entails
   1. A thorough assessment of the situation
   2. Planned strategies that do not attempt to rearrange a person's life
   3. Strategies that increase intellectual understanding, explore current feelings, offer coping mechanisms, and support existing ties and helpful relationships

Crisis of Rape or Incest

Assisting survivors of these violent acts requires substantial time. This intervention begins when the victim calls for help in any form or seeks treatment. There are two possible phases to this violence. One is the acute or immediate phase wherein the victim exhibits fear, confusion, disorganization, and restlessness. The second phase is a long-term process of reorganization and usually begins weeks after the attack.
A. Early relevant feelings include
   1. Physical pain
   2. Anger
   3. Fear of reattack
   4. Outrage at the perpetrator
   5. Total violation of (emotional) space
   6. Fear of involvement with anyone of the same sex as the perpetrator
   7. Emotionally drained

8. Helplessness

9. Fear of pregnancy

B. If these immediate feelings are not externalized and dealt with, the result may be permanent psychologic damage including but not limited to the following psychosexual dysfunctions

1. Sexual arousal disorders

2. Sexual deviations (several varieties)

3. Sexual aversions

4. Delusions of violent sexual behavior, which could be incorporated in the patient's lifestyle

C. Interventions include

1. Assess the victim's safety: Are you in a safe place?; Is there help for you?

2. Listen: accept what is said

3. Respond as appropriate

4. Refer patient to appropriate agency

Suicide Prevention

Suicide ranks as a leading cause of death in the United States. There are specific indicators that assist in assessing suicidal risk. Risk factors include

A. Age and sex: more women attempt suicide; more men are successful

B. Men over 35 are at higher risk; most suicides occur in men between the ages of 35 and 50 years

C. Anxiety and depression: many potential suicide victims report increasing anxiety and depression; most significant is a recent change in these feelings

D. Past coping pattern: not working in the current situation

E. Past suicide attempt is always considered a high-risk factor

F. Alcohol or drug abuse: many suicides are committed by alcoholics

G. Concrete plan: if there is a plan, considerations are

1. Is it set in a current time frame?

2. Is it lethal?

3. Does the potential victim have the necessary resources to carry out the plan?

H. Significant others: often a suicide is committed to communicate with others

I. Interventions include

1. Focus on clear and present danger

2. Reduce present hazards

3. Give clear directions for victim to follow

4. Assign to constant monitoring in a hospital

5. Mobilize significant others when possible

6. Mobilize past coping mechanisms

7. Assign concrete specific tasks

8. Explore positive alternatives to suicide

9. Teach problem-solving techniques

Suicide Intervention

Intervention becomes critical at the point of suicidal ideation. If intervention does not occur, suicide is highly likely. The patient may be having underlying feelings of hopelessness, helplessness, and impending doom. Frequently the patient will verbalize the need to "end it all."

A. Always ask

1. Do I understand that you want to hurt yourself? (confirming suicide ideation)

2. Do you have a plan or how will you hurt yourself? Will you share your plan with me? (suicidal gesturing may be evident)

3. If the specific plan calls for using an enabling device or instrument: May I have the _____ that is included in the plan? (specify item: knife, razor, rope, etc.)

B. Ordinarily a loud cry for help can be heard before the suicide occurs if others are perceptive enough to hear it

NOTE: Severely depressed patients are so physically impaired that they rarely have the energy to commit suicide. As the depression begins to lift, the potential to commit suicide increases, that is, especially if they have communicated that need to "end it all."

Treatment Modalities

PSYCHOTHERAPY

A. Individual psychotherapy: one-to-one relationship between a therapist (physician, psychologist, social worker, nurse clinician) and a patient; sessions of 45 to 50 minutes are usually held weekly or more often; the aim is to improve the functioning of the person; it is most effective with the neuroses and in patients who have good verbal skills and high intelligence

B. Family group therapy: a family is seen as a group by a therapist, based on the premise that disturbance arises as a function of family interactions and that treatment must be aimed at the family as a whole

C. Group therapy: treatment provided to a group of persons related by age, symptom, or other commonality; treatment occurs on a weekly or biweekly basis and may include more than one therapist

D. Behavior modification: techniques based on conditioning; undesired behaviors are ignored and desired behaviors are rewarded

MILIEU THERAPY

Milieu therapy is the use of a controlled environment to influence the treatment of a patient

A. Interactions between patient and staff, as well as interpatient relationships, are used as a basis for treatment

B. Therapeutic communications: behavior modeling and some behavior modification techniques are often used

THERAPEUTIC COMMUNITY

Therapeutic community (Maxwell Jones, 1968) is a method of establishing a milieu for treatment wherein all members, staff as well as patients, have assigned responsibilities in the community and defined roles. The reasoning is that this type of democratic environment prepares the patient for release into the larger community.

ELECTROCONVULSIVE THERAPY

Use of electroconvulsive therapy (shock therapy) has recently increased for patients with severe depression who have not responded to other therapies. It is the application of an electrical current through the brain resulting in a grand mal seizure. Some patients suffer a short-term memory loss as a result of the treatment.

PSYCHOPHARMACOLOGIC THERAPY

Psychopharmacologic agents are used in the treatment of mental health disorders.

NOTE: When administering medication to the mental health patient, remember to use a tongue blade to examine the interior of the mouth if you suspect the patient is "cheeking" the medication.

A. Anti-EPS (extrapyramidal symptoms): EPS, known locally as "pretzeling," is unusual muscle movement that involves the fine muscles of the body; these symptoms are acute and chronic dystonic reactions to the antipsychotic medication.
  1. Frequently EPS appears in the tongue or in the muscles of the upper chest, neck, and shoulders.
  2. Anti-EPS medications used to reverse the muscular effects of the antipsychotics are diphenhydramine hydrochloride (Benadryl) and benztropine mesylate (Cogentin)
B. Refer to Chapter 3 (Pharmacology) for greater detail regarding drugs that are commonly used to treat mental illness.

ADJUNCTIVE THERAPIES

A. Occupational therapy: the use of vocational tasks to allow patients to express various underlying feelings
B. Recreational therapy: the use of recreational activities to allow patients to express feelings
C. Art therapy: the use of the plastic and graphic arts to express feeling
D. Other therapies may include vocational counseling, bibliotherapy (writing or reading), and dance therapy

Ethical Considerations in Patient Care

A. In most places, patients may sue insitutions under habeas corpus proceedings for their release from treatment
B. Laws guarantee rights to patients
C. Nurses and other staff members may be sued for assault and battery for forcing treatments on patients
D. Wrongful death suits have been brought in circumstances where a patient has died
E. There is a narrow line between treatment and abuse
F. Local laws vary in different parts of the country, and nurses should be aware of local statutes
G. Confidentiality is essential in mental health nursing
H. Communications between a patient and a nurse may be considered "privileged," whereas most medical records are open to subpoena
I. Documents should contain only factual material, not conjecture
J. If a patient threatens bodily harm to others, such information is no longer considered privileged and is required to be reported to the authorities
K. Oppressive mental institutions may infringe on a patient's rights, and nurses should be aware of their responsibilities in such situations

Patient's Rights Movement

A. Although patients in psychiatric settings are ill, they retain their civil rights and are often specifically protected under special sections of the law

B. In most places, "commitment" only removes the patient's right to leave the hospital or terminate treatment
C. Recent legal decisions indicate that patients may expect treatment and may not simply be detained in hospitals where there is no active treatment available
D. In recent years, patient and former-patient groups have formed and demanded access to records of treatment rationales

Care and Treatment of Patients

A. Basic needs: the basic needs of patients in psychiatric settings are similar to those of other patients; usually, psychiatric patients do not have the accompanying impairments of the physically ill patient
  1. Most patients are ambulatory
  2. The nurse's role is to guide, encourage, and teach by example
  3. Patients may be socially deteriorated and require assistance in activities of daily living such as how to arrange time to complete their own care
  4. Reward such as praise is helpful in guiding patients in these activities

SUGGESTED READING

American Psychiatric Association Diagnosis and Statistical Manual of Mental Disorders, ed 4, Washington, DC, 1994, The Association.

Carson VB, Arrold EN: *Mental health nursing: the nurse-patient journey,* Philadelphia, 1996, WB Saunders.

Fortinash KM, Holoday-Worret PA: *Psychiatric-mental health nursing,* St Louis, 1996, Mosby.

Haber J et al: *Comprehensive psychiatric nursing,* ed 4, St Louis, 1992, Mosby.

Johnson BS: *Psychiatric-mental health nursing,* Philadelphia, 1993, JB Lippincott.

Keltner NL, Schwecke LH, Bostrom CE: *Psychiatric nursing: a psychotherapeutic management approach,* St Louis, 1991, Mosby.

Rawlins RP, Williams SR, Beck CK: *Mental health-psychiatric nursing: a holistic life-cycle approach,* ed 3, St Louis, 1993, Mosby.

Schuster CS, Ashburn SS: *The process of human development: a holistic life span approach,* ed 3, Philadelphia, 1992, JB Lippincott.

Smeltzer SC, Bare BG: *Brunner and Suddarth's textbook of medical-surgical nursing,* ed 8, Philadelphia, 1996, JB Lippincott.

Stuart GW, Sundeen SJ: *Principles and practice of psychiatric nursing,* ed 5, St Louis, 1995, Mosby.

Varcarolis EM: *Foundations of psychiatric-mental health nursing,* ed 2, Philadelphia, 1994, WB Saunders.

REVIEW QUESTIONS

Answers and rationales begin on p. 317.

1. A patient is admitted to a psychiatric unit following an unsuccessful suicide attempt. He repeatedly tells the nurse, "I want to die, please help me die." The *most* appropriate nursing response is:
   ① "Don't worry, you're safe here."
   ② "Relax, nobody's going to kill you."
   ③ "Why do you want to die?"
   ④ "You must be feeling very sad right now."

2. A short-term goal for a depressed patient is that the patient will interact with two other patients by the end of the week. At the end of the week the patient remains socially withdrawn. The *most* appropriate nursing action should be to:
   ① Reevaluate the problem
   ② Change the goal
   ③ Modify the nursing interventions
   ④ Change the goal to a long-term goal

3. A short-term expected outcome (goal) for a manic patient is that the patient will gain 3 pounds in 1 week. At the end of the week the patient has gained 2 pounds. The nurse should record which of the following outcomes?
   ① Goal met
   ② Goal will be met in 3 more days
   ③ Goal not met
   ④ Goal partially met

4. A patient who has been receiving haloperidol (Haldol) regularly is currently on 5 mg po tid. When he arrives at the medication room for his scheduled Haldol he tells the nurse he has a sore throat. Which of the following nursing actions is *most* appropriate?
   ① Administer the Haldol with plenty of water
   ② Hold the Haldol and notify the physician
   ③ Hold the Haldol and take the patient's temperature
   ④ Administer the Haldol and plan to take the patient's temperature

5. A hospitalized schizophrenic patient who experiences auditory hallucinations is placed on clozapine (Clozaril) by his physician. The nurse knows the medication is effective when the patient reports that:
   ① He no longer hears voices
   ② The voices aren't as loud
   ③ He is too drowsy to concentrate on the voices
   ④ He does not disturb the other patients any more

6. A patient approaches the nurse and says, "I am omnipotent. Some day soon I'm going to take over this unit, you'll see." The appropriate nursing intervention should be to:
   ① Call a code
   ② Tell the patient that no one is omnipotent and to calm down
   ③ Redirect the patient
   ④ Ask the patient why he thinks he is omnipotent

7. During the termination phase of the nurse/patient relationship the patient abruptly gets up and leaves. The *most* appropriate nursing action should be to:
   ① Go after the patient and bring him back
   ② Remain at the interaction site until the end of the contracted time
   ③ Resume her regularly scheduled activities
   ④ Speak with the head nurse about assigning another nurse to the patient

8. A patient is admitted to a psychiatric unit. After completing the nursing history and assessment, the nurse determines that a tour of the unit and explanation of the unit rules and regulations is appropriate. The nurse's rationale for this intervention is to:
   ① Reduce the patient's anxiety
   ② Demonstrate that interaction with others is required
   ③ Assure that patient rights aren't violated
   ④ Make sure all the other patients know who the new patient is

9. The patient does not appear for a contracted interaction with the nurse. The *most* appropriate nursing intervention should be to:
   ① Ignore it and see what evolves
   ② Show up early for the next scheduled interaction
   ③ Remind the patient of contracted interaction times
   ④ Reduce the patient's privileges

10. The nurse uses role playing as a therapeutic intervention for which phase of the nurse/patient relationship?
    ① Preorientation
    ② Orientation
    ③ Working
    ④ Termination

11. A man is angry with and actually hates his boss, but to his co-workers he appears to be the boss's favorite employee. This is an example of:
    ① Repression
    ② Projection
    ③ Reaction formation
    ④ Rationalization

12. On the day before finals a student has sweaty palms and "butterflies" in the stomach. The anxiety level is most probably:
    ① Panic level
    ② Free floating
    ③ Apprehension level
    ④ Alertness level

13. A nursing diagnosis in psychiatric nursing is:
    ① A behavior or problem related to its probable cause
    ② Not used, because nurses do not diagnose
    ③ Based on the medical condition of the patient
    ④ Useful only in general hospital settings

14. Suicide is most likely to occur:
    ① On admission
    ② On discharge
    ③ As the depression deepens
    ④ As the depression lifts

15. You are attempting to communicate with your patient. The patient says, "My car is red, your hair is short, my socks are gold, DeWayne, Jewish, my wife's cooking is awful, she burns." This is called:
    ① Word salad
    ② Ambivalence
    ③ Confabulation
    ④ Flight of ideas

16. Anxiety can be expressed through emotional feelings. Which of the following signs is *least likely* to be observed in the anxious patient?
    ① Fear
    ② Phobias
    ③ Hostility
    ④ Depression

17. A patient tells the nurse that the television is cursing her and that there are electrodes in her head that make her arms and legs burn. The idea of the television cursing the patient is an example of:
    ① Persecutory delusion
    ② Visual hallucination
    ③ Incoherence
    ④ Flight of ideas

18. A patient tells the nurse that there are electrodes in her head that are making her arms and legs burn. Which of the following responses is *most* therapeutic?
    ① "That's silly, your legs are okay."
    ② "Does the fire travel from one leg to the other?"
    ③ "If your legs were burning, I would see it."
    ④ "I understand you feel the fire. How can you stop it?"

19. A newly admitted patient has not bathed in 4 weeks and is extremely disheveled. To help her with her ADLs (activities of daily living) it is appropriate for the nurse to:
    ① Insist that she bathe before she may have recreational privileges
    ② State in a manner-of-fact way that she is expected to bathe each morning at 8 AM, stay with her, and assist her with this task
    ③ Postpone her bath until her symptoms subside as it is not the major concern now
    ④ Tell her she will be excluded from social groups because she is untidy

20. Thorazine is one of the oldest and most widely prescribed antipsychotic medications. The correct generic name for Thorazine is:
    ① Fluphenazine
    ② Mesoridazine
    ③ Chlorpromazine
    ④ Compazine

21. Paranoid thinking is characterized by feelings of:
    ① Anger and aggression
    ② Suspicion and jealousy
    ③ Self-pity and self-centeredness
    ④ Simultaneous hero worship and hero hating

22. The two outstanding examples of paranoia include:
    ① Grandiosity and poverty
    ② Poverty and persecution
    ③ Persecution and poisoning
    ④ Grandiosity and persecution

23. Patients who abuse alcohol may become tremulous and have hallucinations when they stop drinking. This is called:
    ① Tolerance
    ② Abstinence
    ③ Withdrawal
    ④ Dementia

24. Monoamine oxidase inhibitors are dangerous when used with certain foods. The substance in these foods is called:
    ① Histamine
    ② Phenylalanine
    ③ Lysine
    ④ Tyramine

25. Which of the following nursing measures is *most often* recommended when caring for a patient who is aggressive and hyperactive?
    ① Physically restraining the patient
    ② Secluding the patient
    ③ Providing safe, diversional activity
    ④ Explain that this behavior is unacceptable so that the patient can control it

26. The chief defense mechanism used by the alcoholic (addict) is:
    ① Denial
    ② Compensation
    ③ Reaction formation
    ④ Sublimation

27. The medication most frequently given to the bipolar (manic depressive) patient is:
    ① Chlorpromazine (Thorazine)
    ② Perphenazine (Trilafon)
    ③ Imipramine (Tofranil)
    ④ Lithium (Lithane)

28. A patient rushes up to you and says, "They're after me. They want to torture me and kill me." Which of the following is the most appropriate response?
    ① "Tell me who they are."
    ② "There's no one here except you and me."
    ③ "I need to go look for myself."
    ④ "You are safe here. Can you tell me more?"

29. A patient is admitted to a psychiatric unit following attempted suicide by superficially cutting her wrist. She is sullen and angry and has worked as a prostitute. Recently her "man" told her she wasn't needed. She has a history of minor drug abuse and states she's bored with life and doesn't enjoy anything. Which of the following terms *best* describes the patient?
    ① Schizophrenic
    ② Ambivalent
    ③ Borderline personality
    ④ Psychotic

30. A promiscuous drug-dependent adolescent is admitted to a psychiatric hospital after superficially cutting her wrist. Her attempted suicide is an example of:
    ① Poor impulse control
    ② Regressive behavior
    ③ Manipulation
    ④ Depression

31. A 14-year-old girl is admitted to the psychiatric unit after superficially cutting her wrist. She has a history of prostitution and minor drug abuse. An appropriate nursing goal for this patient is to:
    ① Show her that her life of prostitution is immoral
    ② Eliminate self-destructive manipulative behavior
    ③ Get her to settle down with a husband
    ④ Convince her to have a tubal ligation to avoid pregnancy

32. A patient with a personality disorder is brought to the outpatient clinic by her mother, who states her daughter is out of control. The nurse should begin to foster trust by:
    ① Telling her you are available regardless of her behavior
    ② Tell her you care about her but may not always approve of her behavior
    ③ Avoid the establishment of trust because the relationship will eventually be terminated
    ④ Let her know she can call you day or night

33. During the early phase of detoxification, an assessment for physical signs should be made when the patient:
    ① Asks for medication to stop the "shaking"
    ② Vomits
    ③ Complains of a sore throat
    ④ Asks to leave the hospital

34. A key feature of patients with borderline personality disorder is that they:
① Are able to cope successfully in society
② Learn from previous mistakes
③ Are driven by intense hallucinations
④ Manipulate everyone they can

35. A patient approaches you and says, "With all my troubles I feel worthless. I would like to end all this misery. Everyone would be better off if I were gone." Your most appropriate response to this statement would be:
① "Tell me more."
② "Are you thinking of killing yourself?"
③ "I can see that you are very upset."
④ "I have to take blood pressures right now, then we can talk."

36. During a group therapy session, a patient asks you what the difference is between a psychosis and neurosis. Your most correct reply to this question is:
① Psychotics can't think; neurotics can think
② Psychotics are always depressed; neurotics are not depressed
③ Psychotics have disorganized thinking; neurotics' thoughts are organized
④ Psychotics are always in touch with reality; neurotics are not in touch with reality

37. A patient complains of trouble with control of her or his tongue. Also, the neck muscles are beginning to tighten and the patient is having difficulty keeping her or his head in an upright position. Your *first* response should be:
① Check the medication administration record
② Call the physician
③ Draw blood per standing order
④ Fill out an incident report

38. Crisis intervention theory is based on which of the following assumptions:
① Crises lead to long-term damage
② Crises have common elements that are useful to know for intervention
③ A crisis is abnormal and occurs as a sign of deeper trouble
④ A crisis may take years to resolve

39. In a crisis the aim of intervention is to:
① Rearrange life elements of the people involved
② Provide treatment for as long as possible
③ Offer support and explore alternatives
④ Avoid old ties because these led up to the crisis

40. A 46-year-old woman is admitted to the hospital's psychiatric unit because of an increasingly depressed mood. She is unable to care for her house, and her husband reports she stays up late at night, has difficulty getting up in the morning, and complains of abdominal pain, which she states is punishment for her sins. The patient's symptoms are characteristic of:
① Alcoholic psychosis
② Affective disorder
③ Schizophrenia
④ Bipolar illness

41. A depressed psychiatric patient who demonstrates the inability to arise in the morning is often described as having:
① Loose associations
② Difficulty in thinking
③ Psychomotor retardation
④ Mental retardation

42. A 46-year-old patient is admitted to the hospital's psychiatric unit because of an increasingly depressed mood. After a few weeks of treatment you observe that she has started putting on large amounts of makeup, has become seductive with male patients, and stays up very late pacing the floor. You might conclude that the patient:
① Was initially diagnosed incorrectly
② May be having a manic episode as part of her illness
③ Is showing signs of recovery
④ May be having side effects of the medication

43. Four of the major features that clearly distinguish schizophrenia from other mental illness are:
① Low self-esteem, low morals, worthlessness, and poverty
② Fantasy, hallucinations, delusions, and personality flaws
③ Inappropriate affect, autistic behavior, ambivalence, and inability to associate thinking and reality
④ Ambivalence, autism, apathy, and associative looseness

44. Extreme mood swings ranging from deep depression to high activity levels is most often seen in:
① Paranoid disorders
② Bipolar disorders
③ Schizophrenia
④ Eating disorders

45. When dealing with a patient having somatic delusions, it is important to remember that:
① The patient really doesn't feel the delusional sensation
② Touching such a patient may be nontherapeutic, because they may have disturbed personal borders
③ Agreeing with the patient is helpful
④ Placebos can be used to alleviate somatic complaints

46. A patient on suicide precautions reports a recent change in mood. The nurse knows:
① This is a high-risk factor
② The crisis has probably passed
③ The patient may be manic-depressive
④ The patient is responding to the added attention of the precautions

47. In assessing suicidal risk, which of the following is a high-risk factor?
① Long psychotherapeutic treatment
② A concrete plan that is relatively lethal
③ Past attempts, because these usually mean the person is now able to cope better with stresses
④ Deviance in the person's background

48. If you were to select a single identifying characteristic of the obsessive-compulsive patient, it would be:
① Seclusiveness
② Aggression
③ Orderliness
④ Instant gratification

49. A teenager admits to you that he or she is smoking marijuana on a fairly regular basis. You would know that marijuana is considered a(n):
① Highly addictive substance
② Amphetamine
③ Hallucinogen
④ Cannabinol

50. Which of the following statements is most true about the difference between a delusion and a hallucination?
    ① Delusions are false beliefs; hallucinations are projections
    ② Delusions are systems; hallucinations are beliefs
    ③ Delusions are always true; hallucinations are always false
    ④ Delusions are based on fact; hallucinations are based on belief

51. Which of the following statements about suicide is *most* correct?
    ① Suicide is 100% preventable
    ② Suicide is only inherited
    ③ Suicide occurs without any prior warning
    ④ Suicide lethality increases in proportion to the details of the plan

52. Your patient tells you that he or she is depressed over the recent death of a parent. Which response is the best communication intervention for this patient?
    ① Say nothing
    ② "Wouldn't you rather talk about something else?"
    ③ "I have some time. Would you like to tell me more about your feelings?"
    ④ "I don't have time for sad people."

53. You enter a patient's room and stand just inside the door. The patient is obviously agitated and is escalating to the point that physical harm may occur. What is your best action?
    ① Take the patient to the seclusion room
    ② Talk to the patient and try to identify why he or she is so agitated
    ③ Go to the nurses' station and report the patient's behavior
    ④ Call the physician

54. A patient who has just been admitted for polysubstance abuse is demanding to leave. Which of the following is the *best* nursing action?
    ① Ask the patient why he or she wants to leave so soon
    ② Inform the patient that no one is allowed to leave once he or she is admitted
    ③ Take the patient to the seclusion room
    ④ Respond, "I would like you to tell me how you feel. Can you do that?"

55. In working with mental health patients you would know that *all* records are confidential, which means:
    ① Everyone who asks may see the patient's records
    ② Only the medical and nursing staffs may view the records
    ③ Only nurses are allowed to make entries in the records
    ④ The patient may view her or his record on request

56. You are caring for a patient with major depression. When planning activities, you know that the patient needs:
    ① Frequent changes in activities
    ② Constant redirection into numerous activities
    ③ Behavior modification that restructures feelings
    ④ Well-defined, structured interactions at the beginning of treatment

57. The dominant feeling that the patient with major depression is *most* likely to display is:
    ① Agitation
    ② Ambivalence
    ③ Anxiety
    ④ Hopelessness

58. The drug that cannot be given if the patient has consumed alcohol within the past 24 hours is:
    ① Chlorpromazine (Thorazine)
    ② Loxapine succinate (Loxitane)
    ③ Disulfiram (Antabuse)
    ④ Trifluoperazine (Stelazine)

59. To foster feelings that bolster a patient's self-esteem, it is important that the nurse:
    ① Constantly criticize the patient's behavior
    ② Accept and give positive reinforcement for appropriate behavior
    ③ Enforce behavior modification, including ignoring all previous unacceptable behavior
    ④ Remain very strict with unacceptable behavior and structure precise expectations for the patient

60. You have answered a phone call. The caller tells you that he or she is going to commit suicide. What should be your *initial* response?
    ① "People who talk about it, never do it."
    ② "Do you have a plan?"
    ③ "Why would you want to do a thing like that?"
    ④ "Could you tell me your phone number?"

ANSWERS AND RATIONALES

1. Application, implementation, psychosocial (b)
   ❹ It is appropriate to recognize the patient's feelings and encourage him to verbalize those feelings.
   ①,②,③ Nontherapeutic. Patient's feelings are not addressed.

2. Application, implementation, psychosocial (a)
   ❶ When goals are not met, the cyclic nursing process must begin again.
   ②,④ Goals are not changed when they are not met; the nursing process is started again.
   ③ The nursing interventions are appropriate only if the goal is appropriate for the problem statement.

3. Comprehension, evaluation, physiologic (a)
   ❹ 3-pound goal not met but the patient did gain 2 pounds, which is partial goal achievement.
   ① 3-pound goal not met.
   ② Goal isn't changed when it's not met. The nursing process is cyclic and has to be reentered.
   ③ Goal was partially met. To not meet the goal, the patient would have to have gained no weight.

4. Application, implementation, physiologic (c)
   ❸ Sore throat could indicate agranulocytosis. The nurse should take the patient's temperature and report the temperature and the patient's complaint to the physician before administering the next dose.
   ① Although Haldol should be administered with plenty of water, it is not appropriate to administer the Haldol.
   ② Although ultimately correct, the nurse should take the patient's temperature before calling the physician.
   ④ The Haldol should be held, the patient assessed, and the physician notified.

5. Comprehension, evaluation, psychosocial (c)
   ❷ When the antipsychotic is effective, patients report a decrease in the frequency and/or volume of the voices they hear.
   ① The voices do not disappear.
   ③ Drowsiness is an undesirable side effect. The patient should be assessed and findings reported to the physician and documented.
   ④ The nurse needs to clarify what the patient means by this and validate the patient's behavior.

6. Application, implementation, safe, effective care (c)
   ❸ Of the options given, this is the most appropriate. After very briefly acknowledging the patient's feelings (e.g., "This subject seems troubling for you") he should be distracted from his delusion of grandeur and engaged in a less threatening activity or topic.
   ① Measures to reduce the patient's anxiety should be employed at the first sign of discomfort or anxiety.
   ② Never challenge the patient's delusional system; that may force the patient to defend it.
   ④ Reinforces the delusion and further distances the patient from reality.

7. Application, implementation, safe effective care (c)
   ❷ Being dependable is necessary for the patient to trust and feel secure. Contracted time with the patent is for that patient only. Terminating a session early is a patient response that the nurse should understand and be prepared for.
   ① Inappropriate: The patient has to assume responsibility for his behavior.

   ③ Contracted time with the patient is time for that patient only. The nurse should remain for the duration of the contracted time.
   ④ Inappropriate: The focus is always the patient, not the nurse.

8. Knowledge, implementation, psychosocial (b)
   ❶ The unfamiliar is anxiety provoking. A tour and review of expectations will assist with reducing the patient's anxiety.
   ② Patients are free to interact with others but are never required to do so.
   ③ Patients receive a copy of the Patient Bill of Rights on admission, and either a written copy of the unit rules and regulations or a verbal explanation of them. This builds trust and security.
   ④ Not the purpose. The patient will be introduced to the group at the first community meeting.

9. Application, implementation, psychosocial (b)
   ❸ The working phase is usually painful for the patient. It's important to demonstrate caring and interest and to address the patient's responsibility for the contract. There may be a reason the patient couldn't keep the appointment.
   ① The patient's behavior should not be ignored, and the patient needs to know that he has a responsibility to the contract.
   ② This presumes that the patient's behavior was not addressed. Showing up early for the next session will not change the patient's behavior.
   ④ Punitiveness is inappropriate and nontherapeutic. Arrangements for notifying nurse/patient if not able to keep appointments should be discussed when formulating the contract.

10. Knowledge, implementation, psychosocial (b)
    ❸ Purpose of this phase is to assist the patient with positive behavior change. The focus is on the present and role playing can be insightful problem-solving.
    ① Data collection, autodiagnosis, and planning occur during this phase before interaction with the patient.
    ② This is the getting acquainted phase; the contract is formulated and patient problems identified. Usually lasts 2 to 10 sessions.
    ④ Dissolution of the relationship; synthesis of what has occurred and summary of patient progress are discussed.

11. Comprehension, assessment, psychosocial (b)
    ❸ Uses repression in part to rid self of unacceptable feelings, while conscious effort is made to express opposite type of feelings.
    ① A blocking of painful or unacceptable feelings.
    ② Giving of or assigning of unacceptable feelings to someone else.
    ④ Explaining away, via logical construction, unacceptable thoughts, feelings, or acts.

12. Comprehension, assessment, psychosocial (b)
    ❸ Apprehension level; anxiety is related to a concrete future event.
    ① Panic includes loss of control.
    ② Free-floating has no specific object or event.
    ④ Alertness level is less severe, only vague symptoms.

13. Comprehension, planning, psychosocial (b)
   ❶ Correct because nurses diagnose and treat human responses to illness, behaviors, or problems related to their probable causes.
   ② Nurses diagnose responses and not disease entities.
   ③ The medical diagnosis may or may not be related to the nursing diagnosis.
   ④ Nursing diagnosis is useful in many diverse settings.

14. Comprehension, assessment, environment (b)
   ❹ Most authorities agree that as depression lifts the patient is at greatest risk of committing suicide.
   ① The attention of the patient being admitted is diverted and focused on the admission, and he or she is not likely to commit suicide during the admission process.
   ② Discharge will *not* occur if the patient is actively suicidal.
   ③ As the depression deepens, it is less and less likely that suicide will occur, because the patient is experiencing decreasing physical functioning.

15. Comprehension, assessment, psychosocial (a)
   ❹ By definition, the ideas are flying by; hence flight of ideas.
   ① Word salad is a mixture of *just* words.
   ② Ambivalence is "I hate you, I love you"—opposite feelings within the same thought.
   ③ Confabulation is filling in a memory lapse with untrue statements.

16. Comprehension, assessment, psychosocial (c)
   ❹ Anxiousness is characterized by accelerated behavior and activity, hence depression will *least likely* be observed; depression is not exhibited by high levels of activity.
   ① Fear may represent the cause for anxiety.
   ② Phobias always have an anxiety component.
   ③ Hostility may be seen in the anxious patient.

17. Comprehension, assessment, psychosocial (c)
   ❶ Persecutory delusion; the television actually does not curse the patient; she feels persecuted by it.
   ② Not visual hallucination.
   ③ Not incoherent, but structured.
   ④ Not flight of ideas.

18. Comprehension, implementation, psychosocial (c)
   ❹ Accepts reality of her experience and suggests self-control.
   ① Denies reality of her experience.
   ② Enters into the delusion.
   ③ Denies reality of her experience.

19. Comprehension, implementation, physiologic (b)
   ❷ Gives a clear message, helps organize patient.
   ① May lead to a power struggle.
   ③ Not true; she should be encouraged to begin routine self-care as soon as possible.
   ④ Moralizing does not help patient.

20. Knowledge, planning, environment (b)
   ❸ Chlorpromazine is the generic name for Thorazine.
   ① Fluphenazine is the generic name for Proxilin.
   ② Mesoridazine is the generic name for Serentil.
   ④ Compazine is the trade name for prochlorperazine.

21. Comprehension, assessment, psychosocial (b)
   ❷ Suspicion and jealousy are the predominant thoughts of the paranoid patient.
   ① Paranoid patients are so preoccupied with suspicion and jealousy that these are not substantial possibilities.

③ Self-pity and self-centeredness are more closely associated with the depressed patient, who is trying to blame self or relieve feelings of guilt.
   ④ This is the definition of ambivalence.

22. Comprehension, assessment, psychosocial (b)
   ❹ These are the two that satisfy the condition of examples.
   ① Poverty is an economic condition.
   ② See rationale for #1.
   ③ Poisoning is not an example of paranoia.

23. Knowledge, assessment, physiologic (a)
   ❸ Symptoms occur on stopping the drug.
   ① Tolerance means increasing doses to achieve effects.
   ② To abstain is not to drink.
   ④ Dementia is unrelated.

24. Knowledge, implementation, physiologic (a)
   ❹ Tyramine.
   ① Not correct.
   ②,③ An amino acid, but not correct.

25. Comprehension, implementation, physiologic (b)
   ❸ The least restrictive means is always the rule. If the patient is destroying the milieu, herself, or others, then physical restraint would be necessary. Aggression and hyperactivity would best be handled by offering diversional activities.
   ① Will be appropriate if destruction is occurring.
   ② Unless the behavior is destructive, seclusion would be used.
   ④ Depending on the cause of the aggression/hyperactivity, the patient may not be able to control the behavior. It would be more appropriate to say, "You seem really aggressive. Can you tell me why?"

26. Comprehension, assessment, psychosocial (a)
   ❶ Denial is the chief defense mechanism in that the addict can always find a reason to drink.
   ② The addiction is the weakness and has an underlying cause that is uncompensated.
   ③ Underlying feelings of guilt, sadness, etc. are relieved by the addiction, but these feelings return once the drug wears off. The addiction isn't the expression of an opposite attitude; it is relief from the underlying feelings.
   ④ Sublimation does not fit in the discussion of addiction.

27. Comprehension, implementation, psychosocial (c)
   ❹ Lithium is the medication of choice in the treatment of bipolar disorders.
   ① Chlorpromazine (Thorazine) is an antipsychotic. Not used in bipolar disorder.
   ② Perphenazine (Trilafon) is an antipsychotic-neuroleptic.
   ③ Imipramine (Tofranil) is an antidepressant of the tricyclic group.

28. Comprehension, assessment, psychosocial (b)
   ❹ Assurance and willingness to listen are keys to good therapeutic relationships.
   ① You should not acknowledge that you have knowledge and want to know more about "them." Avoid "buying into" the delusion or hallucination.
   ② Avoid denial of what the patient is seeing or doing. Remember to be nonjudgmental and nonthreatening.
   ③ See rationale for #1.

29. Comprehension, assessment, psychosocial (b)
     ❸ Classical symptoms of borderline personality disorder.
     ① No delusions or hallucinations reported.
   ②,④ Not relevant.
30. Comprehension, assessment, physiologic (a)
     ❶ Poor impulse control; superficial wrist-cutting is impulsive behavior.
     ② Regressive is not correct; situation does not indicate earlier, more comfortable behavior.
     ③ May be manipulative, but situation does not indicate this.
     ④ Probably not depressive; situation does not include this.
31. Comprehension, planning, physiologic (b)
     ❷ Clearly a goal that is attainable and appropriate.
   ①,③,④ Unrealistic.
32. Comprehension, implementation, environment (b)
     ❷ This is a realistic, feasible approach.
     ① Blanket approval is unrealistic.
     ③ She should begin to learn to tolerate separation.
     ④ Unrealistic; leads to mistrust.
33. Comprehension, assessment, physiologic (b)
     ❷ Vomiting is the end result of serious physiologic changes occurring as a result of detoxification. Of these answers, it has the most serious consequences and requires measuring the physiologic parameters. The vomiting is uncontrollable and interferes with nutritional and liquid intake. Whatever the patient ingests is vomited within minutes. The offer of an antiemetic would be appropriate *after* blood pressure, pulse, respiration, and temperature are taken.
     ① Usually the "shaking" is internal feelings, not outward signs. Medication is routinely ordered to control this feeling.
     ③ No need to measure vital signs unless there are other accompanying complaints.
     ④ This response is irrelevant.
34. Comprehension, assessment, environment (b)
     ❹ Manipulate and control are key features.
     ① They manage to get by, but tend to cause avoidant behavior among those who know them.
     ② They never seem to learn from previous mistakes. Rather, they repeat them time and time again.
     ③ Delusions maybe, but never hallucinations unless a problem coexists with the borderline personality.
35. Comprehension, planning, environment (b)
     ❷ Identify the plan, then intervene.
     ① "Tell me more" may not identify the plan.
     ③ Although this is true, it does not address the plan.
     ④ Incorrect. If anyone approaches you with statements like the ones in this question, find out if they have a plan.
36. Knowledge, implementation, health (a)
     ❸ Of the choices here, this is the most correct one.
     ① Not true. Psychotics can think; it is disorganized.
     ② Psychotics are rarely depressed; mostly they cannot operate in reality.
     ④ These statements are reversed. The psychotic isn't in reality; the neurotic is in reality, but reality may be distorted.
37. Comprehension, assessment, physiologic (c)
     ❶ This is the correct answer. The patient may be experiencing the beginning effect called EPS (extrapyramidal symptoms). These symptoms are associated with the administration of antipsychotic medications. Incidentally, there will probably be an anti-EPS medication ordered to reverse the EPS effects.
   ②,③ Not appropriate as a *first* response.
     ④ Not a first response, but may be required at some point in the event.
38. Knowledge, assessment, physiologic (a)
     ❷ Basis of theory.
     ① Usually resolve in some fashion without long-term damage.
     ③ False statement.
     ④ Usually resolve in a few weeks.
39. Knowledge, implementation, environment (a)
     ❸ Often a new observer is helpful in sorting out complexities and offering useful solutions.
     ① Not a goal.
     ② Treatment is always time limited.
     ④ Old ties are often strengthened.
40. Comprehension, assessment, psychosocial (b)
     ❶ Affective disorder characterized by depressed mood, low energy, and somatic delusions.
   ①,③ Not indicated in situation.
     ④ Unknown from data given; may or may not be.
41. Knowledge, assessment, psychosocial (b)
     ❸ Psychomotor retardation characterizes low motor activity based on psychologic factors.
   ①,② Irrelevant.
     ④ Not in situation.
42. Comprehension, assessment, psychosocial (a)
     ❷ The behavioral changes indicate mania.
     ① May not be true; diagnosis was accurate for the presenting symptoms.
     ③ Not true; change too rapid and extreme.
     ④ Unrelated.
43. Knowledge, assessment, psychosocial (b)
     ❸ These are the four *As* of schizophrenia.
     ① Poverty is an economic state; hence this answer is incorrect.
     ② Schizophrenic patients may have hallucinations and delusions, but the other parts of the answer are not correct.
     ④ Apathy is not one of the four *As*.
44. Knowledge, assessment, psychosocial (a)
     ❷ Mood swings are the characteristics of bipolar disorder. Manic (elation) and depression are two phases.
     ① Paranoid disorders generally do not involve mood swings at all.
     ③ Schizophrenia is characterized by disorganized thinking.
     ④ Persons with eating disorders do not suffer from mood swings.
45. Comprehension, implementation, psychosocial (b)
     ❷ Patient should be alerted before being touched.
     ① The delusion is very real to patient.
     ③ Agreeing may or may not be helpful.
     ④ Placebo may or may not be helpful.
46. Comprehension, assessment, environment (c)
     ❶ High risk: mood change may signal behavior change.
     ② The nurse should not assume crisis has passed.
     ③ This is a medical diagnosis, not a nursing assessment.
     ④ Not necessarily true.

47. Knowledge, assessment, environment (b)
    ❷ Concrete, lethal plan is a very high-risk factor.
    ① Treatment duration is usually unrelated.
    ③ Past attempt is high risk but not for reason stated.
    ④ Unrelated.
48. Knowledge, assessment, psychosocial (a)
    ❸ Orderliness is the single feature of the obsessive-compulsive disorder; usually done in ritual format.
    ① The obsessive-compulsive patient is so busy thinking and doing, there would be no time for seclusion.
    ② Aggression is not an obsessive-compulsive characteristic.
    ④ Instant gratification is related to poor impulse control. The obsessive-compulsive patient has an overwhelming need to perform activities that release the underlying feelings.
49. Knowledge, assessment, health (a)
    ❹ Marijuana is a cannabinol.
    ① It is not highly addictive; however, a psychologic dependency can develop.
    ② Amphetamine is a class of psychoactive substance that is a cerebral stimulant.
    ③ Marijuana causes impaired brain function, but it is generally not known to generate hallucinations.
50. Knowledge, assessment, psychosocial (a)
    ❶ These are exact definitions of the respective terms.
    ② See rationable for #1.
    ③ Delusions are always false, as are hallucinations.
    ④ See rationale for #3.
51. Comprehension, assessment, environment (c)
    ❹ The more details contained in the plan of self-destruction, the more likely it is to occur.
    ① Suicide is not 100% preventable. Many previous accidental deaths have proven to be suicides. Surviving suicide is increasingly difficult as the instances of attempts increase.
    ② Not a true statement.
    ③ Most suicides occur after ample warnings have been offered.
52. Application, implementation, psychosocial (a)
    ❸ Open-ended question, with ample time to listen, is the best therapeutic technique in this situation.
    ① You should indicate an interest in what the patient has said. Saying nothing is the wrong activity.
    ② The pressing issue is death of parents; diversion of discussion is not appropriate.
    ④ Inappropriate, and it is a put-down.
53. Comprehension, assessment, environment (b)
    ❷ Verbal intervention is always the first course of action.
    ① This action may be required later, depending on the ability to verbally deescalate the situation.
    ③ Go for the underlying feeling *first.*
    ④ Not until it is necessary.
54. Comprehension, assessment, psychosocial (c)
    ❹ Always go for the underlying feeling.
    ① A good second-choice answer.
    ② Not true. This is imprisonment.
    ③ This is viewed as punitive for asking a question and has no foundation in fact for such an action.
55. Knowledge, planning, psychosocial (a)
    ❹ This is true. Patients have the right to view their own medical records.
    ① Not everyone has access to the medical record.
    ② Mental health workers from all disciplines may view the records.
    ③ Mental health workers from all disciplines may make entries into the medical record, provided they are caring for the patient.
56. Comprehension, planning, psychosocial (b)
    ❹ The depressed patient may become overwhelmed if too much is offered too soon. The patient should be engaged in structured, goal-directed activities.
    ① Could lead to withdrawal or seclusive behavior.
    ② Overwhelming to the patient at the beginning of treatment.
    ③ Feelings cannot be restructured, but they can be dealt with if the patient will allow.
57. Knowledge, assessment, psychosocial (b)
    ❹ A key indicator of depression.
    ①,② Not consistent with depression.
    ③ The most distant feeling from depression.
58. Comprehension, assessment, physiologic (a)
    ❸ Disulfiram (Antabuse) causes violent nausea and vomiting if taken within 24 hours of consuming alcohol.
    ① Is a major antipsychotic.
    ②,④ Is an antipsychotic.
59. Comprehension, implementation, psychosocial (b)
    ❷ This is most therapeutic.
    ① This will have a negative effect.
    ③ Previous unacceptable behavior should be challenged and integrated into current behavioral activities.
    ④ This is not therapeutic.
60. Comprehension, assessment, environment (a)
    ❷ The most therapeutic in providing safety from self-destruction.
    ① Not true.
    ③ Inappropriate response.
    ④ Irrelevant and inappropriate.

Chapter 7 — Maternity Nursing

The aim of obstetrics is to offer health services to the childbearing mother, her baby, and her family that will ensure a normal pregnancy and a safe prenatal and postnatal experience. This chapter reviews components of the nursing process. Each topic presents pertinent information helpful in planning the nursing assessment and in analyzing the nursing need of the family. Nursing management is outlined giving options for selecting appropriate plans for action. The evaluation of whether outcomes and goals of maternity nursing have been met completes the nursing process. The information presented in this review will assist the nurse in understanding how to:

- Plan, implement, and evaluate the nursing process as it relates to the maternity patient, her baby, and her family.
- Integrate selected theoretic information into the nursing process to effectively meet the basic aims of maternity nursing.

Brief History

A. Primitive society
   1. Practiced infanticide
   2. Treated mothers with indifference and brutality
   3. Superstitions, incantations, taboos
B. Ancient civilizations
   1. Egypt: first to describe podalic version; first to practice cesarean section, as Egyptian law forbade burial of pregnant mother with infant
   2. China: published manual on obstetrics describing treatment of mother
   3. Greco-Roman: obstetric writings of Soranus of Ephesus (Father of Obstetrics); also wrote on midwifery (AD 200)
C. Evolution of modern obstetrics
   1. Middle Ages and early Christianity: pain of childbirth believed to be a means of expiation for sins
   2. Judaism: contributed to public health through its kosher dietary laws and to hygiene through its ritual of circumcision.
   3. Renaissance: Leonardo da Vinci (Italy, 1452-1519): contributed to understanding human anatomy through his anatomic drawings
   4. Western European influence
      a. Ambroise Paré (France, 1510-1590): started trend of doctors replacing midwives
      b. Peter Chamberlen (England and Holland, 1560-1631): introduced forceps, paving the way for mechanical devices to assist in difficult deliveries
      c. William Smellie (England, 1697-1763): published book on midwifery in 1752 and wrote rules for the use of forceps during a delivery
      d. William Hunter (England, 1718-1783): described placental anatomy
      e. Jean Louis Baudelocque (France, 1746-1810): described positions, presentations, and pelvic measurements
      f. Ignaz Philipp Semmelweiss (Austria, 1818-1865): a pioneer in obstetric asepsis, Semmelweis found that handwashing before attending mothers greatly reduced the incidence of puerperal (child-bed) fever
      g. Louis Pasteur (France, 1822-1895): discovered *Streptococcus* as the causative organism in puerperal fever (1860)
   5. Contributors in the United States
      a. Anne Hutchinson (1634): midwife who delivered many babies of early settlers
      b. William Shippen: established first lying-in hospital and midwifery school in the United States in 1762
      c. Oliver Wendell Holmes (1809-1894): stressed cleanliness and handwashing before caring for new mothers
      d. Margaret Sanger Research Bureau (1923): first organization to address question of contraception and planned parenthood
   6. United States legislation affecting mothers and children
      a. 1921: Sheppard Towner Act: promoted health and welfare for mothers and children
      b. 1936: Social Security benefits begun; later to include entitlement benefits for mothers and their dependent children
      c. 1943: Emergency Maternal and Infant Care Act to assist families of soldiers during World War II
      d. 1973: Supreme Court legalizes abortion
      e. 1974: WIC: federally funded nutritional program providing supplementary food to eligible pregnant, lactating, or postpartum women, their infants, and children under 5 years of age
      f. 1995-1996 Several states enacted legislation to lengthen a postpartum stay to 48 hours for a vaginal delivery and 96 hours for a cesarean birth. Early discharge would be voluntary.

Definitions Commonly Used in Obstetrics

STATISTICS

birth rates   number of live births per 1000 population
fetal death (stillborn)   infant of 20 weeks or more gestational age who dies in utero prior to birth
infant mortality rate   number of deaths before the first birthday per 1000 live births
maternal mortality rate   number of mothers dying in or because of childbearing per 100,000 live births
neonatal death   death within first 4 weeks of life
neonatal death care   number of deaths within the first 4 weeks of life per 1000 live births

ABBREVIATIONS (LIMITED LISTING)

ABC   alternative birthing center
ARM   artificial rupture of membranes
BOW   bag of waters; amniotic sac
CPD   cephalopelvic disproportion
CS   cesarean section
DIC   disseminated intravascular coagulation
EDC   estimated date of confinement; due date for birth
EDD   estimated date of delivery
FHR   fetal heart rate
FHT   fetal heart tone
G   gravida; number of pregnancies
GTPAL   gravida, term, premature, abortions, living children; identification of pregnancy status
HCG   human chorionic gonadotropin
HELLP   hemolysis, elevated liver enzymes, low platelet count; extention of pathology related to severe preeclampsia
HIV   human immunodeficiency virus
LDRP   labor\delivery\recovery\postpartum; all phases of maternal and child care occur in the same room with the same staff member
LGA   large for gestational age
LMP   last menstrual period
P   para; number of viable births
PIH   pregnancy-induced hypertension
PROM   premature rupture of membranes
Q   quadrant; one of four equal parts into which the abdomen is divided to designate position of fetus in uterus
RhoGAM   antibody against Rh factor given early prenatally or within 72 hours postpartum to mother
SGA   small for gestational age
TORCHES   a group of intrauterine infections including: Toxoplasmosis, Rubella, Cytomegalovirus, Herpes, and Syphilis. These are commonly associated with high infant mortality.

COMMON OBSTETRIC TERMINOLOGY

Apgar score   method of evaluating infant immediately after delivery; usually at 1 minute and at 5 minutes

Braxton-Hicks contractions painless uterine contractions felt throughout pregnancy, becoming stronger and more noticeable during second and third trimester

caput head; cephalic portion of infant

cyesis pregnancy

dystocia long, painful labor and delivery

elderly primipara pregnant woman over 35 years of age giving birth to her first child

gestation developmental time of embryo, fetus, in utero

grand multipara more than five children

high risk pregnant woman with preexisting problems that could jeopardize the pregnancy, the fetus, or herself; under 18 years of age or over 35 years of age with no prenatal care (any one or more of these conditions)

lightening dropping of the uterus as the fetal head enters the pelvis during the last 2 weeks before EDC (usually just before labor in multiparas)

low birth weight weight less than 2500 grams because of the baby being preterm (premature) or because of intrauterine growth retardation.

low risk pregnant woman with normal history, between ages 18 and 34, with no medical, psychologic, or other preexisting problems, and under good prenatal care

meconium first bowel movement of the newborn—thick, tarlike, greenish-black substance

multigravida pregnant more than one time

multipara given birth to more than one child

postmature infant one born after 42 weeks' gestation

premature infant one born anytime before 37 weeks' gestation

primigravida pregnant for the first item

primipara giving birth to first child

pseudocyesis false pregnancy

quickening first movements of the fetus felt by the mother (16 to 18 weeks' gestation)

secundines afterbirth of placenta and membranes

term infant one born between 38 and 42 weeks' gestation

vernix caseosa cheesy material covering the fetus and newborn that acts as a protection to the skin

viable ability to live outside uterus; living

vis a tergo external pressure on the fundus to assist in the delivery of the infant

Trends

A. Cost containment: rising health care costs are a national concern; increased home care, shortened stays, and increased emphasis on prenatal care are interventions to help control cost and maintain quality

B. Early discharge: may be discharged home within 12 to 24 hours (uncomplicated labor and delivery) and 3 to 4 days or less for a cesarean. These shortened stays are an attempt to control health care costs. These shortened stays are creating an increased need for prenatal education materials and follow-up phone numbers to reinforce education

C. Prenatal care: Emphasis must be placed on improving access to prenatal care; particularly for low-income women. Prenatal care can avoid many conditions that can be avoided with adequate monitoring during pregnancy

D. Early discharges: These have caused an increased demand for home care and other community services. This home follow-up is especially important for adolescents or other families with psychosocial complications. Nurse entrepreneurs have helped to bridge this gap for many families

E. Changing demographics: Women are waiting longer in life to have their first babies. Nurses need to be familiar with effects of pregnancy on older women

F. Teen pregnancy: Nurses need to identify and implement strategies to decrease incidence of adolescent pregnancy

G. Changing cultures: Nurses need to be sensitive to different cultures' ideas and health practices

H. Prepared childbirth experience: mother and father (or alternate) jointly attend childbirth education classes to prepare for the child and for the childbearing and childbirth experience

I. Alternate birth settings
   1. Birthing centers outside of hospital; ABC (alternate birth centers)
   2. Individual's home
   3. Use of the birthing chair instead of traditional table
   4. Birthing room: labor, delivery, and postpartum hospital stay incorporated into one cheerful, homelike room set up with necessary labor and delivery equipment

J. Variety of positions used to assist labor and delivery (squat, side position, etc.)

K. Showering during first or second stage of labor

L. Inclusion of father or alternate: support person stays in labor and delivery area for both vaginal and cesarean section deliveries

M. Rooming in: allows newborn in room with mother for the day; fathers allowed unlimited visiting time

N. Sibling visits: designated hours that children may visit with mother and see baby (from nursery window)

O. Use of midwives: many hospitals and birthing centers throughout the United States now have nurse-midwives as the primary care person conducting prenatal, labor, delivery, and follow-up care

P. Cesarean sections: more frequent now because of sophisticated fetal monitoring; controversial because of high numbers of sections in recent years

Q. Breast-feeding: accepted and encouraged; societies such as La Leche League and popularity of "natural" foods encourage breastfeeding

R. Genetic counseling: increasingly accurate, safe amniocentesis and advances in genetics encourage counselors to advise couples with genetic problems

S. In vitro method of fertilization to assist pregnancy/fetal development: usually chosen by couples with fertility problems after exploring various methods, including fertility drugs and other insemination practices

Procedures to Determine Maternal/Fetal Problems

A. Alpha fetoprotein (AFP) test
   1. Screening procedure, not diagnostic
   2. Serum from maternal blood sample is tested; best results if sample is taken at 16 to 18 weeks' gestation; identifies unrecognized high-risk pregnancies
   3. Elevated levels of maternal serum indicate 5% to 10% open neural tube defect (spina bifida) in developing fetus
   4. Recommend two samples of test followed by ultrasound and amniocentesis to confirm findings; genetic counseling availability if confirmed
   5. Other causes of elevated AFP levels: multiple gestation, missed abortions, other abnormalities

B. Amniocentesis: invasive procedure during which a needle is inserted through abdomen and uterus to withdraw amniotic fluid; usually done after 14th week
1. Used for determination of sex, defects in fetus (e.g., Down syndrome); fetal status (Rh isoimmunal problem, fetal maturity, other tests as listed below)
2. Lecithin/sphingomyelin ratio (L/S ratio): used to determine fetal maturity by testing surfactant by 35th week of pregnancy; lecithin level two times greater than sphingomyelin level indicates that lungs are mature
3. Creatinine level: used to test fetal muscle mass and fetal renal function; 0.2 mg/100 ml amniotic fluid at 36 weeks is normal level; large amount may also indicate large fetus, such as fetus of diabetic mother
4. Bilirubin level: used for determination of fetal liver maturity; should decrease as term progresses; 450 μm is optimal density
5. Cytologic testing: determines percentage of lipid globules present in amniotic fluid, indicates fetal age

C. Chorionic villi test
1. Permits first-trimester testing for biochemical and chromosomal defects; invasive and high-risk procedure during which a plastic catheter is inserted vaginally into the uterus; ultrasound guides catheter to chorionic frondosum
2. Can be done 9 to 11 weeks after LMP
3. Done earlier than amniocentesis; recent evidence shows that test may increase risk of babies born with missing toes and fingers or shortened digits (Burton, 1992)

D. Fetoscopy: invasive procedure using transabdominal insertion of metal cannula into abdomen; visualization of fetus and placenta for developing abnormalities
1. High-risk procedure; complications include spontaneous abortion and premature labor
2. Has limited usage, only if defect cannot be detected otherwise

E. Estriol level study: 24-hour urinalysis of urine from mother; determines estriol level to ascertain fetal well being and placental functioning
1. Done at third trimester (32 weeks)
2. 12 mg in 24 hours is good; below 12 mg indicates that infant is in jeopardy (related to decreased placental functioning)
3. Decreasing estriol levels can be used in combination with other diagnostic tests to indicate a compromised placenta or fetus

F. Heterozygote testing (mother's blood): done to detect clinically normal carriers of mutant genes
1. Tay-Sachs disease: common fatal genetic disease affecting children of Ashkenazi Jews (Eastern Europe)
2. Sickle cell anemia: common disorder among black Americans of African descent; 1 in 10 American blacks is a carrier
3. Cooley's anemia (beta thalassemia): genetic disorder frequent among Mediterranean ethnic groups: Italians, Sicilians, Greeks, Turks, Middle Eastern Arabs, Asian Indians, Pakistanis

G. Oxytocin challenge test (OCT) or stress test: late trimester test to measure placental insufficiency and measure fetal reaction to uterine contractions
1. Usually done after estimated date of confinement (EDC) has passed
2. Invasive procedure during which IV oxytocin is administered, baseline recorded on monitor; takes 20 minutes to 1 hour
3. Breast stimulation techniques are done in some health care settings in place of oxytocin infusion during a contraction stress test
4. Results: late decelerations during contraction for at least three contractions indicate a positive test; no decelerations during three successive contractions within 10 minutes indicate a negative test; occasionally inconsistent decelerations indicate suspicious conditions

H. Nonstress test (NST): assesses and evaluates fetal heart tone (FHT) response to uterine movement or increased fetal activity

I. Umbilical cord technique: evaluates condition of fetus
1. Superior technique because fetal blood can be analyzed as early as 18th week of gestation
2. Can evaluate blood count, liver function, blood gases, acid-base status
3. Invasive procedure; limited use because of risk of injury to fetus

J. Ultrasound procedure: use of high-frequency sound waves to determine fetal size, estimate amniotic fluid volume, neural tube defects, limb abnormalities, and so forth
1. Usually a second-trimester procedure
2. Risks still under investigation
3. Acoustic sound waves can be used to help stimulate an inactive fetus during a nonstress test

K. Biophysical profile: using ultrasound and a nonstress test, this profile evaluates five fetal variables: breathing movements, body movements, muscular tone, qualitative amniotic fluid volume, and heart rate

Anatomy and Physiology of Reproduction
OBSTETRIC PELVIS
A. Types (Fig. 7-1)
1. Gynecoid: "true" female pelvis
2. Anthropoid: resembles pelvis of anthropoid apes
3. Android: male pelvis
4. Platypoid: flat pelvis

B. Components
1. Ilium: flat or lateral, flaring part of pelvis or hip; iliac crest is top part of ilium
2. Ischium: inferior dorsal or lower part of hip bone; the ischial spines, sharp projections of the ischium, are important in obstetrics because they are landmarks to measure progress of presenting part of fetus
3. Sacrum: triangular bone between the two hip bones; flat part of the lower back (spine)
4. Coccyx: two to five rudimentary vertebrate that are fused and attached to lower part of sacrum (tailbone)

C. Measurements
1. Diagonal conjugate: measured through vagina from lower border of symphysis pubis to promontory of sacrum (12.5 to 13 cm)
2. Conjugate vera (true conjugate): measured from upper margin of symphysis pubis to promontory of sacrum by x-ray examination or sonogram (11 cm)
3. Transverse diameter: distance between inner surfaces of the tuberosities of ischium (13 to 13.5 cm)

PURE TYPES

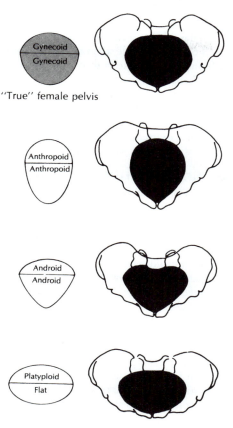

"True" female pelvis

Figure 7-1. Female pelves: pure types. (From Bobak IM, Jensen MD: *Essentials of maternity nursing,* ed 2, St Louis, 1987, Mosby.)

4. Obstetric conjugate: measured by x-ray examination or sonogram or by subtracting 1.5 to 2 cm from diagonal conjugate (9.5 to 11.5 cm)

FERTILIZATION AND IMPLANTATION
A. Definitions
   1. Fertilization: occurs when the sperm and ovum join, usually at the distal third of the fallopian tube within 12 to 48 hours after intercourse
   2. Zygote: product of the union of a sperm and ovum
   3. Implantation: occurs when zygote burrows into the endometrium of the uterus, approximately 7 days after fertilization
   4. Nidation: completion of implantation
B. Processes
   1. Mitosis: rapid cell division
   2. Blastoderm: first division of the zygote
   3. Morula: ball-like structure of the blastoderm; sometimes referred to as mulberry-like
   4. Blastocyst: as morula enters uterus
   5. Trophoblast: as blastocyst implants in the uterus, the wall becomes the trophoblast
   6. Chorionic villi: trophoblasts develop villi that become fetal portion of the placenta
   7. Decidua: endometrium undergoes a change when pregnancy occurs

8. Decidua vera: that portion of the decidua that becomes the lining of the uterus except for around implantation site
9. Decidua basalis: where implantation occurs and where chorionic villi become frondosum or the beginning of the placental formation
10. Decidua capsularis: covers blastocyst and fuses to form fetal membranes
11. Amnion: inner membrane, which comes from the zygote and blends with the cord
12. Chorion: outer membrane, which comes from the zygote and blends with the fetal portion of the placenta

DEVELOPMENT OF HUMAN ORGANISM
A. Ovum stage: preembryonic stage from conception until the primary villi appear (first 14 days)
B. Embryo: end of ovum stage to 8 weeks from LMP; period of rapid cellular development: disruption will cause developmental abnormality
C. Fetus: from end of embryonic stage (8 weeks) to term
D. Placenta: membrane weighing about 450g (1 lb); develops cotyledons that act as areas for nourishing fetus; maternal surface is beefy and red; fetal surface is shiny and gray
E. Amnionic cavity: fills with fluid (1000 ml) that is replaced every 3 hours; shelters fetus

SEX DETERMINATION
A. Normal sperm; carries 22 autosomes and 1 sex chromosome (either an X or a Y chromosome)
B. Normal ovum: carries 22 autosomes and 1 sex chromosome (always an X chromosome)
C. Combined number of chromosomes: 44 autosomes and 2 sex chromosomes (at conception)
D. Genetic component of sperm determines sex of child (see the example below)
E. Chromosome carries genes plus DNA and proteins
F. Genes: factors in chromosomes carrying hereditary characteristics

Example

Sperm supplies 22 autosomes and an X sex chromosome
Ovum supplies 22 autosomes and an X sex chromosome
Result: 44 autosomes and an XX = female
Sperm supplies 22 autosomes and a Y sex chromosome
Ovum supplies 22 autosomes and an X sex chromosome
Result: 44 autosomes and an XY = male

Physiology of Fetus
A. Membranes and amniotic fluid
   1. Protect from blows and bumps mother may experience
   2. Maintain even heat to fetus
   3. Act as an excretory system
   4. Supply oral fluid for fetus
   5. Allow free movement of fetus

B. Placenta
1. Transport organ: passes nutrients from mother to fetus and relays excretory material from fetus to mother
2. Formation completed by 3 months
3. Functions: kidney, lungs, stomach, and intestines
4. Requirement: adequate oxygen from mother to function well
C. Monthly development
1. Embryonic stage (1st to 8th week)
    a. Beginning: pulsating heart, spinal canal formation: no eyes or ears; buds for arms and legs
    b. By end: little over 1 inch (2.5 cm) long; eyelids fused; distinct divisions of arms, legs; cord formed; tail disappears
2. Fetal stage (9th week to term)
    a. 3 months: 3 inches (7.5 cm) long; weighs 1 oz (28 g); fully formed arms, legs, fingers; distinguishable sex organs
    b. 4 months: development of muscles, movement; mother feels quickening; 6 to 7 inches (15 to 17.5 cm) long; weighs 4 oz (112 g); lanugo over body; head large
    c. 5 months: 10 to 12 inches (25 to 30 cm) long; weighs $1/2$ to 1 lb (225 to 450 g); internal organs maturing; lungs immature; FHT heard on examination; eyes fused; rarely survives more than several hours
    d. 6 months: 11 to 14 inches (27.5 to 35 cm) long; weighs 1 to $1^1/2$ lb (450 to 675 g); wrinkled "old man" appearance; vernix caseosa covers body; eyelids separated; eyelashes and fingernails formed
    e. 7 months: begins to store fat and minerals; 16 inches (40 cm) long; may survive with excellent care
    f. 8 months: beginning of month weighs 2 to 3 lb (900 to 1350 g); by end of month, 4 to 5 lb (1800 to 2250 g); continues to develop; loses wrinkled appearance
    g. 9 months: 19 inches (47.5 cm) long; weighs 7 lb (3200 g) (girl) $7^1/2$ lb (3400 g) (boy); more fat under skin; vernix caseosa; has stored vitamins, minerals, and antibodies; fully developed
D. Fetal circulation
1. Special structures
    a. Ductus venosus: passes through liver; connects umbilical vein to inferior vena cava; closes at birth
    b. Ductus arteriosus: shunts blood from pulmonary artery to descending aorta; closes almost immediately after birth
    c. Foramen ovale: valve opening that allows blood to flow from right atrium to left atrium; functionally closes at birth; all three fetal structures listed above allow blood to bypass the fetal lungs and liver
    d. Umbilical arteries (2): transport blood from the hypogastric artery to the placenta; functionally closes at birth
    e. Umbilical vein (1): transports oxygenated blood from placenta to ductus venosus and liver, then to the inferior vena cava (IVC); closes at birth
2. Fetal circulation (Fig. 7-2)
    a. Oxygenated blood from placenta goes through umbilical vein, bypassing portal system of the liver by way of the ductus venosus
    b. From the ductus venosus blood goes to the ascending vena cava (inferior) to the heart, right auricle
    c. From the right auricle through the foramen ovale
    d. To the left auricle, then to the left ventricle
    e. Leaves the heart through the aorta to the arms and head
    f. The blood then returns to the heart, passing through the descending vena cava (superior)
    g. To the right auricle, then to the right ventricle
    h. Blood leaves the heart through the pulmonary arteries, bypassing the lungs
    i. Blood goes through the ductus arteriosus to the aorta and down to the trunk and lower extremities
    j. It then goes through the hypogastric arteries to the umbilical arteries on to the placenta, carrying carbon dioxide and waste materials

Normal Antepartum (Prenatal)
PHYSIOLOGIC CHANGES DURING PREGNANCY
A. Reproductive system
1. External changes
    a. Perineum: increased vasculature; enlarges
    b. Labia majora: change especially in parous woman; separate and stretch
    c. Anal and vulvar varices: caused by increased pelvic congestion
2. Internal changes
    a. Uterus: enlarges to accommodate growing fetus; walls thicken first trimester; *Hegar's* sign (soft, lower lip of uterus)
    b. Cervix: *Goodell's* sign (thickens, softens) 6 weeks from LMP because of vascular changes
    c. Vagina: *Chadwick's* sign (bluish violet color); mucosal changes about 8 weeks from LMP; estrogen activity may cause thick vaginal discharge
B. Other body system changes
1. Breasts
    a. Increased size, tingling sensations, heavy
    b. Increased pigmentation, darkened areolae
    c. Montgomery's tubercles on areolae
2. Cardiovascular changes
    a. Slight enlargement of heart resulting from increased blood volume
    b. Increased circulation (47%)
    c. Cardiac output increased 30% first and second trimester, then levels off until term; during labor and delivery increases; and about 13% above normal during postpartum period
3. Hematologic changes
    a. Increased RBC count; decreased hemoglobin level
    b. Increased tendency for blood to coagulate during pregnancy
    c. Coagulation factors return to normal during postpartum, increasing likelihood of thromboembolism
4. Respiratory/pulmonary changes: enlarging uterus presses on diaphragm, causing difficulty breathing
5. Skin: increased pigmentation
    a. Linea nigra: darkening line from below breast bone (sternum) down midline of abdomen to symphysis pubis
    b. Chloasma gravidarum (mask of pregnancy): dark, frecklelike pigmentation over nose and cheeks; disappears after delivery
    c. Stria gravidarum: stretching of skin with silvery to reddish, bluish stretch marks on breasts, abdomen,

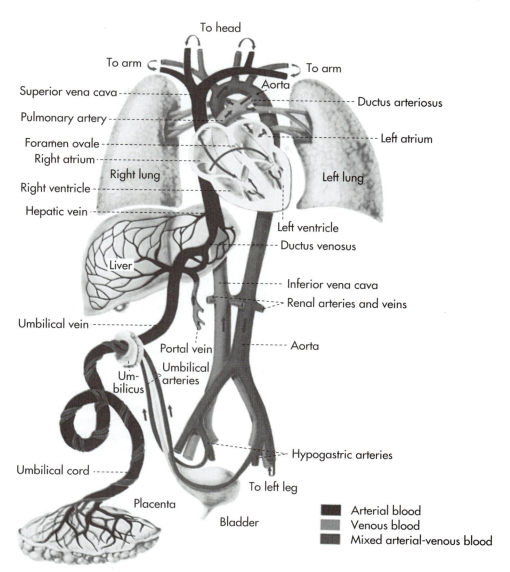

To head

To arm

To arm

Aorta

Superior vena cava

Ductus arteriosus

Pulmonary artery

Foramen ovale

Left atrium

Right atrium

Right lung

Left lung

Right ventricle

Left ventricle

Hepatic vein

Liver

Left ventricle

Ductus venosus

Inferior vena cava

Renal arteries and veins

Umbilical vein

Portal vein

Aorta

Umbilical arteries

Um-bilicus

Hypogastric arteries

Umbilical cord

To left leg

Placenta

Bladder

■ Arterial blood
■ Venous blood
■ Mixed arterial-venous blood

Figure 7-2. **Fetal circulation.** *Before birth.* Arterialized blood from the placenta flows into the fetus through the umbilical vein and passes rapidly through the liver into the inferior vena cava; it flows through the foramen ovale into the left atrium, soon to appear in the aorta and arteries of the head. A portion bypasses the liver through the ductus venosus. Venous blood from the lower extremities and head passes predominantly into the right atrium, the right ventricle, and then into the descending pulmonary artery and ductus arteriosus. Thus the foramen ovale and the ductus arteriosus act as bypass channels, allowing a large part of the combined cardiac output to return to the placenta without flowing through the lungs. Approximately 55% of the combined ventricular output flows to the placenta; 35% perfuses body tissues; and the remaining 10% flows through the lungs (Behrman, Vaughan, 1987). *After birth.* The foramen ovale closes, the ductus arteriosus closes and becomes a ligament, the ductus venosus closes and becomes a ligament, and the umbilical vein and arteries close and become ligaments. (Courtesy Ross Laboratories, Columbus, Ohio.)

thighs, never disappears completely; lotion, cocoa butter lubricants may help

6. Urinary system changes
   a. Traces of sugar in urine resulting from activity of lactiferous ducts
   b. Even though glucosuria is common in pregnancy, all women should be screened for diabetes
   c. Transitory albumin: may be indication of pending pregnancy-induced hypertension
   d. Cystitis: frequent because ureters lose some compliance or elasticity

7. Endocrine system
   a. Variable production of insulin during pregnancy
   b. Mother's cells become more insulin resistant
   c. Thyroid gland increases in size, resulting in increased basal metabolic rate (BMR)

8. Digestive system
   a. Morning sickness: nausea and vomiting common during first trimester
   b. Increased appetite after first trimester
   c. Indigestion (heartburn): caused by increasing upward pressure of enlarging uterus or by relaxin

hormone, which slows metabolism and keeps food in stomach longer in pregnant women

   d. Constipation: caused by changes in organ positions; pressure of growing uterus on sigmoid colon

9. Musculoskeletal system

   a. Normal lumbar curve becomes more pronounced as weight of pelvic contents tilts the pelvis forward

   b. Extra weight may lead to backache experienced in late pregnancy

10. Weight gain: total weight gain varies from 25 to 30 lb (12 to 13.5 kg) (Table 7-1)

DURATION OF PREGNANCY

A. Length in terms of time
1. 9 calendar months
2. 10 lunar months
3. 280 days (266 days from time of ovulation)
4. 40 weeks

B. Nägele's rule: to calculate EDC count back 3 months from the month of the LMP and add 7 days to the first day of LMP

EXAMPLE: first day of LMP was July 17

7	(July)	17	
−3	months	+7	
4th month		24 = EDC April 24	

SIGNS AND SYMPTOMS OF PREGNANCY

A. Presumptive signs (subjective: mother usually notices)
1. Missed menstrual period
2. Breast changes; nipples tingle, fuller, darker areola in about 6 weeks
3. Frequency of urination in about 6 weeks
4. Morning sickness: nausea and vomiting in 4 to 6 weeks
5. Skin changes: chloasma, linea nigra, striae (some authors call this "probable" sign)

B. Probable signs (objective examiner usually notices)
1. Uterus: enlarges; shape changes at 12 to 16 weeks; Hegar's sign: 8 weeks
2. Cervix: Goodell's sign
3. Vagina: Chadwick's sign
4. Implantation site: softens, enlarges (von Fernwald's sign) 6 to 7 weeks
5. Laboratory tests:
   a. Biologic: used before 1960; laboratory animals: Aschheim-Zondek (AZ) test and Friedman's test
   b. Immunologic: widely used today; faster, 90% accurate; beta subunit of HCG can be used even before missed period; home pregnancy tests can be used 9 days after missed period (for names of tests see Prenatal Care)
6. Braxton-Hicks contractions
7. Ballottement

C. Positive signs (by examiner)
1. Palpate: can feel fetal parts
2. Hearing: fetal heart tone
   a. Electronic Doptone scope (audible at 8 to 11 weeks)
   b. Sonogram (can ascertain at 12 weeks)
   c. Auscultation (17 to 24 weeks) with fetoscope (head-scope) or Leff stethoscope
3. Ultrasonographic (echographic) evidence of pregnancy visualized on screen
4. Fetal movement palpable after 20 weeks

PRENATAL CARE

A. Importance
1. Regular assessment and monitoring detect early signs and symptoms disrupting normal, healthy pregnancy
2. Early evaluation of problem permits development of an appropriate plan of action based on findings

B. Visits and examinations
1. Initial visits: establish diagnosis of pregnancy
   a. Latex agglutination inhibition (LAD) test: results in 2 minutes; accurate 4 to 10 days after missed period (e.g., Pregnosticon)
   b. Hemagglutination inhibition (HAD) test: more sensitive; results in 1 to 2 hours; accurate 4 days after missed period
   c. Radioreceptor assay test: serum test; results in 1 hour; accurate at time of missed period (e.g., Biocept G)
   d. Radioimmunoassay (RIA): most sensitive; results can range from 1 to 48 hours (depends on the degree of sensitivity required); can detect pregnancy 2 days after implantation
   e. Commercially sold pregnancy test: an HAI in home test; results in 4 minutes; should be confirmed by a physician (e.g., ept [early pregnancy test])
   NOTE: All tests use urine from the mother
2. Complete medical history
   a. General personal health, habits, diseases, and medical or surgical problems
   b. History of communicable diseases, especially scarlet fever, measles, rubella, *streptococcus* infections, kidney conditions that might adversely affect pregnancy, and sexually transmitted diseases
   c. Psychosocial history: assess substance use or abuse (including alcohol, tobacco, illegal prescription, or over-the-counter drugs), social support, physical abuse, stress, employment, and physical activity
   d. Previous pregnancies, miscarriages, abortions, blood transfusions, gynecologic problems
   e. Family health status: diabetes, tuberculosis, heart disease, cancer, epilepsy, allergies, mental problems
3. Complete examination to include:
   a. Routine laboratory tests
     (1) Matching blood type and Rh factor
     (2) Antibody screen (rubella, sickle cell) if appropriate

Table 7-1	Distribution of Weight Gain During Pregnancy	
Distribution	**Pounds**	**Grams**
Fetus	7½	3400
Placenta	1	450
Amniotic fluid	2	900
Uterus	2½	1125
Increased blood volume	3-4	1350-1800
Breasts	2-3	900-1350
Mother's gain (fat, tissue, etc.)	4-8	1800-3600
Total weight gain	21-28 lb	9.5-12.7 kg

(3) Hemoglobin and hematocrit
(4) Venereal Disease Research Laboratory (VDRL) test (for syphilis)
(5) Herpes 1 and 2 tests
(6) HIV testing for the AIDS virus
(7) Hepatitis A and B tests
(8) Pap smear
(9) PPD test used for tuberculosis
  b. Physical examination to include
    (1) Pelvic examination and measurements
    (2) Abdominal palpation
    (3) Examination of breasts, nipples
    (4) Vital signs: blood pressure, weight, temperature, respirations
    (5) Urinalysis for sugar and albumin
    (6) Smears (Papanicolaou's test) for cytology, gonorrhea, chlamydia
4. Usual schedule for prenatal visits
  a. Every month for 28 weeks
  b. Every 2 weeks thereafter to 36th week
  c. Every week from 37th week to term
  d. Adjusted to individual needs
5. Usual routine for prenatal visits:
  a. Urinalysis each visit for sugar, acetone, albumin
  b. Capillary blood testing on a glucose oxidase strip for gestational diabetes mellitus (GDM); followed by plasma glucose testing at 12 weeks' gestation on all high-risk pregnancies
  c. Check vital signs (especially blood pressure)
  d. Check weight gain every visit
    (1) First trimester: 3 to 4 lb (1.5 to 2 kg) total
    (2) Second trimester: 1 lb (0.5 kg) per week; 12 to 14 lb (6 to 7 kg) total
    (3) Third trimester: 1 lb (0.5 kg) per week; 8 to 10 lb (4 to 5 kg) total
  e. Measure height of fundus to evaluate growth of fetus (Fig. 7-3)
  f. Listen to FHT and FHR by Doptone or auscultation
  g. Ask about fetal activity, attitude of family; answer mother's questions, fears
  h. Recommend childbirth education classes
C. Promotion of positive health
  1. Nutritional counseling
    a. Fetus receives all nourishment from mother
    b. Teenage pregnant mother requires extensive counseling (nutritional pattern poor); focus on positive effect of good nutrition on teenager as well as on fetus
    c. Salt restrictions may be advised in presence of edema, retention of fluids, sudden change in blood pressure
    d. Direct relationship between maternal nutrition and mental development of the child
  2. Nutritional needs during pregnancy: Table 7-2
  3. General health teaching
    a. Daily baths for cleanliness; showers during last 6 weeks for safety's sake
    b. Moderate exercise, especially walking
    c. Douching only on advice of physician
    d. Sexual intercourse permissible as long as it is not uncomfortable and cervix is closed
    e. Good support bra
    f. Unrestrictive comfortable clothing, hose

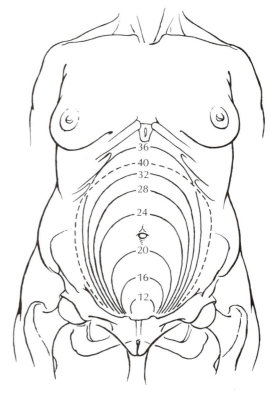

Figure 7-3. **Height of fundus by weeks of normal gestation with a single fetus.** Dotted line indicates height after lightening. (Adapted from Malasanos L et al: *Health assessment,* ed 4, St Louis, 1990, Mosby.)

  g. Good mental attitude; discuss ambivalent feelings
  h. Smoking: nicotine retards growth of fetus, constricts blood vessels in mother, decreases placental function, and may cause premature labor; growing evidence shows that secondary smoking has damaging effects on the mother, fetus, children, and spouses
  i. Alcohol: research has yet to determine minimum safe amounts of alcohol (if any) that can be consumed in pregnancy; caffeine has been shown to cause tetragenic effects in animals; pregnant women should be counseled to avoid foods containing caffeine (found in coffee, tea, chocolate, colas, and some analgesics)
  j. Drugs: May pass placental barrier and affect fetus; greatest danger is during first trimester, but effects may not be evident for years after birth; new evidence shows that crack or cocaine may cause significant complications for mother and newborn; pregnant women should be counseled to avoid over-the-counter or prescription medications without the advice of a physician
4. Childbirth and parent education classes
  a. Dick-Read method ("childbirth without fear") (1944): philosophy of relaxation coupled with abdominal and chest breathing and education
  b. Lamaze method, American Society for Prophylaxis in Obstetrics [ASPO]; psychoprophylactic method [PPM]) 1960: combines breathing techniques with preparation for childbirth by training mother to anticipate various stages of labor and meet each

Table 7-2	Nutritional Needs During Pregnancy			
Nutrient	**Nonpregnant woman (19-22 yr)**	**Pregnant woman**	**Usage**	**Food source**
Protein	44 g	74-100 g; needs twice as much	Growth of fetus Placental growth During labor and delivery During lactation	Milk, cheese, eggs, meat, grains, legumes, nuts
Major minerals Calcium	800 mg	1200 mg; needs one and a half times as much	Fetal skeleton Fetal tooth buds Calcium metabolism in mother	Milk, cheese, whole grains, leafy vegetables, egg yolk
Phosphorus	800 mg	1200 mg; needs one and a half times as much		Milk, cheese, lean meats
Iron (Fe)	18 mg	30-60 mg supplement; needs almost two to three times as much	Increased maternal blood volume Fetus stores iron in third trimester	Liver, meats, eggs, leafy vegetables, nuts, legumes, whole wheat
Vitamin C (not stored in body so pregnant mother should take at least 1 serving per day)	60 mg	80 mg	Tissue formation Increased iron absorption	Citrus fruits, berries, melon, tomatoes, green peppers, green leafy vegetables, broccoli
Vitamin D	5-10 µg*; 200-400 IU†	10-15 µg; 400-600 IU; needs almost twice as much	Tooth buds Mineralize bone tissue Aid absorption of calcium and phosphorus	Fortified milk Fortified margarine
Folic acid	180 µg	400 µg	Increase red blood cell formation; prevention of macrocytic and megaloblastic anemia and neural tube defects	Green leafy vegetables, oranges, broccoli, asparagus and liver

*µg = microgram.
†IU = international units.

stage with practiced relaxation and breathing methods; coach to support mother and direct her if necessary.
  c. Bradley method, 1965: husband-coached childbirth, emphasizing quiet, darkened atmosphere, no stress
 5. Teaching danger signs (those that must be reported to physician immediately)
  a. Persistent, severe vomiting beyond first trimester
  b. Epigastric or abdominal pain
  c. Edema: face, fingers; especially in the morning
  d. Visual disturbances: blurring, double vision, spots
  e. Frequent or continuous headaches
  f. Bleeding or "leakage of fluid" from vagina
  g. Absence of fetal movements (after quickening)
  h. Chills and fever (signs of infection)
  i. Rapid weight gain (signs of possible preeclampsia)

NORMAL DISCOMFORTS OF PREGNANCY
Table 7-3

Abnormal Antepartum
HYPERTENSIVE STATES
A. Definition: a group of conditions that occur during pregnancy usually after 20 weeks' gestation: symptoms can range from high blood pressure (BP) to headaches, blurred vision, and convulsions with ensuing coma

Table 7-3	Normal Discomforts of Pregnancy	
Discomfort	**Probable cause**	**Relief measures**
First trimester		
Breasts: painful	Hypertrophy of glandular tissue Increased blood flow to area Hormonal effects	Firm, supportive bra; even a nursing bra
Urinary frequency	Pressure on bladder from expanding uterus reduces bladder capacity; increased vascular content	Pads if necessary
Yawning (tired, sleepy)	Whether result of relaxin hormone is questionable; possibly caused by sudden chemical changes in body	Frequent rest periods Balanced diet to prevent anemia

Nausea/vomiting	Hormonal changes
	Ambivalent feelings regarding pregnancy
		Small, frequent meals
		Limited fluids
		    Dry crackers with tea
		    Avoid greasy fried foods

Second trimester		
Heartburn (acid taste in mouth)	Relaxin hormone effect Enlarging uterus displaces stomach upward	Avoid fatty foods Antacids: Milk of Magnesia, Gelusil, Maalox, Amphojel
Pigmentation	Hormonal	Reassure mother that it is temporary and will disappear after delivery
Leg cramps	Calcium-phosphorus imbalance	Position relief Calf stretching Calcium supplements, milk
Constipation	Hormonal: slowing down of peristaltic movements Compression of colon by uterus and baby	Adequate fluids, fruits, foods with roughage Exercises Stool softener but no mineral oil
Third trimester		
Urinary incontinence	Lightening/dropping of fetus into pelvic cavity pushes presenting part on bladder	Pelvic floor exercise (Kegel): tighten perineal muscles, relax, then repeat
Hemorrhoids	Pressure from fetal presenting part Increased vascular activity	Knee-chest (elevate hips): Kegel exercises Comfort measures: frequent rest periods; sitting in warm tub; supporting legs with pillows
Low back pain	Increased pressure Fatigue Poor weight distribution	Pelvic exercises Pushing, stretching Comfort massaging Good posture
Insomnia	Increased fetal movements Muscular cramping Frequency Dyspnea	Adequate rest periods Warm milk at bedtime Relaxing shower Support with pillows Deep breathing
Varicosities (leg, vulva)	Hereditary disposition Pelvis vasocongestion Pull of gravity Pressure of uterus Forcing stool (constipation)	Support stockings Changing position frequently Abdominal support Keeping legs uncrossed
Edema (legs, feet)	Immobility (staying in one position for a prolonged time)	Periodic resting Moving around Support stockings Elevating legs Plenty of fluids (to serve as a diuretic)
Dyspnea (shortness of breath)	Pressure on diaphragm from expanding uterus	Sitting erect Deep breathing Putting arms above head Keeping weight down

Table 7-3	Normal Discomforts of Pregnancy—cont'd	
Discomfort	**Probable cause**	**Relief measures**
Leaking of colostrum	Increased blood supply Prominent nipples	Support bra Pads if necessary (keep clean and dry)
Supine hypotension syndrome (feel faint)	Pressure on ascending vena cava by uterus	Lying on left side with legs flexed or semi-sitting position
Vaginal discharge	Hormonal	No douching Keep area clean, dry (perineal care)

1. Frequent in high-risk mothers
2. Greater likelihood during first pregnancies
3. Incidence: 5% to 7% of all pregnancies
B. Types
  1. Pregnancy-induced hypertension (PIH): increase of blood pressure to or above 140/90 mm Hg
    a. Increased BP only symptom
    b. Disappears within 10 days following delivery
  2. Preeclampsia: an acute hypertensive condition resulting in elevated BP and proteinuria; edema may also be present
    a. Mild preeclampsia:
      (1) BP 140/90
      (2) Proteinuria 1+
      (3) Rapid weight gain
    b. Moderate-to-severe preeclampsia
      (1) Hospitalize stat
      (2) BP 160/110
      (3) Albumin 2+ to 4+
      (4) Persistent, severe headaches with visual disturbances
      (5) Epigastric pain (late sign)
      (6) Hyperactive: twitching musculature
  3. Eclampsia
    a. Definition: most severe form of the hypertensive states, characterized by hypertensive crisis, shock, or convulsions and possibly coma
    b. Signs and symptoms
      (1) Alarming weight gain
      (2) Scanty urine (less than 30 ml/hour)
      (3) Proteinuria 4+, red blood cells (RBCs) in urine
      (4) BP 200/100 or higher
      (5) Edema of retina; can cause blindness
      (6) Severe epigastric pain
      (7) Convulsions: tonic and clonic
      NOTE: May start labor prematurely; infant may be severely compromised and die
C. Treatment and nursing management
  1. According to classification and severity of symptoms; varies from home care precautions to absolute bed rest in a hospital with patient lying on left side
  2. Reduce stimuli
  3. Convulsion precautions
  4. Selective antihypertensive and diuretic therapy may be ordered (e.g., hydralazine [Apresoline] hydrochloride, furosemide [Lasix], magnesium sulfate, mannitol); nurse should know effects and untoward symptoms
  5. Monitor edema, BP, FHT, levels of consciousness, reflexes, impending labor signs

HYPEREMESIS GRAVIDARUM

A. Definition: pernicious vomiting of pregnancy lasting into second trimester
B. Signs and symptoms
  1. Excessive nausea and vomiting
  2. Considerable weight loss
  3. Severe dehydration
  4. Depletion of essential electrolytes (sodium and potassium)
  5. Vitamin, glucose, and protein deficiencies
  6. Ketone bodies in urine: 1+ protein
  7. Elevated hemoglobin level, RBC count, and hematocrit
C. Treatment and nursing management: untreated will lead to death of mother, child, or both
  1. Hospitalize in well-ventilated, private, pleasant environment
  2. No visitors, not even husband first 48 hours
  3. Nothing by mouth (NPO) first 48 hours
  4. Record intake and output (I & O)
  5. Intravenous (IV) fluids to replace losses in nutrition
  6. Gradual serving of attractive, small portions of food on china dishes, starting with dry toast and tea
  7. Nonjudgmental nursing attitudes
  8. Refer for psychotherapy when appropriate

HEMORRHAGIC CONDITIONS

A. Abortion (early pregnancy bleeding)
  1. Definition: the expulsion of uterine contents before viability of the fetus for medical reasons or spontaneously
  2. Types
    a. Induced abortion
      (1) Therapeutic: legal aborting of the fetus for medical or psychologic reasons by a licensed physician under controlled, aseptic conditions
      (2) Criminal: an abortion performed under illegal, unsafe conditions
    b. Spontaneous abortion
      (1) Definition: an abortion that occurs naturally (usually in the first trimester)
      (2) Possible causes: hormonal deficiencies, abnormalities of the fetus, incompetent cervix, abnormalities of the reproductive organs, emotional shock, physical injury, acute infections, growths, and so on
  3. Terminology of abortions
    a. Habitual abortion: three or more consecutive spontaneous abortions for unknown reasons
    b. Threatened abortion: minimal signs and symptoms

of abortion such as bleeding and cramping but with no loss of uterine contents

   c. Imminent abortion: considerable blood loss, severe contractions, urge to push that without treatment will result in loss of uterine contents

   d. Inevitable abortion: bleeding, contractions, rupture of membranes, and cervical dilatation in which the uterine contents will be lost, so treatment will concentrate on the mother

   e. Incomplete abortion: part(s) of uterine contents retained, necessitating administration of oxytocins to accelerate expulsion of remaining contents, or dilatation and curettage (D&C; a minor surgical intervention) to prevent prolonged bleeding

   f. Complete abortion: entire uterine contents are expelled

4. Signs and symptoms of abortion
   a. Vaginal bleeding: scant to profuse
   b. Abdominal cramping: slight to severe
   c. Contractions: intermittent, steady, mild, or severe

5. Treatment and nursing management
   a. Prompt and immediate bed rest
   b. Hospitalization when appropriate
   c. Prevention of blood loss and shock
   d. Replacement blood treatment if necessary
   e. Checking vital signs and temperature for 24 hours
   f. Endocrine therapy when appropriate
   g. Surgical intervention when appropriate: Shirodkar operation (purse-string suturing) for known incompetent cervix
   h. Psychotherapy when appropriate
      (1) Prepare for grieving process
      (2) Provide assistance for burial regulations
      (3) Let mother vent feelings of love, loss, guilt
      (4) Quiet, supportive, compassionate nursing care

B. Ectopic pregnancy (early pregnancy bleeding)
1. Definition: an extrauterine pregnancy in which the products of conception are implanted outside the uterine cavity; 90% occur in the fallopian tube (right tube more frequent); other sites include the abdomen or the ovary
2. Signs and symptoms
   a. Abnormal or missed menstrual period
   b. Slight uterine bleeding or spotting
   c. Possible mass on affected side; pain, tenderness, rigid abdomen
   d. If tube ruptures, may be little bleeding externally, but massive internal hemorrhaging with accompanying severe shock
3. Treatment and nursing management
   a. Hospitalization stat
   b. Treat shock (warm, quiet, replacement therapy—IV fluids, oxygen, etc.)
   c. Crossmatch and other blood work: transfusion readiness
   d. Support mother, who will be extremely frightened
   e. Prepare for stat surgery if appropriate
   f. Arrange for baptism of fetus when appropriate
   g. Postsurgical care with IV fluids, medications, other appropriate treatments (RhoGAM if necessary)
   h. Provide emotional support to mother and family; get assistance of clergy when requested

C. Gestational trophoblastic neoplasm (formerly known as hydatidiform mole)

1. Definition: rare degeneration of chorionic villi into a benign neoplasm in which the villi fill with clear viscous fluid and form grapelike clusters; the neoplasm fills the decidua and expands the uterus to larger than normal for gestational age
2. Signs and symptoms
   a. Enlarging uterus, greater than for normal gestation
   b. Missed period; spotting to profuse bleeding
   c. Several shiny, tapioca-like "grape clusters" escape through vaginal tract
   d. Nausea and vomiting
   e. Signs of pregnancy-induced hypertension (PIH); usually before 20 weeks' gestation
   f. No FHT
   g. Ultrasound reveals no fetal structures
   h. Laboratory findings: human chorionic gonadotropin (HCG) titers up to 1 to 2 million (normally 350,000 to 400,000 at 8 weeks)
3. Treatment and nursing management
   a. Termination as soon as diagnosis confirmed
   b. Blood transfusion if indicated
   c. Assistance in grieving process of mother and family
   d. Follow-up very important
      (1) Contraceptive advice (no oral since that will distort HCG titers)
      (2) HCG titers for at least 6 months

D. Placenta previa (third-trimester bleeding)
1. Definition: abnormal implantation of a normal placenta for unknown reasons, usually in the lower segment of the uterus; condition usually occurs in multiparas, and incidence appears to increase with age; may also be caused by fibroids
2. Types (Fig. 7-4)
   a. Partial (incomplete): incomplete coverage of the uterine os
   b. Complete (total): entire uterine os completely covered
   c. Marginal (low lying): located in lower uterine segment but away from the os
3. Signs and symptoms
   a. Painless uterine bleeding: may be intermittent or occur in gushes; scanty to severe; bright red
   b. Third-trimester occurrence
4. Treatment and nursing management
   a. Diagnosis confirmed by ultrasound or x-ray examination
   b. Avoidance of vaginal examinations
   c. Hospitalization stat
   d. Quiet environment; fetus uncompromised; station high
   e. Fowler's position (head at 30-degree angle)
   f. Tocolytic therapy with use of magnesium sulfate to manage uterine irritability under certain circumstances
   g. Have double set-up ready so that if vaginal examination is imperative, emergency cesarean section equipment is available and blood is ready for transfusion
   h. Foley catheter if condition is severe; shock care
   i. Count pads to determine amount, color, duration of bleeding
   j. Monitor vital signs, especially blood pressure
   k. Monitor FHT and FHR
   l. IV fluids

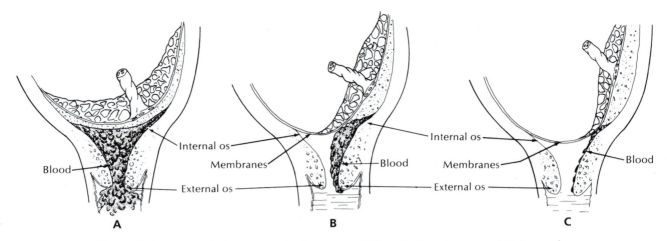

Figure 7-4. **Types of placenta previa after onset of labor. A,** Complete, or total. **B,** Incomplete, or partial. **C,** Marginal, or low-lying. (From Bobak IM, Lowdermilk DL, Jensen MD: *Maternity nursing,* ed 4, St Louis, 1995, Mosby.)

m. Support patient and family; keep them informed

E. Abruptio placentae (third-trimester bleeding)
1. Definition: premature separation of a normally implanted placenta before the birth of the fetus
2. Causes
    a. Trauma
    b. Chronic maternal disease
    c. Grand multipara
    d. Unknown
3. Types (Fig. 7-5)
    a. Complete: separation of the placenta from the uterine wall before birth of the fetus
    b. Partial: separation of a portion of the placenta from the wall of the uterus before the birth of the fetus
4. Signs and symptoms
    a. Severe abdominal pain; sometimes called "exquisite"
    b. Patient is distressed, depressed, and exhibits signs of shock
    c. Painful bleeding: moderate to severe; internal or external; dark red, not clotted; amount varies
    d. Abdomen tense, boardlike; nurse unable to feel contractions; uterus irritable
    e. Hypovolemic shock can result in renal failure
    f. Sudden change in heartbeat or bradycardia, or absence of FHT
5. Treatment and nursing management
    a. Depends on stage and intensity of condition; for reasons not clearly understood, partial abruptio placentae may seal off bleeding spontaneously, and labor will proceed normally
    b. Check coagulation profile: fibrinogen/fibrin, platelets
    c. Prevent hypovolemic shock and fetal hypoxia
    d. Crossmatch, type, readiness for transfusions
    e. Monitor contractions, FHT, and vital signs
    f. Slight or moderate bleeding may indicate artificial rupture of membranes (ARM) to hasten delivery or seal off bleeding
    g. Severe bleeding (dark red) may indicate immediate cesarean section
    h. Support mother and family

i. Continued bleeding after delivery may necessitate hysterectomy

F. Disseminated intravascular coagulation (DIC)
1. Cause
    a. Unknown
    b. Coincidental with abruptio placentae, postabortal infection, amniotic fluid emboli
2. Pathology: not clearly understood; massive clotting, depletion of coagulant factor
3. Signs and symptoms: Excessive bleeding at placental site, incisional site, nose, mouth, gums
4. Treatment and nursing management
    a. Halt or reverse DIC
    b. Eliminate cause
    c. Delivery stat
    d. Blood replacement
    e. IV fibrinogen/heparin

MEDICAL AND INFECTIOUS CONDITIONS

A. Chickenpox (varicella)
1. Causative agent: herpesvirus; varicella zoster virus (VZV)
2. Effect on mother
    a. May manifest itself as herpes zoster (shingles)
    b. May be fatal if severe
    c. May cause abortion
3. Effect on fetus
    a. May cause defects of skin, bones, hydrocephalus if contracted during first trimester
    b. Fetal death

B. German measles (rubella or 3-day measles)
1. Causative agent: virus
2. Effect on mother
    a. Rash, fever, photophobia
    b. Possible abortion
3. Effect on fetus if infected during first trimester
    a. Rubella syndrome: heart defects, blindness, deafness, mental retardation
    b. Delayed effect on brain (15 to 20 years of age)

C. Genital herpes
1. Causative agent: herpes simplex virus 2
2. Effect on mother

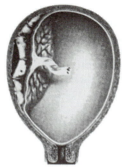
Partial separation
(Concealed hemorrhage)

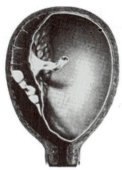
Partial separation
(Apparent hemorrhage)

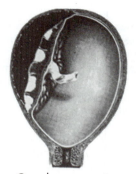
Complete separation
(Concealed hemorrhage)

Figure 7-5.   **Abruptio placentae.** Premature separation of normally implanted placenta. (From Bobak IM, Lowdermilk DL, Jensen MD: *Maternity nursing*, ed 4, St. Louis, 1995, Mosby.)

a. Vaginal discharge
b. Genital blisters, ulcers
c. Fever
d. Painful inguinal lymph nodes
3. Effect on fetus
a. Abortion or premature birth
b. Neonatal infections
c. Survivors may have CNS symptoms
D. Group B *streptococcus*
1. Causative agent: *Streptococcus* bacterium
2. Effect on mother: septicemia
3. Effect on fetus
a. Neonatal death (stillborn)
b. Blindness, deafness, mental retardation
E. Hepatitis A
1. Causative agent: virus
2. Effect on mother
a. Abortion
b. Liver failure
3. Effect on fetus
a. First-trimester infection: fetal anomalies
b. Premature birth
c. Neonatal hepatitis
F. Hepatitis B (serum hepatitis)
1. Causative agent: virus (HBV)
2. Effect on mother
a. Prolonged illness
b. Destruction of liver cells
c. Cirrhosis
3. Effect on fetus
a. Preterm at birth
b. May be asymptomatic at birth
c. May exhibit signs of acute hepatitis
d. Possible carrier
4. Vaccine available for high-risk women and health care workers
G. Influenza
1. Causative agent: virus
2. Effect on mother
a. Pneumonia
b. Abortion

c. Premature labor
3. Effect on fetus
a. Abortion or premature birth
b. Fetal death
4. Vaccine for pregnant women available; live viral vaccine can infect fetus
H. Gonorrhea (clap)
1. Causative agent: *Neisseria gonorrhoeae* bacterium
2. Effect on mother
a. Vaginal discharge
b. Cervical tenderness
c. Dysuria
d. Affects ovaries, tubes, causing sterility
3. Effect on fetus
a. Ophthalmia neonatorum
b. Conjunctivitis
c. Mild-to-severe infections
I. Syphilis (lues)
1. Causative agent: *Treponema pallidum* bacterium
2. Effect on mother (if untreated)
a. Primary chancre
b. Secondary skin rash
c. Latent or tertiary CNS problems
3. Effect on fetus
a. Rhagades of the corners of mouth and anus
b. Snuffles
c. Maceration of palms of hands and soles of feet
d. Congenital syphilis (symptoms appearing later in life)
e. Death (stillborn)
J. Cytomegalovirus (CMV)
1. Causative agent: cytomegalovirus of the herpes group, transmitted by close bodily and sexual contact
2. May be transmitted by asymptomatic woman to fetus causing fetal damage, retardation, or fetal death
3. The infant may acquire the virus by exposure to cervical mucus during vaginal birth
4. No satisfactory treatment for maternal or neonatal CMV
K. Chlamydia
1. Causative agent: bacterial microorganism *Chlamydia trachomatis* (CT)—transmitted by close bodily and sexual contact

2. May initiate pelvic inflammatory disease (PID) leading to ectopic pregnancy and infertility
3. Some evidence suggests relationship between CT and premature rupture of membranes, preterm labor and delivery, low birth weight, increased perinatal mortality, and late onset endometritis
4. Treated with extended erythromycin
5. Transmission from infected birth canal may result in conjunctivitis and/or pneumonia

L. Cardiac disease
1. Classification
   a. Class I: no limitation of activity
   b. Class II: slight limitation of activity
   c. Class III: considerable limitation of even ordinary activity
   d. Class IV: symptoms of cardiac insufficiency even at rest
2. Treatment and nursing management
   a. Close medical and nursing supervision
   b. Watch for signs and symptoms of fatigue, dyspnea, coughing, palpitations, tachycardia
   c. Promote rest
   d. Hospitalize at end of second trimester
   e. Breastfeeding contraindicated
   f. Contraceptive education
   g. Nutrition: offer foods high in iron and protein; avoid raw, deep green vegetables because vitamin K counteracts effects of heparin
   h. Prevent infections: report first signs of exposure
   i. Teach comfortable positions: pillows, support, left side
   j. During labor and delivery: saddle block; caudal block to minimize discomfort on bearing down
   k. Watch for cardiac decompensation (pulse rate over 100 beats/min; respirations, 25+)
   l. Vaginal delivery preferred
      (1) Episiotomy, low forceps
      (2) Oxygen to decrease pulmonary edema
      (3) Medication to regulate heart rate
      (4) Diuretic to reduce fluid retention
   m. Postpartal care
      (1) Hospitalization longer than normal to stabilize cardiac output
      (2) Application of abdominal binder (because of rapid change in intraabdominal pressure)
      (3) Bed rest with progressive bathroom privileges dependent on progress
      (4) Prevent overdistention of bladder
      (5) Encourage bonding; nurse should hold baby at eye level to allow mother to touch and talk to baby
      (6) Inform mother and family of progress

M. Diabetes mellitus
1. Definition: inborn error in the transportation and metabolism of carbohydrates
2. Classification
   a. Class A
      (1) Gestational diabetes mellitus (GDM) occurs with onset of pregnancy or later in pregnancy; caused by an intolerance to carbohydrates
      (2) Classified as *A* according to plasma glucose readings of 140 mg/dL after regular screening procedure

     (3) Return to normal after delivery (usually 6 weeks)
   b. Class B: frank diabetes; duration 9 years; unable to use oral hypoglycemics
   c. Class C: duration 10 to 19 years
   d. Class D
      (1) Duration 20 years or more
      (2) Vascular complications such as retinopathy and calcification of leg muscles
   e. Class E
      (1) Vascular complications
      (2) Calcification in pelvic area
   f. Class F: Same as class E plus retinopathy and kidney complications
3. Effects of diabetes on pregnancy
   a. Difficult to control because of changing patterns of fetal growth and development and maternal demands
   b. Fluctuating insulin requirements
   c. Tendency to develop acidosis (diabetic coma) from lack of insulin
   d. Increased tendency to infection (urinary tract, vaginal tract), preeclampsia, and polyhydramnios
   e. Increased incidence of premature labor
   f. Oversized baby
   g. Possibility of dystocia
   h. Increased danger of placental deterioration causing hypoxia in fetus
   i. Tendency to abruptio placentae
4. Changing insulin requirements during pregnancy
   a. First trimester: insulin requirement decreased
   b. Second trimester: insulin requirement increased
   c. Third trimester: careful regulation (blood sugar); evaluation of placenta, oxytocin challenge test (OCT)
   d. Intranatal: labor depletes glycogen
   e. Postpartum: insulin reaction resulting from sudden drop in need
   f. Watch for hypoglycemia, shock, infection, bleeding
   g. No need for insulin 24 to 48 hours after delivery
   h. Hospitalized until insulin balance restored
5. Early recognition of insulin reaction and diabetic coma
6. Treatment and nursing management
   a. Weekly prenatal visits
   b. Regulation of insulin dosage and dietary management
   c. Mother taught to test blood three or four times a day
   d. Testing for placental adequacy: OCT (stress test) measures fetal response to uterine contractions; late deceleration indicates problem
   e. Teach good nutrition
   f. Help allay fears and anxieties

N. Addiction and pregnancy
1. Drug addition
   a. Effect on mother
      (1) Abortion
      (2) Premature birth
      (3) Stillbirth
   b. Effect on neonate: see Abnormal Newborn
2. Alcohol and pregnancy
   a. Effect on mother
      (1) Poor nutritional habits
      (2) Poor hygiene
      (3) Physical, psychosocial deterioration
   b. Effect on neonate: see Abnormal Newborn

3. Treatment and nursing management
   a. Supervised withdrawal
   b. Substitute therapy

ACQUIRED IMMUNODEFICIENCY SYNDROME (AIDS)

Pregnant women whose partners were drug users sharing common needles, high-risk category men (bisexual or homosexual), or men who were infected with the disease have been known to become infected. Transmission of the HIV virus to the unborn fetus has now been confirmed.
A. Confirmed avenues of transmission
   1. Anal/vaginal intercourse
   2. Drug addicts sharing needles of infected users
   3. Contaminated blood transfusions
   4. Transmission to the fetus or neonate can occur transplacentally or by exposure to blood and vaginal secretions at delivery and or by exposure to maternal secretion such as breast milk
   5. Cesarean section does not appear to prevent the transmission of the virus
B. Treatment and nursing management
   1. Pregnant HIV-infected women should receive pneumovax, influenza, and hepatitis vaccines and should be screened for sexually transmitted diseases
   2. HIV testing is voluntary and must be accompanied by informed consent and counseling; results are confidential
   3. Immune status needs to be monitored; if immune status falls physicians may elect to administer azidothymidine (AZT) to delay onset of illness
   4. HIV-positive women need counseling to practice safe sex to decrease risk of repeatedly exposing fetus
   5. Infants need to be followed and tested for a minimum of 2 years to determine if they have the disease
C. Centers for Disease Control (CDC) guidelines for preventing transmission of the AIDS virus
   1. Wear gloves when in contact with body fluids, mucous membranes, and nonintact skin; wear gloves when performing venipuncture or when handling items soiled with blood or body fluids
   2. Change gloves after caring for each patient; wash hands and most of your exposed surfaces with soap and water
   3. Wear masks, gown, and apron (if available); protect mucous membranes of your mouth, nose, and eyes
   4. Prevent injuries from needles, sharp instruments, toys, and other products; be alert when handling, cleaning, and disposing of instruments
   5. Avoid needle pricks; all sharp items that have been used should be placed in puncture-resistant containers; do not recap needles
   6. To minimize need for emergency mouth-to-mouth resuscitation, keep resuscitation bags, mouthpieces, and ventilation devices in easily located areas
   7. Refrain from direct patient care and do not handle patient care equipment if you have open lesions, weeping dermatitis, and so forth
   8. Pregnant nurses should be especially careful, as an HIV infection could place the fetus at risk
D. Minimum precautions for invasive procedures
   1. Wear gloves, surgical masks, and protective eyewear for all invasive procedures
      a. Prevent skin and mucous membrane contact with blood and other body fluids by using appropriate barrier precautions
      b. Wear protective eyewear or face shields, gowns, or aprons for procedures resulting in splashing to protect from blood or other body fluids
   2. Wear gloves and gowns when handling placenta or the infant until blood and amniotic fluid have been removed from the infant's skin and during postdelivery care of the umbilical cord
   3. Put on new gloves as soon as patient safety permits should you tear a glove or be injured by a needle-stick or other injury; always check gloves for holes

TUBERCULOSIS

Tuberculosis is an increasingly prevalent health problem throughout the world; its resurgence in the United States is attributed to homelessness, drug abuse, poverty, and human immunodeficiency virus (HIV); rates are particularly high among minorities and recent immigrants to the United States.
A. Confirmed avenues of transmission
   1. Airborne: coughs or sneezes of a person with infectious tuberculosis
   2. Shared air: persons in close air contact for a prolonged period of time
B. Treatment and nursing management
   1. Preventive therapy postponed until after delivery
   2. A pregnant woman with active disease needs immediate treatment of 2 to 3 antituberculosis drugs
   3. Breastfeeding is permitted; however, infant still needs to undergo prophylactic treatment

PREMATURE LABOR

A. Definition: labor occurring before 37 to 38 weeks' gestation
B. Effect on family (focus on psychosocial problems)
   1. Mother not ready for delivery: apprehensive and frightened; may feel guilty
   2. Family plus professional staff: restrained, quiet, anticipating complications
C. Effect on fetus: see Preterm Infant (Premature) under Abnormal Newborn, p.349
D. Treatment and nursing management
   1. Usually premature rupture of membranes precedes premature labor; test fluid with nitrazine paper: if alkaline, positive for amniotic fluid
   2. If membranes intact and cervix undilated, halt labor if possible
   3. Bed rest stat
   4. Monitor maternal pulse and blood pressure
   5. Know untoward effects of medications
   6. Prevent infection
   7. Offer constant emotional support to mother and family: inform, reassure, encourage mother and family

Normal Intrapartum (Labor and Delivery)

A. Fetal head (passenger)
   1. Two parietal bones: one each side of head
   2. Two temporal bones: one each side of head near temple
   3. Two frontal bones: one each side of forehead
   4. One occipital bone: lower back of head
   5. Sutures: membranous spaces between bones
      a. Sagittal suture: separates parietal bones and extends longitudinally back to front
      b. Frontal suture: between two frontal bones and is continuation of the sagittal suture

c. Coronal suture: like a crown, separates frontal and parietal bones

d. Lambdoidal suture: separates occipital bone from two parietal bones

6. Fontanels: formed by intersection of sutures; allow head bones to override and accommodate to birth passage

    a. Anterior fontanel: membranous, diamond-shaped space (bregma) formed by intersection of sagittal, frontal, and coronal sutures; called "soft spot"; closes within 12 to 18 months

    b. Posterior fontanel: small, membraneous triangle-shaped space between occipital bone and two parietal bones; closes within 6 to 8 weeks

7. Principal measurements of the fetal head

B. Presentations, positions, station

1. Presentation

    a. Definition: refers to that part of the passenger (fetus) that enters the passage (true pelvis, uterine os, vaginal canal) first

    b. Types of presentations

      (1) Cephalic: head, vertex, occiput (93%)

      (2) Breech: buttocks, sacrum, leg(s), foot (feet) (3%)

      (3) Shoulder: scapula (3%)

2. Lie (Fig. 7-6)

    a. Definition: refers to the relationship between the long axis of the passenger and the long axis of the mother

    b. Types

      (1) Longitudinal (99%)

      (2) Transverse (sideways)

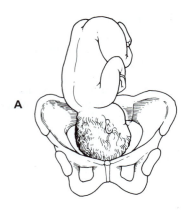

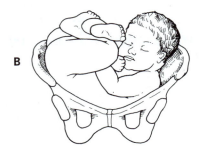

Figure 7-6. **A,** Longitudinal lie. **B,** Transverse lie. (From Philips CR: *Family-centered maternity/newborn care: a basic text,* ed 2, St Louis, 1987, Mosby.)

3. Position (Fig. 7-7)

    a. Definition: the way in which the presenting part of the fetus lies in relation to the four quadrants of the mother's pelvis and to her back (posterior) and her front (anterior)

    b. To determine position, fetal "reference points" are used, and they are

      (1) Occiput (back of fetal head): O

      (2) Chin (mentum): M

      (3) Brow (bregma): B

      (4) Buttocks (sacrum): S

      (5) Shoulder (scapula): Sc

      (6) Transversus

    c. Types of position with occiput presentations: LOA, LOT, LOP, ROA, ROT, ROP (see Fig. 7-7)

4. Attitude

    a. Definition: relationship of the various fetal parts to one another, or the relationship of the fetal extremities to its body (trunk)

    b. Normal attitude: flexed; fetal head on sternum, arms folded against chest; knees bent, pressing abdomen; legs flexed so toes touch arm

5. Station

    a. Definition: degree to which presenting part is located in the true pelvis; points of reference are the ischial spines, which are designated as *0* (zero)

    b. Levels

      (1) Minus: as in −1, −2, −3 station, means that presenting part is above the ischial spines

      (2) Plus: as in +1, +2, +3 station, means that the presenting part is below the ischial spines

      (3) −5 = floating; +5 = presenting part on perineum; or −3 to −5 = floating; +3 to +5 = presenting part on perineum; check with agency for the numbers used

C. Mechanisms and stages of labor: labor cannot progress without power

1. Definition: the steps or maneuvers the fetus must undertake to accommodate to the passage and be delivered

2. Process (mechanisms) (Fig. 7-8)

    a. Engagement: passage of the passenger into the pelvic inlet

    b. Descent: continuous slow progress of the fetus through the pelvis and the birth canal

    c. Flexion: head slowly adapts to birth canal by flexing chin

    d. Internal rotation: fetal head turns in corkscrew maneuver so the long diameter of the head is parallel to the longest diameter of the pelvic outlet

    e. Extension: the back of the fetal head goes under the pubic arch; the spine of the fetus extends to adapt itself to the curvature of the birth canal, and the head is delivered

    f. Restitution: as the head emerges, it rotates back 45 degrees to the position it was before internal rotation, which helps the shoulders accommodate to the outlet

    g. External rotation: the shoulders drop down and turn to the anteroposterior (AP) position, and the head slowly turns so both head and shoulders are aligned

    h. Expulsion: the posterior (underneath) shoulder is delivered by lateral flexion (upward motion); then the anterior upper shoulder will slide out (down-

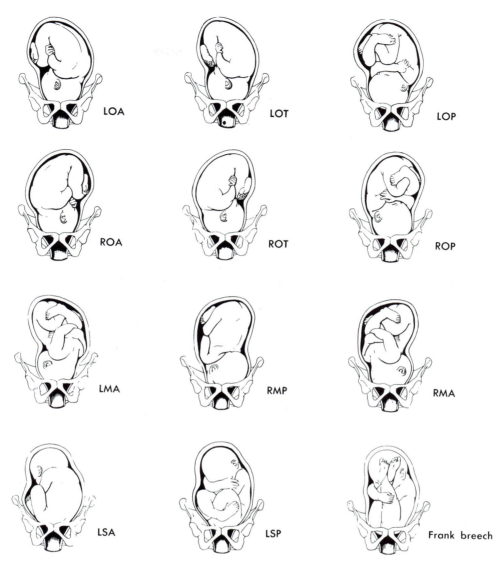

LOA   LOT   LOP

ROA   ROT   ROP

LMA   RMP   RMA

LSA   LSP   Frank breech

Figure 7-7.   **Categories of presentations.** (From Obstetrical presentation and position, Ross Laboratories Nursing Education Service, 1978. Reprinted with permission of Ross Laboratories, Columbus, Ohio.)

ward motion) from under the pubic arch, and the body is easily expelled

3. Stages of labor
   a. First stage: begins with the first true labor contraction; ends with complete dilatation and effacement of the cervix
   b. Second stage (expulsion): from complete effacement and dilatation to expulsion of the infant
   c. Third stage (placental): from delivery of the infant to delivery of the placenta and membranes (5 to 20 minutes)
   d. Fourth stage: from delivery of the secundines and repair of the perineum to 1 hour thereafter

D. Fetal evaluation during labor and delivery and immediately after
   1. During labor
      a. Fetal monitoring devices
         (1) Phonotransducer: amplification of fetal heart activity

         (2) Doppler transducer: ultrasonic device
      b. Special stethoscopes for monitoring FHT
         (1) Headscope (fetoscope): stethoscope on a head device; FHT conducted through monitor's frontal bone
         (2) Leff stethoscope: stethoscope with large, heavy conductor
      c. Direct fetal monitoring: an electrocardiogram (ECG) electrode is placed directly to the fetal head
   2. Evaluation immediately after delivery
      a. Establishment of patent airway
      b. Apgar scoring (Fig. 7-9): system of evaluating newborn response 1 minute after birth and 5 minutes after birth
      c. Observation for any visible anomalies

E. Nursing assessment
   1. Premonitory (impending) signs and symptoms of labor
      a. Lightening: descent of fetus down pelvic cavity

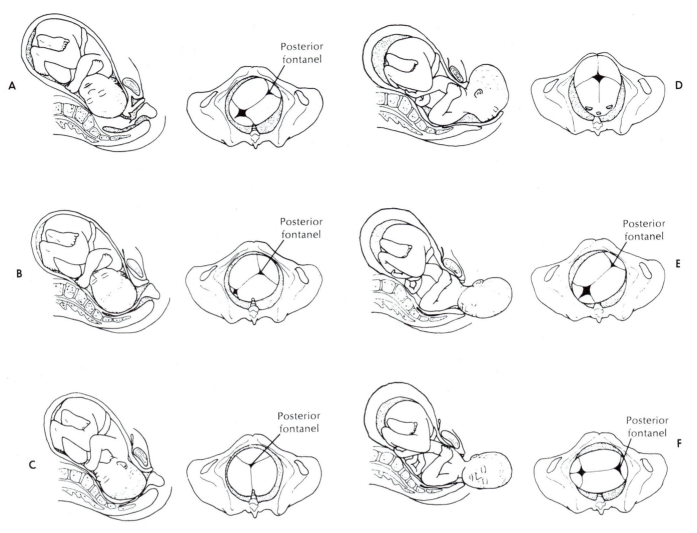

Figure 7-8. **Mechanism of labor in left occipitoanterior (LOA) presentation. A,** Engagement and descent. **B,** Flexion. **C,** Internal rotation to OA. **D,** Extension. **E,** Restitution. **F,** External rotation.

b. Braxton-Hicks contractions: painless contractions more frequent, regular
c. Breathing easier; heartburn disappears; hungry
d. Weight loss (decrease in water retention)
e. Frequency (pressure on bladder by presenting part)
f. Bloody show (slight pinkish discharge with or without discharge of mucous plug)
g. Bag of waters (BOW) ruptures spontaneously without prior contractions

2. Differences between true and false labor
a. False labor
(1) Contractions irregular
(2) No progress in interval or duration of contractions
(3) Some abdominal discomfort
(4) No bloody show
(5) Relief by walking
(6) No cervical change
(7) Discomfort mostly in front (lower abdomen)
b. True labor
(1) Contractions regular and progressive

(2) Not relieved by walking
(3) Cervical changes
(4) Progressive discomfort starting in back, going around lower abdomen, indentable fundus

3. Spontaneous rupture of membranes
a. Note time, amount
b. Prevent infection (handwashing, good hygienic practice)
c. Observe for prolapsed cord (notify physician immediately)
d. If leakage minimal, spontaneous resealing may occur
e. If close to EDC, contractions may begin, usually within 4 to 16 hours

F. Nursing intervention
1. Nursing management during first stage of labor
a. Admit patient to labor room
b. Establish rapport; ask pertinent questions regarding labor; observe reaction to labor process
c. Offer bedpan frequently (keep bladder empty)
d. Usually an IV is started to keep a vein open (KVO) (get equipment, solutions)

APGAR SCORING CHART

Sign	0	1	2
HEART RATE	Absent	Slow (below 100)	Over 100
RESPIRATORY EFFORT	Absent	Weak cry, hypoventilation	Good strong cry
MUSCLE TONE	Limp	Some flexion of extremities	Well flexed
REFLEX RESPONSE 1. Response to catheter in nostril (tested after oro-pharynx is clear)	No response	Grimace	Cough or sneeze
2. Tangential foot slap	No response	Grimace	Cry and withdrawal of foot
COLOR	Blue, pale	Body pink, extremities blue	Completely pink

Figure 7-9. **The Apgar scoring chart.** (From Philips CR: *Family-centered maternity/newborn care: a basic text,* ed 2, St Louis, 1987, Mosby.)

e. Monitor contractions, FHR
  (1) Hook up to fetal monitoring device
  (2) Check every 30 to 60 minutes (depending on progress)
f. Keep mother, father informed on status and progress
  (1) Effacement, dilatation, station
  (2) Encourage father to follow monitor readout
  (3) Encourage father to use comfort measures for mother
2. Nursing management during second stage of labor
  a. Uterine muscles bring about effacement and dilatation; abdominal muscles bring fetus down after dilatation and effacement are complete, and levator ani muscles assist in pushing and expelling fetus
  b. All monitoring equipment removed from mother
    (1) Explain procedures
    (2) Clean perineal area according to hospital policy
    (3) Monitor FHR every 5 minutes with fetoscope; inform physician on rate, strength, position
    (4) Check blood pressure every 15 minutes as necessary
    (5) Prepare necessary equipment for delivery readiness and for reception of baby
    (6) Instruct mother to push with contractions when indicated
    (7) When infant delivered completely, note time
    (8) Establish patent airway
    (9) Encourage mother and father to see, touch, and speak to infant
    (10) Carefully place prophylactic drops in each eye
    (11) Follow proper identification routine
    (12) Transfer infant into warm crib to transport to nursery for further evaluation and care
3. Nursing management during third stage (placental)
  a. Be sure cord blood specimen is taken
  b. Placenta delivered within 5 to 20 minutes from expulsion of infant
  c. Note time and which side of placenta delivered

  (1) Maternal side, raw and meaty: Duncan delivery
  (2) Fetal side, shiny and neat: Schultze delivery
  d. Administer oxytocin immediately following delivery of placenta to contract uterus and prevent hemorrhage
  e. Check blood pressure every 15 minutes
  f. Check fundus for firmness; soft, boggy indicates possible hemorrhaging
  g. Check and clean perineal area; apply sanitary napkin
  h. Mother may experience knees shaking, teeth chattering
    (1) Sudden changes in abdominal pressure plus hormonal changes trigger these symptoms
    (2) Place several warm blankets over mother
    (3) Reassure mother and family that it is a normal physiologic phenomenon
  i. Transfer mother to recovery area (if not in birthing room)
4. Nursing management during fourth stage of delivery
  a. Critical hour after delivery; watch for complications, especially hemorrhaging
  b. Perform fundal check every 5 minutes; massage gently if necessary
  c. Check blood pressure and vital signs every 10 to 15 minutes until stable
  d. Offer warm drink, toast, or even meal tray if mother wishes and physician approves
  e. Offer bedpan frequently to prevent bladder distention, which will impede involution
  f. After 1 hour, when vital signs are stable, give sponge bath to refresh and clean body
  g. Teach perineal care with peribottle
  h. Transfer to postpartum room
  i. Advise mother to request help the first time she wishes to use the bathroom
5. Commonly used medications during labor and delivery: prepared childbirth has greatly diminished use of analgesics and anesthetics during labor and delivery; patients who experience dystocia may need some

medication for relief from exhaustion, fright, or prolonged pain
  a. Amnesic
  b. Tranquilizer
  c. Analgesic
  d. Regional anesthesia
    (1) Paracervical block: anesthetizes cervical area
    (2) Pudendal block: peripheral nerve block; may also block urge to push for 30 minutes
    (3) Caudal block (spinal): used during first and second stages; continuous or one dosage
    (4) Saddle block: third, fourth, or fifth lumbar interspace; anesthetizes saddle area (inner groin, perineal area)
    (5) Epidural: also administered into lumbar interspace: uses less anesthetic than caudal; blocks urge to push
  e. Nursing management
    (1) Flat in bed after spinals
    (2) Observe for headache
    (3) Encourage urination
    (4) Force fluids
  f. General anesthesia: rare

Abnormal Intrapartum

DYSTOCIA
A. Definition: prolonged, difficult, painful labor or delivery involving any one or more problems with the three P's: passage, power, and passenger
B. Problems with passage
  1. Inadequate pelvis
  2. Soft tissue deviation
C. Problems with the power (uterine contractions)
  1. Primary uterine inertia: inefficient contractions from the beginning
  2. Secondary uterine inertia: well-established labor with good contractions at first; then progress suddenly or gradually slows and stops altogether
  3. Hypotonic contractions (atonic uterus); most common; no progress in effacement or dilatation
  4. Hypertonic uterine contractions
    a. Intense, titanic
    b. No interval between contractions
  5. Dystonic contractions
    a. Painful
    b. Ineffective
    c. Asymmetric (contractions in different segments of the uterus)
D. Problems with passenger (fetus)
  1. Excessive size
  2. Fetal anomaly
  3. Fetal malposition or malpresentation
    a. Occiput posterior (most common)
    b. Breech
    c. Transverse
    d. Face
    e. Soldier (military) presentation
  4. Cephalopelvic disproportion (CPD)
    a. Accommodation impossible
    b. May note unusual contour of uterus or abdomen
E. Complications
  1. Premature rupture of membranes
  2. Predisposition to infection
  3. Trauma
  4. Hemorrhage
  5. Prolapse of cord
  6. Hypoxia of fetus
  7. Severe molding of fetal head: danger of intracranial hemorrhage
  8. Extreme backache (posterior positions)
  9. Flowering of anus early because of pressure of occiput on lower sacral region, with subsequent residual of hemorrhoids
  10. Extreme fatigue
F. Treatment and nursing management
  1. Electronic monitoring of fetus and mother
  2. Frequent confirmation of cervical progress
  3. Sterile techniques during vaginal examination
  4. Check status of BOW
  5. Check vital signs
  6. Observe condition of mother
    a. Need for pain relief
    b. Sometimes after a medicated sleep or rest dystocia disappears
  7. Support physical and psychologic needs
  8. Watch for dehydration
  9. Spontaneous rotation toward end of transition may occur in occiput posteriors

SUPINE HYPOTENSIVE SYNDROME
A. Definition: condition caused by compression of vena cava by heavy uterus for a prolonged period; caused by mother's staying in one position for a long time
B. Signs and symptoms
  1. Pallor
  2. Light-headedness
  3. Dizziness
  4. Slight nausea
C. Treatment and nursing management: turn patient on left side to relieve pressure; advise frequent turning and changing of position

RUPTURED UTERUS
A. Causes
  1. Titanic, pauseless contractions for unexplainable reasons
  2. Stretching of uterine walls by extensive, rapid growth of hydatidiform mole
  3. Unmonitored pitocin infusion
B. Treatment and nursing management
  1. Prepare for cesarean section (CS)
  2. Prepare for all anticipatory nursing responsibilities, surgical or medical

PROLAPSED CORD
A. Definition: displacement of the cord below the presenting part and into the vaginal passage before delivery of fetus
B. Causes
  1. Spontaneous rupture of the membranes before engagement
  2. Breech presentations
  3. Prematurity
  4. Polyhydramnios
  5. Abnormal presentations
C. Signs and symptoms
  1. Cord may be seen, felt, or palpated
  2. Fetal heart pattern abnormal

D. Treatment and nursing management
1. Do not compress cord; do not try to reposition it
2. Sterile saline compress to keep cord moist and protected from infection
3. Place mother in knee-chest position or in Trendelenburg's position so presenting part is pushed away from cord by gravity
4. Preparation for cesarean section, blood crossmatch, IV fluids, and so on
5. Check FHR every 5 minutes
6. Support frightened mother and family

MULTIPLE PREGNANCIES
A. Definition: simultaneous gestation; twins, triplets, quadruplets, quintuplets, sextuplets, septuplets
B. Signs and symptoms
1. Not always discernible
2. History of twins (female lineage)
3. Hearing two FHTs, each with own rate
4. Disclosure of multiple limbs, heads, by palpation
5. Larger than normal gestation uterus
6. Weight gain increased more than in normal gestation
7. Striae gravidarum more noticeable early on
8. Confirmation by x-ray examination, sonogram
C. Types (Fig. 7-10)
1. Single-ovum twins (monozygotic, identical)
   a. Union of one sperm with one ovum
   b. During mitosis divides into two embryos
   c. One placenta, two amniotic sacs
   d. Same sex
   e. Heredity a factor
2. Fraternal twins (dizygotic, unidentical)
   a. Union of two sperm with two separate ova
   b. Two amniotic sacs
   c. Separate or fused placenta
   d. Same or different sex
   e. Do not look alike
   f. Age of mother a factor; older women tend to release more than one ovum
3. Formation of triplets and so on is varied
D. Treatment and nursing management
1. Prenatal care
   a. Visits increased
   b. Observe for signs and symptoms of preeclampsia
   c. Premature labor common
   d. Backaches common: support girdle, longer rest periods
   e. Varicosities common
   f. Watch for complications resulting from position, presentation, lie of fetuses
   g. Size of fetuses may cause problems
   h. Be alert for possible cesarean section
2. Natal care
   a. Be prepared for premature labor and premature babies
   b. High-risk second stage
3. Third and fourth stages
   a. Possibility of hemorrhage because of oversized uterus
   b. Blood loss greater than for single births
   c. Oxytocin not administered to mother until all babies delivered
   d. Risk of infection greater than in normal single births
   e. Perinatal mortality greater than in single deliveries

INDUCTION OF LABOR
A. Definition: the use of medication (oxytocin) to stimulate contractions
B. Indications
1. Overdue fetus (over 42 weeks' gestation)
2. Fetal death/uterine death

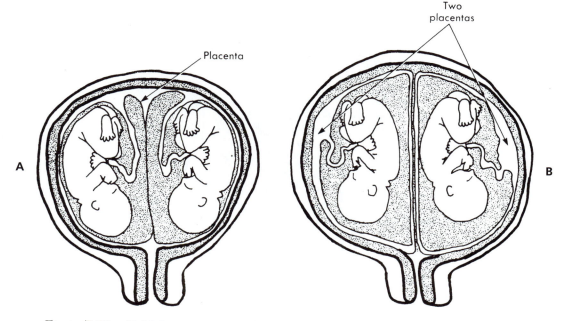

Figure 7-10. **Multiple pregnancy. A,** Identical (monozygotic) twins: two sacs, one placenta. **B,** Fraternal (dizygotic) twins: two sacs, two placentas. (From Philips CR: *Family-centered maternity/newborn care: a basic text,* ed 2, St Louis, 1987, Mosby.)

3. Uterine inertia, primary or secondary
4. Atonic or hypotonic uterine contractions (may be enhanced by a boost of oxytocin)
5. Prolonged rupture of membranes (over 24 hours) if uterine contractions have not begun
6. Diabetic mother
7. Severe preeclampsia (exercise extreme caution)
8. Steeply rising Rh titer

C. Contraindications
1. Cephalopelvic disproportion (CPD)
2. Fetal distress
3. Previous cesarean section
4. Multiple births
5. Heart conditions
6. Prematurity
7. Unengaged presenting part

D. Treatment and nursing management
1. Monitor contractions carefully
2. If there are no intervals between contractions, stop medication drip and call physician immediately
3. Monitor FHR and report any changes stat
4. Check blood pressure: gradual elevation warrants immediate discontinuation of medication and prompt notification of doctor
5. Keep family and mother informed of progress and procedure

OPERATIVE OBSTETRICS

A. Episiotomy
1. Definition: surgical incision of the perineum during delivery to enlarge the vaginal outlet
2. Types (Fig. 7-11)
3. Indications
   a. To avoid tearing
   b. To shorten second stage of labor

c. Fetus or mother is in jeopardy
4. Treatment and nursing management
   a. Comfort measures (promote healing)
   b. Encourage Kegel exercises—lessen pain and promote healing
   c. Apply witch hazel pads to perineal area (decrease swelling, promote healing)

B. Forceps deliveries
1. Definition: an operative procedure using various instruments to deliver the presenting part
2. Indications for use
   a. To shorten second stage
   b. Assist in descent of presenting part when there has been poor progress
   c. Maternal exhaustion
   d. When rotation (of head) is necessary, e.g., left occiput posterior (LOP) to occiput anterior (OA)
   e. To save fetus in jeopardy
3. Requirements for application
   a. No cephalopelvic disproportion
   b. Presenting part engaged and below ischial spines
   c. Full dilatation and effacement
   d. Ruptured membranes
   e. Empty bladder
   f. FHR checked before and after application
4. Complications
   a. Lacerations and tears
   b. Hemorrhage
   c. Rupture of uterus
   d. Facial marks or facial paralysis of fetus
   e. Intracranial hemorrhage or brain damage to fetus

C. Cesarean section
1. Definition: an operative procedure to deliver the fetus through a surgical incision made through the abdominal and uterine walls

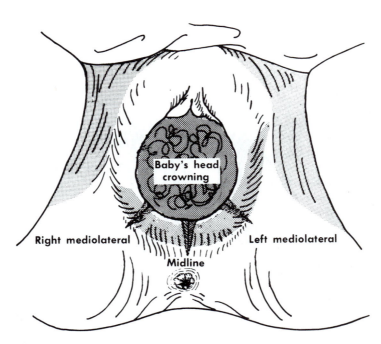

Figure 7-11. Three types of episiotomies. (From Hamilton PM: *Basic maternity nursing,* ed 6, St Louis, 1988, Mosby.)

2. Indications
   a. Cephalopelvic disproportion
   b. Fetal distress
   c. Prematurity
   d. Dystocia
   e. Prolapsed cord
   f. Oversized infant
   g. Positions and presentations undeliverable through the vagina
   h. Some hypertensive states, placenta previa, abruptio placentae, prolapsed cord abnormalities
   i. Maternal exhaustion
3. Types
   a. Elective
      (1) Anticipated difficulties: for example, inadequate pelvis or vaginal deliveries inadvisable because mother has AIDS or herpes
      (2) Previous cesarean sections (selective)
   b. Emergency
      (1) Sudden fetal distress
      (2) Accident
4. Treatment and nursing management
   a. Routine surgical preoperative and postoperative care plus normal postpartum care
   b. Promote involution
   c. Perineal care
   d. Lochia; color amount same as for vaginal delivery
   e. Support mother and family; allay fears
   f. Watch for signs and symptoms of infection (chills, fever)
5. Care of cesarean section newborn
   a. Place in incubator or Isolette for 24 hours
   b. Section babies prone to respiratory distress
   c. Controlled humidity to assist absorption of fluid in lungs
6. Vaginal birth after cesarean (VBAC): vaginal delivery after a cesarean section may be encouraged; depends on reason for cesarean section

Normal Postpartum

A. Definition: period from end of fourth stage of labor to 6 weeks after day of delivery
B. Immediate care following delivery
   1. Continue checking of vital signs
   2. Encourage urination
      a. Full bladder impedes involution
      b. Full bladder may cause excessive bleeding
   3. Offer food: if policy permits, offer food and drink to mother after vital signs are stable
   4. Care of fundus
      a. Check for firmness
      b. Lochia checked for color, amount, and presence of clots
   5. Provide perineal care and care of breasts
   6. General hygiene: shower may be permissible to clean, refresh mother after vital signs are stable (policies vary)
   7. Encourage putting infant to breast for feeding and bonding
C. Physiologic changes during puerperium
   1. Reproductive organs
      a. Uterus: involution (return of uterus to normal size and function)
         (1) Walls of uterus return to normal in 3 to 4 weeks
         (2) Menstruation may return in 3 to 4 weeks

(3) Nursing mothers: menstruation may be delayed several months
(4) Fundus involutes 1 finger width every day if umbilicus is used as point of reference (Fig. 7-12)
   b. Vagina
      (1) Returns to normal within 3 to 6 weeks after delivery, depending on type of delivery, length of labor, lacerations, healing process, and so on
      (2) Cesarean sections: vaginal recovery rapid
   c. Perineal area
      (1) Should be intact and clean
      (2) Complete healing should take 5 to 7 days
   2. Return to normal of body system and functions
      a. Hormonal recovery begins immediately
      b. Lochia: vaginal discharge coming from decidual lining of uterus after delivery
         (1) Lochia rubra: dark red to bright red; occasional clots; flow lasts 2 to 3 days
         (2) Lochia serosa: pale pink to brownish lochia; lighter flow, dependent on ambulation; lasts 2 to 5 days
         (3) Lochia alba: yellowish, creamy discharge consisting of leukocytes and dead cells; lasts 5 to 10 days
         (4) Prolonged or recurring bleeding may indicate a medical problem
      c. Vascular system
         (1) Average loss of blood at delivery: 250 to 400 ml
         (2) Blood loss of 500 ml or more considered hemorrhage
      d. Urinary tract
         (1) Perineal soreness may temporarily reduce voiding reflexes
         (2) Marked diuresis 8 to 12 hours postpartum
D. Treatment and nursing management during postpartum
   1. Objectives for daily care

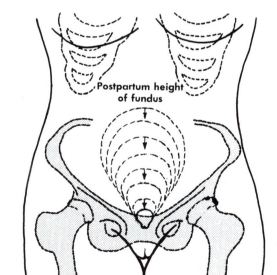

Figure 7-12. Involution. Height of fundus as it descends to prepregnant levels postpartum. (From Hamilton PM: *Basic maternity nursing*, ed 6, St. Louis, 1988, Mosby.)

a. Assist in normal process of involution
b. Prevent infection
c. Promote infant bonding with mother and family
2. Nursing techniques for postpartum care
   a. Vital signs: watch for symptoms of hypovolemic shock and hemorrhage (fainting); stay with mother who is out of bed (OOB) for the first time since delivery
   b. Check breasts
     (1) Should be soft until milk comes in
     (2) Daily cleansing in shower
     (3) Daily breast examination to note any complications; nodules may be felt second or third day as milk production begins; teach breast self-examination; report any abnormalities
   c. Engorgement
     (1) Nursing usually prevents this; breast pump; nipple shield
     (2) Nonnursing mother
      (a) Cold compresses or ice bag on breasts
      (b) Tight binder for 1 to 2 days
      (c) Restrict fluids for 1 to 2 days
      (d) Follow steps a, b, c only if requested
   d. Infections
     (1) Redness, warmth, pain, elevated temperature
     (2) May require minor surgical intervention to release drainage
   e. Check fundus
     (1) Height and firmness for proper involution
     (2) Relaxed fundus may indicate problem (hemorrhage or infection)
   f. Check lochia: color, amount, odor
   g. Check perineal area: healing and cleanliness
   h. Check legs: pain, tenderness, swelling (thrombi); check for Homans' sign
   i. Check urination: overdistention (subinvolution)
   j. Bowels: keep open (encourage fluids with balanced diet): administer stool softener (e.g., docusate sodium sulfosuccinate [Colace])
   k. Afterpains: involution
   l. Postpartum blues (baby blues): possible hormonal transitory depression
3. Teaching: important component of postpartum nursing management
   a. Personal hygiene
   b. Weight loss
     (1) Immediately after delivery, 7- to 10-lb weight loss
     (2) Total weight loss of pregnancy may take 6 weeks to 6 months or more to achieve
   c. PKU tests: requirement by law to test for inborn error of metabolism involving proteins and amino acids
   d. Capacity of newborn and infant stomach:
     (1) At birth can take 1 to 2 oz (30 to 60 ml) per feeding
     (2) By 1 to 2 weeks, can nurse 4 oz (120 ml) per feeding
     (3) Gradual increase to 6 to 8 oz (180 to 240 ml) per feeding in 1 month
   e. Discuss with mother and father
     (1) Importance of bonding
     (2) Readiness for parenthood
   f. Postpartum exercises
   g. Review methods of holding, bubbling, or burping baby

Abnormal Postpartum
POSTPARTUM INFECTION
A. Definition: any infection in the reproductive organs during labor, delivery, or up to 1 month postpartum
B. Signs and symptoms
  1. Chills, fever, localized back pain (kidney involvement)
  2. Malaise
  3. Lower abdominal tenderness, lower back pains
  4. Foul-smelling lochia (retained placental infection)
  5. Fundal height changes abnormal
C. Treatment and nursing management in general
  1. Administration of appropriate antibiotics on time and as directed
  2. Comfort measures appropriate to discomfort
  3. Check vital signs q4h
D. Specific infections
  1. Urinary track infection (cystitis, pyelitis)
    a. Cause: trauma (stretching or tearing) or by an organism
    b. Signs and symptoms
     (1) 3 days postpartum
     (2) Low back pain
     (3) Localized pain (pyelitis)
     (4) Chills, high fever, apprehension
     (5) Frequency and burning urination (cystitis)
     (6) Discomfort
    c. Treatment and nursing management
     (1) Bed rest until symptoms subside (1 day)
     (2) Drugs (antibiotics)
     (3) Force fluids
     (4) Careful handwashing by mother and nursing staff
  2. Mastitis
    a. Definition: inflammation of the glands in the breast(s); if untreated could lead to abscess complications
    b. Cause
     (1) Staphylococcus infection
     (2) Stasis of milk
     (3) Bruising of breast tissue
     (4) Open cuts in nipple or areola
    c. Signs and symptoms
     (1) High fever (103°F; 39.5°C)
     (2) Chills
     (3) Red, tender, painful, hard
    d. Treatment and nursing management
     (1) Support bra
     (2) Antibiotic therapy
     (3) Check incision for drainage
     (4) Reassurance of mother
     (5) Discontinuation of breast-feeding in most cases
  3. Thrombophlebitis
    a. Definition: infection or clot occurring in the deep pelvic veins when placental site becomes infected
    b. Signs and symptoms
     (1) Local tenderness: femoral vein
     (2) 1 to 2 weeks postpartum
     (3) Swelling, chills, fever
    c. Treatment and nursing management
     (1) Administration of anticoagulant
     (2) Bed rest
     (3) Antibiotic therapy
     (4) Elevation of legs
     (5) Warm, wet compresses every 15 to 30 minutes
     (6) Never massage

POSTPARTUM HEMORRHAGE
A. Definition: any loss of 500 ml or more of blood during first 24 hours following delivery
B. Types
1. Early postpartal hemorrhage resulting from uterine atony (1 to 3 days)
2. Late postpartal hemorrhage resulting from subinvolution (inability of the uterus to involute or return to its prepregnant state) or placental infection
C. Causes
1. Mismanagement of the third stage
2. Retained placental fragments
3. Complications of labor and delivery
4. Complications of pregnancy
5. Inversion (uterine)
D. Signs and symptoms
1. Visible blood loss
2. Shocklike symptoms: pale, clammy, hypotensive, apprehensive
E. Treatment and nursing management
1. Warm drink, warm covers
2. IV fluids
3. Replacement transfusion if appropriate
4. Quiet assurance; support to family and mother
5. Medical management of cause

HEMATOMAS
A. Definition: local accumulation of blood caused by
1. Undue pressure of heavy gravid uterus
2. Bearing down inappropriately
3. Long second stage
4. Primigravida's prolonged pushing
B. Signs and symptoms
1. Visible vaginal hematoma
2. Vulvular hematoma
3. Large blood-filled sac visible
C. Treatment and nursing management
1. Ice to area for 24 hours
2. Analgesics if ordered
3. Incision or ligation if necessary
4. Comfort measures similar to episiotomy care, that is, sitz bath

SUBINVOLUTION
A. Definition: inability of the uterus to return to its normal size after delivery
B. Cause
1. Retention of placental pieces
2. Infection (endometrium)
C. Signs and symptoms
1. Involution process abnormal
2. Boggy uterus (not firm); foul odor
3. Intermittent or constant lochia rubra after cycle has passed
D. Treatment and nursing management
1. Surgical intervention (D&C)
2. Support and reassurance to mother and family

Normal Newborn
A. Immediate care following delivery
1. Maintain patent airway
2. Apply cord clamp, check for bleeding, follow procedure for daily cord care
3. Maintain warmth
   a. Wrap in prewarmed receiving blankets
   b. Place in preheated crib
4. Preventive care
   a. Instill prophylactic eye drops to each eye as required by law to prevent ophthalmia neonatorum
   b. Commonly used prophylactic drugs: silver nitrate, erythromycin, penicillin ointments/drops
   c. Administer intramuscular (IM) injection of vitamin K to reduce likelihood of hemorrhage (optional)
5. Identification procedures
   a. Complete identification bands as required
   b. Record footprints of baby and pointer fingerprint of mother
6. Apgar scoring
7. Initial observation of newborn
   a. Is the primary responsibility of physician/pediatrician
   b. Nurse should wear gloves when handling newborn during immediate care and until initial bath; regulations differ for daily routines
   c. Nurse also makes quick observation, checking for visible anomalies such as cleft lip, cleft palate, extra digits, spinal column, limbs, skin, head
   d. Reflexes that nurse may check include Moro's, sucking, rooting, blinking, grasping
8. Encourage bonding
   a. After initial delivery room care, wipe off excess blood and debris from baby; wrap securely in clean, warm receiving blanket and let parents hold baby
   b. Allow time for mother and father to look at, touch, and hold infant
B. Normal physiology of newborn
1. Vital signs
   a. Temperature: 96° to 99° F (35.5° to 37° C); baby loses body heat in delivery room and during transit
   b. Pulse rate: 120 to 160 beats/min
      (1) Apical pulse rate
      (2) Irregular in rate and cadence (normal)
   c. Respirations: abdominal and irregular, 32 to 40 per minute
2. Measurements
   a. Weight
      (1) Girls 7 lb (3100 g)
      (2) Boys 7½ lb (3300 g)
      (3) 5 to 8 lb (2500 to 4000 g) considered normal
      (4) 5% to 10% weight loss in first 2 to 3 days
      (5) Regains birth weight in 5 to 7 days
   b. Length: 18 to 22 inches (45 to 55 cm) long
   c. Head circumference: 13 to 14 inches (33 to 35 cm)
   d. Chest circumference: 12 to 13 inches (30 to 33 cm)
3. Skin
   a. Milia: small, white sebaceous glands visible about nose, forehead, chin
   b. "Stork bites": telangiectasis or capillary hemangiomas
   c. Red nevi: discoloration, circumscribed, blanch on touch, prominent during crying, disappear in 6 months to a year
   d. Mongolian spots: bluish, bruiselike spots on buttocks, back, shoulders; disappear by toddler or preschool age and found in babies of Hispanic, black, Slavic, or oriental background
   e. Erythema toxicum neonatorum (newborn rash):

appears as scratches and pimples; may be nosocomial infection

f. Nevi vasculosus (strawberry mark): bright red or dark capillary hemangiomas with raised, rough surfaces; usually disappear by school age

g. Nevi flammeus (port-wine stain): reddish purple raised capillary hemangiomas; do not blanch on pressure and may not disappear

h. Lanugo: soft, downy hair on top of skin on ears, forehead, neck, shoulders; disappears in weeks

i. Vernix caseosa: cheeselike protective material coating fetus, especially under arms, beneath knees, and in folds of thighs

j. Acrocyanosis: extremities are bluish for several hours after delivery

4. Elimination
   a. Urine: 3 to 4 times a day for first few days; usually urinates after every feeding
   b. Bowel movement: 5 to 6 times a day for first week
      (1) Meconium: expelled within 2 to 12 hours; black, tarry, thick unformed stool
      (2) Transient stool: blackish or greenish stool expelled after first few feedings
   c. Breast-fed stool: yellow, odorless, slightly runny
   d. Bottle-fed stool: formed, brownish yellow, distinct odor
   e. Each infant establishes own pattern of stool movement

5. Hyperestrogenism and its effect on the newborn
   a. Swelling of the breasts in male or female infant because of hormones from mother; the ensuing discharge is called "witches milk"
   b. Swelling of the male scrotum: large, with rugae; disappears within days

6. Reproductive organs of the male newborn
   a. Cryptorchidism: testes have not descended into scrotum; often present in premature infants
   b. Occasionally testes are in inguinal sac at birth but will descend within hours or more; if undescended after 1 month, pediatrician should evaluate
   c. Prepuce (foreskin) should be carefully retracted daily during bath time if newborn is uncircumcised; some prepuces will not retract for months or years

7. Circulatory system: pulmonary circulation established within minutes of birth

8. Digestive system: immature at birth but can metabolize nutrients except fats

9. Visual capabilities: immature coordination and muscle control

10. Hearing capabilities: acute hearing within 2 minutes of birth

11. Taste perception: can distinguish sweet and sour in 1 to 3 days

12. Smelling perception: can distinguish smell of mother at 5 days

13. Sleep patterns
    a. Unstable for 6 to 8 hours after birth
    b. Has regular and irregular sleep cycles

14. Newborn reflexes
    a. Sucking, rooting, swallowing, extrusion reflexes
    b. Tonic neck (fencing) should disappear in 3 to 4 months
    c. Grasping (palmar) lessens in 3 to 4 months
    d. Moro's (startle) disappears in 2 months
    e. Dancing (stepping, walking) disappears in 3 to 4 weeks
    f. Babinski's (plantar): absence indicates CNS damage
    g. Blinking, sneezing

15. Immunity in the newborn
    a. Has 3-month supply from mother if baby is term
    b. Begins own synthesis by 3 months of age

C. Daily observation and nursing care
   1. Newborn nursery care and observation
      a. Constant, careful observation
      b. After transferring infant from delivery room, place in warmer until vital signs are stable
      c. Check temperature; follow agency policy (rectal, axilla, etc.)
         (1) Drops 3° first hour after delivery
         (2) Heat production normal in 2 to 3 days
         (3) Newborn loses heat through convection, conduction, radiation, and evaporation
      d. Check respirations
      e. Place infant on right side to promote expansion of lungs and drain excess mucus
      f. Observe for signs and symptoms of respiratory distress syndrome (RDS)
      g. Check for bleeding
      h. Cord
         (1) Removal of cord clamp within 8 to 24 hours
         (2) Daily application of antigermicidal agent to prevent infections
      i. Check eyes and ears for abnormal drainage
   2. Daily nursery routine
      a. Daily weight and vital signs, especially temperature
      b. Observation and recording condition of skin, cord, eyes, elimination
      c. Daily care and changing of crib linen
         (1) Daily cord care
         (2) General observation
      d. During feeding routine observe infant-mother bonding
   3. Teaching mothers care of newborn: mothers' classes should incorporate the care, handling, and dressing of the newborn in addition to procedures and demonstrations in sponge baths, tub baths, and cord care
   4. Daily bath routine
      a. Purpose
         (1) Cleansing
         (2) Exercise time
         (3) Play, social time with mother (bonding time)
      b. Prepare environment: select safe, convenient, warm area
      c. Select and prepare equipment
         (1) Utensils for sponge or tub bath
         (2) Necessary articles for procedure
         (3) Clean clothing
      d. Sponge baths: recommended for babies with cord intact
      e. Tub baths: recommended for babies whose cord has fallen off—10 to 14 days after birth
   5. Cord care
      a. Wipe base of cord with alcohol or designated antiseptic every time diapers are changed and during bath time
      b. After cord falls off

(1) Wipe with alcohol as instructed after daily bath routine for first day or two

(2) If drainage persists, cleanse with alcohol and notify pediatrician

6. Diaper rash
   a. Change diapers frequently
   b. Wash area with warm tap water
   c. Apply A and D Ointment as a preventative and protective
   d. Expose to air if possible
      (1) Lay infant on abdomen and expose buttocks to air
      (2) Apply Desitin or Balmex if A and D Ointment does not help

7. Circumcision
   a. Definition: the surgical cutting and removal of foreskin; usually done 1 to 3 days after birth
   b. Treatment and nursing management
      (1) Observe for bleeding
      (2) Petrolatum (Vaseline) gauze for 3 days
      (3) Check and record first voiding after procedure
      (4) Complications: rare

8. Facts about feeding the newborn
   a. Newborn metabolic rate twice that of adult
   b. Carbohydrates needed for brain growth and as source of energy
   c. Protein needed for building tissue; inadequacy results in infection, slow growth, flabby muscles
   d. Fat difficult to digest and metabolize but needed to maintain integrity of skin
   e. Iron: continuous supply needed for growth and development; storage from mother depleted in 4 to 6 months

9. Facts about breast milk
   a. Less protein than cow's milk; easier to digest
   b. More lactose than cow's milk, which facilitates metabolism and is good for bones
   c. Lactoferrin decreases dangers to infection
   d. Sucking stimulates posterior pituitary of mother to trigger let-down reflex, which allows milk to flow

10. Guidelines for breastfeeding
    a. A general rule of thumb is to nurse until breasts are soft
    b. To ensure a good supply of breast milk, the mother should
       (1) Have adequate rest
       (2) Drink sufficient fluids
       (3) Eat a balanced, nutritious diet
       (4) Maintain psychologic equilibrium

11. The length of time for breastfeeding varies considerably from infant to infant and is normally 10 to 30 minutes. Limiting the time of nursing on each breast is no longer considered effective in preventing sore nipples. It is more important to use correct technique and empty the breasts completely

Abnormal Newborn

THE PRETERM (PREMATURE) INFANT

A. Definition: a baby born before 37 weeks' gestation and weighing less than 5½ lb (2500 g)

B. Infants may be small for gestational age (SGA) because they are preterm or from genetic or intrauterine causes

C. Statistics
   1. Of all live births 7% are premature
   2. Incidence of prematurity increases to 10% in some minority populations
   3. Prematurity is leading cause of death in infants in the United States

D. Cause
   1. Young, adolescent mothers
   2. Elderly primigravidas
   3. Multiple births
   4. Poor prenatal care
   5. Congenital anomalies
   6. Diseases or conditions that compromise fetus
      a. Pregnancy-induced hypertension
      b. Diabetes
      c. Heart disease
      d. Nutritional deficits
      e. Neglect
      f. Drug or alcohol addictions
      g. Smoking
      h. Placental insufficiency

E. Characteristics of a premature infant
   1. Central nervous system
      a. Poor muscle tone
      b. Poor reflexes
      c. Limp
      d. Assumes froglike position
      e. Weak, feeble cry
      f. Unstable heating mechanism: temperature fluctuates from 94° to 96° F (34° to 36° C)
      g. Poor sucking reflexes
      h. Weak gagging and swallowing reflexes
   2. Respiratory system
      a. Insufficient surfactant
      b. Immature lungs, rib cage, muscles
      c. Prone to respiratory distress syndrome (RDS)
      d. Poor oxygenation
   3. Digestive system: immature gastric system
   4. Integumentary system
      a. Harlequin pattern observed
      b. Veins and capillaries visible
      c. Lanugo prominent
      d. Vernix prominent
      e. No subcutaneous fat
      f. Skin tight, shiny, taut
   5. Circulatory system
      a. Fragile capillaries
      b. Susceptible to hemorrhages (intracranial)
   6. Renal system
      a. Inability to urinate properly
      b. Easily dehydrated
      c. Fragile electrolyte balance
   7. Immune system
      a. Too young to have obtained any immunity from mother
      b. Vulnerable to infection
   8. Endocrine system: a common complication is hypoglycemia
   9. Head
      a. Fontanels large
      b. Suture lines prominent
      c. Old looking in appearance

F. Treatment and nursing management

1. Maintain patent airway
2. Frequently monitor blood gases to determine oxygen need
3. Maintain body temperature by placing in Isolette
4. Conserve energy: basic care only
5. Provide adequate nutrition
   a. Nasogastric feedings
   b. Special soft nipples
   c. Parenteral fluids
6. Prevent infection
   a. Prevent skin breakdown: change positions
   b. Keep dry and clean
7. Length of hospitalization: until a weight of 5½ lb (2500 g) is reached
8. Mothering stimulation taught and practiced
   a. Encourage parents to stroke, cuddle, talk
   b. Feed, diaper infants
   c. Play soft music
   d. Encourage tapping on Isolette and talking
9. Listen to concerns of mothers and fathers

POSTMATURE INFANT

A. Definition: over 43 weeks' gestation
B. Cause: unknown
C. Characteristics of postmature infant
   1. Old looking
   2. No vernix; no lanugo
   3. Color: yellow-green or meconium stained
   4. Desquamation of hands (palms) and feet (soles)
   5. May have respiratory problems
D. Nursing management
   1. Observe for hypoglycemia
   2. Observe for RDS
   3. Look for birth injuries
   4. Symptomatic nursing care

NEONATAL RESPIRATORY DISTRESS SYNDROME

A. Definition
   1. A series of symptoms signifying respiratory distress
   2. Synonyms: RDS, hyaline membrane disease (HMD)
B. Statistics
   1. Common in premature babies
   2. Leading cause of death in infants in the United States
C. Cause
   1. Lack or loss of surfactant in lungs
   2. Immaturity
   3. Hypoxia
   4. Hypothermia
D. Signs and symptoms
   1. Appears within minutes to hours after birth
   2. Grunting, rib retraction, nasal flaring (RDS symptoms)
   3. Inadequate oxygen: 60 or more respirations per minute
E. Diagnosis: x-ray examination shows collapsed portions of lungs; arterial blood gases reveal hypoxia
F. Treatment and nursing management
   1. Transfer to intensive care unit and Isolette care
   2. Initiate oxygen therapy: 60%; hood is best
      a. IPPB (intermittent positive pressure breathing)
      b. CPAP (continuous positive airway pressure)
      c. Monitor blood gases
   3. Endotracheal tube if necessary
   4. IV hydration and nutrition and antibiotic therapy

5. Place in modified Trendelenburg's position
G. Complication
   1. Retrolental fibroplasia
   2. Causes
      a. High arterial oxygen levels
      b. Retinal vascular immaturity

BIRTH INJURIES

A. Normal deviations of the head
   1. Caput succedaneum (Fig. 7-13)
      a. Definition: edema (water) under the scalp
      b. Cause: continuous pressure of the fetal head on cervix
      c. Signs and symptoms
         (1) Crosses suture lines
         (2) Appears at birth
         (3) Disappears in 3 to 4 days
      d. Treatment: none
   2. Cephalhematoma (Fig. 7-13)
      a. Definition: blood between the periosteum and bone
      b. Cause: pressure during delivery (forceps)
      c. Signs and symptoms
         (1) Never crosses suture lines
         (2) Appears several hours to several days after birth
         (3) Disappears within 3 to 6 weeks
      d. Treatment: none
   3. Molding (Fig. 7-14)
      a. Definition: changes in the shape of the head
      b. Cause: accommodation of fetal bones to birth canal during labor and delivery
      c. Signs and symptoms: visual
      d. Treatment: disappears without treatment in 3 days
   4. Soft tissue injuries (subcutaneous fat necrosis)
      a. Definition: pressure necrosis
      b. Signs and symptoms: purplish, movable mass
      c. Treatment: resolves spontaneously
B. Subconjunctival hemorrhage (scleral or retinal)
   1. Definition: rupture of small capillaries in eye
   2. Cause: increased intracranial pressure of birth
   3. Signs and symptoms: small, red pin dots in white of sclera, or hemorrhaging in retina
   4. Treatment: resolves without treatment in 5 days
C. Ecchymosis, petechiae, edema
   1. Definition: blood within tissues; does not blanch with pressure
   2. Cause: forceps, manipulation, pressure
   3. Signs and symptoms: visual in affected areas
   4. Treatment: resolves without treatment in 2 days
D. Skeletal injuries
   1. Skull fracture: rare, and unless blood vessels are involved, heals without treatment
   2. Fracture of the clavicle: most common fracture; usually caused by shoulder impaction
      a. Treatment: handle infant with care
      b. Prognosis: good
   3. Fracture of the humerus or femur: rare
      a. Cause: dystocia and difficult delivery
      b. Treatment
         (1) Immobilize
         (2) Heals rapidly
      c. Complications: rare
E. Neurologic injuries
   1. Brachial paralysis of upper arm: Erb-Duchenne

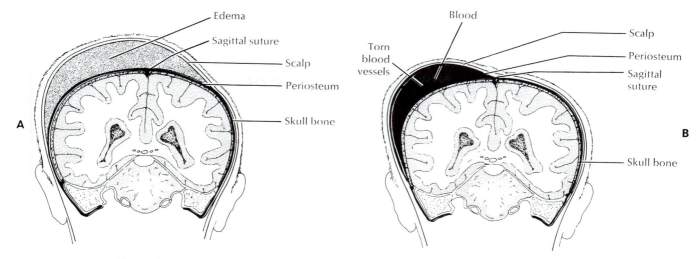

Figure 7-13. **Differences between caput succedaneum and cephalhematoma. A,** Caput succedaneum: edema of scalp noted at birth; crosses suture line. **B,** Cephalhematoma: bleeding between periosteum and skull bone appearing within first 2 days; does not cross suture lines.

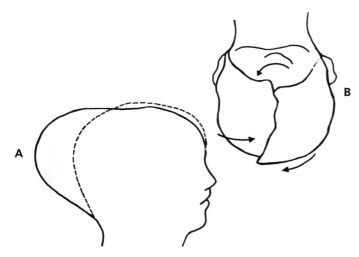

Figure 7-14. **A,** Various types of molding. **B,** Bones overlapping during molding. (From Hamilton PM: *Basic maternity nursing,* ed 6, St Louis, 1988, Mosby.)

a. Definition: nerves of the brachial plexus are crushed or severed
b. Cause
(1) Difficult labor
(2) Shoulder impaction
(3) Malposition of forceps
c. Treatment: immobilize with brace or splint
d. Nursing management
(1) Skin care as necessary
(2) Gentle range-of-motion exercises after healing
2. Brachial paralysis of lower arm: Klumpke's
a. Definition: nerves of hand and wrist crushed or severed
b. Treatment
(1) Pad wrist and fingers

(2) Corrective surgery
(3) Gentle massage after surgery
(4) Range-of-motion exercises when appropriate
c. Prognosis: good
3. Facial paralysis
a. Definition: crushed or severed nerves of face that cause grimacing and distortion, especially when crying; asymmetric paralysis
b. Cause: misapplication of forceps
c. Treatment: condition transitory; reassure parents
F. Central nervous system injuries
1. Definition: injuries causing intracranial hemorrhaging
2. Cause
a. Prematurity
b. Large full-term babies
c. Dystocia
d. Hypoxia
e. Hypovolemia
3. Types
a. In brain itself
b. Subdural hematoma
4. Signs and symptoms
a. Suture line separation
b. Bulging anterior-fontanel
c. High-pitched cry
d. Abnormal respirations
e. Cyanosis
f. Irritability or lethargy
g. Twitching; convulsions
5. Treatment and nursing management
a. Head higher than hips
b. Warmth
c. Oxygen
d. IV therapy
e. Minimal handling
f. Surgical aspiration (if appropriate)
g. Measurement of head size weekly
h. Convulsion precautions

INFECTIONS OF THE NEWBORN

A. Causes
   1. Dystocia
   2. Premature rupture of the membranes of 24 hours or more
   3. Clinical amnionitis
   4. Maternal infection
   5. Nosocomial infection (hospital-based infection; usually staph)
   6. *Monilia* or yeast infection in mother's vagina
B. Signs and symptoms
   1. Appears within first 48 hours
   2. Vague symptoms
   3. Lethargy, irritability, lack of appetite
   4. Low-grade temperature
   5. Diarrhea
   6. Jaundice
C. Treatment and nursing management
   1. Take cultures of blood, urine, throat
   2. Administer antibiotic therapy
   3. Keep warm
   4. Administer oxygen therapy if necessary
   5. Isolate if appropriate
   6. Weigh daily
   7. Watch for signs of jaundice
   8. Keep parents informed of progress

CONGENITAL MALFORMATIONS

A. Perinatal signs
   1. Polyhydramnios: excessive amniotic fluid
   2. Oligohydramnios: scant amniotic fluid; indicates urinary tract anomalies and renal disturbances
B. Postnatal congenital malformations
   1. Choanal atresia (gastrointestinal anomaly)
      a. Definition: postnares obstructed by bone or membrane; unilateral or bilateral condition
      b. Signs and symptoms
         (1) Cyanotic at rest
         (2) Color improves when crying
         (3) Snorts when feeding
      c. Treatment and nursing management
         (1) Physician may pierce obstruction with a probe if it is only a membrane
         (2) Minor surgical repair if bone involved; prognosis excellent
         (3) Feeding problems; positioning important
         (4) Gavage feeding may be necessary
         (5) Watch closely for aspiration
   2. Esophageal atresia: refer to Chapter 8, Pediatric Nursing
   3. Congenital laryngeal stridor
      a. Definition: abnormal condition around larynx that causes noisy respiration, especially a crowing sound on inspiration
      b. Cause:
         (1) Flabby epiglottis
         (2) Extraglotteal structures
         (3) Relaxation of laryngeal wall
         (4) Absence of tracheal rings
         (5) Deformity of vocal cords
      c. Signs and symptoms
         (1) Noisy respirations on inspiration
         (2) Most noticeable when crying

         (3) Mild-to-severe intercostal or supraclavicular retractions
         (4) Cyanosis
         (5) Dyspnea
      d. Treatment and nursing management
         (1) Depends on cause
         (2) Mild stridor may subside in 6 to 18 months
         (3) Mother taught to position baby upright for feeding
         (4) Feed slowly, pausing to let infant catch his breath
         (5) Use small nipple
         (6) Watch for aspiration of feedings
         (7) Prevent respiratory complications
         (8) Keep infant warm, dry, away from drafts
         (9) Oxygen in readiness
         (10) Tracheotomy preparedness
      e. Prognosis: good
   4. Cleft lip and cleft palate
      a. Definition: bilateral or unilateral fissure or opening on the palate or the upper lips resulting from failure of the bony and soft tissue structures to unite
      b. Cause: developmental failure during the embryonic stage because of heredity, age, or a variety of other factors such as radiation or viral infections
      c. Signs and symptoms
         (1) Visual on lips
         (2) Palate more difficult to notice sometimes
         (3) Occurs more frequently in males
         (4) Difficulty feeding
         (5) Choking
         (6) Drooling
         (7) Milk may drain through nostrils
      d. Treatment
         (1) Cleft lips may have butterfly adhesive taping as initial treatment; may be helpful in feeding so milk does not continually drain through fissure
         (2) Cleft lip may be surgically repaired at 1 to 2 weeks of age, or at 12 lb (5.5 kg)
         (3) Cleft palate; first repair usually by 18 months
      e. Nursing management
         (1) Feeding precautions
            (a) Use soft duck nipple, medicine dropper with rubber tip
            (b) Place nipple away from cleft side
            (c) Feed slowly
            (d) Bubble frequently
            (e) Rinse mouth after feedings
            (f) Watch for aspiration, respiratory distress, gastrointestinal disturbances
         (2) Mouth care: prevent cracks, fissures on lips
         (3) Postoperative care for cleft lip
            (a) Place infant on side
            (b) Mouth care important because of Logan bar applied to prevent stretching of sutures
            (c) Prevent crying
            (d) Check swelling (tongue, nose, mouth)
            (e) Watch for hemorrhage
            (f) Apply elbow restraints
            (g) Prevent crust formation
            (h) Feed on opposite side of surgery
            (i) Use rubber-tipped dropper (3 weeks)

5. Diaphragmatic hernia
   a. Definition: herniation of abdominal viscera into the thoracic cavity as a result of incomplete development during embryonic stage, ranging from minimal to complete herniation
   b. Signs and symptoms
      (1) Constant respiratory distress
      (2) Bowels distended
      (3) Bowel sounds heard in chest
      (4) Asymmetric chest contour
   c. Treatment and nursing management
      (1) Early recognition and prompt surgery
      (2) Usual preoperative and postoperative management
   d. Prognosis guarded, depending on severity
6. Omphalocele: see Chapter 8, Pediatric Nursing
7. Imperforate anus: see Chapter 8, Pediatric Nursing
C. Congenital anomalies of central nervous system
   1. Spina bifida occulta
      a. Definition: defect in vertebral column without protrusion of spinal cord and meninges; this is one of three types of spina bifida, which is a malformation of the spine, most common in the lumbosacral region, in which the posterior portion of the vertebrae fails to close
      b. Signs and symptoms
         (1) Dimple in lower lumbosacral skin
         (2) Hair over area sometimes
         (3) X-ray film confirmation
      c. Treatment and nursing management: no treatment necessary unless neurologic symptoms occur
   2. Meningocele (another form of spina bifida)
      a. Definition: defect in spinal cord with protrusion of meninges through an opening in spinal canal
      b. Surgical correction with excellent results
   3. Meningomyelocele
      a. Definition: both spinal cord and meninges protrude through defective bony rings in spinal cord; possible paralysis
      b. Signs and symptoms
         (1) Arnold-Chiari syndrome
         (2) Observe for change in intracranial pressure
         (3) Check head measurements
         (4) Report signs and symptoms of CNS involvement
      c. Preoperative management
         (1) Flat on abdomen with sterile gauze, petroleum jelly (Vaseline), or Telfa pad
         (2) No diapers
         (3) Keep clean
         (4) Use care to prevent sac from breaking
         (5) Prevent infection: sterile technique
         (6) Prevent deformity
         (7) Prevent injury
      d. Postoperative management
         (1) Vital signs
         (2) Symptoms of shock
         (3) Oxygen readiness
         (4) Head measurements
         (5) Cast care if necessary; sometimes casts applied to legs
         (6) Importance of good nutrition
         (7) Orthopedic and urologic habilitation

      (8) Encourage normal use of functions
      (9) Minimize disabilities
      (10) Paralysis (if present) may not be alleviated, but further damage could be prevented; aim of surgery is to give infant opportunity for optimal growth and development
      (11) "Crede" bladder to keep it empty and free from infection
   4. Hydrocephalus: refer to Chapter 8, Pediatric Nursing
   5. Congenital dislocation of the hip: refer to Chapter 8, Pediatric Nursing
   6. Talipes equinovarus (clubfoot): refer to Chapter 8, Pediatric Nursing
   7. Phocomelia
      a. Definition: developmental congenital anomaly in which only stubs or parts of arms and legs are present; degree of severity varies
      b. Cause: interference with embryonic development of long bones; is rare and seen as a result of the drug thalidomide taken during early pregnancy to relieve nausea
      c. Treatment and nursing management
         (1) Psychosocial problems for family and infant
         (2) Body surface limited, so heating mechanism overheats rest of body, causing diaphoresis
         (3) Personal hygiene: frequent baths
         (4) Special education imperative
   8. Polydactyly
      a. Definition: supernumerary fingers or toes
      b. Cause: possibly hereditary
      c. Treatment and nursing management
         (1) Usually no bone or nerve involvement
         (2) Tie digit with silk suture in newborn nursery; it falls off
         (3) Surgical intervention necessary with bone involvement
   9. Exstrophy of bladder
      a. Definition: anomaly of lower urinary tract in which bladder, mucosa, and ureters are exposed, sometimes without a ventral covering
      b. Signs and symptoms
         (1) Lining of posterior bladder exposed and red
         (2) Urine drips into abdominal wall from abnormal ureters
         (3) Ulceration of bladder mucosa from seepage
      c. Treatment and nursing management
         (1) Surgical corrective procedures dependent on extent of exstrophy
         (2) Adequate hydration to keep ureter patent
         (3) Avoid infections
         (4) Good skin care
         (5) Involvement of parents in problems, surgical procedures, nursing care, management, and prognosis
         (6) Long-term hospitalization and care
   10. Hypospadias: refer to Chapter 8, Pediatric Nursing
   11. Epispadias: refer to Chapter 8, Pediatric Nursing

HEMOLYTIC DISEASE OF NEWBORN
A. Hyperbilirubinemia (erythroblastosis fetalis)
   1. Definition: a congenital condition in which red blood cells are broken down by an antigen-antibody reaction

2. Cause: an Rh-negative mother giving birth to an Rh-positive baby
3. Pathophysiology: fetal Rh antigen enters the Rh-negative mother, who then produces anti-Rh antibodies, which return through placenta to the fetal circulation, attach to fetal red blood cells, and destroy (hemolyze) them
4. Signs and symptoms
   a. Jaundice
   b. Anemia
   c. Enlarged liver and spleen
   d. Generalized edema
   e. If untreated, "yellow bodies" will travel to brain, causing brain damage, heart failure, kernicterus, and death
5. Treatment and nursing management
   a. Blood types of mother and father important for anticipatory guidance
   b. Usually first babies do not present a problem
   c. If baby's bilirubin is above 10 or 12 mg/dl, phototherapy may be applied to reduce jaundice; exchange transfusions may be necessary
   d. After birth of Rh-positive baby, an unsensitized Rh-negative mother is given RhoGAM, a specific gamma globulin that will prevent the production of Rh antibodies; this must be given within 72 hours after delivery; the effect is the assurance that subsequent pregnancies will not be harmful to the baby
   e. Rh-antibody titers can be monitored throughout pregnancy (prenatal)
   f. Amniocentesis will reveal, by indirect Coombs' test, if mother has antibodies circulating in the maternal plasma or serum

B. ABO incompatibility
   1. Definition: an incompatibility of blood groups A and B because of the presence of antigens developed and passed on to the fetus by a type O mother
   2. Signs and symptoms
      a. Jaundice: mild, occurring during first day or two
      b. Slight enlargement of liver and spleen
   3. Treatment and nursing management
      a. Phototherapy
      b. If bilirubin is above 20 mg/dl, an exchange transfusion with group O and appropriate Rh type
      c. Observe for progressive lethargy
      d. Level of jaundice (visual and laboratory)
      e. Observe color of urine
      f. Observe for edema
      g. Observe for convulsions
      h. Symptomatic nursing care

DOWN SYNDROME (TRISOMY 21)
Refer to Chapter 8, Pediatric Nursing

DRUG ADDICTION IN NEWBORNS
A. Definition: secondary addiction, caused by drugs being ingested or injected by mother-addict; drugs cross placental barrier and create a drug-dependent newborn (immature liver unable to excrete drug rapidly during fetal life)
B. Signs and symptoms
   1. Low birth weight
   2. Premature
   3. Immature
   4. Withdrawal symptoms within 48 to 72 hours; watch for
      a. Sneezing
      b. Respiratory distress
      c. Excessive sweating
      d. Feeding problems
      e. Frantic sucking of fists
      f. High-pitched cry
      g. Irritable, hyperactive, tremors
      h. Fever
      i. Diarrhea
C. Treatment and nursing management
   1. Prevent infection
   2. Promote good nutrition
   3. Keep quiet (quiet, darkened environment)
   4. Offer loving, soothing, cuddling care
   5. Give medications on time
   6. Monitor vital signs
   7. Keep warm
   8. Protect from injury because child is hyperactive
   9. Good skin care because of excessive sweating and diarrhea
   10. Adequate fluids (prevent dehydration)
   11. Encourage mother to assist in care
      a. Teach holding, diapering, talking, bathing
      b. Encourage visits

INFANTS OF DIABETIC MOTHERS
A. Complications
   1. Delivery date may be recommended before EDC or about 36 to 37 weeks' gestation to prevent:
      a. Oversized baby
      b. High-risk infant (diabetic babies have high rate of infant mortality)
   2. Neonatal hypoglycemia common
   3. RDS complications
   4. Hyperbilirubinemia (severe jaundice)
   5. Intracranial hemorrhage
   6. Congestive heart failure
   7. Congenital anomalies in 5% of infants
   8. Hypocalcemia
B. Signs and symptoms
   1. Lethargic
   2. Plump, puffy face
   3. Long and heavy
   4. Respiratory problems evident
   5. Enlarged heart, liver, and spleen
   6. Symptoms of hypoglycemia
   7. Symptoms of hypocalcemia
C. Treatment and nursing management
   1. Medical management difficult because of rapid, changing growth patterns, nutritional demands, illness
   2. Parents must be taught techniques for blood glucose monitoring
   3. Short-acting insulin best (easier to control)
   4. Treat hypoglycemia and hypocalcemia
   5. Oral feedings when tolerated and blood sugar levels stable

CRETINISM (CONGENITAL HYPOTHYROIDISM)
Refer to Chapter 8, Pediatric Nursing

Family Planning
A. Trends
   1. Smaller families (except for the poor and disadvantaged)
   2. Delayed parenthood by choice

a. Career women
b. Desire for higher education
c. Alternate living arrangements
3. Single parents
a. High divorce rate
b. Expanding role of father as single parent because custody of children, traditionally awarded to mother, is now being awarded to fathers
c. Lessening barriers for adoption by single men and women
d. Cultural and ethnic acceptance of unmarried mothers
e. Opportunities to continue education for pregnant teenager without pressure of forced marriage
B. Communes: labor and delivery in communal community homes
C. Early sexual encounters (teenage pregnancies)
1. Need for referrals to family planning centers for guidance and counseling
a. Teach use of condoms (controversial)
b. Practice abstinence
2. Problems originating from early sexual encounters
D. Surrogate mothers
1. In vitro transplantation of embryo in the uterus of a woman who agrees to have a full-term pregnancy for another woman
2. Moral and legal implications

POSSIBLE INFLUENTIAL FACTORS
A. Sex education: incorporation of sex education in public and parochial schools at an early age
B. Freedom of choice
1. Availability of over-the-counter pregnancy tests
2. Availability of over-the-counter contraceptives
3. Abortions mandated as legal by the United States Supreme Court, 1977
C. Postponement of family: using available contraceptive devices
D. Economic factor: high cost of medical care forces young people to consider waiting until affluent enough to "afford" a family

COMMON METHODS OF BIRTH CONTROL (CONTRACEPTION)
A. Natural
1. Rhythm (calendar) method
a. Based on the principle that ovulation occurs during midcycle of a menstrual period; that is, in a 28-day cycle, ovulation would occur on the 14th day
b. Accordingly the most fertile days are considered to be 3 to 4 days before and 3 to 4 days after ovulation
2. Basal metabolism method: daily monitoring of early morning temperature for a period of several months and entering it on a graph (Fig. 7-15) will establish an ovulation time; "safe" and "fertile" times can be determined, and mother advised on use of this method
B. Coitus interruptus
1. Penis is withdrawn from vagina just before ejaculation
2. Least effective of all methods
C. Condom (sheath, snakeskin, rubbers): thin rubber or plastic sheath that fits over penis and acts as barrier, preventing sperm from entering the vagina
D. Diaphragm: mechanical barrier placed at mouth of cervix; used with contraceptive cream or jelly to be effective; may

engage in intercourse immediately after placement; should be left in place for 6 hours after intercourse; spermicide must be added each time intercourse occurs
E. Chemical agents: foam, creams, jelly, vaginal suppositories, and the newest on the market, sponges, form a chemical barrier in the vagina and render the area unsafe for sperm
F. Intrauterine device (IUD)
1. Devices come in various shapes made of memory plastic; inserted into the uterine cavity by a physician during or immediately following the woman's menstrual cycle
2. Mode of action unclear: thought to interfere with implantation by creating peristaltic waves
3. Disadvantages:
a. Excessive bleeding during menstrual cycle
b. Extremely controversial: Dalkon shield taken off the market because of permanent sterility and multiple gynecologic problems
c. Possible contamination from IUD string hanging in vaginal orifice
4. Advantage: once IUD is inserted, only periodic checking to confirm that it is still intact
G. Oral contraceptives (birth control pill)
1. Most widely used
2. Considered 90% or more effective
3. Prevent anterior pituitary from releasing follicle stimulating hormone (FSH); artificially raises estrogen and progesterone levels and prevents ovulation
4. Stimulates endometrium, creating hostile environment for sperm
5. Minor side effects lasting few weeks to few months: nausea, weight gain, full breasts
6. Major side effects: thrombophlebitis, hypertension, embolism, cardiovascular disturbances
H. Sterilization
1. Surgical procedures for females are permanent

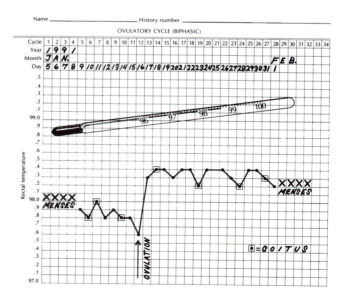

Figure 7-15. Basal temperature record shows drop and sharp rise at time of ovulation. (From Bobak IM, Jensen MD: *Essentials of maternity nursing,* ed 3, St Louis, 1991, Mosby.)

a. Tubal ligation (cutting or tie) most commonly done
b. Hysterectomy (removal of uterus)
c. Oophorectomy (removal of ovaries)
2. Surgical procedure for the male—vasectomy: tying or ligating duct from each testicle so sperm cannot escape
3. Careful consideration of these procedures because they are permanent
I. Newer methods
1. Morning after pill: (diethylstilbestrol [DES]); must be taken orally within 72 hours after intercourse; prevents ovulation, alters endometrium, prevents implantation; not 100% effective; most commonly used in emergencies such as rape
2. Contraceptive sponge: can be worn up to 24 hours; must be left in place for 6 hours after intercourse to be effective; danger of toxic shock syndrome (TTS)
3. RU486: binds progesterone and appears to block its action; widely used in Europe
4. Depo-Provera: injectable progesterone every 3 months
5. Steroid implants: inhibits gonadotropins; not widely used
6. Patches: time-released hormones; experimental

SUGGESTED READING

Anderson B, Shapiro P: *Basic maternal and newborn nursing,* ed 5, Albany, NY, 1989, Delmar.

Bobak IM, Lowdermilk DL, Jensen MD: *Maternity nursing,* ed 4, St Louis, 1995, Mosby.

Dulock DNS: *Hypoglycemia in the newborn,* March of Dimes BFD mod 2, ser 1, ed 2, White Plains, NY, 1990.

Guzzetta C et al: *Clinical assessment tools for use with nursing diagnoses,* St Louis, 1989, Mosby.

Hamilton PM: *Basic maternity nursing,* ed 6, St Louis, 1989, Mosby.

Ingalls JA, Salerno CM: *Maternal and child health nursing,* ed 8, St Louis, 1995, Mosby.

Karch A, Boyd E: *Handbook of drugs and the nursing process,* Philadelphia, 1989, JB Lippincott.

King J: Helping patients choose an appropriate method of birth control, *Matern Child Nurs* 17:91-95, 1992.

Kosanek J: *Manual of labor and delivery nursing procedures,* 1990, ABC Decker.

Lone P: Silencing crack addiction, *Matern Child Nurs* 16:264-266, 1991.

Long JW: *The essential guide to prescription drugs,* New York, 1990, Harper & Row.

Phillips C: *Family centered maternity and newborn care,* St Louis, 1996, Mosby.

Plovie B: *Diabetes in pregnancy, prenatal care,* March of Dimes BDF mod 10, ser 2, White Plains, NY, 1989.

Richardson J, Richardson LI: *The mathematics of drugs and solutions: with clinical applications,* ed 4, St Louis, 1990, Mosby.

Stringer M, Libizzi R, Weiner S: Establishing a prenatal genetic diagnosis: the nurse's role. *Matern Child Nurs* 16:152-156, 1991.

Whaley L, Wong D: *Nursing care of infants and children,* ed 4, St Louis, 1991, Mosby.

REVIEW QUESTIONS

Answers and rationales begin on p. 363.

1. A 38-year-old primigravida is scheduled to undergo an amniocentesis. She and her significant other are very apprehensive and ask the nurse to reinforce the explanation that the physician has already given to them. The nurse should explain:
   ① "It is not my place to explain procedures after the physician has already done so."
   ② "It is a procedure where a small amount of amniotic fluid is withdrawn from the uterus via a needle inserted in the mother's abdomen."
   ③ "Would you like me to ask the physician to explain the procedure to you again?"
   ④ "Don't worry! It is a very short procedure and the risks are minimal."

2. There are three categories of signs of pregnancy: presumptive signs, probable signs, and positive signs. Which of the following would be a positive sign of pregnancy?
   ① An immunologic pregnancy test
   ② Hegar's sign
   ③ Missed menstrual cycle
   ④ Echographic testing

3. Which of the following is considered the most effective method of birth control?
   ① Insertion of intrauterine device (IUD)
   ② Coitus interruptus
   ③ Use of condom
   ④ Oral contraceptives

4. Pregnancy affects every major system in the body. Changes occur to the respiratory, skin, urinary, nervous, and digestive systems. Changes in the digestive system include:
   ① Aggravation of prepregnancy psychosocial problems
   ② Traces of sugar in the urine
   ③ Cholasma gravidarum
   ④ Increased appetite after the first trimester

5. Prenatal care is considered the primary deterrent to complications during pregnancy. Which complication would you consider as most affected by good prenatal care?
   ① Placenta previa
   ② Hyperemesis gravidarum
   ③ Pregnancy-induced hypertension (PIH)
   ④ Abortion

6. A patient who is 2 months pregnant asks the nurse if it is all right to exercise during pregnancy. The nurse's most appropriate answer should be:
   ① "It depends on your previous exercise patterns."
   ② "Absolutely. It will help you and your baby to feel better."
   ③ "Do not do any exercise that will jar the baby, such as horseback riding or skydiving."
   ④ "Make certain that you let your physician know if you experience any pain or discomfort."

7. Mothers are routinely screened during their first prenatal examination for a variety of conditions. One of the most important tests is the alpha-fetoprotein (AFP) test, which:
   ① Determines fetal maturity
   ② Detects a neural tube defect such as spina bifida
   ③ Detects Tay-Sachs disease
   ④ Detects respiratory distress syndrome (RDS) in the newborn

8. A couple is admitted to the maternity care department. The mother-to-be has been having contractions intermittently at 10- to 20-minute intervals for the past 12 hours. The contractions are relieved by ambulation. Her EDC is 2 weeks away. The physician examines her and finds her to be 0 centimeters dilated and just slightly effaced. The nurse should know that these contractions are most likely:
   ① True labor and will progress rapidly
   ② True labor and will progress differently for every woman
   ③ False labor, as they are relieved by activity
   ④ False labor that most likely will change to true labor in 24 hours

9. Which female hormone is said to "hold" the pregnancy?
   ① Estrogen
   ② Luteinizing hormone
   ③ Progesterone
   ④ Human gonadotropic hormone

10. A home care nurse is interviewing and assessing a mother who gave birth 10 days ago. Which of the following items should be reported to the physician?
    ① A fundus that is not palpable
    ② Reports by the mother of problems with constipation
    ③ Reports by the mother of periods when she just cannot stop crying
    ④ Reports of the mother of dark red lochia with small clots

11. Which of the following statements is correct relative to a stress test and a nonstress test?
    ① A nonstress test is done by abdominal palpation by the physician
    ② A nonstress test is done early in pregnancy to determine sex of the infant
    ③ A stress test is usually done late in pregnancy to measure fetal response to uterine contractions
    ④ A stress test is done after the mother has been given orange juice to drink

12. You are to interview several pregnant women in the prenatal clinic. In today's psychosocial climate, which would be an *important* item to include in your initial interview?
    ① Economic and ethnic status
    ② Family and genetic history
    ③ Abuse of drugs or alcohol
    ④ Educational or schooling status

13. Magnesium sulfate is a CNS depressant and should not be given if:
    ① BP is elevated
    ② DTRs are absent
    ③ DTRs are brisk
    ④ Should never be withheld for any reason

14. Magnesium sulfate in 100 ml D5W is due to run out in 1 hour. The administration set has 15 gtt/ml. How many drops per minute would you run the IV?
    ① 15 gtt/min
    ② 18 gtt/min
    ③ 25 gtt/min
    ④ 100 gtt/min

15. A patient appears to be an impending eclamptic. She has complained of visual disturbance and severe epigastric pain. The nurse should observe her closely for signs of:
    ① Seizure
    ② Elevated BP
    ③ Lowered BP
    ④ Labor

16. A home health care provider is assessing a newborn who is 36 hours old and was discharged home from the hospital 12 hours ago. Which of the following should be of concern to the nurse?
    ① The infant produces a greenish tarry stool
    ② A positive Babinski reflex is elicited
    ③ The infant's elbows are fully flexed when lying in a supine position
    ④ A respiratory rate greater than 70 breaths per minute is counted

17. A nurse on a postpartum unit has just completed a parents' class for 6 couples. Which of the following statements should indicate to the nurse that at least one of the partners has understood a major concept of the class?
    ① "This is a lot of work; my partner is going to have to be very organized."
    ② "Having a schedule everyday is extremely important, so that we can keep our life organized."
    ③ "My wife is breastfeeding, so this is something that I can do to help."
    ④ "Staying with the baby and maintaining safety precautions is a top priority."

18. A patient is 36 weeks pregnant and in danger of becoming eclamptic. Delivery is induced. She delivers a 5 lb 8 oz (2500 g) boy after just 6 hours of labor. She must continue to be watched for impending eclampsia for how long?
    ① 1 hour
    ② 2 hours
    ③ 24 hours
    ④ 72 hours

19. What is considered to be a major problem in teaching prenatal care to the pregnant teenager today?
    ① Inability to comprehend the psychosocial impact of her pregnancy on herself and on her unborn child
    ② Nutritional counseling
    ③ Physical immaturity
    ④ Dangers of HIV

20. The patient is 4 weeks pregnant. She is gravida II para I. Her 3-year-old child was born with spina bifida. In addition to regular vitamin supplements, the health care provider prescribes an additional supplement. The nurse should know that this supplement would most likely be:
    ① Vitamin K
    ② Thiamine
    ③ Vitamin E
    ④ Folic acid

21. A newly-arrived immigrant woman is being seen by the health care provider for the first time. It is determined that she is pregnant with her first child. The health care provider is concerned, however, because she is also complaining of fever, weight loss, night sweats, and a persistent cough. A diagnosis of active TB is made. The most appropriate course of action for this patient at this time should be:
    ① Begin a drug treatment regimen according to drug susceptibility and patient's response to treatment
    ② Do nothing until the pregnancy is over because of the risk of injury to the fetus
    ③ Start with a mild drug and monitor the pregnancy carefully for any signs of complications
    ④ Monitor the pregnancy carefully and begin treatment in the third trimester after the major fetal structures are complete

22. Which would be the best source of calcium?
    ① Calcium tablets
    ② Milk
    ③ Greens
    ④ Multivitamin D

23. A patient wants to know what substance in her urine specimen showed she was positive for pregnancy. A nurse should explain that a hormone presents itself at implantation and can be detected in the urine within 42 days after the LMP. It is called:
    ① Estrogen
    ② Progesterone
    ③ Relaxin hormone
    ④ Chorionic gonadotropin

24. A patient is uncertain whether or not she wishes to breast-feed her newborn. Which of these statement should the nurse make to assist the patient in making a choice?
    ① "Breastfeeding is the absolute best !!! There is nothing healthier for the baby."
    ② "Ask your mother. She will help you decide what is best."
    ③ "Research has shown that there is a benefit from breastfeeding for both the mother and the baby. Tell me what questions and concerns you have about breastfeeding."
    ④ "Whatever choice you make, the important thing is that the baby gets enough to eat."

25. A patient is admitted to your med-surg unit after delivering a full-term infant who was stillborn. The husband says to the nurse, "I will see my baby and take care of the arrangements. I don't want anyone to say anything to my wife about what happened." The most appropriate action of the nurse should be to:
    ① Reassure the husband that his wishes will be respected
    ② Explain to the husband that no one will initiate the specific topic with his wife but they will not stop her from talking about it
    ③ Encourage the husband to talk with his wife so that they can support each other through the grieving process
    ④ Explain politely to the husband that his wife is the patient and it is your responsibility to encourage communication in every way possible

26. A patient has learned that the placenta is an all-purpose organ that nourishes the fetus, excretes waste materials, and acts as a respiratory organ. She is curious about the role of the umbilical cord. The best explanation should be:
    ① The cord is the staff of life and is surrounded by Wharton's jelly for protection of its contents
    ② It contains two veins and an artery that carry the vital life-sustaining products to the fetus
    ③ The umbilical cord contains the umbilical vein, which supplies oxygen and nutrients to the fetus while two arteries carry away the waste products
    ④ The oxygen flows from the umbilical vein to the liver through a fetal structure called the ductus venosus; then the arteries go through another fetal structure called the ductus arteriosus into the aorta and eventually back to the umbilical arteries

27. A patient is curious to know when the fetal heart begins to function. The nurse tells her it is usually:

① By the third or fourth week after LMP
② Within 6 weeks after implantation
③ By the first trimester
④ By the time the placenta is formed

28. A patient is a chain-smoker. The prenatal nurse has taught her the effect of nicotine and hazards of passive smoking. She does not drink, but the nurse has taught her that fetal alcohol syndrome is a major concern today. In addressing the abuse of tobacco, the nurse would stress that it:
① Is a dirty, nasty habit that yellows your teeth, can cause lung cancer, and can offend nonsmokers
② Is becoming socially unacceptable and has widespread negative effects on children as well as grown-ups
③ May cause adverse physiologic effects on the fetus
④ Retards fetal growth, constricts blood vessels in the mother, decreases placental function, and may cause premature labor

29. There are identical twins and fraternal twins. How would you distinguish the kind of twins a patient has if she delivered a boy and a girl?
① Monozygotic or single-ovum twins: union of one sperm and one ovum, divides during mitosis into two embryos; one placenta, two amniotic sacs; heredity is a factor
② Dizygotic twins: union of two sperms with two ovas; two amniotic sacs; separate or fused placenta; same or different sex
③ They look exactly alike even though they are of a different sex; blood tests will reveal if they are identical or fraternal
④ DNA will identify the type of twins they are

30. A patient early in her second pregnancy experiences occasional traces of sugar in her urine specimen. What should be the nurse's evaluation of these findings?
① She is eating a diet high in carbohydrates
② She is experiencing pregnancy-induced hypertension
③ This is probably the result of absorption of lactose from the breasts
④ Because she is a multipara there is more absorption of lactose from the breasts

31. A patient who is a mother of a 5-year-old son and is now pregnant again should be classified as:
① Gravida 1 para 1
② Gravida 2 para 2
③ Gravida 2 para 1
④ Gravida 2 nullipara

32. If a blood typing was Rh negative, there would be no complications to the new baby if:
① The patient was Rh negative
② The patient was Rh positive
③ Her son was Rh positive
④ She did not receive RhoGAM after the birth of her first son

33. A patient whose last menstrual period began on May 18 should have an estimated date of confinement (EDC) of:
① February 9
② February 11
③ February 18
④ February 25

34. In her third trimester a patient suddenly notices that she is bleeding. At first the bleeding was scanty but has become heavier. She reports she has no pain. A nurse should suspect:

① Abruptio placentae
② Placenta previa
③ Ruptured uterus
④ Vasa previa

35. To relieve supine hypotensive syndrome in a patient, the nurse should:
① Massage her leg
② Instruct her to breathe deeply
③ Turn her on left side and advise frequent changing of position
④ Advise her to walk slowly and carefully

36. A prenatal patient is experiencing leg cramps. A nursing intervention should include:
① Advising hot compresses bid
② Instructing her to elevate her legs at least 15 minutes 3 times daily
③ Informing her of the cause (excessive phosphorus) and encouraging her to drink milk
④ Advising her to chew Tums for calcium

37. A prenatal patient is complaining of low back pains. A nurse might suggest:
① Sitz baths
② Heating pads to her back
③ Pelvic rocking or pelvic tilting exercises
④ Visits to the chiropractor

38. In looking over a patient's chart a nurse sees that her hemoglobin is 7. What does this mean to the nurse?
① That the patient is anemic and needs treatment stat
② That this is probably resulting from increased blood volume of pregnancy
③ That this must be her baseline
④ That Z-track iron should be administered to this patient

39. To confirm a patient's pregnancy the nurse should give which of the following instructions regarding the required urine specimen:
① Give a voided specimen during her first visit
② Instruct her on how to give a sterile specimen in the office
③ Tell her to withhold fluid intake during the night and bring in the first voided specimen in the morning
④ A catheterized specimen will be required

40. After reviewing prenatal care with a patient the nurse should include an advisory that she notify the physician immediately if she experiences:
① Abdominal pain, discharge of bright red blood, chills, and fever
② Blood-streaked mucus, Braxton-Hicks contractions
③ Constipation, urgency, hemorrhoids
④ Quickening, varicosities, and discomfort

41. Estriol testing is a urine test taken at certain intervals to determine:
① Fetal age
② Lung surfactant of the fetus
③ Uterine nomenclature
④ Placental functioning

42. The communicable (childhood) disease most likely to affect pregnancy, with harmful effects to the fetus is:
① Chickenpox
② Rubella
③ Varicella
④ Rubeola

43. Orders for a patient on the maternity floor include notifying the physician immediately of any changes in status, no vaginal or rectal examinations, fetal monitoring, pad count, oxygen if necessary, and laboratory work (type and cross match, Hgh, Hct). These orders would alert the nurse to prepare for which of the following?
    ① Pending abortion
    ② Ectopic pregnancy
    ③ Third-trimester bleeding
    ④ Postpartum hemorrhage

44. A doctor has just ruptured the patient's membranes. The primary responsibility of the attending nurse is to:
    ① Clean up after the procedure
    ② Note the time of the procedure, color, odor, other pertinent data
    ③ Chart the physician's name and the procedure done, sign your name in full
    ④ Hold patient's hand, reassure her, change the bed

45. The labor-room nurse should encourage a patient to void because a full bladder:
    ① During labor may cause postpartum hemorrhage
    ② May cause a rupture of the bladder during descent of the head
    ③ May cause cystitis
    ④ May impede the progress of labor

46. Nursing management during the first stage of labor includes which of the following?
    ① Admit patient to labor room, establish rapport, monitor FHT, keep patient and significant others apprised of progress
    ② Monitor FHT with fetoscope, monitor blood pressure (BP) q 15 min, give pushing instructions, maintain patent airway for newborn, follow proper identification routine
    ③ Be sure cord blood specimen is obtained, observe time and delivery of placenta, check perineal area, check fundus, administer oxytocin IV after placenta is delivered; check BP and fundus q 5 min
    ④ Watch for hemorrhaging, check fundus q 15 min, monitor BP q 15 min, offer warm food and fluid, offer bedpan for urination, teach perineal care, transfer patient to postpartum room when condition is stable

47. The greatest comfort a nurse can give a patient in labor is to assure her that:
    ① Her progress is normal
    ② She will not be left alone
    ③ Her physician is in the building
    ④ She will be able to hold the baby after delivery

48. Why does a fetal position of left occiput posterior (LOP) create dystocia and severe back pain?
    ① The baby's face is descending, facing toward the spine
    ② The fetus is descending with its occipital bone against the mother's spine
    ③ The left shoulder is against the spine
    ④ The presenting part is pressing against the symphysis pubis

49. After the placenta is delivered and suturing is completed, the nurse notices that the patient has begun to shiver. What should the nurse suspect as the probable cause of the shivering?

① The sudden emptying of the uterine contents, plus the return of the body chemistry and hormones to the prepregnant state, causes a certain shock to the system
② Loss of blood, length of labor, and a certain tiredness cause the lowering of the body temperature; the warm blankets will help
③ Pitocin is given after the delivery of the placenta and may cause the body to respond by shivering
④ The shiver is a normal reaction, since she has been in a cold delivery room, swallowing ice chips, and only covered with a thin sheet

50. What Apgar score would you give a newborn who exhibited the following?
    Heart rate—below 100 beats/min
    Respiratory effort—weak cry
    Muscle tone—some flexion
    Reflex response—cough or sneeze
    Color—body pink; extremities blue
    ① 4
    ② 6
    ③ 7
    ④ 8

51. Of the following newborn conditions, which is *not* normal?
    ① Milia are small, white sebaceous glands found in the chin, forehead, nose, cheek, and upper lip
    ② Mongolian spots are noted as dark pigmented areas on the lower back and buttocks
    ③ Erb-Duchenne, brachial plexus
    ④ Cephalhematoma, molding, or caput succedaneum

52. A couple arrive at the emergency room visibly upset and frightened. She has been in labor for 3 hours and suddenly had a sudden sharp pain that made her gasp for breath. The nurse notices that she is diaphoretic, ashen, cold, and clammy. The nurse also assesses her abdomen to be rigid and boardlike. Judging from the symptoms described, the most likely complication for the nurse to suspect would be:
    ① Low marginal placenta previa
    ② Appendicitis
    ③ Premature separation of the placenta
    ④ Rupture of the uterus

53. A patient in labor is admitted to the emergency department. The physician's diagnosis is abruptio placenta. Her partner asks why she is so pale and weak when there is no significant bleeding. The nurse's explanation should be:
    ① "The bleeding is all internal; perhaps you should line up some blood donors.".
    ② "In this condition, shock is out of proportion to the blood loss, but we are watching her closely and will not leave her bedside."
    ③ "It is a good sign that you cannot see much bleeding."
    ④ "As you can see, we are doing everything to treat the shock. She should be coming out of it soon."

54. A patient is diagnosed with abruptio placenta. The physician is checking the blood every 15 minutes. The partner is frightened and asks the nurse why the physician has to withdraw so much blood. The best answer for the nurse should be:
    ① "Ask the physician yourself."
    ② "Do you want me to ask the physician for you?"

③ "The physician is checking the fibrinogen level to determine the status of the clotting factor so she can plan what further action to take. We will keep you informed."
④ "The physician is finding out whether he should give her a transfusion or whether to operate."

55. A patient is admitted to the labor and delivery room with a diagnosis of abruptio placenta. A nurse responsible for obtaining equipment for the physician should quickly prepare the equipment for a:
① Cesarean section
② Natural vaginal delivery
③ Double set up
④ Precipitate delivery

56. A patient admitted with abruptio placenta delivers a healthy baby girl via cesarean. After the delivery the physician examines the placenta very thoroughly. Why?
① The placenta will reveal a tear where any separation might have occurred
② The placenta will clearly show calcified areas that caused the problem
③ The placenta will be much heavier in weight than normal
④ The placenta will be sent to the laboratory for further analysis

57. A patient is admitted to the emergency department in active labor. She delivers a baby girl spontaneously after 1 contraction. The nurse is still alone; her first responsibility is to:
① Ascertain whether the fundus is likely to hemorrhage
② Establish an airway for the baby by milking the trachea and maintaining the head lower than the body
③ Quickly tie and cut the umbilical cord
④ Look for the uterus to rise, watch the perineum for a trickle of blood, and deliver the placenta

58. The physician arrives after a precipitous delivery. He examines the baby, then examines the mother. He has her wheeled into a delivery room, where he delivers the secundines intact. He reexamines the mother internally, orders oxytocin (Pitocin) IM, and starts an IV with a piggyback of an antibiotic. Because the patient had a precipitous delivery, a nursing responsibility should be to:
① Watch for infiltration of the IV and observe for antibiotic reaction
② Watch for excessive bleeding or signs of hemorrhage
③ Anticipate the patient's legs shaking and chills
④ Watch for sudden elevation of temperature as a forerunner of an infection or infectious process

59. After a delivery termed nonsterile birth (NSB), the responsibilities of the emergency room nurse should include:
① Checking the cord, the Apgar score, making identification bands as for a normal delivery
② Informing the nursery of the baby's status so they will observe predesignated hospital precautions for deliveries performed outside the hospital
③ Ordering an antibiotic because of the circumstances of birth
④ Placing the baby in an Isolette for observation

60. After a particularly stormy labor, posterior presentation, severe back pains, nausea, and vomiting during transition and difficulty pushing, the patient delivered a 9 lb 14 oz

baby boy. The placenta was not yet delivered when suddenly the patient started to hemorrhage profusely from the vaginal orifice. Within minutes the nurse sees blood trickling from her nose and mouth. What can the nurse do to help in alleviating this condition, which the physician has labeled as disseminated intravascular coagulation (DIC)?
① Call the laboratory for blood replacement (fresh whole blood) and assist the physician to deliver the placenta as quickly as possible
② Prepare all necessary equipment for possible blood replacement, get extra IV poles for possible fibrinogen and heparin administration if ordered, get extra warm blankets for both fetus and mother, monitor blood pressure, and prepare dressings as necessary
③ Apply fundal pressure to help deliver the placenta stat
④ Hold patient's hand and reassure her

61. The patient is a primipara. She has passed her due date by 2 weeks. She is apprehensive and does not know why she was instructed to come in for a test. She appears confused and bewildered. How can the nurse help her?
① To ease her distress the nurse could engage her in trivial conversation regarding the weather, current styles, and so forth
② Explain that she will be placed on a monitor for 20 minutes to an hour to see if her baby responds to her drinking water or to gentle external pressure by the nurse on her abdomen. The procedure is called a nonstress test
③ Tell the patient she may have to have an oxytocin challenge test (OCT) at a later date but that it is invasive
④ Tell the patient that many people are often past due, and she probably miscalculated her dates

62. As the nurse watches the monitor during an OCT procedure on a patient, she notes at least 3 late decelerations during at least 3 contractions. What should the nurse do?
① This indicates a positive test; call the head nurse immediately
② This is not a positive test; wait until the pattern changed
③ Stop the oxytocin (Pitocin) and administer nasal oxygen
④ Wheel her into the delivery room for immediate delivery

63. A patient over 35 years of age should be classified as:
① A good candidate for a normal pregnancy and delivery
② A high-risk pregnant mother
③ A candidate for eclampsia
④ A grand multipara

64. The nurse should explain to the patient that the OCT test is an invasive test because medication is given in the veins and it:
① Is uncomfortable for a short while
② Is not painful at all
③ Will take a few minutes to complete
④ Is a routine procedure for all pregnant women

65. If a patient is truly overdue, her newborn baby may have:
① Polydactyly and jaundice
② Desquamated palms of hands and soles of the feet
③ Meconium-stained amniotic fluid
④ Mongolian spots

66. A newborn is diagnosed with pathological jaundice. His sclera is yellow, his bilirubin index is 17, and he is not nursing well. If the newborn's index continues to rise, the nurse should:
    ① Tell the mother the baby will probably need an exchange transfusion and plan a teaching module of pros and cons
    ② Prepare unit for possible exchange transfusion procedure; obtain supplies, review procedure, wait for physician's orders
    ③ Place the baby under phototherapy light for longer periods of time; offer water every 2 hours until jaundice begins to fade
    ④ Suggest that the family all be tested for proper blood type

67. A patient who is 38 weeks pregnant is admitted to the maternity ward complaining of headaches and "blind spots" for about a week. She complained of upper abdominal pain in the AM and a few hours later experienced a convulsion. Her husband brought her to the hospital immediately.

    Admitting record:
    BP 140\112
    Albumin 4+
    FHT 140 strong
    Cervix effaced, dilated 3 cm
    Presenting part; station 0
    Membranes intact

    The admitting nurse, knowing the situation, would place her in:
    ① A semiprivate room with plenty of sunlight and air
    ② A semiprivate room, darkened and quiet; restricted visitors
    ③ A single, darkened room; no visitors, close to nurses' station
    ④ Single room, plenty of sunlight; no visitors, away from the nurses' station

68. The symptom that is often considered a warning sign of an impending convulsion in the toxic mother is:
    ① Headache
    ② Severe epigastric pain
    ③ Scotoma
    ④ Puffy face

69. A patient delivered her first baby, a boy, several hours ago. She has been admitted to her postpartum room in stable condition and is euphoric over her successful implementation of the Lamaze techniques. The nurse finds her uterus firm, slightly above the umbilicus. She has saturated one pad with red lochia. Her episiotomy appears clean, but her labia and perineal area are swollen and slightly black and blue. The nurse's first priority in nursing care should be to:

① Apply an ice glove to the perineal area
② Massage her uterus so it will go down below the umbilicus
③ Administer a tranquilizer because she is so euphoric
④ Watch for hemorrhage because her lochia is so red

70. A patient delivered a macrosomic infant, which means the infant is:
    ① Small for gestational age (SGA)
    ② Large, somewhat lethargic, weighing over 4500 g
    ③ Covered with newborn milia, which will disappear without treatment
    ④ Definitely diabetic and will be insulin dependent

71. The most important precaution that the nurse should follow in working with AIDS or HIV-positive patients is to use:
    ① Frequent handwashing procedures
    ② The designated forms to notify the Centers for Disease Control and report the name of your patient(s)
    ③ Universal precaution protocol
    ④ Masks, gloves, and gowns at all times

72. As a rule, the nurse should schedule the high-risk pregnant mother to be screened for gestational diabetes mellitus (GDM) at:
    ① 12 weeks' gestation
    ② 20 to 24 weeks' gestation
    ③ 32 weeks' gestation
    ④ 40 weeks' gestation

73. Postpartum teaching of a pregnancy-induced diabetic should include which of the following?
    ① Her symptoms should disappear in about 6 weeks
    ② She must be careful because she may become insulin dependent
    ③ She should try not to gain over 25 lb
    ④ She should have her glucose level checked for 5 years

74. A major health concern in women is alcohol consumption. When should nurses ideally direct their efforts toward counseling to prevent fetal alcohol syndrome (FAS)?
    ① Before pregnancy
    ② By the first trimester
    ③ Aggressive counseling during the second trimester
    ④ During the third trimester

75. Cocaine is addictive to newborns because of:
    ① The inability of the newborn's immature liver to excrete the drug rapidly
    ② The mother's long-term use of drugs before conception
    ③ The mother's ingestion of several different drugs is doubly addictive to the newborn
    ④ The mother's impaired uterine growth, resulting in the newborn having respiratory distress syndrome (RDS) after birth

ANSWERS AND RATIONALES

1. Application, implementation, health (a)
   ❷ Gives correct information without raising unnecessary alarm.
   ① It is within the scope of nursing practice to reinforce explanations of diagnostic procedures.
   ③ This is not what they asked the nurse. If they want information from the physician they should be encouraged to ask the physician themselves.
   ④ This does not answer the question and raises unnecessary alarm.

2. Comprehension, assessment, health (b)
   ❹ This is another term for an ultrasonography, which can outline the embryo, the placenta, and fetal parts as early as 4 weeks; this is a positive sign of pregnancy.
   ① Not a positive sign. The human chorionic gonadotropin (HCG) used in pregnancy tests may also emanate from a hydated mole or other nonpregnant sources. This is a probable sign.
   ② This is also a probable sign noted by an examiner. It is a softening of the lower segment of the uterus.
   ③ This is a presumptive sign, which the mother realizes after she has missed a period. Various occurrences from emotional stress to physical stress could cause amenorrhea, so this is not a correct answer.

3. Knowledge, implementation, psychosocial (c)
   ❹ Still considered the most effective method of birth control with very little side effects. This is the best answer.
   ① Incorrect. Intrauterine devices are still controversial. These are devices placed in the uterus to prevent pregnancy; however, there have been cases of extreme irritability to the uterus resulting in excessive bleeding and possible contamination. The jury is still undecided on the efficacy of this insertion method. It is invasive.
   ② Incorrect. Sperm can escape into the vagina if ejaculation is not carefully controlled. Very tenuous method subject to psychosocial factors as well.
   ③ Sheath that prevents sperm from entering the cervix. Must be placed effectively, and must be reliable—made from material that will not tear. Psychosocial factors influence this method. This is the recommended method to prevent spread of AIDS, but for the prevention of pregnancy, not 100% effective.

4. Knowledge, evaluation, physiologic (a)
   ❹ Correct answer. This is a digestive system change that occurs after an episode of morning sickness, which is a particular digestive system change.
   ① This belongs to the nervous system changes.
   ② This is caused by the activity of the lactiferous ducts, which are not a part of the digestive system, and the traces of sugar in the urine are a direct result of the activity of the ducts on the urinary system.
   ③ This is a "mask of pregnancy" and is an integumentary system change.

5. Comprehension, assessment, environment (b)
   ❸ Correct answer. Early, frequent, and continual testing of urine and blood pressure would signal early signs that could be addressed rapidly and appropriately.
   ① This is usually a third-trimester complication and would not be considered a preventable condition.
   ② This is not exactly preventable but can be helped by easing discomfort, teaching, and advising on care.
   ④ Abortions—spontaneous ones might have some early signs and symptoms that alert pending conditions, but this is not the best answer.

6. Application, implementation, physiologic (a)
   ❶ Exercise is generally safe in pregnancy if the woman has exercised previously. Otherwise it may be necessary to begin slowly.
   ②,③ This is true, however, it does not completely answer the question.
   ④ A physician should be consulted before starting exercise. A patient should not wait until pain is experienced.

7. Comprehension, planning, physiologic (a)
   ❷ Correct answer. Elevated levels of AFP indicate up to 5% to 10% of a neural defect, but must be followed by two consecutive AFP tests, ultrasound readings, and an amniocentesis.
   ① Fetal maturity is tested by an L/S ratio that determines lung maturity by measuring the ratio of the two components of surfactant (lecithin and sphingomyelin). An amniocentesis done after the 35th week of pregnancy should show an increase in the amount of lecithin and a decrease in sphingomyelin.
   ③ Genetic work-up, including family history and a series of blood tests, can evaluate risk of disease in offspring.
   ④ Respiratory distress syndrome is most likely to occur in low-birth-weight babies, premature babies, or babies known to be at risk for immature lung development.

8. Knowledge, assessment, physiologic (a)
   ❸ False labor is generally relieved by activity.
   ① True labor will have a regular interval between contractions and progress is shown in effacement and dilation of cervix.
   ② True labor does progess differently; however, this is not true labor.
   ④ There is no way to determine when true labor will occur after an episode of false labor.

9. Knowledge, assessment, physiologic (a)
   ❸ Correct answer. Without this, the embryo and fetus could not survive. This hormone changes the walls of the endometrium to prepare to accept a fertilized ovum.
   ① Stimulates endometrium to thicken; a "preparation" hormone to thicken uterine lining.
   ② Controls ovarian function.
   ④ This is secreted by the fertilized ovum and helps the corpus luteum to produce progesterone for the first trimester. This hormone affects pregnancy testing, and without it there would be no positive test results.

10. Application, implementation, physiologic (b)
    ❹ Return of lochia rubra after its initial cessation may be indicative of uterine subinvolution or hemorrhage.
    ① At ten days postpartum the fundus has returned to its position as a pelvic organ and is no longer palpable.
    ② Mothers commonly experience constipation; simple interventions can be suggested.
    ③ Postpartum blues occur most commonly during the third to tenth day postpartum.

11. Knowledge, comprehension, physiologic (a)
   ❸ Correct answer.
   ① This is ballottement or locating of fetal parts. It is not a part of a nonstress test.
   ② Sex of an infant may be seen on a screen during a sonogram, but not by a fetal monitoring device, which only measures fetal heart tones—strength of contractions and fetal movements through the FHT response.
   ④ Wrong. The mother is given orange juice for a nonstress test; for the stress test she is given oxytocin intravenously.

12. Knowledge, planning, health (b)
   ❸ Correct answer. In seminars by the March of Dimes the single abuse most negatively affecting the pregnant woman is crack and cocaine; alcohol abuse is also important.
   ① Economic and ethnic status does not necessarily affect mother or child negatively. It does affect nutrition and other physical deprivations, but there are social workers, related programs such as WIC, food stamps, and entitlement programs that may help.
   ② These are routine questions included in taking history and are rarely omitted in interviewing.
   ④ This is also included in the initial interviews but not in interviewing techniques. It may affect the ability to learn baby care and self-care. Important, but not current.

13. Comprehension, evaluation, physiologic (c)
   ❷ DTRs are absent; respiratory effort may quickly be impaired.
   ① BP is not affected by the drug.
   ③ It is being given to decrease the DTRs.
   ④ Should use good nursing judgment if DTRs are absent.

14. Knowledge, implementation, environment (b)
   ❸ 100 ml in 1 hr
   $$\frac{\times\ 15\ \text{gtt ml}}{1500\ \text{gtt in 1 hr}}$$
   1500 gtt divided by 60 min = 25 gtt/min
   ①,②,④ Incorrect calculation.

15. Knowledge, implementation, physiologic (b)
   ❶ When the patient becomes eclamptic, she has a seizure.
   ②,③ BP should be watched but is an indication of preeclampsia.
   ④ You should watch all pregnant patients for labor. This does not cause eclamptic conditions.

16. Application, assessment, physiologic (b)
   ❹ This may be a sign of illness.
   ① This is meconium, which is normal stool for about 48 hours.
   ② This is normal for a newborn. In older children and adults it may indicate possible CNS abnormality.
   ③ This is normal for full-term infants.

17. Application, evaluation, health (a)
   ❹ Never leaving the baby alone is essential to prevent injuries.
   ① Organization is important. Both partners are capable of providing the newborn with a bath.
   ② A schedule is not needed. Infants can be bathed any time day or night. Infants do not necessarily need a bath every day. Their face and perineal area have to be washed every day.

   ③ This is true; however, it is not the most important thing that is ascertained from a class.

18. Comprehension, implementation, physiologic (c)
   ❹ Within 72 hours, danger of seizure passes.
   ①,② Danger of seizure lasts longer. Normal recovery may be 1 to 2 hours or more.
   ③ Danger of seizure lasts longer than 24 hours.

19. Comprehension, planning, physiologic (b)
   ❷ Correct answer. Teenage nutritional patterns are poor whether the patient is rich, middle class, or poor.
   ① Incorrect answer. Although this is very important, psychosocial standards vary. A poor teenager brought up by a single, unmarried mother may view her situation as being able to have something (someone) whom she can love and who will love her. The nurse must know her patient's psychosocial background to counsel effectively.
   ③ Incorrect answer. It is true that many very young pregnant patients have underdeveloped pelvic bones and immature physiologic bony development, but this includes only a certain age group. Teenagers vary greatly in developmental maturity.
   ④ Incorrect answer. It is not relevant only to pregnant teenage patients. It is important, but not the major concern.

20. Application, implementation, physiologic (b)
   ❹ Folic acid has been shown to be a benefit in preventing neurological conditions.
   ① Given to newborns to prevent hemorrhaging.
   ② A B-complex vitamin involved in carbohydrate metabolism.
   ③ Useful in preventing certain forms of anemia in newborns.

21. Application, implementation, health (b)
   ❶ A pregnant woman with active disease needs effective treatment to protect herself and her unborn fetus.
   ② Preventive therapy can be postponed until after pregnancy. The risks of doing nothing in active disease are too great.
   ③ Treatment for active disease includes a minimum of 2 to 3 drugs.
   ④ Risk to the mother and fetus is too great to wait until the third trimester.

22. Comprehension, planning, physiologic (a)
   ❷ Milk is high in calcium, and natural sources are absorbed more fully.
   ①,④ Only a small portion of calcium is absorbed from a supplement, compared with a natural source.
   ③ Greens have less calcium than milk.

23. Knowledge, implementation, physiologic (a)
   ❹ This is the correct hormone.
   ① Levels significant toward end of pregnancy.
   ② Levels gradually increase to "hold" pregnancy.
   ③ Hormone that lowers peristalsis of the stomach and slows metabolism during pregnancy.

24. Application, implementation, health (b)
   ❸ Factual information; allows communication to be open.
   ① Factual information; however, does not allow patient to express concerns.
   ② Mothers may have definite feelings, which may or may not be backed up with facts.
   ④ Breastfeeding has advantages for mother and baby.

25. Application, implementation, psychosocial (b)
- ❸ This answer allows for communication that will encourage the couple to deal with their pain as a family unit. Allows for more effective coping with grief.
- ① The patient is an adult who cannot have her rights for appropriate standards of care taken away from her.
- ② Nurses should implement therapeutic methods of communication as an appropriate standard of care.
- ④ Patients exist as part of a family unit. Family members' needs should be considered.

26. Knowledge, comprehension, health (a)
- ❸ Correct and direct answer to the patient's question.
- ① Correct statement, but irrelevant to the question.
- ② Incorrect information.
- ④ Wrong. This is a partial explanation of fetal circulation.

27. Knowledge, assessment, health (b)
- ❶ Heart beating during embryonic period—correct.
- ② Incorrect.
- ③ Is third month; heart and cardiovascular system would have had to been working long before.
- ④ Placenta begins to form shortly after implantation and continues to form for 16 to 20 weeks into gestation, so this answer is wrong.

28. Knowledge, comprehension, physiologic (b)
- ❹ Correct answer.
- ① All true, but not a good answer to a pregnant mother.
- ② Also true, but not the best answer.
- ③ Too vague; not the best answer.

29. Knowledge, assessment, physiologic (b)
- ❷ Because the patient delivered a boy and a girl, they must be fraternal or unidentical. If they had been the same sex, the placenta and sacs would have to be identified.
- ① Monozygotic twins are always the same sex.
- ③ Blood tests are not the *best* answer; as a nurse you should know the status by identifying the placenta and sacs.
- ④ DNA tests are not the *best* answer; as a nurse you should know the status by identifying the placenta and sacs.

30. Comprehension, assessment, physiologic (a)
- ❸ Scientifically established.
- ① Unlikely; has probably had nutritional counseling for both pregnancies.
- ② Further testing needed to confirm this as gestational diabetes.
- ④ False statement.

31. Comprehension, assessment, environment (a)
- ❸ Pregnant twice, one child. Correct.
- ① Pregnant once, one child. Incorrect.
- ② Pregnant twice, two children. Incorrect.
- ④ Twice pregnant, no children. Incorrect.

32. Comprehension, assessment, physiologic (a)
- ❶ Two negatives are compatible.
- ② A negative and a positive are not compatible.
- ③ Her son has nothing to do with the pregnancy.
- ④ RhoGAM prevents problems when given either prenatally or within 72 hours of delivery.

33. Comprehension, planning, environment (a)
- ❷ According to Nägele's formula this is correct.
- ① Wrong according to Nägele's formula.
- ③ Incorrect.
- ④ Do not use the last day of the LMP.

34. Knowledge, assessment, physiologic (c)
- ❷ Correct answer. Signs and symptoms are bright red clots first, then light, painless bleeding.
- ① In abruptio placentae, there is pain, and there may or may not be bleeding. If there is bleeding, it is dark red and usually not clotted.
- ③ Bright red in variable amounts with pain.
- ④ Painless vaginal bleeding with bloody amniotic fluid.

35. Knowledge, implementation, physiologic (b)
- ❸ Correct. Simply relieving pressure by changing positions.
- ① The symptoms are pallor, light-headedness, dizziness, and slight nausea—rubbing the legs does not correct the syndrome.
- ② Incorrect. It is caused by the heavy uterus exerting pressure on the aorta and hampering good circulation. Determine the cause and effect first, then plan the intervention.
- ④ Know cause and effect. Because patient is dizzy, you would not recommend walking.

36. Application, implementation, physiologic (b)
- ❸ Correct information and advice.
- ① This does not alleviate leg cramps.
- ② This is for relief from the discomfort of varicose veins.
- ④ Not incorrect but not best answer.

37. Application, implementation, physiologic (b)
- ❸ Best answer.
- ① Relieve perineal discomfort.
- ② Temporary relief at best.
- ④ Improper advice.

38. Comprehension, assessment, physiologic (b)
- ❷ Correct statement and correct answer.
- ① You would consider doing follow-up tests to determine precise findings, and the physician would consider what medical treatment is needed.
- ③ False assumption.
- ④ Not a part of the nursing process to make this kind of determination.

39. Knowledge, implementation, physiologic (a)
- ❸ Correct instructions.
- ① This is acceptable for a routine urinalysis.
- ② Pregnancy tests do not require a sterile specimen.
- ④ Untrue.

40. Comprehension, planning, health (a)
- ❶ Reportable signs and symptoms which should be taught to the patient.
- ② Usual signs and symptoms and are normal.
- ③ Nonemergency signs and symptoms, which can be addressed during regular visits.
- ④ Later signs and symptoms; nonemergency.

41. Comprehension, planning, physiologic (b)
- ❹ Usually estriol levels are tested for placental functioning in the third trimester; a level of 12 mg is good, but below 12 mg in 24 hours may place the fetus in jeopardy.
- ① Fetal age is determined by uterine height, calculation of EDC.
- ② Amniocentesis procedure may reveal surfactant lecithin/sphingomyelin ratio and help determine lung maturity.
- ③ Human gonadotropin hormonal levels in the urine are tested early on in pregnancy, but the words *uterine nomenclature* are not related to the question.

42. Knowledge, assessment, health (a)
    ❷ German measles have a devastating effect on fetal growth: physical abnormalities, mental retardation, hearing impairment or deafness, blindness.
    ① Chickenpox may have a more severe action on the mother, but will not cause fetal physiologic defects or problems.
    ③ Synonym for chickenpox.
    ④ Regular measles; does not affect the unborn.

43. Knowledge, planning, environment (c)
    ❸ Third-trimester bleeding conditions, particularly because it includes no vaginal/rectal examinations.
    ① The bleeding, pain, or contractions would not be as acute.
    ② The pregnancy in itself would not necessitate these nursing measures unless the mother had symptoms.
    ④ Postpartum hemorrhage most likely would occur in recovery or within an hour or so after delivery. Because the baby is born, there would be no fetal monitoring.

44. Application, evaluation, environment (a)
    ❷ Correct. Responsible nursing procedure.
    ① Done as part of the routine responsibility, but #2 is specific to procedure accomplished.
    ③ Incomplete recording.
    ④ Part of the routine nursing care and not specific to this question.

45. Comprehension, implementation, physiologic (a)
    ❹ As the fetal presenting part descends down the birth canal, a full bladder will create an impediment to descent.
    ①,②,③ Possible but unlikely.

46. Comprehension, planning, physiologic (a)
    ❶ Correct answer.
    ② Incorrect answer. These are nursing responsibilities for the second stage of labor.
    ③ Incorrect answer. These are major nursing interventions for the third stage of labor.
    ④ Incorrect. These are nursing care measures for the fourth stage of labor, or 1 hour after delivery, usually in the recovery room.

47. Knowledge, implementation, environment (a)
    ❷ Fear is a major threat to women in labor.
    ① Whatever progress is made, the fear of facing labor alone is worse.
    ③ This statement is of no help if the physician is not beside her.
    ④ It is during labor she needs support.

48. Knowledge, assessment, environment (b)
    ❷ Correct answer. The LOP position means the bony back of the head presses against the spine, causing lower back pain because it presents bone against bone. The head must turn until the face is against the spine; this may happen spontaneously or by artificial means (maneuvers by the physician). Usually a slow and painful process of descent.
    ① This is a more normal descent and does not present itself to dystocia and pain.
    ③ Almost an impossible vaginal delivery position or lie; most certainly a cesarean section elective.
    ④ Does not describe a presentation.

49. Knowledge, planning, physiologic (b)
    ❶ See text; this is the correct answer.
    ② Does not explain the physiologic dynamics.
    ③ Pitocin is an oxytocic acting on the uterus.
    ④ Does not explain the physiologic dynamics of immediate postpartum phenomenon.

50. Comprehension, assessment, physiologic (a)
    ❷ Correct answer. Apgar score is 6. (See chart on p. 341.)
    Heart rate = 1
    Respiratory effort = 1
    Muscle tone = 1
    Reflex response = 2
    Color = 1
    ①,③,④ Incorrect.

51. Comprehension, evaluation, physiologic (a)
    ❸ Correct answer. Birth injury—occurs when the upper arm has been injured in such a way that the nerves of the brachial plexus are severed or injured, resulting in a paralysis.
    ①,② These are normal.
    ④ Normal cranial deviations resulting from normal vaginal delivery; these conditions occur as the caput descends through the birth canal.

52. Comprehension, assessment, physiologic (a)
    ❸ Symptoms indicative of abruptio placentae.
    ① This would give rise to painless bleeding.
    ② Onset gradual, accompanied by nausea, possibly vomiting, and gradual shock; abdomen tender but not boardlike.
    ④ Not a rigid, boardlike abdomen.

53. Comprehension, implementation, psychosocial (a)
    ❷ Attempts to teach, reassure, and describe condition.
    ① Alarming, senseless, and incorrect response; insensitive as well.
    ③ Inappropriate, incorrect answer.
    ④ Does not reassure or answer the partner's concern.

54. Application, planning, psychosocial (c)
    ❸ Explaining procedure, giving reassurance.
    ① Rude, curt; did not answer question.
    ② The physician was in the room, but he asked you.
    ④ Answer creates unnecessary anxiety with no explanation.

55. Knowledge, implementation, environment (b)
    ❸ In abruptio placentae this is standard practice.
    ① If bleeding subsides or stops, vaginal delivery is preferable.
    ② Should bleeding continue, a vaginal delivery places both mother and fetus in jeopardy.
    ④ Unlikely; emergency delivery tray items limited.

56. Comprehension, evaluation, physiologic (a)
    ❶ True statement. Physician and nurse should check to determine location of tear.
    ② Calcification indicates age, not a tear.
    ③ An abruptio does not preclude size or weight.
    ④ Unlikely. Confirmation by physician sufficient.

57. Comprehension, implementation, physiologic (b)
    ❷ First priority is to establish patent airway so baby can breathe, cry, and fill her lungs with oxygen.
    ① Not first priority.
    ③ Umbilical cord can be left attached; there is no danger in delaying the cutting of the cord while tasks with a higher priority are performed.

④ The delivery of the placenta may take anywhere from 5 to 20 minutes, since it must separate itself from the walls of the uterus; therefore this too is not top priority.

58. Comprehension, assessment, physiologic (b)
❷ The suddenness of precipitous delivery always predisposes the patient to possible hemorrhage.
① Not top priority; usual checking of IV and administration of any drug.
③ Many women experience this after delivery.
④ Precipitous delivery does not of itself cause massive infection.

59. Comprehension, planning, environment (b)
❷ Regulations for NSB clearly outlined in hospital policy.
① Depends on policy and will be determined by nursery supervisor.
③ Varied policies; that is, nursery nurse may be responsible for these procedures.
④ Administration of medication may be ordered and given on admission (to nursery).

60. Comprehension, planning, physiologic (b)
❷ Interpreting what is happening to the patient, the best assistance would be to prepare for medical interventions and anticipate what nursing actions you will implement.
① You will anticipate this, but you will have the necessary equipment ready.
③ You would not intervene unless requested to do so by the physician.
④ With massive bleeding, your patient is probably in shock and needs nursing and medical intervention stat.

61. Comprehension, assessment, psychosocial (b)
❷ Explain procedure.
① She wants to know what is going to happen to her, nothing else.
③ This is an unnecessary anxiety-causing statement, irrelevant at this time.
④ Not a comforting statement; implies stupidity.

62. Comprehension, implementation, physiologic (b)
❶ Your analysis and plan of action are correct.
② It is a positive test for trouble, and waiting for the pattern to change may compromise the fetus.
③ Together with the head nurse you may proceed to this.
④ There is nothing in this situation that tells you of an imminent delivery.

63. Knowledge, assessment, physiologic (a)
❷ From your textbook readings you know this to be true.
① Though the patient may indeed have a normal pregnancy and delivery, she is in a high-risk group.
③ The question asked for "classification."
④ This "grand" refers to pregnancy and children, not "age."

64. Application, planning, psychosocial (a)
❶ Reassurance and explanation.
② Levels of perception of pain differ, so do not promise there will be "no pain."
③ This test takes from 20 minutes to over an hour.
④ Untrue. Most women will never need this test.

65. Knowledge, planning, health (a)
❷ From your readings you know this is true so you will plan your nursing care accordingly.
① These are genetic anomalies not caused by overdue date.

③ An overdue baby may be larger than normal but will not necessarily have meconium-stained fluid.
④ These are normal birthmarks.

66. Application, planning, environment (a)
❷ Best response: preparation is started, so if the procedure is ordered, time is not lost.
① Responsibility is not assumed until order is given by physician.
③ Unless there is a standing order, this would not be appropriate.
④ Alarming family without proper teaching or preparation is inadvisable.

67. Comprehension, implementation, environment (a)
❸ Prevent convulsions; be able to respond stat.
① A severely eclamptic mother should not be in a semiprivate room, and certainly not in a sunny room with visitors.
② Must be quiet with absolutely no visitors.
④ Bright sunshine will aggravate the central nervous system, and being far from the nurses' station will hamper emergency nursing care.

68. Knowledge, assessment, environment (b)
❷ Significant symptom of an impending convulsion.
① Sign of change in blood pressure, preeclampsia.
③ Eye changes would not be noticed by the mother.
④ Not necessarily a sign of impending convulsions; rather of fluid retention.

69. Application, implementation, health (a)
❶ To reduce perineal swelling and edema.
② Normal location of the fundus a few hours after delivery.
③ Natural reaction is to be happy over an apparently successful birthing experience.
④ One pad saturated with red lochia several hours after delivery is normal and not a sign of hemorrhage.

70. Knowledge, evaluation, environment (b)
❷ Correct answer by definition, usually born of patients with gestational diabetes mellitus (GDM).
① *Macro* is large; *micro* is small.
③ Milia are small white visible papules on the face of the newborn and have nothing to do with infant size.
④ Large babies are screened and tested for diabetes, but this does not necessarily mean that they are or will become insulin-dependent diabetics.

71. Comprehension, implementation, environment (b)
❸ Correct answer.
① Incorrect. This is still a procedure used in some nurseries; however, more and more hospitals are using universal precaution protocol.
② Incorrect. It is not the responsibility for a nurse to report to the Centers for Disease Control. The nurse is responsible to the supervisor (or equivalent).
④ The mask, gloves, and gown at all times is not correct because most HIV-positive patients are not necessarily ill with the signs and symptoms of active AIDS. This precaution is for the patient whose immune system places him or her at risk or whose body fluid symptoms are positive.

72. Comprehension, planning, health (c)
    ❶ Correct answer. The sooner the mother is seen and evaluated, the better.
    ② If the opportunity to see the high-risk mother was not before this time (20 to 24 weeks' gestation), by all means see her. It is never too late.
    ③ Although scheduled evaluation should be even before, it is never too late to schedule continuing evaluations.
    ④ Evaluation scheduling should have been started as early as possible and continue at appropriate times throughout pregnancy.

73. Knowledge, planning, health (b)
    ❶ Correct answer: Most patients with pregnancy-induced diabetes or gestational diabetes mellitus (GDM) will return to normal by the 6-week checkup with the obstetrician.
    ② Not a good statement for health teaching. This is a scare tactic and not accurate. Some studies indicate that women who have successive large babies, and gain considerable weight, or are grossly overweight-before and after pregnancy, may experience some problems, but good follow-up teaching with emphasis on weight and nutritional care should help in maintaining sugar-free urine, etc.
    ③ There is no indication that a blanket number ensures against diabetes. There is considerable evidence to support the claim that excess weight is detrimental to health.

④ Unfounded statement. In education of pregnancy-induced diabetes or GDM, teaching mothers to follow up after each pregnancy is a good idea.

74. Comprehension, planning, psychosocial (b)
    ❶ Correct answer. To prevent FAS, the woman who drinks should have early and continuous counseling to prevent FAS and to maintain her psychosocial integrity needs. Record her family history, immediate family circumstances, and social activities.
    ② Fetal damage has already begun.
    ③ Never too late to try, but by the second trimester counseling aims to curb consumption to limit fetal damage.
    ④ Continued counseling; planned care to confront and assist in lowering alcohol dependency.

75. Comprehension, evaluation, psychosocial (c)
    ❶ Correct answer. Because all newborns have an immature liver, putting a drug into the system jeopardizes the infant.
    ② Prolonged use of a drug by the mother just before conception does not necessarily cause newborn addiction unless the mother continues the habit from conception throughout pregnancy to term.
    ③ This answer is itself is not correct. Usage must be continued during pregnancy.
    ④ Drugs may affect uterine growth because the addictive mother seldom has good nutritional habits, but, if carried through term, the infant does not necessarily have RDS.

Chapter 8 Pediatric Nursing

Pediatric nursing includes the care of both well and sick children and covers both preventive health care and restorative nursing care. This chapter is divided into the following age groups: infancy, toddlerhood, preschool, school age, and adolescence. The areas covered include normal growth and development, psychosocial development, health promotion, and health problems specific to each age group. Other topics discussed include the battered child syndrome, hospitalization and the child, and nursing care of the hospitalized child. The information provided in this chapter presents both the physical and psychologic aspects of care necessary in providing pediatric nursing care.

Assessment of Child and Family

A. Functions and structure of family
1. The functions and structure of the family are vital to the normal growth and development of the child
2. Three primary functions of the family are
   a. Providing physical care such as food, clothing, shelter, safety, prevention of illness, and care during illness
   b. Education and training: language, values, morals, and formal education
   c. Protecting psychologic and emotional health
B. Physical assessment of child
1. Performing a health history, including the child's past history as well as current complaints or problems, is done by the nurse, physician, or nurse practitioner
2. Assessment of child's physical growth and development level is done by the physician or nurse practitioner
C. Concepts of child development (Table 8-1)
1. Freud's theory of development is based on the child's psychosexual development
2. Erikson's theory of development is based on psychosocial development as a series of developmental tasks
3. Piaget's theory of development is based on intellectual (cognitive) development: how the child learns and develops his or her intelligence

INFANCY (AGES 4 WEEKS TO 1 YEAR)
Normal Growth and Development
PHYSICAL DEVELOPMENT*

A. 1 month
1. Physical
   a. Weight: gains about 150 to 210 g (5 to 7 oz) weekly during the first 6 months of life
   b. Height: gains about 2.5 cm (1 inch) a month for the first 6 months of life
2. Motor
   a. May lift the head temporarily, but generally the head must be supported
   b. Holds the head parallel with the body when placed prone
   c. Can turn the head from side to side when prone or supine
   d. Asymmetric posture dominates, such as tonic neck reflex
   e. Primitive reflexes still present and strong (grasp, Moro, tonic neck)
3. Sensory
   a. Follows a light to midline
   b. Eye movements coordinated most of the time
   c. Visual acuity 20/100 to 20/50
   d. Quiet when hears a voice
4. Socialization and vocalization
   a. Smiles indiscriminately
   b. Makes small throaty sounds
   c. Watches parent's face when he or she talks to infant
B. 2 to 3 months
1. Physical: posterior fontanel closed
2. Motor
   a. Holds the head erect for a short time and can raise chest supported on the forearms

b. Can carry hand or an object to the mouth at will
   c. Reaches for attractive objects but misjudges distances
   d. Grasp, tonic neck, and Moro reflexes are fading
   e. Can sit when the back is supported; knees will be flexed and back rounded
   f. Step or dance reflex disappears
   g. Plays with fingers and hands
3. Sensory
   a. Follows a light to the periphery
   b. Has binocular coordination (vertical and horizontal vision)
   c. Locates sounds by turning head in direction of the sound
4. Socialization and vocalization
   a. Smiles in response to a person or object
   b. Coos and gurgles; shows pleasure in making sounds
   c. Stops crying when parent enters the room
C. 4 to 5 months
1. Physical: drools because salivary glands are functioning, but the child does not have sufficient coordination to swallow saliva
2. Motor
   a. Balances the head well in a sitting position
   b. Sits with little support; holds the back straight when pulled to a sitting position
   c. Symmetric body position predominates
   d. Can sustain a portion of own weight when held in a standing position
   e. Reaches for and grasps an object with the whole hand
   f. Can roll over from back to side
   g. Lifts the head and shoulders at a 90-degree angle when prone
   h. Primitive reflexes (e.g., grasp, tonic neck, and Moro) have disappeared
3. Sensory
   a. Recognizes familiar objects and people
   b. Beginning eye-hand coordination
4. Socialization and vocalization
   a. Laughs aloud
   b. Definitely enjoys social interaction with people
   c. Vocalizes displeasure when an object is taken away
D. 6 to 7 months
1. Physical
   a. Weight: gains about 90 to 150 g (3 to 5 oz) weekly during second 6 months of life; weight doubles by 6 months
   b. Height: gains about 1.25 cm (½ inch) a month
   c. Teething may begin with eruption of two lower central incisors, followed by upper incisors (Fig. 8-1)
2. Motor
   a. Can turn over equally well from stomach or back
   b. Sits fairly well unsupported, especially if placed in a forward-leaning position
   c. Hitches or moves backward when in a sitting position
   d. Can transfer a toy from one hand to the other
   e. Can approach a toy and grasp it with one hand
   f. Plays with feet and puts them in mouth
   g. When lying down, lifts head as if trying to sit up
   h. Transfers everything from hand to mouth
3. Sensory
   a. Has taste preferences; will spit out disliked foods
   b. Responds to own name

---

*From Saxton DF, Nugent PM, Pelikan PK: *Mosby's comprehensive review of nursing*, ed 15, St. Louis, 1996, Mosby.

Table 8-1	Concepts of Child Development			
Age	Developmental stage	Freud's theory	Erikson's theory	Piaget's theory
4 wk-1 yr	Infancy	Oral stage	Trust vs. mistrust	Sensorimotor phase
1-3 yr	Toddlerhood	Anal stage	Autonomy vs. shame and doubt	Preoperational phase
3-5 yr	Preschool age	Oedipal stage Latency stage	Initiative vs. guilt	Preoperational phase continued
6-12 yr	School age	Latency stage continued Genital stage	Industry vs. inferiority	Concrete operational phase Formal operational phase
13-18 yr	Adolescence	Genital stage continued	Identity vs. identify confusion	Formal operational phase continued

4. Socialization and vocalization
   a. Begins to differentiate between strange and familiar faces and shows "stranger anxiety"
   b. Makes polysyllabic vowel sounds ("baba," "dada")
   c. Plays peekaboo
   d. Responds to word "no"
E. 8 to 9 months
   1. Motor
      a. Sits steadily alone
      b. Has good hand-to-mouth coordination
      c. Developing pincer grasp, with preference for use of one hand over the other
      d. Crawls and then creeps (creeping is more advanced because the abdomen is supported off the floor)
      e. Can raise self to a sitting position but may require help to pull self to feet
   2. Sensory
      a. Depth perception is beginning to develop
      b. Displays interest in small objects
   3. Socialization and vocalization
      a. Shows anxiety with strangers by turning or pushing away and crying
      b. Definite social attachment is evident: stretches out arms to loved ones
      c. Is voluntarily separating self from mother by desire to act on own
      d. Reacts to adult anger: cries when scolded

   e. Dislikes dressing, diaper change
   f. No true words as yet, but comprehends words such as "bye-bye," "no-no"
F. 10 to 12 months
   1. Physical
      a. Has tripled birth weight by 1 year
      b. Upper and lower lateral incisors usually have erupted for total of 6 to 8 teeth
      c. Head and chest circumferences are equal
      d. Lumbar curve develops; lordosis evident when walking
   2. Motor
      a. Stands alone for short times
      b. Walks with help; moves around by holding onto furniture
      c. Can sit down from a standing position without help
      d. Can eat from a spoon and drink from a cup but needs help; prefers using fingers
      e. Can play pat-a-cake
      f. Can hold a crayon to make a mark on paper
      g. Helps in dressing, such as putting arm through sleeve
   3. Sensory
      a. Visual acuity 20/50+
      b. Amblyopia may develop with lack of binocularity
      c. Discriminates simple geometric forms
   4. Socialization and vocalization
      a. Shows emotions such as jealousy, affection, anger

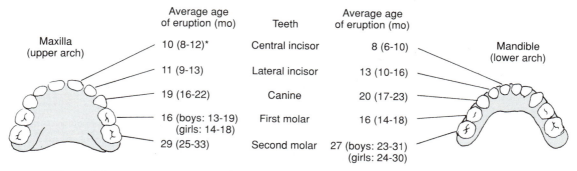

Figure 8-1.   Sequence of eruption of primary teeth. Range represents ± 1 standard deviation or 67% of subjects studied. (Data from McDonald RE, Avery DR: Dentistry for the child and adolescent, ed 6, St Louis, 1994, Mosby.)

b. Enjoys familiar surroundings and will explore away from mother

c. Fearful in strange situation or with strangers; clings to mother

d. May develop habit of "security" blanket

e. Can say 3-5 words besides *Dadda* or *Mama*

f. Understands simple verbal requests, such as "Give it to me"

g. Knows own name

PSYCHOSOCIAL DEVELOPMENT

A. Infants are in Erikson's stage of "trust vs. mistrust." Infants will develop a sense of trust or mistrust depending on how their needs are met by their parents (or other caregivers)

B. As infants grow older, they slowly realize that they are separate from their environment and that they influence their environment with their actions

C. Infants' early activities are mostly reflexes: crying, sucking, kicking, and so on. As the months progress, they learn to move in certain ways, follow with their eyes, and smile in response to a smile and soft words

Health Promotion

A. Immunizations should be given on schedule; Fig. 8-2

B. Nutrition appropriate to the age and needs of the infant should be provided

1. Human milk is the most desirable complete diet for the first 6 months of life

2. Introduction and strained foods may begin at 6 months of age, starting with strained fruits

3. Solid foods should be introduced slowly, in small amounts, and one at a time, to determine the infant's likes and dislikes; this also helps detect possible allergies to certain foods. Allow 4 to 7 days between introduction of each new food

Recommended Childhood Immunization Schedule
United States, January - June 1996

Vaccines are listed under the routinely recommended ages. Bars indicate range of acceptable ages for vaccination. Shaded bars indicate catch-up vaccination: at 11-12 years of age, hepatitis B vaccine should be administered to children not previously vaccinated, and Varicella Zoster Virus vaccine should be administered to children not previously vaccinated who lack a reliable history of chickenpox.

Age ▶ Vaccine ▼	Birth	1 mo	2 mos	4 mos	6 mos	12 mos	15 mos	18 mos	4-6 yrs	11-12 yrs	14-16 yrs
Hepatitis B[1,2]	Hep B-1									Hep B[2]	
		Hep B-2			Hep B-3						
Diphtheria, Tetanus, Pertussis[3]		DTP	DTP	DTP	DTP[3] (DTaP at 15+ m)				DTP or DTaP	Td	
H. influenzae type b[4]		Hib	Hib	Hib[4]	Hib[4]						
Polio[5]		OPV[5]	OPV	OPV					OPV		
Measles, Mumps, Rubella[6]					MMR				MMR[6] or MMR[6]		
Varicella Zoster Virus Vaccine[7]					Var					Var[7]	

Approved by the Advisory Committee on Immunization Practices (ACIP), the American Academy of Pediatrics (AAP), and the American Academy of Family Physicians (AAFP).

[1] **Infants born to HBsAg-negative mothers** should receive 2.5 µg of Merck vaccine (Recombivax HB) or 10 µg of SmithKline Beecham (SB) vaccine (Engerix-B). The 2nd dose should be administered ≥1 mo after the 1st dose.
Infants born to HBsAg-positive mothers should receive 0.5 mL Hepatitis B Immune Globulin (HBIG) within 12 hr of birth, and either 5 µg of Merck vaccine (Recombivax HB) or 10 µg of SB vaccine (Engerix-B) at a separate site. The 2nd dose is recommended at 1-2 mos of age and the 3rd dose at 6 mos of age.
Infants born to mothers whose HBsAg status is unknown should receive either 5 µg of Merck vaccine (Recombivax HB) or 10 µg of SB vaccine (Engerix-B) within 12 hr of birth. The 2nd dose of vaccine is recommended at 1 mo of age and the 3rd dose at 6 mos of age.

[2] Adolescents who have not previously received 3 doses of hepatitis B vaccine should initiate or complete the series at the 11-12 year-old visit. The 2nd dose should be administered at least 1 mo after the 1st dose, and the 3rd dose should be administered at least 4 mos after the 1st dose and at least 2 mos after the 2nd dose.

[3] DTP4 may be administered at 12 mos of age, if at least 6 mos have elapsed since DTP3. DTaP (diphtheria and tetanus toxoids and acellular pertussis vaccine) is licensed for the 4th and/or 5th vaccine dose(s) for children aged ≥15 mos and may be preferred for these doses in this age group. Td (tetanus and diphtheria toxoids, adsorbed, for adult use) is recommended at 11-12 years of age if at least 5 years have elapsed since the last dose of DTP, DTaP, or DT.

[4] Three H. influenzae type b (Hib) conjugate vaccines are licensed for infant use. If PRP-OMP (PedvaxHIB [Merck]) is administered at 2 and 4 mos of age, a dose at 6 mos is not required. After completing the primary series, any Hib conjugate vaccine may be used as a booster.

[5] Oral poliovirus vaccine (OPV) is recommended for routine infant vaccination. Inactivated poliovirus vaccine (IPV) is recommended for persons with a congenital or acquired immune deficiency disease or an altered immune status as a result of disease or immunosuppressive therapy, as well as their household contacts, and is an acceptable alternative for other persons. The primary 3-dose series for IPV should be given with a minimum interval of 4 wks between the 1st and 2nd doses and 6 mos between the 2nd and 3rd doses.

[6] The 2nd dose of MMR is routinely recommended at 4-6 yrs of age or at 11-12 yrs of age, but may be administered at any visit, provided at least 1 mo has elapsed since receipt of the 1st dose.

[7] Varicella zoster virus vaccine (Var) can be administered to susceptible children any time after 12 months of age. Unvaccinated children who lack a reliable history of chickenpox should be vaccinated at the 11-12 year-old visit.

Figure 8-2. Recommended childhood immunization schedule.

4. Weaning from breast or bottle to a cup can begin between 5 and 6 months of age, although the infant cannot be weaned completely until between 12 and 24 months of age

C. Safety and accident prevention includes a safe home environment, safe toys, use of car seats, and close attention to the infant who is crawling or walking

Health Problems

NUTRITIONAL DISORDERS

FAILURE TO THRIVE (FTT)

A. Definition: a state of inadequate growth resulting from inability to obtain and/or use calories; leads to malnutrition

B. Symptoms: below normal weight and height (below 5th percentile for age), listlessness, poor feeding habits, unresponsive to holding and attention, voluntary regurgitation, prolonged periods of sleep

C. Diagnosis
1. Based on symptoms and a continued deviation from an established growth curve
2. Three general categories of FTT
   a. Organic: result of a physical cause such as congenital defects of gastrointestinal (GI) system or heart
   b. Nonorganic: unrelated to a disease; usually caused by psychosocial factors
   c. Idiopathic: unexplained cause; may be grouped with nonorganic FTT

D. Treatment/nursing interventions (directed at correcting the malnutrition)
1. Correction of organic causes, if possible
2. Development of a structured routine
3. Sensory stimulation
4. Adequate food for weight gain; this may include nasogastric feedings as well as bottle feedings during early treatment
5. Tender loving care; holding and cuddling, talking to the infant
6. Teaching and encouraging the mother and father regarding feeding, infant care, and parenting skills
7. Family counseling when needed

COLIC

A. Definition: paroxysmal abdominal pain or cramping that is manifested by crying and drawing the legs up to the abdomen; colic is most commonly seen in infants under the age of 3 months

B. Symptoms: episodes of loud crying accompanied by abdominal cramping; despite obvious indications of pain, the infant usually tolerates feedings well and gains weight

C. Diagnosis: based on symptoms reported by parents/care givers

D. Treatment/nursing interventions:
1. If child is bottle-fed, investigation of possibility of cow's milk allergy; substitution of another formula (such as casein hydrosolate [Nutramigen]) may be tried
2. Comfort measures that can be used by the parents/care givers:
   a. Place infant prone over a covered hot-water bottle or covered heating pad (ensure that hot water bottle is warm, not hot)
   b. Massage infant's abdomen
   c. Change infant's position frequently
   d. Provide smaller, frequent feedings; burp infant during and after feedings, and place infant in an upright seat after feeding
   e. Introduce pacifier for added sucking
3. Pharmacologic agents such as sedatives, antispasmodics, antihistamines, and antiflatulents are sometimes recommended

RESPIRATORY DISORDERS

UPPER RESPIRATORY INFECTIONS (URIs)

A. Definition: viral or bacterial infection affecting the upper respiratory tract; nasopharyngitis or the "common cold" is particularly common in children of all ages

B. Symptoms: fever, sore throat, sneezing, nasal congestion, occasional cough, irritability, anorexia

C. Diagnosis: based on the symptoms

D. Treatment/nursing interventions
1. Bed rest until free of fever
2. Encourage oral fluids
3. Antipyretics for fever (acetaminophen, not aspirin)
4. Nose drops to relieve nasal congestion
5. Oral decongestants as ordered
6. Adequate nutrition for age; high-calorie fluids and soft foods are better tolerated by infants and young children
7. Cool air humidifier for moistened air (to assist in decreasing congestion)

ACUTE OTITIS MEDIA

A. Definition: middle ear infection; frequently caused by nasopharyngeal infections that travel through the infant's shortened, widened eustachian tubes

B. Symptoms: fever, irritability, restlessness, pulling or rubbing of the ears, loss of appetite; otoscopy reveals a bright red, bulging tympanic membrane

C. Diagnosis: based on the symptoms and history of recent URI

D. Treatment/nursing interventions
1. Antibiotics as ordered for bacterial infections (usually oral and/or ear drops)
2. Antipyretics for fever
3. Analgesics/antipyretics for discomfort (acetaminophen, ibuprofen)
4. Encourage oral fluids
5. Promote rest and quiet environment
6. Myringotomy and insertion of polyethylene tubes by the physician, to allow for drainage of fluid
7. Observe for drainage; keep ears clean

LOWER RESPIRATORY INFECTIONS

Respiratory Syncytial Virus (RSV)/Bronchiolitis

A. Definition:
1. Bronchiolitis is an acute viral infection that occurs primarily in winter and spring, and is most common in infants and children 2 years of age; it causes the bronchioles to become plugged with mucus, and the bronchiole mucosa to swell; the mucus traps the air in the lungs, making it difficult for the infant to expel the air
2. RSV is related to the parainfluenza virus; it is responsible for at least 50% of the diagnosed cases of bronchiolitis; the peak incidence for RSV infection is 2 to 5 months of age; it is transmitted predominantly through direct contact with respiratory secretions; RSV has been known to survive for hours on countertops, gloves, and cloth, and for half an hour on skin

B. Symptoms:
1. Usually begins with an upper respiratory infection; symptoms include rhinorrhea, coughing, sneezing, pharyngitis, wheezing, and intermittent fever
2. With progression of the disease, there is increased coughing and wheezing, air hunger, tachypnea, retractions, and cyanosis
3. Symptoms of severe illness include tachypnea of >70 breaths per minute, listlessness, poor air exchange, apneic spells, O$_2$ saturation <95%

C. Diagnosis
1. Based on clinical symptoms
2. RSV can be identified by various tests done on nasal/nasopharyngeal secretions to detect RSV antigen

D. Treatment/nursing interventions
1. Humidified oxygen inhalation (to relieve dyspnea and hypoxia)
2. Elevate head of crib
3. Monitor vital signs and oxygen saturation (via pulse oximeter)
4. Adequate fluid intake, including IV fluids as needed for hydration
5. Allow infant to rest as much as possible
6. Medical therapy for bronchiolitis has not proved to be effective; however, Ribavirin, an antiviral agent, is used specifically for RSV infection
   a. Ribavirin is administered by nebulization via an oxygen hood, tent, or mask for 12 to 20 hours per day, for 3 to 5 days
   b. It is most commonly used in children with RSV infection who are at high risk for complications caused by other conditions, including chronic lung conditions, immunodeficiency, and certain neurologic diseases (such as severe cerebral palsy)

Viral Pneumonia
A. Definition: inflammation of the lung, characterized by interstitial pneumonitis with inflammation of the mucosa and walls of bronchi and bronchioles
B. Symptoms: fever, cough, rapid respiratory rate, listlessness
C. Diagnosis: based on the symptoms and results of chest x-ray films
D. Treatment/nursing interventions
1. Elevate the head of the crib
2. Croup tent for humidified oxygen inhalation
3. Chest physiotherapy and postural drainage
4. Antibiotics as ordered (for bacterial pneumonia)
5. Antipyretics for fever
6. Monitor vital signs frequently
7. Encourage clear fluids by mouth
8. Allow infant to rest to prevent dyspnea

GASTROINTESTINAL DISORDERS
INFECTIOUS GASTROENTERITIS
A. Definition: diarrhea and vomiting that may be caused by viral or bacterial infections
B. Symptoms: frequent, loose stools, irritability, vomiting, abdominal distention, dehydration, sunken fontanel, poor skin turgor, weak, rapid pulse
C. Diagnosis: based on the symptoms; specific bacterial cause can be isolated in a stool culture (most commonly *E. coli* or rotavirus in the infant)

D. Treatment/nursing interventions
1. Oral rehydration therapy (with commercially prepared solutions such as Pedialyte); amount is based on infant's weight, and percentage of dehydration
2. IV fluids with electrolytes as ordered, if oral rehydration therapy is not effective, or if dehydration is severe
3. Return to normal diet (including formula, cow's milk, and age-appropriate solids) should be started as soon as they are tolerated; the "BRAT" diet (bananas, rice cereal, applesauce, tea/toast) is contraindicated for the infant with acute diarrhea because it has little nutritional value
4. Note amount, color, and consistency of stools and emesis
5. Keep accurate intake and output record (if necessary, weigh diapers to measure urine output)
6. Maintain proper isolation technique (enteric precautions)
7. Provide good skin care to buttocks and perineum after each diaper change; cleanse well; leave area open to air when possible; apply ointments as ordered
7. Provide time for stimulation, holding, and cuddling

HYPERTROPHIC PYLORIC STENOSIS
A. Definition: hypertrophy of the pyloric muscle fibers and narrowing of the pylorus, which is at distal end of the stomach (Fig. 8-3)
B. Symptoms: usually appear between 3 and 8 weeks of age; projectile vomiting of formula and mucus, irritability, weight loss, and dehydration; the physician can often palpate the olive-size pyloric mass in the abdomen
C. Diagnosis: based on the symptoms, physical examination, and, if necessary, upper gastrointestinal radiographic or ultrasound studies
D. Treatment/nursing interventions
1. Preoperative
   a. IV fluids with electrolytes as ordered
   b. NPO unless ordered to feed
   c. Nasogastric (NG) tube is often inserted to remove excess stomach contents immediately before surgery (pyloromyotomy)
2. Postoperative
   a. Position the infant on right side or abdomen or in infant seat to prevent aspiration
   b. NPO; first feeding begins about 4 to 6 hours after surgery (glucose water); amounts are increased slowly, to administer small frequent feedings as ordered, formula is started 24 hours postoperatively if clear fluids are retained
   c. General postoperative nursing care

NERVOUS SYSTEM DISORDERS
FEBRILE SEIZURES
A. Definition: seizures caused by high fever (102° to 105° F; 38.8° to 40.5° C); most often seen between 6 months and 3 years of age
B. Symptoms: seizures characterized by stiffening of the body, with jerking movements of the extremities and face, ending with a lapse of consciousness
C. Diagnosis: based on evidence of seizure activity preceded by high fever
1. Simple febrile seizures are brief and generalized
2. Complex febrile seizures are prolonged and may have focal features

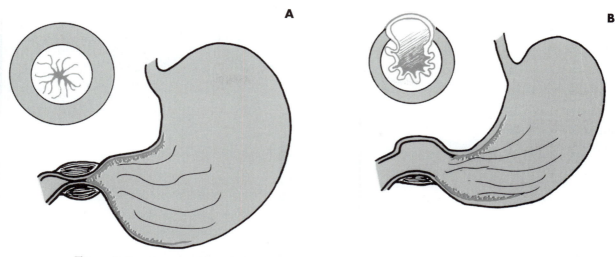

Figure 8-3. **Hypertrophic pyloric stenosis. A,** Enlarged muscular tumor nearly obliterates pyloric channel. **B,** Longitudinal surgical division of muscle down to submucosa establishes adequate passageway. (From Whaley LF, Wong DL: *Nursing care of infants and children*, ed 5, St Louis, 1995, Mosby.)

D. Treatment/nursing interventions
   1. Anticonvulsant (phenobarbital) and antianxiety (diazepam) medications to control the seizures; antipyretics (acetaminophen) to control fever (see Chapter 3, Pharmacology)
   2. Padded side rails
   3. Airway and suction equipment at bedside
   4. During seizure, do not restrain the infant; turn his or her head to the side to allow saliva to drain out of the mouth; *do not* try to insert a seizure stick or airway in the infant's mouth during a seizure; observe the seizure and protect the infant from harm
   5. Documentation: note the kinds of movements, behavior before the seizure (if known), duration of the seizure, skin color and vital signs during and after the seizure, and medications given during the seizure, including the infant/toddler's reaction to the medications
   6. Parent teaching should include care of the infant during a seizure

MENINGITIS

A. Definition: infection of the spinal meninges and fluid; caused by several bacteria and viruses
B. Symptoms: elevated temperature, irritability, poor feeding, high-pitched cry, nuchal rigidity, seizures, bulging fontanel
C. Diagnosis: based on the symptoms and the presence of cloudy spinal fluid when lumbar puncture is performed (increased WBC count; decreased glucose level and increased protein level in the spinal fluid) (Fig. 8-4)
D. Treatment/nursing interventions
   1. Isolation from other children (for bacterial meningitis)
   2. IV antibiotics as ordered
   3. Monitor vital signs, neurologic status, and level of consciousness frequently
   4. IV fluids as ordered
   5. Diet: infant may be NPO at first, until liquids can be tolerated

   6. Antipyretics to reduce elevated temperature
   7. Handle the infant as little as possible when the infant is irritable and uncomfortable; keep room quiet
   8. Seizure precautions (padded side rails)

INTEGUMENTARY DISORDERS
INFANTILE ECZEMA

A. Definition: atopic dermatitis caused by an allergic reaction to some irritant; usually begins between 2 and 6 months of age, and undergoes spontaneous remission around age 3
B. Symptoms: reddened, raised rash starting on cheeks and spreading to arms and legs; itching, oozing of vesicles
C. Diagnosis: based on the story and symptoms; the cause of the eczema (the allergen) must also be determined to control further episodes
D. Treatment/nursing interventions
   1. Good skin care; keep affected areas clean
   2. Tub baths with tepid water, baking soda, and corn starch to relieve the itching
   3. Keep skin well hydrated; various lubricants or moisturizing lotions may be ordered.
   4. Antihistamines and topical steroids as ordered to control itching
   5. "Mittens" to prevent scratching
   6. Elbow restraints to prevent scratching (only if necessary)
   7. Provide for sensory stimulation, holding, and cuddling at frequent intervals

IMPETIGO

A. Definition: infection of the skin caused by *Streptococcus* or *Staphylococcus* bacteria; occurs in nurseries when strict handwashing technique is not followed (impetigo neonatorum); also occurs in preschool and school-age children
B. Symptoms: reddened, vesicular lesions (pustules)
C. Diagnosis: based on the symptoms; specific bacterial cause can be determined by culture of the draining lesions
D. Treatment/nursing interventions
   1. Isolation of infant (child)

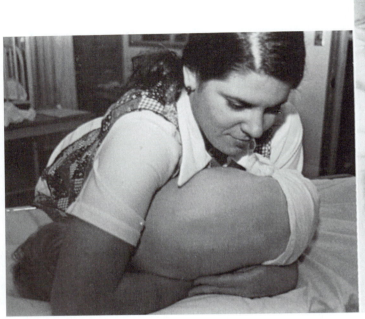
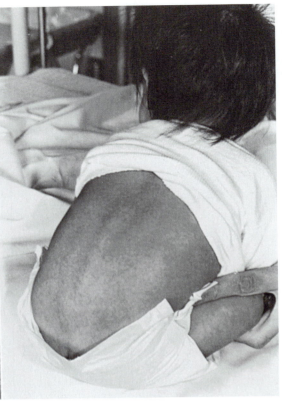

Figure 8-4. **Position for lumbar puncture. A,** Older child. **B,** Infant. (From Whaley LF, Wong DL: *Nursing care of infants and children*, ed 4, St Louis, 1991, Mosby.)

2. Strict handwashing technique by all persons coming in contact with the infant
3. Warm saline compresses to lesions, followed by a gentle cleansing and topical antibiotic ointment
4. Systemic antibiotics and corticosteroids may be ordered for infants/children with widespread lesions

CONGENITAL DEFECTS AND HEREDITARY DISORDERS
GASTROINTESTINAL SYSTEM
Hirschsprung's Disease
A. Definition: distention of a portion of the lower colon caused by a congenital lack of nerve cells in the wall of the colon just below the distended section (Fig. 8-5)
B. Symptoms: constipation (including a lack of meconium stool in the newborn in the first 24 hours), abdominal distention, bile-stained mucus and emesis, inadequate weight gain
C. Diagnosis: based on the symptoms, results of barium enema, rectal biopsy, and/or anorectal manometry
D. Treatment/nursing interventions: based on the type of surgery done (bowel resection, sometimes with temporary colostomy); surgery done in two or three stages
   1. Preoperative
      a. Observation of stools: color, amount, and consistency
      b. IV fluids and electrolytes as ordered
   2. Postoperative
      a. NG tube to low-suction or gravity drainage
      b. General postoperative care
      c. Routine colostomy care as necessary (prn)

d. Vital signs as ordered; axillary temperatures should be taken
e. IV fluids as ordered
f. NPO; resume diet as ordered
g. Record intake and output (I&O) every shift
h. Observe stools and record amount and characteristics
i. Observe for rectal bleeding and abdominal distention
j. Parent teaching and support

Omphalocele
A. Definition: the abdominal organs protrude through an abnormal opening in the abdominal wall and form a sac lying on the abdomen
B. Diagnosis: based on symptoms and physical examination
C. Treatment/nursing interventions
   1. Preoperative
      a. Keep the omphalocele covered with sterile gauze, moistened with normal saline and a plastic drape until surgery can be performed
      b. Maintain sterile technique as much as possible in caring for the omphalocele
   2. Postoperative
      a. Surgery: the organs are returned to the abdominal cavity, and the abdominal wall is closed
      b. General postoperative care, including mechanical ventilation for several days
      c. Parenteral nutrition for several days
      d. Observe stools and record amount and characteristics

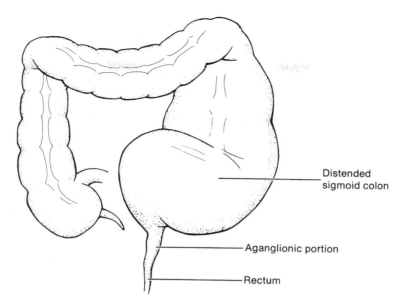

Distended
sigmoid colon

Aganglionic portion

Rectum

Figure 8-5. **Hirschsprung's disease.** (From Whaley LF, Wong DL: *Nursing care of infants and children*, ed 4, St Louis, 1991, Mosby.)

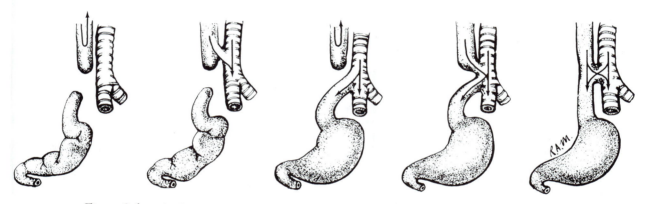

Figure 8-6. **The five most common types of esophageal atresia and tracheoesophageal fistula.** (From Whaley LF, Wong DL: *Nursing care of infants and children*, ed 4, St Louis, 1991, Mosby.)

Imperforate Anus

A. Definition: the rectal pouch ends blindly at a distance above the anus; sometimes there is no anal opening; there are various forms of this defect
B. Symptoms: no stools in the first 24 hours after birth; rectal thermometer cannot be inserted properly
C. Diagnosis: made by digital rectal examination, intestinal x-ray examination, and endoscopy
D. Treatment/nursing interventions
    1. Surgical procedure to reconnect the ends of the rectum and form an anal opening
    2. General postoperative nursing care

Esophageal Atresia

A. Definition: the upper end of the esophagus ends in a blind pouch; the lower end may also end in a blind pouch or may be connected to the trachea by fistula defect (tracheo-esophageal fistula) (Fig. 8-6)

B. Symptoms: excessive salivation and drooling, coughing and choking during feedings, regurgitation of all feedings
C. Diagnosis: based on symptoms as well as passage of an NG tube or catheter down the esophagus to test for patency; exact anomaly is determined by x-ray studies
D. Treatment/nursing interventions
    1. NPO with administration of IV fluids as ordered
    2. Suctioning of nose and mouth as needed
    3. Insertion of an NG tube to drain mucus and fluid from the blind pouch
    4. Antibiotic therapy as ordered (for probable aspiration pneumonia)
    5. Surgical repair to correct the defects and reconnect the ends of the esophagus

Intussusception

A. Definition: telescoping of one portion of the bowel into a distal portion; the most common site is at the ileocecal valve; usually occurs between 3 and 12 months of age

B. Symptoms: appear suddenly; pallor; sharp, colicky pain causes infant to draw up legs and cry out (this occurs every 5 to 10 minutes); vomiting; stools with blood and mucus ("red currant jelly" stools); signs of shock

C. Diagnosis: based on symptoms; definitive diagnosis can be made radiographically with barium enema

D. Treatment/nursing interventions: this is an emergency that requires immediate treatment. The initial treatment of choice is hydrostatic reduction by barium enema; if this is not effective, surgery is necessary

   1. Preoperative
     a. Careful observation and recording of vital signs frequently
     b. IV fluids with electrolytes as ordered
     c. NPO
     d. NG tube to remove gastric contents
     e. Emotional support for parents; explain all procedures; answer questions
     f. Observe for passage of abnormal brown stool (indicates the intussusception has reduced itself); report to physician immediately

   2. Postoperative
     a. General postoperative care
     b. IV fluids as ordered; NPO
     c. Record intake and output
     d. Auscultate for return of bowel sounds
     e. Observe all stools and record
     f. Resume feedings slowly as ordered

NERVOUS SYSTEM

Hydrocephalus

A. Definition: disorder caused by an obstruction of cerebrospinal fluid drainage or by impaired absorption of CSF fluid in the subarachnoid space; characterized by an excess of cerebrospinal fluid (CSF) within the cranial cavity, which causes an enlarged head and potential brain damage or retardation; it occurs in association with several other anomalies

B. Symptoms: bulging of the anterior fontanel, enlargement of the head, irritability, lethargy, opisthotonos, "setting-sun" sign (sclera can be seen above the iris because of increased intracranial pressure); lower extremity spasticity

C. Diagnosis: based on the symptoms, frequent measurements of head circumference, computerized tomography (CT), and magnetic resonance imaging (MRI)

D. Treatment/nursing interventions
   1. Surgical repair is necessary to relieve the obstruction or to shunt the CSF from the ventricles of the brain into the abdomen (ventriculoperitoneal shunt) (Fig 8-7)
   2. Postoperative care includes frequent position changes to prevent pressure on the head, care of the shunt, general postoperative care, and observation for complications (infection, shunt malfunction, return of increased ICP)
   3. Measure head circumference daily

Down Syndrome

A. Definition: an abnormality caused by extra chromosome 21 (trisomy 21). Children with Down syndrome are born to women of all ages. Although there is a higher risk in women over age 35, the majority of infants with Down syndrome are born to women under age 35

B. Symptoms: hypotonia; small, low-set ears; slanted eyes; protruding tongue; small, flattened nose; short, broad neck;

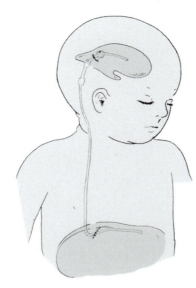

Figure 8-7. Ventriculoperitoneal shunt. Catheter is threaded beneath the skin. (From Whaley LF, Wong DL: *Nursing care of infants and children*, ed 5, St Louis, 1995, Mosby.)

single transverse palmar (simian) crease; dry, cracked skin; congenital heart defects; and mental retardation

C. Diagnosis: based on the physical defects; chromosomal studies are done to determine specific defects

D. Treatment/nursing interventions
   1. Emotional support for parents; they expected a "normal" infant without defects
   2. Assist family in preventing physical problems (respiratory, integumentary, nutrition)
   3. Promote the child's developmental progress, and help parents to set realistic goals for the child
   4. Encourage activity and intellectual stimulation for the child through early intervention programs and school
   5. Genetic counseling for the parents

GENITOURINARY SYSTEM

Epispadias and Hypospadias

A. Definition: congenital conditions in male infants where urethra ends on the under side (hypospadias) or the top side (epispadias) of the penis, rather than at the end

B. Symptoms: obvious physical defects evident on physical examination; abnormal stream of urine

C. Diagnosis: based on physical examination

D. Treatment/nursing interventions
   1. The surgery to extend the urethra to the end of the penis is usually done in several stages when the child is 6 to 18 months of age
   2. Postoperative care includes inspection of the operative site for bleeding, catheter care, and emotional support for the child and parents, as well as general postoperative care

Cryptorchidism

A. Definition: failure of one or both testes to descend into the scrotal sac; sterility may result if not treated

B. Symptoms: testes not palpable in the scrotal sac on physical examination

C. Diagnosis: based on symptoms

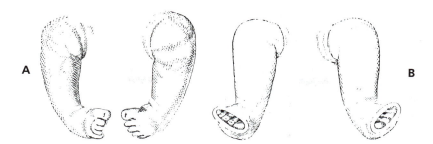

Figure 8-8. Feet casted for correction of bilateral congenital talipes equinovarus. **A,** Before correction. **B,** Undergoing correction in plaster casts. (From Brashear HR Jr, Raney RB: *Shands' handbook of orthopaedic surgery,* ed 10, St Louis, 1986, Mosby.)

D. Treatment/nursing interventions
  1. The testes often descend by 1 year of age
  2. Hormonal therapy (human chorionic gonadotropin [HCG]) may be used at an early age to promote descent of the testes into the scrotum
  3. Surgical intervention (orchiopexy) is usually necessary to bring the testes down the inguinal canal and into the scrotum; routine postoperative care

Wilms' Tumor
A. Definition: tumor (nephroblastoma) in the kidney region
B. Symptoms: occasional hematuria and elevated blood pressure; swelling or mass in the abdomen
C. Diagnosis: the tumor is often palpable through the abdominal wall; it occurs most often in children under 2 years of age and is usually found by the caregiver before the child reaches the age of 3
D. Treatment/nursing interventions
  1. Surgery to remove the tumor is performed within 48 hours of diagnosis; routine postoperative care is given
  2. Radiation therapy is given postoperatively as ordered
  3. Chemotherapy as ordered (see Chapter 3, Pharmacology)
  4. Emotional support/education for parents
E. Prognosis is good with early diagnosis and treatment for children under 2 years of age

MUSCULOSKELETAL SYSTEM
Congenital Clubfoot (Talipes Equinovarus)
A. Definition: defect in which the entire foot is inverted, heel is drawn up, and front of the foot is adducted; can affect one or both feet (Fig. 8-8)
B. Symptoms: obvious physical defect evident on physical examination
C. Diagnosis: based on the presence of the physical defect on examination
D. Treatment/nursing interventions
  1. The deformity is usually repaired in stages; the type of treatment depends on the severity of the defect
  2. Various methods of treatment include manipulation and serial casting, splints, and surgery when necessary to repair the deformities; nursing care depends on method chosen

Developmental Dysplasia of the Hip (DDH)
A. Definition: DDH describes a group of disorders related to abnormal development of the hip, in which there is a shallow acetabulum, subluxation, or dislocation; DDH may result from laxity of the supporting capsule or an abnormality of the acetabulum
B. Symptoms: limited hip abduction, apparent shortening of femur, asymmetry of gluteal and thigh folds (see Fig. 8-9)
C. Diagnosis: symptoms found on physical examination by the physician/nurse practitioner
D. Treatment/nursing interventions
  1. Treatment is started as soon as the defect is diagnosed; the hip is manipulated into proper position and an abduction device (Pavlik harness) or hip spica cast is applied (Fig. 8-10), Bryant's traction, modified Bryant's, or modified Buck's extension may also be used
  2. Nursing care includes parent teaching regarding application of the harness and cast care

CARDIOVASCULAR SYSTEM
Congenital Heart Defects
A. Atrial septal defect (ASD): abnormal opening in the septum between the two atria, or a patent foramen ovale, that causes left-to-right shunting of the blood
B. Ventricular septal defect (VSD): abnormal opening in the septum between the two ventricles that causes left-to-right shunting of the blood
C. Patent ductus arteriosus (PDA): the ductus arteriosus remains open after birth instead of closing off as normal, causing an overload of the left heart and a slight murmur
D. Coarctation of the aorta: constriction of the aortic arch, causing hypertension in the upper body and hypotension in the lower body
E. Tetralogy of Fallot: consists of four congenital defects: pulmonary stenosis, ventricular septal defect, overriding of the aorta, and right ventricular hypertrophy
F. Classic symptoms of congenital heart defects: dyspnea, difficulty with feeding, clubbing of fingers, cyanosis (in certain defects), heart murmurs, rapid pulse, recurrent respiratory infections, edema
G. Diagnosis: based on the symptoms, electrocardiograms, echocardiograms, cardiac catheterizations, and chest x-ray films
H. Treatment/nursing interventions
  1. Most defects must be corrected by surgical intervention, often in stages; some symptoms can be treated with medications as ordered
  2. Nursing care measures depend on the type of treatment or surgery; most often, immediate postoperative care is given in intensive care units

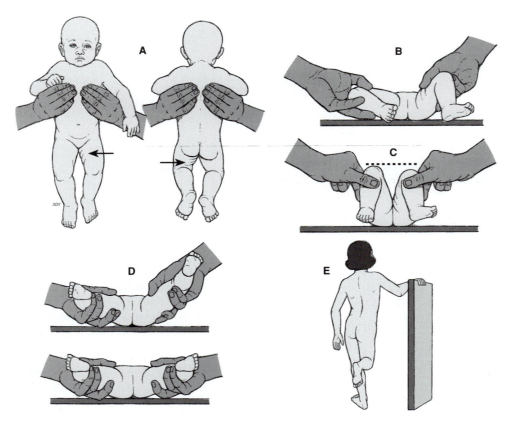

Figure 8-9. **Signs of developmental dysplasia of the hip. A,** Asymmetry of gluteal and thigh folds. **B,** Limited hip abduction, as seen in flexion. **C,** Apparent shortening of the femur, as indicated by the level of the knees in flexion. **D,** Ortolani click (if infant is under 4 weeks of age). **E,** Positive Trendelenburg sign or gait (if child is weight bearing). (From Whaley LF, Wong DL: *Nursing care of infants and children*, ed 5, St Louis, 1995, Mosby.)

Sickle Cell Anemia

A. Definition: autosomal disease occurring mainly in blacks, but also occurs on occasion in whites of Mediterranean descent; causes breakdown of red blood cells carrying an abnormal hemoglobin S, which leads to a severe hemolytic anemia; the disease may not be recognized until the toddler or preschool period.

B. Symptoms: appear only in children who inherit the trait from both parents; fatigue, anorexia, decreased hemoglobin; sickle cell crisis may occur, causing severe joint pain, abdominal pain, fever, and firm and distended abdomen

C. Diagnosis: based on the symptoms, family history of the disease, and specific blood tests including the sickle-cell slide preparation, sickle-turbidity test (Sickledex), and hemoglobin electrophoresis ("Fingerprinting")

D. Treatment/nursing interventions
1. IV fluids and fluids by mouth (PO) as ordered
2. Oxygen therapy, especially during sickle cell crisis
3. Bed rest
4. Electrolyte replacement
5. Analgesics for pain as ordered
6. Blood transfusions as ordered (packed red blood cells)
7. Antibiotic therapy as needed
8. Genetic counseling for parents
9. Proper nutrition, as tolerated
10. Avoid exposure to people with colds and infections

ENDOCRINE SYSTEM

Hypopituitarism (Dwarfism)

A. Definition: growth retardation due to deficiency of the growth hormone (GH)

B. Symptoms: short stature, well-nourished appearance, delayed physical development

C. Diagnosis: based on the family history, child's growth patterns, physical examination, x-ray studies, and endocrine studies

D. Treatment/nursing interventions
1. Replacement of the growth hormone by subcutaneous injections
2. Early diagnosis and treatment help to prevent many physical and emotional problems that occur later in childhood
3. Provide emotional support for the child and parents during diagnostic procedures and early stages of treatment (even after growth hormone therapy is started, growth will be slower than normal)

Congenital Hypothyroidism (Cretinism)

A. Definition: lack of thyroid function resulting from a failure of the embryonic development of the thyroid gland

B. Symptoms: usually do not appear until 6 to 12 weeks of age in bottle-fed infants and after weaning in breast-fed infants; include feeding problems, inactivity, anemia, thick, dry, mottled skin, bradycardia, relaxation of the abdominal

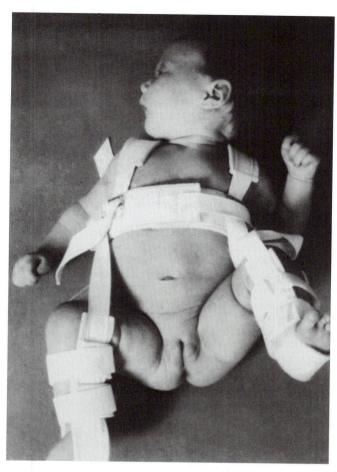

Figure 8-10. **Child in Pavlik harness.** (From Whaley LF, Wong DL: *Nursing care of infants and children*, ed 5, St Louis, 1995, Mosby.)

muscles, and delayed development of the nervous system, which leads to mental retardation
C. Diagnosis: based on the symptoms and tests of thyroid function, such as initial measurement of the newborn's T_4 (thyroxin) and thyroid stimulating hormone (TSH) level
D. Treatment/nursing interventions
1. Early diagnosis and treatment are essential in preventing retardation and other severe physiologic symptoms
2. Treatment is indefinite replacement therapy of the thyroid hormone
3. Parent teaching concerning administration of the thyroid hormone, including signs and symptoms of thyroid overdose

DISORDER OF UNKNOWN ETIOLOGY
SUDDEN INFANT DEATH SYNDROME (SIDS)
A. Definition: sudden death of an infant under 1 year of age that remains unexplained after a complete postmortem examination, including an investigation of the death scene and a review of the infant's clinical history; the leading cause of death in children between 1 and 12 months of age; the peak age for SIDS is 2 to 4 months; 95% of cases occur by the age of 6 months

B. Research: Numerous theories have been proposed regarding the cause of SIDS, but the exact cause is unknown; many researchers believe that it may be related to a brainstem abnormality in the regulation of cardiorespiratory control; other studies have demonstrated that infants sleeping in the prone position are at an increased risk for SIDS; because of these findings, the American Academy of Pediatrics recommends that healthy infants up to 6 months of age sleep on their side or back
C. Emotional support for the parents
1. Parents always feel guilty and must be reassured that SIDS is not their fault
2. Encourage them to allow an autopsy to try to determine a specific cause of death; this helps to allay their guilt and feelings that they could have prevented it
3. Allow parents to spend some time with the child to say goodbye
4. Refer the parents to the SIDS Foundation for counseling and support
5. After the parents return home from the hospital, emotional support should continue to be provided for them by qualified healthcare professionals

TODDLERHOOD (AGES 1 TO 3 YEARS)
Normal Growth and Development
PHYSICAL DEVELOPMENT
A. Toddlerhood shows a decrease in the rate of growth but an increase in the rate of development
B. Toddlers gain approximately 4 to 6 lb (1.8 to 2.7 kg) each year, and add 3 inches (7.5 cm) in height per year
C. They have learned, and continue to learn, to walk between 1 and 2 years of age
D. Visual acuity of 20/20 is achieved during the toddler years
E. Toddlers continue to learn to talk, learning new words and phrases; their favorite word is "no!"

PSYCHOSOCIAL DEVELOPMENT
A. Behavior in the toddler is characterized by several things
1. Negativism: toddlers say "no!" to almost everything; this is part of their becoming an individual person separate from their parents
2. Ritualism: developing and following certain patterns of behavior to develop their own security
3. Temper tantrums: toddlers like to do everything for themselves; when they can't, they are frustrated, and this frustration leads to temper tantrums; tantrums should be ignored as much as possible, and the child should be dealt with after the "storm" is over
B. Toddlers are in Erikson's stage of "autonomy vs. shame and doubt"; they need to develop a sense of autonomy and self-control; to do this, toddlers must be able to make some choices as well as learn to function within the limits set for them
C. Discipline and limit setting must be consistent to be effective; it is also important to remember to criticize the behavior, not the child
D. Toilet training is an important part of the socialization process in toddlers; they should be praised when they use the "potty chair" or toilet properly, rather than being punished for not using it; toilet training should only begin when the toddler is physically capable of controlling bowel and bladder (18 to 24 months)

Health Promotion

A. Nutrition needs change because of change in growth rate; toddlers need less food, and their appetites decrease (18 months of age)
   1. Teach parents that the decrease in food intake is normal
   2. The child is more autonomous now; should be allowed to feed himself or herself as much as possible; "finger foods" are ideal
   3. Snacks should be nutritious; cheese, fruits, and crackers are good choices
   4. Desserts should not be used as rewards; this gets the toddler into a habit of expecting something sweet whenever doing something good
B. Prevention of accidents is a major responsibility with toddlers; keep dangerous items (sharp objects, medications, cleaning supplies) out of their reach; toddlers should not be left unattended near a bathtub, swimming pool, whirlpool bath, or hot objects, such as pans on the stove or open flames
C. Teaching the toddler good oral hygiene habits is necessary to prevent early tooth decay and problems with gums
   1. Brushing the teeth should begin between 12 and 18 months of age
   2. Dental checkups with the dental hygienist or dentist should begin at about 1 year of age
   3. Proper nutrition helps prevent a large amount of early dental caries

Health Problems

RESPIRATORY DISORDERS

EPIGLOTTITIS

A. Definition: one of the croup syndromes; a severely inflamed epiglottis; begins abruptly and progresses rapidly into severe respiratory distress; usually caused by *Haemophilus influenzae* bacteria
B. Symptoms: fever, sore throat, difficulty swallowing; child insists on sitting up, leaning forward with chin thrust out, mouth open, and tongue protruding; drooling is common
C. Diagnosis: based on the symptoms and visualization of enlarged reddened epiglottis on careful throat examination and enlarged epiglottis on lateral neck x-ray examination
D. Treatment/nursing interventions
   1. Do *not* examine throat unless immediate intubation can be performed if necessary
   2. Keep child as quiet as possible; allow child to sit up in bed or on lap of parent
   3. Keep emergency tracheostomy tray (and intubation tray) with patient at all times
   4. Administer IV fluids and antibiotics as ordered
   5. Monitor child closely

CYSTIC FIBROSIS

A. Definition: an autosomal recessive hereditary disease affecting the exocrine glands; the lungs, pancreas, liver and small intestine produce abnormal mucus secretions and become obstructed
B. Symptoms
   1. In newborns: meconium ileus, bile-stained emesis, distended abdomen, no stools, and salty "taste" to the skin resulting from increased sodium in the perspiration
   2. In infants and children: harsh, dry cough, frequent bronchial infections, malnutrition, distended abdomen, barrel chest, clubbed fingers, and bulky, greasy, foul-smelling stools (steatorrhea)

C. Diagnosis: based on family history, a history of FTT, the symptoms, lung changes revealed by chest x-ray films, an elevated sweat chloride level (increased sodium in the perspiration), and stool analysis for fat and enzymes
D. Treatment/nursing interventions
   1. Pancreatic enzymes are given as ordered with food to improve digestion of fats and proteins
   2. High-carbohydrate, high-protein, and low-fat diet
   3. Increased amounts of salt and water-soluble vitamins
   4. Inhalation therapy: nebulizer treatments of bronchodilators (see Pharmacology, Chapter 3) and recombinant human deoxyribonuclease (Dnase) to decrease the viscosity of the mucus
   5. Postural drainage and chest physiotherapy to help in expectoration of mucus
   6. Physical exercise to stimulate mucus secretion
   7. Antibiotics for all pulmonary infections
   8. Parent teaching regarding diet, medications, and inhalation therapy for proper home care after discharge
   9. Referral to the Cystic Fibrosis Foundation for financial or emotional support
   10. Genetic counseling for parents

GASTROINTESTINAL DISORDERS

CELIAC DISEASE (GLUTEN ENTEROPATHY)

A. Definition: a defect of metabolism precipitated by the ingestion of wheat or rye gluten, leading to impaired fat absorption; exact cause unknown
B. Symptoms: usually appear between 1 and 5 years of age; chronic diarrhea with bulky, greasy, foul-smelling stools; malnutrition; anorexia; unhappy disposition; retardation of growth; distended abdomen; and muscle wasting especially of extremities and buttocks
C. Diagnosis: laboratory tests including stool analysis for fecal fat; blood studies for anemia, hypoproteinemia, and serum iron; definitive diagnosis is based on these tests, the symptoms, and a jejunal biopsy to demonstrate changes in the jejunal mucosa
D. Treatment/nursing interventions
   1. Gluten-free, low-fat diet; rice cereal for infants
   2. Parent teaching regarding diet and specific foods to avoid
   3. The child should be protected from respiratory infections, which may lead to exacerbations of the disease known as celiac crisis (characterized by severe vomiting and diarrhea, dehydration, and acidosis)

NEUROSENSORY DISORDERS

EYE DISORDERS

Strabismus (Fig. 8-11)

A. Definition: failure of the eyes to direct and focus on the same object at the same time
B. Symptoms: deviation of one eye to the center (esotropia) or to the other corner (exotropia)
C. Diagnosis: based on the symptoms
D. Treatment/nursing unaffected interventions
   1. Patching of unaffected eye to increase visual stimulation of weaker eye
   2. Glasses and exercise to help improve vision
   3. Surgery to correct the muscle defects is often necessary when conservative treatment is ineffective
   4. Preoperative and postoperative nursing care as indicated

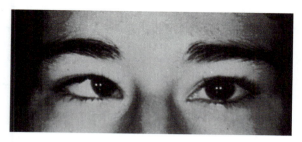

Figure 8-11. Strabismus. Note the obvious malalignment of the eyes. The light reflections are centered in the left cornea and to the side of the right cornea. (From Havener WH et al: *Nursing care in eye, ear, nose, and throat disorders,* ed 4, St Louis, 1979, Mosby.)

Amblyopia ("Lazy Eye")

A. Definition: reduced visual acuity in one eye, usually caused by strabismus; the eyes are unable to focus and work together, and blindness may occur in the weaker eye if there is no treatment
B. Symptoms: blurred vision, double vision, development of a "blind spot"
C. Diagnosis: based on results of Snellen's eye test and the symptoms
D. Treatment/nursing interventions: patching of the unaffected eye so that the child is forced to use and focus the weaker eye; the best time for treatment is during early childhood

CEREBRAL PALSY

A. Definition: a group of nonprogressive disorders caused by a malfunction of the motor centers of the brain; oxygen deprivation (anoxia) damages the brain's motor centers prenatally, during or immediately after delivery, or during childhood after an accident or disease
B. Symptoms: abnormal muscle tone and coordination, delays in development, hearing and vision impairment, seizures, and, in some cases, mental retardation
C. Diagnosis: based on the mother's prenatal history, birth history, history of an accident or disease, presence of delays in growth and development, and abnormal neurologic examination
D. Types of cerebral palsy
   1. Spastic: hypertonicity with poor control of posture, balance, and coordination; impaired motor skills; hypertonicity of muscles and tendon reflexes lead to development of contractures
   2. Dyskinetic: abnormal involuntary movement; athetosis, characterized by slow, writhing movements that involve extremities, trunk, neck, facial muscles, and the tongue
   3. Ataxic: wide-based gait; disintegration of movements of the upper extremities when the child reaches for objects
   4. Mixed type: combination of spasticity and athetosis
E. Treatment/nursing interventions
   1. Treatment and care are supportive to ensure optimal level of development for the child
   2. Physical and occupational therapy to help the child learn some control over muscle movements
   3. Braces/splints as needed to hold extremities in correct positions of function
   4. Use of wheelchairs, walkers, and crutches as needed for ambulation/locomotion
   5. Speech therapy/assistance with feeding as needed

6. Treatment for respiratory problems, seizures, contractures as needed
7. Emotional support for the family and child; most often, cerebral palsy children are of normal intelligence and have only physical handicaps
8. Encourage the child to live as normal a life as possible; refer the family to supportive groups such as the Easter Seal Society

ACCIDENTS

A. Accidents are the major cause of death in children between 1 and 4 years of age, chiefly because of their ability to walk and move about more freely than during infancy, along with their unawareness of danger within the environment
B. Accident prevention during toddlerhood is a major task requiring the involvement of both parents and other family members; following are several basic suggestions for accident prevention
   1. Supervise play, especially around dangerous areas such as cars, swimming pools, and open flames or hot appliances
   2. Use well-designed, safe car seats or restraints
   3. Turn all handles of pots and pans in toward the stove, away from the child's reach
   4. Cover electrical outlets with protective plastic caps
   5. Do not allow the child to play with the bathtub faucets; do not leave the child unattended in the bathroom
   6. Keep all medications and poisonous substances out of the child's reach (preferably in a locked cabinet)
   7. Know the number and location of the nearest poison control center and hospital
   8. Put up gates at the top and bottom of stairwells
   9. Choose well-made toys appropriate for the child's age, without sharp edges or small removable pieces
   10. Store all guns, dangerous tools, and equipment in a locked cabinet
   11. Teach the toddler about common dangers such as "hot" items, looking "both ways" before crossing the street, and water safety
   12. Provide bicycle helmets for toddlers to wear every time they ride a bike

PRESCHOOL AGE (AGES 3 TO 5)
Normal Growth and Development
PHYSICAL DEVELOPMENT

A. Growth is slow during the preschool years; children gain approximately 5 lb (2.3 kg) and 2 to 3 inches (5 to 7.5 cm) in height each year
B. Deciduous teeth are being replaced by permanent teeth; there is a definite need for proper dental hygiene and regular dental checkups at this age level and throughout childhood
C. Language development of preschoolers is rapid; 3 year olds talk to themselves and their toys; 4 year olds begin to talk and communicate more with other people

PSYCHOSOCIAL DEVELOPMENT

A. Preschoolers are in Erikson's stage of "initiative vs. guilt"; at this age level they learn how to interact with other children and adults; they also learn the difference between proper and improper behavior, and the rewards and disciplines associated with each; without proper adult guidance, preschoolers can learn improper behavior and develop a sense of guilt and inferiority rather than a sense of initiative and accomplishment

B. Preschoolers begin to develop their imaginations; they use "magical thinking" and have difficulty distinguishing fantasy from reality

C. Preschoolers become acutely aware of their sexuality, including their roles as boys or girls and their sex organs; parents must work with their children in a positive way to help them develop healthy attitudes toward themselves and their bodies

D. Preschoolers continue to learn through play; they still use parallel play but also begin to use associative play (play with other children) and imitative play (play by imitating the actions of adults or other children)

Health Promotion

A. Immunizations started in infancy and toddlerhood should continue according to schedule (see Figure 8-2)

B. Nutrition should be appropriate to age, keeping in mind that growth is slow during this period; preschoolers should be eating foods from all four basic food groups

Health Problems

COMMUNICABLE DISEASES
See Appendix I

RESPIRATORY DISORDERS: TONSILLITIS AND ADENOIDITIS
A. Definition: inflammation of the tonsils and adenoids caused by chronic upper respiratory infections

B. Symptoms: sore throat, difficulty in swallowing and breathing ("mouth breathers"), hoarseness, harsh cough

C. Diagnosis: based on the symptoms and the presence of swelling and redness of the tonsils and adenoids on examination

D. Treatment/nursing interventions
   1. Acute infections are treated with antibiotics as ordered, increased oral fluids, and warm saltwater gargles
   2. If chronic infections continue after antibiotic treatment, surgery is often indicated (tonsillectomy and adenoidectomy); however, surgery is less common today than in the past
   3. Postoperative nursing care measures include keeping the child in a prone position with head to the side until fully awake; monitoring vital signs frequently; checking the throat and nares for active bleeding; keeping the suction equipment at the bedside for emergency use; observing the child for frequent swallowing (this may indicate oozing of blood in the nasopharynx or pharynx); warm, saltwater gargles; analgesic/antipyretic drugs for discomfort; and encouraging cool, clear oral fluids after the nausea subsides

GENITOURINARY DISORDERS
NEPHROTIC SYNDROME
A Definition: massive proteinuria, hypoalbuminemia, hyperlipemia, and edema; is the most common glomerular injury in children; it can be classified as primary (restricted to glomerular injury) or secondary (when it develops as part of a systemic illness)

B. Symptoms: edema of the face, extremities, and abdomen; proteinuria, hypoalbuminemia, respiratory distress; malnutrition; irritability; increased susceptibility to infection

C. Diagnosis: based on decreased serum protein levels and increased proteinuria, edema, and hypercholesterolemia, and on results of a renal biopsy

D. Treatment/nursing interventions
   1. Nephrotic syndrome is a chronic disorder, with remissions and exacerbations, usually lasting 12 to 18 months; treatment measures continue for an extended period
   2. Corticosteroids as ordered to reduce the edema
   3. Administration of an oral alkylating agent, usually Cytoxan, alternating with prednisone, to reduce the relapse rate and induce long-term remission
   4. Frequent urine testing for protein and albumin
   5. Recording of intake and output
   6. Diuretics as ordered (not always effective)
   7. Low-salt diet during exacerbations
   8. Antibiotics as ordered during exacerbations
   9. Parent teaching for home care regarding medications, diet, and follow-up

ACUTE GLOMERULONEPHRITIS
A. Definition: inflammation of the glomeruli and nephrons of the kidney; it may occur as a primary event, or as a reaction to an infection (most often streptococcal, pneumococcal, or viral)

B. Symptoms: edema of the face and eyes, anorexia, dark-colored ("tea") urine, oliguria, listlessness, irritability, headache, abdominal discomfort, vomiting, slightly elevated blood pressure, proteinuria; if the disease occurs as a result of a systemic infection, the symptoms occur approximately 10 days after the infection

C. Diagnosis: based on the symptoms and a positive recent history of streptococcal or other infection

D. Treatment/nursing interventions
   1. Bed rest for 2 to 4 weeks until the symptoms subside
   2. Antibiotics as ordered (see Chapter 3, Pharmacology)
   3. Liquid diet, progressing to a regular, low-salt diet
   4. Measurement of intake and output and observation of color of urine
   5. Frequent checking and recording of blood pressure
   6. Urine testing for protein and specific gravity
   7. Daily weights
   8. Antihypertensives and diuretics for elevated BP, as ordered.

CIRCULATORY DISORDERS
HEMOPHILIA
A. Definition: an X-linked recessive disorder of metabolism that results in a delayed coagulation of blood; hemophilia is typed according to which clotting factor is affected

B. Symptoms: prolonged bleeding and clotting times; easy bruising and bleeding into tissues and joints; joint pain

C. Diagnosis: based on the symptoms, as well as family health history, and a prolonged clotting time

D. Treatment/nursing interventions
   1. Observations for any signs of internal bleeding and shock
   2. Transfusions as ordered with the missing clotting factor
   3. Frequent laboratory tests, such as partial thromboplastin time (PTT), clotting time, complete blood count (CBC); screening for HIV (from receiving contaminated transfusions or clotting factors)
   4. Corticosteroids and nonsteroidal antiinflammatory drugs as ordered
   5. Exercise and physical therapy to strengthen muscles around joints
   6. Protection of the child from injuries as much as possible
   7. Emotional support and counseling for the child and parents

8. Parent teaching regarding follow-up physical examinations, protecting the child from physical harm, the need for immediate care if any injury occurs, and administering the clotting factor to the child
9. Referrals to community resources, such as the National Hemophilia Foundation
10. Genetic counseling for parents

LEUKEMIA

A. Definition: a broad term given to a group of malignant diseases of the bone marrow and lymphatic system; an unrestricted proliferation of immature WBCs in the blood-forming tissues of the body; classified according to its predominant cell type and level of maturity
B. Symptoms: the three main consequences of bone marrow dysfunction are anemia, infection, and bleeding; other symptoms include lethargy, pallor, anorexia, fever, pain in the bones and joints; petechiae, easy bruising, and sores in the mouth; decreased RBCs and WBCs
C. Diagnosis: made on the basis of history, symptoms, an elevated WBC count, and presence of immature leukocytes and blast cells in a bone marrow biopsy or aspiration
D. Treatment/nursing interventions
   1. Leukemia is a chronic, sometimes fatal disease with remissions and exacerbations; the child and family need a great deal of emotional support from the physician and nursing staff
   2. Chemotherapy drugs and corticosteroids as ordered (see Chapter 3, Pharmacology)
   3. IV fluids and blood transfusions as ordered
   4. Administration of pain medications as ordered; joint pain during exacerbations may be severe, especially in the more advanced stages; higher than normal doses are often required
   5. Proper skin and mouth care
   6. Providing proper nutrition as the child's condition allows
   7. Prevention of infections whenever possible; chemotherapy drugs lower the WBC count, which in turn decreases the child's resistance to infection
   8. Observation for possible side effects of chemotherapy drugs
   9. Bone marrow transplants may be ordered in certain types of leukemia to replace unhealthy bone marrow; an exact "match" is often difficult to find

Musculoskeletal Disorders
MUSCULAR DYSTROPHY
A. Definition: a group of hereditary muscle diseases (recessive trait) characterized by gradual degeneration of muscle fibers, which is evidenced by muscle wasting and weakness and increasing disability and deformity
B. Symptoms: gradual muscle weakness including difficulty walking, standing up, a "waddle" gait, and mild mental retardation; most symptoms appear in children between 3 and 5 years of age
C. Diagnosis: based on the history of the symptoms, family history, muscle biopsy to determine muscle degeneration, electromyography (EMG), and serum enzyme measurement
D. Treatment/nursing interventions
   1. There is no cure for muscular dystrophy, so treatment is supportive

2. Encourage the child to be as active and to lead as normal a life as possible
3. Range-of-motion exercises and physical therapy as ordered to prevent contractures
4. Use of walkers, crutches, braces, and wheelchairs as needed
5. Emotional support for the parents and child; this is a progressive disease, and the family requires ongoing support by the health care team
6. Frequent medical checkups to observe for progressive symptoms such as respiratory distress
7. Genetic counseling for the parents

SCHOOL AGE (AGES 6 TO 12)
Normal Growth and Development
PHYSICAL DEVELOPMENT
A. Growth is slow in children between the ages of 6 and 10 years; the child gains 4½ to 6½ lb (2 to 3 kg) and 2 inches (5 cm) per year
B. Bone growth is slow; the cartilage is replaced by bone at the bone epiphyses
C. Middle childhood (ages 6 to 12) is the stage of development when deciduous teeth are shed

PSYCHOSOCIAL DEVELOPMENT
A. School-age children are in Erikson's stage of "industry vs. inferiority"; an eagerness to develop new skills and interests, and the processes of cooperating and competing with other children are characteristics of this age that engender a sense of accomplishment rather than a sense of inferiority and poor self-worth
B. Children ages 7 to 10 start to become more influenced by their peer group than by their parents; they develop "best friends" and start to separate into boy and girl groups
C. The most significant skill acquired during the school-age period is the ability to read

Health Promotion
A. Communicable disease prevention is accomplished by timely immunizations, proper rest and diet, and frequent medical and dental check-ups
B. Accident prevention remains a major factor at this age level; safety measures should include rules for bicycle and skateboard safety (helmets and pads for safety in competitive sports such as baseball, football, and soccer)
C. Sex education should begin at this age level and should be presented by the parents in simple, honest terms; audiovisual aids such as books and pictures are available to assist parents in presenting the information on the child's level
D. Promotion of a balanced diet continues to be important at this age level; high calorie, low-nutrition snacks are popular with school-age children but often lead to excess weight gain

Health Problems
RESPIRATORY DISORDERS: ALLERGIC CONDITIONS
ASTHMA
A. Definition: an obstructive airway disease caused by spasms of bronchial tubes; results from hypersensitivity of the airways, accompanied by inflammation and edema of the bronchial mucosa and increased production of bronchial mucus; it is often caused by an allergic response to allergens ("triggers") such as pollen, animal fur, food, or irritants,

such as tobacco smoke, exercise, cold air, respiratory infections, and changes in the weather; it is the most common chronic disease of childhood

B. Symptoms: irritability; restlessness; tightness in the chest; hacking, nonproductive cough; dyspnea; wheezing

C. Diagnosis: based on the symptoms, physical examination, the child's history, family history, chest x-ray films that rule out other respiratory diseases, and pulmonary function studies

D. Treatment/nursing interventions
   1. Bronchodilator medications as ordered (administered by inhalation, by mouth, or by injection) (see Chapter 3, Pharmacology)
   2. Antiinflammatory medications, either corticosteroids (prednisone) or nonsteroidal agents (cromolyn sodium) administered by inhalation, by mouth, or by injection
   3. Chest physiotherapy
   4. IV fluids as ordered
   5. Liquid diet, progressing to a regular diet
   6. Identification and removal of the allergens if possible
   7. Parent and child teaching regarding home care including medications, removal of any potential "triggers," use of peak flow meter to measure peak expiratory flow rates, and follow-up examinations

ALLERGIC RHINITIS (HAY FEVER)

A. Cause: an allergy to some pollen, dust, or animal fur

B. Symptoms: sneezing, runny nose, postnasal drip, and watery, itchy eyes

C. Diagnosis: based on the symptoms and results of allergy testing done to discover specific allergen

D. Treatment/nursing interventions
   1. Find and remove the allergen if possible
   2. Antihistamines or decongestants as ordered
   3. Immunotherapy may be necessary if symptoms cannot be controlled

GASTROINTESTINAL DISORDERS

APPENDICITIS

A. Definition: inflammation of the appendix, often following an infection elsewhere in the body

B. Symptoms: pain in the abdomen, migrating to the right lower quadrant; nausea and vomiting, fever, and constipation

C. Diagnosis: based on the symptoms and usually an elevated WBC count

D. Treatment/nursing interventions
   1. Removal of the inflamed appendix (appendectomy), preferably before it ruptures and spreads the infection throughout the abdomen, causing peritonitis
   2. Routine postoperative care, including monitoring vital signs, frequent observation of the incision or dressing for bleeding, careful recording of intake and output, and administration of IV fluids as ordered
   3. Antibiotics may be ordered if there is a possibility of infection (especially with a ruptured appendix)
   4. Pain medication as ordered

PINWORMS

A. Definition: worms that affect the intestine; the worms or eggs are swallowed and are spread easily from person to person by the hands, linen, or food

B. Symptoms; itching around the anus, anorexia, and diarrhea

C. Diagnosis: made by the cellophane tape test; the eggs are captured from the anal area during the night or early morning hours by placing a tongue blade covered with cellophane tape at the anal opening; the worms come out of the intestine at night to lay their eggs, and the eggs are picked up on the tape

D. Treatment/nursing interventions
   1. Good handwashing technique to prevent spread of the worms and reinfection
   2. Frequent changes of underwear and linen
   3. Medication of choice is mebendazole (see Chapter 3, Pharmacology)
   4. Examination and treatment of all family members, since pinworms are easily transmitted

NERVOUS SYSTEM DISORDER: EPILEPSY

A. Definition: chronic seizure disorder with recurrent and unprovoked seizures; although there are many causes for seizures, most are idiopathic

B. Symptoms: classification of seizures (see the box to the right)

C. Diagnosis: based on the evidence of seizures; differentiation of the type of seizure by physical examination, neurologic assessment, patient history, and changes in the electroencephalogram (EEG) (changes in the brain wave patterns)

D. Treatment/nursing interventions
   1. Anticonvulsant medications as ordered (see Chapter 3, Pharmacology)
   2. Parent and child education regarding medications and the necessity of taking them as prescribed; safety factors; actions to take if the child has a seizure at home; the importance of follow-up physical examinations and laboratory work (to measure blood levels of anticonvulsants)
   3. In children with poorly controlled seizures, a ketogenic diet (either with or without the use of anticonvulsants) has been tried with moderate success in some children; children on this strict diet must be followed closely by a dietitian, neurologist, and pediatrician; the length of time of the diet ranges from 1 to 3 years
   4. Community referrals to support groups such as the National Epilepsy Foundation

MUSCULOSKELETAL DISORDERS

SCOLIOSIS

A. Definition: a lateral S-shaped curvature of the spine; it can be congenital, or caused by a variety of conditions, but most often has no known cause (idiopathic); most often seen in young girls, and is most noticeable at the time of the preadolescent growth spurt

B. Symptoms: poor posture; uneven length of legs; asymmetry of shoulder and hip height; pelvic obliquity

C. Diagnosis: based on symptoms, x-ray films, and physical examination

D. Treatment/nursing interventions
   1. A brace (Milwaukee brace or Boston brace) or splint is often used along with exercises to prevent an increase in the degree of curvature; this may be the only treatment, or may be used before surgery
   2. Spinal fusion may be necessary to correct severe scoliosis; postoperative care as indicated

I. Partial seizures (seizures beginning locally)
 A. Simple partial seizures (with elementary symptoms; consciousness unimpaired)
  • With motor symptoms
  • With somatosensory or special sensory symptoms
  • With autonomtic symptoms
  • Compound forms (with psychic symptoms)
 B. Complex partial symptoms (temporal lobe or psychomotor; generally with impaired consciousness)
  • With impairment of consciousness only
  • With cognitive symptoms
  • With affective symptoms
  • With psychosensory symptoms
  • With psychomotor symptoms
  • Compound forms
 C. Partial seizures, secondarily generalized
II. Generalized seizures (bilaterally symmetric; without local onset; with impairment of consciousness)
  • Tonic-clonic (gland mal) seizures
  • Tonic seizures
  • Clonic seizures
  • Absence (petit mal) seizures
  • Atonic seizures
  • Myoclonic seizures
  • Infantile spasms
  • Akinetic seizures
III. Unilateral seizures (those involving one hemisphere)
IV. Unclassified epileptic seizures (incomplete data)

Modified from Commission on Classification and Terminology of the International League Against Epilepsy: Proposal for revised clinical and electroencephalographic classification of epileptic seizures, *Epilepsia* 22:489-501, 1981.

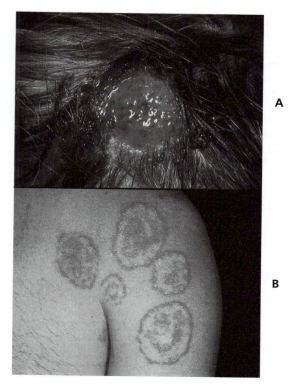

Figure 8-12. **A, Tinea capitis. B, Tinea corporis.** Both infections are caused by *Microsporum canis*, the "kitten" or "puppy" fungus. (From Habif TP: *Clinical dermatology: a color guide to diagnosis and therapy,* ed 2, St Louis, 1990, Mosby.)

INTEGUMENTARY DISORDERS
RINGWORM
A. Definition: a fungal infection transferred from person to person or from animal to person; it can occur on the scalp (tinea capitis), the body (tinea corporis), and the feet (tinea pedis) (Fig. 8-12)
B. Symptoms: small papules, dry, scaly skin, and itching on the affected part
C. Diagnosis: based on the symptoms
D. Treatment/nursing interventions
 1. Washing the affected areas with soap and water and removal of crusts
 2. Antifungal ointment to affected areas as ordered
 3. Antifungal oral medication as ordered (see Chapter 3, Pharmacology)

PEDICULOSIS
A. Definition: infestation by lice of the scalp and hairy areas of the body
B. Symptoms: severe itching in the affected area and appearance of lice on the hair or clothing

C. Diagnosis: based on the symptoms
D. Treatment/nursing interventions
 1. Pediculicide shampoo to hair/scalp as ordered; remaining nits are removed with an extra-fine-tooth comb
 2. Washing of all linens and clothing in hot water to destroy the nits (small lice) and eggs of the lice
 3. Emphasis on importance of follow-up treatment to prevent reinfestation
 4. Examination and treatment of other family members (if affected)
 5. Report to school, day-care facility

HIVES (URTICARIA)
A. Definition: an allergic reaction on the skin, usually caused by an allergy to food or drugs
B. Symptoms: bright red, raised wheals on the skin and itching of the affected areas
C. Diagnosis: based on the symptoms; allergy testing may be done to determine the specific allergen
D. Treatment/nursing interventions
 1. Determination and removal of the allergen
 2. Antihistamines as ordered to decrease the swelling and inflammation
 3. Cool-water soaks to the affected areas to decrease the itching
 4. Local soothing antipruritic lotions to affected areas as ordered
 5. Keep the child's nails short to avoid itching and possible infection

RHEUMATIC FEVER

A. Definition: autoimmune reaction to a group A beta hemolytic streptococcal pharyngitis (strep throat); it involves the joints, skin, brain, and heart

B. Symptoms: begin 2 to 6 weeks after the initial streptococcal infection; lethargy, anorexia, muscle and joint pain, fever, polyarthritis, chorea (muscle tremors and emotional upset), and carditis

C. Diagnosis: based on the symptoms; specific diagnosis based on the Jones criteria (see the box to the right)

D. Treatment/nursing interventions
1. Bed rest to decrease the workload on the heart and help prevent or ease the carditis
2. Feeding meals to the child during strict bed rest
3. Medications as ordered including salicylates for pain, steroids to decrease inflammation of the muscle and connective tissue, and antibiotics to fight infection (penicillin is the drug of choice) (see Chapter 3, Pharmacology)
4. Emotional support and nonstressful diversion for the child during bed rest
5. Monitoring of frequent laboratory tests, including the WBC count and the erythrocyte sedimentation rate (ESR) (elevated in inflammatory diseases)
6. Parent and child teaching for home care, including the need for rest, proper nutrition, proper administration of medications, and the need for prophylactic antibiotic therapy before dental work and invasive procedures

INSULIN-DEPENDENT DIABETES MELLITUS (IDDM)

A. Definition: in insulin-dependent (formerly juvenile-onset) diabetes the beta cells of the pancreas stop producing insulin, which is necessary for the metabolism of fats, carbohydrates, and proteins; peak incidence is 10 to 15 years of age

B. Symptoms: rapid onset of symptoms, including easy fatigability, polydipsia (excessive thirst), polyphagia (increased appetite), polyuria (increased urine output), glycosuria (glucose in the urine), and weight loss

C. Diagnosis: based on the symptoms, blood glucose levels, and the presence of glucose and ketones in the urine

D. Treatment/nursing interventions
1. Daily insulin administration by subcutaneous injections (usually twice a day), or by a means of a portable insulin pump (see Chapter 3, Pharmacology)
2. American Diabetes Association diet as ordered
3. Routine blood sugar monitoring; Chemstrips, Accu-check, or one-touch glucometers are commonly used for this
4. Routine urine testing for glucose and ketones may be done
5. Child and parent teaching regarding insulin injection technique, diet, exercise, urine testing, blood glucose monitoring, signs of hypoglycemia and hyperglycemia, and need for regular follow-up visits to the pediatrician
6. Support group for parents and child

ADOLESCENCE (AGES 13 TO 19 YEARS)
Normal Growth and Development

PHYSICAL DEVELOPMENT

A. During the adolescent period there is a growth spurt. This accelerated growth includes an increase in both height and weight. In girls, this occurs between 10 and 12 years of age; in boys it occurs between 12 and 14 years of age

---

Guidelines for the Diagnosis of Initial Attack of Rheumatic Fever (Jones Criteria, 1992 Update)*

Major Manifestations
Carditis
Polyarthritis
Chorea
Erythema marginatum
Subcutaneous nodules

Minor manifestations
Clinical findings
  Arthralgia
  Fever
Laboratory findings
  Elevated acute phase reactants
    Erythrocyte sedimentation rate
    C-reactive protein
  Prolonged PR interval

Supporting evidence of antecedent group A streptococcal infection
Positive throat culture or rapid streptococcal antigen test
Elevated or rising streptococcal antibody titer

From Guidelines for the diagnosis of rheumatic fever, *JAMA* 268:2070, 1992. Copyright 1992, American Medical Association.
*If supported by evidence of preceding group A streptococcal infection, the presence of two major manifestations or of one major and two minor manifestations indicates a high probability of acute rheumatic fever.

B. Secondary sex characteristics also develop during early adolescence
1. In girls the pelvis widens, the breasts develop and enlarge, and body hair starts to appear
2. In boys the penis and scrotum enlarge and pubic and facial hair start to appear, puberty in boys officially begins with the first nocturnal emission

PSYCHOLOGIC AND EMOTIONAL DEVELOPMENT

A. Adolescence is the time of transition from childhood to adulthood; adolescents are in Erikson's stage of "identity vs. role confusion;" they are in the process of developing a self-image or a sense of identity about who they are and what they want in life; if they do not develop a positive self-image and identity, they may develop a sense of inferiority, or a negative self-image

B. Development of a positive self-image and healthy personality depends a great deal on the adolescents' relationships with their peer group as well as with their family

C. Body image is the major part of adolescents' self-concept; sexuality and sexual feelings are a new part of their body images; physical appearance is important to how they perceive themselves as being accepted by their peer group
1. Boys' responses to puberty include pleasure at becoming a "man" as evidenced by enlargement of the sex organs, being able to shave, and the sexual feelings they begin to have during this stage; because of their strong sex drive,

they often masturbate to relieve themselves of strong sexual tension

2. Girls' responses to puberty include a developing awareness of their bodily changes, both internal and external (such as hormonal changes and menstruation); the sex drive in girls is usually not as strong as it is in boys

Health Promotion

A. Immunizations and physical examinations should continue according to schedule
B. Counseling and sex education, especially concerning AIDS, venereal disease, and birth control, should be made available to all adolescents
C. Counseling regarding drug and alcohol abuse should be presented and readily available to all adolescents who are in need of it
D. Emotional stress is high during adolescence; psychiatric counseling is necessary for some adolescents to work through their stresses and fears
E. Proper nutrition needs may not be met because of increased snacking, especially on high-calorie, high-fat foods; nutritional counseling may be helpful

Health Problems

SUBSTANCE ABUSE (DRUGS, ALCOHOL)
A. Definition: abuse of alcohol or mood-altering drugs, usually because of peer pressure or increased tension and stress
B. Signs of abuse: increased school absences, poor academic performance, changes in behavior patterns, wearing dark glasses inside, wearing long-sleeved shirts/blouses every day, and a sloppy, unclean appearance; signs often depend on drug being used
C. Diagnosis: based on the symptoms (signs of abuse)
D. Substances abused
1. Alcohol
2. Narcotics
3. Psychedelic drugs (LSD, marijuana, PCP)
4. Depressants (barbiturates, methaqualone [Quaalude])
5. Minor tranquilizers (Valium)
6. Hallucinogens (marijuana, LSD, PCP)
7. Analgesics (codeine)
8. Opiates (heroin, morphine, methadone)
9. Valium
10. Organic solvents (e.g., glue, cleaning fluids)
11. Stimulants (amphetamines ["speed"], cocaine)
12. Inhalants
E. Treatment/nursing interventions
1. Prevention of the problem is of course the best treatment
2. Emergency measures when necessary (such as cardiopulmonary resuscitation [CPR] and gastric lavage)
3. Psychiatric counseling as needed for the adolescent and family; identify reason(s) for drug abuse
4. Follow-up health care; group support and counseling as needed for adolescent and family

SUICIDE
A. Definition: the act of taking one's own life voluntarily
B. Etiology: suicide usually does not occur without warning; the adolescent usually has a history of emotional problems, difficult relationships, and emotional upsets including such things as divorce in the family, death of a family member or friend, or a self-identity crisis

C. Treatment/nursing interventions
1. Prevention is the best treatment; listen for verbal clues, such as "after tomorrow, it won't matter anymore"; and watch for warning signs, such as giving away favorite possessions
2. Psychiatric counseling to determine the reasons for the adolescent's actions; this should also include the family members
3. Follow-up medical care as needed
4. Emotional support and counseling for the family members, especially during the crisis stages

ANOREXIA NERVOSA AND BULIMIA
A. Definition (these disorders can occur together or separately)
1. Anorexia nervosa: an eating disorder characterized by a refusal to maintain a minimally normal body weight; most often seen in adolescent females
2. Bulimia: an eating disorder characterized by repeated episodes of "binge eating," followed by inappropriate compensatory measures, such as self-induced vomiting; misuse of laxatives, diuretics, or other medications; fasting; or excessive exercise
B. Symptoms
1. With anorexia nervosa there are three basic psychologic disturbances: the inability to correctly perceive body size, the absence of hunger or inability to perceive hunger, and feelings of inadequacy or lack of self-esteem; other symptoms include amenorrhea, constipation, dry skin, low blood pressure, anemia, and lanugo (fine, soft hair) on the back and arms
2. With bulimia, as the disease increases, the frequency of binges increases; the adolescent loses control over the binge/purge cycle; other symptoms are similar to those seen in anorexia nervosa
C. Diagnosis: based on the symptoms, family history, and psychologic evaluation
D. Treatment/nursing interventions
1. The adolescent is usually hospitalized to correct the malnutrition and to identify and treat the psychologic cause
2. Behavior modification techniques are often used to assist in changing the adolescent's behavior; for example, privileges or visitors are withdrawn until the adolescent begins to gain weight
3. Psychologic counseling for the adolescent and family members to determine the cause

CROHN'S DISEASE
A. Definition: a chronic, recurrent inflammatory disorder of the intestines; it occurs most often in upper-middle-class men and women, aged 15 to 35 years
B. Symptoms: regional ileitis causing acute low abdominal pain, fever, chronic diarrhea, weight loss, abdominal tenderness and distention, anemia, and failure to grow
C. Diagnosis based on the symptoms, x-ray films of the intestine (barium enema), endoscopy, and mucosal biopsy of the intestines
D. Treatment/nursing interventions
1. The goal of treatment is to relieve the symptoms and discomfort
2. Adequate rest and relaxation to alleviate stress
3. Soft, low-fiber diet

4. Corticosteroids as ordered to decrease inflammation of the intestines
5. Sulfasalazine as ordered (as this interferes with the absorption of folic acid, folic acid may be ordered)
6. Antidiarrheal drugs as ordered
7. Antispasmodic drugs as ordered to relieve intestinal spasms
8. Emotional support and psychologic counseling as needed to decrease the stress level

MONONUCLEOSIS

A. Definition: an acute infectious viral disease causing an increase in mononuclear WBCs and signs of general infection; it is usually thought to be only mildly contagious and is spread by oral contact; the Epstein-Barr virus is the principal cause
B. Symptoms: general malaise, sore throat, fever, enlarged lymph glands, lack of energy, headache, red, flat rash on the body, and tonsillitis
C. Diagnosis: based on the symptoms, an elevated WBC count, and a positive Monospot blood test (which indicates increased agglutinins in the blood count)
D. Treatment/nursing interventions
1. Antibiotics as ordered
2. Antipyretics to relieve fever and discomfort
3. Increased oral fluids; IV fluids may be ordered for severe dehydration
4. Gargles or lozenges as ordered for sore throat
5. Adequate rest and sleep
6. Diet as tolerated; if the patient can only tolerate fluids, high-calorie fluids should be provided
7. Patient teaching regarding follow-up care, including the need for adequate rest and sleep

ACNE VULGARIS

A. Definition: a disorder of the sebaceous glands; the glands become irritated with the secretion of sebum and the interaction of the sebum with the hormones; the glands become impacted with sebum and form comedones (noninflamed) and papules and pustules (inflamed)
B. Symptoms: the appearance of the comedones, papules, and pustules on the face; they can also appear on other places on the body such as the chest and back
C. Diagnosis: based on the symptoms
D. Treatment/nursing interventions
1. Cleaning the affected areas with soap or soap substitute and water daily
2. A diet low in greasy foods, chocolate, and nuts may help decrease the amount of oil in the skin, avoid other foods that tend to exacerbate the condition
3. Nonprescription topical creams and lotions have limited effectiveness; retinoic acid and benzoyl peroxide, when used together (one in the morning, the other in the evening), are the most effective
4. Encouraging the adolescent to keep stress levels to a minimum when possible may help in keeping acne to a minimum
5. Patient teaching: papules and pustules should not be squeezed; they can become infected and spread
6. Counseling for the adolescent to maintain a positive body image

ACQUIRED IMMUNODEFICIENCY SYNDROME (AIDS)

A. Definition: an immune disorder caused by a retrovirus, the human immunodeficiency virus (HIV)
1. The AIDS virus is known to be transmitted by blood and other body fluids (semen; saliva) (see Chapter 5, Medical-Surgical Nursing; Chapter 8, Maternity Nursing)
2. Three primary modes of transmission of the AIDS virus in children are prenatal exposure to infected mothers, blood transfusion, and engaging in high-risk activities (sexual or IV drug use, specifically with adolescents)
3. As of 1995, over 4200 children with AIDS have been reported to the Centers for Disease Control (CDC); the majority of children with HIV are less than 5 years of age; the number of adolescents with HIV is increasing rapidly; AIDS is the 6th leading cause of death for people ages 15 to 24 years
B. Symptoms: recurrent or chronic infections (because of decreased number of CD-4 T-cells) including meningitis, pneumonia, and urinary tract infections; fever; weight loss; failure to thrive; anemia; hepatosplenomegaly; persistent lymphadenopathy
C. Diagnosis: abnormal laboratory values, including abnormal T-cell ratio, decreased T-lymphocytes and hypergammaglobulinemia; history of possible exposure to AIDS virus; positive HIV test; and history of recurrent infections
D. Treatment/nursing interventions
1. There is no cure for AIDS, so treatment and nursing care measures are supportive and designed to prevent and alleviate opportunistic infections
2. The drugs azidothymidine (AZT), dideoxycytidine (ddC), and didanosine (DDI) have been approved for use in children to assist in slowing the progression of the disease; protease inhibitors were recently shown to be effective when used in combination with other drugs
3. Antibiotics/antifungal drugs as ordered (see Chapter 3, Pharmacology)
4. IV gamma globulin may be helpful in compensating for the deficiency of B-lymphocytes
5. Adequate nutrition and fluid intake
6. Use of universal precautions when caring for the child in the hospital, clinic, or home
7. Maintenance of an environment as free from infection as possible
8. Immunizations against childhood diseases (as well as the pneumococcal and influenza vaccines) should be given; however, inactivated poliovirus should be given rather than the oral poliovirus
9. Promotion of normal development of the child
10. Education and emotional support for the child and family
E. Prognosis: poor, especially in children with AIDS who are under 1 year of age

The Battered Child Syndrome

A. Definition: abuse of children by parents or other caregivers; the abuse can be physical, sexual, nutritional, or emotional; can occur at any age
B. Characteristics of battered children
1. They are often from an unplanned pregnancy
2. Many of them were premature, had a low birth weight, or had major birth defects

3. They sometimes resemble a person that the parents disliked

C. Characteristics of abusive parents
1. One parent often has a previous emotional problem
2. The abuse is usually done by one parent; the other parent knows about the abuse but usually does not report it
3. Abusive parents often have very high expectations of their children; if they do not "perform" up to these expectations, they are "punished"
4. Abusive parents are often substance abusers
5. The most common characteristic of abusive parents is that often they were abused themselves as children; however, this is not always true
6. They come from all socioeconomic levels

D. Identifying the battered child
1. The child has many unexplained scars, bruises and injuries; many of these markings are characteristic of abuse (Fig. 8-13)
2. Bone fractures may be seen on x-ray examination at various stages of healing
3. The child exhibits signs of physical neglect: malnourishment or improper or dirty clothing
4. The parents' explanations of the child's injury are inconsistent; one parent's explanation differs from the other's, or it changes from one time to the next

5. The child withdraws when approached by the parents, nurse, or physician
6. The parents' emotional reaction is inconsistent with the extent of the child's injury

E. Nursing interventions for the battered child and parents
1. Interview the parents calmly regarding the history of the incident; document all information carefully
2. Nursing personnel must control their own feelings and attitudes toward the parents to work effectively with the family
3. Provide physical care for the child as needed
4. Emotional care for the child should include providing a safe environment, explaining all procedures, providing toys and familiar belongings while the child is hospitalized, and physical cuddling and holding when appropriate
5. Referrals should be made to the hospital social worker, the local department of children and family services, the police, and the psychologist as needed

Hospitalization and the Child

A. Preparation for hospitalization
1. The rationale for preparing children for hospitalization is based on the theory that fear of the unknown is more severe than fear of the known

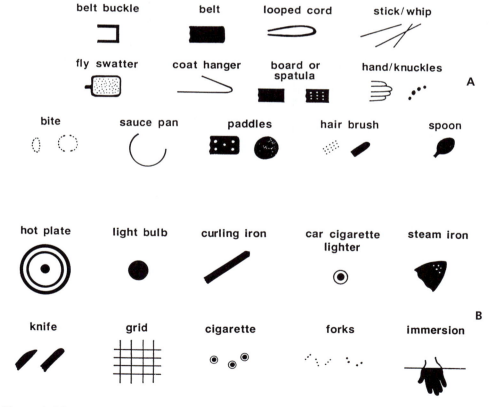

Figure 8-13.   **Characteristic markings often seen in child abuse. A,** Marks from objects. **B,** Marks from burns. (From Reece RM, Smith MK, editors: Inflicted injury versus accidental injury, *Pediatr Clin North Am,* Aug 1990.)

2. Preadmission preparation can be done by both parents and professionals (nurses and physicians) honestly at a level the child can understand

3. Hospital admission procedures include the admission history, blood tests, chest x-ray studies when necessary, physical examination, and placement in the child's room and bed; these should be explained to the child during preadmission preparation

4. In preparing the child for any hospital procedure the nurse or parent should include all necessary information regarding the procedure and any necessary preparation; time should be allowed for questions by the child and parents

B. Hospitalization as a crisis
   1. Children are more vulnerable to the crisis of illness and hospitalization because stress is a change from their usual state of health and routine, and children have a limited number of coping mechanisms to deal with stressful events
   2. Their reactions to stress differ in each developmental age group
      a. Infants and preschoolers: their major stress is separation anxiety (fear of being separated from their parents and family)
      b. Preschoolers: their major stresses are separation anxiety and fear of loss of body control and of bodily injury and pain
      c. School-age children: their major stresses are fear of separation (sometimes more from peers than from family), of loss of body control, and of bodily injury, mutilation, pain, and death
      d. Adolescents: their major stresses are fear of separation from their peer group; of loss of body control, independence and identity; and of bodily injury and pain, especially concerning sexual changes
   3. Nursing measures that can be used to minimize the hospitalized child's fears and stresses
      a. Open visiting for parents and siblings; visiting by peers in the school-age and adolescent groups should be encouraged
      b. Explain procedures or preparation for procedures at the child's age level (medical play)
      c. Allow the child to have favorite toys and games from home
      d. Nursing personnel should not lie to the child about the parents' visits; the visits should not be used as rewards or as something to be withheld if the child does not cooperate or behave
      e. Allow the child as much physical freedom as his or her condition will allow
      f. Allow the child to participate in decision making as much as possible, especially regarding treatments and procedures; this allows the child some control in the situation
      g. Encourage the parents to visit as much as possible; explain all procedures to them and encourage them to assist in their child's care if they are comfortable in doing so
      h. Instruct the parents not to lie to the child; lying only sets up a sense of mistrust among the child, the parents, and the hospital staff
      i. Administer pain medications as ordered whenever necessary; a child's pain response is affected by developmental level
      j. Expect some regressive behavior during the child's hospital stay; tell the parents that this is normal during stressful periods

C. Use of play during hospitalization
   1. Play in the hospital helps relieve tension and anxiety, lessens the stress of separation and feelings of homesickness, and helps the child to relax and feel more secure
   2. The play activities should be based on the child's age, interests, and limitations
   3. Play can be used for diversion, for recreation, and to play out the child's fears and anxieties over his illness and treatment
   4. Toys can come from home or from the hospital play area; they can even be adapted from hospital "stock" supplies
   5. Play therapy can be used to teach the child about procedures and surgery, as well as to help the child work through fears and anxieties about hospitalization

D. Preparation and teaching for discharge
   1. Preparation for discharge should begin during the admission by setting long-term goals concerning discharge
   2. Discharge planning should include several areas
      a. Parent-child teaching regarding home care procedures and medication regimen
      b. Follow-up care including physician appointments and the importance of keeping them
      c. Referrals to community agencies, public health nurses, and other resources as needed

NURSING CARE OF THE HOSPITALIZED CHILD

A. Safety factors
   1. Side rails should be kept up at all times when the child is in bed; if the bed is adjustable, it should be kept in the low position
   2. When restraints are used, they should be applied securely to the child; extremities should be checked frequently for impaired circulation caused by tight restraints; appropriate charting should be done
   3. Small toys, game pieces, and other small objects should be kept away from infants and toddlers who may swallow them
   4. Toddlers and young children should not be left unattended in their rooms or hallways; if they are out of bed, they should be observed continuously to avoid accidents and injuries
   5. Medications, needles, and syringes should be kept out of the reach of all children

B. Medication administration
   1. General guidelines in giving medications to children
      a. Approach the child with a cheerful, positive attitude and explain what you are going to do
      b. Be honest when talking to the child; tell the child it is medicine, not "juice" or "candy"
      c. When necessary, use foods or liquids to disguise the taste of bad-tasting medications
      d. Oral syringes or syringes without needles may be used to deliver oral medications to infants and young children
      e. Allow the child some control in the situation; make sure the question you ask the child is appropriate to the child's age level and the situation
      f. Intramuscular (IM) injections are safer and easier to give to a young child if a second person helps restrain the child

g. Tell the child that it is all right to cry if the shot "hurts"; offer a Band-aid
h. Teach the child to "say no" to street drugs but that the medicines received in the hospital are okay to take

2. Safe IM injection technique includes the same steps used for IM injections in adults
   a. In infants the lateral thigh (vastus lateralis muscle) should be used
   b. In toddlers and preschoolers, the ventrogluteal area is the preferred site (lateral thigh can also be used)

c. In older children and adolescents, other regularly used injection sites may be used (ventrogluteal muscle is the safest; deltoid and dorsogluteal muscles may also be used) (Fig. 8-14)

C. Assisting with treatments and procedures
   1. All tests and procedures should be explained to the child in an honest, simple manner; older children and adolescents should be allowed to ask questions and receive answers
   2. All children should be allowed to say "ouch" or to cry if the procedure is a painful one; rewards are often given

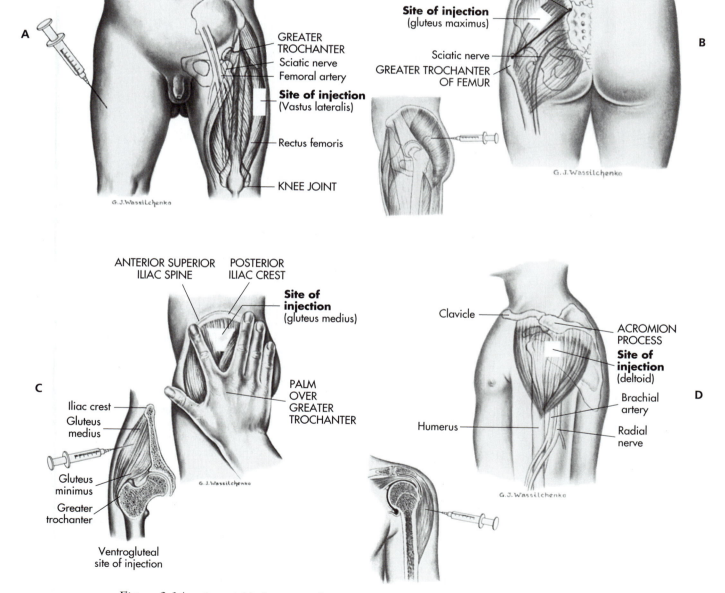

Figure 8-14.   Acceptable intramuscular sites in children. A, Vastus lateralis. **B,** Dorsogluteal. **C,** Ventrogluteal. **D,** Deltoid. (From Whaley LF, Wong DL: *Nursing care of infants and children,* ed 4, St Louis, 1991, Mosby.)

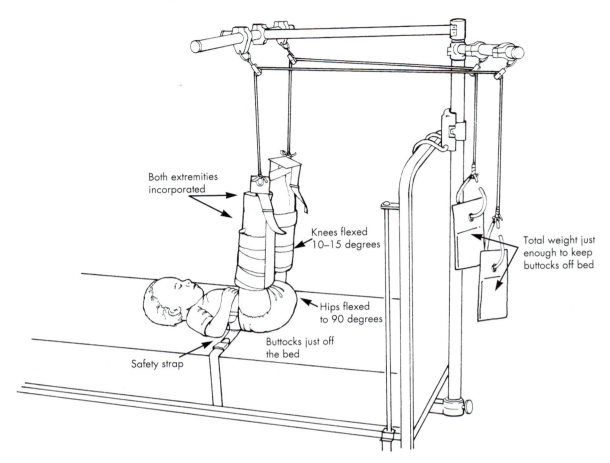

Both extremities
incorporated

Knees flexed
10–15 degrees

Total weight just
enough to keep
buttocks off bed

Hips flexed
to 90 degrees

Buttocks just off
the bed

Safety strap

Figure 8-15. Bryant's traction is used with children under 3 years of age and weighing less than 35 pounds (15.9 kg) who have developmental dysplasia of the hip (DDH). (From Folcik MA, Carina-Garcia G, Birmingham JJ: *Traction, assessment, and management,* St Louis, 1994, Mosby.)

after a painful procedure (a reward sticker, toy, or special food treat)

3. The child may need to be held or restrained in certain positions for procedures; all equipment should be assembled before the procedure is started so that the nurse can stay with the child as much as possible

D. Preoperative teaching
1. Patient teaching in pediatrics should include the child (preschool age and older) and the parents; both should be involved in the teaching and preparation for surgery
2. Use words that the child can understand; audiovisual aids (pictures, dolls, puppets, and bandages) are extremely useful in helping the child understand the procedure or surgery
3. Be honest with the child, especially regarding procedures or treatments that may be uncomfortable or painful
4. Tell the child that he or she will not feel any pain during the surgery because of the "special sleep" of anesthesia and that he or she will wake up after surgery is over in the recovery room
5. Include details specific to the child's surgery such as dressings, tubes, IV fluids, medications, the specific site of the pain or discomfort, and the diet restrictions before and after surgery

E. General postoperative care
1. Basic postoperative care is similar to nursing care of adult postoperative patients
   a. Frequent vital signs; pulse oximetry, as needed
   b. Observation of the incision or dressings
   c. Level of consciousness
   d. Intake and output, IV fluids, Foley catheter, nasogastric (NG) tube
   e. Administer pain medications as needed (IV, PO, epidurals; IM may be used, but should be avoided)
2. Allow the child's parents to assist in the child's care if they desire to do so
3. Explain all postoperative procedures before doing them

F. Care of the child in a cast
1. The cast should be handled lightly with open palms while it is still damp to avoid indentations
2. Observe and record the condition of the skin at the edges of the cast for color, warmth, irritation, sensation, and edema
3. Check the color of the nail beds below the cast; check the pulse in the area below the cast if it is in an accessible area (radial or pedal pulse)
4. Teach the child not to put anything inside the cast or to "scratch" the skin beneath the cast

5. Check the cast for drainage or discoloration; any drainage should be marked, timed, and dated
6. Protect the cast from water, urine, and stool
7. "Petal" the edges of the cast before the patient goes home (if cast is damp, teach parents the proper way to do it)
8. Before discharge, talk to the parents regarding a safe method for restraining the child with a cast while in the car; infants and children in long leg and hip spica casts will need adapted car seats/safety belts

G. Care of the child in traction
  1. Types of traction
     a. Skeletal: uses pins, wires, and tongs
     b. Skin: uses tapes, plastic, and bandages attached to the skin
     c. Bryant's/modified Bryant's: a type of skin traction; it is most commonly used in infants and toddlers for treatment of a fractured femur and congenital hip dislocation (Fig. 8-15)
  2. Nursing care measures for the child in traction
     a. Explain the traction apparatus to the child; allow the child to participate in his or her care as much as possible
     b. Maintain traction alignment; be sure that all ropes are in the center tracks of the pulleys and that the weights are hanging freely
     c. Provide proper skin care; observe for reddened, irritated areas at the edges of the tape and elastic bandages, as well as at other pressure sites
     d. Observe skeletal pin sites for bleeding, inflammation, and signs of infection; provide pin-site care as ordered
     e. Observe affected extremity for skin color, nail bed color, and changes in sensation and mobility
     f. Administer pain medications as ordered and keep the child as comfortable as possible
     g. Provide range-of-motion exercises to the unaffected body parts to help prevent contractures and muscle atrophy
     h. Provide toys and activities appropriate to the child's age level and limited mobility

SUGGESTED READING

Caspe WB: Guidelines for the care of children and adolescents with HIV infection, *J Pediatr* 119(suppl):S1-S68, 1991.

Ingalls AJ, Salerno MC: *Maternal and child health nursing*, ed 7, St Louis, 1991, Mosby.

Jackson PL, Vessey JA: *Primary care of the child with a chronic condition*, ed 2, St. Louis, 1996, Mosby.

Kline MW, Shearer WT: A national survey on the care of infants and children with HIV infection, *J Pediatr* 118:817-821, May 1991.

Physicians' desk reference, Montvale, NJ, Medical Economics (published annually).

Pizzo PA, Wilfert CM: *Pediatric AIDS: the challenge of HIV infection in infants, children and adolescents*, Baltimore, 1991, Williams & Wilkins.

Reece RM, Smith MK: Child abuse, *Pediatr Clin North Am* 37:905-922, Aug 1990.

Whaley LF, Wong DL: *Nursing care of infants and children*, ed 5, St Louis, 1995, Mosby.

Wong DL: *Clinical manual of pediatric nursing*, ed 4, St. Louis, 1996, Mosby

Wong DL: *Whaley and Wong's essentials of pediatric nursing*, ed 4, St Louis, 1993, Mosby.

REVIEW QUESTIONS

Answers and rationales begin on p. 401.

1. A Wilms' tumor is an adenosarcoma found in the:
   ① Brain
   ② Small intestine
   ③ Colon
   ④ Kidney

2. Infancy is that period from:
   ① Birth to 6 weeks of age
   ② Birth to 1 year of age
   ③ 4 weeks to 1 year of age
   ④ 4 weeks to 2 years of age

3. The physician orders meperidine (Demerol) 20 mg with atropine 0.08 mg IM as a preoperative medication. The meperidine is supplied at 50 mg/ml, the atropine at 0.2 mg/ml. The nurse should draw up a total volume of:
   ① 0.4 ml
   ② 0.8 ml
   ③ 1.0 ml
   ④ 1.2 ml

4. Your neighbor, age 7 years, has developed a red, raised rash on her face, neck, and trunk. She also has a temperature of 101.4° F (38.5° C) and whitish spots on the back of her throat. From these symptoms, you know she has:
   ① Chickenpox
   ② Measles (rubeola)
   ③ Mumps
   ④ German measles (rubella)

5. The patient, age 4, was admitted with a diagnosis of possible epiglottitis. If the nurse suspects the patient has epiglottitis, the nurse should:
   ① Check her throat carefully with a flashlight
   ② Increase her oral intake
   ③ Direct warm steam toward the patient
   ④ Have emergency tracheostomy equipment immediately available

6. The symptoms of epiglottitis are caused by:
   ① A bacterial infection; usually *H. influenzae*
   ② Inflammation of the trachea and esophagus
   ③ Spasms of the epiglottis
   ④ Viral upper respiratory infection (URI)

7. The patient, age 3, has to have blood drawn for a CBC. When she asks you if it will hurt to have the blood drawn, the best response would be:
   ① "No, of course it won't hurt!"
   ② "It might hurt for a minute, but I will be here with you, and you can hold my hand if you want to."
   ③ "If you are a big girl, the blood test won't hurt you."
   ④ "It might hurt, but you have to have it done, so try not to cry."

8. The patient, age 3, has an order for sulfisoxasole (Gantrisin) 750 mg po q AM. On hand, you have sulfisoxasole 0.5 g/5 ml. You give the patient:
   ① 2 ml
   ② 4 ml
   ③ 1½ tsp
   ④ 2 tsp

9. Adolescence begins when:
   ① The growth rate increases rapidly
   ② The child develops a positive self-image
   ③ Secondary sex characteristics appear
   ④ The child starts to be attracted to the opposite sex

10. Hospitalized teenagers have the most difficulty with:
    ① Dependency vs. independency
    ② Trust vs. autonomy
    ③ Reality vs. fantasy
    ④ Initiative vs. guilt

11. According to Erikson's theory of psychosocial development, preschoolers are in the stage of:
    ① Trust vs. mistrust
    ② Industry vs. inferiority
    ③ Autonomy vs. shame and doubt
    ④ Initiative vs. guilt

12. The best way for the pediatric nurse to establish a good working relationship with parents is to:
    ① Avoid contact whenever possible
    ② Answer their questions honestly
    ③ Refer all questions to the physician
    ④ Keep them out of their child's room as much as possible

13. Rheumatic fever is caused by:
    ① A fungus
    ② *Staphylococcus* bacteria
    ③ A virus
    ④ *Streptococcus* bacteria

14. The most serious complication of rheumatic fever is:
    ① Endocarditis
    ② Pneumonia
    ③ Arthritis
    ④ Meningitis

15. Which of the following pathophysiologic mechanisms is responsible for respiratory alterations seen in children with cystic fibrosis?
    ① Decreased ciliary action causing stasis of mucus in lungs
    ② Edema of the epiglottis causing upper airway occlusion
    ③ Excessive production of thick mucus leading to airway obstruction
    ④ Laryngeal stricture leading to bronchospasm

16. The child with cystic fibrosis takes pancreatic enzymes with each meal. The purpose of this therapy is to facilitate:
    ① Absorption of vitamins A, C, and K
    ② Increased carbohydrate metabolism for growth
    ③ Digestion and absorption of fats and proteins
    ④ Sodium excretion and electrolyte balance

17. Aerosol treatment, chest physiotherapy, and postural drainage are ordered for children with cystic fibrosis to:
    ① Decrease respiratory effort and mucus production
    ② Dilate the bronchioles and clear secretions
    ③ Increase efficiency of the diaphragm and gas exchange
    ④ Stimulate coughing and arterial oxygen consumption

18. One of the major physical characteristics of the child with Down syndrome is:
    ① Hypertonic musculature
    ② A single transverse crease on palms
    ③ Inflexibility of the joints
    ④ Janeway spots on the palms and soles

19. In caring for a child with Down syndrome, the nurse should be aware that a frequent accompanying defect is:
    ① Congenital heart disease
    ② Congenital hip dysplasia
    ③ Central auditory imperception
    ④ Pyloric stenosis

20. Which of the following statements is appropriate when giving medications to a 5-year-old patient?
    ① "Hi! It's time for your medicine. I know you don't like the flavor of the medicine, so I mixed it in your juice."
    ② "Are you finished with breakfast? I have some candy pills for you to take. They taste just like peppermint."
    ③ "I have a shot to give to you. I know shots hurt, but you need to have the medicine in the shot to make you better. Would you like me to give it to you now or in 5 minutes?"
    ④ "Hi! It's time for your medicine. Your mom has to leave."
21. The safest place to give an infant an intramuscular (IM) injection is the:
    ① Deltoid muscle
    ② Vastus lateralis muscle
    ③ Ventrogluteal muscle
    ④ Dorsogluteal muscle
22. Celiac disease is characterized by disturbance in the absorption of:
    ① Proteins
    ② Carbohydrates
    ③ Vitamins
    ④ Fats
23. Symptoms of celiac disease include which of the following?
    ① Constipation, anorexia, and malnutrition
    ② Malnutrition, distended abdomen, constant appetite for sweets
    ③ Distended abdomen, constipation, anorexia
    ④ Bulky, greasy stools, distended abdomen, and malnutrition
24. The infant with diagnosed celiac disease should be given which cereal?
    ① Rice
    ② Wheat
    ③ Oat
    ④ Barley
25. The best, most reliable method of assessing for pinworms in a child is by:
    ① The history, symptoms, and a stool culture
    ② A blood culture
    ③ Capturing the eggs from the anal edge on cellophane tape
    ④ Sending a stool culture to the laboratory
26. A two-year-old patient is diagnosed as having leukemia. The most common signs and symptoms of leukemia related to bone marrow involvement are:
    ① Headache, papilledema, and irritability
    ② Muscle wasting, weight loss, and fatigue
    ③ Decreased intracranial pressure, psychosis, and confusion
    ④ Anemia, infection, and bleeding
27. The most common method of treatment for an infant weighing more than 30 lb with a simple fractured femur is:
    ① Surgery and placement of a pin to set the fracture
    ② Putting the child in skeletal traction
    ③ Immediate setting and casting of the fractured leg
    ④ Putting the child in Bryant's traction
28. The lateral S-shaped curvature of the spine that most often occurs in school-age girls is:
    ① Scoliosis
    ② Nephrosis
    ③ Lordosis
    ④ Kyphosis

29. A patient, age 17 months, is admitted to the hospital with a diagnosis of meningitis. Which of the following findings would be noted relative to the patient's cerebrospinal fluid (CSF)?
    ① Reduced protein level
    ② Elevated glucose level
    ③ Reduced pressure
    ④ Cloudy color
30. The most notable symptoms the nurse would observe in a toddler with meningitis would be:
    ① Weak or absent cry, coma
    ② Bulging fontanel, irritability
    ③ Absent reflexes, rigid digits
    ④ Dilated and fixed pupils
31. While you are caring for a 2-year-old female patient, she has a complex febrile seizure in her crib. What is the most important nursing activity at this time?
    ① Place a seizure stick between her jaws
    ② Prepare the suction equipment
    ③ Observe the seizure and protect her from harm
    ④ Restrain her to prevent injury
32. A male patient, age 18 months, is admitted to the hospital for a bilateral myringotomy because of frequent occurrences of otitis media. Otitis media occurs more frequently in young children than in older children because of the different position and shape of the young child's:
    ① Esophagus
    ② Tympanic membranes
    ③ External ear canals
    ④ Eustachian tubes
33. When performing a procedure on an uncooperative small child, which of the following actions would be the best for the nurse to try first?
    ① Sedate the child
    ② Use wrist and ankle restraints
    ③ Allow a parent to assist
    ④ Bring in another nurse to assist
34. Which of the following is responsible for airway narrowing characteristic of an asthma episode?
    ① Laryngeal edema, dehydration, and anxiety
    ② Bronchospasm, respiratory mucosal inflammation and edema, and increased production and accumulation of mucus
    ③ Increased negative pleural pressure, laryngospasm, and mucus plugging
    ④ Carbon dioxide retention, pharyngeal hyperemia, and alveolar collapse
35. You are caring for a child who weighs 25 lb. The usual dose for Ampicillin for children is 100 mg/kg/day. Which of the following would be an appropriate order for this child?
    ① Ampicillin 25 mg q4h
    ② Ampicillin 250 mg qid
    ③ Ampicillin 100 mg q6h
    ④ Ampicillin 100 mg qid
36. The physician orders Ampicillin 300 mg IVPB. Ampicillin is supplied as 500 mg/2 ml. What volume of Ampicillin would you draw up from the vial?
    ① 0.6 ml
    ② 0.8 ml
    ③ 1.2 ml
    ④ 1.4 ml

37. Bulimia is an eating disorder characterized by:
    ① Severe weight loss
    ② "Binge" eating followed by induced vomiting
    ③ Sudden weight gain
    ④ Chronic diarrhea

38. The childhood disease that exhibits symptoms of lethargy, muscle pain, polyarthritis, and chorea and is diagnosed by using the Jones criteria is:
    ① Infectious mononucleosis
    ② Muscular dystrophy
    ③ Cystic fibrosis
    ④ Rheumatic fever

39. A 3-month-old infant is admitted to the pediatric unit for treatment of bronchiolitis. Oxygen therapy is ordered for the infant primarily to:
    ① Reduce fever
    ② Allay anxiety and restlessness
    ③ Liquify secretions
    ④ Relieve dyspnea and hypoxemia

40. Fluids by mouth are initially contraindicated for an infant with bronchiolitis because of feeding difficulty caused by:
    ① Tachypnea
    ② Bradycardia
    ③ Irritability
    ④ Fever

41. The stage of development where "parallel play" takes place is:
    ① Infancy
    ② Toddler
    ③ Preschool age
    ④ School age

42. The disorder characterized by a malfunction of the motor centers of the brain (because of lack of oxygen to the brain) is:
    ① Down syndrome
    ② Scoliosis
    ③ Osteomyelitis
    ④ Cerebral palsy

43. Which of the following statements about pain in children is true?
    ① A child's behavioral response to pain is affected by his or her age and developmental stage
    ② Recovery from a painful experience occurs at a faster rate in children than in adults
    ③ Narcotic use in children is dangerous because of the increased risk of addiction and respiratory depression
    ④ Immaturity of the nervous system in young children provides them with increased thresholds for pain

44. The average 2- to 3-month-old infant:
    ① Babbles
    ② Has a crude pincer grasp
    ③ Has a closed posterior fontanel
    ④ Has one lower incisor

45. About 95% of all sudden infant death syndrome (SIDS) cases occur:
    ① In the first 10 weeks of life
    ② In the first 3 months of life
    ③ In the first 6 months of life
    ④ Between 6 and 12 months of age

46. The first immunizations an infant receives at 2 months of age are:
    ① DPT vaccine only
    ② PPD, OPV, first hepatitis B vaccines
    ③ DTP, OPV, MMR
    ④ DTP, OPV, Hib, second hepatitis B vaccine

47. The leading cause of death in children between 1 and 14 years of age is:
    ① Meningitis
    ② Leukemia
    ③ Accidents
    ④ Polio

48. A disorder caused by an obstruction of cerebrospinal fluid drainage is:
    ① Opisthotonos
    ② Wilms' tumor
    ③ Hydrocephalus
    ④ Meningitis

49. Characteristics of an infant diagnosed as failure to thrive (FTT) include:
    ① Sociable smile at 2 month
    ② Weight below twentieth percentile
    ③ Distrust of human contact
    ④ No interest in toys

50. A baby with gastroesophageal reflux and FTT is classified as:
    ① Organic FTT
    ② Nonorganic FTT
    ③ Idiopathic FTT
    ④ Unstable FTT

51. In caring for a child in a full leg cast, which of the following findings should the nurse report to the physician *immediately*?
    ① The cast is still damp after 4 hours
    ② The child's pedal pulse is 80
    ③ The child complains of pain in his leg
    ④ The child is unable to move his toes

52. Of the following, the most important criterion on which to base the decision to report suspected child abuse is:
    ① Inappropriate parental concern for the degree of injury
    ② Absence of the parents for questioning about the child's injuries
    ③ A complaint other than the one associated with the signs of abuse
    ④ Incompatibility between the history given and the injury observed

53. When starting an infant on new foods, it is best to instruct the mother to:
    ① Mix the new food with one that the infant already likes
    ② Mix the new food with breast milk or formula
    ③ Feed the infant one new food at a time, to observe for possible allergic reactions
    ④ Try a new food at each feeding

54. By the end of the school-age years, a child should have developed a sense of:
    ① Initiative, purpose
    ② Industry, competence
    ③ Identity, role
    ④ Intimacy, fidelity

55. Your patient is 2 years old. Her favorite word is "No!" She is in Erikson's developmental stage of:
    ① Trust vs. mistrust
    ② Initiative vs. guilt
    ③ Autonomy vs. shame and doubt
    ④ Industry vs. inferiority

56. A 5-week-old infant is brought to the pediatrician's office with symptoms of irritability, weight loss, and projectile vomiting. On physical examination the infant appears dehydrated. From these symptoms you know that the infant probably has:
    ① Hirschsprung's disease
    ② Pyloric stenosis
    ③ Esophogeal atresia
    ④ Intussusception

57. A 12-month-old female with sickle cell anemia is admitted in sickle cell crisis. Her symptoms might include:
    ① Fever, seizures, coma
    ② Abdominal pain; swollen, painful joints
    ③ Polycythemia, tachycardia
    ④ Severe itching, vomiting

58. Nursing intervention for the child in sickle cell crisis is directed primarily toward:
    ① Maintaining active range of motion
    ② Oxygen therapy
    ③ Administration of blood
    ④ Maintaining adequate hydration

59. A Denis Browne splint is a common method of treatment for:
    ① Scoliosis
    ② Congenital clubfoot
    ③ Developmental dysplasia of the hip (DDH)
    ④ Fractured femur

60. Preparation of a child for surgery should include all of the following *except:*
    ① Explaining all procedures and treatments before they occur
    ② Telling the child not to cry but to "be brave" if something hurts
    ③ Explaining anesthesia as a "special sleep"
    ④ Explaining where the incision or dressings will be after surgery

61. The physician has ordered an IV of D5.2NS to be infused at 100 ml/hr. If the IV tubing delivers 10 gtt/ml, at what rate would you infuse the IV fluid?
    ① 10 gtt/min
    ② 12 gtt/min
    ③ 16 gtt/min
    ④ 18 gtt/min

62. A female patient, 18 months of age, has developmental dysplasia of her right hip, and will be hospitalized for surgery and application of a hip spica cast. Which of the following nursing measures will be necessary in caring for her?
    ① Avoid giving her pain medication as much as possible, to prevent constipation
    ② Limit fluids, so she will be less likely to get the cast wet when she voids
    ③ Tell the parents that they can take her home in the car propped up on pillows, with her legs down
    ④ Assess sensation, circulation, and motion of her feet and toes

63. Many researchers believe that SIDS may be related to a brainstem abnormality in the regulation of cardiorespiratory control. Other recent studies have demonstrated that there is an increased risk of SIDS in infants who:
    ① Breastfeed rather than bottle feed
    ② Sleep in the prone position
    ③ Are over 10 months of age
    ④ Use a pacifier while they sleep

64. The treatment of a child with nephrotic syndrome includes administration of corticosteroids to:
    ① Decrease the amount of proteinuria
    ② Increase the amount of albumin in the blood
    ③ Help control hypertension
    ④ Reduce edema of the face, extremities, and abdomen

65. A ketogenic diet is sometimes used in the treatment of:
    ① Epilepsy
    ② Crohn's disease
    ③ Bulimia
    ④ Acute glomerulonephritis

66. The principal cause of mononucleosis is:
    ① Streptococcus
    ② The Epstein-Barr virus
    ③ Respiratory syncytial virus (RSV)
    ④ *H. influenzae*

67. A child with asthma would most likely present with which of the following symptoms?
    ① Laryngitis, sore throat, and productive cough
    ② Fever, rhinorrhea, and coarse breath sounds
    ③ Tightness in the chest, nonproductive cough, and wheezing
    ④ Rapid respiratory rate, difficulty swallowing, and fever

68. The two main types of medication used to treat asthma are:
    ① Antiinflammatory agents and immunosuppressants
    ② Bronchodilators and antiinflammatory agents
    ③ Antibiotics and bronchodilators
    ④ Decongestants and antihistamines

69. One of the medications approved for use in children with AIDS that assists in slowing the progression of the disease is:
    ① IV gamma globulin (Gamamine N)
    ② Ceftazidime (Fortaz)
    ③ Vancomycin (Vancocin)
    ④ Azidothymidine (Retrovir)

70. The hepatitis B vaccine series should begin at what age?
    ① Newborn
    ② 2 months
    ③ 6 months
    ④ 12 months

71. A female patient, age 2 months, presents at the pediatrician's office with a 2-week history of paroxysmal abdominal cramping. Her mother states that she is very fussy and cries as if she is in pain. She is tolerating her normal amounts of formula well and has gained weight since her last visit. These signs and symptoms indicate that she most likely has:
    ① An intussesception
    ② Colic
    ③ A pyloric stenosis
    ④ Hirschsprung's disease

72. A 5-month-old infant with chronic lung disease is admitted with a severe case of RSV. Treatment for this child will include:
    ① Cromolyn (Intal) nebulizer treatments and IV fluids
    ② Ribavirin (Virazole) and humidified oxygen
    ③ Antibiotics and IV fluids
    ④ Prednisone (LiquiPred) and oxygen

73. Which of the following statements about RSV/bronchiolitis is true?
① It occurs primarily in fall and winter
② Peak incidence for RSV infection is 6 to 18 months of age
③ RSV can survive for hours on gloves, countertops, and skin
④ It causes the bronchioles to plug with mucus, trapping air in the lungs

74. Oral rehydration therapy is the treatment of choice for children with:
① Infectious gastroenteritis
② Hypertrophic pyloric stenosis
③ Viral meningitis
④ Celiac disease

75. At the time of delivery, an infant is born with its abdominal organs, covered by a sac, protruding through an abnormal opening in the umbilical ring. This condition is known as:
① Intussusception
② Diaphragmatic hernia
③ Omphalocele
④ Gastroschisis

ANSWERS AND RATIONALES

1. Knowledge, assessment, environment (b)
   ❹ A Wilms' tumor is found only in the kidney and kidney area.
   ① It is not found in the brain.
   ② It is not found in the small intestine.
   ③ It is not found in the colon.

2. Knowledge, assessment, psychosocial (b)
   ❸ This is the period of life known as infancy.
   ① Birth to 4 weeks is the newborn period; birth to 6 weeks includes newborn and part of infancy.
   ② Birth to 4 weeks is the newborn period and is not considered part of the infancy period.
   ④ After 1 year of age until 3 years of age is considered the toddler period.

3. Application, implementation, environment (b)
   ❷ Meperedine: DD = 20 mg
                        DH = 50 mg
                        V = 1 ml

   $$\frac{DD}{DH} = \frac{20 \text{ mg}}{50 \text{ mg}} \times 1 \text{ ml} = 0.4 \text{ ml}$$

   Atropine: DD = 0.08 mg
                  DH = 0.2 mg
                  V = 1 ml

   $$\frac{DD}{DH} = \frac{0.08 \text{ mg}}{0.2 \text{ mg}} \times 1 \text{ ml} = 0.4 \text{ ml}$$

   0.4 ml + 0.4 ml = 0.8 ml
   ①,③,④ This is not the correct amount.

4. Comprehension, assessment, environment (c)
   ❷ These are symptoms of rubeola.
   ① Symptoms of chickenpox include a clear, vesicular rash, fever, irritability, and pruritus.
   ③ Symptoms of rubella do not include a high fever or white spots at the back of the throat.
   ④ Symptoms of mumps include enlarged parotid glands and fever, with no rash.

5. Application, implementation, environment (a)
   ❹ This equipment may be necessary if the enlarged epiglottis completely obstructs the airway.
   ① Any examination of the throat could lead to laryngospasm.
   ② The child with epiglottitis has difficulty swallowing.
   ③ Warm steam is not a method of treatment in epiglottitis.

6. Comprehension, assessment, environment (b)
   ❶ *H. influenzae* is the responsible organism in most cases of epiglottitis.
   ② The trachea and esophagus are not affected.
   ③ This is not the cause.
   ④ Although the child may have other symptoms of URI, the cause is bacterial, not viral.

7. Application, implementation, physiologic (b)
   ❷ This is the most honest, helpful answer the nurse can give.
   ① This is a lie.
   ③ At 3 years of age she is not a "big girl"; she is a child and should be allowed to act like one.
   ④ She should be allowed to cry if the blood test hurts. Telling her not to cry only gives her something else to worry about.

8. Application, implementation, environment (b)
   ❸ DD = 750 mg
      DH = 0.5 g (500 mg)
      V = 5 ml

   $$\frac{DD}{DH} = \frac{750 \text{ mg}}{500 \text{ mg}} \times 5 \text{ ml} = 7.5 \text{ ml} = 1\frac{1}{2} \text{ tsp}$$

   ①,②,④ This is not the correct amount.

9. Comprehension, assessment, health (b)
   ❸ This is when adolescence is considered to begin in each child's life.
   ① This occurs more than once in childhood.
   ② Developing a self-image is part of adolescence, but it may be positive or negative during the teenage years.
   ④ Adolescent boys are often attracted to adolescent girls at an earlier age than the girls are attracted to the boys.

10. Knowledge, assessment, physiologic (a)
    ❶ Adolescents are at the stage where they are constantly struggling to develop a positive self-image and their own identity and independence.
    ② These are the developmental skills developed during infancy and toddlerhood.
    ③,④ This occurs during the preschool stage.

11. Knowledge, assessment, physiologic (a)
    ❹ Preschoolers are at the stage where they are learning how to interact with other people, as well as proper behavior; this helps them develop a sense of initiative and accomplishment.
    ① This is the stage of infants.
    ② This is the stage of school-age children.
    ③ This is the stage of toddlers.

12. Comprehension, implementation, psychosocial (a)
    ❷ The parents will deal best with a nurse who is open and honest with them.
    ① This will put a strain on the relationship between the parents and the nurse.
    ③ The nurse should answer as many questions as possible and only refer questions that she cannot answer to the physician.
    ④ The parents should be involved as much as possible in their child's care and recovery, and this should be encouraged by the nurse.

13. Knowledge, assessment, environment (b)
    ❹ Rheumatic fever is a chronic disease caused by a streptococcal infection.
    ① It is not caused by a fungus.
    ② It is not caused by *Staphylococcus* bacteria.
    ③ It is not caused by a virus.

14. Comprehension, assessment, environment (c)
    ❶ This is the most common, serious complication of rheumatic fever; the endocardium and valves become inflamed and often are permanently damaged.
    ② This is not a common complication of rheumatic fever.
    ③ Arthritis is a symptom of rheumatic fever but not the most serious complication.
    ④ This is not a complication of rhematic fever.

15. Comprehension, assessment, environment (a)
    ❸ Large amounts of abnormally thick mucus are produced in the lungs, as well as the pancreas and liver. The mucus from the lungs leads to airway obstruction.
    ①,④ This does not occur in cystic fibrosis.
    ② This occurs in epiglottitis.

16. Knowledge, assessment, environment (a)
    ❸ Pancreatic enzymes are given regularly with food to improve the digestion and absorption of proteins and fats in the small intestine.
    ① Pancreatic enzymes do not directly affect vitamin absorption.
    ② Pancreatic enzymes do not affect carbohydrate metabolism.
    ④ Although sodium levels are a problem in the child with cystic fibrosis, pancreatic enzymes do not affect them.

17. Knowledge, assessment, environment (a)
    ❷ The main function of aerosolized bronchodilators and chest physiotherapy is to dilate the bronchioles and loosen and move secretions out of the lungs.
    ① Nothing has been shown to be effective in decreasing mucus production.
    ③ Efficiency of the diaphragm is not a problem in cystic fibrosis.
    ④ Although chest physiotherapy may stimulate coughing to some degree, it is not done to increase oxygen consumption.

18. Comprehension, assessment, environment (a)
    ❷ This is a classic sign seen in children diagnosed with Down syndrome.
    ① These children are hypotonic.
    ③ These children have hyperflexibility of the joints.
    ④ This is a symptom seen in bacterial endocarditis.

19. Comprehension, assessment, environment (a)
    ❶ Some form of congenital heart defect is often seen in children with Down syndrome.
    ②,③,④ This is not frequently seen in children with Down syndrome.

20. Application, implementation, physiologic (a)
    ❸ It is important not to lie to children when a shot or procedure is going to hurt. Allowing them to decide whether to get the shot "now, or in 5 minutes" gives them some control in the situation.
    ① Medicine should not be mixed in juice.
    ② The nurse should always be honest with the child when giving medicine; medicine should never be called candy.
    ④ The parent is the child's support system.

21. Knowledge, implementation, psychosocial (b)
    ❷ This is the best developed muscle in infants and therefore is the safest for IM injections.
    ① This muscle is not well developed in infants, toddlers, or young children.
    ③,④ This muscle is not well developed in infants and toddlers.

22. Knowledge, assessment, environment (a)
    ❹ Celiac disease is a basic defect of metabolism, leading to impaired fat absorption.
    ① Celiac disease does not affect absorption of proteins.
    ② Celiac disease does not affect absorption of carbohydrates.
    ③ Celiac disease does not affect absorption of vitamins.

23. Knowledge, assessment, environment (b)
    ❹ These are all common symptoms of celiac disease.
    ①,③ Constipation is not a symptom of celiac disease.
    ② An appetite for sweets is not a symptom of celiac disease.

24. Comprehension, planning, environment (a)
    ❶ Rice cereal is digested properly in the infant with celiac disease.
    ② Because of the defect in metabolism in the child with celiac disease, ingestion of wheat leads to impaired fat absorption.
    ③ Ingestion of oats leads to impaired fat absorption.
    ④ Ingestion of barley leads to impaired fat absorption.

25. Knowledge, assessment, psychosocial (a)
    ❸ The cellophane tape test is used in diagnosing pinworms.
    ① The child's history and symptoms are not enough to definitely diagnose pinworms; a stool culture will not diagnose pinworms.
    ② A blood culture would not be helpful in diagnosing pinworms.
    ④ A stool culture will not diagnose pinworms.

26. Comprehension, assessment, environment (a)
    ❹ These symptoms of leukemia result directly from changes in the bone marrow.
    ① These symptoms are caused by leukemic effects on the nervous system that lead to increased intracranial pressure.
    ② These symptoms result from the body's increasing need to meet the metabolic needs of the leukemic cells.
    ③ These are not symptoms of leukemia.

27. Comprehension, assessment, environment (b)
    ❹ Bryant's traction is the usual method of treatment for an infant with a fractured femur.
    ① This is more extensive treatment than is usually needed.
    ② Skeletal traction is not usually used for infants with fractured femurs; often used in older children.
    ③ Traction is usually necessary before casting can be done if the fracture is to heal properly.

28. Knowledge, assessment, environment (a)
    ❶ Scoliosis of the spine often occurs because of rapid growth; seen most often in girls.
    ② Nephrosis is a disease of the kidneys, causing edema and proteinuria.
    ③ Lordosis is a concave curvature of the spine; called sway-back.
    ④ Kyphosis is a convex curvature of the spine; called hunchback.

29. Knowledge, assessment, environment (b)
    ❹ The CSF of a child with meningitis is cloudy because of the increased WBC count.
    ① Meningitis causes an increased protein level.
    ② Meningitis causes a decreased glucose level.
    ③ There is an increase in the CSF pressure in meningitis.

30. Comprehension, assessment, environment (b)
    ❷ These signs are the most notable because these symptoms are caused by increased intracranial pressure, a serious complication in meningitis.
    ① The child's cry would be shrill and high pitched.
    ③,④ These are not signs seen in meningitis.

31. Application, implementation, environment (b)
    ❸ Observing the length and type of seizure is important, as is preventing the child from injuring herself.
    ① This could injure the child's mouth.
    ② Suctioning may be needed but would not be feasible until the seizure was over.
    ④ Restraints could lead to severe injury.

32. Comprehension, assessment, environment (a)
    ❹ The eustachian tubes are shorter and wider in the young child than in the older child, which allows for easier introduction of bacteria.
    ① The shape and position of the esophagus do not affect otitis media.
    ② The shape and position of the tympanic membranes do not affect otitis media.
    ③ The external ear canals are basically the same shape and in the same position in young and older children.
33. Application, planning, psychosocial (b)
    ❸ Having a parent assist in procedures often helps to calm the child, making it much easier to perform the procedure.
    ① Sedation is only used as a last resort when absolutely necessary.
    ② Restraints may be needed if assistance by a parent or by another nurse has not been effective.
    ④ Bringing in another nurse may frighten a small child; strange faces may upset the child instead of help calm him or her.
34. Comprehension, assessment, environment (b)
    ❷ These changes in the respiratory system lead to narrowing of the child's airway.
    ①,③,④ This does not occur in asthma.
35. Application, implementation, environment (b)
    ❷ 25 lb = 11.3 kg
    100 mg × 11.3 kg/day = 1130 mg/day
    $\frac{1130 \text{ mg}}{4 \text{ doses}} = 282$ mg
    Appropriate order = 250 mg qid.
    ①,③,④ This is not an appropriate order for this child.
36. Application, implementation, environment (b)
    ❸ DD = 300 mg
    DH = 500 mg
    V = 2 ml
    $\frac{DD}{DH} = \frac{300 \text{ mg}}{500 \text{ mg}} \times 2$ ml = 1.2 ml
    ①,②,④ This is not the correct amount.
37. Knowledge, assessment, environment (a)
    ❷ "Binge" eating followed by induced vomiting is the classic symptom of bulimia.
    ① This is a symptom of anorexia nervosa.
    ③,④ This is not a symptom of bulimia.
38. Comprehension, assessment, environment (a)
    ❹ The Jones criteria are used only to diagnose rheumatic fever.
    ① This is a viral disease diagnosed by the symptoms and the Monospot test.
    ②,③ This is a hereditary disease.
39. Comprehension, assessment, environment (a)
    ❹ The infant with bronchiolitis needs oxygen to relieve his extreme dyspnea and resultant hypoxemia.
    ① Oxygen would not reduce a fever.
    ② This is not the primary reason for oxygen therapy.
    ③ Oxygen would not liquefy secretions.
40. Comprehension, assessment, environment (b)
    ❶ Severe tachypnea seen in bronchiolitis is a contraindication for oral feedings.
    ② Bronchiolitis normally causes tachycardia
    ③,④ This is not a contraindication for oral fluids.

41. Knowledge, assessment, physiologic (b)
    ❷ Toddlers use parallel play when playing with other children.
    ① Infants usually play alone or with an adult.
    ③ Preschoolers use associative play.
    ④ School-age children use associative play.
42. Comprehension, assessment, environment (b)
    ❹ Cerebral palsy is a disorder that affects the motor centers of the brain; it is usually caused by birth trauma or head trauma.
    ① This is a chromosomal abnormality.
    ② This is an S-shaped lateral curvature of the spine.
    ③ This is an infection of the bone.
43. Comprehension, assessment, psychosocial (a)
    ❶ This statement about children's pain is true.
    ② Recovery from a painful experience does not occur faster in children.
    ③ Narcotics are both safe and often necessary in the management of children's pain.
    ④ Children do not have increased pain thresholds.
44. Knowledge, assessment, physiologic (a)
    ❸ The posterior fontanel closes by this age.
    ① This develops at 6 to 7 months of age.
    ② This develops at 8 to 9 months of age.
    ④ This occurs at 7 to 8 months of age.
45. Knowledge, assessment, psychosocial (a)
    ❸ Although some SIDS occur later, most occur by 6 months of age.
    ①,②,④ This is not true of SIDS.
46. Knowledge, assessment, health (a)
    ❹ These are the immunizations normally given at 2 months of age.
    ① The OPV is also given.
    ② The PPD is not given.
    ③ The MMA vaccine is not given.
47. Comprehension, assessment, health (b)
    ❸ Accidents of all types are the leading cause of death in this age level.
    ① Meningitis is seldom fatal.
    ② Leukemia occurs less often than accidents.
    ④ Polio occurs only rarely.
48. Knowledge, assessment, physiologic (a)
    ❸ Hydrocephalus occurs when there is an obstruction of the cerebrospinal fluid drainage pathways.
    ① Opisthotonos is a sign of increased intracranial pressure.
    ② It does not cause the formation of a Wilms' tumor.
    ④ It does not cause meningitis.
49. Knowledge, assessment, environment (a)
    ❸ The infant with FTT is distrustful of people.
    ① This could be a normal characteristic.
    ② This could be caused by other medical conditions/prematurity.
    ④ The infant prefers inanimate objects.
50. Knowledge, assessment, environment (b)
    ❶ Gastroesophageal reflux is an organic (physical) cause of FTT.
    ② Nonorganic FTT is usually caused by psychosocial factors.
    ③ Idiopathic FTT has no explainable cause.
    ④ There is no classification with this name.

51. Comprehension, implementation, environment (b)
   ❹ This may indicate nerve damage at the fracture site or pressure from the cast and should be reported immediately.
   ①,② This is a normal finding.
   ③ This is usually a normal finding; any sudden increase in pain or severe muscle spasms should be reported to the physician.

52. Knowledge, assessment, psychosocial (b)
   ❹ In cases of child abuse, the history given by the caregiver does not fit with the severity or type of injury.
   ① This may occur with other types of injury as well as child abuse.
   ② This is not an indication of abuse; the child may not have been home at the time of the abuse or injury.
   ③ This is not an indication of abuse.

53. Application, implementation, health (b)
   ❸ Introducing new foods one at a time helps to determine the infant's likes, dislikes, and possible allergies to certain foods.
   ① Mixing the food with formula does not allow the infant to taste the new food.
   ② Mixing the food with other foods does not allow the infant to taste the new food.
   ④ New foods should be introduced one at a time for 2 to 3 days to determine possible allergies the infant might have.

54. Knowledge, assessment, physiologic (a)
   ❷ School-age children are in the stage of industry vs. inferiority.
   ① This is the developmental task in the preschooler.
   ③ This is the developmental task in the adolescent.
   ④ This is the developmental task in the young adult.

55. Knowledge, assessment, physiologic (b)
   ❸ Toddlers (age 1 to 3 years) are in the stage of autonomy vs. shame and doubt.
   ① Infants are in the stage of trust vs. mistrust.
   ② Preschoolers are in the stage of initiative vs. guilt.
   ④ School-age children are in the stage of industry vs. inferiority.

56. Comprehension, assessment, environment (b)
   ❷ These are classic symptoms of an infant with pyloric stenosis.
   ① These are not symptoms of Hirschsprung's disease.
   ③ These are not symptoms of esophageal atresia.
   ④ These are not symptoms of intussusception.

57. Knowledge, assessment, environment (a)
   ❷ A child in sickle cell crisis often experiences abdominal pain, swollen, painful joints, and fever.
   ① Seizures and coma do not occur in sickle cell crisis.
   ③ Polycythemia is not a symptom of sickle cell crisis.
   ④ Severe itching and vomiting are not symptoms of sickle cell crisis.

58. Knowledge, implementation, environment (b)
   ❷ Oxygen therapy to prevent tissue deoxygenation is of primary importance in sickle cell crisis.
   ① This is part of the treatment for children with chronic sickle cell disease.
   ③ This may be part of the treatment in chronic sickle cell disease.
   ④ Hydration is important in treating sickle cell crisis; however, oxygen therapy ranks first in order of importance.

59. Comprehension, assessment, environment (b)
   ❷ The Denis Browne splint is often used for the treatment of congenital clubfoot.
   ① It is not used to treat scoliosis.
   ③ It is not used to treat DDH.
   ④ It is not used to treat a fractured femur.

60. Application, planning, health (b)
   ❷ The child should not be told to be brave; children should be allowed to cry if something hurts.
   ①,③,④ Should be covered during preoperative preparation of the child.

61. Knowledge, implementation, environment (b)
   ❸ This is the correct rate of infusion.
   ①,② This rate is too slow.
   ④ This rate is too fast.

62. Application, intervention, environment (a)
   ❹ Assessing sensation, circulation, and motion in affected extremities is necessary for all children in a cast.
   ① Children having pain should be medicated for pain as needed.
   ② Fluids should be encouraged; the cast can be kept dry by careful diapering and padding of the cast.
   ③ The child will need an adapted car seat to take her home safely.

63. Knowledge, evaluation, health (b)
   ❷ Several studies have demonstrated that infants sleeping prone are at a greater risk for SIDS.
   ① This is not applicable to SIDS.
   ③ The peak age for SIDS is 2 to 4 months.
   ④ This is not applicable to SIDS.

64. Comprehension, intervention, physiologic (b)
   ❹ The antiinflammatory effects of corticosteroids will decrease the edema commonly seen with nephrotic syndrome.
   ① Steroids have no affect on proteinuria.
   ② Steroids have no affect on increased albumin levels.
   ③ Steroids are not antihypertensive drugs.

65. Application, intervention, environment (b)
   ❶ In epileptic children with poorly controlled seizures, a ketogenic diet is often suggested as a method of treatment.
   ② Children with Crohn's disease are usually on a soft, low-fiber diet.
   ③ Children with bulimia are not placed on a ketogenic diet.
   ④ Children with acute glomerulonephritis are usually on a low-salt diet.

66. Knowledge, assessment, physiologic (b)
   ❷ Mononucleosis is an acute infectious disease caused by this virus.
   ① Mononucleosis is a viral disease; *Streptococcus* is a bacteria.
   ③ RSV is not the cause of mononucleosis; it is responsible for 50% of the cases of bronchiolitis seen in infants.
   ④ *H. influenzae* is not the cause of mononucleosis.

67. Comprehension, application, physiologic (b)
   ❸ The bronchoconstriction and inflammation of the airways seen in asthma cause these symptoms.
   ① These are symptoms of a cold; a child with asthma has a nonproductive cough.
   ② Asthma does not produce a fever or rhinorrhea.
   ④ These are symptoms of epiglottitis.

68. Comprehension, intervention, physiologic (b)
    ❷ Bronchodilators (to relieve bronchial constriction) and antiinflammatory agents (to relieve inflammation of bronchial mucosa) are used to treat asthma.
    ① Immunosuppressants are not used to treat asthma.
    ③ Antibiotics are not used to treat asthma; they may be used in patients with asthma who have respiratory infections.
    ④ Decongestants and antihistamines are not effective in relieving the bronchoconstriction and inflammation seen in asthma.

69. Knowledge, planning, physiologic (a)
    ❹ Azidothymidine (AZT) (Retrovir) is approved for children and assists in slowing the progression of AIDS.
    ① IV gamma globulin (Gamamine N) may be used in children with AIDS to compensate for B-lymphocyte deficiency.
    ② Ceftazidime (Fortaz) is an antibiotic and does not affect the progression of AIDS.
    ③ Vancomycin (Vancocin) is an antibiotic used for severe staphylococcal infections.

70. Knowledge, intervention, health (b)
    ❶ The first hepatitis B vaccine is given to the newborn infant, usually within the first 24 to 48 hours of delivery.
    ② At 2 months, the infant receives the DTP, Hib, OPV, and the second dose of hepatitis B vaccine.
    ③ At 6 months, the infant receives the DTP, OPV, and the third dose of hepatitis B vaccine.
    ④ At 12 months, the infant receives the MMR, the varicella zoster vaccine, and the DTP.

71. Comprehension, assessment, physiologic (b)
    ❷ The infant with colic demonstrates these signs and symptoms.
    ① Signs and symptoms of intussusception begin suddenly and include vomiting and bloody stools.
    ③ Signs and symptoms of pyloric stenosis include projectile vomiting and weight loss.
    ④ Signs and symptoms of Hirschsprung's disease include abdominal distention, vomiting, and inadequate weight gain.

72. Application, intervention, physiologic (c)
    ❷ Ribavirin (Virazole), an antiviral agent, is used specifically for an RSV infection, especially in children with chronic conditions; humidified oxygen relieves the dyspnea and hypoxia seen with RSV disease.
    ① Cromolyn (Intal), a nonsteroidal antiinflammatory agent, is used in the treatment of asthma.
    ③ Antibiotics are not used for RSV infection.
    ④ Prednisone (LiquiPred) is not used for RSV infection.

73. Knowledge, assessment, physiologic (c)
    ❹ This is the pathophysiology of RSV bronchiolitis.
    ① RSV occurs primarily in the winter and spring.
    ② Peak incidence for RSV infection is 2 to 5 months of age.
    ③ RSV can survive for hours on many surfaces, but for only half an hour on the skin.

74. Comprehension, intervention, environment (a)
    ❶ This type of fluid replacement is favored for treatment of all ages of children with infectious gastroenteritis.
    ②,③,④ Incorrect treatment for this disease.

75. Knowledge, assessment, physiologic (a)
    ❸ An omphalocele is a defect in which the abdominal contents protrude through the abdominal wall in an intact sac.
    ① Intussusception is a telescoping of the bowel and occurs within the abdomen.
    ② A diaphragmatic hernia is a congenital defect in the diaphragm that allows the abdominal contents to enter the thoracic cavity.
    ④ Gastroschisis is a herniation of the abdominal contents, not covered by a peritoneal sac, that herniates lateral to the umbilical ring.

Chapter 9

Nursing Care of the Aging Adult

The percentage of the American population over age 65 is rapidly passing 13% and continues to constitute our fastest-growing age group. As the life expectancy of Americans continues to lengthen, the year 2010 will see the first baby boomers retiring. By the year 2030 we will be challenged to care for an aging adult population that constitutes 20% of the total population. How we address these future trends will be reflected in history as a measure of our civility.

It is nursing's challenge to meet the care needs of our elders, who are so vulnerable to the biases of our fast-paced, youth-oriented society. As nurses we have an opportunity to play a significant role in determining whether these will be years of continued growth and development, years of happiness and accomplishment, or years of forced shame, illness, and neglect.

This chapter focuses on aging as a normal process and strives to increase the practitioner's knowledge of and understanding for a stage of life we will all pass through.

"For age is opportunity no less than youth itself,
though in another dress."

Longfellow

Government Resources for the Elderly

INCOME

A. Social Security (Federal Old-Age, Survivors, and Disability Insurance, FOASDI)
1. Funded by employee and employer payroll taxes
2. Entitlement determined by United States Social Security Administration; benefits are granted in accordance with:
   a. Age
   b. Lifetime earnings record
   c. Free earnings credits for active military service
   d. Whether required number of work credits have been earned (work credits are measured in quarters)
3. Specific maximum benefit amount with cost-of-living protection against inflation
4. Retirement benefits may start at age 62
5. Railroad workers have a separate retirement system; workers who have less than 10 years of railroad service may transfer earnings to Social Security to be counted toward Social Security benefits
6. Federal employees are covered under the Civil Service Retirement System, the Federal Employees Retirement System, and the Thrift Savings Plan
7. Social Security benefits are reduced according to monies earned over a stated maximum annual allowable income
8. No reduction in Social Security benefits for full-time employees over the age of 70
9. Payments are indexed according to inflation rate

B. Supplemental Security Income (SSI)
1. Funded from general tax revenues
2. Cash assistance program
3. Administered by Social Security Administration
4. Designed to provide for disabled, blind, or aged with limited incomes and resources
5. Medicaid eligibility in many states is based on SSI eligibility

HEALTH

A. Medicare (Title XVIII of Social Security Act)
1. Administered by Health Care Finance Administration of U.S. Department of Health and Human Services
2. Designed to help those over 65 years of age and certain disabled people under 65, who are eligible under Social Security, to meet medical care costs regardless of income, and people of any age with permanent kidney failure
3. Major insurance companies in each state handle claims (e.g., Travelers Insurance Company in New York)
4. Do not have to be retired to receive benefits
5. Financed by employer and employee payroll taxes and by self-employment tax monies
6. Everyone over 65 who is entitled to Social Security benefits receives hospital insurance without paying premium charges
7. Automatic hospital insurance is provided to disabled persons who have been entitled to Social Security disability benefits for 24 consecutive months
8. Initial enrollment period begins 3 months before the month individual will become 65 and continues for 4 months after individual turns 65
9. Annual enrollment periods (January 1 through March 31)
10. Premiums generally increase if people do not apply when they are eligible
11. Deductible is applied to each benefit period
12. Two parts
    a. Part A designed as hospital insurance that has certain exclusions
    b. Part B covers physician services and outpatient services; has exclusions and excess charges
    c. If subscribing to part A, automatically enrolled in part B unless it is declined

B. Medicaid (Title XIX of Social Security Act)
1. Purposes
   a. To cover specific expenses not provided for by Medicare
   b. To reduce expenses of those who have exhausted their Medicare benefits
   c. To defray medical expenses of those who cannot afford Medicare premiums
2. Funded by federal and state contributions
3. State-operated programs
4. Other programs
   a. Qualified Medicare Beneficiary (QMB) Program
      1. Annual income must be below or at the national poverty level and additional financial resources may not be more than $6,000/couple or $4,000/single; income cannot be more than $9,190/couple or $6,810/single
      2. Functions like Medigap policy
      3. State Medicaid program helps pay
      4. Pays Medicare Part B premium
      5. Pays Medicare Part A premiums for eligible elderly and disabled persons; Medicare deductible; and co-insurance fees
   b. Specified Low-Income Medicare Beneficiary (SLMB)
      1. Income cannot be more than 20% above the national poverty level
      2. Must be eligible for Medicare Part A
      3. State will pay Medicare Part B premiums
      4. Does not pay Medicare co-insurance or deductibles

C. Private health insurance
1. Medigap
   a. Medicare Supplement Insurance
   b. Regulated by state and federal law
   c. Ten standard plans
   d. Lifetime maximum of $50,000
   e. Not government sponsored
   f. Policies of choice may be purchased from any insurer doing Medigap business in one's state of residency for a 6-month period from date enrolled in Medicare Part B; and age 65 or older
   g. Plans pay all or most medical co-insurance amounts; some policies pay for Medicare deductibles
2. Medicare Select
   a. Purchase of Medicare Select Plan is Medigap insurance
   b. Supplements Medicare's benefits
   c. Sold by insurance companies and HMOs
   d. Difference between Medicare Select and Medigap is that specific doctors and certain hospitals must be used for nonemergent care to qualify for full benefits
   e. Federally approved through 1998 in all states

HOUSING

A. Department of Housing and Urban Development
   1. Rent Supplement Program: rent-subsidized apartments for elderly, disabled, or low-income families
     a. Utility and rent costs in existing buildings
     b. Renovations of existing units
     c. Building of new units
   2. Provides home improvement loans
   3. Provides mortgage insurance
   4. Age, asset, income eligibility requirements
B. Elderly and handicapped housing (Housing Act of 1959)
   1. Funding to private, nonprofit organizations for renovation or building of units for the elderly and handicapped
   2. Low-interest federal loans for same
C. National Housing Act (Housing and Urban Development Act, 1968): funding to private corporations for construction of low- and middle-income housing
D. National Housing Act of 1952: funding to private, profit, or nonprofit groups for nursing home construction or renovation

TITLE XX OF THE SOCIAL SECURITY ACT

A. Federal monies for social programs
B. State administered
C. Individual must be eligible for SSI
D. Many of the programs are suitable and available for the elderly

FOOD STAMP PROGRAM

A. Administered by U.S. Department of Agriculture
B. Eligibility requirement
C. State welfare department determines eligibility
D. Components
   1. Home-delivered meals
   2. Grocery store food purchases

ADMINISTRATION ON AGING

A. State, regional, area, and local units: area units responsible for providing program coordination and development expertise
B. Major services
   1. Nutritional programs
     a. On-site meals
     b. Home-delivered meals
   2. Senior centers
     a. Services
     b. Programs
   3. Home care
     a. Homemaker
     b. Home health aide
     c. Home visits
     d. Telephone calls
     e. Chore maintenance
   4. Information and referral
   5. Transportation
     a. Urban Mass Transit Act
     b. Area agencies on aging

Theories of Aging

SOCIOLOGIC THEORIES

A. Disengagement
   1. Controversial
   2. Mutual withdrawal from social interaction by aged individual and society
   3. Engagement, meaning active occupation and devotion
   4. Supports leisure as a form of activity
   5. Respects individual-initiated withdrawal
B. Activity
   1. Individual remains active and interacts with society's events
   2. Pursues new interests, friends, and roles to substitute for lost roles
   3. Supports social activity as beneficial
C. Continuity or development
   1. Lifelong personality characteristics and coping strategies continue
   2. Sense of inferiority develops
   3. Supportive network of relationships established
D. Passages: life cycle changes can be identified, predicted, planned for, and managed

BIOLOGIC THEORIES

A. Wear-and-tear
   1. Stress and use deplete the body cells of repair ability
   2. Coping mechanisms decline because of decrease in available energy
B. Collagen
   1. Most abundant body protein
   2. Collagen molecules held together by bonds
   3. Chemical reactions cause a switching of bonds between collagen molecules, resulting in structural changes characteristic of the aging process
C. Lipofuscin accumulation
   1. Lipofuscins or age pigments are insoluble end products of cell metabolism
   2. Accumulate in the cell, altering the cell's ability to function normally
D. Immunologic responses
   1. Aging is an autoimmune disease process
   2. Cells change, and the body does not recognize its own cells
   3. Autoimmune responses damage the cells, causing cell death
E. Cell death of genetic programming
   1. Cell reproduction is programmed
   2. The programming determines the rate and time a given species ages and dies
F. Stress adaptation
   1. Damage from stress accumulates
   2. System's resistance to stress steadily declines, leading to death
G. Free radical
   1. Molecules that have an extra electron are free radicals
   2. Free radicals attach to other molecules, altering function or structure
   3. There are internal and external sources of free radicals
   4. It is believed that the free radicals damage membrane function and structure (vitamins A, C, and E are thought to reduce free radical activity)
H. Mutation and error
   1. Cell division errors occur progressively over time
   2. Mutated cells are altered in their function and effectiveness
   3. Error theory expands mutation theory to include errors in interpretation of cell messages

PSYCHOLOGIC THEORIES

A. Freud: did not recommend psychoanalysis for the aged population (see Chapter 6, Mental Health Nursing)

B. Sullivan: see Chapter 6, Mental Health Nursing

C. Maslow: see Chapter 2, Review of the Basics: Nursing Concepts, Process, and Trends

D. Erikson: see Chapter 6, Mental Health Nursing
  1. Eighth stage (65 to 100 years of age) identified as "integrity vs. despair" (Fig. 9-1)
  2. Older adult who views own life as having no meaning ends life's stages in despair; older adult who can review his or her accomplishments and errors derives a sense of integrity

E. Peck
  1. Expanded Erikson's developmental theory
  2. Expanded Erikson's eighth stage into three stages to focus on new roles, alternatives to preoccupation with body changes and illness, thereby achieving life satisfaction (Fig. 9-2)

Role Changes

A. Types
  1. Crisis
    a. Sudden
    b. Not able to plan for appropriate replacement
    c. Substitute not readily available
    d. Stress producing
  2. Gradual
    a. Develops slowly
    b. Time available for preparation, which eases transition
    c. Control over whether to develop a substitute

B. Sufficient preparation and adequate support determine adjustment success or failure

C. Role changes that occur to the older adult are predominantly crisis oriented
  1. Forced retirement
  2. Alteration in income
  3. Loss of spouse
  4. Illness
  5. Friends move away or die
  6. Family members relocate, assume new roles, have increasingly less time for relationships
  7. Society's assigned role of decreased psychologic and physiologic functioning

D. Role losses
  1. Work
    a. No longer the breadwinner
    b. Job-related companionship
    c. Usefulness, competence, identity
    d. Income
    e. Sense of purpose
    f. Self-esteem
  2. Family
    a. Usually no longer the decision maker
    b. Not held in the same esteem
    c. Loss of independence

E. Role gains
  1. Grandparenthood or great-grandparenthood
  2. Family support roles assumed
    a. Economic
    b. Child care
    c. Caring role in illness
    d. House care
  3. Community activities
  4. Religious activities
  5. Recreational activities

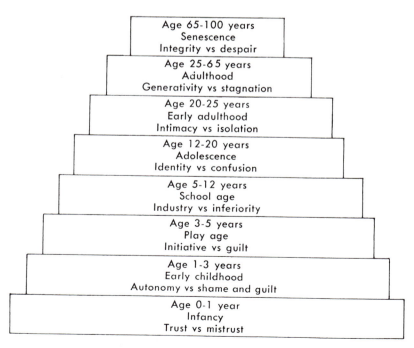

Figure 9-1.   **Erikson: Eight stages of man.** (From Forbes ES, Fitzsimmons VM: *The older adult: a process for wellness*, St Louis, 1981, Mosby.)

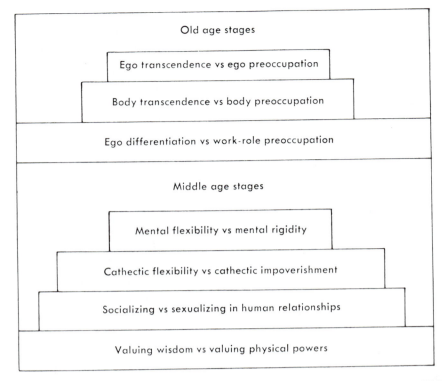

Figure 9-2.   **Peck: Stages of middle age and old age.** (From Forbes ES, Fitzsimmons VM: *The older adult: a process for wellness*, St Louis, 1981, Mosby.)

6. Clubs, organizations, and associations
7. Advisory roles
8. New friends
9. Adult education
10. Volunteerism

Alterations in Lifestyle

EMPLOYMENT

A. Society emphasizes the employed as valuable and the unemployed as useless
B. Increase in the number of older women working
C. Decrease in the number of older men working
D. Part-time employment more common
E. Trend toward early retirement
F. Serial careers emerging in keeping with interest changes
G. More women are joining the workforce at a time when men are winding down their working lives
H. Older worker possesses involuntary limitations
  1. Health problems
  2. Sensory or perceptual alterations, for example, in vision and auditory acuity
  3. Decline in physical strength, endurance, and speed
I. Older workers possess innumerable strengths
  1. Reliability
  2. Dependability
  3. Knowledge
  4. Expertise
  5. Experience

RETIREMENT

A. Mandatory retirement in federal employment eliminated
B. Mandatory retirement age raised to 70 in private employment
C. Changes in the economy leading to forced retirements
D. More people taking advantage of early retirement
E. Health problems are primary reason for voluntary retirement
F. Increase in leisure time
G. Stress-producing event at a time when one's ability to handle stress is diminished
H. Creates tremendous anxiety
I. Some derive an initial feeling of relief, but for most it's a loss that comes at a time of meaningful productivity
J. Adjustment depends on previously established patterns of adjustment, degree of financial security, state of health, and future outlook
K. For most it creates an additional series of losses and problems at a time in life when coping and problem-solving abilities are fragile
L. Job loss
  1. Loss of daily routine
    a. Alters household routine
    b. Alters lifestyle
    c. Creates discouragement, depression, and loneliness
    d. Alters family relationships
    e. Alcohol abuse
  2. Loss of income
    a. Relocation
    b. Daily decision-making determined by economics
    c. Decreases self-esteem
    d. Increases fear and anxiety
    e. Increases insecurity
M. Welcome changes
  1. New friends
  2. New activities

3. New interests
4. Renewal of marriage
5. Seek new and different employment
6. Find purpose and opportunity
7. Rest and relaxation

ECONOMIC CHANGES

A. Most elderly live on fixed incomes
B. Of elderly persons, 1 out of 10 lives below the nation's poverty level
C. Independence declines as costs increase and buying power decreases
D. For many Social Security is the sole source of income
E. Many elderly are not receiving the assistance to which they are entitled
  1. Lack of resource knowledge
  2. Inability to find out about resources
    a. Lack of mobility
    b. Health problems
F. Supplemental Social Security: may qualify for in addition to or instead of Social Security benefits
G. Economic penalties: limit on the amount a Social Security beneficiary can earn annually without losing some monthly payments
H. Income tax reforms: once-in-a-lifetime capital gains tax exemption on sale of personal residence for person over 55 years of age
I. Income sources
  1. Public
    a. Social Security (Federal Old-Age, Survivors, and Disability Insurance)
    b. Supplemental Social Security income
  2. Private (e.g., pensions and investments)
  3. Other (e.g., Railroad Retirement System, Federal Employee's Retirement System, and Civil Service Retirement System)

HEALTH

A. Most elderly have more than one chronic disease
B. Health care needs increase with age
C. Cost of health care is increasing as financial income is either decreasing or fixed
D. Elderly account for one third of the nation's health care costs

HOUSING

A. Most elderly prefer to remain independent as long as family and friends live nearby
B. Most live with spouse, alone, or with family
C. Large percentage continue to own their own home and prefer this lifestyle
  1. Security
  2. Privacy
  3. Independence
  4. Sense of purpose
  5. Familiarity
  6. Household activities
  7. Pride
  8. Socialization
D. Other housing alternatives
  1. Mobile homes
    a. Convenient
    b. Economical
  2. Retirement communities
    a. Minimum age requirement
    b. Different cost levels, for example, houses, apartments, and condominiums
  3. Foster home
  4. Life care facilities: living, recreational, medical facilities on the premises
  5. Nursing homes
  6. Homes for the aged
  7. Convalescent homes
  8. Rest homes
  9. House sharing
  10. Public housing
  11. Rooming houses
  12. Hotels: SROs (single room occupancy)
E. Special assistance needs of the elderly that enable them to remain in their own homes longer
  1. Transportation
    a. Reliable
    b. Nearby
    c. Inexpensive
    d. Safe
  2. Meals available in the event of illness or disability
  3. Health hotlines: most elderly are institutionalized because of health needs and lack of convenient community health services
  4. Housecleaners
  5. Homemaker services
  6. Social services
  7. Home care services
  8. Neighborhood safety

RECREATION

A. Elderly have more time for recreation, but deterring factors exist
  1. Cost
    a. Transportation
    b. Special equipment
    c. Special clothing
    d. Fees for membership and use of facilities
  2. Health problems
  3. Diminished energy level
  4. Lack of incentive
  5. Sensory losses
  6. Lack of environmental aids
  7. Lack of conveniently located facilities, for example, rest rooms
  8. Lack of handicapped facilities
B. Most elderly depend on a family as the major source of activity and interaction
C. Alternatives
  1. Religious activities
  2. Community activities, for example, volunteerism
  3. Day care
  4. Senior citizen centers
  5. Clubs, organizations, and associations
  6. Recreation centers
  7. Adult education
  8. Shopping
  9. Cultural events
  10. Elder hostel

Social Isolation

A. Four classifications (Ebersole and Hess, 1985)
B. Attitudinal: that which is self-imposed and that imposed by society
   1. Self-imposed aloneness, loneliness
   2. Society imposes myths about the aged, perceptions of aging
C. Presentational: set apart or sets one apart
D. Behavioral: exhibits behaviors that are not acceptable to a youth-oriented society, for example, confusion, eccentricity
E. Geographic
   1. Lack of resources to relocate
   2. Psychological safety and security at present location
   3. Fear of being victims of crime
   4. Distance from family and friends who have moved away
F. Rural areas have a higher proportion of older people

DRUG USE

A. Largest users of prescription medications are those over the age of 65
B. Tendency to self-medicate
C. Higher frequency of hospital admissions that are drug-related than that for other age groups
D. Self-administration errors are common
E. Slower ingestion of drug into the system as a result of a decline in gastric acid secretion and decreased gastric motility
F. Circulatory alterations affect drug distribution
G. Drug metabolism altered by such factors as a diminished rate of body metabolism
H. Drug excretion time reduced by illness, disease, and the aging process
I. Management
   1. Patient education
   2. Medication administration times more compatible with lifestyle
   3. Color coding
   4. Larger print on labels
   5. Easily removable bottle and vial caps
   6. Monitoring of drug effectiveness and compatibility
   7. Drug holidays (Box 9-1)

ALCOHOL ABUSE

A. Tolerance to alcohol decreases with age
B. System does not excrete and detoxify as rapidly as that of a younger adult
C. Substitution for unmet psychological needs and untreated physiological problems
D. Cause of accidents, nutritional deficiencies, drug incompatibilities, self-neglect, alterations in self-esteem, psychosocial and physiological health care problems
E. Statistics inaccurate as clients are protected by family
F. Significant number of alcohol abusers are over age 60
G. High-risk group for alcoholism
H. Adult men have a higher incidence of abuse than adult women

ELDER ABUSE (TABLE 9-1)

A. Physical (Box 9-2)
   1. Battering
   2. Neglect
   3. Sexual abuse
   4. Confinement or restraint

Box 9-1.   Drug Holiday

Definition
The planned omission of a specific medication on one or more days each week

Benefits
Reduced risk of drug accumulating to toxic level in bloodstream
Increased mental alertness
Cost savings
Decreased demand on care givers' or staff's time

Requirements
Interdisciplinary support, planning, and thorough assessment of appropriateness of client for drug holiday
Careful selection of drugs
Stabilized blood level for certain drugs
Education of client and family or care givers

Drugs not usually omitted
Antibiotics
Anticoagulants
Anticonvulsants
Antidiabetics
Ophthalmic drops

From Eliopoulos C: *Manual of gerontologic nursing,* St Louis, 1995, Mosby.

B. Psychologic: threatened or forced
   1. Relinquishment of assets
   2. Institutionalization
   3. Loss of control over independent functioning
   4. Social isolation
   5. Sensory deprivation
C. Prevention
   1. Acquire knowledge of family abuse and patterns of violence
   2. Identify predisposing factors
   3. Incorporate assessment tools into interviewing and counseling strategies
   4. Increase public awareness and education
   5. Identify actual and potential sources of emergency protection
   6   Acquire knowledge of community resources

Physiologic Alterations (Normal Aging Process) And Selected Disorders (Abnormal)

Normal aging changes are gradual and begin in early middle age.

INTEGUMENTARY SYSTEM ALTERATIONS

1. Moisture loss; dryness
   2. Epithelial layer thinning; fragility
   3. Shrinkage and rigidity of elastic collagen fibers: sagging and wrinkling
   4. Sweat glands decrease in number, activity, and size: less efficient body cooling system

Table 9-1	Profile of the Violent Family Relevant to Elder Abuse	
Elder abuse		
Identifying data	**Abuser**	**Victim**
Age	40 to 60 yr	60 yr and older
Sex	Female	Not a factor; more elders are female
Relationship	Son/daughter, relative, or caretaker	Parent of abuser most often
Marital status	Married	Widowed
History of childhood sexual abuse	Data not widely available; positive history in some cases	Positive history in some cases; repeated victimization
Socioeconomic status (SES)	Not a factor; evident at all SES levels; cases mostly lower to middle class and found through health care systems	
Occupation	Professional or semi-skilled	Not employed
Employment status	Least violence in homes of retired men; victim often physically or mentally impaired	
Race	Highest; American Indians, Asians/Pacific Islanders, minorities; blacks = 12%, whites = 88%; also reported as no difference	
Religion	Protestant	
Education	High school diploma or some college	
Residence	Limited data, evenly distributed with more reports in large cities	
	Not Southern phenomena	

Adapted from Stuart GW, Sundeen S: Profile of the violent family. In *Principles and practices of psychiatric nursing*, ed 3, St Louis, 1987, Mosby.

5. Subcutaneous fat loss deepening of hollows and more prominent contours
6. Loss of capillaries and melanocytes: skin sallowness
7. Peripheral circulation loss: thick, brittle, split nails
8. Skin pigmentation increases: keratoses (scaly, raised areas), senile lentigines (liver spots: brown or yellow spots)
9. Hair changes in color (gray, white), changes in texture (becomes fine or coarse), and thins (balding)
10. Appearance of facial hair for women; decrease in facial hair for men

MUSCULOSKELETAL SYSTEM
A. Alterations
  1. Loss of lean muscle mass and muscle cells: decreased muscle strength, size, and tone
  2. Loss of elastic fibers in muscle tissue: increased stiffness and decreased flexibility
  3. Thinning of long bones: brittle, porous bones
  4. Thinning of intervertebral disks: height loss and changes in posture
B. Selected disorders
  1. Contributing factors
    a. Poor nutritional patterns
    b. Endocrine system changes: decreased estrogen and testosterone
    c. Gastrointestinal system changes: decreased absorption of vitamins and minerals
    d. Cardiovascular system changes: poor circulation
    e. Neurologic deficits causing safety hazards
    f. Decreased level of activity and periods of prolonged bed rest
    g. Side effects of medications, for example, steroids
  2. Resulting problems
    a. Increased susceptibility to fractures
    b. Altered body image

    c. Pain and discomfort
    d. Decreased mobility
    e. Impaired ability to perform activities of daily living (ADL)
    f. Increasing feelings of dependency
    g. Calcium deposits in blood vessels and renal structures
    h. Weakened muscles affecting other systems
      (1) Diaphragm
      (2) Bladder
      (3) Myocardium
      (4) Abdominal wall
  3. Nursing management
    a. Handle patient gently
    b. Reduce environmental safety hazards
    c. Encourage mobility and exercise
    d. Allow extra time for performing activities
    e. Assist with ADL and exercises as needed
    f. Provide encouragement and support for accomplishments
    g. Prevent deformities
      (1) Proper positioning
      (2) Exercises such as range of motion (ROM)
    h. Alleviate pain
      (1) Rest periods
      (2) Positioning
    i. Encourage liberal fluid intake

PULMONARY SYSTEM
A. Alterations
  1. Structural alterations (scoliosis, kyphosis, osteoporosis): decrease in lung expansion
  2. Alveoli enlarge and thin out: decreased oxygen and carbon dioxide diffusion
  3. Loss of bronchiole elasticity: decreased breathing capacity, increased residual air

Box 9-2. Physical Indicators of Actual or Potential Elder Abuse/Neglect

General appearance
Anxious, fearful, and passive
Poor eye contact
Looks to caregiver for answers
Poor hygiene and inappropriate dress
Underweight or malnourished
Physically handicapped
No glasses, false teeth, or hearing aid despite need

Skin
Contusions, abrasions, burns, and scars in various stages of healing
Decubitus ulcers, urine burns
Rope marks

Abdominal/rectal
Distended
Internal bleeding
Fecal impactions

Musculoskeletal fractures
Evidence of old healed fractures
Current fractures and sprains
Limited range of motion
Contractures

Genital/urinary
Vaginal lacerations, bruises, and infections
Urinary tract infections

Neurologic
Slurred speech
Confusion

From Fortinash KM, Holoday-Worres PA: *Psychiatric-mental health nursing*, St Louis, 1996, Mosby.

4. Diaphragm becomes fibrotic and weakened; diminished efficiency
5. Respiratory muscle structure and function decrease: diminished strength for breathing and coughing
6. Changes in larynx: weaker, higher-pitched voice
7. Decrease in ciliary function: increased susceptibility to upper respiratory tract infection

B. Selected disorders
 1. Contributing factors
    a. Decreased resistance to infection
    b. Musculoskeletal system changes: weakened muscles and postural changes
    c. Longer history of smoking and exposure to pollutants
    d. Periods of prolonged bed rest
    e. Cardiovascular system changes
    f. Side effects of medications, for example, sedatives and hypnotics
 2. Resulting problems
    a. Dyspnea
    b. Chronic cough
    c. Fatigue and debilitation
    d. Cerebral hypoxia
       (1) Confusion
       (2) Restlessness
       (3) Behavioral changes
    e. Decreased activity tolerance
    f. Cardiovascular problems, for example, congestive heart failure
    g. Anorexia
 3. Nursing management
    a. Assist with ADL as necessary
    b. Encourage breathing exercises
    c. Administer oxygen therapy
    d. Change position frequently
    e. Encourage liberal fluid intake
    f. Discourage smoking
    g. Position for maximum comfort and efficiency of respiration, for example, extra pillows, Fowler's position
    h. Allow rest periods
    i. Assess pulmonary status when assessing behavioral changes

CARDIOVASCULAR SYSTEM
A. Alterations
 1. Decrease in enzymatic stimulation: longer and less forceful contractions
 2. Increase in fat and collagen amounts: decline in cardiac output
 3. Increase in oxygen demands of coronary arteries and brain: decreased peripheral circulation
 4. Loss of elasticity of vessel walls; decrease in contraction and recoiling responses
 5. Reduced or unaltered heart rate at rest
 6. Mild tachycardia on activity
 7. Slow increase in serum cholesterol
B. Selected disorders
 1. Contributing factors
    a. Poor nutritional patterns
    b. Anxiety and stress
    c. Decreased activity level
    d. Arteriosclerosis and hypertension
    e. Pulmonary system changes
    f. Side effects of medications
 2. Resulting problems
    a. Fatigue and decreased activity tolerance
    b. Increased anxiety
    c. Edema
    d. Hypertension: increased risk of cerebrovascular accident (CVA)
    e. Behavioral changes
    f. Poor circulation to other systems and extremities: delayed healing
    g. Potential risk for coronary artery disease
 3. Nursing management
    a. Assist with ADL prn
    b. Encourage moderate activity and exercise
    c. Patient teaching considerations
       (1) Confusion
       (2) Forgetfulness
       (3) Resistance to change
    d. Avoid excess pressure on the skin
       (1) Change position frequently

(2) Sheepskin; water mattress

(3) Bed cradle

    e. Assess cardiovascular status when assessing behavioral changes

    f. Avoid tight, constrictive clothing and shoes

    g. Special foot care

(1) Prevent trauma

(2) Prevent infection

GASTROINTESTINAL SYSTEM

A. Alterations

    1. Muscle atrophy in the tongue, cheeks, mouth

    2. Esophageal wall thinning

    3. Decrease in ptyalin and amylase secretion by salivary gland: alkaline saliva

    4. Decrease in saliva secretion: thicker mucus and dryness

    5. Oral sensitivity loss

    6. Ill-fitting dentures, periodontal disease, lack of teeth: nutritional deficiencies

    7. Shrinkage of bony structure of mouth

    8. Gastric mucosa shrinks: decline in digestive enzyme secretion leads to delayed digestion

    9. Decrease in lipase secretion: fat intolerance

    10. Decrease in gastric acid: diminished ability to use calcium

    11. Decrease in intrinsic factor: pernicious anemia

    12. Decrease in iron absorption: iron-deficiency anemia

    13. Internal sphincter muscle tone loss: alterations in bowel evacuation

B. Selected disorders

    1. Contributing factors

      a. Decreased level of activity

      b. Dental problems

      c. Poor nutritional patterns

      d. Weakened muscles

      e. Nervous system changes

      f. Overuse of laxative and enemas

      g. Anorexia

      h. Side effects of medications; for example, opiates and steroids

    2. Resulting problems

      a. Discomfort

      b. Constipation and impaction

      c. Fecal incontinence

      d. Anorexia

      e. Increased risk of aspiration

    3. Nursing management

      a. Promote nutritional intake

(1) Consistency of food

(2) Ability to manage utensils

(3) Extra time for feeding (oral and tube)

      b. Provide good oral hygiene

      c. Encourage mobility and exercise

      d. Provide adequate fluid intake

      e. Educate patient regarding constipation and laxative abuse

      f. Check bowel habits regularly

      g. Give prompt assistance to bathroom or with bedpan

      h. Prevent skin and mucosal breakdown

(1) Prompt, thorough cleansing of anal area

(2) Extra gentleness when inserting rectal and feeding tubes

RENAL SYSTEM

A. Alterations

    1. Decrease in kidney size

    2. Decline in renal blood flow

    3. Reduced ability of nephron to filter urine: decreased clearance

    4. Reduced ability of tubule cells to selectively secrete and reabsorb: fluid and electrolyte alterations

    5. Bladder capacity decreases: frequency and urgency

    6. Loss of muscle tone of bladder and uterus

    7. Loss of pelvic muscle tone

    8. Decreased urine concentration ability

    9. Prostate gland enlargement

B. Selected disorders

    1. Contributing factors

      a. Periods of prolonged bed rest

(1) Increased urinary stasis

(2) Renal calculi formation

      b. Cardiovascular system changes, for example, decreased renal perfusion

      c. Nervous system changes

      d. Decreased fluid intake

      e. Muscle weakness

      f. Social withdrawal and apathy, for example, sensory deprivation

      g. Side effects of medication, for example, diuretics, antiparkinsonian drugs

    2. Resulting problems

      a. Hyperglycemia

      b. Behavioral changes, for example, confusion, elevated BUN, electrolyte imbalance

      c. Interference with sleep and recreational patterns

(1) Urinary frequency

(3) Urinary urgency

(3) Nocturia

      d. Increased chance of skin breakdown; for example, incontinence

      e. Feelings of embarrassment, rejection, and withdrawal

    3. Nursing management

      a. Prevent urinary stasis

(1) Encourage liberal fluid intake

(2) Encourage frequent change of position

(3) Encourage ambulation

      b. Prevent skin breakdown: prompt and thorough cleansing

      c. Bladder retraining

      d. Promptly respond to call for bathroom or bedpan

      e. Leave night light on if patient experiencing nocturia

      f. Assess renal status when assessing behavior changes

      g. Early recognition of urinary tract infection

NEUROLOGIC SYSTEM

A. Alterations

    1. Decrease in weight and size of brain

    2. Decline in number of neurons

    3. Diminished nerve conduction speed

      a. Voluntary movement slower

      b. Increased reaction time

      c. Delayed decisions

    4. Alterations in sleep-wake cycle

a. Less rapid eye movement (REM) sleep
b. Less deep sleep: tendency to catnap
c. Easily awakened
d. Difficulty falling asleep
e. Average 5 to 7 hours sleep at night
5. Brain tissue atrophy and meningeal thickening: short-term memory loss

B. Selected disorders
1. Contributing factors
   a. Poor nutrition patterns
   b. Cardiovascular system changes, for example, decreased circulation
   c. Pulmonary system changes, for example, cerebral hypoxia
   d. Sensory deprivation
   e. Side effects of medications, for example, sedatives
2. Resulting problems
   a. Safety hazards
      (1) Impaired senses, for example, vision, hearing, pain, and temperature
      (2) Forgetfulness and confusion
   b. Anorexia, for example, decreased taste buds
   c. Social isolation and rejection
   d. Impaired ability to perform ADL
      (1) Decreased coordination
      (2) Safety hazards
   e. Increased sense of dependency
   f. Incontinence
   g. Altered self-image and declining confidence
   h. Behavioral changes, for example, forgetfulness and confusion
3. Nursing management
   a. Provide for safety
   b. Establish means of communication if patient has hearing impairment
   c. Assess all systems when assessing behavioral changes
   d. Maintain sense of independence when possible
   e. Assist with ADL only when necessary; allow extra time
   f. Encourage socialization
   g. Provide sensory stimulation
   h. Consider forgetfulness and confusion when teaching
      (1) Be consistent
      (2) Provide repetition when necessary
      (3) Be patient
      (4) Provide positive reinforcement and encouragement
   i. Assess other symptoms carefully when assessing for infection and trauma: decreased temperature control and pain perception mask these symptoms
   j. Carefully check temperature of bath water and forms of heat therapy to avoid burns: discrepancy in sensation of heat and cold
   k. Maximize use of environmental aids

ENDOCRINE SYSTEM
A. Alterations
1. Decline in growth hormone secretion
2. Estrogen secretion diminishes
3. Uterus becomes smaller
4. Fallopian tubes decrease in size and motility
5. Vagina loses elasticity

6. Vulva and external genitalia shrink with loss of subcutaneous fat
7. Vaginal secretions diminish
8. Response to sexual stimulation takes longer
9. Elasticity of breast tissue is reduced
10. Testosterone secretion decreases
11. Testes become smaller and less firm
12. Sperm production is slowed
13. Erection takes longer to achieve and subsides more rapidly
14. Ejaculation is shorter and less forceful
15. Time between erection and orgasm lengthens
16. Basal metabolism rate is decreased
17. Woman loses ability to procreate
18. Glucose metabolism diminishes
19. Pancreatic secretions decrease

B. Selected disorders
1. Contributing factors: glandular changes as result of aging process
2. Resulting problems
   a. Adult-onset diabetes mellitus
   b. Musculoskeletal system changes
   c. Hypothyroidism
3. Nursing management of diabetes mellitus: special considerations
   a. Poor vision
   b. Lack of coordination
   c. Poor nutritional patterns
   d. Forgetfulness and confusion
   e. Resistance to change
   f. Masking of symptoms by physiologic changes of aging and disease
   g. Decreased activity level
   h. Stress and anxiety
   i. Increased susceptibility to complications

AUTOIMMUNE SYSTEM
A. Alterations
1. Diminished immunoglobulin production
2. Weakened antibody response
3. Atypical signs and symptoms frequently a response to infection, for example, subnormal temperature, behavior changes, and decreased pain sensation

B. Selected disorders
1. Contributing factors
   a. Weakened antibody response
   b. Reduced immunoglobulin production
      (1) Thymus gland wasting
      (2) Reticuloendothelial system alterations
2. Resulting problems
   a. Self-destructive autoaggressive phenomenon
   b. Increased susceptibility to infection
   c. Increased susceptibility to disease
   d. Misdiagnosis
3. Nursing management
   a. Be careful in observation and assessment
   b. Be aware that atypical symptoms of infection are common among the elderly; for example, with otitis media, difficulty in hearing is too often dismissed as a typical aging problem
   c. Use early nursing intervention
   d. Educate regarding available vaccines

SENSE ORGANS

A. Vision
  1. Alterations
     a. Pupil size diminishes: loss of responsiveness to light
     b. Decline in peripheral vision
     c. Accommodation ability decreases, causing presbyopia (farsightedness)
     d. Decrease in tear production
     e. Decrease in lens transparency and elasticity
     f. Decline in ability to focus quickly
     g. Decline in color discrimination
     h. Difficulty in adjusting to dark-light changes
     i. Altered depth perception
  2. Selected disorders
     a. Cataracts
     b. Glaucoma
     c. Senile macular degeneration
B. Auditory alterations
  1. Progressive loss of hearing, starting with high-frequency tones
     a. Presbycusis (loss of sound perception)
     b. Otosclerosis (bone cell overgrowth)
     c. Cerumen accumulation
  2. Eardrum thickens and becomes more opaque
C. Taste bud alterations
  1. Number of taste buds decline
  2. Taste sensation is dulled
  3. Taste detection declines
D. Olfactory alterations
  1. Olfactory nerve fibers decrease
  2. Sense of smell diminishes
E. Tactile alterations
  1. Sense of touch dulled
  2. Pain threshold higher
  3. Sense of vibration diminished
F. Vestibular/kinesthetic alterations
  1. Diminished proprioception
  2. Decrease in coordination
  3. Decline in equilibrium

Special Considerations

NUTRITION

A. Diet
  1. Nutrition needs same as those of other adults
  2. Decreased need for calories
  3. Adequate protein to prevent muscle wasting and weakness
  4. Adequate fats for padding, insulation, and energy; low saturated fat intake recommended by physician
  5. Adequate carbohydrates from unprocessed foods for energy: elderly have a tendency to buy high-carbohydrate, empty-calorie foods because they
     a. Are less costly
     b. Are filling
     c. Are easy to chew
     d. Require minimal preparation
  6. Ethnic, cultural, and lifestyle preferences should be encouraged for identity reinforcement and appetite stimulation
  7. Fluid intake should be 1500 to 2000 ml per day: tendency is to reduce intake because of urinary frequency, urgency, and incontinence
  8. Vitamin supplements to prevent deficiencies
  9. Lactose deficiency common: calcium can be obtained from other sources, for example, spinach, asparagus, broccoli, and sardines
  10. Fiber, roughage, bulk to aid elimination
  11. Consistency and preparation in accordance with chewing, swallowing, and digestive abilities
  12. Small, frequent meals are easier to digest and conserve energy
  13. Attention to cholesterol and fat intakes
  14. Awareness of food-drug and food-food interactions
B. Unhurried atmosphere to increase appetite and incentive to eat
C. Caution against food fads and megavitamin therapy
D. Assess facilities for appropriateness
  1. Storage
  2. Cooking
  3. Refrigeration
E. Financial assistance and planning
F. Transporation to and from grocery store
G. Assistance with packages because of weakness and physical disabilities
H. Mealtime socialization
I. Assistance for the confused, forgetful, and ill
J. Encourage regular meals—elderly have a tendency to skip meals
K. Education classes on purchasing healthful foods on limited income
L. Factors that increase risk of nutritional problems in the elderly (Box 9-3)

Box 9-3
Factors That Increase Risk of Nutritional Problems in the Elderly

Physiologic Factors
- Decreased secretion of enzymes; indigestion common
- Decreased absorption of nutrients and minerals
- Reduced mobility of stomach; slowing of peristalsis
- Restricted intake of nutrients caused by problems with teeth and dentures (e.g., ill-fitting dentures, periodontal disease, missing teeth)
- Decrease in production of saliva
- Reduced sensitivity to sweet and salty flavors
- Low activity level
- Disease-related symptoms that can reduce appetite, energy, or ability to ingest food
- Side effects of medications

Psychosocial Factors
- Limited finances that prohibit purchase of proper food
- Lack of knowledge regarding nutritional needs, nutritional value of foods
- Inability to shop, store foods, or cook (e.g., lack of transportation, no kitchen facilities, dementia)
- Personal preferences that violate principles of good nutritional intake
- Loneliness or eating alone
- Mood disturbances (e.g., depression, anxiety)

From Eliopoulos C: *Manual of gerontologic nursing*, St Louis, 1995, Mosby.

HYGIENE

A. Skin
1. Water temperature 100° to 105° F (37.7° to 40.5° C)
2. Daily baths not necessary
3. Oil-base or emollient lotion
4. Alcohol and dusting powder not appropriate because they dry out the skin (dusting powder can be inhaled)
5. Avoid friction
6. Avoid pressure
7. Neutral-reaction or oil-based soap
8. Susceptible to bruising and skin tears

B. Nose: blunt-end scissors to trim nasal hairs that extend beyond nares

C. Oral hygiene
1. Dentures
   a. Take out at night and reinsert the next morning to prevent tissue swelling unless contraindicated by dentist
   b. Frequent cleaning
   c. Proper storage
   d. If patient is institutionalized, make sure dentures are labeled
2. Soft nylon toothbrush, electric toothbrush, or adaptive toothbrush
3. Mouthwash (optional)
4. Lanolin to lips
5. Encourage semiannual dental visits
6. Frequent mouth inspection for food accumulation, injury, disease, and infection (tendency to pocket food can lead to infection)

D. Ears
1. Clean with warm, soapy water and dry with towel
2. Do not use cotton swabs because they force cerumen back against the tympanum
3. Trim ear hair growth in men
4. Hearing aids
   a. Wash mold and receiver with mild soap and warm water
   b. Check cannula for patency, and clean and dry with pipe cleaner
   c. Remove batteries when aid is not in use
   d. Store batteries in refrigerator to retain freshness
   e. Turn aid to off position when inserting in patient's ear
   f. Turn aid on to adjust volume
   g. Store aid in its original box away from cold, heat, and sunlight
   h. Components, styles, nursing care (Box 9-4)

E. Eyes
1. More frequent cleaning of eyeglasses required
2. Use warm water to clean eyeglasses
3. Store only in eyeglass case
4. If patient is institutionalized, make sure glasses are labeled

F. Nails
1. Daily care
2. Use moisturizer on nails and cuticles
3. Encourage circulation with buffing of nails
4. File with emery board (cutting makes them more brittle and risks injury)

G. Hair
1. Use mild shampoo that is not irritating to the eyes
2. Remove facial hair from women with tweezers or waxing
3. Use of a shaving brush is recommended for men
4. Moisturizers are beneficial for men's facial skin

Box 9-4. Hearing Aids

Components
Microphone: converts sounds into electric energy
Amplifier: increases energy
Receiver: converts energy back into sound waves
Volume control
On/off switch

Styles
Behind the ear: limited amplification
In the ear: entire unit worn in the ear; limited amplification
Eyeglass attached: unit built in the frame of the eyeglass; limited amplification
Body aided: amplifier housed in a case worn on body; offers most amplification of all

Nursing Care
- Encourage client to obtain hearing aid from a reputable dealer after a full audiometric examination has been done
- Ensure that batteries are functioning before the aid is applied; it is recommended that batteries be changed weekly
- Identify common hearing aid problems
Whistling sound: bad connection between earpiece and amplifier; excessively high volume
Insufficient amplification: volume set too low; weak or dead battery; blockage from cerumen; disconnected tubing or wiring
Periodic loss of amplification: loose connection; poor battery contact; dirt in switch; cracked case
- Recognize that adjustment to a hearing aid is difficult and may take time, and reassure the client that this is not unusual.

Adapted from Eliopoulos C: *Manual of gerontologic nursing*, St Louis, 1995, Mosby.

H. Feet
1. Give daily care (washing, inspection, skin care)
2. Inspect between and under toes for abrasions, cracking, lacerations, and scaling
3. Clip toenails straight across
4. Pumice stone should be used to remove dry, hard skin
5. Discourage use of irritants
6. Avoid elastic-top socks or knee-high stockings
7. Emphasize the danger of roll garters
8. Recommend properly fitting shoes with low, broad, rubber heels for safety, comfort, and fatigue reduction
9. Special foot/limb care for diabetics, e.g. patients with diabetes mellitus

SAFETY

A. Susceptibility to accidents increased by
1. Decline in sensory acuity
2. Decreased ability to interpret environment
3. Increased reflex time
4. Postural change sensitivity

5. Gait disturbances
6. Muscular weakness
7. Urinary urgency and frequency
8. Confusion
9. Judgment alterations
10. Forgetfulness
11. Proprioceptive inadequacies
12. Improper footwear
13. Depression
14. Environmental hazards
15. Medications that cause drowsiness
B. Accident prevention
   1. Attire
      a. Short or three quarter-length sleeves as opposed to long, loose-fitting sleeves
      b. Avoid long garments
      c. Velcro closures
   2. Furniture
      a. Proper height
      b. Chairs with arms
   3. Floors
      a. No-slip wax
      b. No scatter rugs or deep pile carpeting
      c. Avoid clutter
      d. Rubber tips on ambulation aids
   4. Kitchen
      a. Tong reachers instead of footstools, chairs, and step-ladders
      b. Temperature-controlled faucets
      c. Electric rather than gas stoves
      d. Stoves with controls on the front
      e. Shelves within comfortable reach
      f. Wall cabinets at comfortable height instead of floor-based cabinets to avoid bending and stooping
      g. Avoid trash accumulation
      h. Easy-grip utensils
   5. Bathroom
      a. Nonskid strips or rubber mats in tub and shower
      b. Temperature-controlled faucets
      c. Good soap containers
      d. Tub and toilet handrails
      e. Bathtub seats
      f. Shower chairs
      g. High toilet seats
      h. Colored toilet seats
      i. Night light
   6. Bedroom
      a. Bedside commode
      b. Side rails
      c. Night light
      d. Telephone next to bed (amplifier; dial enlarger)
   7. General
      a. Proper lighting
      b. Railings on stairways
      c. Safe electric appliances
      d. No overloading of electric outlets
      e. No frayed wiring or extension cords
      f. Securely taped cords
      g. Emergency telephone numbers readily available at telephone
      h. Smoke detectors
      i. Crime prevention assessment and implementation

      j. Medications
         (1) Separate from those of other household members
         (2) Internal and external medications in different locations
         (3) Large print labels
         (4) Color coded labels
         (5) Daily supply containers
         (6) Calendar or alarm clock reminders
         (7) Discard outdated medications and prescriptions
      k. Medical emergency alarm system
   8. Mobility aids (Box 9-5)

VISION

A. Bright, diffused light is best
B. Place items on better-vision side
C. Avoid glare
D. Strips on stairs improve depth perception
E. Glasses should be kept clean (the elderly frequently forget or ignore this)
F. Use colors that increase visual acuity, for example, red, orange, and yellow
G. Avoid night driving
H. Use resources and aids for visually handicapped
I. Preserve independence
J. Visual losses increase susceptibility to illusions, disorientation, confusion, and isolation
K. Place objects directly in front of individual with decreased peripheral vision
L. Stimulate other senses

HEARING

A. Elderly usually do poorly on hearing tests because of their cautious responsiveness
B. Reduce distractions
C. Do not fatigue with unnecessary noise and talk
D. Speak in a normal tone of voice; shouting is misinterpreted by those who have normal hearing
E. Observe for signs of developing hearing loss
   1. Leaning forward
   2. Inappropriate responses
   3. Cupping ear when listening
   4. Loud speaking voice
   5. Requests to repeat what has been said
F. Reduce background noise before speaking, for example, television and radio
G. Hearing deficits increase social isolation, suspiciousness, and fears
H. Speak toward the better ear
I. Be sure to have the person's attention before speaking
J. Use resources and aids for the hearing impaired, for example, television and telephone amplifiers, sound lamps, and alarm clocks that shake the bed
K. Keep hands and objects away from mouth when speaking

ACTIVITIES OF DAILY LIVING

A. Elderly may ignore appearance because of fatigue, unawareness, or lack of incentive
B. Clean clothing is essential for maintaining pride and dignity
C. Choosing what to wear provides a source of control over one's life, fosters independence, and increases self-confidence and self-esteem

Box 9-5.   Mobility Aids

Cane

Characteristics

- Assists balance by widening base of support; not intended for weight bearing
- Comes in a variety of styles
  Regular (straight): provides minimal assistance with balance
  Three- and four-point (quad): broader base of support, more cumbersome

Fit

- Length should approximate distance between greater trochanter and floor
- Elbow should be flexed slightly when cane rests 6 inches from side of foot

Use

- Use on unaffected side
- Advance when affected limb advances (i.e., if right leg is weak, the cane is held on the left and moved forward as the right leg steps)
- Hold close to body; do not move forward beyond toes of affected foot
- All canes should have suction grips to prevent slippage on floor

Walker

Characteristics

- Broader base of support; more stability than a cane
- Comes in a variety of styles
  Pickup: assists with weight bearing
  Rolling: pushed on wheels rather than lifted; reduces physical strain; often have seats to allow rest after several steps or propulsion from a sitting position

Fit

- Height equivalent to distance between greater trochanter and floor
- Elbows slightly flexed when hands on sides of walker

Use

- When weight bearing is allowed, advance walker and step normally
- When partial or no weight can be borne on one limb, thrust weight forward, then lift walker and replace all four legs on floor
- Always use both hands when transferring from chair or commode; back walker to seat and use arms of chair or commode to assist in standing

Wheelchair

Characteristics

- Used when client's disability prohibits other walking aids
- Should not be used for convenience or speed of client or staff

Fit

- Individually prescribed based on height, weight, limb use, arm strength, and self-propulsion capacity

Use

- Prepare environment for wheelchair use: widen doorways and toilet stalls; plan a functional furniture layout with no rugs; lower mirrors, telephones, drinking fountains, counters; install ramps
- Use special pads and cushions to reduce pressure damage; shift weight and reposition frequently
- Lock chair and remove footrests when transferring to/from

Crutches

Characteristics

- Frequently difficult for older person to use because of inadequate upper body strength, arthritic hands, and balance problems
- Not as stable as other mobility aids

Fit

- Individually sized
- Length should be equivalent to 2 inches below axilla to point on floor 6 inches in front of client
- Hand bars placement crucial because hands should bear total weight
  Elbow should be flexed, wrist slightly hyperextended
  Axillary pressure can cause radial nerve paralysis

Use

- Tailor gait to client's needs; consult with physical therapist
- Use good posture and pay particular attention to foot position on affected side (walking exclusively on ball of foot or toes can cause footdrop)
- General rule when climbing stairs: stronger foot goes up first, down last
  Upstairs: step up with stronger foot; bring crutches to that step; raise affected foot
  Downstairs: crutches to lower step; lower affected foot; follow with stronger foot
- Eliminate obstacles
  Waxed floors
  Throw rugs
  Extension cords
  Uneven surfaces
  Clutter

From Eliopoulos C: *Manual of gerontologic nursing*, St Louis, 1995, Mosby.

D. Lifelong sleeping attire or lack of attire should be encouraged
  1. Reinforces individuality
  2. Reduces sleep interference
E. Standard clothing sizes no longer fit; loose-fitting, comfortable clothing should be encouraged

F. Front closures are more easily managed
G. Cotton socks absorb perspiration
H. Zippers, Velcro, and large buttons make dressing easier
I. Layering and/or sweat suits provide warmth in cold weather
J. Daily exercise should be encouraged and paced
K. Increase self-awareness with mirrors

L. Use daily living resources and aids
   1. Zipper aids
   2. Extralong shoehorns
   3. Shoelace tiers
   4. Adaptive utensils

SEXUALITY

A. Cultural stereotypes deny freedom of sexual expression for the elderly
B. Lifelong sexual adjustment will determine how the elderly person deals with sexual needs
C. Partner availability is made difficult
   1. More elderly women than men
   2. Social and business roles change
D. Physiologic alterations affect self-image and foster nonparticipation
E. Families of elderly persons tend to discourage sexual relationships because of stereotypes and inheritance threats
F. Sexual focus shifts to companionship
G. Older persons continue to enjoy sexual activity; decrease is primarily a result of declining health or lack of available partner

SPEECH

A. Elderly tend to rely on speech more than action
B. Speak slowly and clearly
C. Allow sufficient time for comprehension and response
D. Speak to and treat the individual as an adult
E. Explanations will reduce fear
F. Recovery of speech is influenced by multiimpairments and dependency

Neurologic System (Selected Disorders)

ORGANIC MENTAL SYNDROMES (BOX 9-6)

A. Onset may be rapid or progressive
B. Cognitive function alterations
   1. Judgment
   2. Memory
   3. Intellect
   4. Orientation
   5. Affect
C. Associated factors (Table 9-2)
D. Cognitive dysfunction dementia

DEMENTIA

A. Alzheimer's disease: progressive, deteriorating, chronic dementia
   1. Types
      a. Senile dementia Alzheimer's type (SDAT): onset over age 65
      b. Presenile dementia: onset between ages 40 and 60
   2. Cerebral pathophysiology
      a. Senile plaques
      b. Neurofibrillary tangles
      c. Neurotransmitter abnormalities
      d. Atrophy
   3. Diagnosis confirmed by above findings on autopsy
   4. Assessment
      a. Personality changes
      b. Memory changes
      c. Behavioral changes
      d. Impaired cognition

Box 9-6. Organic Mental Syndromes

Delirium

A reduced ability to maintain attention to external stimuli and to appropriately shift attention to new external stimuli; disorganized thinking, as manifested by rambling, irrelevant, or incoherent speech; reduced level of consciousness; sensory misperceptions; disturbances of the sleep-wake cycle and level of psychomotor activity; disorientation to time, place, or person; memory impairment

Dementia

Impairment of short- and long-term memory; changes in abstract thinking; impaired judgment

Amnestic syndrome

Impairment in a short- and long-term memory that is attributed to a specific organic factor; immediate memory is not impaired

Organic delusional syndrome

Delusions resulting from specific organic factor such as amphetamine use or cerebral lesions of the right hemisphere

Organic hallucinosis

Hallucinations that are persistent or recurrent and caused by a specific organic factor such as use of hallucinogens that produce visual hallucinations, or alcohol, which induces auditory hallucinations

Organic mood syndrome

Persistent depressed, elevated, or expansive mood caused by a specific organic factor such as a toxic effect of substances, including reserpine or methyldopa, an endocrine disorder such as hyperthyroidism, or structural brain disease that results from hemispheric strokes

Organic anxiety syndrome

Recurrent panic attacks or generalized anxiety caused by a specific organic factor such as endocrine disorder, use of psychoactive substances, brain tumors in the vicinity of the third ventricle, vitamin B_{12} deficiency, aspirin intolerance, heavy metal intoxication

Organic personality syndrome

Persistent personality disturbance caused by a specific organic factor such as structural damage to the brain caused by neoplasms, head trauma, cerebrovascular disease

Intoxication

Maladaptive behavior and a substance-specific syndrome caused by the recent ingestion of a psychoactive substance such as alcohol, cannabis, amphetamine, cocaine

Withdrawal

Development of a substance-specific syndrome that follows the cessation of, or reduction in, intake of a psychoactive substance that the person previously used regularly

Adapted from Haber J et al: *Comprehensive psychiatric nursing,* ed 4, St Louis, 1992, Mosby.

Table 9-2	Factors Associated with Organic Mental Syndromes and Disorders

Influential factors	Examples
Volatile agents	Gasoline, aerosols, glues, paint removers, solvents, lacquers, varnishes, dry-cleaning agents, home cleaning products alone or when mixed
Heavy metals	Lead paints, ceramic glazes, moonshine whiskey, mercury, arsenic, manganese
Insecticides	DDT, parathion, malathion, diazine
Brain trauma	Concussion, contusion, hemorrhage, thrombosis, penetrating wounds, blast effects, electrical trauma; exposure to repeated courses of electroconvulsive therapy; oxygen deprivation
Drugs	Alcohol, barbiturates, opioids, cocaine, amphetamines, cannabis, hallucinogens such as lysergic acid diethylamide (LSD) and phencyclidine (PCP)
Infections	Tuberculous and fungal meningitis, viral encephalitis, neurosyphilis (tabes dorsalis), Jakob-Creutzfeldt disease, human immunodeficiency virus (HIV) related disorders (AIDS, ARC)
Neoplasms, tumors	Astrocytoma, medulloblastoma, meningioma
Metabolic and endocrine disorders	Hepatic disease, uremic encephalopathy, porphyria; thyroid, parathyroid, and adrenal dysfunction; Wernicke-Korsakoff syndrome
Nutritional deficiencies	Lack of protein; deficiencies in vitamin C and the B vitamins (folic acid, niacin, pyridoxine, riboflavin, thiamine, B_{12}); fluid and electrolyte imbalance
Seizures	Petit mal, grand mal, focal seizures, psychic seizures
Hypoxia-ischemia	Anoxia related to delayed or prolonged cardiopulmonary resuscitation
Neurologic disease (possible genetic influence)	Huntington chorea, multiple sclerosis, Pick's disease, cerebral degeneration, Parkinson's disease
Cerebral changes associated with Alzheimer's disease	Loss of neurons, plaques, neurofibrillary degeneration, tangles, amyloid deposits, loss of dentritic tree, choline acetyl transferase, CAT defects, degeneration of basal forebrain, elevated platelet fluidity, inherited genetic factor

From Haber et al: *Comprehensive psychiatric nursing*, ed 4, St Louis, 1992, Mosby.

  e. Late-stage physical alterations affecting mobility and swallowing
 5. Nursing intervention/management
  a. Support independence with ADL
  b. Provide structured, consistent environment
  c. Facilitate sleep-activity balance
  d. Promote bowel and bladder continence
  e. Provide reality orientation, remotivation, reminiscence
  f. Provide for patient safety
   (1) At risk for wandering
   (2) Becomes lost easily
   (3) Fails to recognize environmental hazards
  g. Encourage socialization, because withdrawal and social isolation are common
  h. Reduce anxiety-provoking situations
  i. Provide for nutritional needs
  j. Recognized self-concept needs
  k. Encourage verbal communications
  l. Monitor effectiveness of medications, for example, antidepressants
B. Multi-infarct dementia: cognitive impairment caused by cerebrovascular disease
C. Psychoactive substance–induced mental disorders: chemically induced organic disease

PARKINSONIAN SYNDROME
Progressive neurologic movement disorder
A. Primary
 1. Parkinson's disease

 2. Paralysis agitans
B. Secondary
 1. Tumors
 2. Drugs
 3. Infection
C. Assessment
 1. Slowness of movement
 2. Waxlike rigidity of extremities
 3. Facial masking
 4. Tremors while at rest; characteristic pill-rolling motion
 5. Muscular weakness
 6. Shuffling gait
 7. Stature alterations
 8. Drooling; swallowing difficulties
 9. Cognitive impairment
 10. Mood swings
D. Nursing intervention/management
 1. Foster independence with ADL
 2. Maintain physical mobility
 3. Provide adequate nutrition
  a. Keep swallowing difficulties in mind
  b. May require suction; prone to aspiration
  c. Monitor weight weekly
  d. Provide adaptive eating devices
  e. Provide thick liquids
 4. Prevent constipation
 5. Encourage communication
  a. Be attentive: speech is soft and low pitched
  b. Allow time: speech is slow and monotonous
 6. Enhance self-concept

a. Focus on patient's strengths
b. Encourage activities that foster success
c. Give positive feedback
d. Establish realistic goals
e. Encourage verbalization of feelings
f. Maintain intellectual activity stimulation
7. Monitor effectiveness of medications in controlling tremors and rigidity and alleviating characteristic depression
   a. Tricyclic antidepressants; monoamine oxidase inhibitors (MAOI)
   b. Antihistamines
   c. Anticholinergics
   d. Levodopa (eliminate Vitamin B_6 from diet)
8. Provide safety
9. Decrease stress

Psychologic Alterations (Normal Aging Process)
SELF-IMAGE
A. Physiologic alterations
B. Youth-oriented society
C. Retirement
D. Income alterations
E. Role changes
F. Sexual expression alterations

INTELLIGENCE
A. Verbal ability and retained information remain unchanged
B. Abstract thinking and performance response decline
C. Performance of activities involving neuromuscular learning decline
D. Attention span shortens
E. Literal approach to problem-solving affects ability
F. Fluid intelligence declines after adolescence
G. Crystallized intelligence continues to increase throughout life
H. Learning capacity continues

MEMORY
A. Short term: concentration and retention decline
B. Long term: minimal impairment
C. Remote
   1. Remote memory is better than short-term memory
   2. Involved in reminiscence

MOTIVATION
A. Not risk takers
B. Do not actively seek change
C. Possess fear of failure
D. Self-fulfilling prophecies
E. Competitiveness declines
F. Energy levels decline

ATTITUDES, BELIEFS, INTERESTS
A. General attitude realignment
B. Interests either narrow or expand
C. Tend to keep lifelong beliefs amid rapidly changing society

PERSONALITY
A. Basically unchanged
B. Some exaggeration of behavioral responses is evident

C. Adaptive capacities are diminished
D. Reduced ability to handle stress

Psychologic Disorders (Abnormal)
DEPRESSION
A. Reaction to loss of
   1. Independence
   2. Status
   3. Spouse, relatives, and friends
   4. Possessions
B. Medications can cause depression (e.g., digitalis)
C. Physical illness and changes
   1. Lowered self-esteem
   2. Self-concept alterations
   3. Feelings of hopelessness and worthlessness
D. Types
   1. Exogenous
      a. Referred to as neurotic; external, caused by outside events
      b. Common in the elderly
      c. Usually a reaction to losses
   2. Endogenous
      a. Referred to as psychotic; caused by internal events
      b. Characterized by
         (1) Guilt
         (2) Reduced self-regard
         (3) Early morning awakening
         (4) Slowing of thought, verbalization, and level of activity
      c. Classifications
         (1) Unipolar: life history of depression
         (2) Bipolar (manic-depressive psychosis)
            (a) Mood swings from depression to euphoria
            (b) More likely to have hallucinations and delusions
E. Symptoms: Table 9-3
F. Nursing intervention
   1. Encourage self-expression; increase self-esteem
   2. Improve appearance
   3. Provide structure, routine
   4. Assist with maintaining or regaining control
   5. Have kind, understanding attitude
   6. Provide physical care as needed; encourage independence
   7. Provide safety, security
   8. Reduce environmental stimuli and stress
   9. Continuously test reality perception
   10. Ascertain emotional support network
   11. Prevent isolation and avoidance
   12. Realize potential for suicide exists
      a. Suicide is an act that stems from depression
      b. Approximately 25% of suicides occur in persons over age 65
      c. White males over age 75 have the highest rate
      d. Refer to Chapter 6, Mental Health Nursing, for suicidal risk assessment, crisis intervention, and nursing interventions

AGGRESSIVE BEHAVIOR
A. Abnormal anger, rage, or hostility, which if turned inward would lead to depression and if turned outward would lead to aggressiveness

Table 9-3	Symptoms of Depression as Observed in Cognitive, Affective, and Somatic Changes		
Cognitive	**Affective**	**Somatic**
Indecisiveness	Fear*	Tearful
Confusion*	Anxiety	Crying spells
Impaired thinking*	Sadness	Agitation*
Poverty of thought	Irritability	Anorexia
Hopelessness/ emptiness	Anger*	Weight loss
Suicidal ideation*	Feels distant from others*	Constipation
Guilt	Depersonalized*	Palpitations
Inability to concentrate		Fatigue/weakness
Worry		Insomnia
Believes self a failure*		Restlessness*
Believes self causing harm to others*		
Believes self going crazy*		
Believes self deserving of punishment*		

From Ebersole P, Hess P: *Toward healthy aging: human needs and nursing response*, ed 2, St Louis, 1985, Mosby. Data from Morris J, Wolf R, Kerman L: *J Gerontol* 30:209, 1975; Zung W: *Arch Gen Psychiatry* 29:328, 1973.
*Presence of clinically significant depression.

B. Response to
   1. Anxiety
   2. Stress
   3. Guilt
   4. Insecurity
   5. Loss of self-esteem
   6. Loss of control of destiny
   7. Forced dependency
C. Clinical manifestations
   1. Lack of cooperation
   2. Irritability
   3. Demanding
   4. Hostility
   5. Demonstration of coping mechanisms characteristically used to decrease stress, for example, rationalization and repression
   6. Altered interpersonal relationships
   7. Altered reality testing
D. Nursing intervention
   1. Reduce stress source and sensory overload
   2. Encourage ventilation
   3. Set realistic, reachable goals
   4. Respond to questions directly and briefly
   5. Allow ample time for task completion
   6. Meet physical needs as necessary
   7. Encourage environmental participation and activity involvement
   8. Positively recognize attainments
   9. Set limits on activities
   10. Anticipate hostile, demanding behavior
   11. Allow only the degree of independence that can be successfully handled
   12. Avoid responses and action that could lead to guilt, feelings of rejection, bother, or dislike
   13. Increase feeling of self-worth
   14. Medication
   15. Therapy if indicated

REGRESSION
The display of regressive behavior, an ego defense mechanism, is not an uncommon response in the elderly to external stressors. This return to an earlier behavioral stage (e.g., temper tantrums, rocking, or incontinence) requires prevention, early detection, and prompt intervention (remove source of stress and reverse the behavior).

PARANOID BEHAVIOR
A. Inappropriate attempt of coping with stress
B. Response to
   1. Physical impairments
   2. Sensory deprivation
   3. Loss
   4. Loneliness
   5. Medications
   6. Environmental changes
   7. Isolation
   8. Vision alterations
   9. Auditory alterations
C. Clinical manifestations
   1. Secretiveness
   2. Mistrust
   3. Mood disturbances
   4. Oversensitivity
   5. Insecurity
   6. Superiority attitude
   7. Alterations in behavior
   8. Delusions
   9. Withdrawal
   10. Fearfulness
   11. Aloofness
   12. Refusal to take medications, eat, or carry out normal self-care activities
D. Nursing intervention
   1. Attempt to allay anxiety
   2. Allow patient to refuse treatments
   3. Don't argue with patient
   4. Try not to take patient's anger personally
   5. Administer medication
   6. Don't make promises to patient
   7. Look for alterations in ADL as cues to whether the patient's verbalizations are of real concern or are for attention
   8. Be aware of events precipitated by environment
   9. Use stress management techniques
   10. Patient-predicted events that do not occur should be brought to patient's attention
   11. Encourage independence
   12. Monitor impact on hygiene and nutrition
   13. Encourage socialization

Rehabilitation

REALITY ORIENTATION (TABLE 9-4)

A. First used with disoriented, confused elderly at Veterans Administration Hospital in Tuscaloosa, Alabama, in 1965
B. Emphasizes orientation to time, place, and person
C. Reality orientation boards are used to provide contact with reality; for example, time, date, locations, weather, last meal, and next meal
D. Program success depends on total staff commitment and 24-hour implementation
E. Many facilities that care for the elderly have implemented modified programs
F. Program implementation not limited to an institutional setting
G. Components
  1. Small groups
  2. Formal classroom sessions
    a. 20 to 30 minutes
    b. Morning sessions recommended (elderly are more alert in the morning)
    c. Reality orientation board, calendars, clocks, and other materials used according to instructor plan
    d. Positive verbal feedback emphasized
    e. Confusion never reinforced
H. All personnel who come in contact with patients participating in the program are expected to use reality orientation
  1. Address patient by name and title
  2. Orient patient to time, place, and person
  3. Give positive verbal feedback
  4. Do not reinforce confusion

REMOTIVATION (SEE TABLE 9-4)

A. Similar to reality orientation
B. Normal behavior reinforced through structured group program
C. Stimulating participation and interest in the environment are key components
D. Sessions average 20 to 60 minutes
E. Visual aids used, for example, items that stimulate sensory responses
F. Client behavior recorded
G. Staff support and involvement essential

REMINISCENCE (TABLE 9-5)

A. Small group sessions
B. Based on life review process
C. Elderly with cognitive dysfunction retain long-term memory and through reminiscence can adapt to the aging process
D. Purposes
  1. Conflict resolution
  2. Sharing of memories
  3. Sense of identity and self-importance achieved
  4. Focus is on a life that has meaning as opposed to a life viewed as a waste of time
  5. Natural for elderly persons to reminisce
    a. Feel comfortable

Table 9-4	Differences Between Remotivation and Reality Orientation	
Reality orientation		**Remotivation**
1. Correct position or relation with the existing situation in a community. Maximum use of assets		1. Orientation to reality for community living; present oriented
2. Called reality orientation and classroom reality orientation program		2. Called remotivation
3. Structured		3. Definite structure
4. Refreshments or food may be served for identification		4. Refreshments not served
5. Appreciation of the work of the world. Constantly reminded of who they are, where they are, why they are here, and what is expected of them		5. Appreciation of the work of the group stimulates the desire to return to function in society
6. Classes range from 3 to 5 patients, depending on degree/level of confusion or disorientation from any cause		6. Group size: 5 to 12 patients
7. Meeting ½ hour daily at same time in same place		7. Meeting once to twice weekly for an hour
8. Planned procedures: reality-centered objects		8. Preselected and reality-centered objects
9. Consistence of approach response of resident responsibility of teacher		9. No exploration of feelings
10. Periodic reality orientation test pertaining to residents' level of confusion or disorientation		10. Progress ratings
11. Emphasis on time, place, person orientation		11. Topic: no discussion of religion, politics, or death
12. Use of portion of mind function still intact		12. Untouched areas of the mind
13. Residents greeted by name, thanked for coming, and extended handshake and/or physical contact according to attitude approach in group		13. No physical contact permitted. Acceptance and acknowledgment of everyone's contribution
14. Conducted by trained aides and activity assistants		14. Conducted by trained psychiatric aides

From Barns E, Sack A, Shore H. Reprinted by permission of *The Gerontologist* 13:513, 1973.

Table 9-5	Suggestions for Reminiscent Group Strategies		
	Cognitively impaired	**Psychologically disturbed**	**Depressed**
Patient selection	No more than 5 members Age cohorts Both sexes	10 members Varied ages Both sexes	8 to 10 members Those with similar problems, for example, grieving, retired Both sexes
Structure	Consistent place and time Frequent, 30-minute meetings Co-leaders	Consistent place and time Biweekly, 1-hour meetings One leader consistently	Varied meeting places Weekly, 1-hour meeting Variable leadership
Process	Connect specific events, things, and places common to group	Connect members through shared feelings and survival strategies	Focus members on successful coping during life span; encourage mutuality
Goals	Stimulate memory Enhance identity Raise self-esteem Increase socialization skills	Recognition of feelings and meaning of suppressed conflicts Enlarge coping strategies Integrate self-view Promote universality	Reduce feelings of hopelessness Restore personal control Increase affectual responsiveness Develop a sense of integrity and acceptance of life as lived Promote caring between members
Nurse's function	1. Provide a comfortable, mildly stimulating environment 2. Select props that will stimulate memories 3. Assist members by giving specific information, reminders, and clues 4. Give praise and recognition for any participation	1. Establish a private meeting and a closed group 2. Plan to focus on specific developmental stages or critical life events 3. Accept and validate all expressions of feeling 4. Clarify multiple meanings of events 5. Reduce anxiety	1. Provide a comfortable, stimulating environment 2. Appeal to sensory memories 3. Focus members' attention on evidence of caring and sharing 4. Demonstrate a caring attitude 5. Allow time to verbalize feelings, complain, etc.

Adapted from Ebersole P, Hess P: *Toward healthy aging: human needs and nursing response,* ed 2, St Louis, 1985, Mosby.

  b. They're good at it
  c. Reinforces sense of belonging (everyone talks about life's trials and tribulations)
6. Therapeutic relationship with leader more likely to develop as patients realize their memories are important and valued
7. Depressed patients find a caring listener and an opportunity to externalize their anger
8. Psychologically disturbed patients receive acceptance, group validation, and a forum for expression: encourage active exploration of past strengths
9. Strive to change outlook on the past rather than establishing new future directions
10. Psychologic assessment tool (e.g., insight into past coping mechanisms)
11. Reduces isolation, insecurity, and negative self-esteem
12. Confused patients can be assisted to explore a memory that will stimulate latent thoughts, become more oriented, and improve ability to focus
13. Current circumstances are often reflected through memories
E. If patients have difficulty focusing their thoughts, assist by selecting a specific memory
F. Stimulation of dormant thoughts to the surface decreases disorientation

G. Patients who are reluctant to talk can usually be stimulated with topics of food, movies, or music
H. Program implementation is not limited to institutional settings

COGNITIVE TRAINING
A. Consists of memory exercises, problem-solving situations, and memory training
B. Leader must be familiar with patient's past leisure time utilization, hobbies, and occupations
C. Individual, small, or large groups
D. Purpose is to maintain mental activity

RELAXATION THERAPY
A. Promotes sense of physical well-being, reduces stress, releases tension
B. Small groups
C. Involves rhythmic breathing, tension-relaxation exercises, and altered state of consciousness

BLADDER RETRAINING: URINARY INCONTINENCE
A. Causes
  1. Physiologic changes
    a. Decline in muscle support of pelvis
    b. Reduction in bladder's capacity to hold urine

c. Sphincter weakness
2. Behavioral alterations
   a. Regression
   b. Insecurity
   c. Rebellion
   d. Attention seeking
   e. Dependency
   f. Sensory deprivation
3. Drugs
4. Consciousness alterations
5. Disease
6. Obstruction
7. Trauma
8. Immobility
9. Bedpans and urinals
10. Lack of privacy
11. Lack of time

B. Types
1. Stress or passive
   a. Bladder outlet weakness
   b. Involuntary
   c. Frequency when sneezing, coughing, laughing, and lifting
2. Paradoxical or overflow
   a. Uncontrollable contraction waves
   b. Bladder does not empty
   c. Frequency accompanied by retention
   d. At risk for urinary tract infection
3. Total
   a. Constant dribbling
   b. Storage problem

C. Elderly susceptible to
1. Urinary tract infections
2. Urgency
3. Frequency

D. Patient reactions to incontinence
1. Insecurity
   a. Social withdrawal
   b. Isolation
   c. Sensory deprivation
   d. Avoidance of previously developed relationships
2. Depression
   a. Embarrassment
   b. Guilt
   c. Shame

E. Intervention
1. Pelvic exercises
   a. Bearing down
   b. Push-ups from a chair
2. Indwelling catheter as a last resort if skin integrity threatened
3. Condom drainage
4. Absorbent, waterproof underpants
5. Keep patient clean and dry
6. Skin care
7. Retraining
   a. Assess and record voiding pattern for minimum of 72 hours
      (1) Time
      (2) Place
      (3) Quantity
      (4) Activity
      (5) Patient awareness
      (6) Significant medications
      (7) Character of urine
      (8) Presence or absence of constipation or discharge
      (9) Problems: for example, clothing and ambulation hindrances
   b. Reestablish voiding pattern
      (1) First scheduled voiding of the day should be attempted immediately after awakening in the morning even if bed is wet
      (2) Voiding should be attempted at intervals determined from the assessment period (usually at 1-, 2-, or 3-hour periods; goal is every 4 hours)
      (3) Patient takes one or two 8-oz (240-ml) glasses of fluid 1 hour before attempting to urinate
      (4) No fluids should be taken between 6 PM and 6 AM if no urinating is desired
      (5) Fluid intake should be at least 2000 ml per day
      (6) Alcoholic drinks contraindicated
      (7) Soft drinks, tea, and coffee should be avoided
      (8) All fluid intake should be measured and recorded
      (9) All urine output should be measured and recorded

BOWEL RETRAINING: FECAL INCONTINENCE

A. Causes
1. Physiologic changes
   a. External anal sphincter relaxation
   b. Perineal relaxation
   c. Muscle atony
2. Behavioral alterations
   a. Regression
   b. Rebellion
   c. Dependency
   d. Sensory deprivation
3. Central nervous system injury
4. Obstruction
5. Impaction
6. Consciousness alterations
7. Immobility
8. Trauma

B. Intervention
1. Keep patient clean and dry
2. Absorbent, waterproof underpants
3. Skin care
4. Retraining
   a. Bowel retraining is easier than bladder retraining; if patient is incontinent of urine and stool, start bowel retraining program first
   b. Use no laxatives
   c. Ensure adequate fluid intake (2 L per day)
   d. Fluids and solids that promote patient's bowel movements (e.g., bran and orange juice) and roughage should be included in the diet
   e. Encourage physical activity
   f. Obtain bowel history
   g. Procedure
      (1) Establish regular days(s) and time to assist patient to the toilet for evacuation; preferably after a meal

(2) After 20 minutes if patient has not had a bowel movement, insert a lubricated glycerine suppository
   (a) Do not use directly from refrigerator
   (b) Do not insert into a bolus of stool (ineffective)
   (c) After ascertaining that patient requires the suppository for training, it can be inserted 1 to 2 hours before the scheduled training time and after a meal
(3) Digital stimulation is recommended after 48 hours if the above procedure is not successful
(4) Take patient to the bathroom at the scheduled time daily, even if he or she has had a bowel movement between scheduled times

SUGGESTED READING

Eliopoulus C: *Manual of gerontologic nursing*, St Louis, 1995, Mosby.

Hamdy RC et al: *Alzheimer's disease, a handbook for caregivers*, ed 2, St Louis, 1994, Mosby.

Hogstel MO: *Clinical manual of gerontological nursing*, St Louis, 1992, Mosby.

Morice SV: *Geriatric nursing*, Aurora, Colorado, 1996, Skidmore-Roth Publishing.

Smeltzer SC, Bare BG: *Brunner and Suddarth's textbook of medical surgical nursing*, ed 8, Philadelphia, 1996, JB Lippincott.

Stuart GW, Sundeen SJ: *Principles and practice of psychiatric nursing*, ed 5, St Louis, 1995, Mosby.

REVIEW QUESTIONS

Answers and rationales begin on p. 434.

1. An elderly patient has osteoarthritis and is admitted to the hospital for a total knee replacement. Of the following baseline data, which is most important for the nurse to obtain?
   ① Extent of knee flexion and extension
   ② Food likes and dislikes
   ③ Mental health status and history
   ④ Usual sleeping habits

2. A Parkinson's disease patient has difficulty swallowing. The nurse knows he is able to manage his dietary intake when he can:
   ① Eat solid food
   ② Drink thin liquids
   ③ Eat a meal in 20 minutes
   ④ Swallow without choking

3. Preoperative teaching for a 71-year-old patient scheduled for a total knee replacement should include which of the following?
   ① Cast brace application
   ② Continuous passive motion (CPM) device
   ③ Principles of Buck's extension
   ④ Russell traction

4. Routine nursing care following a total knee replacement should include which of the following?
   ① Elevating affected knee when out of bed
   ② Keeping the head of the bed elevated up to 45 degrees
   ③ Keeping the affected leg in abduction
   ④ Using wedge pillows between patient's legs

5. Which of the following statements is accurate regarding ice application to the affected knee following a total knee replacement?
   ① Increases circulation and movement
   ② Reduces the chance of infection
   ③ Reduces edema and bleeding
   ④ Reduces fluid accumulation in the joint

6. The discharge teaching plan for an elderly patient recovering from a total knee replacement should reinforce which of the following measures?
   ① Full weight bearing in the affected leg
   ② Non-weight bearing in the affected leg
   ③ Weight bearing only as prescribed by his physician
   ④ Weight bearing only as tolerated by the patient

7. An 89-year-old patient is alert and active. On annual physical examination, she complains of hemorrhoids and annoying constipation. Her physician instructs her to increase her fluid and dietary fiber intake. Which of the following snacks, if selected by the patient, would indicate that she can identify food sources high in fiber?
   ① Apple juice
   ② Small banana
   ③ Raspberries
   ④ Cucumber

8. A 62-year-old male patient has a diagnosis of Type I or sliding hiatal hernia. Which of the following nursing measures should be included in his case?
   ① Eat three good meals a day
   ② Eat high-protein, high-fat foods
   ③ Lie down for 1 to 2 hours after meals
   ④ Sleep with the head of the bed elevated

9. A positive diagnosis of Alzheimer's disease can be obtained through which of the following procedures?
   ① Computer tomography scanning (CT)
   ② Positron emission tomography (PET)
   ③ Neural tissue evaluation on autopsy
   ④ Serial evaluations of neuropsychologic testing

10. A 67-year-old patient is admitted to a nursing home with a diagnosis of senile dementia Alzheimer's type (SDAT). He's not there very long when the nurse notices he's headed for the exit door. She catches up with him and asks if he needs help. The patient responds, "You can leave me alone. I'm going home." Which of the following nursing actions is *most* appropriate?
    ① Call the security department
    ② Go with the patient
    ③ Engage him in an activity
    ④ Physically prevent him from leaving

11. An elderly patient with Alzheimer's disease is restless and agitated. Which of the following activities is *most* appropriate for the patient?
    ① Listening to music
    ② Taking a nap
    ③ Taking a walk
    ④ Watching television

12. Which of the following activities is *most* appropriate for an Alzheimer's patient who is demonstrating increasing difficulty with planning and decision making?
    ① Hoeing in the garden
    ② Planning the dinner menu
    ③ Sorting the laundry
    ④ Writing out the grocery list

13. An Alzheimer's patient demonstrates progressive personality changes. When he becomes hostile and combative the nurse should include which of the following in his plan of care?
    ① Decrease environmental stimuli
    ② Simplify daily activity
    ③ Secure doors leading from the house
    ④ Use memory aids

14. When caring for the elderly, the nurse must know that the most common and easily reversed cause of dementia is:
    ① AIDS
    ② Alzheimer's disease
    ③ Drug toxicity
    ④ Parkinson's disease

15. An 82-year-old patient has periods of confusion and disorientation as well as difficulty remembering where the bathroom is. Which of the following nursing actions should be *most* helpful?
    ① Take him to the bathroom every hour
    ② Place a sign saying *Here it is* on the door
    ③ Place a picture of a toilet on the bathroom door
    ④ Tell him if he can't find the bathroom he'll have to wear diapers

16. An elderly nursing home patient with a history of poor nutritional intake takes a few mouthfuls of dinner and then gets up and leaves the table. Which of the following nursing approaches is *most* appropriate?
    ① Apply a vest restraint during meals
    ② Have a staff member feed him his meals
    ③ Offer five to six small feedings daily
    ④ Provide him with a variety of finger foods

17. A 79-year-old nursing home patient is confused. When planning his care, which of the following nursing measures is *most* appropriate?
    ① Explain the planned daily activities to him each morning
    ② Leave him alone and let him do what he wants
    ③ Place a weekly activity calendar in his room
    ④ Speak clearly, calmly, and in short sentences

18. The physician orders a geri chair to be used in accordance with agency policy when an elderly nursing home patient becomes overly agitated and combative. Which of the following statements by the nurse indicates the *best* understanding of the patient's needs?
    ① All agitated patients should be restrained for their own safety
    ② The use of a geri chair causes decubiti
    ③ The use of geri chair can increase a patient's agitation level
    ④ The use of a geri chair fosters incontinence

19. Your are assigned to care for Mr. Walters. His nursing care plan indicates that his first name is Jake. When you enter Mr. Walters' room you recognize him as the school crossing guard everyone calls "Pops." Which of the following greeting is most appropriate?
    ① "Hi, aren't you Pops, the school crossing guard."
    ② "Hi Jake. I'm your nurse, Karen."
    ③ "Hi there, Mr. Walters, remember me?"
    ④ "Mr. Walters. Hello. I'm your nurse, Miss Oats."

20. A nursing home patient puts on his call bell for the nurse. When the nurse responds she finds the patient standing at the bedside in a puddle of urine and his pajamas soaked. Which of the following is the *best* response for the nurse to make?
    ① "Let me help you to the bathroom where you can wash up and put on clean pajamas."
    ② "Next time wait for help before getting out of bed. That's what we're here for."
    ③ "Not again. It's diapers for you for sure now."
    ④ "Now look what you've done. I just changed you ten minutes ago."

21. A patient diagnosed with Parkinson's disease is placed on Sinemet 10/100 PO tid by his physician. As he's leaving the doctor's office, he asks the nurse what the drug will do. Which of the following explanations by the nurse is *most* appropriate?
    ① It can decrease his tremors and improve his gait
    ② It's really very complicated and not necessary for you to know
    ③ It's the carbidopa-levodopa content ratio of the drug
    ④ You'll have to discuss that with the physician

22. Which of the following assessments of a patient on Sinemet should indicate possible drug toxicity to the nurse?
    ① Akinesia and drooling
    ② Muscle stiffness and rigidity
    ③ Muscle and eyelid twitching
    ④ Slow movements and handwriting changes

23. A patient with Parkinson's disease has been on Sinemet 10/100 PO tid for 2 weeks. The patient calls the doctor's office and tells the nurse that he has seen no improvement since the Sinemet was started and perhaps another drug should be tried. Which of the following responses by the nurse is *most* appropriate?

    ① "I'll let the physician know you want a medication change."
    ② "It frequently takes several months to achieve maximum effect."
    ③ "What makes you think you're not improving?"
    ④ "Why don't you call the doctor tomorrow when he's in the office?"

24. A patient on Sinemet reports to the nurse that he really doesn't want to eat and occasionally vomits when he does eat. To reduce the gastrointestinal side effects of Sinemet and enhance its absorption, which of the following instructions should the nurse give the patient?
    ① Administer the medication before meals
    ② Administer the medication after meals
    ③ Crush the medication and mix with his food
    ④ Recommend a lower dosage to the physician

25. Which of the following statements made by a patient with Parkinson's disease would indicate to the nurse that the patient has a basic understanding of his disease process?
    ① Autosomal dominant genetic disorder
    ② Chronic progressive hereditary disease of the nervous system
    ③ Progressive damage to neurons that regulate and control movement
    ④ Progressive, fatal disease caused by a virus

26. A 66-year-old skilled nursing facility (SNF) resident has rheumatoid arthritis resulting in severe deformities of both hands. Her medications consist of prednisone (Prednisone) 5 mg PO qd and auranofin (Ridaura) 2 mg PO tid. She refuses her qd dose of prednisone. Which of the following actions should the nurse take?
    ① Call the physician and get an order for an injectable adrenocorticosteroid
    ② Chart the refusal in the nurses' notes and inform the head nurse
    ③ Return to the patient in a half hour and offer her the medication again
    ④ Chart *refused* on the medication sheet and report it to the physician

27. An elderly nursing home patient has a history of paranoid behavior. When planning care for the patient which of the following demonstrated behaviors should the staff identify as unusual?
    ① Verbalized hallucination
    ② Demonstrated superiority
    ③ Refusal of meals and treatments
    ② Verbalized oversensitivity

28. The nurse is busy caring for an elderly nursing home patient when another patient interrupts and insists on being taken to the bathroom immediately. It is correct for the nurse to:
    ① Stop what she's doing and attend to the second patient
    ② Inform the patient that she'll be with her shortly
    ③ Tell the patient to ask someone else who's free
    ④ Tell the patient that she's busy and will be with her in 10 minutes

29. The nurse brings an elderly hospitalized patient his breakfast tray. The patient says, "Take it away, I don't want it." The *most* appropriate response is?
    ① "I'll tell the dietitian you don't like the food here."
    ② "I'll call the kitchen and order something else for you."

③ "I'll leave the tray here just in case you change your mind."
④ "I'll throw it out and record that you refused your breakfast."

30. An elderly nursing home resident reports that nobody does anything for her, and the staff ignores her needs but takes care of all the other patients. The nurse knows this to be inaccurate and understands that the patient is:
① Looking to cause trouble
② Experiencing active hallucinations
③ Demonstrating manifestations of paranoia
④ Attempting to manipulate the staff

31. The staff decides that a 66-year-old patient with deformities of both hands related to rheumatoid arthritis and who has a history of paranoid behavior needs an activity. Which recommendation should the nurse pursue as therapeutic for the patient?
① Operating the Resident Gift Shop
② Making her own bed daily
③ Independently preparing her meal tray
④ Participating daily in arts and crafts

32. An 80-year-old widower lives with his four cats in a two-bedroom, fourth-floor walkup. His children want him to move to a ground floor smaller apartment. He refuses and says he'll stay where he is until he dies. It is important that his children recognize that their father is:
① Becoming paranoid
② Displaying eccentricity
③ Afraid to move
④ Feeling secure where he is

33. An elderly man falls in the street and is taken to the hospital by EMS (Emergency Medical Service). He is diagnosed with a mild concussion and a fractured left radius. His two children live nearby and are notified of their father's hospitalization. He tells the nurse that he can't stay in the hospital because he lives alone and has four cats that he needs to take care of. Which of the following actions should the nurse take?
① Speak with the patient's children about arranging care for his cats.
② Remind the patient that cats are independent and can care for themselves.
③ Tell the patient that he has too many cats and to give them to the ASPCA.
④ Offer to go to his home once a day to care for the cats.

34. A 78-year-old widow is brought to the local emergency room by the police who found her wandering aimlessly about the street. She is confused, disoriented, and hospitalized for pneumonia. The nurse should recognize that the cause of her confusion and disorientation is:
① Arteriosclerosis
② Organic brain syndrome
③ Infection
④ Unknown

35. An elderly man is hospitalized with pneumonia and has a poor nutritional intake. The nurse is expected to know that his appetite will probably improve if:
① He is served small meals frequently
② His food is blenderized
③ All liquids are served warm
④ A roll is served with each meal

36. An elderly patient hospitalized with pneumonia asks the time of each staff member who enters his room. The nurse knows that this is characteristic of:
① Confusion
② Disorientation
③ Memory deficit
④ Impaired judgment

37. An elderly nursing home patient has wet the bed. The *most* appropriate response by the nurse should be to:
① Admonish him for soiling himself and the bed
② Tell him now he'll have to wear diapers
③ Offer him the urinal
④ Proceed with making him clean and dry

38. An elderly nursing home patient has not had a bowel movement in 3 days. The nurse identifies the problem as constipation and knows that constipation in the elderly is frequently the result of:
① Too much fiber in the diet
② Too much bulk in the diet
③ Lack of daily laxatives
④ Poor eating habits

39. A 78-year-old nursing home patient's bedside stand is found to be full of packets of sugar, salt, jelly, napkins, and straws which he has removed from his meal trays. The nurse understands that this behavior indicates:
① Decreased self-esteem
② Increased insecurity
③ Increased confusion
④ Increased disorientation

40. The night staff in a nursing home expresses concern about an elderly patient who is awake most of the night. The *most* appropriate response by the nurse should be:
① "The elderly require less sleep at night as they rest often throughout the day."
② "I'll get a physician's order for a sedative."
③ "As people get older they require less sleep."
④ "We'll increase his day activities."

41. An elderly stroke survivor is being followed in the Outpatient Clinic. He is on sodium warfarin (Coumadin) daily. His prothrombin times have been unstable and the physician requests the nurse to review the patient's dietary intake for indications of possible food-drug interactions. The nurse ascertains that the patient eats large quantities of the following foods. Which foods high in vitamin K should he avoid ingesting in unusual increases?
① Spaghetti and meatballs
② Broccoli and turnip greens
③ Chicken and rice
④ Rice and beans

42. A 67-year-old woman recently diagnosed with diverticulitis plans to shop for groceries that are appropriate for her prescribed high fiber diet. Her selection of which of the following vegetables indicates that she has a clear understanding of her dietary needs?
① Brussel sprouts
② Asparagus
③ Black-eyed peas
④ Vegetarian baked beans

43. An elderly man with coronary artery disease (CAD) is instructed by his physician to eliminate as much saturated fat as possible from his diet. While dining out at a local restaurant, his selection of which of the following desserts would indicate to the nurse that he has taken his physician's advice seriously?
   ① Angel food cake
   ② Butterscotch brownie
   ③ Baklava
   ④ Apple pie

44. An elderly patient tells the home health nurse that he's always troubled with constipation. To increase fiber and bulk in the patient's diet the nurse should assist the patient with planning which of the following lunches?
   ① Corned beef on rye
   ② Chili with beans
   ③ Chicken with dumplings
   ④ Bean burrito with cheese

45. An elderly patient has developed hemorrhoids and gives a history of chronic constipation and straining on defecation. His doctor tells him to take an over the counter (OTC) bulk forming laxative. Which of the following selections by the patient indicates that he understands his physician's instructions?
   ① Senna (Senokot)
   ② Mineral oil (Petrogalan Plain)
   ③ Glycerin (Glycerin USP)
   ④ Psyllium hydrophilic (Metamucil)

46. Diets low in fat and cholesterol are recommended for all patients, including the elderly, who are at risk for heart disease. Dietary teaching of fast-food addicts at a senior citizen center is effective when the senior citizen selects which of the following fast foods lowest in cholesterol content?
   ① One Taco Bell frijoles and cheese
   ② One Wendy's grilled chicken sandwich
   ③ One Burger King ocean catch fish fillet
   ④ Two slices of Domino's 16″ veggie pizza

47. Which of the following patient concerns would indicate the age-related change of loss of subcutaneous tissue?
   ① Muscle cramps
   ② Foot problems
   ③ Increased susceptibility to infection
   ④ Increased urination at night

48. A 62-year-old patient, diagnosed with hypercholesterolemia, is placed on cholestyramine (Questran Light) by his physician. The nurse concludes that medication teaching has been effective when the patient states:
   ① "I won't forget to take it. I'll take it every day with my water pill."
   ② "I'll sprinkle it over my food so I won't forget to take it."
   ③ "I'll make a batch every other day and keep it in the refrigerator."
   ④ "My memory isn't so good but I'll continue taking it each day I remember."

49. A 90-year-old nursing home patient will be 91 next month. The last couple of months she has been repeatedly asking staff how old she'll be on her next birthday. Today she asked for the fourth time, "How old did you say I'll be next month?" Which response by the nurse indicates the nurse has an appropriate understanding of the patient's behavior?

   ① "You'll be ninety-one next month."
   ② "You'll be ninety-one and don't ask me again today."
   ③ "I just told you 5 minutes ago."
   ④ "Why do you keep asking me the same question?"

50. Age-related eye changes include a yellowing of the lens. When color coding the door to the room of an elderly nursing home patient which of the following colors would be most effective?
   ① Pink
   ② Blue
   ③ Red
   ④ Green

51. An elderly patient is seen in the Outpatient Clinic for routine monitoring of his hypertension. He has lost weight since his last visit and tells the nurse that food just doesn't have much taste anymore. Which recommendation by the nurse indicates the *most* appropriate interpretation of the patient's problem?
   ① Make meals look more attractive
   ② Brush teeth before eating
   ③ Add more salt to the food
   ④ Sprinkle onion pieces in the food

52. To evaluate the judgment of a patient in the early stages of Alzheimer's disease the nurse should pay particular attention to the patient's ability to:
   ① Manage personal finances
   ② Set the dining room table
   ③ Navigate in familiar surroundings
   ④ Cooperate with caregiver

53. The nurse should anticipate early Alzheimer's patients having difficulty with which of the following:
   ① Recalling a telephone conversation right after hanging up the phone
   ② Remembering how to operate an automobile
   ③ Remembering they have put a meal in the oven
   ④ Remembering where they put the house keys the evening before

54. A 69-year-old woman is diagnosed with osteoporosis. Her physician states he's going to start her on daily calcium. The nurse should anticipate the patient's dosage to be:
   ① 400 mg
   ② 800 mg
   ③ 1200 mg
   ④ 1500 mg

55. Which of the following statements by an elderly patient with osteoporosis would indicate to the nurse that the patient has an understanding of her dietary needs?
   ① "I don't know if I can drink two glasses of wine a day."
   ② "How much calcium did you say was in yogurt?"
   ③ "I guess I'll have to start eating liver once a week."
   ④ "Thank goodness I don't have to give up my tea."

56. An elderly patient with osteoporosis is visited by the home care nurse. The nurse's *best* indication that the patient is successfully managing his disease is when the patient states:
   ① "I walk twice a week in the mall with the Senior Citizen's Group."
   ② "I sit out in the sun for 15 minutes every day I can."
   ③ "I walk three times a week for at least 20 minutes, rain or shine."
   ④ "I dust the entire house every day now."

57. An elderly diabetic patient is hospitalized and scheduled for a right below-the-knee amputation. On the fifth post operative day the nurse notices that the stump is edematous. The nurse should plan to:
① Communicate with the physician regarding the application of an ace bandage to the stump
② See if the patient has an order for a diuretic
③ Instruct the patient to sit on the edge of the bed and dangle
④ Elevate the stump on a pillow

58. Which of the following signs/symptoms would be the earliest indication of a postoperative infection following a total knee replacement?
① Fever
② Joint pain
③ Purulent drainage
④ Swelling

59. An elderly diabetic patient who has had a right below-the-knee amputation is discharged from the hospital. Ten days after discharge the visiting nurse goes to the patient's home. The nurse evaluates the achievement of wound healing by observing that the patient:
① Demonstrates increasing independence
② Focuses on future functioning
③ Demonstrates residual limb care
④ Uses appropriate assistive devices

60. A 70-year-old nursing home patient has Parkinson's disease. He has tongue tremors and hesitancy in initiating swallowing. The nursing care plan for this patient should indicate the most appropriate diet to be:
① Thin liquids
② Thick liquids
③ Regular diet
④ Mechanical diet

ANSWERS AND RATIONALES

1. Comprehension, assessment, environment (a)
   ❶ Pain and limited motion occur as the disease progresses. Extent of the knee flexion and extension is essential baseline data to provide a clear understanding of the patient's health status. Your nursing decisions and interventions will be based on this data.
   ②,③,④ Important data, but not initially the most important.

2. Application, evaluation, environment (c)
   ❹ When the patient swallows without choking and takes his time eating, he's safely able to manage his dietary intake.
   ① Solid food is unsafe for a Parkinson's patient who has difficulty swallowing.
   ② Thin liquids are difficult for these patients to swallow and are, therefore, unsafe.
   ③ Parkinson's patients who have difficulty swallowing must take their time eating as they may have tongue tremors, pharynx motility difficulties, swallowing hesitancy, and difficulty forming a bolus.

3. Application, planning, environment (a)
   ❷ Continuous passive motion (CPM) device is used postoperatively to facilitate joint range-of-motion. Equipment to be used postoperatively should be introduced, demonstrated, and made familiar to the patient preoperatively.
   ① Not appropriate; enhances fracture healing.
   ③ Not appropriate; skin traction is used for hip injuries before surgery.
   ④ Not appropriate; used for tibia fractures.

4. Application, implementation, physiologic (a)
   ❶ Routine postoperative total knee replacement (TKR) care to control edema and bleeding.
   ② Not appropriate; used with postoperative total hip replacements (THR) to prevent acute hip flexion.
   ③ Not appropriate; used with postoperative hip replacements.
   ④ Not appropriate; used with postoperative hip replacements to keep hip in abduction.

5. Application, assessment, physiologic (a)
   ❸ Vasoconstriction will control bleeding and edema.
   ① CPM device is used to increase circulation and movement.
   ② Good infection-control measures will reduce the chance of infection.
   ④ Wound suction drain will remove joint fluid accumulation.

6. Comprehension, planning, environment (a)
   ❸ Weight-bearing limits are always determined by the physician and depend on the surgical technique used, the patient's postoperative condition, and the type of prosthesis.
   ①,②,④ Incorrect, because a physician's order is required for postoperative weight-bearing limits.

7. Comprehension, evaluation, health (a)
   ❸ 5.1 fiber g/100 g.
   ① 0.3 fiber g/100 g.
   ② 2.1 fiber g/100 g.
   ④ 0.8 fiber g/100 g.

8. Application, planning, physiologic (a)
   ❹ Head of bed should be elevated to prevent movement of the hernia by gravity and passive reflux.
   ① Management includes frequent small feedings that can readily pass through the esophagus.
   ② Low-fat diets are usually less irritating and more readily digested, reducing discomfort and reflux.
   ③ Patients should sit up for at least 1 hour after eating to prevent hernial movement and reflux.

9. Knowledge, assessment, physiologic (a)
   ❸ Alzheimer's disease is diagnosed by exclusion and confirmed only by autopsy.
   ①,② CT and PET may refute or support a diagnosis, but they are not conclusive.
   ④ Serial neuropsychologic testing will reveal progressive cognitive impairment but is not specific to Alzheimer's disease nor is it in any way diagnostically conclusive.

10. Application, implementation, environment (a)
    ❸ Distraction is facilitated by short-term memory loss and is the least anxiety provoking.
    ① Security department presence implies force and will only increase the patient's anxiety and place him at risk for dysfunctional behavior.
    ② Although this may on occasion be an acceptable intervention, it is not the most appropriate.
    ④ Again, force increases the patient's anxiety and places the patient's physical safety at risk.

11. Application, implementation, environment (b)
    ❸ Restlessness and agitation are best reduced by an active intervention such as walking.
    ①,②,④ All are passive interventions that will not reduce the agitation and restlessness and produce the required calming effect.

12. Application, planning, environment (b)
    ❶ Hoeing is a repetitive action that does not require planning or decision making and therefore is the most appropriate activity.
    ②,③,④ All require either planning and/or decision making and are not the most appropriate.

13. Comprehension, planning, environment (b)
    ❶ Excess environmental stimuli increase anxiety, are upsetting to the patient, and frequently precipitate a combative state.
    ②,④ These maintain cognitive function.
    ③ Promotes physical safety.

14. Knowledge, assessment, environment (b)
    ❸ Drug toxicity is the only reversible state listed.
    ①,②,④ All characterized by progression and are irreversible.

15. Application, implementation, environment (b)
    ❸ Pictures reduce environmental confusion and are good memory aids for the cognitively impaired.
    ① Unrealistic and does not promote independence in self-care activities.
    ② This would add to the patient's confusion.
    ④ Never threaten a patient.

16. Application, implementation, physiologic (b)
    ❹ Convenient method for ensuring nutritional intake when the patient will not sit and eat a meal.
    ① Restraints are totally inappropriate and are used for patient safety only.

② This does not promote independence in self-care activities.

③ Appropriate on a day-to-day basis but not the most appropriate when the patient won't stay seated.

17. Application, planning, environment (b)
❹ Short-term memory loss is characteristic of impaired cognition. If short sentences are used, it is easier for the patient to remember.
① Too much information for the patient to remember.
② This does not support the patient's cognitive function.
③ Again, too much information for the patient to absorb and remember. Patient would also have difficulty remembering to look at the schedule.

18. Comprehension, planning, environment (b)
❸ This is the only answer choice that is accurate and demonstrates knowledge of agitated behavior.
① "All agitated patients" is an inappropriate generalization.
② Properly applied restraints released in accordance with facility policy along with other appropriate nursing measures will prevent decubiti.
④ The use of restraints does not cause incontinence.

19. Application, assessment, psychosocial (a)
❹ This is the only response that demonstrates respect and courtesy.
①,②,③ All inappropriate responses that fail to demonstrate compassion and understanding.

20. Application, implementation, psychosocial (b)
❶ This is the only response that does not chastise and humiliate the patient and that demonstrates an understanding of the situation.
②,③,④ All inappropriate responses that fail to demonstrate compassion and understanding.

21. Knowledge, implementation, physiologic (a)
❶ The patient is asking the reason the drug is being given. This is the only response that answers the question.
②,③,④ Inappropriate; they do not acknowledge what the patient has said, and they turn off communication.

22. Knowledge, assessment, physiologic (c)
❸ Toxic effects of Sinemet.
①,②,④ These are symptoms of Parkinson's disease.

23. Comprehension, implementation, physiologic (b)
❷ This is accurate information and directly addresses the patient's communication.
① Not necessary.
③ Threatening response that turns off communication.
④ Not necessary and inappropriate.

24. Application, implementation, physiologic (a)
❶ Administering medication before meals decreases gastric upset.
② Administering the medication on a full stomach will alter its absorption rate.
③ Medications should never be mixed with a patient's food. Medications that are distasteful will turn the patient off to the food.
④ The level of effectiveness of a medication is recorded and reported to the physician. Physicians prescribe and adjust dosage.

25. Comprehension, evaluation, environment (b)
❸ This is the only appropriate description.
①,② Huntington's disease.
④ Jakob-Creutzfeldt disease.

26. Application, implementation, physiologic (b)
❸ It's not imperative that the patient take a once a day medication at exactly 9 AM. This type of person has mood alterations and often attempts to exert control by refusing medications and treatments and might well take it later if offered.
① A person with paranoid behavior would be threatened by this inappropriate action and might feel that the staff is trying to harm her.
② Appropriate to do this eventually but not until the individual has again been offered the medication.
④ The nurse might have to do this ultimately, but not before the medication has again been offered.

27. Knowledge, assessment, environment (b)
❶ Hallucinations are not usually characteristic of paranoid behavior in the elderly.
②,③,④ All are expected characteristics of paranoid behavior in the elderly.

28. Application, implementation, environment (b)
❷ Demonstrates therapeutic calmness and provides an atmosphere of acceptance of the patient but not of her behavior.
① Not appropriate to reinforce unacceptable behavior.
③ Reinforces beliefs of persecution or mistreatment by staff.
④ Does not accept or acknowledge the patient's problem and reinforces beliefs of persecution or mistreatment by staff.

29. Application, implementation, psychosocial (b)
❸ Refusal is not uncommon as the patient struggles with feelings of powerlessness and unacceptable impulses.
①,② Inappropriate, as you are assuming that the patient doesn't like the food.
④ Inappropriate, as sufficient time is not being provided for the patient to use a more appropriate coping mechanism for whatever is bothering her.

30. Comprehension, evaluation, environment (a)
❸ Characteristically expressed feelings of being taken advantage of or plotted against.
①,②,④ The patient really isn't exhibiting any of these behaviors but rather is displaying subjective data of paranoia.

31. Knowledge, planning, psychosocial (a)
❶ Allows the patient to function independently in an area where she can be successful.
②,③,④ Would not be able to be successful with these activities because of debilitated state of hands, and such activities would most likely increase her paranoia.

32. Comprehension, assessment, psychosocial (a)
❹ Moving at this time would threaten feelings of safety and security, contributing further to his losses.
① Situation does not indicate paranoid behavior.
② Situation does not indicate eccentric behavior.
③ Situation does not indicate that he's afraid to move but rather that he chooses not to experience additional losses.

33. Application, implementation, psychosocial (b)
 ① Informing the family of his concern should be sufficient to activate an appropriate plan of action in this case.
 ② Inappropriate response because it ignores his concern.
 ③ It is inappropriate to suggest he experience another loss.
 ④ Inappropriate nurse-patient relationship.

34. Knowledge, assessment, physiologic (a)
 ④ The situation as presented does not indicate the cause.
 ①,②,③ All are possible causes but inappropriate responses. Thorough assessment is required.

35. Comprehension, assessment, environment (a)
 ❶ Easier to digest and conserve energy.
 ② No indication in the situation for blenderized foods.
 ③ No indication in the situation for warm liquids.
 ④ Rolls do not stimulate the appetite.

36. Knowledge, assessment, environment (b)
 ❷ Impairment in orientation to time, place, and person is disorientation.
 ①,③,④ These are signs of chronic brain syndrome, and the situation specifies a time impairment.

37. Application, implementation, physiologic (a)
 ④ This is the only nursing intervention that meets the patient's needs and that is appropriate.
 ①,② These actions reinforce guilt, shame, and embarrassment, which should never be done.
 ③ If the patient has just voided, it's unlikely he would have to void again so soon—not the most appropriate response.

38. Comprehension, assessment, physiologic (a)
 ❹ This is a common cause of constipation in the elderly.
 ① Too much fiber in the diet does not cause constipation.
 ② Too much bulk in the diet does not cause constipation.
 ③ Daily laxatives are a common cause of constipation in the elderly.

39. Comprehension, assessment, psychosocial (c)
 ❷ Hoarding is a manifestation of insecurity.
 ① Decreased self-esteem is associated with role losses and is not related to hoarding.
 ③,④ Increased confusion and disorientation are symptoms of organic brain syndrome and are not related to hoarding.

40. Comprehension, planning, environment (b)
 ❶ Characteristic of the aging process.
 ② Thorough assessment should be done before medication is given.
 ③ Sleep time does not necessarily change in the elderly but rather the quality and continuity of sleep patterns change.
 ④ This would not be compatible with the rest needs of the patient.

41. Knowledge, assessment, environment (b)
 ❸ In addition to broccoli and turnip greens, spinach, kale, cabbage, cauliflower, green beans, and green leafy vegetables are rich in vitamin K and can interfere with the effectiveness of oral anticoagulants.
 ①,③,④ Not vitamin K–rich foods.

42. Knowledge, evaluation, health (c)
 ❹ One-half cup of vegetarian baked beans contains 5 grams of fiber.
 ① One-half cup of cooked brussel sprouts contains 2 grams of fiber.
 ② One-half cup of cooked asparagus contains 2 grams of fiber.
 ③ One-half cup of cooked black-eyed peas contains 2 grams of fiber.

43. Knowledge, evaluation, health (b)
 ❶ 1/12 of an angel food cake contains no saturated fat and a total fat content of 0.2 grams.
 ③ One piece of baklava contains 7.2 grams of saturated fat and a total fat content of 29.2 grams.
 ② A butterscotch brownie contains 0.7 grams of saturated fat and a total fat content of 1.8 grams.
 ④ One-eighth of an apple pie contains 2.3 grams of saturated fat and a total fat content of 16.9 grams.

44. Knowledge, planning, health (c)
 ❷ One cup contains 6 grams of fiber.
 ①,③ Contains 1 gram of fiber.
 ④ Contains 4 grams of fiber.

45. Knowledge, evaluation, health (b)
 ❹ This is the only bulk-forming laxative. It absorbs water in the intestines, creating expansion and increased peristalsis.
 ① This is a stimulant laxative that acts on the smooth muscle of the intestine to increase peristalsis.
 ② This is a lubricant laxative that coats the stool and prevents absorption of fluid from the stool, resulting in easier defecation.
 ③ This is a hyperosmolar agent that pulls liquid into the colon, creating bowel distention and increased peristalsis.

46. Application, evaluation, health (c)
 ❶ Contains 19 mg of cholesterol and has the lowest cholesterol content of the fast food choices.
 ② Contains 60 mg of cholesterol.
 ③ Contains 57 mg of cholesterol.
 ④ Contains 36 mg of cholesterol.

47. Comprehension, assessment, physiologic (c)
 ❷ Loss of fat tissue on the soles of the feet coupled with the trauma of walking places the patient at risk for foot problems.
 ① With the decrease in muscle mass tendons shrink and sclerose, increasing muscle cramping.
 ③ Respiratory system changes of cilia atrophy and muscle strength reduction alter the body's ability to handle foreign particles and secretions, increasing susceptibility to infection.
 ④ Nocturia is related to reduced bladder muscle tone.

48. Application, evaluation, health (c)
 ❸ Questran Light can be mixed and stored in the refrigerator for up to three days. It should be mixed well each time before drinking.
 ① Questran Light can interfere with other medications, including thiazides. Medications should be taken 1 hour before or 4 to 6 hours after taking Questran Light.
 ② This medication should not be taken dry. It must be mixed with liquid, soups, pulpy fruits, or cereals.
 ④ Compliance is important; toxicity may result if doses are missed.

49. Application, implementation, psychosocial (b)
   ❶ Recent memory (24 hours to 1 week) may be impaired in an elderly patient. As the patient struggles to remember, responding just with the facts will help preserve her self-esteem.
   ②,③,④ All are inappropriate responses; they embarrass the patient and can decrease her self-esteem.
50. Application, planning, physiologic (b)
   ❸ The elderly with yellowing of the lens can see yellows, reds, and oranges best.
   ①,②,④ Lower color tones such as purples, pinks, greens, and blues are more difficult for the elderly to differentiate.
51. Application, planning, health (b)
   ❹ The elderly lose tastebud sensitivity, especially to salt and bitterness. Lemons or other spices can enhance food flavor.
   ① This may make food more appealing but will not affect its taste.
   ② Although frequent oral hygiene will rid the mouth of odors that can mask taste, it's not the appropriate interpretation of the patient's problem. Decreased saliva production is the physiological change for which frequent oral hygiene is recommended to reduce plaque building.
   ③ Although decreased sensitivity to salt occurs, adding excess salt to the food of a hypertensive patient is dangerous.
52. Comprehension, evaluation, environment (c)
   ❶ Difficulty managing personal finances indicates impaired cognition. Because of poor judgment the patient may make unwise financial decisions and have difficulty with bill paying and check-book balancing.
   ② The inability to perform minor tasks even though sensory and motor systems are intact is apraxia. It is evident in early Alzheimer's and is not a cognitive deficit.
   ③ This is visuospatial impairment.
   ④ Resistance to care is an abnormal behavior pattern, not a cognitive deficit.
53. Comprehension, assessment, psychosocial (c)
   ❸ In early Alzheimer's disease short-term memory, which spans a few minutes or hours, is impaired.
   ① This is an example of immediate memory, remembering for a few seconds, which is not impaired in early Alzheimer's.
   ② Long-term memory is preserved in early Alzheimer's.
   ④ This is benign forgetfulness, which is usually limited to trivial matters, tends to occur sporadically, is experienced by normal people, and is not associated with early Alzheimer's.
54. Comprehension, planning, health (b)
   ❹ 1500 mg is the standard dose for postmenopausal women. The elderly have a reduced ability to absorb dietary calcium and tend to excrete it more readily.
   ① 400 mg is required in the 0-6 month age category.
   ② 800 mg is required for children under 10 years of age.
   ③ 1200 mg is recommended for adolescents.

55. Comprehension, evaluation, health (c)
   ❷ Yogurt is an excellent source of calcium. An 8 oz container of plain yogurt made with low fat milk contains 415 mg of calcium. An 8 oz container made with non-fat milk contains 452 mg of calcium.
   ① Alcohol should be eliminated from the diet; it interfers with the metabolism of calcium.
   ③ Liver is not a good source of calcium. Three ounces of fried liver contains 9 mg of calcium.
   ④ Like alcohol, caffeine interferes with calcium metabolism and should be eliminated from the diet.
56. Application, evaluation, health (b)
   ❸ Regular weight-bearing exercise, preferably in the sunshine, 3 times a week, is the recommended measure for managing osteoporosis.
   ① Twice a week is under the recommended number; the walking should be done out in the sun whenever possible. The distractor does not indicate the time element.
   ② The sun enhances vitamin D production, which is necessary for calcium absorption and bone minimalizing action.
   ④ Dusting is not a weight-bearing exercise, which is needed for maintaining bone mass.
57. Application, planning, physiologic (c)
   ❶ An Ace bandage is used to shrink and shape the stump in preparation for prosthesis application.
   ④ The stump is elevated for 12 to 24 hours postoperatively to decrease edema. After 24 hours the stump is not elevated, to prevent hip flexion contractures.
   ② Diuretics promote urine excretion and will not reduce stump edema.
   ③ Dangling will place the limbs in a dependent position, creating further stump edema.
58. Knowledge, assessment, environment (a)
   ❶ Fever (pyrexia) would be the earliest indication of pathogen invasion.
   ② Although pain is a symptom of inflammation, there will be some postoperative pain that would not necessarily indicate infection.
   ③ Purulent drainage would indicate infection but usually is a later sign.
   ④ Swelling, although a symptom of inflammation, would be expected postoperatively and by itself would not necessarily indicate infection.
59. Application, evaluation, health (b)
   ❸ Residual limb care or controlling right limb edema could indicate successful wound healing.
   ① This would indicate impaired body image.
   ② This would indicate resolution of grieving.
   ④ This would indicate self-care independence.
60. Application, planning, environment (c)
   ❷ The swallowing disorder indicates the need for liquids; thick liquids are easiest to swallow.
   ① Thin liquids are difficult to swallow and place the patient at risk for potential respiratory problems.
   ③ The patient would be unable to safely ingest solid food.
   ④ Mechanical diets are ordered for patients with chewing problems. Parkinson's patients with a swallowing disorder require semiliquids and thick liquids.

Chapter 10   Emergency Nursing

This chapter emphasizes the nursing assessments and interventions essential to preserving the lives of victims of acute illness or injury. Rapid clinical assessment emphasizing airway, breathing, and circulation, establishment of care priorities, and implementation of lifesaving measures should be instituted until emergency medical care is available. The most serious and life-threatening injuries should be treated first, and all first aid measures carried out before transporting the victim(s).

Concurrent with emergency management is the practitioner's recognition and understanding of the victim's emotional state. The feelings of the victim's significant others should be acknowledged and responded to realistically, gently, and as expeditiously as possible.

Nurses should be familiar with the extent of protection and legal limitations of practice under the Good Samaritan Act, which varies from state to state.

The incidence of AIDS and hepatitis B indicates that nurses should consider all patients potentially infected; have access to equipment that minimizes the need for mouth-to-mouth, mouth-to-nose, and mouth-to-stoma resuscitation; and implement universal infection control precautions.

Current cardiopulmonary resuscitation literature raises the issues of cardiac pump theory versus thoracic pump theory; the effectiveness of abdominal compressions; and whether synchronized or interposed abdominal and chest compressions are more effective than chest compressions. No new cardiopulmonary resuscitation guidelines specific to these issues have been released by the American Heart Association as of the printing of this text.

Basic Life Support
ARTIFICIAL RESPIRATION

A. Simultaneously shake victim and shout to establish unconsciousness

B. Activate the EMS system (call 9-1-1) immediately when the victim is an adult; if an infant or child, call for help (even if you do not see anyone in the immediate vicinity), give 1 minute of CPR (20 cycles), check for pulse, and then activate EMS.

C. Quickly place victim in supine position

D. Establish airway using the head-tilt–chin-lift maneuver or head tilt–jaw thrust maneuver (Fig. 10-1) if additional forward displacement of the jaw is required; for patients with possible neck or spine injuries, use only jaw-thrust maneuver (Fig. 10-2)
   1. Infant: maintain neck in neutral position
   2. Child: maintain neck slightly further back

E. Put your ear near victim's mouth and look, listen, and feel for breathing

F. Commence mouth-to-mouth, mouth-to-nose, or mouth-to-stoma resuscitation by delivering two breaths (1½ to 2 sec/breath) at the lowest possible pressure

G. Allow for victim's exhalation between breaths by removing your mouth; check the carotid pulse (brachial for infant) for 5 seconds

H. In the presence of a pulse continue to deliver one breath every 5 seconds (12 breaths/min) for the adult and every 3 seconds (20 breaths/min) for the infant and for a child until breathing is restored (rescue breathing)

CARDIOPULMONARY RESUSCITATION (CPR)

A. Follow steps A to G above; be sure victim is on a firm surface

B. In the absence of a pulse, place the heel of one hand on top of the other two finger-breadths above the victim's xiphoid process (Fig. 10-3)
   1. Child (1 to 8 years old): place heel of one hand two finger-breadths above the end of the sternum and deliver 100 compressions per minute
   2. Infant (less than 1 year old): place two fingers one finger-breadth below an imaginary line drawn between the nipples and deliver 100 compressions per minute

C. Compress the **adult** sternum 1½ to 2 inches for 15 compressions; then deliver two breaths

D. Compress the sternum of the **child** 1 to 1½ inches for 5 compressions; then deliver one breath

E. Compress the **infant** sternum ½ to 1 inch for 5 compressions; then deliver one breath

F. Continue the 15 compressions and two breaths sequence in the adult: 5 compressions and one breath sequence for infants and children

G. With two rescuers present for an **adult** deliver 5 compressions and one breath

H. Check the carotid pulse:
   1. After four cycles of 15:2 (1 minute) in the *adult* with one rescuer
   2. After 10 cycles of 5:1 (1 minute) in the *adult* with two rescuers
   3. After 20 cycles of 5:1 (1 minute) in the *child*

I. Check the brachial pulse after 20 cycles of 5:1 (1 minute) in the *infant*

J. If no pulse, resume CPR. If there is a pulse but no breathing, resume artificial respiration (rescue breathing)

HEIMLICH MANEUVER

The Heimlich maneuver is used for management of foreign body airway obstruction (FBAO). Do not interfere if victim can cough, speak, or breathe

A. Conscious adult victim
   1. Stand behind the victim, encircle his or her waist with your arms, place your fist above the umbilicus and

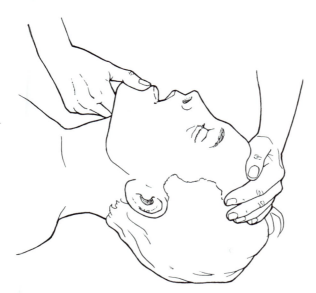

Fig. 10-1.   **Head-tilt–jaw-thrust maneuver.** Pull mandible forward using thumb and forefingers. (From Sheehy SB: *Emergency nursing: principles and practice,* ed 3, St. Louis, 1992, Mosby.)

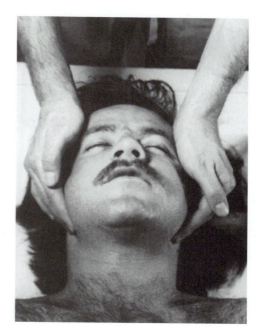

Fig. 10-2.   **Jaw-thrust maneuver.** (Photo by Richard Lazar.) (From Sheehy SB: *Emergency nursing: principles and practice,* ed 3, St Louis, 1992, Mosby.)

below the xiphoid process with your thumb against victim's abdomen; grasp your fist with your other hand and apply pressure with an inward and quick upward motion (Fig. 10-4)
2. Repeat the thrusts until the obstruction is relieved, or switch to procedure for conscious victim who loses consciousness
B. Conscious adult victim who loses consciousness
1. Place victim in supine position, call for help, and activate Emergency Medical Service (EMS)
2. Perform tongue-jaw lift and carefully sweep your curved finger in one direction along the back of the victim's throat to retrieve object
3. Establish airway using the head-tilt–chin-lift maneuver
4. Deliver two breaths
5. Kneel at level of victim's hips or straddle victim to deliver 5 abdominal thrusts by placing the heel of one hand above the umbilicus and below the xiphoid process; place your second hand on top of the first hand and apply pressure with an inward and upward motion

6. Perform the tongue-jaw lift and carefully sweep curved finger in one direction along the back of the victim's throat to retrieve object
7. Establish airway using the head-tilt–chin-lift maneuver
8. Attempt to ventilate: deliver one breath
9. Continue repeating abdominal thrusts, finger sweeps, and breathing attempts in rapid sequence
C. Unconscious adult victim
1. Simultaneously shake victim and shout to establish unconsciousness
2. Activate EMS
3. Quickly place victim in supine position
4. Establish airway using the head-tilt–chin-lift maneuver
5. Put your ear near victim's mouth and look, listen, and feel for breathing
6. Deliver two breaths
7. If unable to ventilate, reposition head and again attempt to deliver two breaths
8. Repeat steps 5 to 8 of *conscious adult victim who loses consciousness* until effective

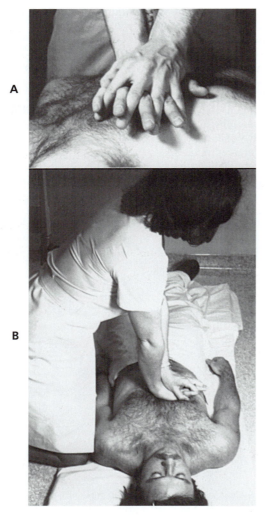

Fig. 10-3. **A,** Hand position for chest compression: no weight on fingers. **B,** Body position for CPR. Rescuer should be kneeling, with knees slightly separated and elbows in straight, locked position. (Photos by Richard Lazar.) (From Sheehy SB: *Emergency nursing: principles and practice,* ed 3, St Louis, 1992, Mosby.)

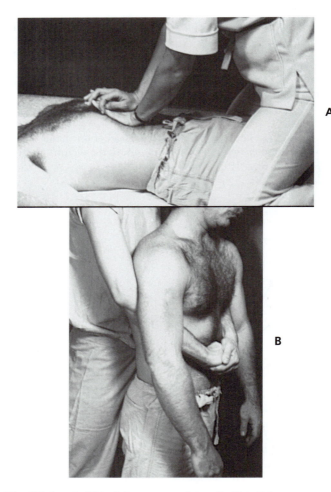

Fig. 10-4. **A,** Heimlich maneuver, lying. **B,** Heimlich maneuver, standing. (Photos by Richard Lazar.) (From Sheehy SB: *Emergency nursing: principles and practice,* ed 3, St Louis, 1992, Mosby.)

D. Child
1. Same as adult, except
2. Provide 1 minute of rescue support, then activate EMS
3. Do not perform finger sweeps; use tongue-jaw lift and remove object only if visualized
E. Obese victim and later stages of pregnancy
1. Conscious victim: deliver chest thrusts (place thumb side of fist on middle of breast bone) until foreign body is expelled or victim becomes unconscious
2. Unconscious victim
   a. Deliver chest thrusts with victim in supine position by placing heel of hand on lower half of sternum with other hand on top (CPR position)
   b. Follow Heimlich maneuver, finger sweep, ventilate sequence
F. Conscious infant
1. Supporting head and neck, position infant face down with head lower than trunk along rescuer's forearm
2. Administer 5 back blows between the shoulder blades with heel of hand
3. Continue to support head and turn infant over, keeping head lower than trunk
4. Compression location is directly below the point where the sternum is bisected by an imaginary line between the nipples
5. Administer 5 chest thrusts with the ring and middle fingers
6. Continue to administer back blows and chest thrusts until airway is cleared or infant becomes unconscious
G. Conscious infant who loses consciousness
1. Place in supine position, call for help, and activate EMS
2. Perform tongue-jaw lift and remove object only if you see it (do not perform finger sweeps)
3. Establish airway using the head-tilt–chin-lift maneuver
4. Attempt to deliver two breaths; if unable to ventilate, reposition head and repeat
5. Administer 5 back blows
6. Administer 5 chest thrusts
7. Perform tongue-jaw lift and remove object only if you see it
8. Establish airway using head-tilt–chin-lift maneuver and deliver two breaths
9. Continue repeating back blows, chest thrusts, tongue-jaw lift, and breathing until effective
H. Unconscious infant
1. Simultaneously shake and tap victim to establish unconsciousness
2. Call for help even if you do not see anyone in the immediate vicinity
3. Quickly place infant in supine position while supporting the head and neck
4. Establish airway using head-tilt–chin-lift maneuver but do not tilt too far
5. Put your ear near victim's mouth and look, listen, and feel for breathing
6. Administer two breaths
7. If unable to ventilate, reposition head and again deliver two breaths
8. Activate EMS
9. Administer five back blows
10. Administer five chest thrusts

11. Perform tongue-jaw lift and remove object only if you see it
12. Attempt to ventilate
13. Repeat steps 9 through 12 until effective

Hemorrhage

A. Description: loss of a large amount of blood in a short period of time either externally or internally
B. Types
1. Venous: dark color; steady flow
2. Arterial: bright color; spurts
3. Capillary: red; oozes
C. Assessment
1. Restlessness
2. Anxiety
3. Rapid, weak pulse
4. Cool, moist, pale skin
5. Rapid respirations
6. Thirst
7. Nausea/vomiting
8. Alteration in level of consciousness
9. Hypotension
10. If bleeding is internal (within a cavity or joint), pain will develop because the cavity is stretched by increasing blood volume
D. Intervention: external
1. Apply direct pressure with a clean cloth for at least 6 minutes (use gloves if available)
2. Elevate injured part above heart level
3. If arterial bleeding does not respond to direct pressure, attempt to control by applying direct pressure on supply artery (Fig. 10-5)
4. Tourniquets are not recommended unless an extremity is amputated or severely mutilated
   a. Leave tourniquet exposed
   b. Tag or label victim with location of tourniquet
   c. Apply proximal to wound
   d. Tourniquet should not be removed except by a physician
5. Cover victim to maintain body temperature; maintain supine position
6. Treat for shock and transport immediately
E. Intervention: internal
1. Cover victim to maintain body temperature
2. Keep in supine position
3. Monitor VS
4. Treat for shock and transport immediately
F. Usual medical care:
1. Replacement of fluids intravenously to expand blood volume
2. Blood transfusions
3. Locate source of and stop hemorrhage

EPISTAXIS (NOSEBLEED)
A. Description: bleeding from the nose caused by trauma, local irritation, violent sneezing, or chronic conditions such as hypertension
B. Assessment: obvious bleeding from one or both nares (most often unilateral)
C. Intervention
1. Sit victim upright, head slightly forward to prevent swallowing blood

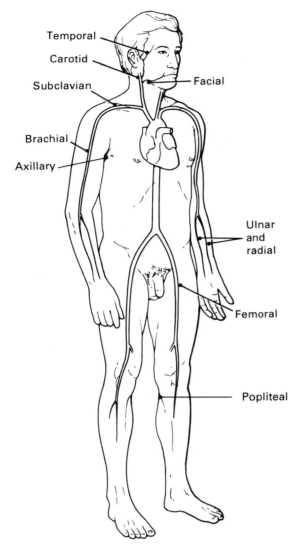

Fig. 10-5. Pressure points for control of hemorrhage. (From Lewis SM, Collier IC: *Medical-surgical nursing: assessment and management of clinical problems,* ed 3, St Louis, 1992, Mosby.)

2. Apply firm, continuous pressure (pinch nose) using thumb and forefinger
3. Ice compress to nose
4. Limit activity; avoid drinking hot or cold liquids
5. Monitor vital signs
D. Usual medical care
1. Nasal pack soaked in a topical vasoconstrictor
2. Cauterization (silver nitrate or electrocautery)

Shock
A. Description: depressed state of vital body functions that, if untreated, could result in death
B. Types: (3 basic types) (Box 10-1)
1. Hypovolemic: primarily a fluid problem caused by a loss of blood or fluid volume (for example: hemorrhage, severe burns, trauma, or dehydration)
2. Cardiogenic: faulty pumping action resulting in reduced cardiac output (for example: myocardial infarction, cardiomyopathy, or diseases of the heart valve)

3. Vasogenic or distributive: a vascular problem or disturbance in tissue perfusion caused by alteration in circulating blood volumes (vasculature dilatation); 3 types are as follows:
   a. Septic: massive bacterial infection resulting in release of endotoxin that causes vasodilatation (e.g., gram-negative organisms)
   b. Neurogenic or spinal: disruption of arterioles and venules resulting in a decrease of circulating blood volume (e.g., spinal cord injury)
   c. Anaphylaxis: severe allergic reaction resulting in histamine release, increased capillary permeability with eventual dilatation of arterioles and venules
C. Assessment: determination of the exact cause is vital to patient survival
1. Shallow, rapid respirations
2. Cool, pale, clammy skin
3. Thirst
4. Tachycardia
5. Decreased blood pressure
6. Weak, thready pulse
7. Restlessness
8. Decreased urine output
9. May become confused or disoriented
D. Intervention: isolation of cause determines specific intervention strategies, which include:
1. Ensure adequate airway and ventilation
2. Control bleeding if present
3. Place in supine position with legs elevated unless contraindicated (e.g., head injuries)
4. Insert urinary catheter
5. Monitor vital signs
6. Cover victim to conserve body heat
7. Remain with victim if possible
E. Usual medical care
1. IV fluids
2. Administer oxygen
3. Medications depending on the type of shock

Anaphylactic Reaction
A. Description: a type of vasogenic or distributive shock (see above)
B. Assessment
1. Pallor
2. Diaphoresis
3. Tachycardia or bradycardia
4. Hypotension
5. Wheezing, dyspnea
6. Anxiety, restlessness
7. Urticaria
8. Edema
9. Pruritus
10. Rash
11. Possible respiratory distress
12. Diffuse erythema
C. Intervention
1. Ensure adequate airway and ventilation
2. Elevate feet slightly unless contraindicated (e.g., head injuries)
D. Usual medical care
1. Administer oxygen
2. Epinephrine

Box 10-1. Causes of Shock

Hypovolemic
External major bleeding
Hemothorax
Hemoperitoneum
Fractures
Gastrointestinal bleeding
Major vomiting
Major diarrhea
Major diaphoresis
Renal failure
Excessive diuretic use
Fluid loss from diabetes
Burns
Ascites

Cardiogenic
Myocardial infarction
Cardiomyopathy
Cardiac contusion
Dysrhythmias
Diseases of heart valve

Distributive
Sepsis
Anaphylaxis
Spinal cord injury
Overdose
Anoxia

Adapted from Sheehy S.: *Emergency nursing principles and practice,* ed 3, St Louis, 1992, Mosby.

3. Antihistamines
4. Steroids
5. IV fluids
6. Drug therapy for cardiovascular support
E. Preventive measures
 1. Allergy history
 2. Medical identification tag for high-risk persons
 3. Sting emergency medical kits
 4. Skin testing when possible
 5. Question previous allergic reactions before administering medications

Head Injuries

Traumatic damage to the head from blunt or penetrating trauma resulting in scalp, skull, and brain injuries

Scalp Injury

Type	Intervention
Abrasion	Wash with soap and water
Hematoma	Apply ice
Laceration	Stop bleeding by compression (only if no depression is present)
	Shave around laceration
	Cleanse wound
	Suture

SKULL FRACTURE

A. Simple: linear crack in surface of skull with no displacement of bone
 1. Observation for alteration of respiration, vision, level of consciousness, pupils (dilated, fixed, pinpoint), motor strength, and speech
 2. X-ray examination
B. Depressed: skull fracture with depressed bone fragments resulting in a "pressed-in" appearance
 1. Intervention
  a. Ensure adequate airway and ventilation
  b. Administer oxygen
  c. Control bleeding
  d. Treat for shock
  e. Observe for alteration of respiration, vision, level of consciousness, pupils (dilated, fixed, pinpoint), motor strength, and speech
  f. Maintain body temperature
  g. Protect cervical spine
  h. Monitor vital signs
 2. Usual medical care
  a. Surgical intervention
  b. Antibiotic therapy
C. Basilar: fracture located along base of skull
 1. Assessment
  a. Periorbital ecchymosis (black eyes)
  b. Cerebrospinal fluid (CSF) leak from nose or ear
  c. Ecchymosis behind ears (Battle's sign)
  d. Blood behind eardrum (hemotympanum)
 2. Intervention: observe for alterations of respiration, vision, level of consciousness, pupils (dilated, fixed, pinpoint), motor strength, and speech; monitor vital signs; if CSF leak noted, *do not* attempt to stop; apply a loose bulky dressing over area; protect cervical spine
 3. Usual medical care
  a. X-ray examination (although usually not visible)
  b. Antibiotic therapy if CSF leak is present

BRAIN INJURY

A. Concussion: temporary alteration of neurologic functioning caused by a blow to the head, which results in jarring of the brain
 1. Assessment
  a. Nausea and vomiting
  b. Headache
  c. Possible brief period of unconsciousness and memory loss
  d. Possible skull fracture
  e. Confusion
 2. Intervention
  a. Observe for alteration of respiration, vision, level of consciousness, pupils (dilated, fixed, pinpoint), and motor strength
  b. Administer nonnarcotic analgesics as ordered
  c. Maintain hydration
  d. Protect cervical spine
B. Contusion: brain surface bruise resulting in structural alteration
 1. Assessment
  a. Nausea and vomiting
  b. Visual alterations (diplopia)
  c. Neurologic alterations (ataxia, confusion)

2. Intervention
   a. Maintenance of adequate airway and ventilation
   b. Observation
   c. Protect cervical spine
   d. Monitor vital signs
3. Usual medical care
   a. Hospitalization
   b. Antiemetics
C. Intracranial bleeding: hemorrhage or bleeding within the cranial vault
  1. Assessment
   a. Epidural (extradural) hematoma; bleeding between skull and dura mater; short period of unconsciousness followed by consciousness; severe headache, hemiparesis if conscious, bradycardia, and increased blood pressure
   b. Subdural hematoma; bleeding between dura mater and arachnoid membrane; can be acute or chronic; loss of consciousness, fixed dilated pupils, hemiparesis, and positive Babinski's sign
   c. Subarachnoid hematoma; bleeding between arachnoid membrane and the pia mater: severe headache, nausea and vomiting, delirium, syncope, or coma
  2. Intervention
   a. Maintenance of adequate airway and ventilation
   b. Administer oxygen
   c. Monitor vital signs
   d. Protect cervical spine
   e. Observe for alterations of respiration, vision, level of consciousness, pupils (dilated, fixed, pinpoint), and decreased motor strength (signs of increased ICP [intracranial pressure])
   f. Maintain body temperature
   g. Treat for shock
  3. Usual medical care
   a. Hospitalization
   b. CT scan
   c. Possible surgery

Eye Injuries

FOREIGN BODY IN EYE
A. Evert eyelid
B. Touch particle gently with sterile swab moistened in sterile saline solution or water (do not remove if particle is on the cornea or if there is eyeball penetration)
C. Apply an eye patch after ensuring that the eye is closed

FOREIGN BODY IN CONJUCTIVA
A. Invert eyelid
B. Remove particle as described above
C. Irrigate with saline solution or water
D. Eye patch may be applied

EYELID CONTUSION (BLACK EYE)
A. Cold compresses or ice pack intermittently for the first 24 hours
B. Warm compresses after 48 hours
C. Bilateral eye patches if intraocular hemorrhage is present

CORNEAL ABRASION
A. Assessment
  1. Pain

2. Photosensitivity
3. Spasms of the eyelid
4. Tearing
B. Intervention: apply eye patch to injured eye
C. Usual medical care: local ophthalmic antibiotics

BURNS
A. Chemical
  1. If action of chemical is not enhanced by water, immediately flush area with copious amounts of normal saline solution or tap water for 15 minutes (damage increases with length of chemical contact)
  2. Usual medical care: topical application of antibiotics, administration of cycloplegic agents, or corticosteroids (alkali burns)
  3. The following solutions will neutralize the following types of burns
   a. Acid: sodium bicarbonate 2% solution
   b. Lime: ammonium tartrate 5% solution
   c. Alkali: boric or citric acid solution
B. Thermal (usually occurs with facial burns)
  1. Irrigate with normal saline solution or tap water
  2. Apply bilateral eye patches
  3. Usual medical care: analgesia, sedation, antibiotics, cycloplegics
C. Radiation
  1. Types
   a. Ultraviolet (sun)–severity depends on period of exposure
   b. Infrared (x-rays)–severity depends on wavelength and period of exposure (may cause loss of vision)
  2. Assessment
   a. Excessive blinking
   b. Tearing
   c. Feeling that something is in the eye
   d. Pain
  3. Intervention
   a. Cold compresses
   b. Bilateral eye patches
  4. Usual medical care
   a. Topical antibiotics
   b. Cycloplegics
   c. Analgesics

PENETRATING INJURIES
A. Place a protective shield, such as a paper cup, over the eye to prevent further damage by pressure (Fig. 10-6)
B. Apply eye patch to the uninjured eye
C. See an ophthalmologist immediately

Spinal Cord Injuries (Table 10-1)
A. Assessment
  1. Pain, tenderness
  2. Numbness, tingling, paralysis
  3. Weakness of extremities
  4. Alterations of sensation and motor function below level of injury
  5. Possible signs and symptoms of shock
B. Intervention
  1. Ensure adequate airway and ventilation; if helmet is on victim, leave it in place if airway is accessible
  2. Treat for shock

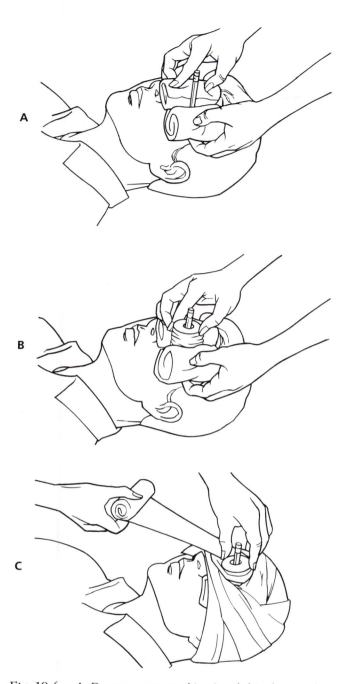

Table 10-1	Cervical Spine and Spinal Cord Lesions and Resultant Physiologic Function	
Lesion	**Resultant function**	
C3, C4, or above	Respiratory arrest; flaccid paralysis; quadriplegia	
C5, C6	Reduced respiratory effort; almost total dependence; flaccid paralysis; quadriplegia	
C7	Reduced respiratory effort; almost total dependence; splints necessary for functioning of forearms; quadriplegia	
T1	Reduced respiratory effort; partial dependence; paraplegia	
T1, T2	Reduced respiratory effort; complete independence; paraplegia	
T7	Complete independence; walking with long-leg braces; paraplegia	
L4	Complete independence; walking with foot braces; paraplegia	

From Sheehy SB: *Emergency nursing: principles and practice*, ed 3, St Louis, 1992, Mosby.

Fig. 10-6. **A,** Do not remove an object impaled in the eye. Place sterile dressings around the object. **B,** Support the object with a paper cup and carefully bandage the cup in place. **C,** Cover the other eye to keep blood, fluid, and dirt out. (Courtesy American Red Cross: *First aid: responding to emergencies,* St Louis, 1991, Mosby.)

Neck Injuries
SOFT TISSUE NECK INJURIES
FRACTURED LARYNX
A. Assessment
   1. Hoarse voice
   2. Cough with hemoptysis
   3. Difficulty breathing; respiratory distress
   4. Subcutaneous emphysema
B. Intervention
   1. Administer oxygen
   2. Observation
C. Usual medical care
   1. Emergency cricothyrotomy or tracheostomy
   2. Broad-spectrum antibiotics

PENETRATING NECK WOUNDS
A. Assessment
   1. Noticeable penetrating wound
   2. Airway obstruction
   3. Signs and symptoms of hypovolemia, hemathorax, or shock
B. Intervention
   1. Ensure adequate airway and ventilation
   2. Control bleeding
   3. Surgery

Chest Injuries
FRACTURED RIB (SIMPLE, UNDISPLACED)
A. Assessment
   1. Chest pain (increases on inspiration), tenderness
   2. Shortness of breath, shallow breathing
   3. Tachycardia
   4. Hypotension
   5. Ecchymosis
B. Intervention (individualized)

   3. Immobilization (movement may cause further damage)
   4. Maintain body temperature
   5. When help (EMS) arrives, place victim on board without flexing neck or back
   6. Transport immediately (EMS)

1. Rest
2. Apply heat locally
3. Observe for signs and symptoms of pneumothorax by monitoring breathing patterns and lung sounds
4. Encourage deep breathing
5. Administer analgesics sparingly

FLAIL CHEST

A. Fracture of several ribs resulting in loss of chest wall stability; pulmonary or myocardial contusion may also be present because of force of injury; may be life threatening
B. Assessment
   1. Pain
   2. Difficulty breathing
   3. Shallow, rapid, noisy respirations
   4. Chest moves in opposite from normal direction: moves in on inspiration, out on expiration
   5. Tachycardia and cyanosis
   6. Possible bruising
C. Intervention
   1. Ensure adequate airway and ventilation
   2. Stabilization of chest wall
   3. Application of pressure dressing
   4. Position victim on affected side in semi-Fowler's position
   5. Monitor vital signs and lung sounds
D. Usual medical care
   1. Pain control
   2. Possible intubation and ventilation with severe flail
   3. Possible traction

SIMPLE PNEUMOTHORAX

A. Description: air enters the pleural cavity; negative pressure is lost resulting in partial or total lung collapse
B. Assessment
   1. Chest pain
   2. Shortness of breath (SOB) and tachypnea
   3. Decreased breath sounds
C. Intervention
   1. Ensure adequate airway and ventilation
   2. Place victim in semi-Fowler's position
   3. Administer oxygen
D. Usual medical care: possible chest tube placement

TENSION PNEUMOTHORAX

A. Description: air enters the pleural cavity on inspiration and is trapped during exhalation, creating pressure that causes eventual collapse of the lung (same side) resulting in a life-threatening condition in which there is mediastinal shift that compresses the heart, great vessels, and the trachea as well as the opposite lung
B. Assessment
   1. Extreme shortness of breath
   2. Observed tracheal deviation
   3. Paradoxic movement of the chest
   4. Neck vein distention
   5. Hypotension
   6. Tachycardia
   7. Restlessness
   8. Cyanosis
   9. Distant breath sounds
   10. History of chest trauma
C. Intervention
   1. Ensure adequate airway, breathing, and circulation

2. Administer oxygen
D. Usual medical care
   1. Needle thoracotomy
   2. Chest tube placement
   3. Intravenous fluids

OPEN PNEUMOTHORAX (SUCKING CHEST WOUND)

A. Description: presence of air in the chest resulting from an open wound in the chest wall
   1. One-way flap: air enters pleural space but cannot escape (tension pneumothorax)
   2. Two-way flap: air enters and leaves pleural space
B. Assessment
   1. Audible sucking noise
   2. Shortness of breath
   3. Chest pain
   4. Cyanosis
   5. Shock
   6. Possible signs and symptoms of tension pneumothorax
C. Intervention
   1. Ensure adequate airway, breathing, and circulation
   2. Cover wound with air-tight dressing (depends on size of wound)
   3. Administer oxygen
   4. CPR may be necessary
D. Usual medical care
   1. Chest tube placement
   2. Antibiotic therapy
   3. Treat for shock

SPONTANEOUS PNEUMOTHORAX

A. Description: presence of air in the intrapleural space resulting from rupture of lung tissue and visceral pleura with no evidence of trauma; can occur during periods of strenuous physical activity
B. Assessment
   1. Sudden, sharp chest pain
   2. Shortness of breath
   3. Diaphoresis
   4. Anxiety
   5. Hypotension
   6. Tachycardia
   7. Cessation of normal chest movement on affected side
C. Intervention
   1. Ensure adequate airway and ventilation
   2. Keep victim quiet
   3. Place in semi- or high-Fowler's position
D. Usual medical care
   1. Needle aspiration
   2. Chest tube
   3. IV fluids
   4. Oxygen

HEMOTHORAX

A. Description: blood in the pleural space from traumatic injury (stabbing) or rupture of congenital blebs
B. Assessment
   1. Chest pain
   2. Shortness of breath
   3. Distant breath sounds
   4. Anxiety
   5. Shock
   6. Cyanosis

C. Intervention
 1. Ensure adequate airway and ventilation
 2. Treat for shock
D. Usual medical care: chest tube placement; thoracentesis

PULMONARY EMBOLISM

A. Description: thrombus becomes detached and lodges in a branch of the pulmonary artery causing a partial or total occlusion resulting in a pulmonary infarct; commonly seen with trauma, surgery, or long-bone fractures
B. Assessment
 1. Sudden, sharp chest pain
 2. Shortness of breath
 3. Pallor, possible cyanosis
 4. Anxiety
 5. Tachycardia
 6. Rapid, shallow respirations (tachypnea)
 7. Possible hypotension, elevated temperature
 8. Possible cough, wheeze, hemoptysis
 9. Possible sudden death if large blood vessel is blocked
C. Intervention
 1. Ensure adequate airway, breathing, and circulation
 2. Treat for shock
 3. Administer oxygen
 4. Keep victim quiet
 5. Place patient in semi- to high-Fowler's position if vital signs permit
D. Usual medical care
 1. Anticoagulant therapy
 2. IV fluids
 3. Surgical intervention in cases of profound shock or cardiovascular collapse

Intraabdominal Injuries

PENETRATING WOUND

A. Description: wounds resulting from stabbings, shootings, impalement
B. Assessment
 1. Hypotension
 2. Shock
 3. Diminished bowel sounds
 4. Pain
 5. Tenderness
 6. Progressive abdominal distention
 7. Nausea or vomiting
C. Intervention
 1. Do not move victim
 2. Ensure adequate airway, breathing, circulation
 3. Control bleeding
   a. Look for entrance and exit wounds
   b. Apply compression for external bleeding
   c. Look for chest injuries
 4. Cover wounds with wet, sterile, or nonadhesive dressing(s) (e.g., saline or plastic wrap)
 5. Monitor vital signs
 6. Treat for shock
 7. Keep victim NPO
D. Usual medical care
 1. IVs
 2. Oxygen
 3. Tetanus prophylaxis
 4. Antibiotics
 5. Analgesics

 6. Indwelling catheter
 7. Nasogastric tube
 8. X-ray examination
 9. Possible surgery

BLUNT WOUND

A. Description: wounds resulting from a motor vehicle accident (MVA), contact sport injury, falls, or physical abuse (domestic violence)
B. Assessment
 1. Observable bruises and abrasions
 2. Abdominal pain, rigidity, palpable masses, or distention
 3. Signs and symptoms of shock
 4. Guarding
 5. Diminished bowel sounds
C. Intervention
 1. Do not move victim
 2. Ensure adequate airway, breathing, circulation
 3. Observe for hemorrhage
 4. Observe for chest injuries
 5. Monitor vital signs
 6. Treat for shock
D. Usual medical care
 1. Oxygen
 2. Nasogastric tube
 3. X-ray examination
 4. Peritoneal lavage
 5. Possible surgery

Burns

A. Depth of Classification

Depth	Degree	Assessment
Superficial partial thickness (involves only the epidermis)	1st	Pain; red; minimal or no edema
Deep partial thickness (involves epidermis and part of the dermis)	2nd	Pain; mottled color; blistering; edema; wet appearance
Full thickness (involves epidermis and damage to subcutaneous layer, muscle and bone)	3rd	Gray, white, brown, leathery, or charred appearance; edema; minor or no pain

B. Surface Area Classification
 1. The greater the body surface area (BSA) affected, the more serious the damage
 2. Use rule of nines (Fig. 10-7) to estimate percent of BSA affected

MAJOR BURNS

A. Burns are considered major or critical if they fulfill the following criteria
 1. Deep partial thickness burns: greater than 25% body surface area (BSA) in adults: greater than 20% in children under 10 and adults older than 40 years of age
 2. Full thickness burns: greater than 10% BSA in adults and children
 3. Electrical burns
 4. Burns involving face, eyes, ears, hands, feet, and perineum
 5. Burns in victims with preexisting chronic conditions (diabetes, cardiac conditions, renal failure)
B. Intervention

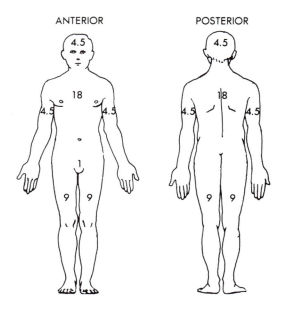

ANTERIOR   POSTERIOR

Fig. 10-7. Rule of nines is used to estimate amount of skin surface burned. (From Phipps WJ et al, eds: *Medical-surgical nursing: concepts and clinical practice,* ed 5, St Louis, 1995, Mosby.)

1. Lay victim flat (standing forces him or her to breathe flames and smoke; running fans flames)
2. Roll victim in carpet or blankets or use water to extinguish fire
3. Remove any smoldering clothing that is nonadherent
4. Ensure adequate airway and ventilation
5. Administer oxygen
6. Assess for inhalation burns
7. Remove nonadherent, tight-fitting clothing
8. Remove tight jewelry
9. Apply cold soaks
10. Cover burns with moist, sterile dressings or clean cloth
11. Elevate affected parts if possible
12. Cover victim
13. Insert indwelling catheter
14. Treat burned areas as ordered by physician
C. Usual medical care
   1. Tetanus prophylaxis
   2. Central venous pressure line
   3. Pain management
   4. Nasogastric tube
   5. Reverse isolation
   6. Intravenous therapy
   7. Antibiotic therapy
D. Warnings
   1. *Do not use salves, ointments, or oils*
   2. *Do not soak large burns unless you can maintain body warmth*
   3. *Do not use ice or ice water on deep partial- or full-thickness burns; causes further injury and promotes hypothermia*

CHEMICAL BURNS
A. Powdered chemicals: sweep off skin
B. Nonpowered chemicals: irrigate with copious amounts of water or saline solution

C. Cover loosely with a clean cloth
D. Usual medical care: treated as thermal burns (cleanse wound, open blisters and remove outer layer, apply topical antibacterial agent)

ELECTRICAL BURNS
A. Assessment
   1. Discoloration
   2. Edema
   3. Cardiac irregularities
   4. Entrance and exit sites of current visible
   5. Confusion
   6. Unconsciousness
   7. Respiratory distress
B. Intervention
   1. Do not touch the victim
   2. Remove electrical source with a nonconductor or shut off current source
   3. If victim has no pulse and is not breathing, institute cardiopulmonary resuscitation
   4. Extremeties should be handled minimally and with extreme caution
   5. Check victim for other injuries
   6. Monitor cardiac and renal function

RADIATION BURNS
A. Intervention
   1. Remove contaminated clothing
   2. Apply cool, moist compresses
B. Usual medical care: possibly antipyretics

SMOKE INHALATION
A. Assessment
   1. History
   2. Singed hair in nares
   3. Mouth burns
   4. Brassy cough
   5. Respiratory distress
   6. Rales, rhonchi, or wheezes
   7. Restlessness
   8. Cyanosis
B. Intervention
   1. Ensure adequate airway and ventilation
   2. Administer oxygen
   3. Be prepared to initiate cardiopulmonary resuscitation
C. Usual medical care
   1. Hospitalization for 24 to 48 hours
   2. IV fluids
   3. Chest physical therapy
   4. Possible endotrachial intubation or tracheostomy
   5. Use of bronchodilators, steroids
   6. Nasogastric tube

Wounds

A. Open (break in skin integrity)
   1. Laceration: jagged cut through the skin and underlying tissue
   2. Abrasion: skin scrape or "brush burn"
   3. Avulsion: flap of skin and subcutaneous tissue torn loose
   4. Puncture: tissue penetration by a sharp object
   5. Abscess: localized pus formation
B. Closed (no break in skin integrity; e.g., contusion): injury to underlying tissue by blunt object

C. General management
  1. Stop bleeding
    a. Apply pressure dressing
    b. Elevate affected part
    c. Use digital pressure on supply artery
    d. Apply tourniquet only as a lifesaving measure and leave tourniquet visible
  2. Treat shock
  3. Control infection
    a. Wounds requiring medical care: it is generally recommended not to clean them until they are seen by a physician
    b. Cover open wounds with a clean, nonadhesive dressing
    c. Apply ice during the first 24 to 48 hours for closed wounds
    d. Minor wounds being treated at home: clean well with soap and water; thoroughly rinse; approximate wound edges with adhesive; cover with a clean dressing; seek medical care for signs of infection
  4. Puncture wounds
    a. Impaled object should be stabilized and left in place
    b. Medical attention should be sought
D. Special wounds
  1. Human bites
    a. May be self-inflicted or inflicted by another; evidenced by teeth marks and often by knuckle lacerations (occurs when fist hits another person's teeth during a fight)
    b. Intervention
      (1) Clean with soap and water
      (2) Rinse thoroughly
      (3) Apply clean dressing
      (4) Keep injured part elevated
    c. Usual medical care
      (1) Tetanus prophylaxis
      (2) Antibiotic therapy
      (3) Observe closely for systemic responses to bite: toxic shock syndrome, hepatitis, HIV (occurs during healing phase or post injury)
  2. Animal bites: potential for contracting rabies must be seriously considered with any animal bite
    a. Dog bites are most common, causing crushing injury to skin and underlying tissue or avulsion injuries should the victim attempt to pull away
    b. Cat bites are more likely to cause puncture wounds
    c. Intervention
      (1) Obtain history of bite
      (2) Clean minor wounds with soap and water
      (3) Rinse thoroughly
      (4) Flush with povidone-iodine (Betadine) or other cleansing solutions (hydrogen peroxide) if allergic to Betadine
      (5) Apply clean dressing
      NOTE: major wounds (severe bleeding) require control of bleeding and medical attention
    d. Usual medical care
      (1) Antibiotic therapy for large, contaminated bites
      (2) Tetanus prophylaxis
      (3) Rabies prophylaxis if necessary
  3. Snakebites
    a. Assessment
      (1) Teeth marks; possibly fang marks
      (2) Edema
      (3) Pain
      (4) Ecchymosis
      (5) Bleeding
      (6) Numbness of affected part
    b. Intervention
      (1) Have victim lie quietly in shaded area
      (2) Clean wound
      (3) Suction
        (a) Do not use mouth suction if you have open sores in your mouth
        (b) Suction wound using snakebite kit
        (c) Use mouth suction only if no other means is available
      (4) Apply clean dressing
      (5) Immobilize affected limb
      (6) Affected limb should be in dependent position
    c. Usual medical care
      (1) Analgesics
      (2) IV fluids
      (3) Tetanus prophylaxis
      (4) Antivenom therapy
  4. Insect bites (bees, wasps, hornets)
    a. Assessment
      (1) Obtain detailed medical and activity history
      (2) Pruritus
      (3) Burning
      (4) Swelling
    b. Intervention
      (1) Remove the stinger by scraping; do not pull out because this releases more toxin; do not squeeze
      (2) Clean with soap and water
      (3) Apply ice (DO NOT apply heat)
      (4) Apply ammonia diluted with warm water or a paste of baking soda and water
    c. Usual medical care
      (1) Epinephrine
      (2) Antihistamines
      (3) Steroids
  5. Tick
    a. Attaches to host with its teeth
    b. Releases a toxin that may cause tick paralysis or Lyme disease
    c. Squeezing tick releases more toxin
    d. If paralysis progresses to bulbar, respiratory failure and subsequent death may occur
    e. Paralysis will disappear after tick is removed
    f. Intervention
      (1) Grasp tick with tweezers and pull slowly and steadily (Fig. 10-8)
      (2) Wash with soap and water
      (3) Seek medical treatment

Fracture

A. Description: a complete or incomplete break in bone continuity
  1. Fracture without displacement presents normal alignment despite the fracture
  2. Fracture with displacement presents a separation of bone fragments at fracture site
  3. Compound or open: bone protrusion through skin
  4. Simple or closed: no bone protrusion through the skin
  5. Incomplete: part of bone is broken
  6. Complete: breakage producing two fragments

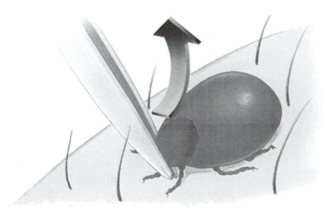

Fig. 10-8. Remove a tick by pulling steadily and firmly with fine-tipped tweezers. (Courtesy American Red Cross: *First aid: responding to emergencies,* St Louis, 1991, Mosby.)

B. Types of fractures (Box 10-2)
C. Assessment
   1. Five *P*s (*p*ain, *p*allor, *p*ulses, *p*aresthesia, and *p*aralysis)
   2. Discoloration; ecchymosis
   3. Swelling
   4. Deformity, possible limb shortening and external rotation
   5. Crepitus (characteristic grating sound)
   6. Possible bone snap heard by victim
   7. External bleeding from associated wounds
   8. Tenderness (pain) relative to specific area of the body (sacrum, hip, symphysis pubis)
D. Intervention
   1. Control bleeding if necessary
   2. Treat for shock
   3. Immobilize affected part
   4. Splint above and below the fracture
   5. Apply ice
   6. Elevate affected part, if possible
   7. Observe for changes in sensation, temperature, and color (indicate nerve injury or circulation interference)
E. Usual medical care
   1. X-ray examination
   2. Possible cast application
   3. Possible surgery
   4. Analgesics
   5. Traction

Dislocation

A. Description: joint injury and bone displacement
B. Assessment
   1. Pain, tenderness
   2. Swelling
   3. Deformity
   4. Alterations in function
   5. Discoloration
C. Intervention
   1. Control hemorrhage if present (not usually seen with a simple dislocation)
   2. Immobilize the affected part
   3. Apply sterile dressing to any open wounds
   4. Splint in the position found above and below the site

Box 10-2. Types of Fractures

Typical complete fractures

Closed (simple) fracture—Noncommunicating wound between bone and skin
Open (compound) fracture—Communicating wound between bone and skin
Comminuted fracture—Multiple bone fragments
Linear fracture—Fracture line parallel to long axis of bone
Oblique fracture—Fracture line at 45-degree angle to long axis of bone
Spiral fracture—Fracture line encircling bone
Transverse fracture—Fracture line perpendicular to long axis of bone
Impacted—Fracture fragments are pushed into each other
Pathologic—Fracture occurs at a point in the bone weakened by disease, for example, with tumors or osteoporosis
Avulsion—A fragment of bone connected to a ligament breaks off from the main bone
Extracapsular—Fracture is close to the joint but remains outside the joint capsule
Intracapsular—Fracture is within the joint capsule

Typical incomplete fractures

Greenstick fracture—Break on one cortex of bone with splintering of inner bone surface
Torus fracture—Buckling of cortex
Bowing fracture—Bending of bone
Stress fracture—Microfracture
Transchondral fracture—Separation of cartilaginous joint surface (articular cartilage) from main shaft of bone

(From McCance KI, Huether SE: *Pathophysiology: the biological basis for disease in adults and children,* ed 2, St Louis, 1994, Mosby.)

---

   5. Apply ice
   6. Elevate affected part, if possible
   7. Check for fractures
   8. Monitor neurologic status (check pulses distal to the injury)

Sprain

A. Description: stretched or ruptured ligaments; *sprain should be considered a fracture until proven otherwise by x-ray examination*
B. Assessment
   1. Pain, tenderness
   2. Discoloration
   3. Swelling
   4. Alterations in function
C. Intervention
   1. Elevate affected part
   2. Apply ice intermittently for 72 hours
   3. Apply elastic (Ace) bandages
   4. Immobilize affected part

Strain

A. Description: muscle or tendon damage caused by excessive physical use
B. Assessment
    1. Pain
    2. Discoloration
C. Intervention
    1. Bed rest
    2. Heat application

Hyperthermia

HEAT STROKE

A. Description: life-threatening emergency; body's mechanism for heat regulation breaks down, and excessive body heat is retained; occurs with overexposure to high environmental temperatures, especially those accompanied by high relative humidity and low wind
B. Assessment
    1. Hyperpyrexia to 106° or 107° F (41.1° to 41.6° C)
    2. Flushed, hot, dry skin or clammy and diaphoretic
    3. Dizziness
    4. Headache
    5. Confusion
    6. Nausea
    7. Tachycardia
    8. Hypotension
    9. Fixed and diluted pupils
    10. Seizures
    11. Possible altered level of consciousness
    12. Shallow, rapid breathing
    13. Delirium
C. Predisposing factors are:
    1. Age (elderly)
    2. Obesity
    3. Alcoholism
    4. Preexisting illness (cardiovascular or neurological dysfunctions)
    5. Prescription medications that decrease perspiration (anticholinergics such as antihistamines and antispasmodics; diuretics and beta blockers such as propranolol)
    6. Excessive strenuous exercise
D. Intervention
    1. Ensure adequate airway, breathing, and circulation
    2. Move victim out of sun
    3. Loosen or remove clothing
    4. Provide rapid cooling, for example, immerse in cold water; apply towels soaked in cold water; air conditioning, fanning, and cool-water sponge
    5. If conscious, provide cool water
    6. Control shivering (this causes body temperature to increase)
    7. Advise victim to avoid reexposure and warn of possible lowered tolerance to heat for a long time or indefinitely
E. Usual medical care
    1. Oxygen
    2. IV therapy

HEAT EXHAUSTION

A. Description: ineffective circulating blood volume caused by excessive fluid loss and exposure to heat without sufficient fluid and electrolyte replenishment
B. Assessment
    1. Headache
    2. Dizziness, faintness
    3. Nausea and vomiting
    4. Marked diaphoresis
    5. Cool, pale, damp skin
    6. Muscle cramps
    7. Possible temperature elevation
    8. Orthostatic hypotension
    9. Tachycardia
    10. Dehydration
    11. Anxiety
    12. Anorexia, thirst
C. Especially at risk are
    1. The elderly
    2. The very young
D. Intervention
    1. Move victim to cool, quiet area
    2. Loosen or remove constricting clothing
    3. Administer salted water if vomiting absent
    4. Provide rest
    5. Relieve muscle cramps (firm pressure against muscle with palm of hand)
    6. Advise victim of preventive measures: drink plenty of fluids and curtail activity on hot days

Cold Injuries

FROSTBITE

A. Classification
    1. Superficial: superficial tissue below the skin freezes
    2. Deep: deep subcutaneous tissue freezes, and temperature of affected part is lowered
B. Most frequently affected areas: ears, nose, cheeks, fingers, and toes
C. Assessment
    1. Superficial
        a. Numbness, tingling, burning
        b. Gray-white appearance of affected parts
    2. Deep
        a. Hyperemic skin
        b. Edema
        c. Blister formation
        d. Discoloration
        e. Numbness
D. Intervention
    1. Superficial
        a. Remove wet, constricting clothing
        b. Give warm-water soaks
        c. Advise victim of preventive measures
    2. Deep
        a. Remove wet, constricting clothing
        b. Give warm-water soaks only if continuously available; otherwise keep area dry, place sterile gauze between affected fingers and toes, cover, and elevate frozen part
        c. If conscious, give warm liquids
        d. Do not allow use of frostbitten part
    3. Usual medical care
        a. Tetanus prophylaxis
        b. Analgesics
        c. Antibiotic therapy
E. Warnings
    1. *Do not rub area with snow or ice*
    2. *Do not massage*

IMMERSION FOOT
A. Cause: wet foot in continuous contact with cold temperatures
B. Assessment
   1. Foot is cold and damp
   2. Foot appears shriveled
   3. Gangrene (if conditions were prolonged and repeated)
C. Intervention
   1. Dry footwear
   2. Warm-water soaks

CHILBLAIN
A. Description: localized redness and swelling of the skin resulting from excessive exposure to cold
B. Commonly affected areas: fingers, toes, and earlobes
C. Assessment: burning, itching, blistering, and ulceration (similar to thermal burn) are possible
D. Intervention
   1. Protect part from cold and further injury
   2. Gentle warming
   3. Avoid use of tobacco products

HYPOTHERMIA
A. Description: exposure to cold resulting in heat loss and reduction in body temperature below the average normal range
B. Assessment (Table 10-2)
C. Intervention
   1. Ensure adequate airway and ventilation
   2. Administer oxygen
   3. Remove wet clothing and cover victim
   4. Give warm beverages high in sugar content
   5. Warm body gradually
      a. Passive rewarming: warm room, blankets, and draft prevention (mild hypothermia)
      b. Active external rewarming: heat packs, warming blankets, and overhead radiant warmers (mild to moderate hypothermia)
D. Usual medical care: (moderate to severe hypothermia— active internal warming)
   1. Warmed humidified oxygen
   2. Warmed gastric and peritoneal lavage
   3. Warmed intravenous fluids
E. *Warnings: Do not rub or massage the skin*

Poisoning

FOOD
A. Cause: pathogenic organisms tranferred to victim from contaminated food; illness is caused by toxins produced by the organism
B. Botulism (*Clostridium botulinum*)
   1. Causes
      a. Improperly canned food
      b. Improperly cured food
   2. Assessment
      a. Headache
      b. Fatigue
      c. Nausea and vomiting
      d. Double vision
      e. Muscle incoordination
      f. Difficulty swallowing, talking, and breathing
   3. Intervention
      a. Ensure adequate airway and ventilation

Table 10-2	Stages, Signs, and Symptoms of Hypothermia	
Stage	**Core temperature**	**Symptoms**
Mild	90-95°F (32-35° C)	Tachypnea, tachycardia, ataxia, shivering, lethargy, confusion, occasional atrial fibrillation
Moderate	86-90° F (30-32.2° C)	Rigidity, hypoventilation, decreased level of consciousness, increased myocardial irritability, hypovolemia, blood sludging with metabolic acidosis, Osborne or J wave (positive deflection in the RT segment)
Severe	<86° F (30° C)	Loss of reflexes, coma, hypotension, acidosis, apnea, cyanosis, ventricular fibrillation, asystole

From Kidd PS, Sturt P: *Mosby's emergency nursing reference*, St Louis, 1996, Mosby.

   b. Be prepared to administer cardiopulmonary resuscitation
   c. Induce vomiting if consumption was recent, if victim has clinical and neurologic symptoms, no seizure activity, and no alterations in level of consciousness
   d. Usual medical care: antitoxin
C. *Staphylococcus aureus*
   1. Causes
      a. Respiratory tract and skin of food handlers
      b. Unrefrigerated cream-filled foods
      c. Fish
      d. Meat
   2. Assessment
      a. Nausea and vomiting
      b. Diarrhea
      c. Abdominal cramps
      d. Weakness
   3. Intervention
      a. Fluids
      b. Bed rest
   4. Usual medical care
      a. Possible IV therapy
      b. Antiemetics
      c. Antidiarrheals
D. *Salmonella*
   1. Causes: inadequately cooked meat, poultry, and eggs
   2. Assessment
      a. Nausea and vomiting
      b. Diarrhea
      c. Weakness

d. Abdominal pain
e. Elevated temperature
f. Chills
3. Intervention
   a. Bed rest
   b. Fluids
4. Usual medical care
   a. Possible IV therapy
   b. Antiemetics
   c. Antidiarrheals

ACCIDENTAL POISONING

A. Description: ingestion, inhalation, or absorption of toxic substances or substances such as drugs, which when taken in large amounts, are toxic to the body
B. Assessment: signs and symptoms will vary according to cause
   1. General
      a. Nausea and vomiting
      b. Abdominal pain
      c. Convulsions
      d. Change in level of consciousness
      e. Decreased pulse and respirations
   2. Drug poisoning: coma; flaccid muscles; hypotension
   3. Chemical poisoning
      a. Burns around lips and mouth
      b. Excessive salivation
      c. Difficulty swallowing
      d. Breath odor (from cleaning or petroleum products)
   4. Inhalation poisoning
      a. Coughing and choking
      b. Headache; bright red skin (carbon monoxide—late indicator)
   5. Absorption poisoning: localized itching and burning (poison)
C. Intervention: see Box 10-3
D. Usual medical care
   1. IV fluids (severe cases)
   2. Hyperbaric oxygenation (carbon monoxide poisoning)

Diabetes Mellitus and Hypoglycemia

A. Ketoacidosis: acute insulin deficiency (develops over a period of 2 to 3 days)
   1. Assessment
      a. Polydipsia
      b. Weak, rapid pulse
      c. Hypotension
      d. Dry, warm, flushed skin
      e. Pallor
      f. Diaphoresis
      g. Acetone odor on breath
      h. Kussmaul's respiration
      i. Nausea and vomiting
      j. Alterations in consciousness
      k. Dehydration
      l. Weakness
      m. Headache
      n. Abdominal tenderness
   2. Intervention
      a. Ensure adequate airway and ventilation
      b. Monitor vital signs, fluid intake and output, and level of consciousness

---

Box 10-3.   Guidelines to Stop Absorption of Poisons

Inhaled poison
Remove victim from source of toxic gas.
Assess cardiopulmonary status and give artificial ventilation if possible.
Give oxygen, if available.

Contact poison
Rinse skin with copious amount of water.
Remove garments and rinse skin again.

Ingested poison
If person is conscious:
a. Call physician or poison control center for assistance
b. Substances other than caustics or hydrocarbons:
   (1) Induce emesis by giving 15 to 30 ml syrup of ipecac; follow with full glass of warm water.
   (2) Inactivate poison by giving activated charcoal (especially after drug ingestion).
c. Caustics or hydrocarbons (petroleum products):
   (1) Give nothing by mouth.
   (2) Seek immediate medical attention.
   (3) Do not induce emesis.
If person is unconscious, transport without delay to medical facility.

From Phipps WJ et al, eds: *Medical-surgical nursing: concepts and clinical practice*, ed 5, St Louis, 1995, Mosby.

---

   c. Provide fluids if conscious, for example, broth
   3. Usual medical care
      a. Regular insulin
      b. IV therapy: normal saline solution or 0.45% saline solution
      c. Monitor blood sugar
B. Hypoglycemia (low blood sugar; insulin reaction)
   1. Assessment
      a. Sudden onset of symptoms
      b. Weakness
      c. Pallor
      d. Hunger
      e. Nervousness; irritability
      f. Cool, moist skin
      g. Tachycardia
      h. Tremors
      i. Dizziness, syncope
      j. Headache
      k. Visual disturbances
      l. Drowsiness
      m. Confusion
   2. Intervention
      a. Ensure adequate airway and ventilation
      b. Administer quick-acting carbohydrate, for example, orange juice with sugar, honey, lump sugar, cola beverage, hard candy

3. Usual medical care: if unconscious
   a. IV therapy: 50% glucose
   b. Monitor blood sugar

Drowning

A. Description: asphyxiation that results from aspiration of fluid into the lungs, which is inhaled as individual panics or gasps for breath
B. Causes
   1. Accidental, for example, exhaustion, inability to swim, panic, injury, medical incident such as a seizure
   2. Intentional: suicide attempt
C. Intervention
   1. Remove victim from water
   2. If victim is not breathing, commence artificial respiration (may need to be instituted while victim is being removed from the water)
   3. If there is no carotid pulse, commence cardiopulmonary resuscitation
   4. Observe for pulmonary edema
D. Usual medical care
   1. IV fluids
   2. Oxygen under pressure

Drug Abuse

A. Description: Use of a substance in a manner or in amounts or in situations in which the drug use causes problems or greatly increases the chance of problems occurring
B. Assessment
   1. Needle marks on the body along the veins (many addicts wear long-sleeved shirts to conceal mainlining)
   2. Anorexia
   3. Abdominal cramping
   4. Constipation
   5. Nutritional deficiencies
   6. Watery, reddened eyes
   7. Runny nose
   8. Dilated or constricted pupils
   9. Central nervous system alterations (agitation, euphoria, seizures)
   10. Poor personal hygiene
   11. History of difficulty in school, on job, with interpersonal relationships
   12. Accident-prone
   13. History of personality change
   14. Possibly hepatitis
C. Effects of frequently abused drugs (Table 10-3)
D. Intervention
   1. Ensure airway, breathing, and circulation
   2. Administer oxygen
   3. Insert indwelling catheter
   4. Monitor vital functions and neurologic status
   5. Take seizure precautions
E. Usual medical care
   1. Arterial blood gases
   2. Specific drug antagonist (e.g., naloxone hydrochloride [Narcan])
   3. IV therapy
   4. Central venous pressure line
   5. Possible dialysis
   6. High-protein, high-calorie diet
   7. Vitamin supplements

8. Psychotherapy
9. Withdrawal treatment: methadone hydrochloride (Dolophine) ; usually used for heroin addiction
   a. Legal synthetic drug addiction
   b. Supervised administration
10. Rehabilitation

Acute Alcoholism

A. Description: large alcohol intake in a short time
B. Assessment
   1. Alcohol on breath
   2. Slurring of speech
   3. Ataxia
   4. Agitation
   5. Belligerence
   6. Vomiting
   7. Drowsiness to stuporousness to unconsciousness
   8. Respiratory failure
   9. Death
C. Intervention
   1. Protect airway
   2. Observe for respiratory embarrassment (depression)
   3. Monitor cardiac status
   4. Assess for head injury
D. Usual medical care
   1. Hydration
   2. Vitamin supplements
   3. High-protein diet
   4. Anticonvulsants to control or prevent seizures

Mild Alcohol Withdrawal

A. Assessment
   1. Nausea and vomiting
   2. Shaking
   3. Headache
   4. Ataxia
B. Intervention
   1. Rest
   2. Quiet environment
C. Usual medical care
   1. Analgesics
   2. Hydration

Delirium Tremens

A. Assessment
   1. Tachycardia
   2. Insomnia
   3. Hypertension
   4. Tremors
   5. Anxiety
   6. Hallucinations (auditory, visual, tactile, and [rarely] olfactory)
   7. Disorientation
   8. Amnesia
   9. Seizures
B. Intervention
   1. Ensure adequate airway and ventilation
   2. Treat for shock
   3. Hydration
   4. Monitor vital signs
   5. Crisis counseling
C. Usual medical care

Effects of Frequently Abused Drugs

Drug	Psychologic effects	Physiologic effects	Effects of overdose	Withdrawal syndrome
Stimulants Cocaine, amphetamines, methylphenidate, phenmetrazine, other stimulants	Elation, psychomotor agitation, grandiosity, talkativeness, ↑ alertness, mood swings	Dilated pupils, ↑ blood pressure, ↑ TPR, diaphoresis, nausea, vomiting, insomnia, loss of appetite	Agitation, increased body temperature, hallucinations, convulsions, possible death	Severely depressed mood, prolonged sleep, apathy, irritability, disorientation
Depressants Chloral hydrate, barbiturates, methaqualone, benzodiazepines, alcohol	Disorientation, euphoria, emotional lability, ↑ sexual and aggressive drives with intoxication (↓ with increased doses), talkativeness	Slurred speech, staggering, constricted pupils, ↓ respirations, sedation, nausea	Shallow respiration, cold and clammy skin, weak and rapid pulse, coma, possible death	Anxiety, insomnia, tremors, delirium, convulsions, possible death
Narcotics Opium, morphine, codeine, heroin, methadone, other narcotics	Euphoria, ↓ sexual and aggressive drives	↓ Respiratory rate, nausea, "nodding out," insensitivity to pain, constricted pupils	Slow and shallow breathing, clammy skin, constricted pupils, coma, possible death	Watery eyes, runny nose, yawning, loss of appetite, tremors, panic, chills and sweating, cramps, nausea
Hallucinogens LSD, psilocybin, mescaline, peyote, amphetamine variants, phencyclidine	Hallucinations, illusions, altered body and time perception, mood swings, suspiciousness, confusion, anxiety, panic, intense emotions, depersonalization	Lack of coordination, dilated pupils, ↑ blood pressure, tremors, blurred vision, nausea, dizziness, ↓ weakness response to pain	More prolonged episodes, possibly resembling psychotic states	N/A
Cannabis Marijuana, tetrahydrocannabinol, hashish	Euphoria, impaired memory and attention, relaxation, poor judgment, apathy, abrupt mood changes, slowed time sensation	↑ Appetite, tachycardia, reddened eyes	Fatigue, paranoia; hallucinogen-like psychotic state (at very high doses)	Insomnia, hyperactivity (rare syndrome)
Inhalants Glues, aerosols, cleaning solutions, nail polish removers, lighter fluids, paints and paint thinners, other petroleum products, halothane, nitrous oxide, amyl nitrite, butyl nitrite	Giddiness, light-headedness, decreased inhibitions, floating sensation, illusions, clouding of thoughts, drowsiness, amnesia	Eye irritation, sensitivity to light, double vision, ringing in ears, irritation in lining of nose and mouth, cough, nausea, vomiting, diarrhea, faint heart beat, cardiac irregularities or dysrhythmias	Anxiety, mental impairment, depressed respiration, cardiac dysrhythmias, sudden death	No clinically relevant syndrome, development of tolerance likely at high doses

From Lewis SM, Collier IC: *Medical-surgical nursing: assessment and management of clinical problems*, ed 3, St Louis, 1992, Mosby.
↑, Increased; *TPR*, temperature, pulse, respirations; ↓, decreased; *LSD*, lysergic acid diethylamide; *N/A*, no data available.

1. Treatment for seizures
2. Anticonvulsant drugs
3. IV therapy
4. Sedation
5. Vitamin therapy
6. High-protein diet

Disulfiram (Antabuse) Reactions

A. Assessment
   1. Nausea and vomiting
   2. Diaphoresis
   3. Hypotension
   4. Consciousness alterations
   5. Tachycardia
   6. Headache
   7. Facial flushing
   8. Reddened conjunctiva
B. Intervention
   1. Ensure adequate airway, breathing, and circulation
   2. Administer oxygen
C. Usual medical care
   1. IV therapy
   2. Diphenhydramine hydrochloride (Benadryl)
   3. Chlorpheniramine maleate (Chlor-Trimeton)
   4. Ascorbic acid

Sexual Assault

A. Victim should be examined and treated as quickly as possible
B. Notify police
C. Victim should not be left alone
D. Victims should be asked who they wish to have stay with them; offer to call family member, friend, or rape crisis center advocate
E. Provide immediate privacy
F. Kindness and support are crucial
G. Obtain history
H. Assess acuteness of physical and psychologic needs
J. Assess victim's readiness for physical examination
G. Explain all procedures and encourage questions
K. Obtain necessary written permissions
L. Assist victim to undress
M. Observe for and ask about other possible injuries
N. Assist with physician's examination
   1. A water-moistened speculum is used
   2. History will indicate the body orifices from which specimens for semen analysis will be required
   3. Pubic hair is combed for foreign hairs
   4. Clothing is usually saved for analysis, and replacement clothing will be necessary
   5. Testing done for sexually transmitted disease (STDs), including HIV; follow-up testing done at appropriate intervals
   6. STD prophylaxis
   7. Pregnancy prophylaxis if contraception not in effect at time of attack: DES (diethylstilbestrol) treatment and side effects should be thoroughly explained
   8. If possible and desired, offer accommodations for bathing and douching
   9. Care for tissue trauma: immediate and follow-up
   10. Care for psychologic trauma: immediate and follow-up
   11. If present, family and friends often require assistance and counseling

Disaster

A. Definition: catastrophic event
   1. Natural, for example, flood, earthquake, hurricane
   2. Man-made, for example, riot, fire, train accident
B. May involve as few as 10 or more than 100 victims
C. Prevention
   1. Community planning
   2. Public education
D. Assessment
   1. Civilian triage: care priority to those whose life is threatened
   2. Military triage: care priority to those most likely to survive
E. Planning: the most capable person is designated to sort casualties
F. Intervention
   1. First aid should be rendered before victims are transported
   2. Care priorities
      a. Ensure airway, breathing, and circulation
      b. Control bleeding
      c. Treat for shock
         (1) Whole blood
         (2) IV fluids
         (3) Parenteral medications
         (4) Pain relief
         (5) Emergency wound care
      d. Preserve motor and sensory functioning
      e. Provide psychologic support
      f. Treat and transport

SUGGESTED READING

American Heart Association: *Heartsaver manual,* Dallas, 1993, The Association.

American Red Cross: *First aid, responding to emergencies,* St. Louis, 1991, Mosby.

Coleman E: Cardiac issues in CPR: what the future might hold, *Nursing 92,* 22(4):54, 1992.

Ignatavicius DD, Bayne MV: *Medical-surgical nursing: a nursing process approach,* Philadelphia, 1991, WB Saunders.

Kidd PS, Sturt P: *Mosby's emergency nursing reference,* St Louis, 1996, Mosby.

Mosby's medical, nursing & allied health dictionary, ed 4, St Louis, 1994, Mosby.

Oakley R, Ksir C: *Drugs, society and human behavior,* ed 6, St Louis, 1993, Mosby.

Phipps WJ, et al: *Medical-surgical nursing: concepts and clinical practice,* St Louis, 1995, Mosby.

Sheehy SB: *Emergency nursing: principles and practice,* ed 3, St Louis, 1992, Mosby.

Sheehy SB, Lombardi JE: *Manual of emergency care,* ed 4, St. Louis, 1995, Mosby.

Smeltzer SC, Bare BG: *Brunner and Suddarth's textbook of medical surgical nursing,* ed 7, Philadelphia, 1992, JB Lippincott.

Stuart GW, Sundeen, SJ: *Principles and practice of psychiatric nursing,* ed 4, St Louis, 1991, Mosby.

REVIEW QUESTIONS

Answers and rationales begin on p. 462.

1. At your 12-year-old son's baseball game, you see the center fielder slump to the ground. As a nurse, you run to him and determine that he is not breathing and has no pulse. You place your hand in position to deliver chest compressions. The correct depth of compression would be:
   ① ½ to 1 inch
   ② 1 to 1½ inches
   ③ 1½ to 2 inches
   ④ 2 to 2½ inches

2. A motor vehicle accident (MVA) victim is admitted to the hospital with an unstable fracture of the pelvis. As part of the initial assessment of this patient, it is important the nurse identify which of the following?
   ① Bowel sounds
   ② External rotation
   ③ Pain on defecation
   ④ Symphysis pubis tenderness

3. A resident of a nursing home has been found in cardiac arrest. You arrive with another nurse and 2-rescuer CPR is begun. The nurse administering ventilations must give a breath:
   ① Whenever possible
   ② Immediately before the 5th compression
   ③ During the pause after the 5th compression
   ④ During the compression phase of every 5th compression

4. For the rape survivor treated in the emergency room, an appropriate short-term expected outcome (goal) would be to:
   ① Initiate social interaction
   ② Regain control over her life before she leaves the ER
   ③ Return to her pretrauma level of functioning
   ④ Verbalize two methods of stress management

5. In caring for an unconscious victim of an airway obstruction, the nurse should take which of the following actions first?
   ① Immediately start cardiopulmonary resuscitation
   ② Open the airway using the head-tilt–chin-lift maneuver
   ③ Place victim in supine position on a firm, flat surface
   ④ Remove any foreign object obstructing the airway

6. An 18 year old was on a rock-climbing expedition with his class when he fell 8 feet onto gravel. He is complaining of pain in his left elbow. It is obviously deformed when he presents to the emergency room. Which of the following should be included in the assessment of this patient's condition?
   ① Level of consciousness
   ② Presence of a radial pulse
   ③ Ability to adduct the elbow
   ④ Presence of ecchymosis on the upper arm

7. The presence of human immunodeficiency virus infection is increasing. Which of the following measures is essential for the nurse to incorporate into her care?
   ① Ask the patient his or her HIV status
   ② Have an HIV-positive health care worker attend to the patient
   ③ Strictly adhere to universal infection control precautions
   ④ Take infection control precautions only if exposure to blood or body fluids is obvious

8. You are caring for a rape trauma survivor. Your initial assessment indicates that the patient appears calm and very much in control. Which characteristic psychologic reaction best describes the patient's behavior?
   ① Denial
   ② Humiliation
   ③ Hyperalertness
   ④ Reorganization

9. During an intake interview in the ER, the nurse asks the patient if he is on any medication. He reports that he is on Methadone. The nurse knows that this patient is being treated for withdrawal from:
   ① Alcohol
   ② Heroin
   ③ Barbiturates
   ④ Benzodiazepines

10. You are alone, caring for a neighbor's infant. When you check the napping baby, you see that she is limp and has a bluish tint. You commence CPR. After 20 cycles of compressions and ventilations, you should:
    ① Activate EMS
    ② Check for breathing
    ③ Check for return of carotid pulse
    ④ Check for return of brachial pulse

11. A 79-year-old female comes to emergency clinic appearing very anxious and complaining of nausea, headache, and muscle cramping. Suspecting heat exhaustion from history given by the patient, the nurse's *first* action would be to:
    ① Call the physician immediately
    ② Monitor the patient's temperature
    ③ Administer an oral balanced salt solution
    ④ Move the patient to a cool quiet room

12. A nurse witnesses a motorcycle accident in which the victim is thrown forcefully from the vehicle to the pavement. Upon initial assessment of the patient, the nurse notes a crack in the helmet. When administering care to this accident victim, which of the following should receive *priority*?
    ① Maintain an open airway
    ② Maintain normal body temperature
    ③ Minimize movement of the head
    ④ Monitor respirations

13. While making midmorning rounds the nurse finds a 60-year-old diabetic patient unconscious on the floor next to his bed. The nurse's *immediate* action should be to:
    ① Call the physician and prepare IV glucose
    ② Establish an airway
    ③ Administer regular insulin
    ④ Commence mouth-to-mouth resuscitation

14. In the presence of a pulse and a patent airway but the absence of respirations, which of the following actions would be *most appropriate* for an adult?
    ① Compress the sternum 1½ to 2 inches (3.75 to 5 cm)
    ② Turn the patient on his or her side
    ③ Sweep the back of the patient's throat
    ④ Continue to deliver breaths

15. While sitting in the park in the midafternoon, you hear cries for help from a young mother. When you run to her side, you see her infant is not breathing and has no pulse. To commence CPR you place 2 fingers:
    ① At the nipple level
    ② The top half of the sternum
    ③ One finger width below the nipple level
    ④ Two finger widths above the xiphoid process

16. A 21-year-old unconscious male is brought to the ER by a friend. His breath smells of alcohol and the friend reports that they were at a fraternity party where there was heavy drinking. The nurse should:
    ① Treat for shock
    ② Ensure adequate airway and ventilation
    ③ Recommend rest in a quiet environment
    ④ Administer disulfiram (Antabuse) immediately

17. The police deliver to the ER a panicky man experiencing tremors, chills and sweating, intestinal cramps, and nausea. His eyes are watery and his nose is running. The nurse should suspect:
    ① Stimulant withdrawal
    ② Narcotics withdrawal
    ③ An overdose of narcotics
    ④ An overdose of an inhalant

18. A mother reports that her 5-year-old son was found drinking from a bottle of wine. On the way to the hospital, he fell asleep. The nurse's *first* priority is to:
    ① Protect the airway
    ② Monitor cardiac status
    ③ Take seizure precautions
    ④ Provide vitamin supplements

19. A 23-year-old female arrives at the hospital in an agitated state, an elevated blood pressure, a temperature of 100.1 degrees (F), and reports having hallucinations. The nurse should suspect that the patient has consumed:
    ① Inhalants
    ② Stimulants
    ③ Depressants
    ④ Hallucinogens

20. Which of the following patients would be most at risk for mortality following burn injury?
    ① A 5-year-old male
    ② A 38-year-old female
    ③ A 12-year-old female
    ④ A 78-year-old male

21. You are driving in a rural area on an isolated country road. You see a child, approximately 12 to 15 years of age, lying in the middle of the road with an overturned bicycle not far away. Which of the following nursing actions should you take *immediately*?
    ① Keep driving to the nearest gas station and telephone for an ambulance
    ② Turn around and go back to the nearest main highway and hail a police car
    ③ Proceed with a rapid clinical assessment with emphasis on ABCs
    ④ Check with local authorities for specifics on the state's Good Samaritan law

22. A child has a bleeding occipital laceration; pain discoloration and swelling of the right ulna; and right-sided chest pain that increases on inspiration. Which of the following nursing actions will have the *highest priority*?
    ① Immobilization of the right arm
    ② Elevation of the right arm and head
    ③ Applying ice to the right side of the chest
    ④ Stopping the bleeding and treating for shock

23. An acquaintance known to be taking lithium and under psychiatric care has taken cocaine. She telephones you with abdominal cramps and extreme anxiety and asks you what to do. Your *best* response would be to:

① Refer her to the local emergency room
② Refer her to her psychiatrist
③ Refer her to the cocaine hotline number
④ Tell her you cannot get involved right now

24. You come across a multiple trauma scene. Priority care should be given to the victim:
    ① With cyanosis of earlobes and nailbeds
    ② Who is hemorrhaging
    ③ Who appears to be in a daze
    ④ With a suspected fracture of the femur

25. Running to catch a bus you trip, fall, and sprain your wrist. Which of the following nursing interventions would be *most appropriate*?
    ① Application of dry heat
    ② Splinting above and below the wrist
    ③ Application of ice for 24 hours
    ④ Observation for sensation changes

26. Which of the following would be your priority nursing concern for a victim with severe burns?
    ① Administering cardiopulmonary resuscitation
    ② Relieving pain
    ③ Stopping the burning process
    ④ Tetanus prophylaxis

27. The nurse knows that oils or ointments are not applied to severe burns. What is the chief reason for this principle?
    ① Burn areas should be left open to the air
    ② These products impede ice application to burn areas
    ③ These products prevent blisters from being broken
    ④ These products seal in heat

28. Two teenagers are playing Frisbee in the park. Suddenly one of them sustains a blow to the nose from the Frisbee, resulting in rapid epistaxis. To prevent aspiration of blood, the victim should be placed in which of the following positions?
    ① Side-lying
    ② Supine
    ③ Upright with head tilted backward
    ④ Upright with head tilted forward

29. The mother of a 3-year-old tells you that her daughter has swallowed bleach, which was stored under the kitchen sink. A rapid assessment reveals no evidence of acute airway swelling. Which of the following interventions should the nurse take?
    ① Absorb the poison with activated charcoal
    ② Give nothing by mouth
    ③ Give water or milk
    ④ Induce vomiting with syrup of ipecac

30. A laboratory employee has sustained chemical burns to his left forearm, thigh, and foot. Which of the following nursing actions should be taken *initially*?
    ① Apply ice to the burns immediately
    ② Cover the burns with wet, sterile dressings
    ③ Flush burns with cool, running water
    ④ Treat the victim for shock and tend to the burns later

31. To stop the bleeding from an occipital laceration the *best* nursing action would be to:
    ① Apply pressure to the site
    ② Apply ice to the site
    ③ Elevate the head
    ④ Elevate the extremities

32. Assessment protocol for a fracture of the right ulna should include which of the following nursing actions?
    ① Ascertaining range-of-motion (ROM) limitations
    ② Observing for changes in sensation, temperature, and color
    ③ Determining the presence of crepitus
    ④ Preventing limb shortening

33. A 10 year old is stabbed in the abdomen on the school playground. You respond to the other children's cries for help. By the time you reach the child he has a rapid pulse, his lips are cyanotic, and he is pale and diaphoretic. Your *priority* nursing action would be to:
    ① Elevate his feet to promote venous return
    ② Ensure a patent airway and maintain breathing
    ③ Administer fluids rapidly to restore blood volume
    ④ Cover him with a jacket to maintain body temperature

34. Your neighbor shouts to come quickly, that her child has been stung by a bee. Which of the following skin manifestations would indicate that a general systemic reaction is developing?
    ① Body itching
    ② Facial pallor
    ③ Localized redness
    ④ Localized swelling

35. A 30-year-old male sustains a crush injury to his left lower arm in a tractor accident. Unable to palpate a radial pulse, you should take which of the following actions?
    ① Check for a pulse in another major artery
    ② Commence cardiopulmonary resuscitation
    ③ Prepare to commence rescue breathing
    ④ Run to the phone and call 9-1-1

36. A 40-year-old female is admitted to the ER bleeding profusely from an injury on the lower portion of her right arm. Emergency management of hemorrhage requires the nurse to implement which of the following actions *first*?
    ① Apply pressure to the bleeding area
    ② Apply a pressure dressing to the bleeding area
    ③ Elevate the injured area
    ④ Immobilize the injured area

37. When one rescuer is performing cardiopulmonary resuscitation on an adult, the rate of cardiac compressions is:
    ① 80 times per minute
    ② 5 times per minute
    ③ 60 times per minute
    ④ 15 times per minute

38. When one rescuer is performing cardiac compressions, the hands should be placed:
    ① Directly over the xiphoid process
    ② 2 inches below the xiphoid process
    ③ Two finger breadths above the xiphoid process
    ④ Two finger breadths to the left of the xiphoid process

39. When two rescuers are performing cardiopulmonary resuscitation, the ratio of compressions to respirations is:
    ① 15:2
    ② 5:2
    ③ 15:1
    ④ 5:1

40. When performing adult mouth-to-mouth resuscitation, the rescuer should deliver breaths that are:
    ① Full and quick
    ② Deep and forceful
    ③ Every 4 seconds
    ④ Every 5 seconds

41. A patient comes to the emergency room with a thermal burn to the left hand. The burned skin is red in color, does not blanch, is not painful, and is leathery in nature. You would classify this burn as:
    ① Minor
    ② Moderate
    ③ Full thickness
    ④ Partial thickness

42. A patient comes to the emergency room with signs and symptoms associated with food poisoning. The patient states he consumed hotdogs, potato salad, potato chips, and carbonated beverages during his picnic lunch. Which of the following foods is the most likely source of his food poisoning?
    ① Hotdogs
    ② Potato salad
    ③ Potato chips
    ④ Carbonated beverages

43. A patient dialed 911 after collapsing with a headache, dizziness, and nausea. The ambulance personnel found him unconscious but breathing. They suspect the victim was overcome by carbon monoxide as the result of a faulty furnace. Initial treatment for this patient should include the administration of oxygen at:
    ① 2 liters/minute via nasal cannula
    ② 5 liters/minute via nasal cannula
    ③ 40% per mask
    ④ 100% per mask

44. A male, age 29, had been under stress from his job and has been having trouble sleeping. In an attempt to relax before bedtime, he drank 2 beers, then became confused, and accidentally overdosed himself with Restoril (temazepam) 45 mg. His wife became concerned and brought him to the emergency room. Which of the following assessments should the nurse complete *first*?
    ① Respiratory rate
    ② Temperature
    ③ Auscultation of lungs
    ④ Determination of pupil size

45. A 26-year-old female has come to the emergency room with lower right quadrant abdominal pain. She complains of feeling thirsty and is requesting a drink of water. To appease her thirst the nurse should:
    ① Provide ice chips
    ② Provide a glass of water
    ③ Provide orange juice
    ④ Withhold fluids until tests are complete

46. A housewife and mother of 2-year-old twin boys was working in her garden and accidentally stepped on a nail as she ran to see why her children were crying. The nail is still embedded in her foot when she comes to the emergency room. When assessing the nature of the injury, the nurse should *first*:
    ① Remove the nail and cleanse the wounds with hydrogen peroxide
    ② Secure the nail with tape until the physician sees the patient
    ③ Administer tetanus toxoid 0.5 cc IM
    ④ Copiously irrigate the foot with normal saline

47. A new employee was opening cartons with a razor-sharp box-opener when he slashed a 6-inch gash across his abdomen. A loop of his intestines is protruding through the wound. Which of the following interventions should the nurse do *first* for this patient while waiting for the doctor?
    ① Cover the wound with a sterile dressing
    ② Apply sterile towels moistened with sterile saline
    ③ Establish a large-bore IV
    ④ Tuck the loop of bowel back into the body

48. A 52-year-old dockworker has come to the emergency room complaining of severe crushing sternal pain that radiates to his left arm. He is cool, pale, and diaphoretic. He believes he is having a heart attack. The first priority of nursing care for this patient is:
    ① Application of the cardiac monitor
    ② Administration of nitroglycerine 0.4 mg sublingually
    ③ Administration of oxygen at 5 L/min
    ④ Insertion of a large-bore IV

49. A 21-year-old construction worker was brought to the emergency room when he was found unconscious but breathing in a roadside ditch. He smells strongly of beer. His vital signs are stable. Initial treatment of this patient should include:
    ① Stabilization of the cervical spine
    ② Insertion of endotracheal tube
    ③ Use of painful stimuli to rouse the patient
    ④ Insertion of a large-bore IV

50. The ER physician orders epinephrine (adrenaline) for a patient whom he suspects is going into anaphylactic shock. The nurse is to avoid IM administration of this parenteral suspension into the buttocks because:
    ① Gas gangrene may occur
    ② Necrosis or pain may occur
    ③ It is to be given subcutaneous only
    ④ This site can cause more adverse reactions

51. A 19-year-old male arrived at the emergency room by a Life-Star helicopter. He had first, second, and third degree burns over seventy percent of his body. He had been on a bass-fishing trip and was smoking a cigarette. Apparently, there was a small gasoline leak in the motor of the boat causing an explosion and fire. The nurse knows that during initial management of a burn victim the first step to take is:
    ① Immediately begin intravenous fluids
    ② Establish and maintain an adequate airway
    ③ Assess if a cutdown for intravenous fluids is necessary
    ④ Give the burned areas initial care and cover with sterile dressings

52. One morning a young mother was making chocolate chip cookies. She used one package mix that called for adding 3 eggs. She mixed the dough and was interrupted by a phone call. Her children, age 7 and 9, helped themselves to the cookie dough. That night both children were complaining of severe stomach cramps, vomiting, headaches, and fever. The nurse, in checking what the children ate that day, recognizes this could be:

① Botulism
② Salmonella
③ Trichinosis
④ Perfringens

53. A male, age 7, is brought to the emergency room on July 4th. A firecracker was thrown at him and it exploded as it hit his bare left arm, in the deltoid area. The nurse noted that the epidermis, dermis, and subcutaneous tissues were burned about 2.5 centimeters in diameter. There were also reddened areas all around the deltoid area. The child states that it doesn't hurt very much. This burn would be characterized as:
    ① First-degree burn
    ② Second-degree burn
    ③ Third-degree burn
    ④ Fourth-degree burn

54. A 20-year-old accident victim arrives at the emergency room after a bad car accident. He has lost so much blood that he is going into shock. The nurse knows that this type of shock is known as:
    ① Septic shock
    ② Neurogenic shock
    ③ Cardiogenic shock
    ④ Hypovolemic shock

55. Your neighbor comes to the emergency room with a partial airway obstruction following ingestion of sirloin steak for dinner. Which of the following assessments would be consistent with a partial obstruction?
    ① Hacking cough and lethargy
    ② Absent respiratory effort
    ③ Flared nostrils and deep cough
    ④ Anxiety and labored use of accessory muscles

56. A competitive racer had a near drowning accident when the canoe she was paddling tipped over and struck her on the head. Her lips and nails are cyanotic. Immediate emergency care for this patient's hypoxia includes:
    ① Insertion of chest tubes to drain the water
    ② Cricothyroid puncture to assure a patent airway
    ③ Placing her in Trendelenburg position to facilitate fluid drainage
    ④ Bag-valve-mask resuscitation

57. A 42-year-old insurance broker sustained severe full thickness burns to his pelvis and legs when he was trapped in a burning car. He was admitted to the ER and has been urinating red urine for several hours. The presence of red urine indicates this patient has possibly sustained:
    ① Kidney damage
    ② Liver damage
    ③ Muscle damage
    ④ Integumentary damage

58. A 32-year-old insulin-dependent diabetic comes to the emergency department in ketoacidosis. Which of the following signs and symptoms should the nurse expect to observe?
    ① Sweating and tremors
    ② Increased hunger and thirst
    ③ Dry skin and mucous membranes
    ④ Anxiety and nervousness

59. The new CPR recommendations for calling for help suggest "Phone first" for an adult and "Phone fast" for a child. The best explanation for this rule is:
① Children can go longer without oxygen
② An arrest in an child is usually caused by cardiac arrest
③ An arrest in an adult is usually caused by cardiac arrythmias
④ It is usually too late by the time you find an adult

60. A 58-year-old executive is admitted to the ER with a myocardial infarction. The nurse assesses the patient for signs of shock. Because the blood pressure is stable the nurse should check:
① For tachycardia and skin temperature
② Pupils every 30 minutes
③ For elevated temperature
④ For mental confusion and slurred speech

ANSWERS AND RATIONALES

1. Knowledge, implementation, physiologic (a)
   ❷ Standard CPR guidelines state that the child's chest should be compressed 1 to 1½ inches, or ⅓ to ½ of chest's total height.
   ① This is appropriate depth for infants.
   ③ This is appropriate depth for adults.
   ④ This is too deep for CPR compressions.

2. Comprehension, implementation, physiologic (a)
   ❶ Hemorrhage is a serious, life-threatening complication of pelvic fractures, and the physician should be notified immediately of the observation.
   ② Although the physician may order a stool guaiac reaction test, the priority is to notify the physician of the observation.
   ③ Not a priority in a life-threatening situation.
   ④ To wait for the next stool specimen would be a highly inappropriate delay in essential medical care.

3. Comprehension, implementation, physiologic (a)
   ❸ The compression:ventilation ratio is 5:1 with a pause for ventilation of 1½ to 2 seconds consisting primarily of inspiration.
   ② With the correct ratio being 5:1, the fifth compression must occur prior to the respiration.
   ①,④ Ventilation (inspiration) must occur during a pause; exhalation occurs during chest compression.

4. Comprehension, planning, psychosocial (c)
   ❷ The only appropriately written short-term goal: patient centered, realistic, reachable, time oriented.
   ①,③,④ These are long-term goals.

5. Application, implementation, physiologic (c)
   ❸ With an unconscious victim, the priority is airway. To open the airway, the victim first has to be properly positioned.
   ①,②,④ Appropriate, but not done first.

6. Application, assessment, physiologic (c)
   ❷ Determining the presence of the pulse is an indication of vascular intactness.
   ① If he is complaining of pain, he is alert.
   ③ The elbow is only capable of extension and flexion.
   ④ Bruising on the upper arm is likely as a result of the fall.

7. Application, planning, environment (b)
   ❸ CDC recommends using universal precautions at all times.
   ① In emergency situations, patients are often not able to provide accurate information.
   ② Highly impractical.
   ④ Inappropriate to rely on only the obvious.

8. Comprehension, assessment, psychosocial (b)
   ❷ Acute disorganization that characteristically follows sexual assault is either verbally expressed or hidden. Regardless of the manner of expression, the survivor experiences feelings of shock, anger, guilt, humiliation, and even fear.
   ①,③ Usually follows acute disorganization and precedes reorganization.
   ④ Reorganization indicates that the survivor has put the event in perspective and moves toward some degree of recovery.

9. Knowledge, assessment, physiologic (a)
   ❷ Methadone is used only for heroin withdrawal.
   ① Alcohol withdrawal is sometimes facilitated by administration of Valium, not Methadone.
   ③ Phenobarbitol is used for barbiturate withdrawal.
   ④ Withdrawal from benzodiazepines (Valium, Lithium) is done by administering progressively smaller doses of the drugs, not by substitution of another drug.

10. Knowledge, implementation, physiologic (a)
    ❶ Standard infant CPR procedure requires 1 minute of CPR, then activation of EMS.
    ②,④ After activation of EMS, the rescuer should resume CPR by checking for return of breathing and brachial pulse.
    ③ Carotid pulse is not used in infant CPR.

11. Application, implementation, physiologic (b)
    ❹ Heat exhaustion occurs when a prolonged fluid loss is caused by perspiration, diarrhea, or diuretics and warm to hot temperatures without adequate fluid replacement. The fastest action is to remove one of the causes (the hot environment), call the physician, monitor vital signs, and replace fluid as ordered.
    ①,②,③ These are appropriate, but not first action that the nurse can implement that will eliminate one of the causes.

12. Application, implementation, physiologic (c)
    ❶ The priority is always ABC: airway, breathing, and circulation.
    ② Although important, not the priority.
    ③ Necessary and important, but not the priority.
    ④ A person cannot breathe unless the airway is patent.

13. Application, implementation, physiologic (a)
    ❷ With an unconscious victim the priority is always airway, breathing, circulation.
    ① This assumes that the patient is in insulin shock.
    ③ This assumes that the patient is in diabetic coma.
    ④ Mouth-to-mouth resuscitation cannot be given until a patent airway has been established.

14. Application, implementation, physiologic (a)
    ❹ Always continue breathing until help arrives or victim spontaneously resumes breathing.
    ① You do not compress the sternum in the presence of a pulse.
    ② The victim must be in a supine position.
    ③ This measure is performed in the presence of an upper airway obstruction only.

15. Knowledge, implementation, physiologic (a)
    ❸ Sternal compression is performed approximately the width of one finger below the nipple level.
    ①,② These positions are too high.
    ④ This is the position for children and adults.

16. Knowledge, implementation, physiologic (a)
    ❷ Vomiting from acute alcoholism can cause aspiration and the depressed central nervous system can lead to respiratory arrest.
    ① Shock is associated with delirium tremens, not acute alcoholism.
    ③ This is appropriate for mild alcohol withdrawal; acute alcoholism requires observation.
    ④ Disulfiram (Antabuse) may be recommended as part of an aftercare program for the alcoholic who has already dried out.

17. Comprehension, assessment, physiologic (b)
    ❷ Watery eyes and runny nose are telltale signs of narcotic withdrawal and are not associated with any other drug classification.
    ①,④ These two situations would not cause the watery eyes and runny nose.
    ③ There would not be chills, sweating, or intestinal cramps; and the patient would be near coma.

18. Application, implementation, physiologic (a)
    ❶ The risk is that the child will vomit and aspirate.
    ②,③,④ These are appropriate actions, but not as a first priority.

19. Comprehension, assessment, physiologic (b)
    ❷ Effects of stimulant overdose include agitation, increased body temperature, and blood pressure, hallucinations, convulsions, and possible death.
    ① Inhalant overdose will cause anxiety, but respirations will be depressed.
    ③ Depressants will not cause any of these symptoms.
    ④ Hallucinogens will cause hallucinations and elevated blood pressure, but not agitation.

20. Application, assessment, physiologic (b)
    ❹ The very young and the elderly are at greatest risk.
    ①,②,③ Neither very young nor elderly.

21. Comprehension, assessment, physiologic (b)
    ❸ Emergency nursing calls for a rapid clinical assessment with emphasis on airway, breathing, circulation, establishing priorities, and then the instituting of life-saving measures.
    ① Although calling for help is important, it is not the priority.
    ② Not a priority action.
    ④ The Good Samaritan Law provisions should be known before traveling out of the home state.

22. Application, implementation, physiologic (c)
    ❹ Priority is always airway, breathing, and circulation.
    ①,②,③ Appropriate, but not the highest priority.

23. Application, implementation, environment (b)
    ❶ Victim requires immediate medical care.
    ② Appropriate, but not the first priority.
    ③ Inappropriate, as victim needs immediate medical care.
    ④ Referring a victim to a physician does not put you at legal risk; not referring a victim to a physician could result in legal action being initiated against you.

24. Application, planning, physiologic (a)
    ❶ Oxygenation *is* compromised in this situation and airway is always the priority.
    ② Oxygenation *will be* compromised if the hemorrhaging is not controlled or stopped.
    ③ No immediate problem with airway, breathing, or circulation.
    ④ Fractures are suspected at multiple trauma scenes; the priorities are always airway, breathing, and circulation, in that order.

25. Knowledge, assessment, physiologic (a)
    ❸ Prevents edema, facilitates vasoconstriction, increases blood viscosity, and acts as a local anesthetic.
    ① Treatment of a strain.
    ②,④ Treatment of a fracture.

26. Application, implementation, physiologic (a)
    ❸ The hemodynamic instability following burn injury must be stopped to proceed with airway, breathing, and circulation and to prevent further trauma to the victim.

① Situation does not indicate that CPR is necessary.
②,④ Appropriate, but not the priority.

27. Comprehension, implementation, physiologic (a)
    ❹ These products seal in the heat, causing further trauma to the victim.
    ① Burns left open place the victim at further risk for infection.
    ② Ice should not be applied because it causes body heat loss, thereby placing the victim at further risk.
    ③ Blisters should not be broken; intact skin prevents infection.

28. Application, implementation, physiologic (b)
    ❹ This is the only position that will prevent the victim from swallowing blood and being at risk for aspiration.
    ①,②,③ Victim at risk for aspiration in any of these positions.

29. Application, implementation, physiologic (a)
    ❸ Bleach is a corrosive substance that should be diluted only if the victim is conscious.
    ①,② Do not do anything besides call the poison control center if you are not absolutely sure of the antidote.
    ④ Do not induce vomiting; this could cause burning of the esophagus, throat, and mouth.

30. Application, implementation, physiologic (a)
    ❸ The chemical will continue to burn the victim as long as it remains on the skin.
    ① Ice or ice water should not be used in the treatment of burns because the burn has decreased the body's ability to retain heat. Overcooling will further increase metabolic demands.
    ② Appropriate, but not the priority.
    ④ Stop the burning first; then proceed with airway, breathing, and circulation.

31. Knowledge, implementation, physiologic (a)
    ❶ The first step in treating hemorrhage is to apply pressure for at least 6 minutes.
    ② Application of ice is not an emergency measure.
    ③ Elevating the affected part aids in controlling the bleeding, but would not stop the bleeding.
    ④ This action would have no effect on occipital bleeding.

32. Knowledge, implementation, physiologic (b)
    ❷ These are appropriate assessments of circulation.
    ①,③ This may cause further damage to the ulna.
    ④ Prevention is not part of assessment.

33. Application, implementation, physiologic (a)
    ❷ Victim is displaying signs of respiratory distress; airway and breathing are the priorities.
    ①,③,④ These are interventions for shock that follow establishment of airway, breathing, and circulation.

34. Comprehension, assessment, physiologic (a)
    ❶ Body itching is the only systemic sign listed.
    ②,③,④ Identified as localized signs.

35. Application, implementation, physiologic (a)
    ❶ Radial artery can be sufficiently damaged in a crush injury so that it will not be palpable. Whenever a pulse cannot be palpated, move on to the next major artery to check circulation.
    ②,③ No indication of need in this situation.
    ④ Take care of airway, breathing, and circulation first; send another person to activate EMS if you can.

36. Comprehension, implementation, physiologic (a)
    ❶ All are correct interventions for hemorrhage, but the priority is to stop or control the bleeding.
    ② Appropriate intervention after bleeding is under control.
    ③ After applying the pressure dressing, the affected body part should be elevated to further aid in control of hemorrhage.
    ④ Movement stimulates circulation; immobilization will also aid in controlling hemorrhage.

37. Knowledge, planning, physiologic (a)
    ❶ Standard CPR procedure calls for a 15:2 count for 60 seconds providing 80 compressions in one-rescuer CPR.
    ②,③,④ Inadequate compressions when administering CPR on an adult.

38. Knowledge, implementation, environment (b)
    ❸ This distance prevents damage to ribs and internal structures while providing adequate cardiac output.
    ① May cause lower rib damage and low cardiac output.
    ② May cause internal organ damage and no cardiac output.
    ④ May cause left lower rib damage.

39. Knowledge, planning, physiologic (a)
    ❹ In two-rescuer CPR the standard ratio of compressions to breaths is 5:1.
    ① 15:2 is correct for one-rescuer CPR.
    ② Overventilation.
    ③ Too many compressions for two-rescuer CPR.

40. Knowledge, planning, physiologic (b)
    ❹ Standard rescue breathing procedure.
    ① Breaths should be full but at 1½ to 2 seconds per breath, allowing the lungs to deflate between breaths.
    ② Breaths should be given at the lowest possible pressure to avoid gastric distention.
    ③ Not standard rescue breathing procedure.

41. Application, assessment, physiologic (c)
    ❸ The painless nature of this burn in conjunction with a lack of capillary refill and red, leathery skin are characteristics of a full thickness burn.
    ① A minor burn is normally painful and will blanch when the skin is compressed.
    ② A moderate degree burn is normally painful in nature, with blistered skin and may or may not blanch.
    ④ A partial-thickness burn, similar in severity to a moderate burn, is normally painful and blistered.

42. Comprehension, assessment, physiologic (b)
    ❷ Potato salad is made with salad dressing or mayonnaise, which are egg products. Salmonella poisoning is the most frequent cause of food-borne illness and is caused by contaminated eggs or egg spoilage.
    ① Hotdogs are highly processed/preserved meat products which are normally not associated with food-borne illness.
    ③ Potato chips are normally not associated with food-borne illness.
    ④ Carbonated beverages are normally not associated with food-borne illness.

43. Comprehension, planning, physiologic (b)
    ❹ Saturating the blood with oxygen may allow the body's tissues to remain oxygenated.
    ① This rate of flow would allow the carboxyhemoglobin to remain in place.
    ② This rate of flow would not provide adequate tissue oxygenation.
    ③ This rate of flow would not break the affinity of carbon monoxide for hemoglobin.

44. Comprehension, assessment, physiologic (b)
    ❶ Sedatives combined with alcohol cause respiratory depression.
    ② Temperature is not affected by these drugs.
    ③ Lung sounds should be included in the baseline assessment.
    ④ Pupil size and reactivity are included in a neurologic assessment.

45. Comprehension, assessment, environment (b)
    ❹ The patient should be kept NPO because the pain may require immediate surgery.
    ① The physician should provide an order for oral fluids.
    ② Ingestion of water could delay surgery, if the physician believes the patient needs abdominal surgery.
    ③ Clear liquids should be tried first and there is no physician order for liquids.

46. Comprehension, assessment, physiologic (b)
    ❷ The nail may be tamponading a major blood vessel.
    ① Impaled objects should not be removed until a doctor sees the patient.
    ③ Determining if the patient has recently had a tetanus shot is required.
    ④ Once the nail has been removed, irrigation will be necessary.

47. Comprehension, implementation, physiologic (c)
    ❷ Sterile towels moistened with saline will prevent the mucous membranes from drying out.
    ① A dry dressing may adhere to the bowel and cause more damage.
    ③ Preventing further damage to the bowel is the primary concern.
    ④ Only a physician should return body parts to their proper position.

48. Comprehension, implementation, physiologic (b)
    ❸ Immediate oxygen may prevent pain and tissue damage.
    ① It is more important to try to save tissue.
    ② Further assessment needs to be done before pain medicine can be given.
    ④ An IV line should be inserted after assessment is completed.

49. Comprehension, implementation, physiologic (b)
    ❶ Because the nature of the injury is unknown, protection of the cervical spine is imperative.
    ② An endotracheal tube is not recommended; he is breathing on his own and his vital signs are stable.
    ③ Determining level of consciousness is secondary to preserving function.
    ④ Because his vitals are stable, insertion of an IV is not a priority.

50. Knowledge, implementation, physiologic (c)
    ❶ Gas gangrene may occur because epinephrine reduces oxygen tension of the tissues, encouraging the growth of contaminating organisms.
    ② Necrosis caused by vasoconstriction usually occurs from repeated local injections.

③ Epinephrine can be given IM with massaging at the site to counteract possible vasoconstriction, but the nurse is to avoid IM administration of the parenteral suspension into the buttocks.

④ This site does not necessarily affect the adverse reactions to a drug that an individual may have. If an adverse reaction occurs, the physician will adjust the dosage or discontinue the drug.

51. Application, implementation, physiologic (b)
   ❷ An open airway always takes first priority in any situation.
   ① Beginning intravenous fluids is the next step, after establishing airway and circulation maintenance.
   ③ Assessing for a cutdown for IV fluids can be done after determining the need for IV fluids.
   ④ Covering the burned areas with sterile dressings and gauze is done after airway maintenance and fluid maintenance are established.

52. Application, assessment, physiologic (b)
   ❷ Salmonella is caused by eating raw eggs contaminated with the salmonella bacteria. This organism can cause the symptoms of stomach cramps, vomiting, headaches, and fever.
   ① Botulism is caused by toxins produced by *Clostridium botulinum* bacteria and is characterized by double vision and respiratory difficulties.
   ③ Trichinosis is caused by a parasite, *Trichinella spiralis,* which is found in undercooked pork. The symptoms include vomiting, fever, chills, and muscle pain.
   ④ Perfringens is a type of poisoning caused by *Clostridium perfringens* bacteria, which is found in soil and on foods. It causes nausea and diarrhea.

53. Knowledge, assessment, physiologic (b)
   ❸ When the epidermis, dermis, and subcutaneous tissues are involved, the burn is classified as a third-degree burn. Colors may vary in this type of burn, and there is little or no pain because nerves have been destroyed.
   ① A first-degree burn involves the epidermis with a red and pink color.
   ② A second-degree burn involves the epidermis and dermis. The color ranges from mottled pink to red, and there is usually some blistering.
   ④ The top three layers of skin are involved in a fourth-degree burn, and may include fat, muscle, and bone.

54. Knowledge, assessment, physiologic (b)
   ❹ Hypovolemic shock results in loss of blood volume in blood vessels.
   ① Septic shock results from complications of septicemia, a condition in which infectious agents release toxins into the blood.
   ② Neurogenic shock results from widespread dilation of blood vessels, caused by an imbalance in autonomic stimulation of smooth muscles in vessel walls.
   ③ Cardiogenic shock results from any type of heart failure.

55. Comprehension, assessment, physiologic (b)
   ❹ Accessory chest muscles will aid in bringing oxygen to the lungs. Anxiety is common with air hunger.
   ① Lethargy is inconsistent with partial obstruction.
   ② Absence of spontaneous respirations indicates total airway occlusion.
   ③ A deep cough requires deep inspiration.

56. Comprehension, assessment, physiologic (b)
   ❹ Bag-valve-mask ventilation or AMBU ventilation provides oxygen to correct the hypoxia.
   ① Chest tubes only drain the pleural space.
   ② Cricothyroid puncture would be indicated if there were upper airway injury.
   ③ Trendelenburg position may assist with fluid drainage but will not help correct hypoxia. It may also cause dyspnea.

57. Comprehension, assessment, physiologic (c)
   ❸ The presence of myoglobin in the urine indicates muscle damage.
   ① Renal failure is not indicated by the color of the urine.
   ② Hepatic failure is uncommon with these types of injuries.
   ④ Red urine is not associated with skin damage.

58. Comprehension, assessment, physiologic (b)
   ❸ These are signs of dehydration seen in DKA.
   ① Dryness is seen.
   ② These are signs of diabetes.
   ④ Lethargy is more common.

59. Knowledge, implementation, physiologic (b)
   ❸ An arrest in an adult is usually caused by a cardiac arrythmia such as ventricular fibrillation. Early defibrillation is necessary to revive the patient.
   ① Lack of oxygen will cause brain damage.
   ② Children need to be ventilated as quickly as possible, because an arrest in a child usually results from choking or suffocation. The child may revive quickly after CPR is begun.
   ④ Adults can be resuscitated many times, especially if defibrillation is done early. You must always try, unless the patient has obviously been without oxygen for a long time.

60. Application, implementation, physiologic (c)
   ❶ Blood pressure does not always drop immediately. Increased heart rate and cold, clammy skin are signs of shock.
   ② Pupils will not indicate shock until the very late stages, after brain damage has occurred.
   ③ Elevated temp will be a sign of cardiac damage, but not in the first 24 to 48 hours. It is not an indication of shock.
   ④ Mental confusion is a late sign of shock.

Appendix A

NANDA-approved nursing diagnoses and definitions*

Activity intolerance
The state in which an individual has insufficient physiological or psychological energy to endure or complete required or desired daily activities.

Activity intolerance, risk for
The state in which an individual is at risk of experiencing insufficient physiological or psychological energy to endure or complete required or desired daily activities.

***Adaptive capacity, decreased: intracranial**
A clinical state in which intracranial fluid dynamic mechanisms that normally compensate for increases in intracranial volumes are compromised, resulting in repeated disproportionate increases in intracranial pressure (ICP) in response to a variety of noxious and nonnoxious stimuli.

Adjustment, impaired
The state in which an individual is unable to modify his/her lifestyle/behavior in a manner consistent with a change in health status.

Airway clearance, ineffective
The state in which an individual is unable to clear secretions or obstructions from the respiratory tract to maintain airway patency.

Anxiety
A vague, uneasy feeling, the source of which is often nonspecific or unknown to the individual.

Aspiration, risk for
The state in which an individual is at risk for entry of gastric secretions, oropharyngeal secretions, or exogenous food or fluids into tracheobronchial passages due to dysfunction or absence of normal protective mechanisms.

Body image disturbance
Disruption in the way one perceives one's body image.

Body temperature, altered, risk for
The state in which an individual is at risk for failure to maintain body temperature within normal range.

Bowel elimination, altered
See Bowel incontinence; Constipation; Constipation, colonic; Constipation, perceived; Diarrhea.

Bowel incontinence
The state in which an individual experiences a change in normal bowel habits characterized by involuntary passage of stool.

Breastfeeding, effective
The state in which a mother-infant dyad/family exhibits adequate proficiency and satisfaction with the breastfeeding process.

Breastfeeding, ineffective
The state in which a mother, infant, and/or family experiences dissatisfaction or difficulty with the breastfeeding process.

Breastfeeding, interrupted
A break in the continuity of the breastfeeding process as a result of inability or inadvisability to put the baby to the breast for feeding.

Breathing pattern, ineffective
The state in which an individual's inhalation and/or exhalation pattern does not enable adequate ventilation.

Cardiac output, decreased
The state in which the blood pumped by an individual's heart is sufficiently reduced that it is inadequate to meet the needs of the body's tissues.

Caregiver role strain
A caregiver's felt difficulty in performing the family caregiver role.

Caregiver role strain, risk for
Vulnerability for feeling difficulty in performing the family caregiver role.

Comfort, altered
See Pain; Pain, chronic.

Communication, impaired verbal
The state in which an individual experiences a decreased or absent ability to use or understand language in human interaction.

***Confusion, acute**
The abrupt onset of a cluster of global, transient changes and disturbances in attention, cognition, psychomotor activity, level of consciousness, and/or sleep/wake cycle.

***Confusion, chronic**
An irreversible, long-standing and/or progressive deterioration of intellect and personality characterized by decreased ability to interpret environmental stimuli, decreased capacity for intellectual thought processes and manifested by disturbances of memory, orientation, and behavior.

Constipation
The state in which an individual experiences a change in normal bowel habits characterized by a decrease in frequency and/or passage of hard, dry stools.

Constipation, colonic
The state in which an individual's pattern of elimination is characterized by hard, dry stool that results from a delay in passage of food residue.

Constipation, perceived
The state in which an individual makes a self-diagnosis of constipation and ensures a daily bowel movement through use of laxatives, enemas, and suppositories.

***Coping, community: potential for enhanced**
A pattern of community activities for adaptation and problem solving that is satisfactory for meeting the demands or needs of the community but can be improved for management of current and future problems/stressors.

***Coping, ineffective community**
A pattern of community activities for adaptation and problem solving that is unsatisfactory for meeting the demands or needs of the community.

*New diagnosis approved at the eleventh NANDA conference, 1994.
Adapted from *Mosby's medical, nursing, and allied health dictionary*, ed 4, St Louis, 1994, Mosby.

Coping, defensive
The state in which an individual experiences falsely positive-self-evaluation based on a self-protective pattern that defends against underlying perceived threats to positive self-regard.

Coping, family: potential for growth
Effective managing of adaptive tasks by family member involved with the client's health challenge, who now is exhibiting desire and readiness for enhanced health and growth in regard to self and in relation to the client.

Coping, ineffective family: compromised
Insufficient, ineffective, or compromised support, comfort, assistance, or encouragement usually by a supportive primary person (family member or close friend); client may need it to manage or master adaptive tasks related to his/her health challenge.

Coping, ineffective family: disabling
Behavior of significant person (family member or other primary person) that disables his/her own capacities and the client's capacities to effectively address tasks essential to either person's adaptation to the health challenge.

Coping, ineffective individual
Impairment of adaptive behaviors and problem-solving abilities of a person in meeting life's demands and roles.

Decisional conflict (specify)
A state of uncertainty about the course of action to be taken when choice among competing actions involves risk, loss, or challenge to personal life values. (Specify focus of conflict, e.g., choices regarding health, family relationship, career, finances, or other life events.)

Denial, ineffective
A conscious or unconscious attempt to disavow the knowledge or meaning of an event to reduce anxiety/fear to the detriment of health.

Diarrhea
The state in which an individual experiences a change in normal bowel habits characterized by the frequent passage of loose, fluid, unformed stools.

Disuse syndrome, risk for
The state in which an individual is at risk for deterioration of body systems as the result of prescribed or unavoidable inactivity.

Diversional activity deficit
The state in which an individual experiences a decreased stimulation from or interest or engagement in recreational or leisure activities.

Dysreflexia
The state in which an individual with a spinal cord injury at T7 or above experiences or is at risk of experiencing a life-threatening uninhibited sympathetic response of the nervous system to a noxious stimulus.

*Energy field disturbance
A disruption of the flow of energy surrounding a person's being which results in a disharmony of the body, mind, and/or spirit.

*Environmental interpretation syndrome, impaired
Consistent lack of orientation to person, place, time, or circumstances over more than three to six months necessitating a protective environment.

Family processes, altered
The state in which a family that normally functions effectively experiences a dysfunction.

*Family processes, altered: alcoholism
The state in which the psychosocial, spiritual, and physiological functions of the family unit are chronically disorganized, leading to conflict, denial of problems, resistance to change, ineffective problem-solving, and a series of self-perpetuating crises.

Fatigue
An overwhelming sense of exhaustion and decreased capacity for physical and mental work regardless of adequate sleep.

Fear
Feeling of dread related to an identifiable source that the person validates.

Fluid volume deficit (1)
The state in which an individual experiences vascular, cellular, or intracellular dehydration related to failure of regulatory mechanisms.

Fluid volume deficit (2)
The state in which an individual experiences vascular, cellular, or intracellular dehydration related to active loss.

Fluid volume deficit, risk for
The state in which an individual is at risk of experiencing vascular, cellular, or intracellular dehydration.

Fluid volume excess
The state in which an individual experiences increased fluid retention and edema.

Gas exchange, impaired
The state in which an individual experiences an imbalance between oxygen uptake and carbon dioxide elimination at the alveolar-capillary membrane gas exchange area.

Grieving, anticipatory
Intellectual and emotional responses by which individuals work through the process of modifying self-concept based on the perception of potential loss.

Grieving, dysfunctional
Extended, unsuccessful use of intellectual and emotional responses by which individuals attempt to work through the process of modifying self-concept based on the perception of loss.

Growth and development, altered
The state in which an individual demonstrates deviations in norms from his/her age group.

Health maintenance, altered
Inability to identify, manage, and/or seek out help to maintain health.

Health-seeking behaviors (specify)
The state in which a client in stable health is actively seeking ways to alter personal health habits and/or the environment in order to move toward optimal health. (*Stable health status* is defined as age-appropriate illness prevention measures achieved; the client reports good or excellent health, and signs and symptoms of disease, if present, are controlled.)

Home maintenance management, impaired
Inability to independently maintain a safe growth-promoting immediate environment.

Hopelessness
The subjective state in which an individual sees limited or no alternatives or personal choices available and is unable to mobilize energy on own behalf.

Hyperthermia
The state in which an individual's body temperature is elevated above his/her normal range.

Hypothermia
The state in which an individual's body temperature is reduced below his/her normal range but not below 35.6° C (rectal)/ 36.4° C (rectal, newborn).

*New diagnosis approved at the eleventh NANDA conference, 1994.

Incontinence, bowel
See Bowel incontinence.

Incontinence, functional
The state in which an individual experiences an involuntary, unpredictable passage of urine.

Incontinence, reflex
The state in which an individual experiences an involuntary loss of urine occurring at somewhat predictable intervals when a specific bladder volume is reached.

Incontinence, stress
The state in which an individual experiences a loss of urine of less than 50 ml occurring with increased abdominal pressure.

Incontinence, total
The state in which an individual experiences a continuous and unpredictable loss of urine.

Incontinence, urge
The state in which an individual experiences involuntary passage of urine occurring soon after a strong sense of urgency to void.

*Infant behavior, disorganized
Alteration in integration and modulation of the physiological and behavioral systems of functioning (i.e., autonomic, motor, state, organizational, self-regulatory, and attentional-interactional systems).

*Infant behavior, disorganized, risk for
Risk for alteration in integration and modulation of the physiological and behavioral systems of functioning (i.e., autonomic, motor, state, organizational, self-regulatory, and attentional-interactional systems).

*Infant behavior, organized, potential for enhanced
A pattern of modulation of the physiological and behavioral systems of functioning of an infant (i.e., autonomic, motor, state, organizational, self-regulatory, and attentional-interactional systems) that is satisfactory but that can be improved resulting in higher levels of integration in response to environmental stimuli.

Infant feeding pattern, ineffective
A state in which an infant demonstrates an impaired ability to suck or coordinate the suck-swallow response.

Infection, risk for
The state in which an individual is at increased risk for being invaded by pathogenic organisms.

Injury, risk for
The state in which an individual is at risk of injury as a result of environmental conditions interacting with the individual's adaptive and defensive resources. See also Poisoning, risk for; Suffocation, risk for; Trauma, risk for

Knowledge deficit (specify)
Absence or deficiency of cognitive information related to specific topic.

*Loneliness, risk for
A subjective state in which an individual is at risk of experiencing vague dysphoria.

*Management of therapeutic regimen (community), ineffective
A pattern of regulating and integrating into community processes programs for treatment of illness and the sequelae of illness that are unsatisfactory for meeting health-related goals.

*Management of therapeutic regimen (families), ineffective
A pattern of regulating and integrating into family processes a program for treatment of illness and the sequelae of illness that is unsatisfactory for meeting specific health goals.

*Management of therapeutic regimen (individual), effective
A pattern of regulating and integrating into daily living a program for treatment of illness and its sequelae that is satisfactory for meeting specific health goals.

*Management of therapeutic regimen (individual), ineffective
A pattern of regulating and integrating into daily living a program for treatment of illness and the sequelae of illness that is unsatisfactory for meeting specific health goals.

*Memory, impaired
The state in which an individual experiences the inability to remember or recall bits of information or behavioral skills. Impaired memory may be attributed to pathophysiological or situational causes that are either temporary or permanent.

Mobility, impaired physical
The state in which an individual experiences a limitation of ability for independent physical movement.

Noncompliance (specify)
A person's informed decision not to adhere to a therapeutic recommendation.

Nutrition, altered: less than body requirements
The state in which an individual experiences an intake of nutrients insufficient to meet metabolic needs.

Nutrition, altered: more than body requirements
The state in which an individual is experiencing an intake of nutrients that exceeds metabolic needs.

Nutrition, altered: risk for more than body requirements
The state in which an individual is at risk of experiencing an intake of nutrients that exceeds metabolic needs.

Oral mucous membrane, altered
The state in which an individual experiences disruptions in the tissue layers of the oral cavity.

Pain
The state in which an individual experiences and reports the presence of severe discomfort or an uncomfortable sensation.

Pain, chronic
The state in which an individual experiences pain that continues for more than 6 months.

*Parent/infant/child attachment, altered, risk for
Disruption of the interactive process between parent/significant other and infant that fosters the development of a protective and nurturing reciprocal relationship.

Parental role conflict
The state in which a parent experiences role confusion and conflict in response to a crisis.

Parenting, altered, risk for
The state in which the ability of nuturing figure(s) to create an environment that promotes the optimum growth and development of another human being is altered or at risk.

*Perioperative positioning injury, risk for
A state in which the client is at risk for injury as a result of the environmental conditions found in the perioperative setting.

Peripheral neurovascular dysfunction, risk for
A state in which an individual is at risk for experiencing a disruption in circulation, sensation, or motion of an extremity.

Personal identity disturbance
Inability to distinguish between self and nonself.

Poisoning, risk for
Accentuated risk of accidental exposure to or ingestion of drugs or dangerous products in doses sufficient to cause poisoning.

Posttrauma response
The state in which an individual experiences a sustained painful response to (an) overwhelming traumatic event(s).

*New diagnosis approved at the eleventh NANDA conference, 1994.

Powerlessness

Perception that one's own action will not significantly affect an outcome; a perceived lack of control over a current situation or immediate happening.

Protection, altered

The state in which an individual experiences a decrease in the ability to guard the self from internal or external threats, such as illness or injury.

Rape-trauma syndrome

Forced, violent sexual penetration against the victim's will and consent. The trauma syndrome that develops from this attack or attempted attack includes an acute phase or disorganization of the victim's life-style and a long-term process of reorganization of life-style.

Rape-trauma syndrome: compound reaction

An acute stress reaction to a rape or attempted rape, experienced along with other major stressors, that can include reactivation of symptoms of a previous condition.

Rape-trauma syndrome: silent reaction

A complex stress reaction to a rape in which an individual is unable to describe or discuss the rape.

Relocation stress syndrome

Physiological and/or psychosocial disturbances as a result of a transfer from one environment to another.

*Role performance, altered

Disruption in the way one perceives one's role performance.

Self-care deficit, bathing/hygiene

The state in which an individual experiences an impaired ability to perform or complete bathing/hygiene activities for oneself.

Self-care deficit, dressing/grooming

The state in which an individual experiences an impaired ability to perform or complete dressing and grooming activities for oneself.

Self-care deficit, feeding

The state in which an individual experiences an impaired ability to perform or complete feeding activities for oneself.

Self-care deficit, toileting

The state in which an individual experiences an impaired ability to perform or complete toileting activities for oneself.

Self-concept, disturbance in

See Body image disturbance; Personal identity disturbance; Self-esteem disturbance.

Self-esteem disturbance

Negative self-evaluation/feelings about self or self-capabilities, which may be directly or indirectly expressed.

Self-esteem, chronic low

Long-standing negative self-evaluation/feelings about self or self-capabilities.

Self-esteem, situational low

Negative self-evaluation/feelings about self that develop in response to a loss or change in an individual who previously had a positive self-evaluation.

Self-mutilation, risk for

The state in which an individual is at high risk to perform an act on the self to injure, not kill, that produces tissue damage and tension relief.

Sensory/perceptual alterations (specify) (visual, auditory, kinesthetic, gustatory, tactile, olfactory)

The state in which an individual experiences a change in the amount or patterning of incoming stimuli accompanied by a diminished, exaggerated, distorted, or impaired response to such stimuli.

Sexual dysfunction

The state in which an individual experiences a change in sexual function that is viewed as unsatisfying, unrewarding, or inadequate.

Sexuality patterns, altered

The state in which an individual expresses concern regarding his/her sexuality.

Skin integrity, impaired

The state in which an individual's skin is adversely altered.

Skin integrity, impaired, risk for

The state in which an individual's skin is at risk of being adversely altered.

Sleep pattern disturbance

Disruption of sleep time causes discomfort or interferes with desired life-style.

Social interaction, impaired

The state in which an individual participates in an insufficient or excessive quantity or ineffective quality of social exchange.

Social isolation

Aloneness experienced by an individual and perceived as imposed by others and as a negative or threatened state.

Spiritual distress (distress of the human spirit)

Disruption in the life principle that pervades a person's entire being and that integrates and transcends one's biological and psychosocial nature.

*Spiritual well-being, potential for, enhanced

Spiritual well-being is the process of an individual's developing/unfolding of mystery through harmonious interconnectedness that springs from inner strengths.

Suffocation, risk for

Accentuated risk of accidental suffocation (inadequate air available for inhalation).

Swallowing, impaired

The state in which an individual has decreased ability to voluntarily pass fluids and/or solids from the mouth to the stomach.

Thermoregulation, ineffective

The state in which an individual's temperature fluctuates between hypothermia and hyperthermia.

Thought processes, altered

The state in which an individual experiences a disruption in cognitive operations and activities.

Tissue integrity, impaired

The state in which an individual experiences damage to mucous membrane or corneal, integumentary, or subcutaneous tissue. See also Oral mucous membrane, altered.

Tissue perfusion, altered (specify type) (renal, cerebral, cardiopulmonary gastrointestinal, peripheral)

The state in which an individual experiences a decrease in nutrition and oxygenation at the cellular level due to a deficit in capillary blood supply.

Trauma, risk for

Accentuated risk of accidental tissue injury (e.g., wound, burn, fracture)

Unilateral neglect

The state in which an individual is perceptually unaware of and inattentive to one side of the body.

Urinary elimination, altered patterns

The state in which an individual experiences a disturbance in urine elimination. See also Incontinence (functional, reflex, stress, total, urge)

*New diagnosis approved at the eleventh NANDA conference, 1994.

Urinary retention
The state in which an individual experiences incomplete emptying of the bladder.

Ventilation, inability to sustain spontaneous
A state in which the response pattern of decreased energy reserves results in an individual's inability to maintain breathing adequate to support life.

Ventilatory weaning process, dysfunctional (DVWR)
A state in which an individual cannot adjust to lowered levels of mechanical ventilator support, which interrupts and prolongs the weaning process.

Violence, high risk for: self-directed or directed at others
The state in which an individual experiences behaviors that can be physically harmful either to the self or others.

Appendix B

Classification of nursing diagnoses by human response patterns (NANDA Taxonomy I-revised)

I. Exchanging
Altered nutrition: more than body requirements
Altered nutrition: less than body requirements
Altered nutrition: high risk for more than body requirements
High risk for infection
High risk for altered body temperature
Hypothermia
Hyperthermia
Ineffective thermoregulation
Dysreflexia
Constipation
Perceived constipation
Colonic constipation
Diarrhea
Bowel incontinence
Altered patterns of urinary elimination
Stress incontinence
Reflex incontinence
Risk for poisoning
Risk for trauma
Risk for aspiration
Risk for disuse syndrome
Altered protection
Impaired tissue integrity
Altered oral mucous membrane
Impaired skin integrity
Risk for impaired skin integrity
Decreased adaptive capacity: energy field disturbance

II. Communicating
Impaired verbal communication

III. Relating
Impaired social interaction
Social isolation
Risk for loneliness
Altered role performance
Altered parenting
Risk for altered parenting
Risk for altered parent/infant/child attachment
Sexual dysfunction
Altered family processes
Caregiver role strain
Risk for caregiver role strain
Altered family processes: alcoholism
Parental role conflict
Altered sexuality patterns

IV. Valuing
Spiritual distress (distress of the human spirit)
Potential for enhanced spiritual well-being

V. Choosing
Ineffective individual coping
Impaired adjustment
Defensive coping

Ineffective denial
Ineffective family coping: disabling
Ineffective family coping: compromised
Potential for enhanced community coping
Ineffective community coping
Family coping: potential for growth
Ineffective management of therapeutic regimen (individuals)
Noncompliance (specify)
Ineffective management of therapeutic regimen: families
Ineffective management of therapeutic regimen: community
Effective management of therapeutic regimen: individual
Decisional conflict (specify)
Health-seeking behaviors (specify)

VI. Moving
Impaired physical mobility
Risk for peripheral neurovascular dysfunction
Activity intolerance
Urge incontinence
Functional incontinence
Total incontinence
Urinary retention
Altered (specify type) tissue perfusion (renal, cerebral, cardiopulmonary gastrointestinal, peripheral)
Fluid volume excess
Fluid volume deficit (1)
Fluid volume deficit (2)
Risk for fluid volume deficit
Decreased cardiac output
Impaired gas exchange
Ineffective airway clearance
Ineffective breathing pattern
Inability to sustain spontaneous ventilation
Dysfunctional ventilatory weaning response (DVWR)
Risk for injury
Risk for suffocation
Risk for activity intolerance
Fatigue
Sleep pattern disturbance
Diversional activity deficit
Impaired home maintenance management
Altered health maintenance
Feeding self-care deficit
Impaired swallowing
Ineffective breastfeeding
Interrupted breastfeeding
Effective breastfeeding
Ineffective infant feeding pattern
Bathing/hygiene self-care deficit
Dressing/grooming self-care deficit
Toileting self-care deficit
Altered growth and development
Relocation stress syndrome

Risk for disorganized infant behavior
Disorganized infant behavior
Potential for enhanced organized infant behavior

VII. **Perceiving**

Body image disturbance
Self-esteem disturbance
Chronic low self-esteem
Situational low self-esteem
Personal identity disturbance
Sensory/perceptual alterations (specify) (visual, auditory, kinesthetic, gustatory, tactile, olfactory)
Unilateral neglect
Hopelessness
Powerlessness

VIII. **Knowing**

Knowledge deficit (specify)
Impaired environmental interpretation syndrome

Acute confusion
Chronic confusion
Altered thought processes
Impaired memory

IX. **Feeling**

Pain
Chronic pain
Dysfunctional grieving
Anticipatory grieving
High risk for violence: self-directed or directed at others
High risk for self-mutilation
Post-trauma response
Rape-trauma syndrome
Rape-trauma syndrome: compound reaction
Rape-trauma syndrome: silent reaction
Anxiety
Fear

Appendix C

Classification of nursing diagnoses by functional health pattern

Health perception-health management pattern
Altered health maintenance
Altered protection
Ineffective management of therapeutic regimen
Noncompliance (specify)
High risk for infection
High risk for injury
High risk for trauma
High risk for poisoning
High risk for suffocation
Health-seeking behaviors (specify)

Nutritional-metabolic pattern
Altered nutrition: high risk for more than body requirements
Altered nutrition: more than body requirements
Altered nutrition: less than body requirements
Effective breastfeeding
Ineffective breastfeeding
Interrupted breastfeeding
Ineffective infant feeding pattern
High risk for aspiration
Impaired swallowing
Altered oral mucous membrane
Potential fluid volume deficit
Fluid volume deficit (1)
Fluid volume deficit (2)
Fluid volume excess
High risk for impaired skin integrity
Impaired skin integrity
Impaired tissue integrity
High risk for altered body temperature
Ineffective thermoregulation
Hyperthermia
Hypothermia

Elimination pattern
Constipation
Perceived constipation
Colonic constipation
Diarrhea
Bowel incontinence
Altered patterns of urinary elimination
Functional incontinence
Reflex incontinence
Stress incontinence
Urge incontinence
Total incontinence
Urinary retention

Activity-exercise pattern
High risk for activity intolerance
Dysfunctional ventilatory wearing response

Inability to sustain spontaneous ventilation
High risk for peripheral neurovascular dysfunction
Activity intolerance
Impaired physical mobility
High risk for disuse syndrome
Fatigue
Bathing/hygiene self-care deficit
Dressing/grooming self-care deficit
Feeding self-care deficit
Toileting self-care deficit
Diversional activity deficit
Impaired home maintenance management
Ineffective airway clearance
Ineffective breathing pattern
Impaired gas exchange
Decreased cardiac output
Altered (specify type) tissue perfusion (renal, cerebral, cardiopulmonary, gastrointestinal, peripheral)
Dysreflexia
Altered growth and development

Sleep-rest pattern
Sleep pattern disturbance

Cognitive-perceptual pattern
Pain
Chronic pain
Sensory perceptual alterations (specify) (visual, auditory, kinesthetic, gustatory, tactile, olfactory)
Unilateral neglect
Knowledge deficit (specify)
Altered thought processes
Decisional conflict (specify)

Self-perception–self-concept pattern
Fear
Anxiety
Hopelessness
Powerlessness
Body image disturbance
High risk for self-mutilation
Personal identity disturbance
Self-esteem disturbance
Chronic low self-esteem
Situational low self-esteem

Role-relationship pattern
Anticipatory grieving
Dysfunctional grieving
Altered role performance
Caregiver role strain
High risk for caregiver role strain
Social isolation

Based on Gordon M: *Manual of nursing diagnoses*, St Louis, 1993, Mosby.

Impaired social interaction
Relocation stress syndrome
Altered family processes
High risk for altered parenting
Altered parenting
Parental role conflict
Impaired verbal communication
High risk for violence: self-directed or directed at others
Sexuality-reproductive pattern
Sexual dysfunction
Altered sexuality patterns
Rape-trauma syndrome
Rape-trauma syndrome: compound reaction

Rape-trauma syndrome: silent reaction
Coping-stress tolerance pattern
Ineffective individual coping
Defensive coping
Ineffective denial
Impaired adjustment
Post-trauma response
Family coping: potential for growth
Ineffective family coping: compromised
Ineffective family coping: disabling
Value-belief pattern
Spiritual distress (distress of the human spirit)

Appendix D

Guide to common drug interactions

Drug	Interacting drug	Effect
Over-the-counter drugs and substances		
Antacids		
Alumina and magnesia		Effects of dicumarol may be faster and/or increased
Dihydroxaluminum sodium carbonate		
Magnesia	Digoxin	Effects of digoxin may be reduced
	Tetracyclines Doxycycline Tetracycline	Effects of tetracyclines may be reduced Should be taken 1-3 hours apart
Painkillers		
Acetaminophen	Alcoholic beverages	May cause liver damage
Buffered acetaminophen		
	Blood-thinning drugs Warfarin sodium	High doses of acetaminophen may increase blood-thinning effects of these drugs
	Tetracycline	Buffered form may cancel the effects of tetracyline Should be taken 1 hour apart
Ibuprofen	Alcoholic beverages	May cause internal bleeding or ulcers
	Blood-thinning drugs Heparin Warfarin sodium	May cause internal bleeding or ulcers
	Salicylates Aspirin Aspirin and caffeine Buffered aspirin	May cause stomach upset without relieving symptoms
Salicylates	Alcoholic beverages	May cause stomach ulcers or internal bleeding
Aspirin		
Aspirin and caffeine	Antidiabetics Chlorpropamide Tolazamide	May cause blood sugar level to drop too low
Buffered aspirin		
	Blood-thinning drugs Heparin Warfarin sodium	Increases risk of internal bleeding
	Ibuprofen	May cause stomach upset without relieving symptoms
	Tetracycline	Effects of tetracycline are reduced
Other substances	Acetaminophen	May cause liver damage
Alcoholic beverages	Buffered acetaminophen	

This table includes only common over-the-counter and prescription drugs. Some of these drugs may also interact with less common drugs and substances not described. When using any drug, always consult your doctor or pharmacist about possible interactions with other drugs, substances, or foods.

Continued

	Guide to common drug interactions—cont'd	
Drug	**Interacting drug**	**Effect**

Over-the-counter drugs and substances—cont'd
Other substances—cont'd
Alcoholic beverages—cont'd

Drug	Interacting drug	Effect

	Antidiabetics
	    Chlorpropamide
	    Tolazamide
		Stomach upset, vomiting, cramps, headaches, low blood sugar

	Antiseizure drugs
	    Carbamazepine
	    Chlordiazepoxide
	    Diazepam
	    Phenytoin
		May cause extreme drowsiness

	Barbiturates
	    Pentobarbital
	    Phenobarbital
	    Secobarbital
	    Secobarbital and amobarbital
		May cause drowsiness, increase effects of either drug, cause breathing to fail, or cause blood pressure to drop too low

	Ibuprofen	May cause internal bleeding or ulcers

	Narcotic analgesics
	    Acetaminophen and codeine
	    Meperidine
	    Propoxyphene
		May depress nervous system and breathing or cause blood pressure to drop too low

	Reserpine	May increase effects of alcohol and reserpine

	Salicylates
	    Aspirin
	    Aspirin and caffeine
	    Buffered aspirin
		May cause stomach ulcers or internal bleeding

	Tricyclic antidepressants
	    Amitriptyline
	    Amoxapine
	    Doxepin
		May cause extreme drowsiness

Sodium chloride (salt)	Lithium	Low-salt diet causes lithium to build up in body and is not advised
Tobacco (smoking)	Birth control pills Norethindrone with ethinyl estradiol	May increase chances of blood clot or heart attack

Tyramine-containing foods
    Avocados, bananas, beer, caffeine, cheese, chicken liver, chocolate, fava beans, fermented sausages (salami, pepperoni, bologna, etc.), canned figs, pickled herring, pineapple, raisins, red wine, sauerkraut, soy sauce, yeast extract, yogurt
	MAO inhibitors
	    Isocarboxazid
	    Phenelzine
	    Tranylcypromine
		May cause severe and sometimes fatal high blood pressure
		Headache, vomiting, fever, and high blood pressure are warning signals

Prescription drugs
Antibiotics
Erythromycins

Drug	Interacting drug	Effect

Erythromycins
    Erythromycin
    Erythromycin lactobionate
	Penicillins
	    Amoxicillin
	    Ampicillin
		Could interfere with the effects of penicillins

This table includes only common over-the-counter and prescription drugs. Some of these drugs may also interact with less common drugs and substances not described. When using any drug, always consult your doctor or pharmacist about possible interactions with other drugs, substances, or foods.

Continued

Guide to common drug interactions—cont'd

Drug	Interacting drug	Effect
Prescription drugs—cont'd		
Antibiotics		
Penicillins		
Amoxicillin	Birth control pills	May interfere with and result in unplanned pregnancy or menstrual problems
Ampicillin	Norethindrone with ethinyl estradiol	
	Blood-thinning drugs	May increase blood thinning effects of these drugs
	Warfarin sodium	
	Erythromycins	May interfere with effects of penicillins
	Erythromycin	
	Erythromycin lactobionate	
	Tetracyclines	May interfere with effects of penicillins
	Doxycycline	
	Tetracycline	
Tetracyclines	Acetaminophen	
Doxycycline	Buffered acetaminophen	
Tetracycline	Antacids	May decrease effects of tetracyclines and should be taken 1 to 3 hours apart
	Alumina and magnesia	
	Dihydroxaluminum sodium carbonate	
	Magnesia	
	Barbiturates	May decrease effects of doxycycline
	Pentobarbital	Other tetracyclines can be used
	Phenobarbital	
	Secobarbital	
	Secobarbital and amobarbital	
	Penicillins	May interfere with effects of penicillins
	Amoxicillin	
	Ampicillin	
	Salicylates	Effects of tetracyclines are reduced
	Aspirin	
	Aspirin and caffeine	
	Buffered aspirin	
Antidepressants		
Lithium	Sodium chloride (salt)	Low-salt diet causes lithium to build up in body and is not advised
	Thiazide diuretics	May cause lithium to have toxic effect
	Furosemide	
	Methyclothiazide	
Tricyclic antidepressants	Alcoholic beverages	May cause extreme drowsiness
Amitriptyline	Antiseizure drugs	Effects of antiseizure drug may be decreased
Amoxapine	Carbamazepine	Dosage should be adjusted
Doxepin	Chlordiazepoxide	
	Diazepam	
	Phenytoin	
	Blood-thinning drugs	May cause internal bleeding
	Warfarin sodium	

This table includes only common over-the-counter and prescription drugs. Some of these drugs may also interact with less common drugs and substances not described. When using any drug, always consult your doctor or pharmacist about possible interactions with other drugs, substances, or foods.

Continued

Guide to common drug interactions—cont'd

Drug	Interacting drug	Effect
Prescription drugs—cont'd		
Antidepressants—cont'd		
Tricyclic antidepressants—cont'd	MAO inhibitors Isocarboxazid Phenelzine Tranylcypromine	Severe seizure and death could result Should be taken 14 days apart
	Narcotic analgesics Acetaminophen and codeine Meperidine Propoxyphene	May depress nervous system and breathing and cause blood pressure to drop too low
Antidiabetics Chlorpropamide Tolazamide	Alcoholic beverages	May cause stomach upset, vomiting, cramps, headaches, low blood sugar
	Beta-adrenergic blockers Metoprolol Propranolol	May increase risk of either high or low blood sugar levels May mask symptoms
	Blood-thinning drugs Warfarin sodium	Blood-thinning effect will be increased at first, later it will be decreased May also cause low blood sugar and become toxic
	MAO inhibitors Isocarboxazid Phenelzine Tranylcypromine	Can cause extreme low blood sugar level
	Salicylates Aspirin Aspirin and caffeine Buffered aspirin	May cause blood sugar level to drop too low
Isophane insulin suspension	Beta-adrenergic blockers Metoprolol Propranolol	These may mask symptoms of low blood sugar
	Birth control pills Norethindrone with ethinyl estradiol	May increase risk of high blood sugar levels Dosages should be adjusted
	MAO inhibitors Isocarboxazid Phenelzine Tranylcypromine	May cause extreme low blood sugar level
Antiseizure drugs Carbamazepine Chlordiazepoxide Diazepam Phenytoin	Alcoholic beverages	May cause extreme drowsiness
	Beta-adrenergic blockers Metoprolol Propranolol	Could decrease the effect of beta-blockers
	Birth control pills Norethindrone with ethinyl estradiol	Phenytoin and carbamazepine may interfere and increase risk of unplanned pregnancy May increase effect of diazepam

This table includes only common over-the-counter and prescription drugs. Some of these drugs may also interact with less common drugs and substances not described. When using any drug, always consult your doctor or pharmacist about possible interactions with other drugs, substances, or foods.

Continued

Guide to common drug interactions—cont'd

Drug	Interacting drug	Effect
Prescription drugs—cont'd		
Antiseizure drugs—cont'd	Tricyclic antidepressants Amitriptyline Amoxapine Doxepin	Effects of antiseizure drug may be decreased Dosage should be adjusted
Barbiturates Pentobarbital Phenobarbital Secobarbital Secobarbital and amobarbital	Alcoholic beverages	May cause drowsiness, increase effects of either drug, cause breathing to fail, or cause blood pressure to drop too low
	Birth control pills Norethindrone with ethinyl estradiol	Barbiturates may interfere with and result in unplanned pregnancy
	Blood-thinning drugs Warfarin sodium	May decrease blood-thinning effects of these drugs
	Doxycycline	May decrease effects of doxycycline Other tetracyclines can be used
Birth control pills Norethindrone with ethinyl estradiol	Antiseizure drugs Carbamazepine Chlordiazepoxide Diazepam Phenytoin	Will increase the sedative effects of these drugs May decrease the effects of other anti-seizure drugs
	Barbiturates Pentobarbital Phenobarbital Secobarbital Secobarbital and amobarbital	Barbiturates may interfere with birth control pills and result in unplanned pregnancy
	Isophane insulin suspension	May increase risk of high blood sugar levels; dosages should be adjusted
	Penicillins Amoxicillin Ampicillin	May interfere with birth control pills and result in unplanned pregnancy
	Tobacco (smoking)	May increase chances of blood clot or heart attack
Blood pressure drugs Thiazide diuretics Furosemide Methyclothiazide	Beta-adrenergic blockers Metoprolol Propranolol	Can cause extremely low blood pressure
	Digitalis glycosides Digoxin	Can cause irregular heartbeat, which can be fatal Can cause extremely low blood pressure
	Lithium	May cause lithium to have toxic effect
	Reserpine	Can cause extremely low blood pressure
Rauwolfia alkaloids Reserpine	Alcoholic beverages	May increase effects of alcohol May increase effects of rauwolfia alkaloids

This table includes only common over-the-counter and prescription drugs. Some of these drugs may also interact with less common drugs and substances not described. When using any drug, always consult your doctor or pharmacist about possible interactions with other drugs, substances, or foods.

Continued

Guide to common drug interactions—cont'd

Drug	Interacting drug	Effect
Prescription drugs—cont'd		
Blood pressure drugs—cont'd		
Rauwolfia alkaloids—cont'd		

Reserpine—cont'd	Beta-adrenergic blockers
	  Metoprolol
	  Propranolol
		May cause extremely slow heartbeat and low blood pressure

	Digitalis glycosides Digoxin	May cause irregular heartbeat

	MAO inhibitors
	  Isocarboxazid
	  Phenelzine
	  Tranylcypromine
		May cause slight to sudden and severe high blood pressure
		May cause extreme high fever
		Either effect could be life-threatening

	Thiazide diuretics
	  Furosemide
	  Methyclothiazide
		Can cause extreme low blood pressure

Blood-thinning drugs Warfarin sodium	Acetaminophen Buffered acetaminophen	High doses of acetaminophen may increase blood-thinning effects of these drugs

	Antacids
	  Alumina and magnesia
	  Dihydroxyaluminum sodium
	    carbonate
	  Magnesia
		Effects of dicumarol may be faster and may also be increased

	Antidiabetics
	  Chlorpropamide
	  Tolazamide
		Blood-thinning effect will be increased at first, later it will be decreased
		May also cause low blood sugar and become toxic

	Barbiturates
	  Pentobarbital
	  Phenobarbital
	  Secobarbital
	  Secobarbital and amobarbital
		Decreases blood-thinning effect

	Heparin	May cause increased risk of internal bleeding
	Ibuprofen	May cause internal bleeding or ulcers

	Penicillins
	  Amoxicillin
	  Ampicillin
		May increase blood-thinning effects of these drugs

	Salicylates
	  Aspirin
	  Aspirin and caffeine
	  Buffered aspirin
		Blood-thinning effects will be increased
		May cause ulcers or internal bleeding

	Tricylic antidepressants
	  Amitriptyline
	  Amoxapine
	  Doxepin
		May cause internal bleeding

Heparin	Blood-thinning drugs Warfarin sodium	May cause increased risk of internal bleeding

This table includes only common over-the-counter and prescription drugs. Some of these drugs may also interact with less common drugs and substances not described. When using any drug, always consult your doctor or pharmacist about possible interactions with other drugs, substances, or foods.

Continued

Guide to common drug interactions—cont'd

Drug	Interacting drug	Effect
Prescription drugs—cont'd		
Blood-thinning drugs—cont'd		

Heparin—cont'd	Salicylates
	   Aspirin
	   Aspirin and caffeine
	   Buffered aspirin
		Blood-thinning effects will be increased
		May cause ulcers or internal bleeding

Heart drugs		

Beta-adrenergic blockers
   Metoprolol
   Propranolol
	Antidiabetics
	   Chlorpropamide
	   Tolazamide
		May increase risk of either high or low
		   blood sugar levels
		May mask symptoms

	Antiseizure drugs
	   Carbamazepine
	   Chlordiazepoxide
	   Diazepam
	   Phenytoin
		Could decrease the effect of beta blockers

	Digitalis glycosides
	   Digoxin
		May cause extremely slow heartbeat with a
		   chance of heart block

	Isophane insulin suspension	Beta blockers may mask symptoms of low blood sugar May also cause low blood sugar
	Reserpine	May cause extremely slow heartbeat and low blood pressure

	Thiazide diuretics
	   Furosemide
	   Methyclothiazide
		Can cause extremely low blood pressure

Digitalis glycosides
   Digoxin
	Antacids
	   Alumina and magnesia
	   Dihydroxaluminum sodium
	      carbonate
	   Magnesia
		Effects of digoxin may be reduced

	Beta-adrenergic blockers
	   Metoprolol
	   Propranolol
	Reserpine
		May cause extremely slow heartbeat with a
		   chance of heart block
		
		May cause irregular heartbeat

	Thiazide diuretics
	   Furosemide
	   Methyclothiazide
		May cause extreme low blood pressure;
		   may cause digitalis to become toxic

Monoamine oxidase inhibitors
(MAO inhibitors)
Isocarboxazid
Phenelzine
Tranylcypromine
	Antidiabetics
	   Chlorpropamide
	   Isophane insulin suspension
	   Tolazamide
		Can cause extreme low blood sugar level

	Narcotic analgesics
	   Acetaminophen and codeine
	   Meperidine
	   Propoxyphene
		May cause severe and sometimes fatal
		   reactions

This table includes only common over-the-counter and prescription drugs. Some of these drugs may also interact with less common drugs and substances not described. When using any drug, always consult your doctor or pharmacist about possible interactions with other drugs, substances, or foods.

Continued

Guide to common drug interactions—cont'd

Drug	Interacting drug	Effect
Prescription drugs—cont'd *Monoamine oxidase inhibitors (MAO inhibitors)—cont'd*	Reserpine	May cause slight to sudden and severe high blood pressure May cause extreme high fever Either effect could be life-threatening
	Tricyclic antidepressants Amitriptyline Amoxapine Doxepin	Severe seizure and death could result Should be taken 14 days apart
	Tyramine-containing foods Avocados, bananas, beer, caffeine, cheese, chicken liver, chocolate, fava beans, fermented sausages (salami, pepperoni, bologna, etc.) canned figs, pickled herring, pineapple, raisins, red wine, sauerkraut, soy sauce, yeast extract, yogurt	May cause severe and sometimes fatal high blood pressure Headache, vomiting, fever, and high blood pressure are warning signals
Painkillers Narcotic analgesics Acetaminophen and codeine Meperidine Propoxyphene	Alcoholic beverages	May depress nervous system and breathing May cause blood pressure to drop too low
	MAO inhibitors Isocarboxazid Phenelzine Tranylcypromine	May cause many severe and sometimes fatal reactions
	Tricyclic antidepressants Amitriptyline Amoxapine Doxepin	May depress nervous system and breathing May cause blood pressure to drop too low

This table includes only common over-the-counter and prescription drugs. Some of these drugs may also interact with less common drugs and substances not described. When using any drug, always consult your doctor or pharmacist about possible interactions with other drugs, substances, or foods.

Appendix E

Commonly used medications: trade to generic name listing

Trade name	Generic name	Trade name	Generic name
Abbokinase	urokinase	Ascorbic Acid	vitamin C
Accutane	isotretinoin	Ascriptin	buffered aspirin
Achromycin	tetracycline	aspirin	acetylsalicylic acid (ASA)
ACTH	corticotropin	Asthmanefin	racepinephrine
Acthar	corticotropin	Atabrine	quinacrine
Actidil	triprolidine	Atarax	hydroxyzine HCl
Actifed	triprolidine and pseudoephedrine	Ativan	lorazepam
Actigall	ursodiol	Atromid-S	clofibrate
Activase	t-PA	Atrovent	ipratropium
Adapin	doxepin HCl	Augmentin	amoxicillin and clavulanate
Adrenalin	epinephrine	Aventyl	nortriptyline
Adriamycin	doxorubicin HCl	Axid	nizatidine
Advil	ibuprofen	Azactam	aztreonam
Afrin	oxymetazoline, nasal	Azene	chlorazepate, monopotassium
Akineton	biperiden	Azo-Gantrisin	phenazopyridine and sulfisoxazole
Aldactazide	hydrochlorothiazide and spirono-lactone	Azolid-A	phenylbutazone
		AZT	zidovudine
Aldactone	spironolactone	Azulfidine	sulfasalazine
Aldomet	methyldopa	Bactrim	sulfamethoxazole and trimethoprim
Alka-2	calcium carbonate	Beclovent	beclomethasone
Alkeran	melphalan	Benadryl	diphenhydramine
Alupent	metaproterenol	Benemid	probenecid
Amcil	ampicillin	Bentyl	dicyclomine
Americaine	benzocaine	Betadine	povidone-iodine
Amicar	aminocaproic acid	Bicillin	penicillin and benzathine
Amikin	amikacin	BiCNU	carmustine
Amoxil	amoxicillin	Blenoxane	bleomycin
Amphogel	aluminum hydroxide gel	Blocadren	timolol maleate
Amytal	amobarbital	Bonine	meclizine
Anacin-3	acetaminophen	Brethine	terbutaline
Anaprox	naproxen sodium	Bretylol	bretylium tosylate
Ancef	cefazolin	Bricanyl	terbutaline
Ancobon	flucytosine	Bronkosol	isoetharine HCl
Anectine	succinylcholine	Bufferin	aspirin, buffered
Ansaid	flurbiprofen	Bumex	bumetanide
Anspor	cephradine	Buprenex	buprenorphine
Antabuse	disulfiram	Bupropion	wellbutrin
Antilirium	physostigmine	Buspar	buspirone
Antivert	meclizine	Butazolidin	phenylbutazone
Apresoline	hydralazine	Butisol	butabarbital
Aquamephyton	phytonadione (vitamin K_1)	Calan	verapamil
Aralen	chloroquine	Calcimar	calcitonin
Aramine	metaraminol	Capoten	captopril
Arfonad	trimethaphan	Carafate	sucralfate
Aristocort	triamcinolone	Cardene	nicardipine
Arlidin	nylidrin	Catapres	clonidine
Artane	trihexyphenidyl HCl	Ceclor	cefaclor

Adapted from *Mosby's medical, nursing, and allied health dictionary*, ed 4, St Louis, 1994, Mosby.

Continued

Commonly used medications: trade to generic name listing—cont'd

Trade name	Generic name	Trade name	Generic name
Cedilanid	lanatoside C	DES	diethylstilbestrol
Cedilanid-D	deslanoside	Desenex	undecylenic acid
Cee Nu	lomustine	Desyrel	trazodone
Cefadyl	cephapirin	Diabeta	glyburide
Cefatrex	cefapirin	Diabinese	chlorpropamide
Cefizox	ceftizoxime	Diamox	acetazolamide
Cefobid	cefoperazone	Diamox Sequels	acetazolamide
Ceftin	cefuroxime	Dianabol	methandrostenolone
Celestone	betamethasone	Diapid	lypressin
Cerespan	papaverine	Dicodid	hydrocodone
Chloromycetin	chloramphenicol	Didronel	etidronate
Chloroptic	chloramphenicol	Dilantin	phenytoin
Chlortrimeton	chlorpheniramine	Dilaudid	hydromorphone
Choledyl	oxtriphylline	Dilaudin cough syrup	hydromorphone and guaifenesin
Chronulac	lactulose syrup	Dimetane	brompheniramine
Cinobac	cinoxacin	Disalcid	salsalate
Cl	potassium chloride	Diuril	chlorothiazide
Claforan	cefotaxime	Dobutrex	dobutamine
Clavulanate-Timentin	ticarcillin disodium	Dolobid	diflunisal
Cleocin-T	clindamycin	Dolophine	methadone
Clinoril	sulindac	Donnatal	belladonna alkaloids and phenobarbital
Clomid	clomiphene		
Cogentin	benztropine	Dopar	levodopa
Colace	docusate sodium (DSS), dioctyl sodium sulfosuccinate (DSS)	Dopram	doxapram
		Doriden	glutethimide
Colestid	colestipol	Dramamine	dimenhydrinate
Compazine	prochlorperazine	Dristan Long Lasting	oxymetazoline, nasal
Corgard	nadolol	Dulcolax	bisacodyl
Cortone	cortisone acetate	Duracillin	penicillin procaine
Cosmegen	dactinomycin	Duramorph	morphine sulfate
Cotazym	pancrelipase	Duricef	cefadroxil
Coumadin	warfarin	Dyazide	hydrochlorothiazide and triamterene
Crysticillin	penicillin procaine	Dymelor	acetohexamide
Crystodigin	digitoxin	Dyrenium	triamterene
Cuprimine	penicillamine	Ecotrin	aspirin, enteric coated
Cyanocobalamin	vitamin B_{12}	Edecrin	ethacrynic acid
Cylert	pemoline	Effersyllium	psyllium hydrocolloid
Cytadren	aminoglutethimide	Elavil	amitriptyline
Cytomel	liothyronine	Elixophyllin	theophylline
Cytotec	misoprostol	Elspar	asparaginase
Cytoxan	cyclophosphamide	Emeta-Con	benzquinamide
Dalmane	flurazepam	Emetrol	phosphated carbohydrate solution
Danocrine	danazol	Endep	amitriptyline
Dantrium	dantrolene sodium	Enkaid	encainide
Daraprim	pyrimethamine	Epsom salt	magnesium sulfate
Darvon	propoxyphene	Equanil	meprobomate
Datril	acetaminophen	Ergomar	ergotamine
Davocet-N	propoxyphene, napsylate, acetaminophen	Ergostat	ergotamine
		Ergotrate	ergonovine
Decadron	dexamethasone	Erythrocin	erythromycin
Declomycin	demeclocyline	Esidrex	hydrochlorothiazide
Delta Cortef	prednisolone	Euthroid	liotrix
Deltalin	vitamin D	Eutonyl	pargyline
Demerol	meperidine	Ex-Lax	phenolphthalein
Depakene	valproic acid	Feen-A-Mint	phenolphthalein

Adapted from *Mosby's medical, nursing, and allied health dictionary*, ed 4, St Louis, 1994, Mosby.

Continued

Commonly used medications: trade to generic name listing—cont'd

Trade name	Generic name	Trade name	Generic name
Feldene	piroxicam	Keflex	cephalexin
Femiron	ferrous fumarate	Keflin	cephalothin
Feosol	ferrous sulfate	Kefzol	cefazolin
Fergon	ferrous gluconate	Kemadrin	procyclidine
Flagyl	metronidazole	Kenacort	triamcinolone
Fleet enema	phosphate enema	Klonopin	clonazepam
Flexeril	cyclobenzaprine	Klorvess	potassium chloride
Florinef	fludrocortisone	Kondremul	mineral oil emulsion
Fluothane	halothane	Kwell	lindane
Folvite	folic acid	Lanoxin	digoxin
Fulvicin P/G	griseofulvin	Larodopa	levodopa
Fungizone	amphotericin B	Larotid	amoxicillin
Furadantin	nitrofurantoin	Lasix	furosemide
Gantanol	sulfamethoxazole	Leucovorin calcium	folinic acid
Gantrisin	sulfisoxazole	Leukeran	chlorambucil
Garamycin	gentamicin	Levo-Dromoran	levorphanol
Gelusil	aluminum-magnesium suspension	Levophed	levarterenol, norepinephrine
Geocillin	carbenicillin	Libritab	chlordiazepoxide
Geopen	carbenicillin	Librium	chlordiazepoxide
Halcion	triazolam	Lidex	fluocinonide
Haldol	haloperidol	Limbitrol	chlordiazepoxide and amitriptyline
Halotex	haloprogin	Limbrax	chlordiazepoxide and clidinium
Herplex	idoxuridine	Lioresal	baclofen
Hexabetalin	vitamin B_6	Lipo-Hepin	heparin
Hexadrol	dexamethasone	Liquaemin	heparin
Hiprex	methenamine hippurate	Lithane	lithium carbonate
Hismanal	astemizole	Lithobid	lithium carbonate
Hurricaine	benzocaine	Lodosyn	carbidopa
Hycodan	hydrocodone and homatropine	Lomotil	diphenoxylate HCL with atropine
Hydergine	ergoloid mesylates	Loniten	minoxidil
HydroDiuril	hydrochlorothiazide	Lopid	gemfibrozil
Hygroton	chlorthalidone	Lopressor	metoprolol
Hyper-tet	tetanus immune globulin	Lorelco	probucol
Hyperstat	diazoxide	Lotrimin	clotrimazole
Ilosone	erythromycin estolate	Loxitane	loxapine succinate
Ilotycin	erythromycin	Ludiomil	maprotiline
Imferon	iron dextran	Lufyllin	dyphylline
Imodium	loperamide	Luminal	phenobarbital
Imuran	azathioprine	Lysodren	mitotane
Inderal	propranolol	Maalox	aluminum-magnesium suspension
Indocin	indomethacin	Magnesium Hydroxide	milk of magnesia (MOM)
Intal	cromolyn	Mandelamine	methenamine mandelate
Intropin	dopamine	Mandol	cefamandol
Inversine	mecamylamine	Marezine	cyclizine
Ismelin	guanethidine	Matulane	procarbazine
Isoptin	verapamil	Maxzide	triamterene and hydrochloro-thiazide
Isoptocarpine	pilocarpine		
Isordil	isosorbide dinitrate	Mebaral	mephobarbital
Isuprel	isproterenol	Meclomen	meclofenamate
K-Lor	potassium chloride	Mefoxin	cefoxitin
Kantrex	kanamycin	Megace	megestrol
Kaon	potassium gluconate, potassium chloride	Mellaril	thioridazine
		Menadione	vitamin K_2
Kaopectate	kaolin-pectin	Mephyton	phytonadione (vitamin K_1)
Kayexalate	sodium polystyrene sulfonate	Mesantoin	mephenytoin

Adapted from *Mosby's medical, nursing, and allied health dictionary*, ed 4, St Louis, 1994, Mosby.

Continued

Commonly used medications: trade to generic name listing—cont'd

Trade name	Generic name	Trade name	Generic name
Mestinon	pyridostigmine	Norpramin	desipramine
Meticortelone	prednisolone	Novocain	procaine
Mevacor	lovastatin	Nubain	nalbuphine
Mexitil	mexiletine	Numorphan	oxymorphone
Mezlin	mezlocillin	Nupercainal	dibucaine
Micro K	potassium chloride	Nupercaine	dibucaine
Micronase	glyburide	Nydrazid	INH (isoniazid)
Midamor	amiloride	Omnipen	ampicillin
Miltown	meprobamate	Oncovin	vincristine
Minipress	prazosin	Optimine	azatadine maleate
Minocin	minocycline	Orinase	tolbutamide
Mithracin	methramycin	Orudis	ketoprofen
Moban	molindone	Pamelor	nortriptyline
Mol-iron	ferrous sulfate	Paral	paraldehyde
Monistat	miconazole	Paregoric	camphorated tincture of opium
Motrin	ibuprofen	Parlodel	bromocriptine
Moxam	moxalactam	Parnate	tranylcypromine sulfate
Mucomyst	acetylcysteine	Pavabid	papaverine
Mustargen	nitrogen mustard, mechlorethamine	Pavulon	pancuronium
Myclex	clotrimazole	Pen-Vee K	penicillin V potassium
Mycostatin	nystatin	Penicillin VK	phenoxymethyl penicillin
Mylanta	aluminum-magnesium suspension	Pentam	pentamidine isethionate
Myleran	busulfan	Penthrane	methoxyflurane
Mylicon	simethicone	Pentid	penicillin G potassium
Mysoline	primidone	Pepcid	famotidine
Mytelase	ambenonium	Percocet	oxycodone, acetaminophen
Nalfon	fenoprofen	Percodan	oxycodone, ASA
Naprosyn	naproxen	Periactin	cyproheptadine
Narcan	naloxone	Pericolace	dioctyl sodium sulfosuccinate with casanthranol
Nardil	phenelzine sulfate		
Navane	thiothixene	Peritrate	pentaerythritol tetranitrate
Nebcin	tobramycin	Persantine	dipyridamole
Neg Gram	nalidixic acid	Pertofrane	desipramine
Nembutal	pentobarbital	Pfizepen	penicillin G potassium
Neosynephrine	phenylephrine	Phenergan	promethazine
Niacin	vitamin B_3	Phytonadione	vitamin K_1
Nicobid	niacin (nicotinic acid)	Pipracil	piperacillin
Nicolar	niacin (nicotinic acid)	Pitocin	oxytocin
Nicotinic Acid	vitamin B_3	Pitressin	vasopressin
Nilstat	nystatin	Placidyl	ethchlorvynol
Nipride	nitroprusside	Platinol	cisplatin
Nitrobid	nitroglycerin	Polycillin	ampicillin
Nitrogen Mustard	mechlorethamine	Polymox	amoxicillin
Nitrospan	nitroglycerin	Pontocaine	tetracaine
Nitrostat	nitroglycerin	Preludin	phenmetrazine
Nizoral	ketoconazole	Premarin	estrogens, conjugated
Noctec	chloral hydrate	Primaxin	imipenem-cilastatin
Noludar	methyprylon	Prinivil	lisinopril
Nolvadex	tamoxifen	Probanthine	propantheline
Norflex	orphendrine	Procardia	nifedipine
Norlutate	norethindrone acetate	Proglycem	diazoxide
Norlutin	norethindrone	Prolixin	fluphenazine
Normodyne	labetalol	Proloid	thyroglobulin
Noroxin	norfloxacin	Proloprim	trimethoprim
Norpace	disopyramide	Pronestyl	procainamide

Adapted from *Mosby's medical, nursing, and allied health dictionary*, ed 4, St Louis, 1994, Mosby.

Continued

Commonly used medications: trade to generic name listing—cont'd

Trade name	Generic name	Trade name	Generic name
Prostaphlin	oxacillin	Sufenta	sufentanil
Prostigmin	neostigmine	Sumycin	tetracyline
Proventil	albuterol	Suprax	cefixime
Provera	medroxyprogesterone	Surfak	dioctyl calcium sulfosuccinate (DOCS), docusate calcium
Prozac	fluoxetine		
Pyopen	carbenicillin	Sus-Phrine	epinephrine
Pyribenzamine (PBZ)	tripelennamine	Symmetrel	amantadine
Pyridium	phenazopyridine HCl	Synalar	fluocinolone acetonide
Pyridoxine	vitamin B_6	Synkayvite	menadiol
Quarzan	clidinium	Synthroid	levothyroxine
Questran	cholestyramine	Tace	chlorotrianisene
Quinaglute	quinidine gluconate	Tagamet	cimetidine
Quinamm	quinine sulfate	Talwin	pentazocine
Quinora	quinidine sulfate	Tambocor	flecainide
Raudixin	rauwolfia serpentina	Tandearil	oxyphenbutazone
Redisol	vitamin B_{12}	Tapazole	methimazole
Regitine	phentolamine	Taractan	chlorprothixene
Reglan	metoclopramide	Tavist	clemastine
Restoril	temazepam	Tegretol	carbamazepine
Retrovir	zidovudine	Temaril	trimeprazone
Riboflavin	vitamin B_2	Tenex	guanfacine
Rifadin	rifampin	Tenormin	atenolol
Rimactane	rifampin	Tensilon	edrophonium
Riopan	magaldrate	Terramycin	oxytetracycline
Ritalin	methylphenidate	Theo-Dur	theophylline
Robaxin	methocarbamol	Thiamine	vitamin B_1
Robinul	glycopyrrolate	Thorazine	chlorpromazine
Robitussin	guaifenesin (glyceryl guaiacolate)	Thyrolar	liotrix
		Ticar	ticarcillin
Rocephin	ceftriaxone	Tigan	trimethobenzamide
Roxanol	morphine sulfate	Timolide	hydrochlorothiazide and timolol
Rufen	ibuprofen	Timoptic	timolol maleate
Sanorex	mazindol	Titralac	calcium carbonate
Sansert	methylsergide	Tobrex	tobramycin
Seconal	secobarbital	Tofranil	imipramine
Seldane	terfenadine	Tolinase	tolazamide
Selsun	selenium sulfide	Tonocard	tocainide
Selsun Blue	selenium sulfide	Torecan	thiethylperazine
Senokot	senna	Tracrium	atracurium besylate
Serax	oxazepam	Trandate	labetalol
Serentil	mesoridazine	Transderm-Scop	scopolamine
Serpasil	reserpine	Tranxene	chlorazepate, dipotassium
Silvadene	silver sulfadiazine	Tremin	trihexphenidyl HCl
Sinemet	carbidopa and levodopa	Trental	pentoxifylline
Sinequan	doxepin HCl	Tridione	trimethadione
Slow K	potassium chloride	Trilafon	perphenazine
Solu-Cortef	hydrocortisone	Trimpex	trimethoprim
Sorbitrate	isosorbide dinitrate	Trinalin	azatadine maleate
Sparine	promazine	Tums	calcium carbonate
Stadol	butorphanol	Tuss-Ornade	caramiphen and phenyl-propanolamine
Staphcillin	methicillin		
Stelazine	trifluoperazine	Tylenol	acetaminophen
Stilbestrol	diethylstilbestrol	Tylox	oxycodone, acetaminophen
Stoxil	idoxuridine	Unasyn	ampicillin and sulbactam
Streptase	streptokinase	Urecholine	bethanechol chloride
Sublimaze	fentanyl		

Adapted from *Mosby's medical, nursing, and allied health dictionary*, ed 4, St Louis, 1994, Mosby.

Continued

Commonly used medications: trade to generic name listing—cont'd

Trade name	Generic name	Trade name	Generic name
Urex	methenamine hippurate	Virazole	ribavirin
V-cillin	phenoxymethyl penicillin	Visken	pindolol
V-cillin K	penicillin V potassium	Vistaril	hydroxyzine pamoate
Valisone	betamethasone	Vitamin C	ascorbic acid
Valium	diazepam	Vitamin K	menadiol
Vanceril	beclomethasone	Voltaren	diclofenac
Vancocin	vancomycin	Wellcovorin	leucovorin
Vaponefrin	racepinephrine, ephedrine	Wycillin	penicillin procaine
Vasodilan	isoxsuprine HCl	Wydase	hyaluronidase
Vasotec	enalapril	Wytensin	guanabenz
Velban	vinblastine	Xanax	alprazolam
Velosef	cephradine	Xylocaine	lidocaine
Ventolin	albuterol	Yutopar	ritodrine
Vepesid	etoposide	Zantac	ranitidine
Vermox	mebendazole	Zaroxolyn	metolazone
Versapen	hetacillin	Zestril	lisinopril
Vibramycin	doxycycline	Zovirax	acyclovir
Viokase	pancrelipase	Zyloprim	allopurinol
Vira-A	vidarabine		

Adapted from *Mosby's medical, nursing, and allied health dictionary*, ed 4, St Louis, 1994, Mosby.

Appendix F

Tables of weights and measures

Metric system

Length	Weight	Volume
meter (m) basic unit	gram (g or gm) basic unit	liter (L) basic unit
1 micrometer (μm) = 0.000001 meter	1 microgram (mgc or μg) = 0.000001 gram	1 milliliter* (ml) = 0.001 liter
1 millimeter (mm) = 0.001 meter	1 milligram (mg) = 0.001 gram	1 centiliter (cl) = 0.01 liter
1 centimeter (cm) = 0.01 meter	1 centigram (cg) = 0.01 gram	1 deciliter (dl) = 0.1 liter
1 decimeter (dm) = 0.1 meter	1 decigram (dg) = 0.1 gram	1 dekaliter (Dl) = 10 liters
1 dekameter (Dm) = 10 meters	1 dekagram (Dg) = 10 grams	1 hektoliter (Hl) = 100 liters
1 hectometer (Hm) = 100 meters	1 hektogram (Hg) = 100 grams	1 kiloliter (kl) = 1000 liters
1 kilometer (km) = 1000 meters	1 kilogram (kg) = 1000 grams	

Apothecary system

Weight	Volume
20 grains (gr) = 1 scruple (Э)	60 minims (♏) = 1 fluidram (f℈ or ℈)
3 scruples (Э) = 1 dram (℈)	8 fluidrams (f℈) = 1 fluidounce (f℥ or ℥)
8 drams (℈) = 1 ounce (℥)	16 fluidounces (f℥) = 1 pint (O or pt)
12 ounces (℥) = 1 pound (lb)	2 pints (O) = 1 quart (qt)
	4 quarts (qt) = 1 gallon (C, Cong, or gal)

Household equivalents

Household equivalents	Other commonly used equivalents (approximate)			
	Weight		**Volume**	
1 teaspoonful (tsp)	= 5 milliliters (ml)	1 grain (gr) = 60 to 65 milligrams (mg)	1 minim (♏) = 0.06 milliliter (ml)	
1 dessertspoonful	= 10 milliliters (ml)	15 grains (gr) = 1 gram (g)	16 minims (♏) = 1 milliliter (ml)	
1 tablespoonful (tbsp)	= 15 milliliters (ml) or ½ ounce (℥)	1 kilogram (kg) = 2.2 pounds (lb)	1 fluidram (f℈) = 1 teaspoonful (tsp)†	
1 teacupful	= 120 milliliters (ml) or 4 ounces (℥)		1 fluidounce (f℥) = 30 milliliters (ml)	
1 cupful	= 240 milliliters (ml) or 8 ounces (℥)		1 pint (pt) = 500 milliliters	

*1 ml is considered equivalent to 1 cubic centimeter (cc).
†In medication orders, ℈i is commonly used to designate 1 tsp (5 ml).

Appendix G

EXCHANGE LIST FOR MENU PLANNING

MILK EXCHANGE LIST

Skim milk (12 g carbohydrate, 8 g protein, 0 g fat, 90 kcal)

1 cup	Skim or nonfat milk (½% and 1%)
⅓ cup	Powdered (nonfat dry, before adding liquid)
½ cup	Canned, evaporated skim milk
1 cup	Buttermilk made from skim milk
1 cup	Yogurt made from skim milk (plain, unflavored)

Low-fat milk (12 g carbohydrate, 8 g protein, 5 g fat, 120 kcal)

1 cup	2% fat milk
1 cup	Plain nonfat yogurt (added milk solids)

Whole milk (12 g carbohydrate, 8 g protein, 8 g fat, 150 kcal)

1 cup	Whole milk
1 cup	Custard-style yogurt made from whole milk (plain, unflavored)

VEGETABLE EXCHANGE LIST

(5 g carbohydrate, 2 g protein, 0 g fat, 25 kcal). 1 exchange equals ½ cup cooked vegetables or vegetable juice and 1 cup raw vegetables

Artichoke (½ medium)	Mushrooms (cooked)
Asparagus	Onions
Beans (green, wax, Italian)	Pea pods
Bean sprouts	Sauerkraut
Beets	Spinach (cooked)
Broccoli	Squash, summer, zucchini
Brussels sprouts	String beans (green, yellow)
Cabbage, cooked	Tomato
Carrots	Tomato juice
Cauliflower	Turnips
Eggplant	Vegetable juice
Green pepper	Zucchini (cooked)
Greens	

FRUIT EXCHANGE LIST

(15 g carbohydrate, 0 g protein, 0 g fat, 60 kcal).
1 fruit exchange equals:

1	Apple (2 in diameter)
4 rings	Dried apple
½ cup	Apple juice
½ cup	Applesauce (unsweetened)
½ cup	Apricots, canned
7 halves	Apricots, dried
4	Apricots, fresh
½	Banana, 9 in
¾ cup	Blackberries
¾ cup	Blueberries
1 cup	Raspberries
1¼ cup	Strawberries
⅓ melon	Cantaloupe (5 in diameter)
½ cup	Cherries, canned
12	Cherries, (large, raw)
½ cup	Cider
⅓ cup	Cranberry juice cocktail
2½ medium	Dates
1½	Figs, dried
2	Figs, fresh (2 in diameter)
⅓ cup	Grape juice
½	Grapefruit
½ cup	Grapefruit juice
15	Grapes
⅛ melon	Honeydew melon (7 in diameter; cubes = 1 cup)
1	Kiwi (large)
¾ cup	Mandarin oranges
½ small	Mango
1 small	Nectarine (1½ in diameter)
1 small	Orange (2½ in diameter)
½ cup	Orange juice
½ cup or 2 halves	Peach, canned
1 medium or ¾ cup	Peach, fresh (2¾ in diameter)
½ cup or 2 halves	Pear, canned
1 small or ½ large	Pear, fresh
1/3 cup	Pineapple, canned
¾ cup	Pineapple, raw
½ cup	Pineapple juice
2	Plums (2 in diameter)
⅓ cup	Prune juice
3	Prunes, dried
2 tbsp	Raisins
2	Tangerine (2½ in diameter)
1¼ cups	Watermelon (cubes)

STARCH/BREAD EXCHANGE LIST

(15 g carbohydrate, 3 g protein, 0 g fat, 80 kcal) 1 starch/bread exchange equals:

Bread

½ (1 oz)	Bagel, small
2 (⅔ oz)	Bread sticks (crisp, 4 in long, ½ in wide)
3 tbsp	Dried bread crumbs
½	English muffin
½ (1 oz)	Frankfurter bun
½ (1 oz)	Hamburger bun
½	Pita (6 in diameter)
1 (small)	Plain roll
1 slice	Raisin (unfrosted)

Adapted from Williams S: *Nutrition and diet therapy*, ed 7, 1993, St Louis, Mosby.

1 slice	Rye or pumpernickel
1	Tortilla (6 in diameter)
1 slice	White (including French and Italian)
1 slice	Whole wheat

Cereal/Grains/Pasta

½ cup	Bran flakes
½ cup	Cereal (cooked)
2½ tbsp	Cornmeal (dry)
2½ tbsp	Flour (dry)
3 tbsp	Grapenuts
¾ cup	Other ready-to-eat unsweetened cereal
½ cup	Pasta (cooked spaghetti, noodles, macaroni)
1½ cups	Puffed cereal (unfrosted)
⅓ cup	Rice or barley (cooked)
½ cup	Shredded wheat
3 tbsp	Wheat germ

Crackers/Snacks

8	Animal
3	Graham (2½-in square)
¾ oz	Matzoh (4 × 6 in)
5 slices	Melba toast
24	Oyster
3 cups	Popcorn (popped with no added fat)
¾ oz	Pretzels
4	Rye crisp (2 × 3½ in)
6	Saltines

Dried Beans/Peas/Lentils

¼ cup	Baked beans
⅓ cup	Dried beans, such as kidney, white, split, blackeye (cooked)
⅓ cup	Lentils (cooked)

Starchy Vegetables

½ cup	Corn
1	Corn on the cob (6 inches)
½ cup	Lima beans
½ cup	Peas, green (canned or frozen)
½ cup	Potato, mashed
1 small	Potato, white (3 ounces baked)
1 cup	Winter squash, acorn or butternut
⅓ cup	Yam or sweet potato

Starch Group (with Fat)

1 starch/bread exchange
1 fat exchange

1	Biscuit (2½ in across)
1 (2 oz)	Corn bread (2-in cube)
6	Cracker, round butter type
10 (1½ oz)	French fries (2-3½ in)
1	Muffin, plain, small
2	Pancake (4 in diameter)
¼ cup	Stuffing, bread (prepared)
2	Taco shell (6 in across)
1	Waffle (4½ in square)
4-6 (1 oz)	Whole-wheat crackers (such as Triscuits)

MEAT EXCHANGE LIST

Lean (0 g carbohydrate, 7 g protein, 3 g fat, 55 kcal)

Beef	1 oz	Baby beef (lean), chipped beef, chuck, flank, steak, tenderloin, plate ribs, round (bottom, top), all cuts rump, spare ribs, tripe
Cheese	1 oz	Cottage, farmer's, or pot (low-fat), grated parmesan
Fish	2 oz	Fresh or frozen, any type canned salmon, tuna, mackerel, crab, or lobster
Pork	1 oz	Leg (whole rump, center, shank), ham (center slices), USDA good or choice grades such as round, sirloin, flank, and tenderloin
Poultry	1 oz	Chicken, turkey, cornish hen (without skin)
Veal	1 oz	Leg, loin, rib, shank, shoulder, chops, roasts, all cuts except cutlets (ground or cubed)

Medium Fat (0 g carbohydrate, 7 g protein, 5 g fat, 75 kcal)

Beef	1 oz	All ground beef, roast (rib, chuck, rump), steak (cubed, porterhouse, T-bone), meat loaf
Cheese	¼ cup or 1 oz	Cottage (creamed), mozzarella with skim milk), ricotta, Neufchatel
Egg	1	Egg
Fish	¼ cup	Tuna (canned in oil); salmon (canned)
Lamb	1 oz	Leg, rib, sirloin, loin (roast and chops), shank, shoulder
Organ meat	1 oz	All types
Other	4 oz	Tofu
Pork	1 oz	Loin (all cuts tenderloin), chops, roast, Boston butt, cutlets
Poultry	1 oz	Capon, duck (domestic), goose, ground turkey, chicken with skin
Veal	1 oz	Cutlets

High Fat (0 g carbohydrate, 7 g protein, 8 g fat, 100 kcal)

Beef	1 oz	Brisket, corned beef (commercial), chuck (ground commercial), roasts (rib), steaks (club and rib); most USDA prime cuts of beef
Cheese	1 oz	All regular cheeses (American, blue, brick, Camembert, cheddar, Gouda, Limburger, Muenster, Swiss, Monterey), all processed cheeses
Cold cuts	1 oz	Bologna, salami, pimento loaf
Frankfurter	1 oz	Turkey, chicken
Lamb	1 oz	Patties (ground lamb)
Peanut butter	1 tbsp	
Pork	1 oz	Spare ribs, loin (back ribs), pork (ground), country-style ham, deviled ham, pork sausage
Sausage	1 oz	Polish, Italian

Adapted from Williams S: *Nutrition and diet therapy*, ed 7, 1993, St Louis, Mosby.

FAT EXCHANGE LIST

(0 g carbohydrate, 0 g protein, 5 g fat, 45 kcal)

⅛ medium	Avocado
1 strip	Bacon, crisp
1 tsp	Butter, margarine
1 tbsp	Cream, heavy
2 tbsp	Cream, light
2 tbsp	Cream, sour
1 tbsp	Cream cheese
10 small or 5 large	Olives

Dressing

2 tsp	All varieties
	Mayonnaise type
1 tbsp	Gravy, meat
1 tbsp	Reduced kcalorie

Nuts

6	Almonds, whole, dry roasted
1 tbsp	Cashews, dry roasted
1 tbsp	Other
20 small or 10 large	Peanuts, Spanish, whole
10	Peanuts, Virginia, whole
2 large	Pecans, whole
2 tsp	Pumpkin seeds
1 tbsp	Seeds (pine, sunflower)
2 whole	Walnuts

Oil

1 tsp	Corn, cottonseed, safflower, soy, sunflower, olive, peanut, canola

FREE FOODS

A free food is any food or drink that contains less than 20 kcal per serving. You can eat as much as you want of those items that have no serving size specified. You may eat two or three servings per day of those items that have a specific serving size. Be sure to spread them out through the day.

Drinks

Bouillon or broth without fat
Bouillon, low-sodium
Carbonated drinks, sugar-free
Carbonated water
Club soda
Cocoa powder, unsweetened (1 tbsp)
Coffee/tea
Drink mixes, sugar-free
Tonic water, sugar-free

Nonstick pan spray

Fruit

Cranberries, unsweetened (½ cup)
Rhubarb, unsweetened (½ cup)

Vegetables

(raw, 1 cup)
Cabbage
Celery
Chinese cabbage
Cucumber
Green onion
Hot peppers
Mushrooms (fresh)
Radishes
Zucchini

Salad greens

Endive
Escarole
Lettuce
Romaine
Spinach

Sweet substitute

Candy, hard, sugar-free
Gelatin, sugar-free
Gum, sugar-free
Jam/jelly, sugar-free (2 tsp)
Pancake syrup, sugar-free (1-2 tbsp)
Sugar substitutes (saccharin, aspartame)
Whipped topping (2 tbsp)

Condiments

Catsup (1 tbsp)
Horseradish
Mustard
Pickles, dill, unsweetened
Salad dressing, low kcalorie (2 tbsp)
Taco sauce (3 tbsp)
Vinegar

Seasonings

Basil (fresh)	Lemon pepper
Celery seeds	Lime
Cinnamon	Lime juice
Chili powder	Mint
Chives	Onion powder
Curry	Oregano
Dill	Paprika
Flavoring extracts (vanilla, almond, walnut, peppermint, butter, lemon, etc.)	Pepper
	Pimento
	Soy sauce
Garlic	Soy sauce, low-sodium (lite)
Garlic powder	Spices
Herbs	Wine, used in cooking (¼ cup)
Hot pepper sauce	Worcestershire sauce
Lemon	
Lemon juice	

Adapted from Williams S: *Nutrition and diet therapy,* ed 7, 1993, St Louis, Mosby.

Appendix H

STATE, TERRITORIAL, AND PROVINCIAL BOARDS OF PRACTICAL/VOCATIONAL NURSING

State and Territorial Boards of Nursing

ALABAMA
Board of Nursing
RSA Plaza, Ste 250
770 Washington Ave
Montgomery, AL 36130

ALASKA
Board of Nursing Licensing
Department of Commerce & Economic Development
Division of Occupational Licensing
PO Box 110806
Juneau, AS 99811-0806

ARIZONA
Board of Nursing
2001 W Camelback Rd, #350
Phoenix, AZ 85015

ARKANSAS
Board of Nursing
University Tower Building, Ste 800
1123 S University Ave
Little Rock, AK 72204

CALIFORNIA
Board of Vocational Nurses and Psychiatric Technical Examiners
1020 N Street, Room 406
Sacramento, California 95814

COLORADO
Board of Nursing
1560 Broadway, Ste 670
Denver, CO 80202

CONNECTICUT
Board of Examiners for Nursing
150 Washington St
Hartford, CT 06106

DELAWARE
Board of Nursing
Margaret O'Neill Bldg
Federal & Court St
PO Box 1401
Dover, DE 19903

DISTRICT OF COLUMBIA
Board of Nursing
614 H Street NW
Washington, DC 20001

FLORIDA
Board of Nursing
111 E Coastline Dr, Ste 516
Jacksonville, FL 32202

GEORGIA
State Board of Licensed Practical Nurses
166 Pryor Street, SW
Atlanta, Georgia 30303

GUAM
Board of Nurse Examiners
Box 2816
Agana, Guam 96910

HAWAII
Board of Nursing
Box 3469
Honolulu, HI 96801

IDAHO
Board of Nursing
2800 N 8th St, Ste 210
Boise, ID 83720

ILLINOIS
Department of Professional Regulation
320 W Washington St
Springfield, IL 62786

INDIANA
State Board of Nursing
Health Professions Bureau
402 W Washington St, Room 041
Indianapolis, IN 46204

IOWA
Board of Nursing
1223 E Court
Des Moines, IA 50319

KANSAS
State Board of Nursing
Landon State Office Building
900 SW Jackson, Room 551
Topeka, KS 66612

KENTUCKY
Board of Nursing
4010 Dupoint Circle, Ste 430
Louisville, KY 40207

LOUISIANA
State Board of Practical Nurse Examiners
Tidewater Place
1440 Canal Street, Suite 2010
New Orleans, Louisiana 70112

MAINE
Board of Nursing
State House Station 158
Augusta, ME 04333

MARYLAND
Board of Nursing
Metro Executive Center
4201 Patterson Ave
Baltimore, MD 21215

MASSACHUSETTS
Board of Registration in Nursing
100 Cambridge St, Room 1519
Boston, MA 02202

MICHIGAN
Board of Nursing
PO Box 30018
Lansing, MI 48909

MINNESOTA
Board of Nursing
2700 University Av W, #108
St Paul, MN 55114

MISSISSIPPI
Board of Nursing
239 N Lamar St, Ste 401
Jackson, MS 39201

MISSOURI
Board of Nursing
3605 Missouri Blvd
PO Box 656
Jefferson City, MO 65102

MONTANA
Board of Nursing
Department of Commerce
Arcade Building, Lower Level
111 N Jackson
Helena, MT 59620

NEBRASKA
Board of Nursing
Box 95007
Lincoln, NE 68509

NEVADA
Board of Nursing
1281 Terminal Way, Ste 116
Reno, NV 89502

NEW HAMPSHIRE
Board of Nursing
Division of Public Health Services
Health & Welfare Building
6 Hazen Dr
Concord, NH 03301

NEW JERSEY
Board of Nursing
1100 Raymond Blvd, Room 508
PO Box 45010
Newark, NJ 07101

NEW MEXICO
Board of Nursing
4253 Montgomery NE, Ste 130
Albuquerque, NM 87109

NEW YORK
NYS Board for Nursing
NYS State Education Department
Cultural Education Center
Albany, NY 12230

NORTH CAROLINA
Board of Nursing
Box 2129
Raleigh, NC 27602-2129

NORTH DAKOTA
Board of Nursing
919 S 7th St, Ste 504
Bismarck, ND 58504

OHIO
Board of Nursing
77 S High St, 17th Floor
Columbus, OH 43266-0316

OKLAHOMA
Board of Nursing
2915 N Classen Blvd, Ste 524
Oklahoma City, OK 73106

OREGON
Board of Nursing
800 NE Oregon St, #25-465
Portland, OR 97232-2162

PENNSYLVANIA
Board of Nursing
PO Box 2649
Harrisburg, PA 17105-2649

PUERTO RICO
Board of Nurse Examiners
Call Box 10200
Santurce, PR 00908-0200

RHODE ISLAND
Board of Nurse Registration and Education
Cannon Health Building, Room 104
3 Capitol Hill
Providence, RI 02908

SOUTH CAROLINA
Board of Nursing
220 Executive Center Dr, Ste 220
Columbia, SC 29210

SOUTH DAKOTA
Board of Nursing
3307 S Lincoln Ave
Sioux Falls, SD 57105

TENNESSEE
Board of Nursing
Bureau of Manpower and Facilities
283 Plus Park Blvd
Nashville, TN 37247

TEXAS
Board of Vocational Nurse Examiners
1300 East Anderson Lane
Building C, Suite 285
Austin, Texas 78752

UTAH
Board of Nursing
Heber M. Wells Building, 4th Floor
160 E 300 S
PO Box 45805
Salt Lake City, UT 84145

VERMONT
Board of Nursing
109 State St
Montpelier, VT 05602

VIRGIN ISLANDS
Board of Nurse Licensure
Kongens Gade #3
PO Box 4247
St Thomas, VI 00803

VIRGINIA
Board of Nursing
1601 Rolling Hills Dr
Richmond, VA 23229

WASHINGTON
State Board of Practical Nursing
PO Box 9649
Olympia, Washington 98504

WEST VIRGINIA
State Board of Examiners for Practical Nurses
922 Quarrier Street
Embleton Building, Suite 506
Charleston, West Virginia 25301

WISCONSIN
Board of Nursing
Room 174, 1400 E Washington Ave
PO Box 8935
Madison, WI 53708

WYOMING
Board of Nursing
Barrett Building, 2nd Floor
2301 Central Ave
Cheyenne, WY 82002

PROVINCIAL BOARDS OF NURSING
CANADIAN NURSES ASSOCIATION/ASSOCIATION DES INFIRMIERES ET INFIRMIERS DU CANADA
50, The Driveway
Ottawa, Ontario
K2P 1E2

NURSES ASSOCIATION OF NEW BRUNSWICK/ ASSOCIATION DES INFIRMIERES ET INFIRMIERS DU NOUVEAU-BRUNSWICK
231 Saunders Street
Fredericton, New Brunswick
E3B 1N6

ASSOCIATION OF NURSES OF PRINCE EDWARD ISLAND
PO Box 1838, 17 Pownal Street
Charlottetown, Prince Edward Island
C1A 7N5

YUKON NURSES SOCIETY
PO Box 5371
Whitehorse, Yukon
Y1A 4Z2

COLLEGE OF NURSES OF ONTARIO
101 Davenport Road
Toronto, Ontario
M5R 3P1

Appendix I

COMMON COMMUNICABLE DISEASES

To prevent the spread of infection, any person with symptoms suggestive of a communicable disease should be kept away from others. Measures for control of communicable diseases are established either by law or by regulation in various states and communities. As these may vary, practical nurses should keep in touch with local health authorities and cooperate with them in preventing the spread of disease.

Contagious diseases

Disease and synopsis of symptoms	Incubation period	Mode of transmission	Period of communicability
Actinomycosis Chronic disease most frequently localized in jaw, thorax, or abdomen; septicemic spread with generalized disease may occur. Lesions are firmly indurated areas of purulence and fibrosis.	Irregular; probably years after colonization in oral tissues, plus days or months after precipitating trauma and actual penetration of tissues.	Contact from person to person as part of normal oral flora.	Time and manner in which *A. israelii* becomes part of normal flora is unknown.
Amebiasis Infection with a protozoan parasite that exists in two forms: the hardy, infective cyst and the more fragile, potentially invasive trophozoite. Parasite may act as a commensal or invade tissues, giving rise to intestinal or extraintestinal disease.	Variation—from a few days to several months or years. Commonly 2 to 4 weeks.	Contaminated water or food containing cysts from feces of infected persons, often as complication of another infection such as shigellosis.	During period of cyst passing, which may continue for years.
Ascariasis (roundworm infection) Helminthic infection of small intestine. Symptoms are variable, often vague or absent, or ordinarily mild; live worms, passed in stools or regurgitated, are frequently first recognized sign of infection.	Worms reach maturity about 2 months after ingestion of embryonated eggs.	By ingestion of infective eggs from soil contaminated with human feces containing eggs, but not directly from person to person.	As long as mature female worms live in intestine. Maximum lifespan of adult worms is under 18 months; however, female produces up to 200,000 eggs a day that can remain viable in soil for months or years.
Balantidiasis Disease of colon characteristically producing diarrhea or dysentery accompanied by abdominal colic, tenesmus, nausea, and vomiting.	Unknown; may be only a few days.	By ingestion of cysts from feces of infected hosts; in epidemics, mainly by fecally contaminated water.	As long as infection persists.
Candidiasis (monilliasis, thrush, candidosis) Mycosis usually confined to superficial layers of skin or mucous membranes with patients who have oral thrush, intertrigo, vulvovaginitis, paronychia, or onychomycosis.	Variable, 2 to 5 days in thrush of infants.	Through contact with excretions of mouth, skin, vagina, and especially feces from patients or carriers; from mother to infant during childbirth; and by endogenous spread.	Presumably for duration of lesions.

Adapted from *Mosby's medical nursing and allied health dictionary*, ed 4, St Louis, 1994, Mosby.

Continued

Contagious diseases—cont'd

Disease and synopsis of symptoms	Incubation period	Mode of transmission	Period of communicability
Carditis, Coxsackie (viral carditis, enteroviral carditis) Acute or subacute myocarditis or pericarditis, which occurs as the only manifestation, or may occasionally be associated with other manifestations.	Usually 3 to 5 days.	Fecal-oral or respiratory droplet contact with infected person.	Apparently during acute stage of disease.
Chickenpox, herpes zoster (varicella shingles) Acute generalized viral disease with sudden onset of slight fever, mild constitutional symptoms, and a skin eruption that is maculopapular for a few hours, vesicular for 3 to 4 days, and leaves a granular scab.	From 2 to 3 weeks; commonly 13 to 17 days.	From person to person by direct contact, droplet, or air-borne spread of secretion of respiratory tract of chickenpox cases or of vesicle fluid of patients with herpes zoster.	As long as 5 days but usually 1 to 2 days before onset of rash, and not more than 6 days after appearance of first crop of vesicles.
Cholera Acute intestinal disease with sudden onset, profuse watery stools, occasional vomiting, rapid dehydration, acidosis, and circulatory collapse. Death may occur within a few hours.	From a few hours to 5 days, usually 2 to 3 days.	Through ingestion of food or water contaminated with feces or vomitus of infected persons or with feces of carriers.	Thought to be for duration of stool-positive stage, usually only a few days after recovery. Carrier stage may last for several months.
Conjunctivitis, acute bacterial Clinical syndrome beginning with lacrimation, irritation, and hyperemia of the palpebral and bulbar conjunctivae of one or both eyes, followed by edema of lids, photophobia, and mucopurulent discharge.	Usually 24 to 72 hours.	Contact with discharges from conjunctivae or upper respiratory tract of infected persons through contaminated fingers, clothing, or other articles.	During course of active infection.
Conjunctivitis, epidemic hemorrhagic (Apollo 11 disease) Virus infection with sudden onset of pain or sensation of a foreign body in eye. Disease rapidly progresses (1 to 2 days) to full case of swollen eyelids, hyperemia of the conjunctivae, often with a cirumcorneal distribution, seromucous discharge, and frequent subconjunctival hemorrhages.	1 to 2 days or even shorter.	Through direct or indirect contact with discharge from infected eyes and possibly by droplet infection from those with virus in throat.	Unknown, but assumed to be for period of active disease, usually 1 to 2 weeks.
Dermatophytosis A. Ringworm of scalp and beard (tinea capitis, tinea kerion, favus) Begins as small papule and spreads peripherally, leaving scaly patches of temporary baldness. Infected hairs become brittle and break off easily. Kerions sometimes develop.	10 to 14 days.	Direct or indirect contact with articles infected with hair from humans or infected animals.	As long as lesions are present and viable fungus persists on contaminated materials.
B. Ringworm of nails (tinea unguium, onychomycosis)	Unknown.	Presumably by direct extension from skin or nail lesions of infected persons. Low rate of transmission.	Possibly as long as infected lesion is present.

Adapted from *Mosby's medical nursing and allied health dictionary*, ed 4, St Louis, 1994, Mosby.

Continued

Contagious diseases—cont'd

Disease and synopsis of symptoms	Incubation period	Mode of transmission	Period of communicability
Dermatophytosis—cont'd Chronic infectious disease involving one or more nails of hands or feet. Nail thickens, becoming discolored and brittle with an accumulation of caseous-appearing material beneath nail. C. Ringworm of groin and peri-anal region (dhobie itch, tinea cruris) D. Ringworm of the body (tinea corporis) Characteristically appears as flat, spreading, ring-shaped lesions. Periphery is usually reddish, vesicular, or pustular and may be dry and scaly or moist and crusted.	4 to 10 days.	Direct or indirect contact with skin and scalp lesions of infected persons or animals.	As long as lesions are present and viable fungus persists on contaminated materials.
E. Ringworm of the foot (tinea pedis, athlete's foot) Scaling or cracking of skin, especially between toes, or blisters containing this watery fluid are characteristic. In severe cases vesicular lesions appear on various parts of body.	Unknown.	Direct or indirect contact with skin lesions of infected persons or contaminated floors or shower stalls.	As long as lesions are present and viable spores persist on contaminated materials.
Diphtheria Characteristic lesion marked by patch or patches of grayish membrane with surrounding dull red inflammatory zone. Throat is moderately sore in faucial diphtheria, with cervical lymph nodes enlarged and tender; occasionally swelling and edema of neck.	2 to 5 days, sometimes longer.	Contact with patient or carrier; more rarely with articles soiled with discharges from lesions of infected persons. Raw milk has been a vehicle.	Variable, until virulent bacili have disappeared from discharge and lesions. Usual period is 2 to 4 weeks but chronic carriers may shed organisms for 6 months or more.
Gastroenteritis, viral A. Epidemic viral gastroenteritis Usually self-limited mild disease that often occurs in outbreaks with clinical symptoms of nausea, vomiting, diarrhea, abdominal pain, myalgia, headache, malaise, low-grade fever, or a combination thereof.	24 to 48 hours; in volunteer studies with Norwalk agent range was 10 to 51 hours.	Unknown; probably by fecal-oral route. Several recent outbreaks strongly suggest food-borne and water-borne transmission.	During acute stage of disease and shortly thereafter.
B. Rotavirus gastroenteritis (sporadic viral gastroenteritis of infants and children) Sporadic severe gastroenteritis of infants and young children characterized by diarrhea and vomiting, often with severe dehydration and occasional deaths.	Approximately 48 hours.	Probably fecal-oral and possibly respiratory routes.	During acute stage of disease and later while virus shedding continues. Virus is not usually detectable after eighth day of illness.

Adapted from *Mosby's medical nursing and allied health dictionary*, ed 4, St Louis, 1994, Mosby.

Continued

Contagious diseases—cont'd

Disease and synopsis of symptoms	Incubation period	Mode of transmission	Period of communicability
Giardiasis (Giardia enteritis, lambliasis)			
Protozoan infection principally of upper small bowel; often asymptomatic, it may also be associated with a variety of intestinal symptoms such as chronic diarrhea, steatorrhea, abdominal cramps, bloating, frequent loose and pale, greasy, malodorous stools, fatigue, and weight loss.	In a water-borne epidemic in United States, clinical illnesses occurred 1 to 4 weeks after exposure; average 2 weeks.	Localized outbreaks occur from contaminated water supplies. By ingestion of cysts in fecally contaminated water and occasionally by fecally contaminated food.	Entire period of infection.
Hepatitis, viral			
A. Viral hepatitis A (infectious hepatitis, epidemic hepatitis, epidemic jaundice, catarrhal jaundice, Type A hepatitis) Onset is usually abrupt with fever, malaise, anorexia, nausea, and abdominal discomfort, followed within a few days by jaundice.	From 15 to 50 days, depending on dose; average 28 to30 days.	Person to person by fecal-oral route. Common-vehicle outbreaks have been related to contaminated water and food.	Studies indicate maximum infectivity during latter half of incubation period, continuing for a few days, after onset of jaundice.
B. Viral hepatitis B (Type B hepatitis, serum hepatitis) Onset is usually insidious with anorexia, vague abdominal discomfort, and nausea and vomiting, sometimes arthralgias and rash, often progressing to jaundice. Fever may be absent or mild.	Usually 45 to 160 days, average 60 to 90 days. Variation is related in part to amount of virus in inoculum, mode of transmission, and host factors.	HB_sAg, the infectious agent, has been found in virtually all body secretions, but only blood, saliva, and semen have been shown to be infectious. Transmission usually by percutaneous inoculation of infected blood and blood products; contaminated needles, syringes, and IV equipment.	From several weeks before onset of symptoms through clinical course of disease; carrier state can last for years.
C. Hepatitis, non-A, non-B (non-B transfusion–associated hepatitis, hepatitis C) Chronic infection may be symptomatic or asymptomatic. Differential diagnosis depends on exclusion of hepatitis types A and B.	2 weeks to 6 months, model 6 to 8 weeks.	Most common posttransfusion hepatitis in United States and is more common when paid donors are used. Percutaneous transmission documented and other modes similar to those of hepatitis B virus are suspected.	Degree of immunity following infection is not known.
Herpangina, hand-foot-and-mouth disease, acute lymphonodular pharyngitis			
Herpangina—grayish papulovesicular phryngeal lesions on an erythematous base. *Hand-foot-and-mouth disease*—more diffuse oral lesions on buccal surfaces of cheeks, gums, and tongue. *Acute lymphonodular pharyngitis*—lesions are firm, raised, discrete, whitish to yellowish nodules.	3 to 5 days for herpangina and hand-foot-and-mouth disease. 5 days for acute lymphonodular pharyngitis.	Direct contact with nose and throat discharges and feces of infected (possibly asymptomatic) persons and by droplet spread.	During acute stage of illness and longer because virus persists in stools for as long as several weeks.

Adapted from *Mosby's medical nursing and allied health dictionary*, ed 4, St Louis, 1994, Mosby.

Continued

Contagious diseases—cont'd

Disease and synopsis of symptoms	Incubation period	Mode of transmission	Period of communicability
Herpes simplex Viral infection characterized by localized primary lesion, latency, and a tendency to localized recurrence. In perhaps 10% of primary infections overt disease may appear as illness of varying severity marked by fever and malaise lasting 1 week or more.	2 to 12 days.	HSV Type 1: Direct contact with virus in saliva of carriers. HSV Type 2: Sexual contact.	Secretion of virus in saliva has been reported for as long as 7 weeks after recovery from stomatitis. Patients with primary lesions are infective for about 7 to 12 days, with recurrent disease for 4 days to 1 week.
Influenza Acute viral disease of respiratory tract characterized by fever, chilliness, headache, myalgia, prostration, coryza, and mild sore throat. Cough is often severe and protracted.	Usually 24 to 72 hours.	By direct contact through droplet infection; probably airborne among crowded populations in enclosed spaces.	Probably limited to 3 days from clinical onset.
Measles (rubeola, hard measles, red measles, morbilli) Acute, highly communicable viral disease with prodromal fever, conjunctivitis, coryza, bronchitis, and Koplik's spots on the buccal mucosa. A characteristic red blotchy rash appears on third to seventh day, beginning on face, becoming generalized, lasting 4 to 7 days and sometimes ending in branny desquamation. Leukopenia is common.	About 10 days varying from 8 to 13 days from exposure to onset of fever; about 14 days until rash appears; uncommonly longer or shorter human normal immune globulin (IG), given later than third day off incubation period for passive protection, may extend the incubation period to 21 days instead of preventing disease.	By droplet spread or direct contact with nasal or throat secretions of infected persons. Measles is one of most readily transmitted communicable diseases.	From slightly before beginning of prodromal period to 4 days after appearance of rash; communicability is minimal after second day of rash.
Meningitis, meningococcal (cerebrospinal fever, meningococcemia) Characterized by sudden onset of fever, intense headache, nausea and often vomiting, stiff neck, and frequently a petechial rash with pink macules or, very rarely, vesicles. Delirium and coma often appear; occasional fulminating cases exhibit sudden prostration.	Varies from 2 to 10 days, commonly 3 to 4 days.	By direct contact, including droplets and discharges from nose and throat of infected persons, more often carriers than cases.	Until meningococci are no longer present in discharges from nose and throat. If organisms are sensitive to sulfonamides, meningococci usually disappear from nasopharynx within 24 hours after institution of treatment. They are not fully eradicated from oronasopharynx by penicillin.
Meningitis, hemophilus (meningitis caused by *Haemophilus influenzae*) Most common bacterial meningitis in children 2 months to 3 years old in U.S. Otitis media or sinusitis may be precursor. Almost always associated with bacteremia. Onset is sudden with symptoms of fever, vomiting, lethargy, and meningeal irritation.	Probably short—within 2 to 4 days.	By droplet infection and discharges from nose and throat during infectious period. May be purulent rhinitis. Portal of entry is most commonly nasopharyngeal.	As long as organisms are present, which may be for prolonged period even without nasal discharge.

Adapted from *Mosby's medical nursing and allied health dictionary*, ed 4, St Louis, 1994, Mosby.

Continued

Contagious diseases—cont'd

Disease and synopsis of symptoms	Incubation period	Mode of transmission	Period of communicability
Mononucleosis, infectious (glandular fever, EBV mononucleosis) Characterized by fever, sore throat (often with exudative pharyngotonsillitis), and lymphadenopathy (especially posterior cervical). Jaundice occurs in about 4% of infected young adults and splenomegaly in 50%. Duration is from 1 to several weeks.	From 4 to 6 weeks.	Person-to-person spread by oropharyngeal route via saliva. Spread may also occur via blood transfusion to susceptible recipients.	Prolonged; pharyngeal excretion may persist for 1 year after infection; 15% to 20% of healthy adults are oropharyngeal carriers.
Mumps (infectious parotitis) Acute viral disease characterized by fever, swelling, and tenderness of one or more salivary glands, usually parotid and sometimes sublingual or submaxillary glands.	About 2 to 3 weeks, commonly 18 days.	By droplet spread and by direct contact with saliva of an infected person.	Virus has been isolated from saliva from 6 days before salivary gland involvement to as long as 9 days thereafter; but height of infectiousness occurs about 48 hours before swelling begins. Urine may be positive for as long as 14 days after onset of illness.
Paratyphoid fever Frequently generalized bacterial enteric infection, often with abrupt onset, continued fever, enlargement of spleen, sometimes rose spots on trunk, usually diarrhea, and involvement of lymphoid tissues of mesentery and intestines.	1 to 3 weeks for enteric fever; 1 to 10 days for gastroenteritis.	Direct or indirect contact with feces or urine of patient or carrier. Spread by food, especially milk, milk products, and shellfish. Flies may be vectors.	As long as infectious agent persists in excreta, which is from appearance of prodromal symptoms, throughout illness, and for periods up to several weeks or months. Commonly 1 to 2 weeks after recovery.
Pediculosis (lousiness) Infestation of head, hairy parts of body, or clothing with adult lice, larvae, or nits (eggs), which results in severe itching and excoriation of scalp or scratch marks of body.	Under optimum conditions, eggs of lice hatch in 1 week, reach sexual maturity in approximately 2 weeks.	Direct contact with infected person and indirectly by contact with personal belongings, especially clothing and headgear. Crab lice are usually transmitted through sexual contact.	Communicable as long as lice remain alive on infested person or in clothing, and until eggs in hair and clothing have been destroyed.
The pneumonias A. Pneumococcal pneumonia Acute bacterial infection characterized by sudden onset with single shaking chill, fever, pleural pain, dyspnea, cough productive of "rusty" sputum and leukocytosis.	Not well determined; believed to be 1 to 3 days.	By droplet spread; by direct oral contact or indirectly, through articles freshly soiled with respiratory organisms is common.	Presumably until discharges of mouth and nose no longer contain virulent pneumococci in significant numbers. Penicillin will render patient noninfectious within 24 to 48 hours.
B. Mycoplasmal pneumonia (primary atypical pneumonia) Predominantly afebrile lower respiratory infection. Onset is gradual with headache, malaise, cough often paroxysmal, and usually substernal pain (not pleuritic). Sputum, scant at first, may increase later.	14 to 21 days.	Probably by droplet inhalation, direct contact with infected person or with articles freshly soiled with discharges of nose and throat from acutely ill and coughing patient.	Probably less than 10 days; occasionally longer with persisting febrile illness or persistence of the organisms in convalescence (as long as 13 weeks is known).

Adapted from *Mosby's medical nursing and allied health dictionary*, ed 4, St Louis, 1994, Mosby.

Continued

Contagious diseases—cont'd

Disease and synopsis of symptoms	Incubation period	Mode of transmission	Period of communicability
The pneumonias—cont'd C. Pneumocystis pneumonia (interstitial plasma cell pneumonia) Acute pulmonary disease occurring early in life, especially in malnourished, chronically ill, or premature infants. Characterized by progressive dyspnea, tachypnea, and cyanosis; fever may not be present.	Analysis of data from institutional outbreaks among infants indicates 1 to 2 months.	Unknown.	Unknown.
D. Chlamydial pneumonia (pertussoid eosinophilic pneumonia) Subacute pulmonary disease occurring in early infancy, primarily in infants of mothers with infection of uterine cervix with causative organism.	Not known, but pneumonia may occur in infants from 1 to 18 weeks of age (more commonly between 4 and 12 weeks).	Presumed to be vertically transmitted from infected cervix to infant during birth, with resultant nasopharyngeal infection.	Unknown, but length of nasopharyngeal excretion can be at least 2 months.
Poliomyelitis (infantile paralysis) Acute viral infection whose symptoms include fever, malaise, headache, nausea, vomiting, and stiffness of neck and back with or without paralysis.	Commonly 7 to 14 days for paralytic cases, with a range from 3 to possibly 35 days.	Direct contact through close association. In rare instances milk, foodstuffs, and other fecally contaminated materials have been incriminated as vehicles. Fecal-oral is major route when sanitation is poor, but during epidemics and when sanitation is good, pharyngeal spread becomes relatively more important.	Not accurately known. Cases are probably most infectious during first few days after onset of symptoms.
Respiratory disease (excluding influenza) A. Acute febrile respiratory disease Viral diseases of respiratory tract are characterized by fever and one or more constitutional reactions such as chills or chilliness, headache, general aching, malaise, and anorexia; in infants by occasional gastrointestinal disturbances.	From a few days to 1 week or more.	Directly by oral contact or by droplet spread, indirectly by hands or other materials soiled by respiratory discharges of infected person.	For duration of active disease; little is known about subclinical or latent infections.
B. Common cold (acute coryza) Acute catarrhal infections of upper respiratory tract characterized by coryza, sneezing, lacrimation, irritated nasopharynx, chilliness, and malaise lasting 2 to 7 days. Fever is uncommon in children and rare in adults.		Presumably by direct oral contact or by droplet spread; indirectly by hands and articles freshly soiled by discharges of nose and throat of infected person.	

Adapted from *Mosby's medical nursing and allied health dictionary*, ed 4, St Louis, 1994, Mosby.

Continued

Contagious diseases—cont'd

Disease and synopsis of symptoms	Incubation period	Mode of transmission	Period of communicability
Rubella (German measles) A. Congenital rubella Mild febrile infectious disease with diffuse punctate and macular rash. Sometimes resembling that of measles, scarlet fever, or both. May be few or no constitutional symptoms in children but adults may experience 1- to 5-day prodrome characterized by low-grade fever, headache, malaise, mild coryza, and conjunctivitis. As many as 20% to 50% of infections may occur without evident rash; overall 50% are not recognized. B. Erythema infectiosum (fifth disease) Mild nonfebrile erythematous eruption occurring as epidemics among children. Characterized by striking erythema of cheeks, reddening of skin, and lacelike serpiginous rash of body. C. Exanthema subitum (roseola infantum) Acute illness of probable viral cause characterized by high fever that suddenly appears and lasts 3 to 5 days. A maculopapular rash on trunk and later on rest of body ordinarily follows lysis of fever.	From 16 to 18 days with a range of 14 to 21 days.	Contact with nasopharyngeal secretions of infected person. Infection is by droplet spread or direct contact with patients and indirect contact.	For about 1 week before and at least 4 days after onset of rash. Highly communicable. Infants with congenital rubella syndrome may shed virus for months after birth.
Shigellosis (bacillary dysentery) Acute bacterial disease primarily involving large intestine, characterized by diarrhea, accompanied by fever, nausea, sometimes vomiting, cramps, and tenesmus. In severe cases stools contain blood, mucus, and pus.	1 to 7 days, usually 1 to 3 days.	By direct or indirect fecal-oral transmissin from patient or carrier. Infection may occur after ingestion of very few organisms.	During acute infection and until infectious agent is no longer present in feces, usually within 4 weeks of illness.
Staphylococcal disease A. Staphylococcal disease in community, boils, carbuncles, furuncles, impetigo, cellulitis, abscesses, staphylococcal septicemia, staphylococcal pneumonia, osteomyelitis, endocarditis Staphylococci produce variety of syndromes with clinical manifestations that range from single pustule to impetigo to septicemia to death. Lesion or lesions containing pus are primary clinical finding, abscess formation is typical.	Variable and indefinite. Commonly 4 to 10 days.	Major site of colonization is anterior nares. Autoinfection is responsible for at least one third of infections. Person with draining lesion or any purulent lesion or who is asymptomatic (usually nasal) carrier of pathogenic strain. Air-borne spread is rare.	As long as purulent lesions continue to drain or carrier state persists.

Adapted from *Mosby's medical nursing and allied health dictionary*, ed 4, St Louis, 1994, Mosby.

Continued

Contagious diseases—cont'd

Disease and synopsis of symptoms	Incubation period	Mode of transmission	Period of communicability
Staphylococcal disease—cont'd			
B. Staphylococcal disease in hospital nurseries, impetigo, abscess of breast Characteristic lesions develop secondary to colonization of nose or umbilicus, conjunction, circumcision site, or rectum of infants with pathogenic strain.	Commonly 4 to 10 days but may occur several months after colonization.	Spread by hands of hospital personnel is primary mode of transmission within hospitals; to a lesser extent, air-borne.	Same.
C. Staphylococcal disease in medical and surgical wards of hospitals Lesions vary from simple furuncles or stitch abscesses to extensively infected bedsores or surgical wounds, septic phlebitis, chronic osteomyelitis, fulminating pneumonia, endocarditis, or septicemia.	Variable and indefinite. Commonly 4 to 10 days.	Major site of colonization is anterior nares. Autoinfection is responsible for at least one third of infections. Person with a draining lesion or any purulent lesion or who is an asymptomatic (usually nasal) carrier of a pathogenic strain. Air-borne spread is rare.	As long as purulent lesions continue to drain or carrier state persists.
Streptococcal sore throat Fever, sore throat, exudative tonsillitis or pharyngitis, and tender anterior cervical lymph nodes.	Short, usually 1 to 3 days, rarely longer.	Transmission results from direct or intimate contact with patient or carrier, rarely by indirect contact through objects or hands. Nasal carriers are particularly likely to transmit diseases.	In untreated uncomplicated cases 10 to 21 days; in untreated conditions with purulent discharges, weeks or months.
Syphilis, nonvenereal endemic Acute disease of limited geographical distribution, characterized clinically by eruption of skin and mucous membranes, usually without evident primary sore.	2 weeks to 3 months.	Direct or indirect contact with infectious early lesions of skin and mucous membranes. Congenital transmission does not occur.	Until moist eruptions of skin and mucous patches disappear—sometimes several weeks or months.
Trachoma Communicable keratoconjunctivitis characterized by conjunctival inflammation with papillary hyperplasia, associated with vascular invasion of cornea, and in later stages by conjunctival scarring that may eventually lead to blindness.	5 to 12 days (based on volunteer studies).	By direct contact with ocular discharges and possibly mucoid or purulent discharges of nasal mucous membranes of infected persons or materials. Flies (*Musca sorbens*) may contribute to spread of disease.	As long as active lesions are present in the conjunctivae and adnexal mucous membranes.
Tuberculosis Mycobacterial disease. Initial infection usually goes unnoticed; tuberculin sensitivity appears within a few weeks; lesions commonly heal, leaving no residual changes except pulmonary or tracheobronchial lymph node calcification. May progress to pulmonary tuberculosis or, by lymphohematogenous dissemination of bacilli, to produce miliary, meningeal, or other extrapulmonary involvement.	From infection to demonstrable primary lesion, about 4 to 12 weeks. Whereas subsequent risk of progressive pulmonary or extrapulmonary tuberculosis is greatest within 1 or 2 years after infection, it may persist for a lifetime as latent infection.	Exposure to bacilli in air-borne droplet nuclei from sputum of persons with infectious tuberculosis. Bovine tuberculosis results from exposure to tubercular cattle and ingestion of unpasteurized dairy products.	As long as infectious tubercle bacilli are being discharged.

Adapted from *Mosby's medical nursing and allied health dictionary*, ed 4, St Louis, 1994, Mosby.

Continued

Contagious diseases—cont'd

Disease and synopsis of symptoms	Incubation period	Mode of transmission	Period of communicability
Typhoid fever (enteric fever, typhus abdominalis) Systemic infectious disease characterized by sustained fever, headache, malaise, anorexia, relative bradycardia, enlargement of spleen, rose spots on trunk, nonproductive cough, constipation more common than diarrhea, and involvement of lymphoid tissues.	Depends on size of infecting dose; usual range 1 to 3 weeks.	By food or water contaminated by feces or urine of patient or carrier.	As long as typhoid bacilli appear in excreta; usually first week throughout convalescence; variable thereafter. About 10% of untreated patients will discharge bacilli for 3 months after onset of symptoms; 2% to 5% become permanent carriers.
Whooping cough (pertussis) Acute bacterial disease involving tracheobronchial tree. Initial catarrhal stage has insidious onset with irritating cough that gradually becomes paroxysmal, usually within 1 to 2 weeks, and lasts for 1 to 2 months.	Commonly 7 days; almost uniformly within 10 days, and not exceeding 21 days.	Primarily by direct contact with discharges from respiratory mucous membranes of infected persons by air-borne route, probably by droplets. Frequently brought into home by older sibling.	Highly communicable in early catarrhal stage before paroxysmal cough stage. For control purposes, communicable stage extends from 7 days after exposure to 3 weeks after onset of typical paroxysms in patients not treated with antibiotics; in patients treated with erythromycin, period of infectiousness extends only 5 to 7 days after onset of therapy.
Acquired immunodeficiency syndrome (AIDS) Acute viral infection characterized by breakdown and failure of immune system, opening body to often lethal infections and disorders such as Kaposi's sarcoma, pneumonia, and meningitis. Symptoms begin with fever, weight loss, fatigue, shortness of breath, diarrhea, and neurologic disorders.	Variable.	By direct sexual contact and transmission of semen, saliva, blood, or other body fluids. Also by blood transfusion or contaminated syringes.	For duration of infection.
Chancroid (ulcus molle, soft chancre) Acute, localized, genital infection characterized by single or multiple painful necrotizing ulcers at site of inoculation, frequently accompanied by painful inflammatory swelling and suppuration of regional lymph nodes. Extragenital lesions have been reported.	From 3 to 5 days, up to 14 days.	By direct contact with discharges from open lesions and pus from buboes; suggestive evidence of asymptomatic infections in women. Multiple sexual partners and uncleanliness favor transmission.	As long as infectious agent persists in original lesion or discharging regional lymph nodes; usually until healed—a matter of weeks.
Conjunctivitis, inclusion (swimming pool conjunctivitis, paratrachoma) In the newborn, acute papillary conjunctivitis with abundant mucopurulent discharge. In children and adults, acute follicular conjunctivitis with preauricular lymphadenopathy, often with superficial corneal involvement.	5 to 12 days.	During sexual intercourse; genital discharges of infected persons are infectious.	While genital infection persists; can be longer than 1 year in female.

Adapted from *Mosby's medical nursing and allied health dictionary*, ed 4, St Louis, 1994, Mosby.

Continued

Contagious diseases—cont'd

Disease and synopsis of symptoms	Incubation period	Mode of transmission	Period of communicability
Cytomegalovirus infections, congenital cytomegalovirus infection, cytomegalic inclusion disease			
Most severe form of disease occurs in perinatal period, following congenital infection, with signs and symptoms of severe generalized infection especially involving central nervous system and liver.	Information inexact. 3 to 8 weeks following transfusion with infected blood. 3 to 12 weeks after birth.	Intimate exposure to infectious secretions or excretions. Virus is excreted in urine, saliva, cervical secretions, breast milk, and semen.	Virus is excreted in urine or saliva for months and may persist for several years following primary infection.
Gonococcal infections			
A. Gonococcal infection of genitourinary tract (gonorrhea, gonococcal urethritis) *Males*—purulent discharge from anterior urethra with dysuria appears 2 to 7 days after infecting exposure. *Females*—few days after exposure initial urethritis or cervicitis occurs, frequently so mild as to pass unnoticed. About 20% of patients have uterine invasion at the first, second, or later menstrual period with symptoms of endometritis, salpingitis, or pelvic peritonitis.	Usually 2 to 7 days, sometimes longer.	By contact with exudates from mucous membranes of infected persons, almost always result of sexual activity.	May extend for months if untreated, especially in females who frequently are asymptomatic. Specific therapy usually ends communicability within hours except with penicillin-resistant strains.
B. Gonococcal conjunctivitis neonatorum (gonorrheal ophthalmia neonatorum) Acute redness and swelling of conjunctiva of one or both eyes, with mucopurulent or purulent discharge in which gonococci are identifiable by microscopic and cultural methods.	Usually 1 to 5 days.	Contact with infected birth canal during childbirth.	While discharge persists if untreated; for 24 hours following initiation of specific treatment.
Granuloma inguinale (donovanosis)			
Mildly communicable, nonfatal, chronic and progressive, autoinoculable bacterial disease of skin and mucous membranes of external genitalia, inguinal, and anal region. Small nodule, vesicle, or papule is present.	Unknown; probably 8 to 80 days.	Presumably by direct contact with lesions during sexual activity.	Unknown and probably for duration of open lesions on skin or mucous membranes.

Adapted from *Mosby's medical nursing and allied health dictionary*, ed 4, St Louis, 1994, Mosby.

Continued

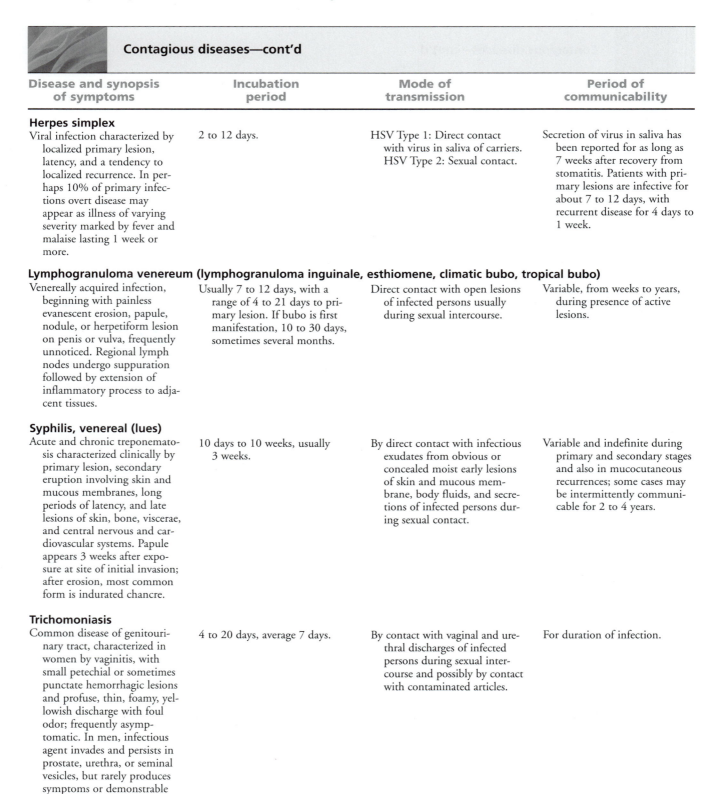

Contagious diseases—cont'd

Disease and synopsis of symptoms	Incubation period	Mode of transmission	Period of communicability
Herpes simplex Viral infection characterized by localized primary lesion, latency, and a tendency to localized recurrence. In perhaps 10% of primary infections overt disease may appear as illness of varying severity marked by fever and malaise lasting 1 week or more.	2 to 12 days.	HSV Type 1: Direct contact with virus in saliva of carriers. HSV Type 2: Sexual contact.	Secretion of virus in saliva has been reported for as long as 7 weeks after recovery from stomatitis. Patients with primary lesions are infective for about 7 to 12 days, with recurrent disease for 4 days to 1 week.
Lymphogranuloma venereum (lymphogranuloma inguinale, esthiomene, climatic bubo, tropical bubo)			
Venereally acquired infection, beginning with painless evanescent erosion, papule, nodule, or herpetiform lesion on penis or vulva, frequently unnoticed. Regional lymph nodes undergo suppuration followed by extension of inflammatory process to adjacent tissues.	Usually 7 to 12 days, with a range of 4 to 21 days to primary lesion. If bubo is first manifestation, 10 to 30 days, sometimes several months.	Direct contact with open lesions of infected persons usually during sexual intercourse.	Variable, from weeks to years, during presence of active lesions.
Syphilis, venereal (lues) Acute and chronic treponematosis characterized clinically by primary lesion, secondary eruption involving skin and mucous membranes, long periods of latency, and late lesions of skin, bone, viscerae, and central nervous and cardiovascular systems. Papule appears 3 weeks after exposure at site of initial invasion; after erosion, most common form is indurated chancre.	10 days to 10 weeks, usually 3 weeks.	By direct contact with infectious exudates from obvious or concealed moist early lesions of skin and mucous membrane, body fluids, and secretions of infected persons during sexual contact.	Variable and indefinite during primary and secondary stages and also in mucocutaneous recurrences; some cases may be intermittently communicable for 2 to 4 years.
Trichomoniasis Common disease of genitourinary tract, characterized in women by vaginitis, with small petechial or sometimes punctate hemorrhagic lesions and profuse, thin, foamy, yellowish discharge with foul odor; frequently asymptomatic. In men, infectious agent invades and persists in prostate, urethra, or seminal vesicles, but rarely produces symptoms or demonstrable lesions.	4 to 20 days, average 7 days.	By contact with vaginal and urethral discharges of infected persons during sexual intercourse and possibly by contact with contaminated articles.	For duration of infection.

Adapted from *Mosby's medical nursing and allied health dictionary*, ed 4, St Louis, 1994, Mosby.

Continued

Contagious diseases—cont'd

Disease and synopsis of symptoms	Incubation period	Mode of transmission	Period of communicability
Urethritis, chlamydial urethritis, nongonorrheal and nonspecific			
Sexually transmitted urethritis of males caused by chlamydial agent. Clinical manifestations are usually indistinguishable from gonorrhea but are often milder and include opaque discharge of moderate or scanty quantity, urethral itching, and burning on urination. Infection of women results in cervicitis and salpingitis.	5 to 7 days or longer.	Sexual contact.	Unknown.

Adapted from *Mosby's medical nursing and allied health dictionary*, ed 4, St Louis, 1994, Mosby.

Appendix J

Comparison of selected effects of commonly abused drugs

Drug category	Physical dependence	Characteristics of intoxication
Opiates	Marked	Analgesia with or without depressed sensorium; pinpoint pupils (tolerance does not develop to this action); patient may be alert and appear normal; respiratory depression with overdose
Barbiturates	Marked	Patient may appear normal with usual dose, but narrow margin between doses needed to prevent withdrawal symptoms and toxic dose is often exceeded and patient appears "drunk," with drowsiness, ataxia, slurred speech, and nystagmus on lateral gaze; pupil size and reaction normal; respiratory depression with overdose
Nonbarbiturate sedatives; glutethimide (Doriden)	Marked	Pupils dilated and reactive to light; coma and respiratory depression prolonged; sudden apnea and laryngeal spasm common
Antianxiety agents ("minor tranquilizers")	Marked	Progressive depression of sensorium as with barbiturates; pupil size and reaction normal; respiratory depression with overdose
Ethanol	Marked	Depressed sensorium, acute or chronic brain syndrome, odor on breath, pupil size and reaction normal
Amphetamines	Mild to absent	Agitation, with paranoid thought disturbance in high doses; acute organic brain syndrome after prolonged use; pupils dilated and reactive; tachycardia, elevated blood pressure, with possibility of hypertensive crisis and CVA; possibility of convulsive seizures
Cocaine	Possible	Paranoid thought disturbance in high doses, with dangerous delusions of persecution and omnipotence, tachycardia, respiratory depression with overdose
Marijuana	Absent	Milder preparations: drowsy, euphoric state with frequent inappropriate laughter and disturbance in perception of time or space (occasional acute psychotic reaction reported); stronger preparations such as hashish: frequent hallucinations or psychotic reaction; pupils normal; conjunctivas injected (marijuana preparations frequently adulterated with LSD, tryptamines, or heroin)
Psychotomimetics: LSD, STP, tryptamines, mescaline, morning glory seeds	Absent	Unpredictable disturbance in ego function, manifest by extreme lability of affect and chaotic disruption of thought, with danger of uncontrolled behavioral disturbance; pupils dilated and reactive to light
Phencyclidine	Unknown	Disinhibition, agitation, confusion, chaotic thought disturbance, unpredictable behavior, hypertension, meiosis, respiratory collapse, cardiovascular collapse, death
Anticholinergic agents	Absent	Nonpsychotropic effects such as tachycardia, decreased salivary secretion, urinary retention, and dilated, nonreactive pupils plus depressed sensorium, confusion, disorientation, hallucinations, and delusional thinking
Inhalants*	Unknown	Depressed sensorium, hallucinations, acute brain syndrome; odor on breath, often glassy-eyed appearance

Adapted from *Mosby's medical, nursing, and allied health dictionary*, ed 4, St Louis, 1994, Mosby.

*The term *inhalant* is used to designate a variety of gases and highly volatile organic liquids, including the aromatic glues, paint thinners, gasoline, some anesthetic agents, and amylnitrite. The term excludes liquids sprayed into the nasopharynx (droplet transport required) and substances that must be ignited before administration (such as marijuana).

Comparison of selected effects of commonly abused drugs—cont'd

Characteristics of withdrawal	"Flashback" symptoms	Masking of symptoms of illness or injury during intoxication
Rhinorrhea, lacrimation, and dilated, reactive pupils, followed by gastrointestinal disturbances, low back pain, and waves of gooseflesh; convulsions not a feature unless heroin samples were adulterated with barbiturates	Not reported	An important feature of opiate intoxication, resulting from analgesic action, with or without depressed sensorium
Agitation, tremulousness, insomnia, gastrointestinal disturbances, hyperpyrexia, blepharoclonus (clonic blink reflex), acute brain syndrome, major convulsive seizures	Not reported	Only in presence of depressed sensorium or after onset of acute brain syndrome
Similar to barbiturate withdrawal syndrome, with agitation, gastrointestinal disturbances, hyperpyrexia, and major convulsive seizures	Not reported	Same as in barbiturate intoxication
Similar to barbiturate withdrawal syndrome, with danger of major convulsive seizures	Not reported	Same as in barbiturate intoxication
Similar to barbiturate withdrawal syndrome, but with less likelihood of convulsive seizures	Not reported	Same as in barbiturate intoxication
Lethargy, somnolence, dysphoria, and possibility of suicidal depression; brain syndrome may persist for many weeks	Infrequently reported	Drug-induced euphoria or acute brain syndrome may interfere with awareness of symptoms of illness or may remove incentive to report symptoms of illness
Similar to amphetamine withdrawal	Not reported	Same as in amphetamine intoxication
No specific withdrawal symptoms	Infrequently reported	Uncommon with milder preparations, stronger preparations may interfere in same manner as psychotomimetic agents
No specific withdrawal symptoms; symptoms may persist for indefinite period after discontinuation of drug	Commonly reported as late as 1 year after last dose	Affective response or psychotic thought disturbance may remove awareness of or incentive to report symptoms of illness
No specific withdrawal symptoms	Occasionally reported	Same as in LSD intoxication
No specific withdrawal symptoms; mydriasis may persist for several days	Not reported	Pain may not be reported as a result of depression of sensorium, acute brain syndrome, or acute psychotic reaction
No specific withdrawal symptoms	Infrequently reported	Same as in anticholinergic intoxication

Comprehensive Exams

COMPREHENSIVE EXAMINATION 1: PART 1

This examination contains individual questions, each containing a relevant clinical situation. Read all questions carefully. There is only *one best answer* for each question.

Test time allotment (Part 1): approximately 2 hours
Answers and rationales begin on p. 552

1. Three days after admission, a patient becomes confused. The nurse's care plan should recommend:
   ① Ambulation and maintaining mobility by ROM exercises
   ② Moving the patient to the psychiatric ward
   ③ Reviewing the medication regimen with the physician
   ④ Obtaining an order for medication to decrease confusion

2. While preparing to administer digitalis to a newly admitted patient, the nurse counted an apical pulse rate of 52 beats/min. The nurse would be correct to:
   ① Give the drug as usual
   ② Omit the drug and report it to the physician
   ③ Give the patient half the dosage
   ④ Give the drug but with twice as much water as usual

3. A patient undergoes a cholecystectomy and duct exploration. She returns to the floor with an IV, nasogastric tube to low suction, and a T-tube in place. The purpose of the T-tube is to:
   ① Remove serous fluid from the abdominal cavity
   ② Provide an access to irrigate the operative area
   ③ Remove excessive bile from the intestines
   ④ Promote bile duct patency until edema subsides

4. In planning care for a patient with arteriosclerosis obliterans, the nurse would consider which of the following?
   ① Direct application of heat to improve circulation to the affected area
   ② Giving instructions in avoiding injury and maintaining circulation
   ③ Elevating the foot of the bed to increase arterial circulation
   ④ Massaging the extremities several times a day to improve circulation

5. If a patient is dissatisfied with his or her physician, the nurse may:
   ① Report the matter to the head nurse or team leader
   ② Suggest three other physicians to the patient
   ③ Report the matter to the medical director
   ④ Report the matter to the patient's family

6. In providing health education to a patient with sarcoidosis, the nurse should most appropriately include:
   ① Ways to determine if the pulmonary system is getting more involved
   ② Agencies and methods to use to quit smoking
   ③ Methods to self-test for mediastinal node involvement
   ④ Symptoms of fibrosis of the advanced stage of disease

7. The patient is to receive ASA 600 mg. The label reads gr V. How many tablets should be given?
   ① 1.5
   ② 2
   ③ 2.5
   ④ 3

8. A patient complains of tenderness at her IV puncture site. On assessment the nurse notes redness and swelling. The nurse should first:
   ① Stop the flow of the IV fluids, and report this to your head nurse
   ② Notify the physician, and fill out an incident report
   ③ Elevate the arm, and apply warm compresses to the puncture site
   ④ Change the dressing over the puncture site using sterile technique

9. Following a cholecystectomy, a patient asks the nurse, "Will I have to stay on a fat-free diet for the rest of my life?" The *best* response would be:
   ① "You need to talk to your physician about that."
   ② "A fat-free diet will always be necessary if you wish to stay well."
   ③ "After you have completely recovered you will probably be able to eat a normal diet without excessive fat."
   ④ "Complications of this type of surgery might cause you to have to abstain from all fats."

10. The function of the state board of nursing is to:
    ① Establish specific nursing procedures in the state
    ② Legislate and execute laws pertaining to nursing
    ③ Operate schools of nursing in the state
    ④ Establish in-service programs in the state

11. The primary purpose of states requiring nurses to be licensed to practice nursing is to:
    ① Protect the employer and nurse
    ② Protect the patient and nursing practice
    ③ Protect the patient and employee
    ④ Protect the nurse from malpractice

12. When assessing a patient's chest pain, the nurse should note which of the following characteristics?
    ① Elevation of temperature
    ② Respiratory rate
    ③ Presence of incontinence
    ④ Radiation of pain to the jaw or arm

13. A patient has a diagnosis of primary dysfunction of the adrenal cortex. The physician has ordered replacement therapy. Which of the following is an important point to stress in patient teaching?
    ① The hormones will have to be taken for the rest of her life
    ② The hormones must be taken until the body's stores have been replenished
    ③ The hormones will only need to be taken during periods of stress
    ④ Daily visits to the physician will be necessary as the dose will be adjusted daily

14. The nutritional requirements of a diabetic patient:
    ① Are the same as for a nondiabetic patient
    ② Will be lower in calories than for a nondiabetic patient
    ③ Will be lower in carbohydrates than for a nondiabetic patient
    ④ Will be higher in protein than for a nondiabetic patient

15. You work in an internist's office. Morning office hours are from 8:30 AM to 11:30 AM. The physician always arrives promptly at 7:45 AM and lives two blocks from the office. At 7:30 AM a patient presents with symptoms of lower right-sided chest pain, pallor, and slight shortness of breath. A *priority* nursing action would be to:
    ① Tell the patient the physician will be in shortly
    ② Start nasal oxygen immediately
    ③ Telephone the physician at home
    ④ Place the patient in high-Fowler's position

16. The nurse's immediate intervention with a victim of sexual assault should be to ensure:
    ① The victim is examined and treated as quickly as possible
    ② The victim is left alone to seek medical care when desired
    ③ Privacy and solitude are rapidly provided the victim
    ④ Accommodations for bathing and douching are offered promptly

17. A patient has sustained burns on the front and back of both her legs and her right arm. What percent of her body would you estimate has been involved?
    ① 45%
    ② 54%
    ③ 72%
    ④ 18%

18. A neighbor runs into your yard screaming hysterically and you see that her bathrobe is on fire. The *immediate* nursing action you should take is to:
    ① Instruct Ms. Stephens to remove her bathrobe
    ② Call the fire department
    ③ Roll her in a blanket
    ④ Tell her to lie down

19. The nurse should know that the purpose of Good Samaritan laws is to:
    ① Mandate nurses and physicians to stop and render care at accident sites
    ② Encourage emergency aid at accident sites
    ③ Prevent any liability arising from care rendered at accident sites
    ④ Have universal laws mandating emergency aid at accident sites

20. Within the first few hours after treating a severe burn patient, the nurse should observe for which of the following?
    ① Laryngeal and tracheal edema
    ② Eschar formation
    ③ Absence of pain
    ④ Leathery appearance to skin

21. A 42-year-old female who has had progressive renal problems since childhood is diagnosed as having end-stage renal disease. She is scheduled for hemodialysis. When preparing the patient for hemodialysis, the nurse will:
    ① Record her weight
    ② Restrict visitors
    ③ Keep her NPO until after the procedure
    ④ Monitor catheter drainage

22. To relieve pruritus from uremic frost the appropriate nursing intervention would be to:
    ① Add mineral oil to the bathwater
    ② Use no soap in bathing
    ③ Use hot water in bathing
    ④ Add a weak vinegar solution to the bathwater

23. In planning nursing care for a patient with end-stage renal disease, which goal would have priority?
    ① Providing rest
    ② Maintaining fluid balance
    ③ Preventing infection
    ④ Preventing contractures

24. Which of the following will aid in early detection of scoliosis?
    ① Complete blood count
    ② Screening programs
    ③ Pneumography tests
    ④ Bone marrow aspirations

25. In preparing a patient for surgery, which of the following laboratory values would concern the nurse enough to call the physician?
    ① WBC, 10,000
    ② Hemoglobin level, 9 g/dl
    ③ Urine pH, 8.5
    ④ Hematocrit, 42%

26. Instructions to prepare a postmastectomy patient for going home would include cautioning her against:
    ① Wearing loose rubber gloves when washing dishes
    ② Allowing blood to be drawn from the arm of her operative side
    ③ Wearing a thimble when sewing
    ④ Allowing pulse to be taken in affected area

27. A small southern town has been devastated by a hurricane that has blown out to sea. You're part of a volunteer rescue team searching for local missing persons. The team splits up; you're alone and you find a man lying on his back moaning. Rapid assessment reveals a questionable back injury. Which of the following nursing actions should have the highest priority?
    ① Keeping the victim in supine position
    ② Positioning the victim in a side-lying position
    ③ Permitting the victim to assume the most comfortable position
    ④ Sitting the victim up to properly assess his pulmonary status

28. A patient has tachycardia. The nurse would expect the pulse rate to be in which range?
    ① 40 to 60 beats/min
    ② 60 to 80 beats/min
    ③ 80 to 100 beats/min
    ④ 100 to 120 beats/min

29. While bathing a patient, the nurse notices a reddened area on the right hip. The appropriate nursing action is to:
    ① Massage the area every 2 hours and keep him off his right side
    ② Clean with alcohol and apply a sterile dressing
    ③ Apply warm, moist compresses intermittently
    ④ Apply lotion and powder before turning him on the right side

30. A 37-year-old AIDS patient who is homosexual has increased susceptibility to disease because of:
    ① Immune suppression
    ② His age
    ③ His sexual orientation
    ④ Side effects of medication

31. The diagnosis of AIDS is confirmed on a patient and isolation precautions must be taken. The nurse understands how the disease is transmitted and as his nurse explains that he will require:

① Complete isolation precautions
② Reverse isolation and room restriction
③ Room restriction and restriction of visitors
④ Body fluids and respiratory isolation

32. A patient has returned to his room after a bronchoscopy. A priority in care would be for the nurse to:
① Explain that bed rest is necessary
② Observe for an allergic reaction
③ Test gag reflex before giving oral food or fluids
④ Force fluids to loosen secretions

33. A new patient needs instructions regarding the proper administration of Synthroid. Patient teaching should include:
① Withholding medication if pulse rate is below 60 beats/min
② Taking the medication at bedtime
③ Discontinuing drug therapy when all symptoms have subsided
④ Withholding medication and calling the physician if the pulse rate is over 100 beats/min

34. A patient who has a diagnosis of hypothyroidism is placed on a thyroid replacement drug called Synthroid. He will return to the clinic in 2 weeks for follow-up laboratory studies. Which of the following classic symptoms of hypothyroidism might the nurse anticipate this patient displaying?
① Hirsutism, buffalo hump between the shoulder blades, hypertension
② Thirst, dry skin, urinary frequency
③ Fatigue, hypotension, urinary frequency
④ Muscle cramping, weakness, slow response time

35. The nutritional status of the institutionalized elderly requires regular monitoring. A patient is 86 years old; it's important for the nurse to know that her:
① Caloric requirements are greater than when she was younger
② Caloric requirements are less than when she was younger
③ Caloric requirements are the same as when she was younger
④ Nutritional requirements are greater now that she's advancing in age

36. A patient is hospitalized and the physician orders an indwelling Foley catheter to be inserted before the scheduled surgical procedure. The nurse needs to take the following precaution while doing this procedure:
① Strict reverse isolation
② Medical asepsis
③ Surgical asepsis
④ Good handwashing

37. A 72-year-old male patient returned to the floor after having surgery on his gallbladder. The patient's wife asks the nurse why her husband cannot have a regular diet instead of clear liquids, because the surgery is over. The nurse's most appropriate response is to explain that the diet will:
① Activate the colon
② Help him lose weight
③ Reduce peristalsis
④ Rest his throat

38. A patient undergoing chemotherapy treatment for osteosarcoma has been vomiting every 2 to 3 hours during the course of the treatment. Which of the following nursing diagnoses is the most pertinent for this patient at this time?
① Self-care deficit
② Alteration in elimination
③ Alteration in tissue perfusion
④ Alteration in fluid and electrolytes

39. A patient has a radioactive device implanted to treat carcinoma of the bladder. Of the following approaches, which would best address the safety of the nurse in performing daily care?
① Perform nursing measures as quickly and completely as possible
② Enter the patient's room frequently to assess the implanted device
③ Perform skills slowly to facilitate discussion of the patient's disease
④ Spend as much time with the patient as possible to decrease feelings of loneliness in the patient

40. A nurse is preparing to administer an injection to a patient. Which of the following is the first step in infection control for this procedure?
① Donning clean gloves
② Donning sterile gloves
③ Swabbing the site with alcohol
④ Washing hands for 30 seconds

41. Which of the following chambers of a chest tube management system would allow air to exit from the lung but also prohibit air from entering the lung?
① Suction chamber
② Water seal chamber
③ Drainage chamber
④ Air chamber

42. A nurse is examining a patient's restrained extremity. Which of the following would indicate compromised circulatory status?
① A bounding pulse
② A warm extremity
③ Capillary refill > 3 seconds
④ Perceives the feeling of light touch

43. Which of the following statements would indicate to the nurse that a postoperative patient is ready to begin an oral intake?
① "I feel hungry."
② "My stomach feels bloated."
③ "I had a bowel movement this morning."
④ "My stomach is really rumbling this morning."

44. A patient with Alzheimer's is unable to recognize a cup as a receptacle to hold fluids. The nurse recognizes this as:
① Agnosia
② Projection
③ Displacement
④ Confabulation

45. A patient scheduled for abdominal surgery tells the nurse that he is a strict vegetarian and would like to continue this lifestyle while hospitalized. When planning for the nutritional needs of this patient, which of the following nutrients may be deficient in his diet, which would interfere with the normal healing process?
① Fat
② Protein
③ Disaccharides
④ Monosaccharides

46. A nurse is caring for a patient admitted with a medical diagnosis of congestive heart failure. In anticipating the patient's needs, which of the following nursing diagnosis will be of primary importance?
    ① Knowledge deficit
    ② Fluid volume excess
    ③ Fluid volume deficit
    ④ Alteration in thought processes

47. A male patient, age 53, slipped on icy steps and fractured his left tibia and fibula. He is in a long leg cast. Injury to the peroneal nerve as a result of pressure from the cast may cause:
    ① Numbness of the dorsal surface of the foot
    ② Volkmann's contracture
    ③ Dupuytren's contracture
    ④ Compartment syndrome

48. When caring for a patient with a blood sugar of 310, which one of the following is of highest priority for nursing care?
    ① Ensuring adequate rest
    ② Protecting patient safety
    ③ Checking nutritional intake
    ④ Bedrest because of potential dizziness

49. The nurse, while making rounds, notices that a 59-year-old male patient is very anxious and unable to relax. He states that his blood pressure was just checked and it is very high, 190/105. He says he just took his medicine 15 minutes ago. The nurse states that his blood pressure will be rechecked in 15 minutes. Which additional comment is best for the nurse to make next?
    ① "That is not really too high to worry about."
    ② "You're in a hospital. This is a safe place to be."
    ③ "I will stay with you until I can recheck it again."
    ④ "Maybe your medicine is not working or has not had enough time to bring it down."

50. A 77-year-old retired executive reports that he has had trouble swallowing food the last 2 weeks. The nurse knows that there are distinct phases for swallowing and dysphagia can be classified by the phase it affects. The patient states that he chews normally and chokes when he begins to swallow, which the nurse recognizes as:
    ① Phase one
    ② Phase two
    ③ Phase three
    ④ Phase four

51. A 53-year-old executive has been put on diuretics by his physician to help decrease edema problems caused by congestive heart failure. Because diuretics can cause hypokalemia, the nurse advises the patient to make sure he selects fruits that are rich sources of potassium. Fruits the nurse can suggest are:
    ① Apples or plums
    ② Canned fruit cocktail
    ③ Oranges, prunes, bananas
    ④ Grapes, pears, and all berries

52. A male patient, age 45, has been put on a sodium-restricted diet because of edema and hypertension. Foods the nurse can teach the patient to avoid or limit are:
    ① Rice, hard candies, fresh fish, fruit
    ② Vinegar, shredded wheat, herbs, honey
    ③ Dried peas and beans, skim milk, plain pasta
    ④ Cheese, bouillon, luncheon meats, sauerkraut

53. In 1989, the Centers for Disease Control and Prevention published a plan to eliminate tuberculosis by the year 2010. Unfortunately, tuberculosis is increasing in both sexes, and especially in persons infected with human immunodeficiency virus (HIV). The greatest obstacle to eliminating TB is:
    ① Noncompliance with prescribed therapy
    ② Crowded cities and homeless street people
    ③ Wrong medicines being prescribed for the disease
    ④ An increase in smog and air pollution in the industrial areas

54. A female patient, age 42, calls the office for an appointment. She has noticed a red "butterfly" pattern over her cheeks and part of her nose. She also complains of soreness in walking and moving and is running an intermittent slight fever. All these symptoms and signs have occurred in the last 6 to 8 weeks. The nurse knows that one possible system disorder that can cause the above is:
    ① Scleroderma
    ② Reynauds disease
    ③ Periarteritis nodosa
    ④ Systemic lupus erythematosus

55. Your new neighbor asks you if a certain surgeon is good, because her husband will soon need surgery on his knee. As a nurse, you know that the surgeon she asked about does not have a good reputation in town. There are rumors that this surgeon would not recognize a "sterile field" anywhere. In addition to this, some OR personnel have reported a recent surgery where this surgeon's glasses fell off his nose into the open wound of a patient. If the nurse offers this information it could be considered:
    ① Libel
    ② Assault
    ③ Slander
    ④ Defamation

56. In caring for an AIDS patient on AZT (zidavudine), the nurse needs to monitor the patient for toxic effects caused by this drug. These toxic effects include:
    ① Stomatitis and fevers
    ② Painful peripheral nerves
    ③ Headache, malaise, fatigue, fever
    ④ Painful peripheral nerves and anemia

57. In a patient with extensive burns from a gas explosion, the nurse must watch for electrolyte disturbances. In major burns the nurse knows that:
    ① Sodium (Na^+) levels may initially decrease
    ② Sodium and potassium levels are not affected
    ③ Potassium (K^+) levels are usually decreased
    ④ Potassium (K^+) levels are initially increased

58. A 78-year-old woman was brought to the clinic by her two children. They tell the nurse that they are concerned because their mother is suffering from memory loss, impaired logic, and the ability to reason. She neglects grooming and eating, and is beginning to exhibit antisocial behavior. The nurse suspects this as which of the following stages of Alzheimer's disease?
    ① First
    ② Second
    ③ Third
    ④ Fourth

59. A 73-year-old female patient complains that she can't hear as well as she used to. The nurse knows that hearing loss

because of nerve impairment is common in the elderly and that this is a condition known as:
① Tinnitus
② Presbycusis
③ Otosclerosis
④ Ménière's disease

60. When caring for an individual with AIDS, the nurse must be aware of standard (universal) precautions. These include:
① Sterile gloves and gown
② Gloves when in contact with blood or any body fluids
③ Mask and gloves at all times when caring for any HIV+ client
④ Gloves at all times when in contact with any patient in the hospital

61. The nurse needs to remember that during the life cycle the body's chemical composition is not precisely the same for every individual. Also, this pattern can change for a given person at different times under various circumstances. The term for this concept is:
① Metabolism
② Deamination
③ Basal metabolism
④ Biochemical individuality

62. A patient with advanced cancer of the liver is admitted to the hospital for oxygen and chemotherapy. When planning his care, the nurse needs to consider adequate amounts of food and fluids to keep him:
① Free from pain
② As comfortable as possible
③ Active and able to perform ADL
④ From developing side effects of chemotherapy

63. While following the physician's orders to do passive range of motion to the left arm and leg of a patient who suffered a slight stroke, the nurse notices that the patient is showing no improvement after 2 weeks. In application of the nursing process, this falls under:
① Assessment
② Planning
③ Implementation
④ Evaluation

64. While visiting a patient's home to check on his blood pressure, the nurse determines that the patient needs further teaching on medications. Which statement below made by the patient indicated this need to the nurse?
① "I try to not use so much salt in cooking any more."
② "I walk around the neighborhood when the weather is nice."
③ "I am trying to lose weight and have cut extra fats from my foods."
④ "Sometimes when I feel sort of dizzy or anxious about something, I take an extra pill."

65. A female, age 30, has been told that her cholesterol and triglyceride levels are high and that she needs to alter her diet to try to lower them. She tells the nurse that she does not eat much fat and does not understand why her levels are so high. The nurse needs to check the foods she has eaten the last several days, paying special notice to her intake of:
① Liquid vegetable oil
② Soft margarine
③ Animal foods
④ Oat bran

66. A patient scheduled to have a creatinine clearance test asks the reason for the test. The nurse tells her that this test is used to determine:
① Proteinuria
② Urine concentration
③ BUN (blood-urea-nitrogen)
④ Overall kidney function

67. When visiting a home health care patient recently discharged from the hospital where he was treated for DVT (deep vein thrombosis), the nurse notes that he is still taking warfarin sodium (Coumadin). Which assessment needs to be brought to the physician's attention immediately?
① He is still smoking and has a cough
② He has some nasal congestion
③ He has bruises on his upper arms
④ He has lost some weight recently, about 3 pounds

68. A 92-year-old female nursing home resident has been diagnosed with pneumonia. She has signed a living will and her physician has given the order "no code." When the nurse checks on her during rounds, she assesses the respiratory rate at 32 BPM. Breathing sounds are labored with deep breaths that resemble sighs; respirations are fast, deep, and without pauses. The nurse knows this type of breathing pattern as:
① Eupnea
② Hyperpnea
③ Cheyne-Stokes
④ Kussmaul's respirations

69. A 58-year-old female is hospitalized with a diagnosis of FUO (fever of unknown origin). She has a urine specific gravity of 1.115. The nurse needs to include which of the following in the plan of care?
① Monitor for jaundice
② Encourage adequate fluid intake
③ Active and passive range of motion
④ Analgesics for pain per physician order

70. When taking an axillary temperature, the nurse should:
① Use no special care in the axilla area
② Rub the axilla area until it is very dry, using a dry washcloth
③ Position the thermometer in the axilla with the tip pointing down to the extremities
④ Position the thermometer in the axilla with the tip pointing toward the patient's head

71. In reviewing the plan of care for a 24-year-old schizophrenic with regressive behavior, the nurse notes the following outcome (goal): patient will complete all ADLs and be neatly groomed within 2 days. The nurse may conclude:
① The goal is appropriate
② The goal is too broad
③ The goal is unrealistic
④ It is a long-term goal

72. According to Maslow's hierarchy, which basic needs must be met first?
① Esteem
② Love and belonging
③ Physiologic
④ Safety and security

73. Causes of mental illness are generally considered to be:
    ① Purely biochemical
    ② Essentially unresolved conflicts of early childhood
    ③ Culturally influenced
    ④ Interaction among biologic, psychologic, and cultural influences

74. Freud's understanding of human behavior is based on:
    ① Nine stages of ego development
    ② Sexuality and aggression
    ③ Cultural and environmental factors
    ④ Interpersonal conflict

75. A 28-year-old male stockbroker claims that he is the richest man in Michigan and a genius. He may be exhibiting:
    ① Tactile hallucinations
    ② Flight of ideas
    ③ Delusions of grandeur
    ④ Neurosis

76. A 42-year-old man has ingested 18 Valium (diazepam) tablets and 18 unidentified capsules. He is in the ER and is now alert after gastric lavage. He is calling his son to come and take him home. He is exhibiting which of the following defenses:
    ① Sublimation
    ② Projection
    ③ Denial
    ④ Regression

77. An 18-year-old woman, states, "It's such a beautiful day; will my new dog learn to sit up; give me some fruit." She is exhibiting:
    ① Confusion
    ② Flight of ideas
    ③ Delusions
    ④ Hallucinations

78. A patient who has been receiving antipsychotic drugs reports that he has a dry mouth, tight throat, and mouth movements. The nurse should consider that:
    ① These may be somatic delusions
    ② The patient is probably manipulating for more medication
    ③ These are transitory reactions that will disappear
    ④ These may be extrapyramidal reactions that require intervention

79. In community mental health programs, patients are:
    ① Not hospitalized
    ② Hospitalized near their homes
    ③ Treated in large mental hospitals
    ④ Hospitalized for more than 6 months

80. Mental health and mental illness are defined:
    ① In scientific studies
    ② In cultural settings
    ③ By behavior
    ④ By feelings

81. A new patient was diagnosed with lung cancer 1 week ago. She uses her call light for multiple small requests and verbalizes dissatisfaction with the care she has been receiving since her diagnosis. The nurse recognizes this behavior as which of the following stages of grieving?
    ① Denial
    ② Anger
    ③ Depression
    ④ Acceptance

82. A 56-year-old male has been admitted to have a biopsy of the bladder for a suspected malignancy. He tells the nurse: "I probably won't leave here alive." The nurse's *best* response is:
    ① "You will get better."
    ② "That's ridiculous. Don't even think that way."
    ③ "What does your family think and feel about all this?"
    ④ "You may feel that way now, but there is still a lot that can be done to help one fight this."

83. An alcoholic patient was admitted for upper GI bleeding. GI and lab tests were ordered by the physician. The patient refused to sign the permission forms, became angry, and stated that he was walking out. The nurse should:
    ① Detain him
    ② Yell for help and put him in restraints
    ③ Try to reason with him until the physician can be notified for proper discharge
    ④ Tell him that leaving against medical advice (AMA) is breaking the law

84. It is recommended that nurses working on stressful units get adequate rest, proper nutrition, exercise, and have enjoyable activities. This is to help prevent a condition known as "burnout" which means:
    ① Physical exhaustion
    ② Acting in hostile manners
    ③ Being overwhelmed by stress
    ④ Making wrong decisions during crisis situations

85. A 32-year-old working mother, was admitted for an evaluation of problems caused by severe anxiety. The nurse knows that anxiety is different than fear, in that anxiety:
    ① Is a response to an obvious threat
    ② Is a response to an unknown stimulus
    ③ Can usually result from an external threat
    ④ Only occurs in people who have mental health problems

86. A 14-year-old boy scout dove into a shallow pond while on a camping expedition. Friends rescued him from drowning when they saw he was in difficulty. When the emergency team arrived, they placed him on a stretcher, being especially careful *not* to:
    ① Move his extremities unnecessarily
    ② Flex his head
    ③ Put pressure on his diaphragm
    ④ Strap him to the stretcher too tightly

87. Oxygen therapy for the newborn must be administered with caution to prevent:
    ① Ophthalmia neonatorum
    ② ABO incompatibility
    ③ Respiratory distress syndrome
    ④ Retrolental fibroplasia

88. An important nursing goal in caring for the newborn with a myelomeningocele is to:
    ① Maintain the newborn in a prone position
    ② Observe the lower extremities for movement
    ③ Promote wound healing
    ④ Prevent infection and harm to the meningocele sac

89. During the postoperative period following repair of a myelomeningocele, signs of increased intracranial pressure the nurse must observe for are:
    ① Increased blood pressure and pulse and decreased pulse pressure
    ② Bulging fontanelles, high-pitched cry, and separated cranial sutures

③ Cheyne-Stokes respirations, hypotension, and increased pulse pressure

④ Decreased reflexes, bulging fontanelles, weak cry, and hypotension

90. An 11-year-old female patient has an order for prochlorperazine (Compazine) 4 mg IM. On hand is Compazine 10 mg/ml. The nurse gives this patient:
① 0.2 ml
② 0.4 ml
③ 0.8 ml
④ 1.2 ml

91. Using Clark's rule, answer the following problem:
Child's weight: 30 lb
Average adult dose: 10 mg
What is the child's dose?

$$\text{Clark's rule:}\ \frac{\text{Weight in pounds} \times \text{Adult dose}}{150}$$

① 1 mg
② 2 mg
③ 2.5 mg
④ 3 mg

92. A 4-week-old boy is admitted to the hospital with a diagnosis of pyloric stenosis. A classic symptom of pyloric stenosis is:
① Projectile vomiting
② Diarrhea
③ Sharp, colicky abdominal pain
④ Distended abdomen

93. To obtain a urine specimen from an infant, the nurse would:
① Clean and dry genitalia, perineum, and skin; apply a self-adhesive plastic bag (urine strap)
② Clean and dry perineum; catheterize infant with sterile infant feeding tube
③ Apply disposable diaper; aspirate urine from diaper with needle and syringe
④ Place infant on small fracture pan, pour urine into specimen container

94. A 4-year-old boy has developed small, reddish blisters on his face and trunk. He has a headache, a slight fever, and complains of itching. These symptoms suggest:
① Measles
② Chickenpox
③ Scarlet fever
④ Rubella

95. A 3-year-old girl has a possible diagnosis of pinworms. The pediatrician has ordered the "cellophane tape test" to attempt to capture the eggs around the anal area. The best time for you to perform this test is:
① After breakfast
② Before her nap
③ After a bowel movement
④ During the early morning hours

96. Treatment for a toddler with nephrotic syndrome will include:
① High-Fowler's position
② Regular diet
③ Diuretics as ordered
④ Sodium and potassium supplements

97. The cause of sudden infant death syndrome (SIDS) is:
① A respiratory viral infection
② Obstruction of the airway by a small foreign body
③ Hypertrophy of the larynx
④ Unknown

98. Freud's theory of child development states that infants are in the:
① Anal stage
② Oedipal stage
③ Genital stage
④ Oral stage

99. Normal nutritional requirements of a preschooler include food from the Food Guide Pyramid. As a result of severe burns, a 3-year-old patient would need a diet:
① High in proteins, carbohydrates, and calories
② High in proteins, iron, and calcium
③ Low in sodium and cholesterol
④ Low in calcium and high in carbohydrates

100. When changing the burn dressing, the nurse would help a young patient control his feelings of fear and pain by:
① Having another nurse restrain the patient until the treatment is over
② Explaining firmly what is to be done and how he can help
③ Allowing the patient to cry until he is tired and less combative
④ Repeating administration of the prescribed pain medication

101. An 18-month-old infant is to have a long-acting antibiotic given IM. The nurse selects the best muscle or site to use, which is:
① Deltoid
② Gluteus maximus
③ Vastus lateralis
④ Ventrogluteal area

102. A 7-year-old girl is admitted with a tentative diagnosis of encephalitis. She recently had chickenpox. The nurse needs to focus care on:
① Monitoring for jaundice
② Monitoring blood sugars
③ Monitoring blood pressure
④ Monitoring neurological status

103. A 4-year-old boy is admitted to a pediatric unit for initial IV treatment of osteomyelitis. The nurse knows that the peak incidence in children occurs between the ages of 3 and 15. It affects boys twice as often as girls. The nurse also knows that the bones most commonly affected are:
① Tibia, fibula, femur
② Fibula, tibia, patella
③ Patella, radius, ulna
④ Femur, tibia, humerus

104. An 18-month-old infant is admitted to a pediatric unit for recurring respiratory infections. She lives in a poor area of town. The physician orders a TB skin test. The nurse knows that best site for this intradermal skin test is:
① Upper arm
② Scapular area
③ Ventral forearm
④ Lateral aspect of the thigh

105. A patient with cystic fibrosis is intubated, on a ventilator, and must be suctioned every 2 to 3 hours for secretion control. Which of the following would be the most important goal for this patient at this time?
① Patient will be free of infection
② Patient will not experience arrhythmias
③ Patient will maintain a patient airway
④ Patient will have an equal intake and output

106. An 18-year-old girl who has been on a diet to lose weight complains to the office nurse that her periods have stopped. The nurse knows the term for this is:
① Amenorrhea
② Menorrhagia
③ Dysmenorrhea
④ Metrorrhagia

107. The nurse asks an 18-year-old girl about her weight loss. The patient states that she fasts for several days at a time on water and juices because she is so fat. The patient is 5′2″ and weighs 120 pounds. The nurse suspects that this patient is experiencing:
① Dysphagia
② Bulimia
③ Anorexia
④ Anorexia nervosa

108. A "chubby" 15-year-old girl asks the office nurse for advice in losing weight, and if there is any "magic" way to lose weight. The nurse advises her that the key to losing weight is:
① Revised eating habits
② Lose fast to keep it off
③ Periods of fasting for few days
④ Drinking diet sodas and a large amount of water

109. A 15-year-old girl asks the nurse how many calories will equal one pound. The nurse answers:
① 500 kcal
② 6500 kcal
③ 1000 kcal
④ 3500 kcal

110. A 23-year-old mother states that her 5-day-old baby girl was born with a wryneck and had to have corrective surgery. The nurse knows that the muscle involved was the:
① Trapezius muscle
② Temporalis muscle
③ Latissimus dorsi muscle
④ Sternocleidomastoid muscle

111. A patient is having contractions 2 minutes apart, of 45 seconds duration, and of moderate intensity. Fetal heart tones at this time should be monitored:
① During contractions
② Simultaneously with the mother's vital signs
③ Between contractions, every 30 minutes
④ Immediately following each contraction

112. The husband of a patient in labor is worried that the increased bloody show is a warning of an impending hemorrhage. The best nursing action would be:
① To reassure the father by reviewing how bloody show develops (since he has been Lamaze trained) and the normal sequence of progress
② Call the physician immediately to examine the mother once more for possible abruptio placentae
③ Take blood pressure and report any changes
④ Apply extra perineal pads to the perineum

113. Placenta previa is characterized by which of the following problems?
① Painless vaginal bleeding and boardlike rigidity over the abdomen
② Vaginal bleeding and fetal distress
③ Severe, sudden abdominal pain and shock
④ Hidden vaginal bleeding and severe abdominal pain

114. If you are pregnant and work in the labor and delivery room, what should you know about your vulnerability to the AIDS virus?
① You are at a greater risk of contracting the HIV virus
② Nurses are not known to be at greater risk of contracting the HIV infection
③ Strict adherence to precautions will not protect you from contracting the infection
④ An HIV infection during pregnancy will put the infant at risk, so do not care for AIDS patients

115. How should a mother who is breast-feeding adjust her diet to meet the nutritional demands of breast-feeding?
① Higher in iron and lower in fluids
② Lower in fats and sodium
③ Lower in cellulose and carbohydrates
④ Higher in calories and proteins

116. Patients receiving oxytocin (Pitocin) to induce labor must be carefully observed for:
① Hypotension
② Hyperstimulation of the uterus
③ Prolapse of the umbilical cord
④ Maternal exhaustion

117. A 32-year-old woman, in her last trimester, was admitted for induction of labor. She complains of feeling faint, particularly in a prone position, during labor. You know that the failure of venous return of blood from the legs and pelvis may be caused by compression of the inferior vena cava by the uterus, so you would:
① Take her blood pressure stat
② Place her in Trendelenburg's position
③ Turn her on her left side
④ Start suction machine; have intubation equipment ready

118. Classes in psychoprophylactic or Lamaze method of natural childbirth education are usually begun:
① As soon as the pregnancy is diagnosed
② Shortly after quickening
③ After lightening
④ 8 to 10 weeks before EDC (expected date of confinement)

119. How would you explain natural childbirth education to parents?
① "It is a method free from the use of drugs during labor and delivery."
② "Basically, it is preparation for labor and delivery by teaching relaxation exercises and breathing exercises to be used during pregnancy, labor, delivery, and postpartum."
③ "It prepares young couples to be good parents by teaching about newborns, nutrition, exercises, labor and delivery, and child care."
④ "It is preparing to have your baby in as natural a setting as you can, free from noise, in a quiet environment with soft music."

120. A postpartum patient complains that her left leg aches. The nurse notes that it is warm to the touch. What should the nurse do while awaiting the arrival of the physician?
① Apply ice bags to the leg
② Apply heat to the leg
③ Exercise the leg vigorously
④ Elevate the leg on pillows

121. A 23-year-old woman has discovered that she is about 3 months pregnant. She asks the nurse if it is safe for her to drink socially, about 3 to 4 drinks per week. The nurse's best response is:
① "Only 1 drink per week is advisable."
② "What you drink does not affect the baby."
③ "If you drink 5 or less drinks per week, it should be safe."
④ "The best thing you can do for your baby is to avoid any alcoholic beverages during the pregnancy."

122. A 31-year-old patient is having a difficult pregnancy and is 4 weeks from her due date. The office physician asks the nurse to instruct the patient on doing a "kick" count at home daily. The nurse needs to advise the patient to call immediately if her kick count is:
① Under 3
② Seven or more
③ In the 4 to 6 range
④ In the 6 to 7 range

123. A pregnant patient tells the nurse that she has not been taking her prenatal vitamins because she believes she can meet the increased nutritional needs of pregnancy by eating a varied diet. Which of the following should the nurse counsel her on as being an increased need that can't normally be met by diet alone?
① Iron
② Sodium
③ Calcium
④ Magnesium

124. A pregnant patient is diagnosed with pica. The nurse recognizes that pica is characterized by:
① Abnormal vaginal bleeding
② The ingestion of nonfood items
③ An abnormally high systolic blood pressure
④ The presence of a high serum blood glucose

125. An unmarried 18-year-old female suspects that she is pregnant and comes to the clinic. She does not remember her LMP (last menstrual period). Because Nägele's rule can't be used to determine EDC (expected date of confinement), the nurse expects that the delivery date will be determined by:
① Weight gain
② Serial estriols
③ First audible fetal heart rate
④ Fetal movement felt by the mother

COMPREHENSIVE EXAMINATION 1: PART 2

This examination contains individual questions, each containing a relevant clinical situation. Read all questions carefully. There is only *one best answer* for each question.

Test time allotment (Part 2): approximately 2 hours

Answers and rationales begin on p. 561

1. Following a transurethral resection of the prostate (TURP) the most common postoperative complication the nurse would assess for is:
   ① Hemorrhage
   ② Pneumonia
   ③ Thrombophlebitis
   ④ Fluid imbalance

2. A patient, age 54, underwent surgery for a suprapubic prostatectomy. Three days after surgery the cystotomy tube was removed. A specific nursing responsibility at this time is to:
   ① Force fluids
   ② Keep dressing dry
   ③ Encourage ambulation
   ④ Monitor fluid balance

3. A patient, 34 years of age, is complaining of infertility, metrorrhagia, and dyspareunia. Examination reveals endometrial-like cells growing elsewhere in her pelvic cavity. The nurse knows this condition as:
   ① Endometriosis
   ② Endometritis
   ③ Pelvic inflammatory disease
   ④ Paraphimosis

4. An 86-year-old retired school nurse is admitted to a nursing home following hospitalization for a fractured left wrist sustained from a fall in her garden. Her medical diagnoses are chronic brain syndrome, arteriosclerotic heart disease, and status post left wrist fracture. The nurse observes the patient to be withdrawn, frequently nonresponsive to conversation directed to her, complaining that everyone mumbles, and believing that others are talking about her. The nurse should suspect that the patient is experiencing:
   ① Psychosis
   ② Presbycusis
   ③ Presbyopia
   ④ Presbyophrenia

5. To promote retraining of the affected side and a faster return to independence, CVA patients should be encouraged to:
   ① Comb their hair, wash their face, brush their teeth
   ② Participate actively in physical therapy
   ③ Perform daily push-ups
   ④ Use a pen with the affected hand

6. The nurse is bathing a 37-year-old female woman, who was admitted for observation after sustaining a head injury in an automobile accident. The nurse is concerned when the patient:
   ① Vomits her breakfast
   ② Insists on giving self-care
   ③ Refuses to take any medications
   ④ Cries after talking on the phone with her children

7. During preoperative teaching the nurse explains why a local anesthetic will be given for removal of a cataract. The correct explanation is:

① This is an individual physician's preference
② Recovery time is shorter with local anesthesia
③ Local anesthetic lessens postoperative bleeding
④ General anesthetic frequently causes vomiting, which puts stress on the sutures in the eye

8. In caring for patients taking Coumadin it is important for the nurse to:
   ① Change the IV site every 48 hours
   ② Record intake, output, and daily weight
   ③ Observe mucous membranes, urine, and stools
   ④ Observe skin texture and turgor

9. A patient's wife reports upon admission that her husband has complained of headaches and has had three black-out spells in the past 6 months. He has complained of numbness and tingling on his right side at intervals but has refused to see his physician since the symptoms have subsided. Previous symptoms experienced by the patient indicate transient ischemic attacks (TIAs), which are caused by a:
   ① Complete obstruction in oxygen supply to the brain, resulting in necrosis
   ② Decreased amount of circulating oxygen
   ③ Complete obstruction in the afferent nerve tracts
   ④ Temporary lack of oxygen to an area of the brain

10. Coumadin is a possible drug of choice in the treatment of TIAs. It is important the nurse instruct patients taking Coumadin to:
    ① Increase their intake of vitamin K
    ② Use razors and sharp instruments with care
    ③ Massage and exercise their legs daily
    ④ Take aspirin four times daily

11. To avoid urinary complications associated with decreased mobility the nurse should encourage patients to:
    ① Increase intake of citrus fruits
    ② Decrease intake of fluids
    ③ Decrease intake of dairy products
    ④ Increase urine acidity

12. To prevent constipation in CVA patients, the nurse should encourage them to:
    ① Take daily enemas
    ② Use a daily laxative
    ③ Increase fruits and fluids in their diet
    ④ Plan a bowel movement for early morning

13. To *best* assist a patient who has been on bed rest to prepare for ambulation, the nurse should:
    ① Dangle the patient's legs and swing them back and forth daily
    ② Have him push his popliteal space against the bed to the count of 5, several times daily
    ③ Perform passive range of motion exercises 3 times daily
    ④ Have him perform push-ups and use the bed trapeze bar as much as possible

14. When teaching an AIDS patient's family about his decreasing resistance to infection, the nurse explains:
    ① The need to remain in the hospital indefinitely
    ② How the patient will be of great danger to those with whom he or she comes in contact
    ③ The expense of being maintained on antibiotics
    ④ That the patient will have to take measures to avoid exposure to new organisms

15. Nursing assessment must be accurately documented. The charted observation states that a patient had tachypnea. The nurse knows that respirations were:
    ① Increased in rate and depth
    ② Slow and regular in rate
    ③ Deep and fast, then shallower and slower with apneic periods
    ④ Increased in rate and decreased in depth

16. A patient who recently had a below-the-knee amputation (BKA) tells the nurse that he feels a burning sensation in the toes of the leg that was amputated. In developing a reply to his statement, the nurse should consider which of the following?
    ① He is probably imagining the sensation as a result of all the medication he has received
    ② He is probably trying to deny having had the surgery by thinking that the leg was not removed
    ③ The complaint is a common one in persons developing a flexion contracture
    ④ The sensation is valid and known to develop following an amputation

17. In caring for a patient who has undergone a midthigh amputation, the nurse should *not* elevate the residual limb after the first 24 hours. This precaution is to prevent:
    ① Phantom limb pain
    ② Circulatory embarrassment
    ③ A hip flexion contracture
    ④ Damage to the peroneal nerve

18. A patient has had an above-the-knee amputation (AKA) because of complications stemming from long-standing, uncontrolled diabetes mellitus. Following an amputation, the *immediate,* most serious postoperative complication(s) is (are):
    ① Infection
    ② Hemorrhage
    ③ Contractures
    ④ Pneumonia

19. A 36-year-old female has had a total hip replacement. The postoperative orders include aspirin, grains 5, PO, daily. The nurse is aware that the rationale for this treatment is to:
    ① Prevent joint inflammation
    ② Produce a mild anticoagulant effect
    ③ Provide better pain-control
    ④ Maintain normal body temperature

20. A 75-year-old female who slipped and fell while working in her yard is admitted to the orthopedic unit. Her diagnosis is subcapital fracture of the right hip. She is scheduled for surgery in the morning. The nurse is aware that until the time of surgery the fracture must be reduced. The nurse will anticipate using which of the following devices?
    ① Buck's extension
    ② Bryant's traction
    ③ Hodgen splint
    ④ Thomas splint with a Pearson attachment

21. Which of the following descriptions of an injured area on a diabetic patient's right leg would be most appropriate for the nurse to chart?
    ① Large excoriated area on anterior aspect of the shinbone
    ② 50-cent size area on anterior aspect of lower leg with moderate amount of serous drainage
    ③ 5-cm abraised lesion with small amount of serous drainage noted on right lower leg

④ Severe injury with minimal amount of drainage noted on right lower leg

22. A newly admitted patient has had insulin-dependent diabetes for 20 years. Now at age 68 she has begun to notice that her right foot and leg get numb and the skin is shiny. Last week she bumped her right leg while making her bed. The injured area has not healed and has worsened. During initial assessment of the patient the nurse discovers that she is wearing garters. It would be appropriate for the nurse to:
    ① Make a note of this on the chart
    ② Notify the physician immediately
    ③ Explain that garters retard circulation and should not be worn
    ④ Explain that garters are better than girdles because they are not so restricting to circulation

23. In caring for a patient with COPD, the nurse notes that the patient is more comfortable after:
    ① Being placed in the low-Fowler's position
    ② Having postural drainage
    ③ Fluids are restricted
    ④ He has provided all his own care

24. A patient with a diagnosis of sarcoidosis wants to know why the physician is planning to perform a biopsy of the lymph node. The nurse's most appropriate reply is:
    ① "He wants to see how far the sarcoidosis has spread."
    ② "Has the physician explained the procedure to you?"
    ③ "That is the way to definitely diagnose this disease."
    ④ "He can find out why your glands are swollen."

25. Frequent assessment of a patient with a fractured left leg would include maintaining proper alignment and:
    ① Checking sensation and circulation in the leg
    ② Increasing the weight of traction as necessary to maintain countertraction
    ③ Taking the apical pulse every 2 hours
    ④ Checking temperature and range of motion in his right leg

26. A patient receiving chlorpromazine (Thorazine) should be instructed to:
    ① Avoid certain foods containing tyramine
    ② Use a sunscreen when outdoors
    ③ Take medication with milk
    ④ Use prophylactic antacid

27. Which of the following statements regarding glycerin suppository insertion is the nurse expected to know to be true?
    ① Glycerin suppositories should be warmed to room temperature before insertion
    ② It is not necessary to lubricate glycerin suppositories before insertion
    ③ Glycerin suppositories should be inserted into a bolus of stool
    ④ Glycerin suppositories should be inserted before an attempt is made to toilet a patient in a bowel-retraining program

28. When preparing a patient for a bowel-retraining program, it is important for the nurse to understand that the most important factor for a successful retraining program is:
    ① Establishing regular day(s) and time to assist the patient to the toilet
    ② Making sure the patient understands the purpose of the program
    ③ Regular administration of a mild laxative
    ④ Skipping a day in the program if the patient has had more than one bowel movement the day before

29. Because respiratory embarrassment could occur following a subtotal thyroidectomy, it is advisable to:
    ① Have an IPPB machine in the room
    ② Place the patient in an oxygen tent for the first 48 hours
    ③ Keep a respiratory stimulant at the bedside
    ④ Keep a tracheostomy tray in the room until all danger has passed

30. A retired schoolteacher whose husband is on a low-cholesterol diet following a heart attack says she is totally confused about cholesterol and its importance in the diet. Of the following statements about cholesterol which should the nurse know to be true?
    ① It is best to be totally eliminated from the diet
    ② It is a normal component of blood and all body cells
    ③ It is not necessary for normal body functions
    ④ It is found in increased amounts in grain products

31. Assuming that the nurse's first action to control bleeding from a slashed wrist was correct but unsuccessful, the nurse should then:
    ① Apply a tourniquet
    ② Apply direct pressure for an additional 6 minutes
    ③ Apply pressure to the brachial artery
    ④ Apply pressure to the carotid artery

32. A patient with advanced cirrhosis of the liver asks the nurse what type of food he might expect to find limited in his diet. The nurse would be correct if she responded:
    ① Fruits
    ② Vegetables
    ③ Meats
    ④ Grains

33. A patient with a diagnosis of peptic ulcer disease develops symptoms of pain, abdominal distention, and projectile vomiting. The nurse knows these symptoms suggest:
    ① Cholecystitis
    ② Hemorrhage
    ③ Peritonitis
    ④ Obstruction

34. A young male, age 20 years, has been admitted to the hospital with a diagnosis of hepatitis. To plan patient care, the nurse should be aware that the primary mode of transmission by which hepatitis A virus (HAV) is passed is:
    ① Contaminated needles
    ② Blood transfusions
    ③ Fecal-oral route
    ④ Misuse of drugs and chemicals

35. The primary purpose of instituting bed rest for a patient with hepatitis is to:
    ① Rest the liver by reducing the metabolic demands
    ② Control the spread of the disease
    ③ Reduce the risk of developing cardiac problems
    ④ Reduce the risk of hepatic coma

36. The nurse is responsible for making the initial emergency room triage following a bus accident. There are 65 victims who will need assistance. According to the principles of triage, which group of victims will receive medical care last?
    ① Victims with minor injuries
    ② Victims with serious but not life-threatening injuries
    ③ Victims with life-threatening injuries
    ④ Victims with little chance of survival

37. A patient had abdominal surgery to relieve a bowel obstruction caused by adhesions and has a urinary catheter in place. The nurse has been measuring his urinary output hourly. Which of the following findings should the nurse report to the physician?
    ① 30 ml at 7 PM; 26 ml at 8 PM
    ② 40 ml at 7 PM; 35 ml at 8 PM
    ③ 60 ml at 7 PM; 100 ml at 8 PM
    ④ 100 ml at 7 PM; 150 ml at 8 PM

38. A 44-year-old woman had a cholecystectomy yesterday. She now has a temperature of 38° C (99.5° F). Which of the following interventions would be most appropriate when caring for this patient's elevated temperature?
    ① Give patient a tepid bath
    ② Apply cool compresses to patient's forehead
    ③ Administer ibuprofen (Motrin) 400 mg po
    ④ Encourage coughing and deep breathing

39. The primary reason that adverse drug reactions occur frequently in elderly patients is because the elderly have a:
    ① Higher percentage of body water
    ② Higher percentage of lean muscle
    ③ Lower percentage of body fat
    ④ Higher percentage of body fat

40. A patient with Alzheimer's disease is attempting to leave a long-term care facility. The most appropriate intervention for this patient would be to:
    ① Reorient the patient to time, place, and person and then escort the patient back to his or her room
    ② Validate the patient's feelings, but distract the patient with another activity
    ③ Call Security and seek assistance to physically restrain the patient from leaving the facility
    ④ Allow the patient to leave the facility and bring the patient back to the facility when he or she becomes fatigued

41. The physician has just ordered meperidine (Demerol) 75 mg IM for a patient complaining of a migraine headache. Which of the following nursing interventions will minimize the pain of the injection?
    ① Insert the needle quickly
    ② Use an 18-gauge needle
    ③ Insert the needle at a 45° angle
    ④ Use a 2-inch needle

42. A patient has been taking Lasix (furosemide) for many years to help control her congestive heart failure. The nurse is administering the drug when the patient says, "This doesn't look like my pill." Which of the following is the most appropriate response by the nurse?
    ① "It's probably just a different brand."
    ② "It is the same thing, so please take the pill."
    ③ "I'll double check this with the nurse in charge."
    ④ "Let me recheck this before you take it."

43. An elderly patient is hospitalized with a bowel obstruction. He has a nasogastric tube to decompress the gastrointestinal tract. In the last 8 hours, the NG tube has removed 525 cc of green fluid. The patient has a maintenance IV running at 75 ml/hr. The physician has ordered cc for cc fluid replacement for the NG drainage over the next 8 hours. He also ordered to maintain the current base rate. Calculate how fast the IV should run if the tubing delivers 10 gtts/ml:

① 13 gtts/min
② 23 gtts/min
③ 33 gtts/min
④ 43 gtts/min

44. A 38-year-old female has been admitted to the hospital with congestive heart failure. She weighs 320 pounds, is very cyanotic and dyspneic with the exertion of talking and is spitting up frothy pink sputum. The nurse notes she has 15-second periods of apnea while she sleeps. When prioritizing this patient's needs, which of the following nursing diagnoses is most urgent?
① Alteration in nutrition, more than body requirements related to imbalances between caloric intake and energy expenditure
② Low self-esteem related to feelings of self-degradation and the response of others to obesity
③ Activity intolerance related to insufficient oxygen for activities of daily living
④ Fluid volume excess related to venous congestion

45. A 24-year-old mother of two comes to the clinic to obtain birth control information. The nurse tells her that the most reliable method of birth control is:
① Condom use
② Coitus interruptus
③ Oral contraceptives
④ Intrauterine device (IUD)

46. A 28-year-old married female is admitted for SOB, dizziness, and fatigue. The patient is 5 feet tall, weighs 315 pounds, and needs total assist with her bath. The nurse needs to wash and dry thoroughly the many folds of skin to help prevent:
① Intertrigo
② Pemphigus
③ Stasis ulcers
④ Decubitus ulcers

47. When caring for an active yet anxious 75 year old who just had cataract surgery, the nurse needs to include which of the following instructions in her discharge care plan?
① "If you bend over, do so slowly."
② "You can only lift up to 20 pounds."
③ "Avoid any sudden movement of the head."
④ "Wearing dark glasses will not be necessary."

48. The physician orders an injection of iron dextran to be given by Z-track method. The nurse knows that this procedure requires careful attention to technique because:
① It stings the patient more
② It has to go between the dermis and epidermis
③ It is used in adult patients with well-developed muscles
④ Leakage into subcutaneous tissue can cause patient discomfort and staining

49. A nurse is preparing to insert an over-the-needle IV catheter that will be used for the administration of blood. Which of the following intravenous catheter sizes would the nurse choose?
① 18 gauge
② 20 gauge
③ 22 gauge
④ 24 gauge

50. Nurses caring for geriatric patients know that common factors associated with major depression in the elderly include which of the following?
① Adverse effects of medications
② Electrolyte balance
③ Occasional feelings of sadness
④ Nutritional supplements

51. Which of the following individuals would most likely develop rheumatoid arthritis?
① A 40-year-old white woman
② A 15-year-old white boy
③ A 65-year-old Hispanic man
④ A 30-year-old African-American woman

52. A 48-year-old rabbi has just been diagnosed with glomerulonephritis. He states he has never heard of it before and asks you what it is. The nurse's *best* initial reply would be which of the following statements?
① "It is an infectious disease that causes varying symptoms, primarily fatigue."
② "It is sometimes caused by a drug reaction and causes kidney damage."
③ "It is an inherited disease and the cause is unknown. It can cause kidney damage."
④ "It is caused by your immune system's negative reaction to a previous infection."

53. A 70-year-old female has been hospitalized several times in the past year with complications from chemotherapy for metastatic breast cancer. She is placed on an antidepressant medication the day of her discharge. Discharge teaching for the patient should include which of the following:
① Fluids should be limited to three glasses a day while taking the antidepressant
② Call the physician immediately if dry mouth or orthostatic hypotension occurs
③ It may take 3 or more (even up to 12) weeks before symptoms improve
④ If this antidepressant fails to control depression, others won't be effective either

54. It is important that the nurse recognize which of the following as a recommendation made by the FDA and JCAHO about restraints?
① Restraints can be used indefinitely once the need for them has been documented
② Alternatives to restraints should be developed and implemented before using restraints
③ Restraints should be removed every 4 hours to allow for activities of daily living
④ Restraints should be tied with a square knot to the immovable part of the bed

55. An 87-year-old male who has Alzheimer's disease had a herniorrhaphy last night. When assessing this patient for postoperative pain the nurse would:
① Repeat the explanation of a pain rating scale until he understands it
② Ask open-ended questions to elicit the information needed
③ Rephrase questions and speak more loudly until he responds
④ Be aware of nonverbal behavior suggestive of pain

56. A 31-year-old female has had multiple sclerosis for 5 years. She tells the nurse she feels worthless and "wants to do everyone a favor by checking out." The best approach for the nurse to take would be to:
   ① Ignore what she said and change the subject
   ② Arrange for her to speak with a social worker
   ③ Use therapeutic communication techniques to explore what she means
   ④ Be sure to avoid asking her if she has a specific plan

57. Nurse Practice Acts are passed by state legislatures to:
   ① Accredit nursing programs
   ② Define legal standards of nursing
   ③ Ensure minimal safety performance of nurses
   ④ Set ethical standards for nurses

58. A 67-year-old male is admitted to the hospital with neurogenic atony of the bladder with urinary retention. The nurse knows that an effective acetylcholine derivative useful in managing nonobstructive urinary retention is known as:
   ① Mestinon
   ② Urecholine
   ③ Pilocarpine
   ④ Pro-Banthine

59. A patient is being admitted to the cardiac unit with ventricular arrhythmias. The nurse knows that the drug of choice for this condition is:
   ① Inderal
   ② Digoxin
   ③ Lidocaine
   ④ Morphine sulfate

60. A patient who is an alcoholic is to be started on Antabuse (disulfiram). The nurse knows that this drug, used to reinforce abstinence, can cause:
   ① Acne
   ② High-level energy
   ③ A sugar taste to foods
   ④ Insomnia and nightmares

61. An elderly patient who is going to have GI testing done has hematuria. The nurse needs to take a complete medication history because this condition can be caused by:
   ① Diuretics
   ② Pyridium
   ③ Macrodantin
   ④ Anticoagulants

62. A patient is admitted to a medical-surgical unit for observation of injuries sustained in a car accident. He was given a citation for DWI (driving while intoxicated). The nurse knows that about 7% of alcoholics are on Skid Row. The remaining 93% are found:
   ① In blue collar jobs
   ② In white collar jobs
   ③ In upper class society
   ④ In every level of society

63. When caring for a patient who has just returned to the floor after having a cystoscopy, the nurse should instruct him to:
   ① Eat a soft diet for 2 days
   ② Decrease his fluid intake for 2 days
   ③ Take a warm sitz bath for discomfort
   ④ Decrease his fluid intake for 24 hours

64. A 25-year-old female was admitted to the hospital where she underwent an emergency appendectomy, during which it was discovered that appendix had become gangrenous. The nurse knows that the organism that causes gas gangrene is:
   ① E. coli
   ② Salmonella
   ③ Clostridium botulinum
   ④ Clostridium perfringens

65. Carefully examining a patient's urine specimen can give the nurse an important clue as to any underlying problems. Urine that shows a possible bacterial infection, vegetarian diet, or a glomerular nephritis appears:
   ① Cloudy
   ② Dark amber color
   ③ Green-green color
   ④ Red or brown color

66. When the nurse enters the patient's room, she finds a 22-year-old male with cystic fibrosis very short of breath. The first step the nurse should take is to:
   ① Take vital signs
   ② Call for help immediately
   ③ Raise the head of the bed
   ④ Obtain a brief health history

67. While the nurse is visiting a patient's home, the wife of a diabetic elderly man tells the nurse that he has been "crankier than usual" the last few days. He is also "moody and hungry as a horse." Which of the next following statements tells the nurse that she needs to check his blood sugar?
   ① He refuses to take a bath and stinks
   ② He has had a cough the last 3 or 4 days
   ③ He had diarrhea once last week in the middle of the night
   ④ He has been in the bathroom off and on all morning urinating

68. The nurse is teaching a 20-year-old male, who has been diagnosed with renal disease, about diet planning. The nurse knows that the patient with a chronic renal disease will possibly have potassium and phosphorus restricted, as well as sodium and:
   ① Fats
   ② Calcium
   ③ Protein
   ④ Carbohydrates

69. An elderly patient comes into the emergency room complaining of pain and nausea and vomits 15 minutes after admission. The nurse suspects he has a gastric outlet obstruction possibly from a gastric tumor or ulcer. What did the nurse observe in the emesis?
   ① Blood
   ② Bright red blood
   ③ Undigested food
   ④ Brown vomitus with fecal odor

70. Persons who have had sexual contact with someone who has AIDS will be tested for the AIDS virus. The nurse lessens their anxiety by explaining:
   ① AIDS is rarely transmitted in monogamous relationships
   ② Infection with HIV does not always result in the AIDS disease

③ Many people have a natural immunity to AIDS

④ Measures can be taken to prevent the disease in someone recently exposed to the virus

71. When caring for a patient who has just completed an electroconvulsive therapy treatment, an important nursing action is to:
① Obtain consent
② Give a complete bed bath
③ Keep accurate input and output data
④ Provide patient with orienting data on awakening because memory may be disturbed

72. An elderly patient who has a diagnosis of chronic brain syndrome approaches the nurse's station and says to the nurse, "Could you please show me where I can get the bus home to Poughkeepsie?" Which response by the nurse would be most therapeutic?
① "Go straight down the hall and turn right."
② "Do you have money for the bus?"
③ "The last bus to Poughkeepsie left 10 minutes ago; you'll have to come back tomorrow."
④ "You don't live in Poughkeepsie anymore, Mr. Z. You live here with us in New York City."

73. A staff nurse on the psychiatric unit insists that her patient be up and bathed by 9 AM. The patient has difficulty complying, saying that she becomes flustered and nervous. This violates which of the following principles?
① Be aware of your own resources and limitations
② Respect the patient as a person; take time to listen to what is being said
③ Be honest
④ Help reduce anxiety by making few demands on the patient

74. A 62-year-old male was admitted 2 days ago with a diagnosis of CVA. His wife tells you, "Every time I go into the room he cries. I am afraid I have done something to upset him." The best response is:
① "He is trying to get your sympathy. You must ignore the crying and talk about other things."
② "He has no control over his crying. It is a symptom of his illness and does not mean that he is unhappy."
③ "He needs some time alone to sort out his feelings. You should consider staying away for a few days."
④ "He might benefit from a psychiatric consultation. Perhaps you could talk to your physician."

75. It is important for the nurse to know that a deprivation particular to the elderly is:
① Nutritional diet
② Touch
③ Intellectual stimulation
④ Olfaction

76. A supportive nurse must recognize that a patient's first reaction to a diagnosis of AIDS will be:
① Anger
② Bargaining
③ Denial
④ Depression

77. According to the theorist Erik Erikson, the first stage of development is focused on:
① Autonomy vs. shame and doubt
② Pleasure principle
③ Anal gratification
④ Trust vs. mistrust

78. A patient needs to see her dentist, but is very frightened. She finally makes an appointment and writes it in her calendar. On the day of the appointment, she looks at the wrong day in her calendar and misses the appointment. This is an example of:
① Repression
② Projection
③ Displacement
④ Rationalization

79. A nurse interacts with a patient who persistently moves his leg in a tapping motion. The psychiatric principle that applies here is:
① Be honest
② The nurse-patient relationship is professional and realistic
③ The staff is viewed as role models
④ There is a reason for all behavior

80. An 84-year-old patient is a former WW II veteran who is experiencing extreme disorientation and agitation. A *priority* intervention for the nurse to implement is which of the following?
① Let the patient make his own care decisions
② Ask the physician for a temporary restraint order
③ Keep orienting the patient to time, place, and person
④ Limit the staff that is caring and talking with the patient

81. A 52-year-old male is admitted for chronic alcoholism. His family tells the nurse that he now has had several episodes of short-term memory loss, is unable to learn new skills, and cannot hold a job because of these problems. The nurse recognizes this as:
① Addiction
② Habituation
③ Korasakoff's psychosis
④ Wernicke's encephalopathy

82. A patient on the mental health unit exhibits involuntary serpentine movements of the face, trunk, and extremities. This individual has been taking Thorazine for 6 years. Which of the following conditions is this individual exhibiting?
① Cowling's rule
② Chvostek's sign
③ Tardive dyskinesia
④ Sjögren's syndrome

83. A 26-year-old woman is admitted for AIDS-related *Pneumocystis carinii* pneumonia and dehydration. She states to the nurse that she feels depressed and is afraid of dying. The best therapeutic response for the nurse to make is:
① "You are afraid of dying?"
② "Does your family know how you feel?"
③ "Would you like me to call your pastor or priest?"
④ "Depression is sometimes repressed anger. Talking about it will help you feel better."

84. An 81-year-old male was admitted to the geriatric ward for diagnostic testing. His wife complained that his memory was becoming a problem. A sample question the nurse can ask to determine long-term memory loss is:
① "What is your age?"
② "What kind of work did you do?"
③ "What did you do last night?"
④ "What state are you and your wife living in?"

85. Following a normal delivery of a fine, healthy little girl weighing 8 lb (3600 g), the parents first touch the child with their fingertips, then palm, then have body contact. The baby receives routine delivery room care followed by routine nursery care. It is important that the parents get to hold their newborn:
    ① Within 24 hours
    ② After the first hour
    ③ As soon as possible
    ④ After the baby is weighed

86. One important complication to avoid following a cesarean section is a pelvic thrombosis. The nursing care plan would therefore include:
    ① Teaching good perineal care
    ② Encouraging early ambulation
    ③ Splinting the lower abdomen when coughing
    ④ Keeping the urinary and bowel tracts emptied by forcing fluids and offering stool softeners

87. If the amniotic sac is to be ruptured by the physician, what is the priority nursing responsibility?
    ① Time and check contractions afterward and report
    ② Note time and instrument used and check FHT after procedure
    ③ Note amount and characteristics of fluid, test with nitrazine, and report
    ④ Note time and amount and place pad on perineum

88. Four days before the EDC a patient's bag of waters ruptured spontaneously at 3:45 AM. Because she had a physician's appointment at 9 AM and did not experience any contractions, she kept the appointment. In the office she had several contractions 6 to 7 minutes apart. She was 65% effaced and 2 cm dilated. She was hospitalized, prepped, and placed on a fetal monitor. FHT are 146, strong, and regular. Strong contractions occur every 2 to 3 minutes. She is hungry and asks for lunch. The most appropriate response by the nurse would be:
    ① "I will make you some lunch if you will wait a few minutes."
    ② "You cannot eat anything, but I will ask the physician if I should start parenteral fluids."
    ③ "Nothing by mouth, sorry."
    ④ "Because you are in active labor, our policy is only liquids you can see through; however, perhaps you would prefer ice chips?"

89. A patient's last menstrual period, which lasted 5 days, began April 24. Using Nägele's rule, when would her EDC (estimated date of confinement) be?
    ① January 17
    ② March 3
    ③ February 17
    ④ January 31

90. A patient is pregnant for the second time and has a 4 year old at home. She would be considered a:
    ① Gravida I para 0
    ② Gravida II para I
    ③ Gravida I para I
    ④ Gravida II para II

91. A young couple, ages 26 and 28 years, respectively, have decided to have their second baby. Their first child is 4 years old. The wife has been on norethynodrel (Enovid) for the past several years; however, after deciding to expand their family, she stopped taking her Enovid and has been trying to conceive. She has not been successful. The probable cause for the delay in conception may be that:
    ① They are too old; especially the wife at 26
    ② It takes time for some individuals to adapt to the normal menstrual cycle after being on oral contraceptives
    ③ They are both anxious to have another child and are therefore anxious and tense
    ④ Four years is a long time to wait between babies, so the body does not respond quickly

92. Nurses working in the labor and delivery room should be familiar with the AIDS protective procedures outlined by the Centers for Disease Control and Prevention. What precautions would the nurse implement when caring for an active labor patient with a diagnosis of AIDS?
    ① Mask and gloves with blood and body fluid precautions for caring for the newborn and the mother
    ② Gloves with blood and body fluid precautions for caring for the mother and baby
    ③ Gown, mask, and gloves with blood and body fluid precautions during labor and delivery
    ④ Reverse isolation techniques when caring for AIDS-infected patients

93. A patient contracted AIDS from sharing contaminated needles with her husband. They have one 15-month-old child, whom her mother is caring for. She has just discovered that she is 5 months pregnant. To guide and help this patient and her husband, what is important for the nurse to know about AIDS?
    ① It is a highly contagious disease so patients must be isolated
    ② It is likely that her unborn child will be infected with the HIV virus and may have a shortened life expectancy
    ③ It is unlikely that her unborn child will be infected and may expect to enjoy a normal life
    ④ Read all you can about the etiology of the disease

94. In the prenatal clinic the nurse observes a patient being examined by the physician. He says, "Hmm, your uterus is at the level of your umbilicus." After the examination, the patient asks what the physician meant by that statement. The nurse's best answer would be:
    ① "It means you have just passed your first trimester of the pregnancy."
    ② "You are approximately in your sixth month of pregnancy."
    ③ "You should be feeling your baby drop soon."
    ④ "You are about 6 weeks from delivery now."

95. A mother is concerned about her 19-year-old pregnant daughter, who has a history of crack-cocaine abuse and who she suspects may be using again. The nurse knows that babies born to crack-cocaine users are born with signs of lethargy, have hypersensitivity to noises or stimuli, have diarrhea, and cannot focus visually. Crack-cocaine use also brings about dangerous changes in the mother's:
    ① Pulse
    ② Temperature
    ③ Respirations
    ④ Blood pressure

96. A 16 year old is pregnant and unmarried. The nurse knows that one of the concerns in dealing with adolescent pregnancies is that adolescents:
    ① Have limited life experiences to draw on
    ② Quickly accept the reality of their pregnancy
    ③ Are eager and ready to accept their pregnancy
    ④ Tend to seek early care the minute they suspect that they may be pregnant

97. A 22-year-old Gravida I Para 0 has gone three weeks over her expected delivery date. She is admitted to the obstetrical floor and an IV oxytocin drip is started. The nurse will need to pay special attention to:
    ① Monitoring intake
    ② The mother's nausea
    ③ Monitoring of the mother's vital signs
    ④ Monitoring contractions and FHTs.

98. An individual with sickle cell disease marries an individual with sickle cell trait. What percentage of their children will have sickle cell disease?
    ① 25%
    ② 50%
    ③ 75%
    ④ 100%

99. While the nurse is teaching a group of single, pregnant teenage mothers about nutritional problems of pregnancy one of the young mothers states that fat intake is only a problem if you eat a lot of meat. The nurse tells the group about other sources of fat that are "hidden" in such foods as:
    ① Tuna, banana, grapes, melons
    ② Apples, oranges, skim milk, rice
    ③ Creamed cottage cheese, ice cream, cashew nuts, chocolate
    ④ English muffins, water packed tuna, uncreamed cottage cheese

100. A nurse observing a 2-day-old, full-term infant girl in the nursery notices that her hands and feet are cyanotic but that her body and cheeks are pink. She has passed greenish black stool and has lost several ounces since birth. This baby is:
    ① Premature
    ② Immature
    ③ Normal
    ④ Slightly abnormal

101. A 9 year old was admitted to the hospital in sickle-cell anemia crisis. Symptoms of sickle-cell crisis include all of the following *except:*
    ① Severe abdominal pain
    ② Elevated temperature
    ③ Joint pain
    ④ Elevated hemoglobin

102. A pneumoencephalogram is ordered for a patient. The nurse explains that this procedure includes having x-ray films taken:
    ① And there will be no discomfort
    ② After an injection of dye into an artery
    ③ After an injection of a radioisotope
    ④ After an injection of air via a lumbar puncture

103. A 15-year-old boy who was recently fitted with a full back brace asks the nurse, "May I leave this brace off for school parties?" The nurse's best response would be:
    ① "Every now and then as long as your back doesn't bother you."
    ② "Your brace shouldn't be off at all, only when bathing."
    ③ "It is most important for you to have it on when taking long walks."
    ④ "After a couple of weeks you should be able to wean yourself from the brace."

104. Erikson's theory of child development is based on:
    ① The child's psychosexual development
    ② Intellectual (cognitive) development
    ③ Psychosocial development as a series of developmental tasks
    ④ The child's sensorimotor development

105. A nurse is working in the newborn nursery when a baby that one of his colleagues is feeding begins to choke on the formula. Immediately he assesses the situation and begins the procedure for obstructed airway on a *conscious infant.* To perform the procedure correctly, the nurse knows that he has to administer:
    ① Eight back blows and eight chest thrusts
    ② Six back blows and six chest thrusts
    ③ Five back blows and five chest thrusts
    ④ Four back blows and four chest thrusts

106. On arrival at the emergency room, the 3-year-old burn patient is semiconscious, whining, and calling for his mother. Once he has been transferred to the trauma room, the nurse begins to obtain baseline data—radial pulse rate, 160 beats/min; respirations, 32/min; and BP, 60/30. Based on the initial data, the nurse would report vital signs to the physician and assist as ordered in initiation of:
    ① Removal of clothing
    ② Central venous line
    ③ IV fluids
    ④ Antibiotics

107. Immediate physical observations of a burn patient would most importantly include:
    ① Physical development
    ② Head circumference
    ③ Height and weight
    ④ Quality of respirations

108. Normally preschoolers have little interest in eating and the anorexia associated with burns presents a problem of nutrition. A 3-year-old patient, whose parents have recently died, would most likely eat better if:
    ① Other children ate with him
    ② His grandmother ate with him
    ③ You fed him
    ④ Tube feedings were given when he did not eat

109. To help a 4-year-old boy adjust to the newborn baby, the parents should be taught to:
    ① Make a plan to have him do simple chores around the house to increase his self-esteem and growing independence
    ② Buy him lots of presents too, since obviously the newborn will be getting presents
    ③ Make him cuddle and kiss the baby to teach him the concept of love
    ④ Include him in the care of the baby and plan to spend some time with him alone

110. Assessment of a child with acute glomerulonephritis would include assessing for:
    ① Pyuria, oliguria, and hypotension
    ② Hematuria, hypotension, and headaches
    ③ Polyuria, tachycardia, and hypertension
    ④ Orbital edema, hypertension, and albuminuria

111. A nurse observes that a patient has sustained a contusion to the left eye from a recent fall. The *initial* nursing intervention should be to:
    ① Apply a sterile patch immediately
    ② Apply an ice pack immediately
    ③ Apply warm compresses immediately
    ④ Irrigate the eye with saline solution

112. Your son is out in the yard with his 10-year-old friend practicing for the Little League game. His friend runs into the house and tells you, a nurse, that your son is hurt and to come quick. Your *priority* action should be to:
    ① Call EMS immediately, then bring him into the house
    ② Tell the friend to stay in the house and go outside to your son
    ③ Take the friend with you and go outside to attend to your son
    ④ Send his friend outside to stay with your son while you call EMS

113. A 14-year-old girl had a spina bifida repaired at birth. She has since developed a marked scoliosis and is now admitted to the hospital for spinal fusion and instrumentation. During her admission procedure the primary goal is to provide:
    ① Privacy
    ② Orientation to ward
    ③ Her mother's presence
    ④ Introduction to her roommates

114. An infant's mother wishes to bathe her baby before surgery. While caring for her baby, the nurse should:
    ① Support the mother emotionally
    ② Clean the utility room
    ③ Take a break
    ④ Prepare chart for the OR

115. A 4-week-old infant is admitted to the unit for a cleft lip repair. He has a bilateral cleft lip and palate. His mother states that he has been a problem to feed and that she has found an Asepto syringe to be best. She says the baby has had the sniffles. His vital signs are temperature, 100.8° F (38.2° C); pulse rate, 90 beats/min; respirations, 36/min; BP, 70/35. The nurse should know that a common complication in children with his diagnosis is:
    ① UTI
    ② URI
    ③ PID
    ④ SOB

116. A 14 year old is a newly diagnosed diabetic. He is just beginning to learn how to give himself injections. He asks the nurse why only certain areas of the body can be used for injections. The nurse answers that in giving insulin injections it is necessary to use:
    ① Muscle tissue
    ② Adipose tissue
    ③ Subcutaneous layer
    ④ Right under the epidermis layer

117. A 19-year-old college student tells the school nurse that she has been having headaches at the back of the head. When asked what she does for them she states that aspirin or Tylenol helps to relieve the pain. The nurse knows that the headache may be caused by:
    ① A brain tumor
    ② Hypertension
    ③ Migraine vascular headaches
    ④ Muscle contractions or tension

118. A foreign exchange student from Egypt visits the school clinic with complaints of nausea and fatigue. The nurse determines there is a need to check for jaundice. She should do this by examining:
    ① Sclera
    ② Overall skin color
    ③ The outer ears and back of neck
    ④ The tongue and inside of the buccal area

119. A 16-year-old student asks the nurse teaching her health class how one would recognize Kaposi's sarcoma. The nurse answers that Kaposi's sarcoma:
    ① First appears as raised purple papules
    ② Begins as hard, raised, and painless nodules
    ③ Begins as lesions that first occur on the upper face of a person and are papules that erode in the center
    ④ Consists of moles that become darker and then begin to spread over the body; the moles are also referred to as pigmented nevi

120. A 15 year old who is trying to lose weight tells the nurse that her friends suggested OTC pep pills (amphetamines) to help her lose weight. She states that they help reduce the appetite. She asks the nurse if this would work for her. The nurse answers that she should avoid them because their effectiveness is short-lived, they can cause nervousness and insomnia, and they can become habit forming. In addition to caffeine and artificial sweeteners, pep pills also contain:
    ① Alcohol
    ② Diuretics
    ③ Laxatives
    ④ Phenylpropanolamine

121. A 12 year old has suffered head trauma from a serious car accident. The pituitary was damaged causing diabetes insipidus, resulting in high urinary output and excessive thirst. The nurse knows that the name of the hormone that is produced by the pituitary gland, which causes the nephrons in the kidneys to reabsorb water is:
    ① Albumin
    ② Aldosterone
    ③ Vasopressin
    ④ Parahormone

122. An 18 year old, recently diagnosed with kidney failure, asks the nurse if he can use salt substitutes because he salts everything. The nurse answers:
    ① "No, it is not safe."
    ② "No, salt substitutes have phosphorus."
    ③ "Yes, it is safe if you drink water with it."
    ④ "Yes, if you limit its use and don't go overboard."

123. A 2-month-old infant is diagnosed with an ear infection. While showing the proper method of administering ear drops to the mother, the nurse needs to place the infant on his:

① Back, and pull the ear auricle up and back
② Side, and pull the ear auricle down and back
③ Back, and place the drops into his lower ear canal
④ Side, and place the drops straight into his ear, one at a time

124. A young mother of a 1-month-old infant comes to the clinic for a well-baby checkup. She tells the nurse that the baby takes formula well, but spits a lot of it up and is very messy. The best response is for the nurse to say:
① "You need to check the nipples you are using."
② "Don't worry. This is normal for new babies."
③ "Try not to feed her so fast as she may be swallowing air."
④ "Can you estimate about how much of the formula that you are using she actually spits up?"

125. A new mother asks the nurse at what age is it best to hang a new, colorful mobile for her newborn baby boy. The nurse can answer that newborns can follow bright and colorful objects at:
① One year of age
② First week of life
③ 9 to 10 months of life
④ Two or three weeks of life

COMPREHENSIVE EXAMINATION 2: PART 1

This examination contains individual questions, each containing a relevant clinical situation. Read all questions carefully. There is only *one best answer* for each question.

Test time allotment (Part 1): approximately 2 hours

Answers and rationales begin on p. 569

1. A patient asks the nurse if her lochia will be heavier because of her cesarean section. The most appropriate answer would be:
   ① "Lochia after a cesarean section will be bright red longer and will be more copious than after a vaginal delivery."
   ② "The characteristics will be the same except that the flow will be for a longer duration than the flow after vaginal delivery."
   ③ "The amount, duration, and characteristics of the lochia are the same for a cesarean section as for a vaginal delivery."
   ④ "The flow will be of a much shorter duration because the vaginal tract was not used."

2. A patient is in transition. What are the major signs and symptoms that will confirm she is indeed at that stage?
   ① Desire to push, slight bloody show, veins in neck bulging, 6 cm dilated
   ② Legs shaky, feels slightly nauseated, strong contractions, mood change, 8 cm dilated, needs reassurance, guidance
   ③ Pressure on perineum, 10 cm, grunting, needs guidance, direction
   ④ Titanic, pauseless contractions; use comfort measures, rub back, guide breathing; start oxytocin (Pitocin)

3. During a patient's tenth week of pregnancy, while the nurse is weighing and taking her vital signs, the patient expresses concern regarding weight gain related to her pregnancy. The *most appropriate* response by the nurse to the patient's concern would be to explain that during pregnancy:
   ① Weight gain should not exceed 22 pounds
   ② Proper nutrition is more important than the actual number of pounds gained
   ③ Caloric intake need not be restricted because metabolic needs increase
   ④ Only individuals who are greatly overweight need to be concerned about excessive weight gain

4. A pregnant patient delivers quickly and without complications. The patient's husband arrives and is taken to the recovery room to see his wife. After visiting with her for a while, he asks to see the baby. It would be *best* for the nurse to suggest that:
   ① He go to the nursery to see the baby and let his wife sleep
   ② He visit with his wife for a while, then go home and see both his wife and the baby the next morning
   ③ The baby can be brought to the parents so they can begin the attachment process
   ④ Both parents go to the nursery to see the baby

5. When caring for a newly delivered infant, the nurse administers antibiotic ointment or silver nitrate eye drops to prevent blindness, which may occur as a result of maternal exposure to:
   ① Herpes type II
   ② Gonococcus
   ③ Syphilis
   ④ Cytomegalovirus

6. A patient has just delivered her third child, a healthy 10-pound (4500 g) baby boy. The baby's Apgar score was 9/9. Because of the baby's birth weight, the nurse should anticipate that the patient will have tests to rule out:
   ① Cardiac problems
   ② Hypothyroidism
   ③ Diabetes mellitus
   ④ Cushing's syndrome

7. A newborn's breasts appear to be enlarged. During a physical assessment of this infant, the nurse knows this to be:
   ① Normal because of fat deposits due to the weight of the baby
   ② Abnormal because the infant is a male
   ③ A normal response to hormones transferred from the mother through the placenta
   ④ Abnormal and probably related to an endocrine disorder

8. A patient whose baby was delivered by cesarean section asks the nurse why her baby has to stay in the Isolette when other babies in the nursery, who are smaller, are not in an Isolette. The *most appropriate* response by the nurse would be:
   ① "Babies delivered by cesarean section are more likely to become chilled because they were removed from the uterus more suddenly."
   ② "Babies delivered by cesarean section may experience difficulty in breathing and are observed closely as a precaution."
   ③ "Babies delivered by cesarean section have a greater incidence of nervous system disorders and must be watched closely for symptoms."
   ④ "Babies delivered by cesarean section are always immature and therefore require special nursing attention."

9. One complication that is more common in cesarean section deliveries is ileus with abdominal distention. To reduce the likelihood of this, the nursing care plan for a patient who has had a cesarean section should include:
   ① A well-balanced diet with adequate bulk
   ② Splinting of the abdomen when deep breathing and coughing
   ③ Early ambulation
   ④ Kegel exercises

10. A young female patient comes to the clinic stating that she has missed a menstrual period. During her visit she tells the nurse that her last menstrual cycle was normal with a moderate amount of flow. It began on February 5th and ended February 11th. Using Nägele's rule, the nurse is able to calculate that her EDC (estimated date of confinement) would be:
    ① November 18th
    ② November 12th
    ③ November 4th
    ④ October 29th

11. Following initial emergency nursing intervention for a child who has sustained an eye injury, the next priority would be to:
    ① Have the patient lie down in a darkened room
    ② Take the patient to the local emergency room

③ Call your pediatrician for the name of an optician
④ Monitor the patient's level of consciousness

12. A 4-year-old boy has become a "picky eater," a fact that is a constant concern to his mother. What might be suggested as acceptable ways to increase the nutritional content of his diet?
① Large servings that make him feel older
② Coaxing him to eat by offering after-dinner rewards
③ Offering "finger foods" such as celery sticks with peanut butter as snacks
④ Making sure that he finishes everything on his plate

13. While obtaining a throat culture, the structure to *avoid* touching with the swab is the:
① Nasal turbinate
② Posterior pharynx
③ Tonsil
④ Uvula

14. Your 17-year-old patient has just received the diagnosis of chickenpox. You should place your patient in which category-specific isolation?
① Drainage/secretion
② Respiratory
③ Strict
④ Universal blood and body fluid

15. A patient returns to her room from the ICU where she was nursed for 24 hours postoperatively. She is allowed to eat but must have a high-protein intake. Which of these foods is highest in protein content?
① Dried beans and peas
② Eggs and cheese
③ Fresh vegetables
④ Cooked cereals

16. A mother states that her 3-week-old infant has not been taking his formula well and is listless and unresponsive when she holds and cuddles him. He has lost 5 oz since birth. He is otherwise healthy and has no congenital defects. The pediatrician diagnoses the infant's condition as:
① Celiac disease
② Failure to thrive
③ Hirschsprung's disease
④ Pyloric stenosis

17. A nurse is on her way to work at a nearby hospital when she spots a child lying on the side of the road. No one appears to be nearby. She calls out for help and proceeds to assess the child, who appears to be about 6 years old. The nurse determines that the child is unresponsive, is not breathing, and does not have a pulse. She then proceeds to:
① Perform one minute of cardiopulmonary resuscitation (CPR) only
② Activate the emergency medical system (EMS) only
③ Perform one minute of CPR, then activate the EMS
④ Activate the EMS, then perform one minute of CPR

18. The care plan for a 42-year-old patient with asthma indicates he has orthopnea; appropriate nursing intervention will include:
① Keeping the bed in the high-Fowler's position
② Maintaining oxygen at 40% by Venturi mask
③ Taking vital signs q2h
④ Using log-rolling technique to turn him to his side

19. On return from the recovery room your infant patient (4 weeks old) appears to be hungry. The order reads, "Return to diet for age when fully awake." What would you give the infant first?
① Formula
② Cereal
③ Fruit
④ Water

20. A 6 week old is admitted for surgical repair of a cleft lip. Vital signs are temperature, 100.8° F (38.2° C); pulse rate, 90 beats/min; respirations, 36/min; BP, 70/35. Which vital sign is abnormal and what would you do about it?
① Respirations: call anesthesia
② Pulse rate: notify anesthesia
③ Temperature: notify admitting physician
④ Blood pressure: notify admitting physician

21. A 4-year-old boy was accidentally shot with a BB gun. His older brother was shooting the gun at an old metal clothesline pole and a BB hit the patient in the right eye. The physician gave the order to prepare the child for emergency surgery as he could not save the eye. The nurse knows that the term for surgical removal of an eye is:
① Enucleation
② Electrodiathermy
③ Scleral buckling
④ Phacoemulsification

22. A 2-day-old infant is jaundiced and phototherapy is ordered by the physician. The nurse needs to:
① Put the diaper and clothes on loosely
② Assess the axillary temperature at least every 4 hours
③ Turn the baby's head so the eyes are away from the phototherapy light
④ Avoid exposure of the skin temperature probe to the phototherapy lights

23. A 16-year-old patient tells the nurse that every time he has an antibiotic IM injection, it is "extremely" painful. One thing the nurse can consider doing is:
① Tell him to relax and it won't hurt as much
② Tell him that it will only hurt a minute or so
③ Numb the area with ice after cleaning the site
④ Numb the area before cleaning it by holding ice on it for several seconds

24. A 4-year-old patient needs an antibiotic IM given that was ordered by the physician for a major inner ear infection. The best thing for the nurse to say to the patient before giving the injection is:
① "I have to give you an injection."
② "I have to give you a 'little shot.'"
③ "I need to put some medicine under your skin."
④ "I have to give you a shot that may sting a little bit."

25. An 18-year-old patient had a full body cast applied 3 days ago. He is complaining he feels "full" and his cast is too tight. The patient is also complaining of nausea and abdominal discomfort. The nurse recognizes that the patient is most likely experiencing:
① Pneumonia
② A claustrophobic reaction
③ An anxiety reaction
④ Decreased intestinal motility

26. A 16-year-old girl broke her left forearm during a roller-blading accident 6 weeks ago. She has had the left arm casted the entire time. She returned to the doctor with complaints of continued discomfort in her arm. The physician orders an x-ray because the patient may have:
    ① Developed compartment syndrome
    ② Developed thrombophlebitis
    ③ Experienced a new fracture
    ④ Experienced a delayed union

27. A 17 year old fell while horseback riding, fracturing her left radius. The physician applied a short-arm plaster cast. Which of the following instructions on cast care should the nurse include when discharge teaching?
    ① Elevate the fingers above the level of the heart
    ② Keep the cast clean by wrapping it in plastic
    ③ If itching begins, insert a flat object, such as a ruler, to scratch
    ④ After the cast hardens, you may shower

28. A newborn baby has been diagnosed with phenylketonuria. As the child begins to eat solid food, which of the following foods will the family need to be taught to restrict in the child's diet?
    ① Bread
    ② Tomato
    ③ Chicken
    ④ Asparagus

29. A 10-year-old male has been diagnosed with bacterial conjunctivitis and is being treated with polymyxin B sulfate (Polysporin Ophthalmic) ointment. The nurse is reinforcing home care instructions. Which of the following activities should the nurse include in her instructions?
    ① Irrigate the eye with boric acid solution before each dose of medication
    ② Massage eyes to enhance blood flow before instilling medication
    ③ Keep personal washcloth and towel separate from those of others in the household
    ④ Wipe secretions from the lateral to medial canthus with a disposable tissue

30. A 2 year old has just been diagnosed with cystic fibrosis (CF) and is being placed on pancrelipase (Pancrease). The nurse is reinforcing teaching about administration of the drug. Which of the following statements by the mother indicates she understands how to administer the drug?
    ① "I will give the medicine every 4 hours during the day and at bedtime."
    ② "I will give the medicine with every meal and with snacks."
    ③ "I will give the medicine only when I notice my child is having more stools."
    ④ "I will give the medicine 2 hours after each meal."

31. A mother, who is also 2 months' pregnant, brings her child to the clinic with a temperature of 100.5° and a rash. She is concerned that her child has a communicable disease that may affect her unborn child. Which of the following can the nurse tell the mother has been identified as having harmful effects on a fetus during the first trimester of pregnancy?
    ① Roseola
    ② Rubeola
    ③ Rubella
    ④ Varicella

32. A 16 year old has just been diagnosed with diabetes mellitus. When planning care for this patient, the nurse must take into consideration that management of diabetes mellitus is most difficult during which of the following developmental stages?
    ① Toddler
    ② Preschool child
    ③ School-age child
    ④ Adolescent

33. An 18-year-old patient needs to have a nasogastric tube inserted to aid in the treatment of a small bowel obstruction. The patient states he is very afraid the procedure will hurt. Which of the following would be the most appropriate statement for the nurse to make to help decrease the patient's anxiety?
    ① "Breathe deeply and relax. It'll be over soon."
    ② "This is a simple procedure and will be over soon."
    ③ "You may feel pressure and be uncomfortable, but it shouldn't hurt."
    ④ "You will be sedated before the tube is inserted."

34. A popular 14-year-old female has just been diagnosed as having an extensive case of acne vulgaris and is concerned about her appearance. She asks the nurse why this happened. The nurse's *most appropriate* response should be:
    ① "It is caused primarily by overactivity of the sebaceous glands."
    ② "It is caused by overactivity of the sex glands during the adolescent period."
    ③ "It is caused by overactivity of the apocrine glands."
    ④ "It is caused by overactivity of bacterial growth on the skin."

35. A 12-year-old boy has a serious allergy to bee stings. Epinephrine is prescribed by his physician for possible anaphylaxis and instructions are given to the patient and his family. Which of the following responses indicate they understand these instructions?
    ① "He must avoid bees and beehives."
    ② "Epinephrine acts by stimulating alpha and beta adrenergic receptors within the sympathetic nervous system."
    ③ "He must always find a parent or another adult to give the injection if needed."
    ④ "Epinephrine has an expiration date on the carton."

36. A 14-month-old has been brought to the emergency room by his mother, who tells the nurse that her son has had a fever of 103° F for the past 2 days. She also states that the child has been very irritable, has had diarrhea, and has had very little urine output. The child is admitted with moderate dehydration and a diagnosis of infectious diarrhea. IV therapy and monitoring of fluids is ordered. As rehydration occurs, the child is given oral feedings of an electrolyte solution. When caring for this child during the latter stage of the rehydration process it is important that the nurse:
    ① Force fluids
    ② Allow the child to drink ad lib
    ③ Monitor intake and output
    ④ Monitor the child's ability to retain fluids

37. A 14 year old is admitted to the pediatric unit with a diagnosis of leukemia. He is pale, lethargic, and withdrawn. The most important and essential nursing measure that the nurse must provide when caring for this patient while he receives chemotherapy is:

① Monitoring for nausea and vomiting
② Performing good handwashing before care
③ Offering emotional support
④ Positioning for comfort

38. A hip spica cast was applied to a 5 year old 2 hours ago. The nurse is assisting with care plan development. Which of the following activities is appropriate for the plan?
① Turning the child every 4 hours
② Drying the cast with a hair dryer
③ Checking the movement and sensation of toes
④ Ambulating the child 3 times per day

39. The nurse is assisting in developing the care plan for relieving symptoms in an infant with colic. Which of the following activities should be included in the plan?
① Apply warmth to the abdominal area
② Schedule feedings every 4 hours
③ Elevate the head of the bed after meals
④ Add rice cereal to the formula with each bottle

40. A 5 year old has been receiving Aminophylline (theophylline ethylenediamine) for asthma. Which of the following signs and symptoms should the nurse expect to observe if the medication is effective?
① Decreased wheezing
② Decreased oxygen saturation
③ Prolonged period of expiration
④ Decreased secretions

41. Awakening in the recovery room following a right-sided mastectomy the patient grabs at the operative site and moans, "It's gone. It's all over." She pleads with the nurse to "let me die." Even though the patient was prepared by the surgeon for the possible removal of her breast, the nurse must be aware that it is common to react with anger, withdrawal, depression, or other emotions. The next day when the patient cries during her morning care, the nurse should say:
① "Don't cry. You're not going to help yourself by doing this."
② "Go ahead and cry. Get it all out. You'll feel better afterward."
③ "It must be very upsetting for you right now. Let me get your husband."
④ "It must be very upsetting for you right now. Would you like me to stay with you awhile?"

42. A 22-year-old woman has a medical diagnosis of anorexia nervosa. One element of her care plan would include:
① Weighing patient daily at the same time dressed in pajamas without shoes
② Offering frequent snacks
③ Offering large meals and firmly suggest she eat them
④ Offering prn medications before mealtimes

43. A man arrives in the emergency room seeking help. When asked the date, he says it is April 1886. He also speaks rapidly and changes the topic frequently. John is best described as:
① Oriented × 3
② Not oriented in time
③ Confused
④ Dishonest

44. The elder of two girls in a family recently went away to college. The younger sister is still at home. The mother has grown increasingly anxious and depressed, saying that she can't manage the large house and all its problems. The younger sister, a typical teenager, is frequently upset over demands made by her mother that she considers unfair. The father finally brings them to the clinic because he is fed up with all the wrangling. An appropriate intervention strategy might be:
① Get the mother some temporary housekeeping help
② Suggest that the younger sister, as the problem focus, enter long-term therapy
③ Suggest that the physician start the mother on tranquilizers
④ Since the father asked for help, suggest he enter therapy

45. A 14-year-old female patient refuses to participate in unit activities in the adolescent psychiatric unit. When the patient is on the unit, she badgers the other patients and is uncooperative with the staff. The nurse needs to incorporate into the care plan:
① Letting the patient know the unit rules
② Letting the patient continue to isolate herself
③ Demanding that the patient participate in activities
④ A conference with the patient, the staff, and psychiatrist

46. One possible nursing diagnosis for a patient experiencing a myocardial infarction expressed in correct NANDA format may be anxiety related to:
① Myocardial infarction
② Threat of death
③ Chest pain
④ Role performance, altered

47. An alcohol and drug abuser is admitted to a substance abuse floor. When working on the care plan, the nurse should have an expected outcome of:
① No negative behaviors
② Observation for defining characteristics and coping behaviors
③ Successful coping with all problems without the use of drugs or alcohol
④ Successful coping is evident, 1 day at a time, without drug and/or alcohol use

48. An elderly patient's son comes to the nurses' station and inquires why his mother can't remember what she had for dinner but can clearly remember a wedding that occurred 30 years ago. The nurse's best response to his question would be:
① That "This is unusual: there is normally long-term memory loss in the elderly."
② That "This is normal: there is normally short-term memory loss in the elderly."
③ That "This is unusual: there is normally no memory deficit in the elderly."
④ That "This is usual, given the underlying physical condition of your mother."

49. A 32-year-old recovering alcoholic arrives at the clinic. She tells the nurse that she feels "nervous, sad, and anxious." Her husband left her one month ago and took her two daughters with him. She states that she is broke, feels out of control, and is depressed. She asks for something to help her sleep. Initially, the nurse needs to assess the patient's:
① Financial ability
② Living situation
③ Suicide potential
④ Future legal problems

50. A 15 year old has been giving several prized possessions to her friends "to remember me." You would interpret this to mean:
    ① She is a teenager attempting to make decisions in her life
    ② She is attempting to "buy" loyalty and friendship
    ③ She is simply giving away things she no longer wants or needs
    ④ She may be suicidal and may require mental health intervention

51. The foundation of the nursing process is assessment. The nurse understands that the purpose of a psychiatric nursing assessment is to:
    ① Establish measurable patient goals
    ② Identify activities with the patient that address causes of the patient's problems
    ③ Obtain an overview of the patient's functional problems and strengths
    ④ Synthesize information and develop a statement about the patient's health

52. The nurse knows that the diagnosis and treatment of human responses to actual or potential health problems are the responsibility of which of the following members of the mental health team?
    ① Clinical psychologist
    ② Psychiatric nurse
    ③ Psychiatric social worker
    ④ Psychiatrist

53. The nurse is expected to know that Wernicke-Korsakoff syndrome is associated with which of the following psychiatric disorders?
    ① Alcoholism
    ② Motor aphasia
    ③ Tardive dyskinesia
    ④ Agoraphobia

54. Which of the following persons is at highest risk for suicide?
    ① Female, age 45, married, no children
    ② Female, age 17, pregnant, minimal social supports
    ③ Male, age 30, single, lacks a significant other
    ④ Male, age 59, divorced, diagnosed with emphysema

55. An appropriate nursing intervention for a depressed patient who has little interest in eating should be to:
    ① Have food and liquids available at all times
    ② Inform the patient of the dangers of not eating
    ③ Limit the patient's intake to three meals a day
    ④ Tell the patient where food is kept on the unit so he may help himself/herself

56. A patient's ostomy is producing a soft, formed stool once or twice per day. Which of the following sections of the bowel is the most likely site of the ostomy?
    ① Ileum
    ② Sigmoid
    ③ Ascending
    ④ Transverse

57. A patient is to receive Prednisone 15 mg PO qd. The label reads: 5 mg tablets. How many tablets would you give?
    ① 1
    ② 2
    ③ 2.5
    ④ 3

58. A 32-year-old construction worker has been hospitalized for the past 4 weeks with a compound fracture of the distal tibia. His physician anticipates that he will be immobilized for another month while the fracture mends. Extended periods of immobility can create many complications, including constipation. To prevent constipation, a diet containing adequate cellulose is recommended. Cellulose is found primarily in:
    ① Refined cereals
    ② Milk products
    ③ Lean tender meats
    ④ Raw fruits and vegetables

59. A 21 year old with recurrent ulcerative colitis is admitted to your unit because of increasing frequency of her diarrheic stools. She is to graduate from college in 2 months. Because her chief complaint is frequent diarrheic stools you would include which of the following in your initial assessment?
    ① Symptoms of fluid and electrolyte imbalance
    ② Urinalysis for presence of urobilinogen
    ③ Pupil check
    ④ Clinitest and Acetest

60. Which of the following symptoms would indicate that a patient with ulcerative colitis suffers from electrolyte imbalance secondary to diarrhea?
    ① Serum potassium level of 3 mEq/L and muscle weakness
    ② Serum sodium level of 135 mEq/L and convulsions
    ③ Serum potassium level of 3.8 mEq/L and diarrhea
    ④ Serium sodium level of 120 mEq/L and edema of feet

61. While changing your patient's abdominal dressing it is most important for you to:
    ① Use forceps
    ② Touch sterile articles with sterile articles only
    ③ Replace all unused 4 × 4s in their package
    ④ Apply ice packs to the incision to decrease swelling

62. A man, 82 years old, heavyset, and unconscious has recently arrived on your unit. He is breathing normally with occasional snoring. His right cheek puffs out with each expiration. His preliminary diagnosis is left-sided CVA. Neurologic assessments necessary to obtain a Glasgow Coma Scale score include:
    ① Vital signs and pupil response
    ② Facial symmetry and motor responses
    ③ Eye opening, verbal responses, and motor responses
    ④ Handgrip and pupil response

63. The nurse's instructions to her patient concerning a glucose tolerance test (GTT) should be that she will be NPO from 12 midnight until the test is over in the morning and that she will have:
    ① One blood sample drawn and a urine specimen collected, after which she will receive a loading dose of glucose solution to drink; then four blood samples and urine specimens will be collected 30 to 60 minutes apart
    ② A blood sample drawn and a 24-hour urine sample collected
    ③ A blood sample drawn 2 hours after each meal and at bedtime with a urine sample collected at the same time
    ④ A loading dose of glucose solution to drink and blood and urine samples taken 2 hours later

64. A patient's FBS level was 300 mg/dl, which indicates she had:
    ① Nothing to eat for 12 hours
    ② Too little glucose in her blood
    ③ Too much insulin in her blood
    ④ Difficulty using the glucose in her blood properly

65. A patient is discharged on a regimen of Coumadin. He is to wear antiembolism stockings and avoid situations that hamper circulation. What instructions will the nurse include in the teaching plan concerning the drug Coumadin?
    ① If pain should develop, aspirin may be taken
    ② The stockings should be taken off for bathing and reapplied in a sitting position
    ③ Instruct the patient to carry a medical identification tag while on anticoagulants
    ④ There will be no restrictions regarding activity

66. Initial treatments that the nurse may anticipate for a patient with thrombophlebitis include:
    ① Warm, moist heat applications to the affected extremity
    ② Exercise to the affected leg four times daily
    ③ Keeping the affected leg lower than the rest of the body
    ④ Administering Coumadin to help dissolve the clot

67. A 59-year-old truck driver came to the emergency room with a right leg that was reddened, warm, and tender. A diagnosis of thrombophlebitis was made. Thrombophlebitis can be precipitated by which of the following conditions?
    ① Early ambulation following surgery
    ② The use of elastic stockings after surgery
    ③ Prolonged standing or sitting
    ④ Range-of-motion exercises during periods of bed rest

68. The evening shift nurse is administering the 10 PM medications. A patient is to receive Nembutal 15 mg at bedtime. When the nurse enters her room, she is talking on the telephone. The nurse should:
    ① Leave the medication at her bedside for her to take when she is finished with her phone conversation
    ② Omit the drug because the patient appears relaxed talking on the phone and won't need a sedative to sleep
    ③ Leave the medication at her bedside and tell her to let the night shift nurse know that she took the medication
    ④ Instruct her to call for the medication when she is finished with her conversation

69. A patient's abdomen feels distended, and she complains of nausea. Her nasogastric tube appears to be in place. Your first action would be to:
    ① Notify the physician
    ② Administer the prescribed antiemetic
    ③ Irrigate the tube with 10 ml of sterile normal saline, if ordered
    ④ Inject 50 ml of air into the tube to check for patency

70. You come across a number of injured people. You have to determine the care priorities and know that civilian triage gives care priority to those whose life is threatened. The victims who need immediate care are those with:
    ① Sucking chest wounds
    ② Closed or simple fractures
    ③ First-degree burns of 25% of the body
    ④ Concussions

71. A patient is receiving the anticoagulant Coumadin, and the physician orders the antidote. The nurse prepares to give:
    ① Protamine sulfate
    ② Vitamin K
    ③ Heparin
    ④ Embolex

72. A 45-year-old executive for a major computer firm has been hospitalized for the past week with the diagnosis of myocardial infarction (MI). During the days immediately following his MI, the patient was on a soft diet. For what reason did his physician probably order this diet?
    ① To reduce the caloric intake of his diet because the patient is overweight
    ② To increase the amount of high-protein foods necessary for tissue repair
    ③ For easy digestion to rest the heart as much as possible
    ④ To promote the healing of the gastric mucosa

73. A patient developed stomatitis as a side effect of chemotherapy. When planning care for this patient, the nurse should include which of the following measures to decrease discomfort?
    ① Frequent mouth rinses with warm water
    ② Use of a firm toothbrush
    ③ Encourage eating of a high-fiber diet
    ④ Administer ASA gr. x qid as ordered

74. A 70-year-old female with osteoporosis is ready for discharge. She plans to return to her home. Which of the following topics should be included in the discharge teaching plan?
    ① Low-calcium foods
    ② Home safety measures
    ③ Sun protection clothing
    ④ Limiting weight-bearing exercise

75. A 71-year-old woman is admitted with a suspected fracture of the left hip. Nursing assessment findings that are indicative of a hip fracture include:
    ① Shortening of the affected leg and external rotation of the foot
    ② Lengthening of the affected leg and muscle spasm
    ③ Weakness and internal rotation of the affected leg
    ④ Pain on the affected side and difficulty in walking

76. A patient has been admitted for a right femoral bone fracture and is placed in balanced suspension traction. Twenty-four hours after admission, the nurse notes that the patient's respirations have increased from a normal of 18 to 46 and the pulse has increased from 88 to 120. The patient does not appear to be in respiratory distress but is slightly apprehensive. What is the *most appropriate* action for the nurse to take?
    ① Briefly examine the patient for signs of cyanosis
    ② Release the traction weights slowly
    ③ Ask the patient who is the current president of the United States
    ④ Ask the patient to talk about what is so upsetting

77. A nursing intervention appropriate for the plan of care of a patient with hyperthyroidism would include:
    ① Providing a cool, quiet environment
    ② Encouraging a decreased caloric intake
    ③ Testing the urine for presence of glucose
    ④ Applying emollients to soothe dry skin

78. A patient, unconscious and vomiting, is admitted to the emergency room after he was thrown from a horse. The nurse suspects increased intracranial pressure. What is the best position in which the nurse should place the patient?
    ① Lateral recumbent with the neck in extension
    ② Trendelenburg's with the neck in extension
    ③ Prone with the neck hyperextended
    ④ High Fowler's with the neck hyperextended

79. Heparin sodium is ordered for a patient because of the potential for developing a blood clot because of immobility. To correctly administer heparin the nurse would:
    ① Administer the heparin deep IM
    ② Aspirate before administering the heparin to ensure the injection is not in a blood vessel
    ③ Administer the heparin in the same site each time
    ④ Refrain from massaging the area after the injection

80. A patient has dysuria and tells the nurse she needs to urgently void frequently. A urinalysis reveals greater than 100,000 colonies of gram-negative bacteria present. The physician has ordered antibiotics for the infection. Which of the following would the nurse include when teaching the patient about urinary tract infections?
    ① Monitor urinary output until symptoms subside
    ② Wipe with toilet tissue from front to back
    ③ Take the antibiotics every 4 to 6 hours
    ④ Make sure to empty the bladder every 2 hours

81. A 30-year-old patient with a history of diabetes and hypertension is to begin hemodialysis because of end-stage renal disease. She tells the nurse that she is upset about having to depend on some machine for the rest of her life. The *most appropriate* response by the nurse is:
    ① "It sounds as though you are in denial and for the time being this is okay."
    ② "Have you talked about these feelings of dependency with your family?"
    ③ "You appear to be angry that you will need to rely on the dialysis machine."
    ④ "A lot of people feel this way when they start hemodialysis treatments, but they adjust."

82. The nurse is reviewing the teaching plan for the long-range care of a patient with Alzheimer's disease. The spouse of the patient asks for advice related to nutrition and meal planning. Which of the following recommendations should be included in the teaching plan?
    ① Provide three well-balanced meals with a variety of choices at each meal
    ② Allow additional time to eat and reminders during the meal to chew and swallow
    ③ Plan mealtimes around the individual's favorite television or radio programs
    ④ Have the individual, at the beginning of each week, plan the daily menus for the upcoming week

83. A patient has been placed on a low-sodium diet following a recent massive myocardial infarction. Which of the following foods should the nurse instruct the patient to avoid?
    ① Canned peaches
    ② Dill pickles
    ③ Fresh peaches
    ④ Fresh cucumbers

84. A patient has insulin-dependent diabetes mellitus. Her glucose level at 8 AM was 204 mg/dl, and she received 4 units of NPH insulin. The nurse plans to evaluate for "onset of action" of the NPH insulin between:
    ① 9 AM - 10 AM
    ② 7 PM - 8 PM
    ③ 12 noon - 1 PM
    ④ 10 AM - 11 AM

85. A 37-year-old woman has undergone arthroscopic surgery to remove loose cartilage from her right knee. The physician has ordered an ice pack to be applied to the knee postoperatively. The nurse explains the rationale for this action to the patient with which statement?
    ① "The cold dilates superficial blood vessels."
    ② "The cold increases blood flow to the knee."
    ③ "The cold will help reduce muscle spasms."
    ④ "The cold helps reduce pain sensitivity."

86. A patient has developed idiopathic thrombocytopenic purpura (ITP). Because of the potential problems associated with this condition, the nurse should instruct the patient to:
    ① Take aspirin for mild discomfort
    ② Avoid persons with infectious diseases
    ③ Sleep with the head of the bed elevated
    ④ Use an electric razor when shaving

87. A 78-year-old patient has been told by her doctor that her breast cancer has now metastasized to the liver. The patient only has a fourth-grade education. She asks the nurse to define metastasis to her. The nurse can best explain this by saying:
    ① "The tumor size has increased."
    ② "The cancer has now spread to the liver."
    ③ "The cancer originally started in the liver and has spread to the breast."
    ④ "There are now two different types of cancer growing in you."

88. A patient with COPD and pneumonia is unable to walk 20 feet without becoming severely dyspneic. His oximeter drops to 79% with activity. His nursing diagnosis is activity intolerance related to insufficient oxygen to meet body requirements. Which of the following would be an appropriate goal for activity intolerance?
    ① Lips are cyanotic after ambulation
    ② Pulse returns to baseline within a half hour of ambulating
    ③ Respiratory rate returns to baseline within a half hour after walking
    ④ Oxygen saturations remain greater than 90% after walking

89. An elderly nursing home resident fractures her hip and becomes bedridden. She complains of constipation. As the nurse assigned to her, what measures would you perform to improve her situation?
    ① Start her on a bowel and bladder program
    ② Increase fluid and fiber in her diet
    ③ Ask the physician for a laxative order
    ④ Increase active range-of-motion activities

90. An elderly nursing home resident has a poor appetite and refuses to eat at times. Which of the following measures would it be most important for the nurse to take to improve his appetite?

① Provide soft, bland foods
② Allow small frequent meals
③ Avoid unpleasant activities at mealtimes
④ Assist the resident to his room to eat alone

91. A patient is concerned about her family history of colon cancer. She has asked for help in decreasing her risk for cancer development. The nurse includes which of the following dietary instructions when assisting this patient?
① Decrease intake of wild rice
② Increase consumption of corn oil
③ Reduce consumption of smoked meats
④ Avoid foods with a high vitamin B content

92. A patient has an IV of 5% dextrose in water running at 150 cc/hr through a 20-gauge needle in his left cephalic vein. Despite having the roller clamp wide open, the nurse is having trouble maintaining the IV at the prescribed rate. The needle insertion site appears normal. For the nurse to maintain the IV at the ordered rate, the nurse should:
① Decrease the height of the infusion
② Increase the height of the infusion
③ Change the tubing to one that delivers 60 gtts/ml
④ Restart the IV using a 22-gauge needle

93. A 41-year-old woman was an unrestrained passenger in a motor vehicle accident. She sustained a displaced fracture of her left femur. To meet this patient's hygienic needs, the nurse may remove which of the following traction devices?
① Crutchfield tongs
② Thomas Pearson splint
③ Buck's extension traction
④ External fixators

94. A 78-year-old woman who had a right total hip arthroplasty done 2 years ago fell yesterday and fractured the left trochanter. She returned from surgery with an order for ketorolac (Toradol) 60 mg IM q4h. Which of the following sites would be recommended for the Toradol injection?
① Left ventral gluteal
② Left dorsal gluteal
③ Right dorsal gluteal
④ Right vastus lateralis

95. Following a fall, a patient arrived at the emergency room with complaints of right shoulder pain and inability to raise her arm above her head. She is able to move the right hand and fingers. An x-ray revealed a fractured clavicle, and a shoulder brace was applied. Which of the following instructions should the nurse include in the discharge teaching?
① You may continue to hang out your laundry
② You may continue to play tennis weekly
③ Exercise your elbow, wrist, and fingers frequently
④ Begin range-of-motion exercises to your shoulder tomorrow

96. An insulin-dependent diabetic was involved in a construction accident and fractured his left humerus and tibia. He is in skeletal traction, and his left arm is immobilized. He needs his morning insulin dose. Identify the site in which his insulin could safely be given:
① Abdomen
② Right deltoid
③ Left vastus lateralis
④ Right ventral gluteal

97. A patient, age 31, has terminal brain cancer. He is 5 feet, 10 inches tall and weighs 92 pounds. The patient is very frail appearing and needs help with bathing and toileting. He eats very little because of complaints of nausea. The term which best describes his condition is:
① Ascitic
② Cachexic
③ Aphasic
④ Dysphagic

98. A patient has been receiving theophylline (Aminophylline) 80 mg per hour intravenously for exacerbation of acute asthma. He states he is feeling "jittery." His pulse is 120 beats per minute, respirations are 22 breaths per minute, and his lungs are clear to auscultation. The physician has ordered a theophylline level to be drawn. Which of the following titers are within therapeutic range?
① 4 mg/dl
② 14 mg/dl
③ 26 mg/dl
④ 34 mg/dl

99. A patient who has been receiving antibiotics for a postoperative wound infection is complaining that her ears are ringing. The nurse recognizes that tinnitus is a side-effect of which category of antibiotics?
① Aminoglycosides
② Penicillins
③ Cephalosporins
④ Tetracyclines

100. A patient has been receiving heparin (Heparin sodium) for a deep vein thrombophlebitis in the left leg. One of the following laboratory tests aids in determining correct dosage of heparin. Which one of these should the nurse report to the physician?
① Prothrombin time (PT)
② Direct Coombs test
③ Indirect Coombs test
④ Partial thromboplastin time (PTT)

101. A patient has been receiving vancocin hydrochloride (Vancomycin) intravenously for five days for a multiple resistant staph aureus (MRSA) infection following a craniotomy for a benign growth. With regard to the vancocin hydrochloride, the nurse should report which of the following lab results to the physician?
① Hemoglobin 12.4 G
② Sodium 137 mEq
③ Potassium 4.2 mEq
④ Creatinine 2.6 mg

102. An 82-year-old patient is receiving oxygen at 8 liters per minute via mask for lung cancer. Her breakfast tray has arrived, but she is unable to eat because of extreme dyspnea when the oxygen is removed. Which of the following nursing interventions would be most effective in aiding this patient?
① Wait until later when the patient is less dyspneic
② Place the patient on a full-liquid diet
③ Ask the physician for a nasal cannula
④ Hold the mask near her face while eating

103. A 51-year-old mechanic has been diagnosed with a grade IV adenocarcinoma of the rectum. The nurse explains that grade IV is:
    ① The depth of tumor penetration
    ② The extent of the spread of the tumor
    ③ The length of time the tumor has been present
    ④ The degree of cell variation from normal

104. In instructing a patient with Parkinson's disease concerning his dietary intake, the nurse will suggest that the patient:
    ① Consume extra raw fruits and vegetables
    ② Consume a large amount of protein
    ③ Eat small, frequent meals
    ④ Eat only home-cooked meals

105. A patient has recurring active genital herpes and is extremely uncomfortable. In assisting this patient with pain relief, the nurse will instruct her in the use of:
    ① Neosporin ointment
    ② Warm, moist dressings
    ③ Campho-Phenique
    ④ Condoms

106. A 22-year-old patient has Crohn's disease. In preparing the patient for self-management of his diet at home, the nurse will instruct him to:
    ① Eat a high-protein and high-calorie diet
    ② Consume adequate prune juice and other intestinal stimulants
    ③ Eat pureed foods and baby foods to enhance digestion
    ④ Consume minimal green, leafy vegetables and citrus fruit

107. A 24-year-old patient is to receive discharge information concerning home management following an appendectomy. In order for the patient to care for her wound, the nurse will instruct her to:
    ① Inspect her incision every 4 hours for signs of infection
    ② Gently wash the incision with soap and water daily and dry
    ③ Resume normal household activities upon her return home
    ④ Replace Steri-Strips with pieces of paper tape as needed

108. A patient has a cervical radiation implant. She is in a private room. Visitation is limited to her spouse and immediate family. A 22-year-old friend comes to the nurse and says, "There is a 'no visitors' sign on my friend's door. I want to see her." The nurse should respond by stating:
    ① "I understand how you feel, but it's doctor's orders that she have no visitors."
    ② "It's against hospital policy for patients receiving radium therapy to have visitors."
    ③ "I understand how you feel. I can take a message to her if you would like me to."
    ④ "If there is any chance that you might be pregnant, your baby would be at risk."

109. A patient has a suspected intestinal obstruction. He has a Miller-Abbott tube for intestinal decompresion in place. He has had no drainage from the tube in 4 hours despite gentle attempts at irrigation with 30 ml of normal saline. In caring for this patient the nurse will:
    ① Tape the tube to the patient's nose to promote drainage
    ② Notify the doctor of the decrease in drainage
    ③ Attach the tube to high suction to promote drainage
    ④ Irrigate the tube with 50 ml normal saline to promote drainage

110. A patient has just returned to his room following a surgical trabeculectomy of his right eye. He is still groggy from the anesthesia but is complaining of severe pain at the operative site. His vital signs are 130/78, 98.2 - 88 - 20. The nurse should:
    ① Administer the ordered Tylenol
    ② Call the doctor immediately
    ③ Position him on his left side
    ④ Position him on his right side

111. A patient tells the nurse that she is unable to take flu shots because they give her the flu. The nurse should reply:
    ① "Many infections that people have in the winter are caused by other viruses, not the flu virus."
    ② "I will call the doctor and tell him that you are unable to take the vaccine."
    ③ "Eggs are used to make the vaccine. Are you allergic to eggs, also?"
    ④ "Would you mind describing for me what your illness was like after your flu shot?"

112. A 24-year-old patient has undergone a bronchoscopy this morning. What should the nurse assess prior to administering fluids by mouth?
    ① Level of alertness
    ② Request for something to drink
    ③ Return of gag reflex
    ④ Presence of breath sounds

113. When the nurse notes an obvious eyelid or eye laceration, the first and best action to take before contacting the physician is to:
    ① Loosely patch the eye
    ② Irrigate the eye with running water
    ③ Administer an eye antibiotic ointment
    ④ Put in 3 to 4 normal saline drops

114. You arrive at the scene of a car accident to find one passenger thrown from the car. He is unconscious, but a pulse is present. You should:
    ① Perform 5 chest compressions, then 1 breath
    ② Perform 15 chest compressions, then 2 breaths
    ③ Perform rescue breathing at 12 to 15 times per minute
    ④ Perform rescue breathing at 10 to 12 times per minute

115. A 65 year old diagnosed with acute MI is admitted to the cardiac care unit. You are the nurse assigned to his care. The highest priority nursing diagnosis is:
    ① Activity intolerance related to prescribed bed rest
    ② Altered tissue perfusion related to myocardial ischemia
    ③ Alteration in comfort: chest pain related to reduced coronary blood flow
    ④ Self-care deficit related to fear of dying

116. Structural defects of the myocardium in which chambers, septum, or large vessels are not normal is known as:
    ① Congestive heart failure
    ② Endocarditis
    ③ Coronary heart disease
    ④ Congenital heart disease

117. A nurse is teaching a newly diagnosed diabetes patient about the importance of diet. Which statement by the nurse indicates proper nutritional management strategies?
    ① "All diabetics must never eat sweets because it increases the blood sugar."
    ② "All diabetics should eat a diet high in fat and protein."

③ "A total calorie intake is individualized but should be comprised of 60% carbohydrates."

④ "Diabetic patients should never eat out."

118. A patient was admitted to the neurological unit 5 days ago with a suspected cerebrovascular accident. He is stuporous and cannot follow simple commands. The physician has ordered a feeding tube to be inserted and tube feedings started at 25 cc/hour. When the nasogastric feeding tube is inserted, the patient develops persistent coughing. The nurse should:

① Stop advancing the tube for a minute and let the patient rest

② Encourage the patient to swallow

③ Remove the tube immediately

④ Elevate the patient's head and flex his neck

119. A patient is scheduled to have a glycosylated hemoglobin test. He asks the nurse to explain the test. The nurse explains that:

① It is a blood test which determines glucose control over a period of time

② The test is the most accurate indicator of diabetes mellitus

③ The test monitors for glycosuria

④ The test will determine how much insulin he will receive

120. A physician is performing CPR and a second rescuer (a nurse) arrives on the scene. The first rescuer completes a cycle of 15 compressions and gives 2 ventilations. If, after a pulse check, no pulse is present, the second rescuer should:

① Perform 15 compressions, then 2 ventilations

② Resume chest compressions preceded with ventilation

③ Resume chest compressions and not precede this with ventilation

④ Take his position at the head of the victim and prepare to ventilate

121. A 24 year old was admitted with acquired immunodeficiency syndrome (AIDS). He has lost 30 pounds and appears emaciated. An appropriate nursing diagnosis for him would be:

① Impaired gas exchange related to impending death

② Anticipatory grieving related to impending death

③ Self-esteem disturbance related to weight loss and general appearance secondary to having AIDS

④ Ineffective individual coping related to loss of friends and family due to the disease process

122. Nursing interventions related to postop care of the patient who has just had a thyroidectomy performed include:

① Immediately report a moderate drop in body temperature less than 98.6° F, heart rate less than 80 beats per minute, and lethargy

② Place in Fowler's position, support head with sand bags, obtain vital signs every 2 to 4 hours

③ Report any signs of redness or discomfort to the physician

④ Assess for hypercalcemia, return of voice, and restlessness

123. A 65-year-old female is 3 days postop hip replacement. Her nursing diagnosis is potential for infection related to surgical incision. Identify the data that best reflects an evaluation statement:

① Temperature 100.9° F, white blood count 12,000, incision with small amount of redness, moderate swelling

② Temperature 99.0° F, white blood count 13,000, incision red with small amount of drainage

③ Temperature 99.0° F, white blood count 9,800, incision with redness or swelling with small amount of serosanguineous drainage

④ Temperature 98.6° F, white blood count 10,000, incision red, large amount of swelling with purulent drainage

124. A patient on a medical-surgical floor is 3 days postop with a history of long-term alcohol use. The nurse is in the patient's room when suddenly he states: "I smell roses." The nurse understands the patient may be experiencing a(n):

① Aura that precedes seizure activity

② Olfactory hallucination

③ Petit mal seizure

④ Pleasant aroma from flowers in his room

125. The coronary arteries supply the heart muscle with oxygen. In coronary artery disease the arteries fail to supply the heart muscle with adequate oxygen. The nurse knows that the result is:

① General hypoxia of the tissues

② The heart gives out and beats at a slower rate

③ Decreased blood pressure

④ Cerebral hypoxia only

COMPREHENSIVE EXAMINATION 2: PART 2

This examination contains individual questions, each containing a relevant clinical situation. Read all questions carefully. There is only *one best answer* for each question.

Test time allotment (Part 2): approximately 2 hours
Answers and rationales begin on p. 578.

1. A patient is a gravida 1, para 0, admitted to the labor unit in beginning labor. She is accompanied by her husband who appears to be very excited about the upcoming delivery. He tells you that they have been attending Lamaze classes in preparation for childbirth. True labor is best characterized by which of the following?
   ① Braxton-Hicks contractions and pinkish vaginal discharge
   ② Regular, forceful contractions and cervical dilation
   ③ Spontaneous rupture of the amniotic membrane (sac) and abdominal pain
   ④ Descent of the presenting part into the pelvis

2. The physician informs you that her patient is completely dilated and effaced. The fetal heart tones and maternal vital signs are within safe limits. The patient says she feels the urge to push with contractions. The most important nursing action to perform at this time is to:
   ① Prepare the delivery room and equipment
   ② Increase frequency of monitoring fetal heart tones and maternal vital signs
   ③ Place the patient's legs in stirrups and apply wrist restraints
   ④ Assist the physician to gown and glove

3. According to the history of maternity care in the United States, the single greatest deterrent to maternal complications, particularly pregnancy-induced hypertension (PIH), has been:
   ① Discovery and use of antihypertensive drugs
   ② Good prenatal care
   ③ The advocation of salt-free diet
   ④ The age of the mother

4. If a patient is to have a forceps delivery, the physician would be sure that the bag of waters has ruptured and that the head is engaged. The nursing responsibility would be to check that:
   ① Sterile forceps are available
   ② Forceps are well lubricated
   ③ The bladder is empty; catheterize if necessary
   ④ The fetal heart tones are regular

5. A couple who wish to have children have been married 5 years and have no demonstrable physical impairments. The wife has read that all IUDs are dangerous and are being recalled. She says she knows several friends who are using them and wonders if she should alert them. Your best response would be:
   ① "IUDs often cause pelvic inflammatory disease."
   ② "Only the Dalkon shield has been recalled; other types of IUDs are still used with an 80% or higher success rate. However, other options are available. Would you like me to tell you about them?"
   ③ "There are other alternatives to IUDs. Would you like me to explore them with you?"
   ④ "It is none of your business what other people use."

6. You work in an obstetrics clinic, and your patient and her husband wish to know about rhythm or a safe method of contraception, even though their problem is fertility and not family planning per se. You would teach them that:
   ① Investigations by the woman and her husband to determine the time of ovulation are necessary
   ② Abstinence from coitus for 10 days before and after the calculated date of ovulation is imperative
   ③ A record of her menstrual cycle for at least 3 months is necessary before initiating the method
   ④ Regular 30-day menstrual cycles are necessary for the method to be useful

7. A 19 year old enrolled in a childbirth class asks the nurse when the preembryonic stage is over. The nurse replies:
   ① At birth
   ② At 9 weeks
   ③ About 3 weeks
   ④ Between the fourth and eighth week.

8. A patient, pregnant for the fifth time, asks the nurse to refresh her memory and explain how waste products and nutrients are transmitted between the mother and the fetus. The nurse explains that the placenta is the organ primarily responsible for the exchange and that the connecting link is the umbilical cord which is comprised of:
   ① Two arteries and one vein
   ② One artery and one vein
   ③ Two veins and one artery
   ④ Two veins only

9. When discussing nutrition with a 3-month pregnant gravida 1, para 0, the nurse explains that the most important consideration in her prenatal diet is to provide:
   ① An adequate diet to assure optimum nutrition for mother and fetus
   ② A low-calorie diet to maintain the mother's weight
   ③ Limited fluid intake to prevent edema in the body tissues of both the mother and the fetus
   ④ A diet high in protein for nourishment of the fetus

10. A patient comes to the prenatal clinic stating she has not had her menstrual period for the last 2 months. The nurse should always consider amenorrhea as an important sign of pregnancy during the assessment process because:
    ① It is very commonly the reason that women seek prenatal care
    ② It offers positive proof that the woman is pregnant
    ③ It really is not important because there are other changes that the doctor can see
    ④ It is important only if it occurs with nausea and quickening

11. A young patient is reluctant to attend the parent's class. She tells the nurse assigned to her, "I know everything I need to know and besides my mother is going to take care of him anyway." The *most appropriate* response for the nurse may be:
    ① "It is great that you have help. However, it is your responsibility to care for this baby. Can you tell me what you know?"
    ② "Grandmothers are fine for cuddling and spoiling. However, you have to learn about this child yourself."
    ③ "I am sure you think that you know a great deal. However, come to the class anyway and see if you can pick up a few new tricks."

④ "All right, if you don't want to go you really don't have to. However, your mother may not always be available to care for this child."

12. A 17-year-old primigravida is 2 days postpartum. She has a healthy baby boy who weighs 8 pounds 3 ounces. When the nurse makes rounds she finds the patient feeding the baby appropriately. However, the new mother says, "Isn't he beautiful? He is never going to cry, only when he is hungry." The nurse's *most appropriate* response at this time should be:
① "Yes, he is beautiful. However, you really are being foolish if you think he will never cry except when he is hungry."
② "If you attend our bath class you will learn the basics about how to take care of your baby."
③ "Yes, he is beautiful. Babies cry for many reasons and hunger is one of them, along with being wet and being lonely."
④ "Yes, he is beautiful. Is your mother going to help you care for the baby when you get him home?"

13. A patient delivers her first child, a normal 7-pound 8-ounce male. The nurse knows the physician will clamp and cut the umbilical cord:
① When it stops pulsating
② Immediately after birth
③ Fifteen minutes after birth
④ Thirty minutes after birth

14. The patient asks the nurse, "Why does my baby have these white spots on his nose?" The best response for the nurse would be:
① "These are called 'stork bites.' Don't worry. They usually disappear within a year."
② "These are called milia. They are caused by clogged follicles and are very common in newborns."
③ "They are nothing to worry about. However, your doctor will explain how to treat them."
④ "We will have to watch them very carefully. They could be a sign of infection."

15. Psychiatric nursing is a field in which:
① Nurses are not sued because patients are not legally competent
② Suits may be brought by patients who believe they have not been actively treated
③ Nurses are not called on to testify in legal cases because there is no "hands-on" care
④ Few cases are tried because patients lose their civil rights

16. A man reports that he has been using "crack" (a form of cocaine) for the last 3 days, has slept very little, and is afraid "they are out to get him." The nurse may conclude:
① His paranoid thoughts are probably psychotic delusions
② He may be in realistic danger from drug dealers
③ Crack users are rarely functionally psychotic
④ Drug use must be reported to legal authorities

17. A wife is angry with her husband. When he comes home, she accuses him of being angry. This is an example of:
① Repression
② Projection
③ Displacement
④ Rationalization

18. A necessary part of communication in mental health nursing is:
① The ability to argue logically
② To ask many questions
③ To allow feedback
④ To give advice

19. An 18 year old is admitted to the hospital with a diagnosis of anorexia nervosa. Her symptoms would most likely include which of the following?
① Dysmenorrhea
② Periods of hyperactivity
③ Tachycardia
④ Diarrhea

20. Treatment and nursing interventions for a patient with anorexia include all the following *except:*
① Reinforcement of her present self-image
② Identification of the psychologic cause
③ Correction of malnutrition
④ Use of behavior modification techniques

21. The nurse might infer that a patient's thought processes were scattered based on:
① Frequent changes of topic
② The rapidity of speech
③ Physical appearance
④ Recent history

22. A nursing observation that would support evidence of the therapeutic effects of antianxiety drug therapy would be:
① Crying, facial grimaces, rigid posture
② Anger, aggressive behavior
③ Decrease in blood pressure, pulse, respirations
④ Verbal statements such as "more worried" or "resting poorly"

23. A 15 year old becomes embarrassed when you attempt to do her perineal care 2 days after her surgery for a spinal fusion. You can best handle this situation by:
① Telling her you will do it today and she can do it next time
② Postponing it until her mother comes in so she can do it
③ Allowing her to participate while you assist
④ Leaving the room so she can do it without embarrassment

24. A 12-year-old patient studies every evening. He carries a 4.0 grade average and takes several foreign language courses. When questioned by the nurse, the patient states that he is shorter than any of the other kids at school and they tease him. The nurse recognizes the patient's interest in excelling in academics as a type of defense mechanism known as:
① Denial
② Conversion
③ Projection
④ Compensation

25. The high school nurse notices that several of the students wear T-shirts of a popular rock band star almost every day. The nurse recognizes this as a possible defense mechanism known as:
① Projection
② Compensation
③ Identification
④ Rationalization

26. A nurse just passed boards and is oriented to the adolescent psychology unit where she accepted a job. The unit stresses to the new nurse that they use behavior modification. She knows that in order to change an undesirable behavior by behavior modification the nurse needs to:
    ① Set limits
    ② Confront the client
    ③ Reprimand the client for inappropriate behavior
    ④ Remove the reward for the inappropriate behavior

27. A patient, age 36, has been admitted to the drug-alcohol rehabilitation unit. When asked why he was admitted, the patient stated to the nurse that his family members forced him to come. He stated that he did not drink what they accused him of. The nurse should respond:
    ① "No one can force you to be here."
    ② "Exactly how much do you drink?"
    ③ "Tell me more about what you mean."
    ④ "It is really for your own good and protection."

28. A family was involved in a car accident. The resulting explosion and fire killed the parents. A 3-year-old boy sustained a fractured left femur and second- and third-degree burns over 43% of his body. The emergency medical technician advised the hospital that the child was burned on both anterior and posterior aspects of his torso, arms, and hands. As part of the emergency team, you would help prepare for the patient's arrival by obtaining a:
    ① Tracheostomy tray
    ② Stretcher with sterile sheets
    ③ Cardiac defibrillator
    ④ Sterile dressing tray

29. The physician chooses the closed method of dressing the burned areas. On the pediatric ward, your patient's room would be set up to provide which type of isolation?
    ① Enteric
    ② Strict
    ③ Reverse
    ④ Respiratory

30. Your 3-year-old patient has been placed in Russell traction and keeps tugging at the pulley ropes. To help him cope with being immobilized, you can:
    ① Play Chinese checkers with him as a diversional activity
    ② Apply Russell traction to his favorite teddy bear
    ③ Place mitten restraints on his hands
    ④ Retie the pulley ropes out of his reach

31. A 5-year-old patient has not had a bowel movement in 3 days. The nurse can promote elimination by encouraging the patient to eat:
    ① Eggs and cheese toast
    ② Popsicles and oranges
    ③ Apples and carrot sticks
    ④ Chicken and whole grain cereal

32. Your patient is in the fourth grade at school. According to Erikson's theory of psychosocial development, the patient is in the stage of:
    ① Autonomy vs. guilt
    ② Industry vs. inferiority
    ③ Initiative vs. guilt
    ④ Trust vs. mistrust

33. As you assess a 12-year-old patient for signs of increased intracranial pressure, you would be concerned on observing:
    ① A change in level of consciousness
    ② Anorexia and thirst
    ③ Increased pulse and respiration rates
    ④ Blurred vision and halos around lights

34. Your teenage patient is scheduled for spinal fusion and instrumentation in the morning. The evening before surgery she comes to the nursing station making demands. You understand this behavior is primarily a result of:
    ① Maladjustment to hospitalization
    ② Stress of pending surgery
    ③ Past hospital experiences
    ④ Inadequate preparation for surgery

35. A 5 year old is admitted to the hospital with a possible diagnosis of acute glomerulonephritis. Symptoms of acute glomerulonephritis include which of the following?
    ① Severe edema, proteinuria, fever
    ② Distended abdomen, decreased serum protein
    ③ Hematuria, fever, elevated BUN level
    ④ Respiratory distress, oliguria, malnutrition

36. A 19 year old is admitted to the hospital after briefly losing consciousness when he was tackled during the Thanksgiving Day football game. During the neurologic assessment the nurse is careful to note and report the following response by the patient:
    ① He did not know the name of the hospital
    ② He could not remember the name of the nurse
    ③ He said the month was June
    ④ He could not remember the incident on the football field

37. Treatment measures for a patient with acute glomerulonephritis include all of the following *except:*
    ① Bed rest for 2 to 4 weeks
    ② Antibiotics as ordered
    ③ Corticosteroids to reduce edema
    ④ Urine testing for protein and specific gravity

38. A patient's diagnosis of acute glomerulonephritis was most likely preceded by:
    ① A streptococcal infection
    ② *H. influenzae* meningitis
    ③ An injury to one or both kidneys
    ④ An allergic reaction to a food or medication

39. Which of the following behaviors is appropriate for the stage identified?
    ① An infant wants to be left alone
    ② Toddlers want to do things for themselves
    ③ A school-age child cries continuously for the mother
    ④ A 4 year old does not talk

40. A mother brings her 2-year-old child to the clinic because of diarrhea. Which of the following statements indicate a need for teaching before sending the patient home?
    ① "I need to stop feeding solid foods and give her only liquids for 8 hours."
    ② "She can eat anything she wants as long as she takes her medication as ordered."
    ③ "It is ok to give her Gatorade to drink."
    ④ "I need to encourage fluid intake while she has diarrhea."

41. A 4 year old has a cold and a runny nose. Which of the following statements by the mother to her daughter may indicate a need for more health teaching?

① "Close off one nostril and blow through the other one."

② "Wash your hands after blowing your nose."

③ "Rub a little ointment around your nose."

④ "You can get an ear infection when you have a cold."

42. When treating a severely dehydrated infant, the nurse should:

    ① Infuse IV fluids as rapidly as possible

    ② Monitor IV fluids closely and give slowly

    ③ Keep NPO until intravascular and intracellular fluids equalize

    ④ Offer PO fluids every hour rather than start an IV

43. The nurse is gathering data related to the growth and development of a 3-week-old infant. The nurse should expect to observe which of the following behaviors in the infant?

    ① Moro "startle" reflex

    ② Cooing and babbling

    ③ Recognizing a familiar face

    ④ Holding head erect

44. Which of the following activities *increases the risk* for development of urinary tract infection (UTI) in the *normal* female pediatric patient?

    ① Restricting fluids after supper to prevent bedwetting

    ② Taking daily tub baths

    ③ Using a front to back motion when wiping for toileting

    ④ Wearing tight panties or diapers

45. A 5 year old was bitten by a raccoon suspected of having rabies. He was taken to the pediatric clinic and received an intramuscular injection of HRIG (human rabies immune globulin) and HDCV (human diploid cell rabies vaccine). The nurse is reinforcing information about discharge instructions. Which of the following discharge instructions is *most* important?

    ① Cleanse wound b.i.d. with betadine solution

    ② Return to the clinic for suture removal in 7 days

    ③ Administer antipyretics for temperature elevation

    ④ Return to clinic *on exact scheduled dates* for HDCV injections

46. A mother must suction her five-year-old son's tracheostomy. Which of the following statements by the mother indicates she has correct understanding of suction technique?

    ① Instill small amounts of hydrogen peroxide into the tube if the tube has caked secretions

    ② Set suction machine at 160 mm Hg pressure when suctioning

    ③ Insert the catheter no more than 0.5 cm beyond the tip of the tube

    ④ During each pass of the catheter, the catheter should remain in the tube no longer than 15 seconds

47. Which of the following activities may *precipitate* an asthma attack in a *pediatric* patient?

    ① Cleaning with an ammonia-based cleaner

    ② Learning a pet mouse died

    ③ Swimming laps at a pool

    ④ Using a fine cool mist humidifier in the house

48. The nurse is assisting with the development of dietary guidelines for a 4-week-old breastfed infant. Which of the following guidelines should be included in this plan?

    ① Breast milk exclusively should be fed to the infant for the first 4 to 6 months

② Formula per bottle should be substituted for breast milk when the father wants to feed the infant

③ Rice cereal mixed with breast milk should be offered 2 × day at 2 months of age

④ The infant should receive multivitamins daily

49. A 2-month-old infant is to receive his/her first immunizations for diphtheria, pertussis, and tetanus. The nurse is assisting with instructions to the parents about these immunizations. Which of the following information should be included with the information?

    ① This single injection will offer lifetime immunity against pertussis, diphtheria, and tetanus

    ② The infant should avoid contact with other children for 2 weeks

    ③ Infants may run a fever and be irritable during the first 24 hours after the injection

    ④ Seizure activity is a common side-effect of this immunization

50. The nurse is assisting with screening for idiopathic scoliosis at the local health department. Which of the following groups is at the greatest risk for development of idiopathic scoliosis?

    ① Preadolescent females

    ② Infants under 6 months

    ③ College-age females

    ④ Toddlers

51. In a child with a cyanotic congenital heart defect, the nurse would expect to observe which of the following signs/symptoms?

    ① Neck vein distention

    ② Plethora

    ③ Peripheral edema

    ④ Adventitious breath sounds

52. The nurse is assisting with the development of a nursing care plan for an infant with bronchiolitis caused by respiratory syncytial virus. Which of the following activities is appropriate for this care plan?

    ① Restrict all fluids

    ② Place infant in strict isolation

    ③ Suction infant prn and before all feeds

    ④ Position infant in prone position after feeding

53. Which of the following behaviors indicates a child *may be ready* to start toilet training?

    ① Able to sit for 2 minutes on the toilet without fussing

    ② Imitates toileting activities of older siblings

    ③ Tolerates soiled diaper/pants without complaint

    ④ Stays dry during naps once per week

54. A 15 year old is post-op day one from knee tendon surgery following a soccer accident. Which of the following methods would *most accurately* determine the patient's level of pain?

    ① Observe the patient for physical signs of pain such as facial grimacing, moaning, and increased blood pressure

    ② Ask the patient to describe her/his pain in words

    ③ Ask the parents of the patient what level of pain she/he has

    ④ Using a pain scale such as 0-10, ask the patient to rate her/his level of pain

55. A 19 year old fractured his left femur in a skiing accident three days ago. His condition has been stable following surgery. Since 2 PM, he has been restless and tachypneic and his nails beds are becoming cyanotic. Of the following signs and symptoms noted by the nurse, which one is most specifically diagnostic of the patient's condition?
    ① The presence of bilateral crackles and wheezes
    ② The presence of petechiae on the eyelids and bucchal surfaces
    ③ The absence of a fever
    ④ A falling blood pressure

56. A 19-year-old patient has her call light on because her IV has run dry and the fluid has stopped halfway down the tubing. Which of the following interventions would be most effective in relieving the IV problem?
    ① Discontinue the IV
    ② Change the IV bag and resume the rate
    ③ Change the IV bag and lower the bag until the fluid in the tubing refills the drip chamber
    ④ Change the IV bag, disconnect the tubing, purge the air, and reconnect to the patient

57. A 16-year-old student tells the school nurse her mother told her not to use tampons anymore because they can lead to a condition known as toxic shock syndrome (TSS). The student asks the nurse to explain what causes this. The nurse can begin by saying that the organism that causes TSS is:
    ① *Chlamydia trachomatis*
    ② *Staphylococcus* strains
    ③ *Neisseria gonorrhoeae* (coccus)
    ④ Group A beta-hemolytic streptococci

58. A patient asks a question about the Recommended Dietary Allowances (RDA) that she sees listed on packaging. Which of the following responses given by the nurse is most appropriate?
    ① "They are used as requirements for individuals with specific nutritional deficiencies."
    ② "They are also called the food pyramid guide."
    ③ "They were developed by the U.S. Department of Agriculture to discourage excesses in the diet."
    ④ "They are suggested levels of essential nutrients to meet the nutritional needs of most healthy individuals."

59. The nurse observes a child's developing awareness of his genital area and learning sexual identity. According to Freud's stages of psychosexual development, the child is in which of the following age groups?
    ① Birth to 18 months
    ② Eighteen to 36 months
    ③ Three to 6 years
    ④ Six to 12 years

60. A 30-year-old mother of an 8 month old is breast-feeding. What would you suggest as an appropriate source of high-quality iron for her infant?
    ① Raisins
    ② Carrots
    ③ Egg yolks
    ④ Yogurt

61. A child has suffered a burn to his/her hand after touching a hot stove burner. Which of the following activities should be performed *immediately* following the injury?

① Apply petroleum jelly to the burned area
② Immerse the hand in cool water
③ Apply a dry sterile gauze to the area
④ Apply an ice pack to the area

62. A 30-year-old female has a history of waking up at midnight with severe pain in the epigastrium. Her skin has a slight yellow cast. She reports noticing a darkening of her urine over the past few weeks. She also reports experiencing intermittent nausea, vomiting, and some moderate epigastric pain over the past 3 months. She is hospitalized for evaluation of the gallbladder. If her pain is of gallbladder origin, the pain would probably be precipitated by:
    ① Excessive exercise
    ② Emotional stress
    ③ Ingestion of protein
    ④ High fatty diet

63. Which would be the most beneficial intervention in dealing with your patient's mobility impairment while unconscious?
    ① Get the patient out of bed to a chair for 2 hours
    ② Turn and reposition patient q2h
    ③ Give passive range-of-motion exercises twice each shift
    ④ Place the patient in Fowler's position once each shift

64. While assessing your patient's ankle edema, in addition to inspection, which other technique would you use?
    ① Auscultation
    ② Evaluation
    ③ Palpation
    ④ Percussion

65. The nurse needs to obtain a 24-hour urine specimen from a patient. Which of the following best describes the proper method for this procedure?
    ① Have him void at 8 AM: then have him void again at 8 AM the following day; send both specimens to the laboratory
    ② Have him void at 8 AM, discarding the specimen: then collect all urine for 24 hours; at 8 AM the following day have him empty his bladder, again discarding the specimen; send the collected urine to the laboratory
    ③ Have him empty his bladder at 8 AM, discarding the specimen; collect all urine for the next 24 hours; have him void again at 8 AM the following day, adding this specimen to the container; send urine to the laboratory
    ④ Have him void at 8 AM; include this specimen in the container: collect all urine for 24 hours; at 8 AM the following day have him void and add this specimen to the container; send to the laboratory

66. Which of the following symptoms should the nurse include in explaining insulin shock to a recently diagnosed diabetes patient?
    ① Drowsiness, weakness, thirst, nausea and vomiting, dry skin, and flushed face
    ② Rapid pulse and respirations, restlessness, dizziness, headache, elevated temperature, and pain
    ③ Low blood pressure, rapid pulse, confusion, and pale, moist skin
    ④ Trembling, irritability, confusion, hunger, profuse perspiration, blurred or double vision, and poor concentration

67. A 67-year-old woman with a diagnosis of congestive heart failure is on a 500-g sodium-restricted diet. Which tray would be most appropriate for her?

① Fresh beef, salt-free cottage cheese, one small sweet potato, and one large tangerine
② Smoked fish, prepared muffins, frozen lima beans, and an apple
③ Corned beef on rye sandwich, dill pickle, and pear
④ Ham and cheese on regular bread, unsalted hard-boiled egg, and an orange

68. A patient has been admitted with right upper quadrant pain and has been placed on a low-fat diet. Which of the following trays would be acceptable for her?
① Whole milk, veal, rice, and pastry
② Liver, fried potatoes, gelatin, and avocado
③ Skim milk, lean fish, tapioca pudding, and fruit
④ Ham, mashed potatoes, creamed peas, and gelatin

69. A 72-year-old man has bladder and bowel incontinence. At a nursing care planning conference the staff decides to proceed with a bowel-retraining program. Bowel retraining is initiated before bladder retraining because:
① Bowel retraining is easier than bladder retraining
② Bowel incontinence is more demoralizing to the patient
③ Bowel retraining may solve the patient's urinary incontinence
④ The patient is usually more cooperative

70. Your patient is to receive Lanoxin 0.125 mg PO qid. Available are 0.25 mg tablets. How many tablets do you give?
① 0.5
② 5
③ 2
④ 1

71. A patient has a diagnosis of leukemia. Tylenol 650 mg is ordered prn. For which of these reasons is Tylenol ordered rather than aspirin?
① Aspirin is less effective than Tylenol in relieving pain that caused this disease
② Tylenol is absorbed in the stomach more rapidly than aspirin
③ Aspirin preparations interfere with prothrombin formation
④ Aspirin preparations have a long therapeutic effect

72. Your patient's chart reveals hypokalemia. The patient should be assessed for:
① Bleeding tendency
② Cardiac dysrhythmias
③ Nausea and vomiting
④ Thirst

73. A patient with spinal cord injury has a sudden extreme elevation in blood pressure, a throbbing headache, nasal stuffiness, sweating and flushing, and chills and pallor. These symptoms indicate:
① Urinary tract infection
② Autonomic dysreflexia
③ Transient ischemic attack
④ Septicemia

74. You have volunteered to teach a class on nutrition at the local community church. Your students range from mothers with young children to retired senior citizens. All are extremely interested in what constitutes good nutrition and ask a variety of questions on the subject. A woman states that she should increase her intake of potassium. You would state that which of the following are good sources of potassium?
① Whole grain breads, oranges, and bananas
② Egg yolk, green leafy vegetables, and raisins
③ Citrus fruits, strawberries, and green peppers
④ Sunshine, fortified milk, and fish liver oils

75. An alert 90 year old came to the hospital after falling at home and scraping her elbow. She has a history of slight vertigo for which she takes meclizine and benzodiazepine. The physician notes a cardiac murmur and orders digoxin and propranolol. Before developing the nursing care plan for this patient, the nurse should obtain:
① A history of her activities of daily living at home
② A family history of diabetes mellitus
③ A list of nursing homes that will accept her
④ The address of her children for an emergency

76. In assisting a patient who has recently suffered a CVA to improve cognitive skills, the nurse would:
① Provide memory aids and stimuli
② Provide range-of-motion exercises
③ Initiate bowel and bladder training
④ Provide leisurely, recreational activities so he doesn't have to think

77. The nurse is assisting with the development of a nursing care plan for a patient who is comatose following a stroke. Which of the following goals should have the highest priority?
① Preventing skin breakdown
② Facilitating therapeutic communication
③ Maintaining a patent airway
④ Maintaining musculoskeletal integrity

78. In observing a patient who is newly diagnosed with Parkinson's disease, the nurse should expect to find which of the following signs/symptoms?
① Ptosis and diplopia
② Blurred vision and loss of balance
③ Tremor and bradykinesia
④ Chorea and slurred speech

79. The nurse is reinforcing teaching about pulmonary tuberculosis to a newly diagnosed patient. Which of the following statements indicates the patient has a good understanding of her/his disease?
① "I cannot return to work until I have finished my entire course of medication."
② "I will take this medication until I stop coughing so much, then I can quit taking it."
③ "I suppose my children, husband, and co-workers will need to be tested for TB."
④ "I will have a positive skin test for TB until my medication is finished; then it will be negative."

80. A 36 year old has been admitted with sickle cell (SC) crisis (vasoocclusive type). Which of the following signs/symptoms would be the nurse expect to observe?
① Severe pain
② Jaundice
③ Plethora
④ Hemarthrosis

81. A 74 year old has been admitted with excessive weight loss related to Parkinson's disease. The nurse is assisting in developing a plan of care to address the patient's nutritional problems. Which of the following activities/techniques should be included in the plan of care?
① Offer a high calorie regular diet
② Encourage the patient to eat in the dining area with other patients
③ Offer a semisolid diet with thick liquids
④ Encourage the family to feed the patient

82. A 67-year-old woman has been admitted to the hospital following a syncopal episode during her weekly card game. She is alert, oriented, and pain free. Her vitals are stable but her pulse is very irregular. Which of the following cardiac rhythms is this patient experiencing?
    ① Sinus bradycardia
    ② Sinus tachycardia
    ③ Atrial fibrillation
    ④ Ventricular fibrillation

83. A patient is receiving oxygen at 50% per Venturi mask. He is a diabetic and has lung cancer. It is suppertime. His glucose check shows a blood sugar of 85. In order for the patient to eat his meal the nurse should:
    ① Assist the patient with eating by administering oxygen between bites
    ② Hyperoxygenate the patient just before the meal and then remove the mask
    ③ Apply a nasal cannula at 5 L/min during the meal
    ④ Remove the oxygen until the patient finishes his meal after obtaining an order

84. A 22 year old has been told by her physician that her physical problems of fatigue and weight loss result from a mild deficiency of daily carbohydrate intake. She asks the nurse for advice on foods to eat. The nurse tells her that about one half of a person's daily energy requirements should come from carbohydrates. The nurse advises the patient to correct her diet because a mild deficiency can lead to a serious deficiency causing:
    ① Overweight and obesity
    ② Ketosis and dehydration
    ③ Dental caries or tooth decay
    ④ Gas in the colon, known as flatulence

85. A 65-year-old woman who retired six months ago is now suffering from problems of constipation. In analyzing her diet, the nurse notices she does not walk as much as she did while working. The nurse also notes that the patient lacks dietary fiber and roughage in her daily food intake. Foods the nurse may suggest to provide bulk for stool formation and to stimulate peristalsis are:
    ① Bananas, cherries, potatoes
    ② Macaroni, pastries, noodles, potatoes
    ③ Tuna, turkey, chicken, lean meats, lobster
    ④ All-bran foods, beans, peas, popcorn, berries

86. A 30-year-old woman has been told her cholesterol level needs to be lower. She tells the nurse that she does not eat foods with cholesterol and doesn't understand why her level is so high. The nurse checks her food list for the foods she has eaten in the last week, and especially notices the following high fat foods:
    ① Homemade pizza using olive oil
    ② Liquid vegetable oils
    ③ Oat brans, few fruits and legumes
    ④ Tuna salad and ham salad sandwiches

87. A 35-year-old woman had surgery 10 hours ago for an incarcerated umbilical hernia. Now her temperature has risen to 99.2° F. Of the following possible nursing interventions, which one is *most appropriate* for the patient at this time?
    ① Offer analgesics
    ② Encourage coughing and deep breathing
    ③ Call the physician immediately
    ④ Change the abdominal dressing

88. When a medication is being administered, the safest and most accurate way for the nurse to verify a patient's identification is to:
    ① Ask the patient to state his name
    ② Ask another nurse to identify the patient
    ③ Call the patient by the name on the Kardex or the drug card
    ④ Check the patient's identification bracelet and/or the name band

89. A 36-year-old woman who has been put on thyroid hormones by the physician asks the nurse when the best time would be to take the medication. The nurse answers that thyroid hormone drugs should be administered:
    ① In divided doses, after meals
    ② In divided doses, before meals
    ③ As the patient's energy level decreases
    ④ In a single dose, normally before breakfast

90. While administering morning care to a patient with a cervical radiation implant, the nurse finds an unfamiliar metal object in the bed. The nurse will *first*:
    ① Place the object in the hazardous waste box
    ② Notify the radiation department
    ③ Notify the physician
    ④ Reinsert the implant

91. A patient who received penicillin approximately 5 minutes ago states that he feels warm and is itching. The nurse will notify the doctor immediately and then:
    ① Administer Benadryl as ordered
    ② Take vital signs every 5 minutes
    ③ Administer oxygen as ordered
    ④ Apply cool compresses to skin

92. A patient who was in a motor vehicle accident 2 days ago has a spinal cord injury at C2-C3. The patient with spinal cord injury must be observed for dysreflexia, which can be life threatening. A precursor to dysreflexia is frequently related to a problem with:
    ① Elimination
    ② Mobility
    ③ Comfort
    ④ Nutrition

93. The nurse positions the patient who had a cervical laminectomy yesterday on his back with the knee gatch up. This position is comfortable for the patient because it:
    ① Promotes tension on the lumbar area, which in turn relaxes the cervical vertebral area
    ② Relieves tension in the back muscles as it promotes tension in the lower leg
    ③ Lengthens the muscles of the back and legs to prevent muscle spasm
    ④ Shortens muscles in the scapular and neck regions, thereby relieving muscle spasms in the cervical area

94. A patient had a urinary diversion 2 days ago. His output is 50 ml for the past 2 hours. He is currently complaining of left flank pain. He has orders for morphine every 4 hours. His last dose was 5 hours ago. The nurse will:
    ① Administer the morphine
    ② Call the doctor
    ③ Assess the respirations
    ④ Turn the patient to his right side

95. In preparing a patient who has a continent urinary diversion for self-management at home, the nurse will instruct him to:

① Drink a maximum of 6 glasses of water per day
② Perform the Valsalva maneuver when catheterizing the pouch
③ Test urine pH weekly
④ Take 1500 mg of vitamin C daily

96. In providing postoperative care to a patient who had an open cholecystectomy 2 days ago, the nurse will:
① Clamp the T-tube every 4 hours for 15 minutes
② Report bile drainage of over 500 ml in 24 hours
③ Maintain tension on the T-tube
④ Report normal colored urine and stools

97. The wife of a patient who is receiving continuous feedings per gastric tube questions the nurse concerning the bright green color of her husband's stools. The nurse will inform her that the color is caused by:
① Blue food coloring
② Green food coloring
③ Multiple vitamins
④ Green vegetables

98. A patient with a gastrostomy is receiving continuous drip tube feeding. The nurse is preparing to refill his bag. His feedings are ordered at 50 ml per hour. The formula container holds 240 ml. The nurse will fill the bag with:
① 2 cans
② 200 ml
③ 1 can
④ 50 ml

99. A patient who has been taking erythromycin (EES) for an upper respiratory infection is now complaining of an upset stomach. The nurse should advise her to:
① Take the erythromycin with meals
② Take the erythromycin on an empty stomach
③ Discontinue taking the medication
④ Take the erythromycin with milk

100. A patient who has had a total thyroidectomy has a large dressing on her throat. In the immediate postoperative phase, the nurse assesses the patient frequently. Which of the following assessments warrants notifying the physician immediately?
① Serosanguineous drainage on the dressing
② A respiratory rate of 24 breaths per minute
③ Cerumen in the auditory canal
④ The patient's hoarse voice

101. A 36-year-old woman is concerned that she may be HIV positive because of her history of multiple sexual partners. Which of the following is an early symptom of HIV infection?
① Cytomegalovirus infection
② Lymphadenopathy and fever
③ *Pneumocystis carinii* pneumonia
④ Multiple resistant *Staph aureus* infection

102. A 57-year-old woman has recently been diagnosed with osteoporosis. Where is she most likely to have compression fractures as the result of her osteoporosis?
① The tibia
② The calcaneous
③ The ribs
④ The vertebrae

103. The nurse suspects that a 24-year-old motorcyclist with bilateral femoral fractures may be experiencing a fat embolus. Which of the following questions should be included in the assessment of the patient at this time?

① "Can you wiggle your toes?"
② "What is today's date?"
③ "How do you rate your pain?"
④ "How many fingers am I holding up?"

104. Two weeks after receiving chemotherapy, the patient has developed petechiae on her abdomen. Her gums and nose tend to bleed easily now. She also has a large ecchymotic area on her right arm where she bumped into a door yesterday. Which of the following laboratory findings would be consistent with this patient's condition?
① An elevated leukocyte count
② A decreased serum calcium
③ A decreased platelet count
④ An elevated blood urea nitrogen

105. A 66-year-old woman needs to have a bowel resection for cancer. She weighs 93 kg and is 150 cm tall. She is taking digoxin (Lanoxin) 0.125 mg daily. Her potassium level is 4.0 mEq/L. Which of the above factors increases this patient's risk for postoperative complications?
① Her age
② Her weight
③ Her daily medication
④ Her potassium level

106. A woman has just been told that there is no more medical treatment for her ovarian cancer. She has been withdrawn and quiet the past few days. The nurse can best help this patient cope with her depression by:
① Advising her to telephone her family
② Asking the physician to prescribe antidepressants for the patient
③ Suggesting she focus on the happier times in her life
④ Allowing the patient time to express her feelings

107. A 32-year-old farmer who sustained a traumatic amputation of his left hand in a corn picking accident 2 weeks ago has verbally expressed acceptance of his altered body image. The nurse overhears the patient yelling at his wife to leave and get herself "a real man." Nursing assessment of this situation is:
① The patient is still in the grieving process
② The patient has serious marital problems
③ The patient is anxious today
④ The patient is depressed today

108. A patient has been admitted to the hospital with acute pancreatitis. The primary reason for the nurse asking the patient questions about home living arrangements during the initial admission assessment is to:
① Develop rapport with the patient
② Identify potential discharge problems
③ Identify areas needing lifestyle changes
④ Assess self-care deficits

109. A patient with a dislocated left shoulder, which was reduced in the emergency room by an orthopedist, received a prescription for acetamenophin with codeine (Tylenol #3) for pain. How many milligrams of codeine are there in each pill?
① 15 mg
② 30 mg
③ 45 mg
④ 60 mg

110. A 77 year old has been receiving heparin sodium (Heparin) to prevent deep vein thrombosis following surgery. Which of the following would be a safe place for an injection of Heparin?
    ① Bruised tissue
    ② Scar tissue
    ③ Freckles
    ④ Moles

111. A 55-year-old patient is beginning a course of radiation to his abdomen in hopes of shrinking his tumor. The nurse anticipates which of the following side-effects from abdominal radiation?
    ① Stomatitis
    ② Thrombocytopenia
    ③ Alopecia
    ④ Nausea

112. A 60-year-old man has been admitted to the hospital with gastroenteritis and dehydration. The physician has ordered the IV to run at 125 cc/hr. The nurse utilizes tubing that delivers 10 gtts/ml. The amount of drops per minute for this order is:
    ① 8 gtts/min
    ② 12 gtts/min
    ③ 15 gtts/min
    ④ 21 gtts/min

113. A 35-year-old patient has a subclavian IV site following traumatic bilateral arm amputation. He is complaining of shortness of breath, and his lips and nailbeds are cyanotic. Upon examination, the nurse notes his IV has a loose connection and a stream of small bubbles is entering the IV system. The nurse should:
    ① Not be concerned as they are only small bubbles
    ② Position the patient on his left side
    ③ Elevate the head of the bed
    ④ Discontinue the IV

114. A 62-year-old woman is receiving radiation therapy to her left humerus for a metastatic bone lesion. Following her first treatment, she shows the nurse pen marks on her arm. When caring for the arm, the nurse should:
    ① Apply lotion twice daily to prevent dryness
    ② Apply baby oil twice daily to remove the marks
    ③ Remove the marks with nail polish remover
    ④ Sponge the area with plain water daily

115. A 44-year-old woman needs to have abdominal surgery. The nurse explains and demonstrates coughing and deep breathing exercises preoperatively to the patient. The rationale for splinting the abdomen during these exercises is that it:
    ① Prevents vomiting and aspiration
    ② Decreases postoperative pain
    ③ Prevents rib fractures
    ④ Increases bowel motility

116. A 47-year-old patient received an injection of meperidine (Demerol) in her right gluteus medius muscle. The nurse administering the injection carefully located the posterior superior iliac spine, the iliac crest, and the head of the greater trochanter to prevent injury to the:
    ① Brachial nerve plexus
    ② Femoral artery
    ③ Sciatic nerve
    ④ Greater saphenous vein

117. A 78 year old has fractured his left femur in a fall. He will have a total hip arthroplasty in the morning. The physician has ordered the patient to be NPO after midnight. The nurse explains this order to him as:
    ① "You can't have anything to eat after midnight."
    ② "The doctor says you may have nothing per orifice since midnight."
    ③ "You can't have anything to drink after dinner."
    ④ "You may not eat or drink anything after midnight."

118. A 55-year-old patient has been receiving an IV of 0.45% normal saline at 500 cc/hr for diabetic ketoacidosis. She is complaining that the IV site is painful. Upon inspection, the nurse notes the site is swollen, red, and warm to the touch. The nurse analyzes the patient's problem as:
    ① Thrombophlebitis at the IV site
    ② IV infiltration
    ③ Circulatory overload
    ④ Speed shock

119. A 22 year old who injured his right knee when playing football is scheduled for an arthroscopy. The nurse explains to him that this procedure involves:
    ① An x-ray using radiographic dye
    ② Visualization of the joint with a small instrument
    ③ Obtaining a bone biopsy
    ④ Aspiration of the synovial fluid from the capsule

120. A 21-year-old college student has been diagnosed with a gastric ulcer. The nurse has included in the discharge instructions a warning to avoid antiinflammatory drugs. Which of the following drugs would be safe for her to take for mild discomfort?
    ① Aspirin
    ② Ibuprofen (Motrin)
    ③ Naproxen (Naprosyn)
    ④ Acetaminophin (Tylenol)

121. A cancer patient is to begin a regimen of three chemotherapeutic drugs for her cancer. The nurse explains the rationale for the multiple drug regimen as:
    ① "Combinations of drugs allow easier access to the blood/brain barrier."
    ② "It is beneficial for end-stage cancer to use any combination of drugs."
    ③ "Combinations of drugs affect different parts of cell reproduction."
    ④ "The more aggressive the tumor, the more aggressive the treatment."

122. A patient with pneumococcal pneumonia has been prescribed cephalexin (Keflex) 240 mg PO qid for 10 days. The nurse explains that he must take all of the pills for the full 10 days. The rationale for this is:
    ① Discontinuing the prescription may allow the bacteria to continue growing
    ② The symptoms of pneumonia won't resolve until all the medication is gone
    ③ Cephalexin has a cumulative effect
    ④ The pneumococcal virus may live for 10 days

123. A patient has had an IV in her left hand for several days. The nurse determined that the IV had infiltrated. To care for the left hand following IV infiltration, the nurse should:
    ① Apply ice for 40 minutes every hour for 24 hours
    ② Elevate the right hand on a pillow
    ③ Apply a warm, moist compress
    ④ Place the left hand in a dependent position

124. A 44-year-old man who has been receiving radiation for his astrocytoma is experiencing stomatitis. To ease his stomatitis, the nurse should:
① Assist the patient with oral care after meals
② Offer the patient support regarding his changed body image
③ Request an antiinflammatory drug from the doctor
④ Request that the dietitian enhance the flavor of his food with spices

125. A 92-year-old man tripped over his sleeping dog and fractured his right trochanter. While waiting for surgery, what type of traction should the nurse expect to apply to the patient?
① Buck's traction
② Crutchfield tongs
③ Bryant's traction
④ Russell's traction

ANSWERS AND RATIONALES FOR COMPREHENSIVE EXAMINATIONS

COMPREHENSIVE EXAMINATION 1: PART 1

1. Comprehension, planning, environment (c)
   - ❸ Abrupt onset of confusion relates to side-effects of antihistamine, benzodiazepine, beta blocker, and cardiac glycoside combination.
   - ① Would not resolve situation.
   - ② Would not resolve situation and is not necessary.
   - ④ Not necessary.

2. Application, assessment, environment (a)
   - ❷ Pulse rate is below 60 beats/min.
   - ①,③,④ Could lead to adverse reactions.

3. Comprehension, planning, physiologic (a)
   - ❹ When the bile duct is explored for stones, edema could ensue and block the duct, hindering bile flow. The T-tube maintains patency.
   - ①,③ The tube is not placed in the abdominal cavity nor in the intestines.
   - ② Not the primary purpose of the tube in this situation.

4. Comprehension, planning, health (b)
   - ❷ Injury could lead to infection. The tissues are already compromised of oxygen and nutrients; certain positions (legs crossed, knees flexed) hamper circulation.
   - ①,③,④ Measure could lead to greater compromise in circulation and burns.

5. Knowledge (a)
   - ❶ The matter must be brought to the attention of the supervisor, since the supervisor is responsible for the patient's welfare.
   - ② The nurse must inspire the patient to have confidence in his physician and must never advocate dismissal or replacement of a physician.
   - ③,④ Not proper chain of command.

6. Application, implementation, health (a)
   - ❷ Smoking decreases pulmonary function; sarcoidosis compromises lung capacity.
   - ① Focus treatment on healing; patient cannot assess pulmonary function.
   - ③ Physician will monitor any increased involvement; too involved for patient.
   - ④ Focus treatment on positive aspects of healing because course of disease is to resolution.

7. Application, planning, environment (a)
   - ❷ 60 mg = 1 gr
     60 × 5 = 300 mg/tablet: 2 tablets = 600 mg.
   - ①,③,④ Incorrect dose.

8. Comprehension, implementation, environment (a)
   - ❶ Stop the flow of the IV fluids to prevent further swelling and report to charge nurse.
   - ②,③,④ Inappropriate responses that will not correct the stated situation.

9. Knowledge, evaluation, health (b)
   - ❸ Following cholecystectomy, most patients can return to a normal diet as long as they avoid excessive fat intake.
   - ①,②,④ Incorrect response related to diet as indicated above.

10. Comprehension (a)
    - ❷ The board of nursing implements the laws governing the practice of nursing.
    - ① Defines the practice of nursing; does not establish nursing procedures.
    - ③ Accredits schools of nursing based on predetermined established standards.
    - ④ Does not oversee in-service programs. Documentation of continuing education required in some states for license renewal.

11. Knowledge (a)
    - ❷ Possession of a nursing license means the nurse has met the requirements of minimal safe practice, which primarily protects the public and nursing practice.
    - ① Employer required to employ only licensed nurses or new graduate scheduled to take next exam.
    - ③ See rationale for #2.
    - ④ Nursing malpractice is failure to possess and exercise the knowledge and skills of a reasonable and prudent nurse.

12. Comprehension, assessment, environment (b)
    - ❹ Chest pain that radiates is a significant finding.
    - ①,③ Not associated with chest pain.
    - ② Increases in respiration caused by anxiety is common.

13. Application, planning, health (a)
    - ❶ In primary hypofunction (not the result of a pituitary disturbance), the therapy is lifelong.
    - ②,③,④ Hormonal therapy is not classically adjusted on a day-to-day basis, nor is hormonal therapy, in this case, temporary or intermittent.

14. Knowledge, assessment, physiologic (a)
    - ❶ Dietary requirements for a diabetic patient are calculated on the basis of age, sex, body build, weight, and activity. They should be the same as those of a nondiabetic patient.
    - ② Diet will be lower in calories only if the diabetic patient is overweight.
    - ③ Diabetic diet contains approximately 50% to 60% carbohydrates, equal to a well-balanced diet of a nondiabetic patient.
    - ④ Should be equal in protein to that of a nondiabetic patient.

15. Comprehension, implementation, physiologic (c)
    - ❷ Airway is compromised; administer oxygen to prevent shock.
    - ① Not the priority.
    - ③ Should be done but not the first priority.
    - ④ Not the priority, and vital signs should be taken before placing patient in high-Fowler's position.

16. Comprehension, planning, environment (b)
    - ❶ Expedient examination and treatment are appropriate for an already traumatized victim.
    - ② Inappropriate, because victim should never be left alone and if left to own devices may not seek medical care.
    - ③ Privacy should be provided but victim should not be left alone.
    - ④ Accommodations for bathing and douching should not be offered until examination and treatment are completed.

17. Knowledge, assessment, environment (b)
    ❶ Follow rule of nines.
    Left leg = 18%
    Right leg = 18%
    Right arm = 9%
    Total = 45%
    ②,③,④ Does not follow rule of nines.
18. Application, implementation, environment (b)
    ❸ Roll victim in carpet or blankets to extinguish fire or use water.
    ①,④ Victim is screaming hysterically and should not be relied on to hear or follow instructions.
    ② Extinguish the fire and have someone call the fire department.
19. Comprehension, planning, environment (a)
    ❷ Many states have Good Samaritan laws to encourage medical aid at the scene of an accident by limiting the legal liability that might arise.
    ① It is not mandatory for nurses or physicians to render emergency aid.
    ③ It is expected that the person rendering aid will act as a reasonable, prudent person would act under similar circumstances. A higher standard of medical aid would be expected of a nurse, physician, and members of a first-aid squad than that of the average general public.
    ④ Laws vary in each state.
20. Comprehension, evaluation, environment (b)
    ❶ Victim should be observed for laryngeal and tracheal edema because the degree of inhalation burns is unknown.
    ②,③,④ Characteristic of second-degree burns; previously determined that victim has second-degree burns.
21. Application, assessment, physiologic (a)
    ❶ The patient has little or no renal function; most of the fluid intake is retained and will be indicated in the weight; after the procedure, fluid removed will be reflected in the weight.
    ② Visits from people with infections must be avoided; others are allowed.
    ③ The patient may eat; meals are served in the dialysis unit.
    ④ A catheter will not be in place; there is no (or scant) urine output to measure; voiding is not the problem.
22. Knowledge, implementation, physiologic (c)
    ❹ This dissolves uric acid crystals; specific for pruritus in uremia.
    ①,② Nursing intervention for dry skin.
    ③ Water should be tepid in the bath; hot water is drying.
23. Comprehension, planning, health (b)
    ❸ Has increased susceptibility to infection; may be life threatening.
    ① Important but not first priority.
    ② Goal of the dialysis procedure, not the nurse.
    ④ Only for immobile (comatose) patient.
24. Comprehension, assessment, health (a)
    ❷ Developed in the 1960s and routine in most public schools.
    ①,③,④ Not relevant diagnostic tests for scoliosis.
25. Knowledge, assessment, environment (a)
    ❷ Normal hemoglobin level for women: 12 to 16 g/dl.
    ①,③,④ Normal values.

26. Application, implementation, health (a)
    ❷ Drawing blood could lead to serious infection.
    ①,③,④ Appropriate instructions allowing blood pressure (not pulse) to be taken on affected side.
27. Application, planning, environment (b)
    ❶ A victim suspected of having an injury to the spine is never moved because of the risk of causing paralysis.
    ②,③ Any movement may cause further damage.
    ④ This is not the proper procedure for assessing pulmonary status.
28. Knowledge, assessment, physiologic (a)
    ❹ Tachycardia is a heart rate greater than 100 beats/min.
    ① Bradycardia.
    ② Normal rate.
    ③ Higher than bradycardia; lower than tachycardia.
29. Knowledge, implementation, health (a)
    ❶ Massaging the area and avoiding repeated pressure will enhance circulation.
    ②,③,④ Inappropriate nursing action for pressure areas.
30. Comprehension, planning, environment (a)
    ❶ The AIDS virus attacks the immune system.
    ② His age, 37, would not be a factor—immunity is lessened in the elderly.
    ③ Immunity has no relationship to one's sexual preference.
    ④ No medication given to this patient with bone marrow suppression.
31. Comprehension, implementation, environment (a)
    ❹ These are the modes of transmission.
    ①,②,③ Not necessary to contain the virus.
32. Application, implementation, environment (a)
    ❸ Local anesthesia is given before bronchoscopy. During the procedure the gag reflex is absent and may not have returned when the patient is returned to his room.
    ① Activity is not restricted.
    ② No dye used in procedure.
    ④ NPO until gag reflex returns.
33. Comprehension, implementation, health (b)
    ❹ May indicate that too much thyroid hormone is in the system.
    ① Not a standard aspect of teaching for a thyroid medication.
    ②,③ See rationale for #1.
34. Knowledge, assessment, physiologic (b)
    ❹ Classic symptoms of hypothyroidism.
    ① Symptoms of Cushing's disease.
    ② Seen in diabetes mellitus.
    ③ Frequency is not a classic symptom.
35. Knowledge, assessment, physiologic (b)
    ❷ Elderly have a decreased need for calories.
    ①,③ Caloric needs are decreased.
    ④ Nutritional needs are the same as those for other adults.
36. Knowledge, implementation, physiologic (a)
    ❸ In a hospital setting, insertion of a Foley catheter must always be done with sterile technique.
    ① Strict reverse isolation is not appropriate here.
    ② Medical aseptic technique can be used by clients in their home setting.
    ④ Good handwashing is always a priority, but the actual Foley insertion must be done with sterile technique.

37. Application, planning, physiologic (b)
    ❸ Clear liquids help reduce peristalsis and are usually given postop for 1 to 3 days after bowel sounds are heard.
    ① A clear liquid diet slows down the activity in the colon, not to activate or speed it up.
    ② One is not put on a clear liquid diet to lose weight after surgery.
    ④ It is not necessary to rest the throat after gallbladder surgery. Clear liquids help keep the throat comfortable.

38. Comprehension, assessment, physiologic (c)
    ❹ The patient's fluid and electrolyte status would be the most important diagnosis at this time, because of the client's repeated emesis.
    ① The patient may or may not be experiencing a self-care deficit at this time.
    ② It is not known whether the patient is suffering an alteration in elimination patterns.
    ③ The patient may or may not be experiencing alterations in tissue perfusion.

39. Application, planning, environment (c)
    ❶ This allows the nurse to perform skills completely, yet decreases the amount of time that the nurse must spend in the radioactive environment.
    ② Entering the patient's room frequently exposes the nurse to the radioactive environment: the implant should not be visible for the nurse to assess.
    ③ This increases the amount of time the nurse spends in the radioactive environment.
    ④ Although it is important to decrease the loneliness of an isolated patient, this measure would increase the amount of time the nurse is in the radioactive environment.

40. Knowledge, implementation, environment (a)
    ❹ Handwashing is the first step in infection control for any nursing skills.
    ① Although donning clean gloves is an important step in infection control for this procedure, it is not the first step.
    ② Sterile gloving is not necessary for the administration of an injection.
    ③ Swabbing the site with alcohol is an important step in infection control for this procedure, but it is not the first step.

41. Knowledge, assessment, physiologic (b)
    ❷ The water seal chamber is designed to allow air to exit from the lung, but does not allow air to enter the lung.
    ① The suction chamber applies suction pressure to the chest tube to facilitate drainage of the chest tube.
    ② The drainage chamber's only function is that of a collection chamber for drainage.
    ④ There is no such chamber in chest tube management systems.

42. Comprehension, assessment, physiologic (c)
    ❸ Capillary refill times exceeding 3 seconds are indicative of compromised circulatory status.
    ① A bounding pulse is indicative of good circulatory status.
    ② Good circulatory status is manifested by a warm extremity.
    ④ Perceiving light touch is indicative of intact circulatory status.

43. Comprehension, assessment, physiologic (b)
    ❹ The patient indicates that his stomach is rumbling, which indicates that normal peristalsis has resumed and an oral intake can be started.
    ① Patients may feel hungry regardless of peristalsis.
    ② The patient who feels bloated is most likely unable to tolerate oral feeding because of abdominal discomfort.
    ③ The stool the patient passed may have been in the bowel before the surgery. This is not an accurate indicator for readiness of oral intake.

44. Knowledge, assessment, environment (b)
    ❶ Agnosia is the inability to recognize commonly used objects of daily living.
    ② Projection is a defense mechanism manifested by blaming another for one's own faults.
    ③ Displacement is a defense mechanism characterized by the rationalization of one's own actions.
    ④ Confabulation is a technique used by demented patients to fabricate explanations for events that they may not remember.

45. Comprehension, planning, health, (b)
    ❷ Strict vegetarians may lack protein in their diet because they do not consume meat or meat products.
    ① Fats are permitted in a strict vegetarian diet.
    ③ Disaccharides are a form of carbohydrate, which is abundant in a strict vegetarian diet.
    ④ Monosaccharides are a form of carbohydrate, which is abundant in a strict vegetarian diet.

46. Comprehension, planning, physiologic (c)
    ❷ The patient with congestive heart failure will have a pronounced fluid volume excess stemming from the inability of the heart to pump effectively.
    ① A knowledge deficit has not been identified for this patient.
    ③ Patients with congestive heart failure normally have fluid overload and not fluid volume deficit.
    ④ Although altered thought processes may occur in a patient with congestive heart failure, this problem has not been identified in the question.

47. Application, assessment, physiologic (b)
    ❶ Paresthesia may result from pressure on a nerve.
    ② Volkmann's contracture affects the arm.
    ③ Dupuytren's contracture affects the hand.
    ④ Compartment syndrome occurs when there is increased fluid in an encapsulated muscle.

48. Comprehension, assessment, environment (b)
    ❷ Protecting patient safety is the highest priority, and steps need to be taken immediately with a blood sugar this high. The nurse needs to call the physician stat.
    ① Ensuring adequate rest is not a high priority when a blood sugar is too high.
    ③ Checking nutritional intake can be done after notifying physician of patient's blood sugar and getting orders for insulin.
    ④ Bed rest does not take priority over taking steps to notify physician.

49. Application, assessment, physiologic (b)
    ❸ Offering to stay with the patient is the best choice and will help to reduce his anxiety, knowing that the nurse is in the room with him.
    ① That is not comforting. Most people today know that a diastolic reading over 100 is a concern.

② This is not necessarily true or comforting to a patient, especially if the nurses are busy or slow in answering call lights.

④ Never suggest to an anxious patient that their medicine may not be working. That will raise the patient's anxiety level.

50. Comprehension, assessment, physiologic (c)
❷ Phase two is the transport phase. Problems swallowing here can indicate spasms or carcinoma.
① Phase one is the transfer phase, consisting of chewing and moistening of the food with saliva.
③ Phase three is the entrance phase, where the food moves through the esophageal sphincter into the stomach. Problems here may indicate esophageal narrowing and other disorders.
④ Phase four does not exist. There are only three phases concerned with swallowing.

51. Knowledge, implementation, health (a)
❸ These fruits are excellent sources of potassium and contain only negligible amounts of sodium.
① Apples and plums are not a source of potassium.
② Canned fruit cocktail is not a decent source of potassium; it also has extra sugar and sodium.
④ Berries, grapes, and pears are sources of vitamins, but not rich sources of potassium.

52. Knowledge, planning, health (b)
❹ These foods are particularly high in sodium and should be avoided by a patient with edema and hypertension.
① These foods are low in sodium and are acceptable.
② These foods have very little sodium and are acceptable.
③ These foods have very little sodium and are recommended for a patient who needs to cut down on sodium.

53. Knowledge, implementation, physiologic (b)
❶ Noncompliance with prescribed therapy is the number one reason that tuberculosis is on the increase. Many refuse to take the medicines or stop taking them because of their unpleasant side-effects.
② Crowded cities and homeless street people also contribute to the increase in TB, but the number one factor is noncompliance with prescribed therapy.
③ The medicines being prescribed are: isoniazid (INH) with rifampin (RIF), streptomycin (SM), ethambutol (EMB), or parazinamide (PZA) given for 9 to 12 months. Failure to remain on these medications is a problem because of the side-effects suffered.
④ Population and smog are not factors in the rise of TB.

54. Knowledge, assessment, physiologic (b)
❹ Systemic lupus erythematosus causes a red "butterfly" pattern on the face, as well as a slight fever and soreness in joints. It is believed to be an autoimmune disorder and affects collagen.
① Scleroderma is a condition in which the skin becomes tight and smooth. Movement becomes difficult. It is thought to be an autoimmune disorder.
② Raynaud's disease is a cardiovascular problem characterized by periodic constriction of arteries usually manifested in the fingers. It can occur in the toes, causing them to become red and eventually cyanotic.
③ Periarteritis nodosa is a disorder that causes nodules that appear along a course of arteries. The nodules cause muscle and joint pain.

55. Application, planning, environment (b)
❸ Offering negative opinions about the level of a physician's expertise is a type of slander. This character attack is uttered orally in the presence of others.
① Libel is a damaging statement that is written and then read by other people.
② Assault is an act in which there is a threat or an attempt to do bodily harm to another person.
④ Defamation is an act in which untrue information that harms a person's reputation is passed on.

56. Knowledge, evaluation, physiologic (c)
❸ These are the symptoms of toxicity effects that may be experienced from a client on AZT (zidovudine).
① Stomatitis and fevers are toxic effects of ddC (dideoxycytidine).
② Painful peripheral nerves are caused by ddI (dideoxyinosine).
④ Painful peripheral nerves and anemia are caused by d4T (dideoxythymidine).

57. Application, assessment, physiologic (c)
❹ Increased potassium levels (hyperkalemia) are noted because the ions move from damaged cells to the bloodstream.
① Sodium levels are initially increased. This condition is known as hypernatremia.
② Both sodium and potassium levels are initially affected. They both increase.
③ No. Potassium levels are initially increased as the ion moves from damaged cells to the bloodstream.

58. Knowledge, assessment, physiologic (b)
❷ The behaviors listed above describe the second stage of Alzheimer's disease.
① The first stage is described as a slight memory loss and disorientation, with mild behavior changes.
③ The third stage of Alzheimer's disease is when the patient may not recognize family members, is incontinent, and walks with an unsteady gait.
④ The fourth stage results in the patient having incoherent speech, total incontinence, and inability to ambulate well or not at all.

59. Knowledge, implementation, physiologic (b)
❷ Presbycusis is progressive hearing loss and is associated with aging.
① Tinnitus is a ringing in the ear that has various causes.
③ Otosclerosis is an inherited bone disorder impairing conduction by causing structural irregularities in the stapes.
④ Ménière's disease is the term for the episodic symptoms created by fluctuations in the production or reabsorption of fluid within the inner ear lobe.

60. Application, implementation, environment (a)
❷ Standard (universal) precautions advise that gloves are to be worn whenever one comes into contact with blood or any body fluid.
① It is not necessary to wear sterile gloves; one cannot keep them sterile anyway. A gown is not necessary unless the patient is also in wound/drainage isolation.
③ A mask is not necessary unless the AIDS patient has active tuberculosis or an MRSA infection.
④ Gloves are not necessary unless one will come into actual contact with any body secretion.

61. Knowledge, comprehension, physiologic (b)
    ❹ Biochemical individuality is the term described in the question.
    ① Metabolism means the sum of all chemical changes that take place in the body.
    ② Deamination is the process of nitrogen converting to ammonia (NH_3).
    ③ Basal metabolism is the term used to define the amount of energy needed by the body for maintenance of life.

62. Application, planning, physiologic (b)
    ❷ Liquids help keep one hydrated and comfortable. Food also provides needed energy, although with this diagnosis the patient will usually only take 1 or 2 bites of food. Liquids should be high in calories to give the patient energy.
    ① Medications will have to be used to keep the patient free from any pain.
    ③ With advanced cancer of the liver, most patients become bedfast and need help with all ADLs.
    ④ Side effects from chemotherapy usually occur with most patients and have to be addressed. Planning of food and fluids has to consider whether or not the patient is nauseated.

63. Knowledge, comprehension, health (a)
    ❹ Evaluation consists of noting how the patient is doing and whether or not the planned care is working.
    ① Assessment is the initial overall view of the patient and what the patient is able to do after having a stroke.
    ② Planning is the care to be carried out by the nurse.
    ③ Implementation is the actual care plan being carried out by the nurse.

64. Application, assessment, health (b)
    ❹ This could be a dangerous practice. Hypertensive medications are to be taken on a schedule.
    ① Cutting down on salt should be encouraged and is recommended for those with hypertension.
    ② Walking and exercise should be encouraged and have been shown to benefit hypertensive patients.
    ③ Losing weight and reducing fats are good for the patient and should be encouraged.

65. Knowledge, assessment, health (b)
    ❸ Animal foods have high levels of cholesterol in their tissue.
    ① Liquid vegetable oils are recommended for cooking.
    ② Soft margarine can be substituted for butter and has less cholesterol than butter.
    ④ This food binds with cholesterol-containing substances and prevents reabsorption by the blood.

66. Knowledge, implementation, physiologic (b)
    ❹ The creatinine clearance test is used to determine kidney function.
    ① Protein in the urine is detected by dipping a test reagent such as an Albustix in urine and comparing color changes with the provided color chart.
    ② Urine concentration is determined by a specific gravity test.
    ③ The BUN (blood-urea-nitrogen) is determined by blood chemistries.

67. Knowledge, assessment, physiologic (a)
    ❸ Bruises on his upper arms indicates bleeding and the physician needs to be notified to order lab tests.
    ① Smoking and a cough go hand in hand and have nothing to do with taking warfarin sodium.
    ② Nasal congestion needs to be reported only if the nurse notes blood in it.
    ④ This weight loss is not significant, unless the client reports blood in the stools. Three pounds could be water loss. The nurse would want to recheck this on the next visit.

68. Knowledge, assessment, physiologic (a)
    ❹ Kussmaul's respirations are faster and deeper than normal respirations. They are without pauses. They are labored and resemble sighs.
    ① Eupnea is a term that refers to a normal rate and rhythm.
    ② Hyperpnea is a term that means respirations are deeper than normal. They are at a normal rate.
    ③ Cheyne-Stokes refers to respirations that are fast and deeper than normal. They are followed by slower respirations over 30- to 170-second periods. One also sees periods of apnea lasting 20 to 60 seconds.

69. Knowledge, planning, physiologic (b)
    ❷ The specific gravity indicates dehydration. Six to 8 glasses daily are recommended for this.
    ① Jaundice is not related to specific gravity.
    ③ Range of motion will not help dehydration problems.
    ④ Dehydration is uncomfortable, but not painful. The most important thing for the nurse to do in this case is encourage fluid intake.

70. Knowledge, assessment, physiologic (b)
    ❹ Positioning the thermometer in the axillar area with the tip pointing toward the patient's head is the correct procedure.
    ① The axilla needs to be patted gently dry. Heat travels through moisture.
    ② Never rub the axillar area dry, as rubbing generates heat and will give a false temperature.
    ③ The tip should point up toward the patient's head.

71. Comprehension, evaluation, environment (c)
    ❸ The goal is inappropriate and too difficult for the type of patient.
    ① See rationale for #3.
    ② The goal itself is not too broad, just unrealistic.
    ④ It is not long term as stated (24 hours).

72. Knowledge, planning, environment (a)
    ❸ First level of the hierarchy.
    ①,② High level of the hierarchy.
    ④ Second level of the hierarchy.

73. Comprehension, assessment, psychosocial (a)
    ❹ Causes of mental illness are considered to be multifactorial.
    ① There is incomplete evidence of the biochemical basis of mental illness.
    ② There is incomplete evidence that developmental conflicts are the only causative agents.
    ③ Although true, it does not sufficiently explain the causes of mental illness.

74. Knowledge, assessment, psychosocial (a)
    ❸ Freud believed the struggle between internal forces to be the basis of human behavior.

① Freud theorized that there are three stages of ego development.

② Freud did not take environmental factors into consideration to any great extent.

④ Freud did not give much consideration to interpersonal conflict.

75. Comprehension, assessment, environment (a)

❸ Exaggerated ideas of one's power or influence are usually delusions of grandeur.

① Tactile hallucination refers to the false sense that there is something on one's skin.

② Flight of ideas refers to scattered thoughts, which are manifested by illogical connections made during verbalization.

④ Neurosis is not usually characterized by delusion.

76. Comprehension, assessment, psychosocial (a)

❸ Denial is indicated by the patient's inability to recognize the seriousness of his act and his belief that he can go home.

① Sublimation is the process by which negative impulses are channeled into more acceptable outlets.

② Projection is the placing of unacceptable impulses onto another person.

④ Regression is the moving back to an earlier time or developmental level during periods of stress.

77. Comprehension, assessment, psychosocial (a)

❷ Flight of ideas refers to scattered thoughts, as evidenced by illogical connections made during verbalizations.

① Confusion is usually a matter of being disoriented as to time, place, or person.

③ Delusions are fixed false beliefs.

④ Hallucinations are the perceptions of sensory stimuli when no external objects are present.

78. Knowledge, assessment, health (a)

❹ Correct assessment.

① Not likely to be delusions.

② Unlikely.

③ Incorrect; symptoms may worsen.

79. Knowledge, assessment, psychosocial (a)

❷ A goal of community mental health is to maintain patients in the community.

① Some patients are hospitalized.

③ Usually treated in general hospital units in the community.

④ Hospitalizations are usually short term.

80. Knowledge, assessment, psychosocial (b)

❸ Behavior, because behavior ultimately defines health.

① Scientific studies in psychiatry are often inconclusive.

② Culture plays a role but is not an overriding factor.

④ Feelings are not observable; therefore they cannot be used to define.

81. Application, assessment, physiologic (b)

❷ Petty complaints usually indicate that the person is angry at the situation.

① Patients in denial usually go on believing that everything is all right.

③ Patients who are depressed are usually quite withdrawn.

④ Acceptance of the disease usually results in a calm, positive approach.

82. Application, assessment, psychosocial (b)

❹ The nurse needs to respond to the patient's feelings and thoughts as well as giving hope. The prognosis for bladder cancer can be good depending on the stage of the tumor.

① This is false reassurance, and the nurse does not know what the outcome may be.

② This is a put-down and belittles the patient. It also makes light of the patient's fears.

③ Changing the subject by referring to his family is not appropriate at this point. The patient's feelings and thoughts need to be addressed first.

83. Knowledge, comprehension, psychosocial (b)

❸ Trying to reason with him is the best and most difficult step, because alcoholics who are not recovering are unreasonable. If he leaves, the nurse needs to notify the physician immediately.

① Detaining him would violate the patient's legal rights.

② Restraints require a physician order as well as being a rights violation.

④ It is not against the law for a patient to leave. The nurse needs to point out to the patient that many insurances will not pay for this admission or future admissions when one goes AMA.

84. Knowledge, assessment, psychosocial (b)

❸ Burnout occurs when one becomes overwhelmed by a stressor. It occurs on stressful nursing units.

① Physical exhaustion is being tired and feeling fatigued to the point that one can no longer function.

② Acting in a hostile manner, as well as being forgetful, can happen to one approaching burnout.

④ This does not define burnout. Even well-adjusted persons may have trouble thinking clearly or making constructive decisions during a crisis.

85. Knowledge, assessment, psychosocial (b)

❷ An unknown stimulus is known to cause anxiety. Stress reactions happen when there is a source believed to be threatening and when it is not obvious to the person involved.

① An obvious threat causes fear, not anxiety.

③ Fear usually results from external threats.

④ No. Everyone experiences anxiety at some point in their lives. This can be mild, moderate, or severe.

86. Knowledge, implementation, physiologic (a)

❷ Suspected spinal cord injuries should be handled with care to prevent further damage to the spinal cord.

① Spinal cord injury is main concern; fractures of extremities are secondary.

③,④ Not relevant to situation.

87. Knowledge, planning, environment (a)

❹ Oxygen therapy for the newborn must be administered with great caution to prevent retrolental fibroplasia. This condition is caused by high levels of oxygen concentration and may result in blindness.

① Purulent gonococcal conjunctivitis.

② Hemolytic disease, which is hereditary.

③ Acute lung disease of newborn, caused by deficiency of pulmonary surfactant.

88. Knowledge, planning, environment (b)
❹ Any trauma to the meningocele sac can cause further neurologic damage and infection.
① Nursing action for meeting nursing goal.
② A nursing observation specific to an infant with a myelomeningocele.
③ Not applicable at this time.

89. Knowledge, assessment, environment (b)
❷ As the cerebrospinal fluid accumulates, the neonate's or infant's head increases in size (noted by separation of cranial sutures and increased head circumference), and intracranial pressure increases.
①,③,④ Not all reflective of signs and symptoms of increased intracranial pressure.

90. Application, implementation, environment (a)
❷ DD = 4 mg
DH = 10 mg
V = 1 ml

$$\frac{DD}{DH} = \frac{4 \text{ mg}}{10 \text{ mg} \times 1 \text{ ml}} = 0.4 \text{ ml}.$$

①,③,④ This is not the correct amount.

91. Application, implementation, environment (a)
❷ $$\frac{\text{Weight in pounds (30)} \times \text{Adult dose (10 mg)}}{150} =$$

$$\frac{300}{150} = 2 \text{ mg}.$$

①,③,④ This is not the correct answer.

92. Knowledge, assessment, physiologic (a)
❶ The most common classic sign of pyloric stenosis is projectile vomiting.
②,③,④ These are not common symptoms of pyloric stenosis.

93. Application, implementation, environment (b)
❶ To be adhesive and to seal, the self-adhesive plastic bag must be applied to a clean, dry area.
②,③,④ Incorrect procedure for obtaining urine specimen from infant.

94. Comprehension, assessment, environment (a)
❷ These are symptoms of chickenpox.
① Symptoms of measles include a red, slightly raised rash with no itching.
③ Symptoms of scarlet fever do not include reddish blisters on the trunk.
④ Symptoms of rubella do not include a fever or reddish blisters on the trunk.

95. Comprehension, implementation, environment (a)
❹ The pinworms lay their eggs near the anal opening during the night, so they are most easily captured in the early morning hours.
①,② This would be too late in the day.
③ Any eggs near the anal opening would probably be expelled along with the stool.

96. Application, implementation, physiologic (b)
❸ Use of diuretics is necessary because of the patient's edema.
① Semi-Fowler's is the most comfortable position to facilitate respiration.
② The normal diet for a child with nephrotic syndrome is a high-protein diet.
④ Sodium and potassium supplements are not usually given; sodium is limited.

97. Knowledge, assessment, physiologic (a)
❹ The specific cause of SIDS is presently unknown.
① SIDS is not caused by a respiratory virus.
② SIDS is not caused by an obstruction of the airway by a foreign body.
③ SIDS is not caused by hypertrophy of the larynx.

98. Knowledge, assessment, psychosocial (a)
❹ Freud's theory states that infants are in the oral stage.
① Toddlers are in the anal stage.
② Preschoolers are in the oedipal stage.
③ Adolescents are in the genital stage.

99. Knowledge, planning, physiologic (b)
❶ The diet provides essential nutrients that encourage tissue repair and replacement, energy for increased metabolic demands, and carbohydrates to prevent utilization of protein for energy.
②,③,④ Inappropriate diet for situation.

100. Comprehension, implementation, psychosocial (a)
❷ Informing the patient of what is expected of him during the procedure will lessen his anxiety and increase his capability to control his feelings.
①,③,④ Inappropriate response indicating lack of understanding and concern.

101. Knowledge, implementation, physiologic (b)
❸ The vastus lateralis is the recommended muscle and site to be used for a patient this age.
① The deltoid muscle is not developed enough to safely give an IM in a patient this age.
② The gluteus maximus should not be used because it is not developed enough, and also the sciatic nerve and artery are in this area.
④ The patient should really be over age 2 years to use the ventrogluteal area.

102. Knowledge, implementation, physiologic (b)
❹ The nurse needs to monitor the neurological status of one suspected of having encephalitis. The patient may have a seizure or go into a coma.
① Jaundice is not a problem with encephalitis.
② Blood sugars are not a problem with encephalitis unless the patient is a diabetic.
③ Blood pressure, like ALL vital signs, needs to be monitored closely, but the neurological status takes priority.

103. Knowledge, planning, physiologic (c)
❹ The femur, tibia, and humerus are the bones in which osteomyelitis occurs in children.
① Not commonly found in the fibula.
② Not commonly found in the fibula or patella.
③ Not commonly found in the patella, radius, and ulna.

104. Application, implementation, physiologic (b)
❸ This is the preferred primary site for a TB skin test.
① The upper arm has the deltoid muscle and is not used for intradermal testing.
② The scapular area is a second choice or a secondary site if for some reason the ventral forearm cannot be used.
④ The lateral aspect of the thigh should not be used. The medial aspect of the thigh can be used, but it is also a second choice.

105. Comprehension, planning, physiologic (c)
❸ Because of the large amount of secretions, the maintenance of a patent airway is the most important goal for this patient.

① Although the frequent suctioning could lead to respiratory infections, this is not the most pressing need at this time.

② Although a problem associated with repeated suctioning, arrhythmias are not the most pressing need at this time.

④ An equal intake and output is important to maintain liquification of secretions; however, this is not the primary concern.

106. Knowledge, assessment, physiologic (a)
❶ Amenorrhea is the absence of menstrual flow and is seen in anorexics or with rapid weight losses.
② Menorrhagia is excess bleeding at the time of normal menstruation.
③ Dysmenorrhea is painful menses.
④ Metrorrhagia is vaginal bleeding at a time other than a menstrual period.

107. Comprehension, assessment, physiologic (b)
❹ Anorexia nervosa is a psychiatric eating disorder resulting in morbid fear of fatness, in which the person's distorted body image is reflected as fat. It is common in teenage girls.
① Dysphagia is difficulty in swallowing, associated with obstructive or motor disorders of the esophagus.
② Bulimia is a psychiatric eating disorder in which a person gorges on large quantities of food followed by self-induced vomiting and the use of laxatives to maintain normal weight.
③ Anorexia is loss of appetite and can be caused by a variety of factors.

108. Comprehension, planning, health (b)
❶ Revised eating habits are the key to losing and keeping weight off. These habits must be truly revised and permanent or lost weight will return.
② Losing weight quickly does not help keep it off. One should only lose 1 to 2 pounds per week.
③ Periods of fasting are not recommended, especially for a motivated 15-year-old girl. The best weight reduction is the food guide pyramid with the calorie content controlled.
④ Drinking water is acceptable, but drinking diet soda is not good advice. Diet soda may pacify the appetite for dieters, but many kinds can cause diarrhea. There is also a question of artificial sweeteners being safe for human use.

109. Knowledge, implementation, health (b)
❹ 3500 kcal amounts to 1 pound.
① 500 kcal is too low.
② 6500 kcal is too high.
③ 1000 kcal is too low.

110. Knowledge, assessment, physiologic (c)
❹ A baby born with a wryneck (torticollis) has sometimes suffered a difficult birth, and one of these muscles may be injured and develop spasms.
① The trapezius muscles are the most superficial muscles of the posterior neck and upper trunk.
② The temporalis muscle is a fan-shaped muscle overlying the temporal bone.
③ The latissimus dorsi muscle is the large flat muscle pair that covers the lower back.

111. Knowledge, implementation, environment (a)
❸ Fetal heart tones are most accurately measured between contractions. During the early stages of labor, monitoring is generally done every 30 minutes.
① True rate not attainable since FHTs normally decrease during contractions.
② Inappropriate—need to be taken more often as indicated above.
④ May be necessary, especially closer to delivery.

112. Comprehension, implementation, psychosocial (a)
❶ Increased flow progressive; reaches peak about transition.
② Physician has just examined patient; unnecessary to call. Abruptio placentae is accompanied by pain.
③ Normal sequence of bloody show; not necessary to take blood pressure for that.
④ Pads rarely used; source of discomfort and contamination.

113. Knowledge, assessment, environment (a)
❷ Vaginal or hidden bleeding and fetal distress are problems seen in patients with placenta previa.
① Abdominal rigidity is common to abruptio placentae.
③ Symptoms of a ruptured uterus.
④ Severe abdominal pain not symptomatic of placenta previa.

114. Comprehension, assessment, health (c)
❷ You comprehend the CDC statements and analyzed and chose this correct answer.
① Pregnant nurses are not known to be at greater risk than any other nurse.
③ False. Strict adherence to precautions should protect you from contracting the infection.
④ The first part is true, but the second part is not based on any medical or scientific proof.

115. Knowledge, evaluation, health (a)
❹ Additional protein and calories are needed for the overall lactation process, including milk content and production.
① Increased fluids are needed to produce milk, a fluid tissue.
② Maintenance of sodium intake and fats is needed.
③ Additional carbohydrates are needed to provide the additional calories necessary for lactation.

116. Application, evaluation, environment (b)
❷ Major adverse reaction.
① Unlikely to occur.
③,④ Complications that should be the concern with every patient in labor.

117. Application, implementation, physiologic (b)
❸ Best and simple nursing measure for comfort and relief.
①,②,④ Inappropriate nursing action that is unnecessary and would not correct situation.

118. Knowledge, planning, health (b)
❹ Ideal time.
① Too early; would not retain instructions.
② Too early; may forget or become bored if too early.
③ Too late; classes are usually once a week for 5 to 6 weeks.

119. Knowledge, implementation, health (a)
    ❷ True; includes all pertinent phases of childbearing.
    ① Untrue; drugs may be requested or even given when necessary, such as with dystocia.
    ③ Preparation for labor and delivery; not necessarily "young" parents; does not include child-rearing classes.
    ④ This is more a description of the Bradley method.

120. Comprehension, implementation, health (a)
    ❹ Will encourage circulation and alleviate pain; symptoms may be indicative of a femoral vein thrombus.
    ① This treatment has not been ordered.
    ② An unauthorized treatment.
    ③ Should be aware of possibility of thrombus in postpartum patient; should not move leg until the physician examines it.

121. Knowledge, implementation, physiologic (b)
    ❹ This is the best advice to give any pregnant woman, because many birth anomalies have been associated with alcohol.
    ① No alcohol during pregnancy is best. Fetal alcohol syndrome is always a potential problem with drinking during pregnancy.
    ② As stated in #4, no alcoholic beverages are recommended during pregnancy. Alcohol is a drug and CNS depressant.
    ③ No alcohol during pregnancy is best. Statistics show a high incidence of birth defects with moderate drinking.

122. Knowledge, implementation, physiologic (b)
    ❶ If the fetal movements felt in 1 hour while resting and doing a kick count are 3 or under, the client needs to phone immediately. This is serious and hypoxia may be developing.
    ② Seven or more kicks are normal, but unusual when the mother is resting.

③ This is a safe range.
④ This, too, is a safe range.

123. Application, implementation, physiologic (c)
    ❶ Iron needs increase during pregnancy, and the normal maternal diet may not be adequate in iron.
    ② Sodium needs increase slightly during pregnancy; however, these needs can be met by the maternal diet.
    ③ Calcium needs do increase during pregnancy but can usually be met by increasing the intake of milk and milk products.
    ④ Magnesium needs also increase during pregnancy but can normally be met by the maternal diet.

124. Knowledge, assessment, physiologic (a)
    ❷ Pica is manifested by the ingestion of nonfood items such as dirt, laundry starch, etc., during pregnancy.
    ① Pica is not characterized by vaginal bleeding.
    ③ PIH, not pica, is manifested by increased blood pressure in pregnant women.
    ④ Gestational diabetes is characterized by the presence of a high serum blood glucose.

125. Knowledge, planning, environment (b)
    ❸ The most accurate method to determine the EDC when the LMP is not known is when the first heartbeats are heard. These occur between the 20th and 22nd week of gestation.
    ① Weight gain is not a reliable way to determine EDC; there are too many variables.
    ② Serial estriols are done in late pregnancy as a method of determining fetal status or well-being.
    ④ Relying on fetal movement felt by the mother is not as accurate as hearing the first fetal heartbeats, especially in a first pregnancy.

COMPREHENSIVE EXAMINATION 1: PART 2

1. Knowledge, planning, health (b)
   ❶ The most common problem after TURP.
   ②,③,④ These are nonspecific, common postoperative problems.
2. Comprehension, planning, physiologic (b)
   ❷ A wet dressing must be changed as soon as possible because it will be a source of infection and is irritating.
   ①,④ Not specifically related to the question.
   ③ The patient should be ambulatory before removal of tube.
3. Knowledge, assessment, physiologic (b)
   ❶ Correct response.
   ②,③,④ Incorrect responses; these are inflammatory conditions; #2 and #3 are related to the female, and #4 to the male.
4. Knowledge, assessment, environment (a)
   ❷ Hearing impairment common with advancing age.
   ① Personality and reality contact alterations.
   ③ Loss of visual accommodation in advancing age.
   ④ Cognitive dysfunction characterized by disorientation and confabulation.
5. Application, planning, physiologic (a)
   ❶ These activities will put the arm through range of motion (ROM) as the patient assumes some responsibility for personal care.
   ② Part of daily routine in rehabilitation.
   ③ Inappropriate activity.
   ④ Too fine a movement and one that does not allow full ROM.
6. Comprehension, assessment, physiologic (c)
   ❶ This could be a manifestation of increased intracranial pressure.
   ② No reason to restrict self-care; can be accomplished when restricted to bed rest.
   ③ A patient has the legal right to refuse medication.
   ④ Appropriate to show emotional reaction when separated from children.
7. Application, implementation, environment (c)
   ❹ Correct.
   ①,②,③ Not correct—do not pertain to eye surgery.
8. Knowledge, planning, physiologic (a)
   ❸ Patients taking Coumadin should be monitored for any signs of bleeding. The mucous membranes, intestines, and urinary tract are common sites.
   ① Inappropriate unless necessary.
   ②,④ Actions do not allow total observation for signs of bleeding.
9. Knowledge, assessment, physiologic (a)
   ❹ Transient ischemic attacks (TIAs) are temporary neurologic disturbances, manifested by sudden loss of motor, sensory, or visual function and lasting a few minutes to several hours. The cause is a temporary lack of blood flow to the area.
   ① Indicative of a CVA.
   ②,③ Not necessarily applicable to situation.
10. Knowledge, planning, environment (a)
    ❷ Coumadin interferes with blood-clotting mechanisms by blocking the synthesis of vitamin K in the liver. Even minor injuries may result in hemorrhage in the patient taking Coumadin.
    ① Counteracts purpose of drug.
    ③ Light exercise is fine; no massage.
    ④ Counteracts purpose of drug, and patients are never to take medications unless ordered by the physician.
11. Knowledge, planning, physiologic (a)
    ❸ Ingestion of dairy products increases calcium intake. Excessive calcium in the body during periods of decreased mobility increases the chance of kidney stone formation.
    ①,②,④ Incorrect response, not applicable to kidney stone formation.
12. Knowledge, planning, physiologic (a)
    ❸ An increase in fruits in the diet will increase bulk in the intestines. Increasing bulk and fluids in the intestines will promote normal elimination.
    ①,② Not appropriate means of encouragement as a routine to follow.
    ④ This may or may not be possible.
13. Comprehension, planning, physiologic (b)
    ❷ Quadriceps setting exercises improve the strength of muscles needed for walking.
    ①,③,④ Actions will not strengthen muscles as indicated above.
14. Application, implementation, health (b)
    ❹ A major aspect in care is to prevent additional infections.
    ① Ideally the patient can and should return to the community and can have a productive lifestyle.
    ② The patient can only be of danger through the exchange of body fluids.
    ③ Health care is provided by third-party payments and community agencies. The expensive drugs are those specifically for AIDS.
15. Knowledge, assessment, physiologic (a)
    ❹ Correct.
    ① Hyperventilation.
    ② Bradypnea.
    ③ Cheyne-Stokes.
16. Comprehension, assessment, physiologic (a)
    ❹ Phantom limb sensation sometimes occurs after this type of surgical procedure.
    ①,②,③ The sensation is not imaginary, is not related to a side effect of medication, and is not a reflection of the grieving process.
17. Comprehension, implementation, health (b)
    ❸ Hip and knee contractures can occur after surgery.
    ①,②,④ Not generally the prime consideration for the identified nursing measure.
18. Comprehension, assessment, environment (a)
    ❷ The *foremost* complication is hemorrhage.
    ① Is possible during the postoperative period.
    ③ Is possible if an exercise regimen is not adhered to.
    ④ Is possible after any surgery.
19. Comprehension, planning, physiologic (a)
    ❷ Thromboembolic problems are a postoperative complication of hip surgery. Low-dose aspirin reduces the risks of this complication.
    ① Dose is too low for an antiinflammatory effect.
    ③,④ Not the primary purpose behind such an order.

20. Comprehension, planning, physiologic (b)
   ❶ Used to immobilize the leg when internal fixation is to be done within a short time.
   ② Pediatric traction used in femoral fractures.
   ③,④ Similar traction devices used for providing balanced traction in injuries where internal fixation cannot be performed within a short time period.

21. Comprehension, assessment, environment (c)
   ❸ Size, location, and character of drainage should be noted on the chart; provides a reference for future evaluation of wound progress.
   ①,②,④ Description lacking adequate information.

22. Knowledge, implementation, health (a)
   ❸ Any type of constriction about the lower extremities will decrease venous return.
   ① Not most appropriate response.
   ② Not necessary.
   ④ Incorrect information.

23. Application, evaluation, physiologic (b)
   ❷ Postural drainage helps drain sections of the lung, aids in coughing and removing secretions, and improves breathing.
   ① High-Fowler's position (45- to 90-degree elevation) is most effective in relieving dyspnea.
   ③ Fluids should be forced to liquefy secretions.
   ④ Patient should have rest and conserve energy.

24. Comprehension, implementation, health (a)
   ❸ Lymph node biopsy is the most definitive diagnostic procedure for sarcoidosis.
   ① Would give patient false sense of spreading disease.
   ② The question was not understood properly.
   ④ Swollen glands are symptomatic of sarcoidosis.

25. Comprehension, assessment, physiologic (a)
   ❶ Circulation and sensation are periodically assessed to determine the presence of pressure areas that may obstruct circulation and nerve pathways.
   ②,③,④ Inappropriate action.

26. Knowledge, implementation, health (a)
   ❷ Chlorpromazine makes skin sensitive to sunlight.
   ① Related to monoamine oxidase (MAO) inhibitor.
   ③,④ Not related.

27. Knowledge, assessment, environment (b)
   ❶ Never use a suppository directly from refrigerator, because cold causes constriction.
   ② Lubrication ensures easy, painless insertion.
   ③ Ineffective when inserted into a bolus of stool.
   ④ Glycerin suppositories are inserted after 20 minutes if patient has not had a bowel movement.

28. Comprehension, planning, physiologic (a)
   ❶ Pattern is essential with retraining.
   ② Not necessary for the patient to understand the program for the program to be successful.
   ③ Laxatives never used with bowel retraining.
   ④ Regular days and times must be strictly followed to establish a pattern.

29. Comprehension, planning, environment (a)
   ❹ Hemorrhage could occur within 12 to 24 hours. The risk of bleeding and edema makes it necessary that a tracheostomy tray be available at the bedside.
   ① Not a classic intervention.
   ②,③ Would not prevent bleeding or edema.

30. Knowledge, assessment, environment (a)
   ❷ Cholesterol is found in blood and body cells, especially brain and nervous tissue.
   ① It should not nor can it be eliminated totally from the diet.
   ③ It is necessary for normal body functioning.
   ④ It is mainly through animal sources—meat, eggs, and saturated fats.

31. Comprehension, planning, physiologic (c)
   ❸ Brachial artery is the supplying artery; this is done when application of direct pressure does not control bleeding.
   ① Tourniquets are not recommended unless an extremity is amputated or severely mutilated.
   ② Direct pressure has already been applied unsuccessfully.
   ④ Not the immediate supplying artery.

32. Knowledge, planning, physiologic (b)
   ❸ Protein sources (meat, fish, poultry, and eggs) are often restricted for a person with liver disease in order to limit the end products of protein metabolism.
   ① Fruits are not protein.
   ② Vegetables are not protein sources.
   ④ Carbohydrates are not protein.

33. Comprehension, assessment, physiologic (a)
   ❹ Result from mechanical barrier to gastric flow usually caused by scarring.
   ① Gallbladder disorder does not occur as a result of peptic ulcers.
   ② Coffee ground emesis would be a key symptom.
   ③ Signaled by fever and abdominal rigidity.

34. Knowledge, implementation, environment (a)
   ❸ Virus is found in blood and feces; primary mode of spread is by food, drink, or water.
   ① Associated with HBV.
   ② Associated with HBV, non-HAV, and non-HBV.
   ④ Associated with toxic hepatitis.

35. Comprehension, planning, physiologic (a)
   ❶ Promotes liver regeneration and increased blood filtration through the liver.
   ② Enteric precautions and proper hygiene prevent the spread of the virus.
   ③ Cardiac effort is reduced, but the primary aim is to rest the liver.
   ④ Will not reduce the risk of hepatic coma.

36. Application, assessment, physiologic (c)
   ❹ Those with little chance of survival must wait until those with survivable injuries are treated first.
   ① Patients with minor injuries can be rapidly treated.
   ② Serious but non–life-threatening injuries require care and time.
   ③ These victims may be saved if the medical staff and supplies aren't depleted caring for those with little chance of survival.

37. Application, assessment, physiologic (b)
   ❶ Urine output of 30 cc/hr or less for more than 1 hour may indicate hypovolemia and cause renal damage.
   ② These urine outputs would bear continued monitoring.
   ③ These urine outputs are satisfactory.
   ④ These urine outputs indicate the patient is well hydrated.

38. Application, intervention, physiologic (b)
   ❹ Atelectasis and pneumonia are frequent complications of upper abdominal surgery.

① The patient's temperature is not high enough to warrant tepid baths.

② Cool compresses are not effective in fever reduction.

③ Although Motrin does have antipyretic effects, it is usually given for its antiinflammatory effects.

39. Comprehension, assessment, physiologic (c)

❹ The elderly have a higher percentage of body fat, which affects the metabolism and storage of medications.

① The elderly have a lower percentage of body water.

② The elderly have a decrease in lean muscle mass.

③ The elderly have a higher percentage of body fat.

40. Application, planning, environment (c)

❷ Validating the feelings that are being manifested by the wandering behavior allows the client to feel understood. Distraction allows the client to expend energy in something other than wandering.

① Reality orientation is not effective in demented clients.

③ Attempting to restrain the client will lead to a catastrophic event.

④ Safety needs of the individual can not be met in an open, free environment.

41. Knowledge, implementation, environment (b)

❶ Rapid needle insertion irritates fewer nerve fibers.

② Large-bore needles such as an 18-gauge needle are used for IVs.

③ An IM injection should have a 60° to 90° angle of entry.

④ A 1½-inch needle is less likely to strike bone or nerves.

42. Knowledge, implementation, environment (b)

❹ This response will prevent a possible medication error.

① The patient may be given an incorrect medication.

② This response could cause a medication error to occur.

③ It would be better to double-check with the pharmacy.

43. Application, implementation, physiologic (c)

❷ To calculate this problem, divide 525 cc by 8 hours. That equals 65 cc/hr of NG replacement fluid. 65 cc + 75 cc/hr maintenance = 140 cc/hr. 140 × 10 divided by 60 = 23 gtts/min.

① This rate would deliver 75 cc/hr.

③ This rate delivers 195 cc/hr.

④ This rate delivers 255 cc/hr.

44. Application, planning, physiologic (b)

❹ Problems associated with airway and breathing are always a priority.

① The obesity is a long-term management problem.

② Self-esteem may remain low until weight is lost.

③ Excess fluid needs to be removed before activity tolerance improves.

45. Knowledge, implementation, physiologic (c)

❸ Oral contraceptives are considered the most effective method of birth control if taken correctly. They also have few side-effects.

① Condoms are sheaths that prevent sperm from entering the cervix and have been known to tear or leak. Some find putting them on correctly a problem. Condoms are recommended to prevent spread of AIDS. They are not 100% effective for birth control.

② Coitus interruptus is difficult to control and sperm can escape.

④ Intrauterine devices are controversial. There is some danger that the device can dislodge and remain in the vagina so a woman may think she is fully protected. There is also literature addressing infections and other problems caused by IUDs.

46. Knowledge, implementation, physiologic (c)

❶ Intertrigo describes a superficial dermatitis that occurs in obese patients.

② Pemphigus is an uncommon skin disorder characterized by blisters and is thought to be an autoimmune disorder.

③ Stasis ulcers result from inadequate or poor circulation in legs.

④ Decubitus ulcers are pressure ulcers caused by one's inability to move or change positions, depriving tissues of blood supply.

47. Comprehension, planning, physiologic (b)

❸ The patient should be advised to avoid any sudden movement or jarring of the head. This will help prevent hemorrhage in the eye or opening of the incision.

① Patients are advised *not* to do *any* bending over until checked and given permission to do so by the physician.

② Most patients are given lifting restrictions of 5 pounds or less.

④ This is not true. Most patients need to wear dark glasses for awhile after surgery. Light can cause great discomfort. Many eye surgeons provide dark glasses for patients to wear over eyeshields or eyeglasses.

48. Application, implementation, physiologic (b)

❹ Iron dextran as well as some other medications can cause staining and irritation of the surrounding tissues. The reason the Z-track method is used is to deposit the medication into deep muscle tissues to decrease this irritation and staining.

① All vitamin and mineral injections sting when given.

② This refers to injections given intradermally.

③ Z-track is used for many iron, vitamin, and some antibiotic medications. It is used widely in the elderly with decreased muscle mass.

49. Application, planning, environment (a)

❶ An 18-gauge catheter is the only choice that has a large enough lumen to accommodate the viscosity of blood and blood products.

② A 20-gauge catheter may be used for this purpose but it is generally not the best choice in this situation.

③ A 22-gauge IV catheter is too small for administration of blood or blood products.

④ A 24-gauge IV catheter is too small for administration of blood or blood products.

50. Comprehension, evaluation, health (b)

❶ Many elderly clients take multiple medications, many of which can be associated with depression.

② Electrolyte balance is not associated with depression.

③ Fleeting feelings of sadness are not associated with depression; prolonged periods of feelings of sadness may be.

④ Nutritional supplements would not contribute to depression.

51. Knowledge, implementation, health (n)

❶ The peak incidence of rheumatoid arthritis is between 30 and 50 years of age.

② Women are much more likely to have rheumatoid arthritis than men.

③ Women are more likely to have rheumatoid arthritis than men until men are in their 70s.

④ Rheumatoid arthritis is more common among whites than among African-Americans.

52. Comprehension, implementation, health (b)
   ❹ Glomerulonephritis usually results from an immune reaction to a strep infection.
   ① Glomerulonephritis is not an infectious disease.
   ② Glomerulonephritis is not caused by a drug reaction.
   ③ Glomerulonephritis is not an inherited disease.
53. Comprehension, implementation, health (b)
   ❸ It may take as long as 12 weeks for antidepressants to achieve their full therapeutic effect.
   ① There is no reason to limit fluids while taking antidepressants.
   ② Dry mouth and orthostatic hypotension are common bothersome side-effects of antidepressants.
   ③ If the first antidepressant fails to control depression, other effective medications are available.
54. Knowledge, planning, environment (c)
   ❷ Alternatives to restraints should be tried before resorting to restraints.
   ① Restraints are to be used only for a specific period of time.
   ③ Restraints should be removed at least every 2 hours to allow for activities of daily living.
   ④ Restraints should be tied with knots that can be quickly released and secured to parts of the bed that move with the patient.
55. Application, assessment, physiologic (b)
   ❹ Nonverbal communication is very important with this patient. He may not be able to process a complaint of pain.
   ① Short, simple messages are understood better by this patient; a pain rating scale may be too difficult to process.
   ② Closed questions are least upsetting to this patient.
   ③ There is no reason to speak more loudly, and rephrasing may increase his confusion.
56. Application, assessment, environment (b)
   ❸ You want to determine if this is a suicide threat and if she's done any planning.
   ① You don't ignore what could be a suicide threat.
   ② She's verbalized to you. The subject needs more exploration before a referral is made.
   ④ If it is a suicide threat, questioning her about a plan would be the next step.
57. Knowledge, assessment, environment (b)
   ❷ Legal standards of nursing are developed by legislative actions.
   ① State boards of nursing and other agencies accredit nursing programs.
   ③ Licensure ensures minimal safety performance of nurses.
   ④ Professional organizations set ethical standards for nurses.
58. Knowledge, planning, physiologic (c)
   ❷ Urecholine (bethanechol chloride) is a cholinergic that has side usage for urinary bladder retention, as long as the cause is not an obstruction.
   ① Mestinon is a cholinergic drug used in myasthenia gravis.
   ③ Pilocarpine is a cholinergic used in the treatment of glaucoma.
   ④ Pro-Banthine is used in adjunctive therapy to treat peptic ulcer.

59. Comprehension, planning, physiologic (b)
   ❸ Lidocaine is the drug of choice for ventricular arrhythmias; it depresses ventricular irritability.
   ① Inderal is a beta-adrenergic blocking agent that depresses cardiac function. It is contraindicated in ventricular arrhythmias.
   ② Digoxin is a drug used to strengthen ventricular contractions.
   ④ Morphine sulfate will not prevent or help arrhythmias.
60. Knowledge, assessment, physiologic (c)
   ❶ Antabuse has been known to cause acne. This is a common side effect that will usually disappear as the body adjusts to the drug.
   ② Antabuse usually causes fatigue and energy loss.
   ③ Antabuse gives foods a metallic aftertaste.
   ④ Antabuse causes drowsiness and is not known to cause nightmares or sleep disturbances.
61. Comprehension, assessment, physiologic (b)
   ❹ Anticoagulants can cause blood to show up in urine.
   ① Diuretics alter the urine quantity output.
   ② Pyridium will alter the urine color to a red or orange color but will not test positive for blood.
   ③ Macrodantin alters the color of urine to a harmless brown.
62. Knowledge, assessment, health (a)
   ❹ There are alcoholics in every social class and every occupation.
   ① This is not true.
   ② Although there are many white-collar alcoholics, they do not constitute the majority.
   ③ All social classes have alcoholics.
63. Application, implementation, environment (b)
   ❸ A warm sitz bath is recommended to help with pain and comfort after a cystoscopy.
   ① There are no diet restrictions after having had a cystoscopy.
   ② One is to increase fluid intake after a cystoscopy.
   ④ One is to increase fluid intake after a cystoscopy, not decrease the fluid intake.
64. Knowledge, assessment, physiologic (a)
   ❹ *Clostridium perfringens* is the organism that causes gas gangrene.
   ① *E. coli* is found in the intestine and stools and is considered part of the normal flora.
   ② *Salmonella* is an organism that causes gastroenteritis, and is found in poultry, raw eggs, and fecal-contaminated meats.
   ③ *Clostridium botulinum* is the spore organism that causes food poisoning.
65. Comprehension, assessment, physiologic (b)
   ❶ A cloudy color in the urine may suggest a possible bacterial infection, vegetarian diet, or glomerular nephritis.
   ② A dark amber color suggests a low fluid intake or fluid loss. It can also suggest an acute febrile disease.
   ③ A green-brown color suggests a bile duct obstruction.
   ④ A red or red-brown color may be caused by porphyria hemorrhage; some drugs such as phenazopyridine or sulfobromopthalein can color the urine.
66. Application, assessment, physiologic (b)
   ❸ Raise the head of the bed first, because many times this will bring a patient back in control of his respirations. It will make breathing easier.

① Take vital signs after raising the head of the bed, or the shortness of breath will continue.

② It is not necessary to call for help unless he does not respond to raising the head of the bed.

④ His health history should already be documented and on the chart. To determine if he has been short of breath before is not necessary, as this goes along with the disease process of cystic fibrosis.

67. Application, assessment, physiologic (b)

❹ Excessive urination is one of the classic signs and symptoms that blood sugar may be off.

① Refusing to bathe is no indication that diabetes is out of control.

② A cough does not indicate that diabetes needs to be checked.

③ One diarrhea stool last week does not need further assessment.

68. Comprehension, planning, physiologic (b)

❸ Protein is limited to help to reduce the amount of excretory work demanded of the kidneys.

① Fats are not restricted. They are necessary to fulfill energy requirements and should be polyunsaturated.

② Calcium supplements may be prescribed to prevent osteomalacia. Calcium is not restricted.

④ Carbohydrates are not restricted and are used to fulfill energy requirements. If energy requirements are not met by fats and carbohydrates, ingested protein or body tissue will be metabolized for energy.

69. Application, assessment, physiologic (b)

❸ Undigested food is caused by a possible gastric outlet obstruction. A gastric tumor or ulcer can lead to this.

① Blood can be seen with upper gastrointestinal bleeding or gastritis.

② Bright red blood is usually seen with peptic ulcers.

④ Brown vomitus with fecal odor is usually seen in intestinal obstructions.

70. Application, evaluation, psychosocial (b)

❷ The finding of antibodies means that the person has been infected with the HIV at some time, but may not have the AIDS disease.

① Not correct.

③ No immunity known.

④ No prevention after exposure; only to prevent exposure.

71. Comprehension, implementation, environment (b)

❹ Memory is usually disturbed.

① Not a nursing responsibility.

②,③ Not necessarily needed.

72. Application, implementation, psychosocial (a)

❹ Reality orientation—only response that does not reinforce confusion and disorientation.

①,②,③ Reinforce disorientation and confusion.

73. Comprehension, implementation, psychosocial (b)

❹ The demands of the nurse lead to increased anxiety rather than a reduction of it.

① The patient may not be aware of her limitations.

② Not specifically related to the situation.

③ Not related to situation.

74. Comprehension, evaluation, psychosocial (a)

❷ Depression is a natural response to catastrophic illness. Other psychologic problems manifested by cerebral damage include emotional lability, hostility, frustration, and noncooperation.

①,③,④ Inappropriate nursing response showing clearly that the nurse lacks understanding of the disease process.

75. Knowledge, planning, psychosocial (a)

❷ Touch, because of relational losses.

① May be deprived, but not the most correct answer.

③,④ May or may not be true.

76. Comprehension, assessment, psychosocial (c)

❸ The first stage toward final acceptance.

① Second stage.

② Third stage.

④ Fourth stage.

77. Knowledge, assessment, psychosocial (b)

❹ Trust vs. mistrust is Erikson's first stage.

① Appropriate for a later stage.

② Sullivan's theory, not Erikson's.

③ Freudian theory.

78. Comprehension, assessment, psychosocial (a)

❶ Repression is unconsciously pushing something from one's conscious awareness.

② Projection is the assignment of one's feelings to others.

③ Displacement is the acting out of feelings on a less threatening object.

④ Rationalization is finding explanations for one's behavior.

79. Comprehension, assessment, psychosocial (b)

❹ The nurse must know behavior is meaningful, regardless of how apparently insignificant.

① The situation does not describe the nurse's behavior.

②,③ Nurse's reactions are not described.

80. Application, implementation, psychosocial (c)

❹ Yes. The best thing a nurse can do for disorientation and anxiety is limit the staff and people who have contact with him.

① When a client is agitated and disoriented, he is not capable of making his own care decisions.

② Asking the physician for a restraint order or medications should be done only as a last resort.

③ Orienting the client to time, place, and person can add to their agitation.

81. Knowledge, assessment, psychosocial (c)

❸ Korsakoff's psychosis is a form of amnesia. It is seen in advanced alcoholism. The person is unable to learn new skills and suffers from short-term memory loss.

① Addiction is defined as compulsive, uncontrollable dependence on a substance or habit.

② Habituation is defined as a psychological and emotional dependence on a drug, tobacco, or alcohol substance without the need to increase the dosage.

④ In Wernicke's encephalopathy there are lesions in several areas of the brain that cause the brain to deteriorate.

82. Comprehension, assessment, physiologic (b)

❸ Tardive dyskinesia is an irreversible syndrome of involuntary movements of the face, trunk, and extremities associated with antipsychotic medications.

① Cowling's rule is a method of calculating pediatric drug dosages.

② Chvostek's sign is a spasm of facial muscles when the cheek is stroked; it is seen in tetany.

④ Sjögren's syndrome is a group of symptoms including rheumatoid arthritis and xerostomia seen in postmenopausal women.

83. Application, implementation, psychosocial (b)
    ❶ Using open-ended questions by picking a key word used by the patient (dying) is a good way to lead to more sharing.
    ② The patient said this to the nurse, not the family. The nurse needs to pursue fears here and now. Many AIDS patients are abandoned by their families, and the nurse does not know the situation here.
    ③ This would be a cop-out by the nurse and is not an appropriate response at this time.
    ④ This is not true. Depression may be repressed anger. Talking may or may not help one feel better when dealing with death.

84. Application, planning, psychosocial (a)
    ❷ Asking about past employment is a question that would give a clue to the patient's long-term memory.
    ① Asking an age is considered a short-term memory question.
    ③ This is an example of a short-term question.
    ④ This is an example of a short-term question, asking for information from the present.

85. Knowledge, planning, physiologic (a)
    ❸ When the baby is stable, which is frequently moments after birth.
    ①,②,④ Parental contact should not be on a schedule.

86. Comprehension, planning, environment (b)
    ❷ Stimulates circulation and prevents the formation of thrombi, besides aiding in breaking up clots.
    ① This is to relieve pain, promote healing, and prevent infection.
    ③ Helps to diminish pain and discomfort.
    ④ Keeping urinary functions at a maximum aids in promoting involution, and offering stool softeners relieves initial pain and discomfort during the postpartum period.

87. Knowledge, implementation, physiologic (a)
    ❷ First priority.
    ① Not first priority.
    ③ Physician knows; not necessary to do test unless you are asked.
    ④ Pads not used during labor and delivery.

88. Application, implementation, environment (a)
    ❹ Best response: explanation and valid reason given; kind and courteous.
    ① Wrong. No solids given during active labor; prevents vomiting and thus aspiration, especially if anesthesia is necessary.
    ② Too technical and flippant; no jokes.
    ③ Abrupt; no compassion; no explanation.

89. Comprehension, assessment, physiologic (a)
    ❹ Nägele's rule: subtract 3 months and add 7 days to LMP.

    $$\begin{array}{cc} 4 & 24 \\ -3 & +7 \\ \hline 1 & 31 \end{array}$$

    Answer: 1   31 (January 31)—correct:
    ① 4 + 9 = 13 = January
       24 − 7 = 17
       Answer: January 17—wrong.
    ② 10 lunar months—February
       February does not have 31 days, so 24 + 7 = 31
       Answer: March 3—wrong.
    ③ Using 10 lunar months:
       4 + 10 = 14 or February 24 − 7 = 17
       Answer: February 17—wrong.

90. Knowledge, assessment, physiologic (a)
    ❷ Correct.
    ① Wrong; she has been pregnant twice and has delivered one child.
    ③ Wrong; pregnant twice.
    ④ Wrong; pregnant twice but has only delivered one child.

91. Knowledge, evaluation, health (a)
    ❷ Best possible answer.
    ① Both at an ideal age.
    ③ Nothing in the situation or question itself suggests this.
    ④ The length of time between pregnancies does not alter the ability to conceive in this case.

92. Comprehension, implementation, environment (c)
    ❸ This is the guideline from the CDC.
    ① Must have gown as well, not just mask and gloves.
    ② Must have gown besides.
    ④ The AIDS victim needs as much protection as the caretaker.

93. Knowledge, comprehension, psychosocial (b)
    ❷ True statement.
    ① Though highly contagious, there must be direct bloodstream contact with the HIV virus.
    ③ The fetus of an HIV-infected pregnant mother is likely to become infected.
    ④ It is important that all nursing personnel familiarize themselves with all aspects of AIDS.

94. Comprehension, implementation, physiologic (b)
    ❷ Uterus at umbilicus at 24 weeks or 6 months.
    ① Fundal height at 12 to 13 weeks (3 months) is just above symphysis pubis.
    ③ At 16 to 20 weeks mother first experiences fetal movement.
    ④ Engagement occurs about 2 weeks before EDC in nullipara; not before labor in parous woman.

95. Knowledge, assessment, physiologic (c)
    ❹ Crack cocaine use causes a surge in the systolic, resulting in many small strokes in the developing fetus, as well as in utero brain hemorrhage.
    ① The pulse can increase with this drug use, but doesn't cause the damage to the fetus that the rise in blood pressure does.
    ② Body temperature is not dangerously affected by crack cocaine use and does not affect the developing fetus.
    ③ Respirations increase because crack cocaine is a stimulant that affects the central nervous system.

96. Knowledge, assessment, physiologic (a)
    ❶ This is true.
    ② Adolescents do not have reality acceptance, and most have a concept of having a live baby doll fantasy.
    ③ Adolescents are not eager or ready to accept their pregnancy and tend to strongly deny being pregnant.
    ④ Adolescents do not seek early care. Statistics show that many teens wait until the third trimester to seek care.

97. Knowledge, implementation, physiologic (b)
    ❹ Oxytocin is used to stimulate uterine contractions. The nurse needs to monitor the fetal heart tones and the length and duration of contractions to pick up any fetal distress. There are many dangers in inducing labor, such as the umbilical cord being wrapped around the baby's neck.
    ① The patient will be NPO and should not have any intake.

② Nausea is a possible side-effect and does not become a major problem unless the mother begins to vomit.

③ The nurse will be monitoring the mother's vital signs, but the best answer and the one to take priority is the monitoring of fetal heart tones and the length and duration of contractions.

98. Comprehension, planning, psychosocial (c)
❷ If an individual with sickle cell disease has children with an individual with sickle cell trait, 50% of the children will have sickle cell disease and 50% will have sickle cell trait.

① If both mother and father have sickle cell trait, 25% of their children will have sickle cell disease.

③ There is no possibility that 75% of these individuals' children will have sickle cell disease.

④ If both mother and father have sickle cell disease, then 100% of their children will have sickle cell disease.

99. Knowledge, implementation, health (a)
❸ These foods, including favorites of teenagers, are very high in fat. The fat is known as invisible or hidden fat because one cannot see it.

① These foods are very low sources of fat.

② These foods have only a trace of fat.

④ These foods have 1 gram total fat per serving.

100. Comprehension, assessment, physiologic (a)
❸ These signs are normal for a 2-day-old newborn.

① This is a full-term infant, so she cannot be premature.

② There is no indication in the situation that the infant is immature.

④ Nothing abnormal is reported in the situation.

101. Knowledge, assessment, physiologic (b)
❹ The hemoglobin is decreased, not increased, in sickle cell crisis.

①,②,③ Common symptom of sickle cell crisis.

102. Knowledge, implementation, environment (a)
❹ Correct description.

① Frequent and severe headaches follow.

② Angiography.

③ Isotope not used.

103. Application, implementation, health (b)
❷ Best response; presenting and reinforcing information already given patient.

①,③,④ Contradicting information given; offering incorrect information.

104. Comprehension, assessment, psychosocial (b)
❸ Erikson's theory is based on the child's psychosocial development.

① This is Freud's theory.

② This is Piaget's theory.

④ This is a portion of Piaget's theory.

105. Application, implementation, physiologic (b)
❸ Correct per the 1993 changes instituted by the American Heart Association.

① Incorrect; eight back blows and eight chest thrusts were never a recommended sequence for obstructed airway in an infant.

② Incorrect; six back blows and six chest thrusts were never a recommended sequence for obstructed airway in an infant.

④ Incorrect; four back blows and four chest thrusts were the recommended sequence for obstructed airway in an infant *before the changes instituted early in 1993.*

106. Application, implementation, physiologic (b)
❸ In assisting the physician you would prepare an IV fluid administration set and fluids (as ordered) for the immediate replacement of fluids lost from the burn site(s).

①,②,④ Yes, but not vital at this point in time.

107. Comprehension, assessment, physiologic (a)
❹ An immediate physical observation of a person burned in the area of the face is assessment of respiration (difficulty, rate, sound).

①,②,③ Not immediate physical observation during an emergency.

108. Comprehension, assessment, physiologic (a)
❷ A preschooler enjoys the close family relationship of mealtimes. Parents are usually the significant persons during the preschool years. Since his parents are dead, his grandmother will become the significant person in his life now.

① Not for his age group.

③,④ Inappropriate before attempting above.

109. Knowledge, planning, psychosocial (a)
❹ Lets him share, yet gives him his own special time.

① Don't separate him from the major activity (newborn) at this time; poor timing of such a plan.

② Presents will not substitute for presumed neglect or inattention.

③ Never force a child to cuddle and kiss someone he feels is threatening.

110. Knowledge, assessment, physiologic (b)
❹ Patient problems are related to glomerulonephritis.

① Pyuria and hypotension are not problems; hypertension is a problem.

② Polyuria is not a problem.

③ Hypotension is not a problem; hypertension is.

111. Knowledge, implementation, physiologic (a)
❷ Prevents edema, facilitates vasoconstriction, increases blood viscosity, acts as local anesthetic.

① No indication for an eye patch.

③ Inappropriate to promote vasodilation and reduce blood viscosity at this time.

④ No indication for irrigation.

112. Comprehension, implementation, physiologic (a)
❸ His friend is old enough to understand and follow instructions you may give him.

① Rapid assessment emphasizing airway, breathing, and circulation is the first priority.

② His friend should be with you in the event you need assistance.

④ Both of you should go outside to your son. After you have done a rapid assessment emphasizing airway, breathing, and circulation, give his friend instructions to assist you.

113. Comprehension, planning, psychosocial (c)
❶ Modesty and sensitivity are of prime importance to this age group.

②,④ This is part of the normal admission procedure for any age group.

③ Not so for this age group.

114. Application, implementation, psychosocial (b)
❶ The mother needs support to help replenish her emotional strength and to know she is helping her baby.

②,③ Inappropriate action.

④ Can be done at a later time.

115. Comprehension, assessment, environment (c)
    ❷ Upper respiratory infection (URI) occurs frequently in children with cleft palate.
    ① Urinary tract infection.
    ③ Pelvic inflammatory disease.
    ④ Shortness of breath.

116. Comprehension, implementation, physiologic (a)
    ❸ The subcutaneous layer is a source of major blood vessels and rich blood supply. This tissue also has a loose, spongy texture, which results in rapid and relatively painfree absorption of injected material.
    ① Muscle tissue has a slow absorption rate and does not work for insulin.
    ② Adipose tissue does not have a good blood supply for the absorption of insulin.
    ④ Right beneath the epidermis is not a good blood supply. One needs to hit subcutaneous tissue.

117. Comprehension, assessment, physiologic (b)
    ❹ Headaches caused by muscle contractions or tension usually respond to aspirin, Tylenol, or analgesics. This is the most common type of headache and accounts for approximately 80% of all headaches.
    ① A brain tumor tends to cause a deep-seated dull pain that is most intense in the mornings.
    ② Hypertension can cause a slightly throbbing occipital headache that is noticed most when first waking up.
    ③ Migraine vascular headaches are not relieved by aspirin. Pain is severe and may last for hours or days.

118. Application, assessment, physiologic (b)
    ❶ The sclera are the best place to check for yellow and jaundice color, especially in a student with darker skin color.
    ② A student from Egypt will usually have a darker skin color and jaundice would be hard to determine.
    ③ The outer ears and back of neck are not appropriate places to check for jaundice.
    ④ The tongue and buccal area are not appropriate places to check for jaundice. The sclera are the first place to check; then look at the palms of the hands and the soles of the feet.

119. Knowledge, assessment, physiologic (a)
    ❶ This is a true description of Kaposi's sarcoma. It quickly spreads to lymph nodes and internal organs.
    ② This describes squamous cell carcinoma.
    ③ This describes basal cell carcinoma.
    ④ This describes malignant melanoma.

120. Application, planning, health (c)
    ❹ Phenylpropanolamine is in amphetamines, and this can damage blood vessels.
    ① Alcohol is not contained in amphetamines.
    ② Amphetamines do not contain diuretics, except for caffeine.
    ③ Laxatives are not in amphetamines, nor do these pills act as a laxative.

121. Comprehension, assessment, physiologic (a)
    ❸ Vasopressin (ADH) is an antidiuretic hormone produced by the pituitary gland. This hormone is triggered to conserve vital body water in any threatened or real loss of body water.
    ① Albumin is a major protein in many animal or plant tissues, as well as a specialized plasma protein maintaining normal blood pressure.
    ② Aldosterone is a hormone produced by the adrenal gland, which is located on the top of each kidney, and causes reabsorption of sodium.
    ④ Parathyroid hormone is produced by the parathyroid gland. It regulates metabolism of calcium and phosphorus.

122. Knowledge, planning, health (b)
    ❶ Salt substitutes are not safe because the sodium in these products is replaced with potassium. Potassium is eventually restricted to reduce the workload of the kidneys.
    ② Salt substitutes contain potassium, not phosphorus.
    ③ They are not safe because of the potassium in them.
    ④ Even a limited use of a salt substitute is not recommended for patients with chronic renal failure.

123. Application, implementation, environment (b)
    ❷ This is the appropriate technique for placing ear drops into an infant's ears. The infant may also be placed on his back with the head turned for this procedure.
    ① This technique is appropriate for placing ear drops in an adult.
    ③ This is incorrect technique; the ear auricle needs to be pulled down and back for the drops to enter where they need to be.
    ④ This is incorrect; the ear needs to be pulled down and back because of the anatomical structure of the ear.

124. Application, implementation, environment (b)
    ❹ The nurse needs to determine the quantity of formula that the baby is spitting up. Conditions such as pyloric stenosis and allergies can cause this to happen.
    ① The nurse would advise the mother to check the holes in the nipples only after determining whether or not the baby had normal spitting and burping.
    ② It is normal for babies to spit small amounts, but the nurse needs to determine this.
    ③ This is a suggestion that should be made after the nurse has determined that there is not a medical problem.

125. Knowledge, implementation, physiologic (a)
    ❹ At this age, the baby should be able to follow bright lights and objects.
    ① Vision is 20/100 at 1 year of age. Because it is not yet normal, this is the age at which babies keep bumping into things.
    ② Visual acuity is about 20/300, and babies can see only at a very close range.
    ③ By 9 to 10 months of age, depth perception is developing.

ANSWERS AND RATIONALES FOR COMPREHENSIVE EXAMINATIONS

COMPREHENSIVE EXAMINATION 2: PART 1

1. Comprehension, implementation, physiologic (a)
   ❸ Discharge materials are from the uterine wall and are the same for vaginal delivery as for cesarean delivery.
   ①,②,④ False. Because lochia is the discharge from the uterus after delivery of its contents, the lochia would be different only if there were internal hemorrhage or some untoward complication.

2. Comprehension, assessment, physiologic (b)
   ❷ Correct.
   ① Transition occurs between 8 and 10 cm, not 6.
   ③ These are some common symptoms of transition.
   ④ Oxytocin (Pitocin) never given with titanic contractions.

3. Comprehension, implementation, physiologic (b)
   ❷ Proper nutrition during pregnancy is critical. The exact number of pounds gained may depend on many other variables.
   ① This is the approximate average weight gain resulting from pregnancy; individuals vary significantly.
   ③ If there is no control of intake, many individuals will gain excessively.
   ④ Even nonpregnant individuals may find it difficult to lose excessive weight gained.

4. Comprehension, implementation, psychosocial (b)
   ❸ It is important to promote attachment of the family to the infant. This is best done by providing an environment in which the family is able to touch the infant and to interact as a unit.
   ①,②,④ This does not promote family interaction and sharing.

5. Comprehension, implementation, physiologic (a)
   ❷ Prophylactic eyedrops or ointment is effective in preventing gonococcal infection of the eyes.
   ①,③,④ Antibiotic ointments and silver nitrate solution are not effective against these causative organisms.

6. Comprehension, planning, health (b)
   ❸ High blood sugar levels in utero may result in infants who are large for gestational age. Women who deliver large infants are frequently tested for diabetes mellitus.
   ① Increased birth weight does not indicate cardiac problems.
   ② Increased birth weight does not indicate maternal hypothyroidism.
   ④ Increased birth weight does not indicate maternal Cushing's syndrome.

7. Knowledge, assessment, physiologic (a)
   ❸ Hormone transfer through the placenta can cause breast enlargement in both male and female newborns.
   ① Tissue enlargement of the breast can be seen even in small infants.
   ② Maternal hormones transfer to either sex.
   ④ This is normal and does not indicate endocrine problems.

8. Comprehension, implementation, physiologic (b)
   ❷ Size is not the main reason for special care and observation. The newborn delivered by cesarean section is at an increased risk for respiratory distress because of predelivery complications and increased likelihood of aspiration of amniotic fluid during delivery.
   ① Chilling is no more likely than with a vaginal delivery.
   ③ There is no greater incidence of neurological damage due to cesarean section.
   ④ Maturity relates to the length of gestation, not to the method of delivery.

9. Comprehension, planning, health (b)
   ❸ Early ambulation helps promote the return of intestinal peristalsis, thereby decreasing the likelihood of ileus.
   ① Until bowel sounds are present, the patient should not receive solid food.
   ② Splinting of the abdomen will do nothing to promote normal bowel function.
   ④ Kegel's exercises promote urinary control and do not affect the intestines.

10. Application, assessment, health (b)
    ❷ Using Nägele's rule, add 7 days to the first day of the last menstrual period, then subtract 3 months.
    ① This calculation incorrectly started using the last day of the menstrual cycle.
    ③ This calculation incorrectly subtracted 7 days instead of adding 7 days.
    ④ This date has no relation to the application of Nägele's rule.

11. Comprehension, planning, health (b)
    ❷ Medical care should be sought for all childhood injuries.
    ① Rest and quiet is appropriate but not the first priority.
    ③ Opticians make optical apparatus and is an inappropriate answer choice.
    ④ The major priority is medical care.

12. Knowledge, planning, physiologic (a)
    ❸ Toddlers enjoy eating finger foods. Many nutrients can be added to a child's diet in this way.
    ① Large servings discourage a child from eating.
    ② Coaxing or bribing a child to eat places unnecessary attention on not eating and may lead to more serious problems later.
    ④ A child should be allowed to choose between several foods with none being forced on him or her.

13. Application, assessment, physiologic (b)
    ❹ Touching the uvula causes the patient to gag or vomit.
    ① The nasal turbinates are located in the nasal passages, not the throat.
    ②,③ The posterior pharynx and tonsils are areas where throat microorganisms are located.

14. Knowledge, implementation, environment (c)
    ❸ Strict isolation is used for diseases like chickenpox, which are transmitted through the air.
    ① Drainage/secretion isolation is used only to prevent contact with infected drainage.
    ② Respiratory isolation is used for diseases spread by air droplets.
    ④ Universal blood and body fluid isolation is used to prevent contact with infected body fluids or blood.

15. Comprehension, assessment, physiologic (a)
    ❷ High in protein as well as calcium.
    ① Provides protein but little else.
    ③,④ Does not provide any protein.

16. Comprehension, assessment, environment (b)
   ❷ These are classic signs and symptoms of the condition known as failure to thrive.
   ① These are not symptoms of celiac disease.
   ③ These are not symptoms of Hirschsprung's disease.
   ④ These are not symptoms of pyloric stenosis.

17. Application, implementation, physiologic (b)
   ❸ The most common cause of arrest in the pediatric age group is primary respiratory arrest or an obstructed airway; it is thought that this age group will benefit from 1 minute of rescue support before entry into the EMS.
   ① This is only partially correct; it is also necessary that the rescuer activate the EMS.
   ② This is only partially correct: it is also necessary that the rescuer perform 1 minute of CPR before entry into the EMS.
   ④ Both are correct, but in the wrong order; see rationale for #3.

18. Knowledge, implementation, physiologic (a)
   ❶ High-Fowler's position allows better lung expansion, thus promoting better oxygenation.
   ② Oxygen therapy would require a physician's order.
   ③ Vital sign frequency is determined by a complete assessment of the patient.
   ④ Log-rolling technique is used to turn a patient whose back cannot be flexed.

19. Knowledge, planning, environment (a)
   ❹ If a baby vomits water, it is less likely than other choices to cause aspiration pneumonia.
   ①,②,③ Inappropriate *first* foods.

20. Comprehension, implementation, environment (c)
   ❸ Patient scheduled for OR with an elevated temperature; admitting physician should be notified.
   ① Respirations are within normal limits; physician should be notified of abnormal vital signs, not anesthesia.
   ② Pulse is within normal limits; physician should be notified of abnormal vital signs, not anesthesia.
   ④ Blood pressure is within normal limits.

21. Knowledge, assessment, physiologic (b)
   ❶ Enucleation is the term for eye removal. It is necessary in some eye injuries, diseases, and rare tumors.
   ② Electrodiathermy is a surgical intervention for retinal reattachment.
   ③ Scleral buckling is a surgical intervention for retinal reattachment.
   ④ Phacoemulsification is a procedure used to break the cataract lens. The procedure uses ultrasound.

22. Application, implementation, physiologic (b)
   ❹ The nurse needs to keep the temperature probe out of the light, because it can give a false temperature resulting from warming.
   ① Clothes are not kept on a baby under the phototherapy light. Diapers are permitted by some physicians to help keep the baby's skin dry.
   ② The axillary temperature should be monitored every 2 hours and PRN.
   ③ The baby should have eye shields put on for safety.

23. Application, planning, physiologic (c)
   ❹ Numb the area *before* cleaning it may help lessen the pain. Do this before cleaning to avoid contaminating the site.

① This is not realistic. The client is 16, and has already experienced pain in previous injections.
② The patient has already stated that injections cause him pain. It is possible to numb the area with ice to lessen the pain as well as showing a caring attitude.
③ If one numbs the area after cleaning it, it will contaminate the area.

24. Knowledge, implementation, physiologic (b)
   ❸ This is the least threatening thing you can say to a 4 year old.
   ① A 4 year old does not have the vocabulary to understand the term injection.
   ② There is no such thing as a "little shot" to a 4 year old.
   ④ This is not quite truthful; most antibiotics sting considerably.

25. Comprehension, assessment, physiologic (b)
   ❹ Compression of the messenteric blood supply can cause constipation.
   ① Pneumonia usually presents with fever and coughing.
   ② Body casts may cause a claustrophobic reaction, but this patient's symptoms are more consistent with constipation.
   ③ Anxiety reactions usually produce sweating, tacchycardia, and a general feeling of unease.

26. Comprehension, assessment, physiologic (c)
   ❹ Delayed union may cause continued pain past the expected healing time.
   ① Symptoms of compartment syndrome would most likely develop within 48 hours of cast application.
   ② Thrombophlebitis in the casted arm is extremely rare.
   ③ A new fracture could occur if there was trauma to the casted arm again.

27. Comprehension, planning, safe effective care (b)
   ❶ Swelling can be prevented if the limb is elevated above the heart.
   ② Enclosing a plaster cast may cause thermal burns because the plaster generates heat when drying.
   ③ Nothing should be inserted into a cast because of the chance of breaking skin integrity.
   ④ Water will cause the plaster to crumble.

28. Comprehension, planning, physiologic (b)
   ❸ Phenylketonurics cannot metabolize the amino acid phenylalanine. Protein foods are high in the amino acid phenylalanine, and chicken is a high-protein food.
   ① Bread is low in phenylalanine and may be ingested in measured amounts.
   ② Tomatoes are also low in phenylalanine and may be consumed in measured amounts.
   ④ Asparagus is a vegetable and therefore low in phenylalanine; it may be consumed in measured amounts.

29. Application, implementation, physiologic (b)
   ❸ Bacterial conjunctivitis is contagious. Bathing linens should be kept separate to prevent the spread of the infection to others in the household.
   ① Secretions should be cleansed before instilling medication so that the medication can contact the infected mucosal surface. However, boric acid should not be used because of irritation and potential drug interaction. Normal saline is preferred.
   ② Massaging eyes will increase irritation and cause more itching.
   ④ Secretions should be cleansed from medial to lateral canthus to prevent recontamination.

30. Application, evaluation, physiologic (c)
    ❷ The pathophysiologic changes in CF cause blockage of the pancreatic ducts resulting in decreased pancreatic enzymes reaching the gastrointestinal tract. These patients must receive enzyme replacement to digest food. These enzymes must be given within 1 hour before, during, or 1 hour after meals and snacks to be effective.
    ① Same as #2.
    ③ Additional enzymes may be ordered when stools increase; however, the dosing with meals and snacks should continue.
    ④ Giving the medication 2 hours after each meal or snack will not be effective; see #2.

31. Knowledge, implementation, safe environment (a)
    ❸ Rubella, commonly known as German measles, may affect the fetus if contracted during the first trimester of pregnancy.
    ① Roseola is uncommon in children greater than 2 years of age and is not known to affect the fetus.
    ② Contraction of rubeola (measles) by a pregnant woman does not endanger the fetus.
    ④ Varicella (chickenpox) has no effect on the unborn fetus.

32. Comprehension, planning, psychosocial (b)
    ❹ Adjusting to the disease and the management thereof tends to be most difficult during this time. Adolescence is a time when there is a great deal of stress on being perfect and being like peers. This is a period of increased body changes, self-image, and need for independence.
    ①,②,③ Young children usually adjust well to problems related to disease. With toddlers and preschoolers, injections and glucose testing may be difficult at first, but adjustment is fairly rapid as long as parents treat these procedures as routine. During the years before adolescence adjustment appears to be easier, although there is still need for considerable parental involvement.

33. Comprehension, implementation, psychosocial (b)
    ❸ It is beneficial to discuss procedures beforehand so that patients can reason out the extent of discomfort.
    ① This may increase the patient's fear by implying that it is a painful procedure.
    ② This statement does not acknowledge the patient's concerns.
    ④ Sedation is usually not done before the insertion of nasogastric tubes because the tube may be aspirated into the lungs.

34. Knowledge, implementation, health (a)
    ❶ Disturbance of androgen-estrogen balance affects the activity of the sebaceous glands.
    ② Sex glands do not have a direct relationship; it is the androgen-estrogen balance.
    ③ Secretory cells are not the direct cause of the condition.
    ④ The bacteria is not the direct cause; the condition of the androgen-estrogen balance causes this to occur.

35. Comprehension, evaluation, physiological (c)
    ❹ Epinephrine prescriptions need to be refilled on or before the expiration date on the carton.
    ① It is not always possible to avoid bees.
    ② This is a true statement, but a foreign language to those without a background in health.

③ The patient needs to be instructed to self-inject epinephrine. There may not be time to find a parent or an adult to give the injection.

36. Comprehension, planning, physiologic (c)
    ❹ The GI tract will not tolerate a full liquid diet immediately. The intestine is rested by eliminating solid foods. Fluids are given slowly to determine the individual's ability to tolerate and retain.
    ① The GI tract would not tolerate forcing fluids.
    ② Fluids should initially be given in sips.
    ③ Monitoring intake and output has been an ongoing process and part of the plan of care since the child was admitted for treatment.

37. Comprehension, implementation, physiologic (b)
    ❷ All individuals coming into contact with this patient must adhere to meticulous handwashing technique to prevent infection because the body system is immunosuppressed.
    ① Not the most important nursing measure at this time, but important. Nausea and vomiting are side-effects of chemotherapy.
    ③,④ Not the most important nursing measure at this time.

38. Comprehension, planning, physiologic (b)
    ❸ The cast may put pressure on blood vessels and nerves, causing damage and circulatory impairment. Changes in sensation or movement may indicate early injury to nerves or circulatory impairment.
    ① The child should be turned every 2 hours to facilitate drying of cast, prevent pulmonary complications, and reduce risk of pressure ulcer development.
    ② A hair dryer should never be used to dry a cast because it results in a dry outer cast and wet inner cast.
    ④ Conditions that warrant hip spica application (i.e. reduction of hip dislocation) contraindicate ambulation.

39. Comprehension, planning, physiologic (b)
    ❶ The warmth of the pad and its position on the abdomen may decrease pain by decreasing abdominal spasms.
    ② Feedings should be offered more frequently in smaller amounts.
    ③ The position will not harm the infant but will not relieve symptoms of colic.
    ④ The exact cause of colic is unknown, but some experts relate it to a food allergy or sensitivity. Therefore, supplemental foods should not be introduced.

40. Knowledge, evaluation, physiologic (b)
    ❶ Wheezing is produced by air moving through a restricted space such as constricted bronchi. Aminophylline relaxes the smooth muscle of airways, resulting in easier airflow and therefore decreased wheezing.
    ② Oxygen saturation should increase to normal or closer to normal with aminophylline because oxygen flow through the airways is less restricted.
    ③ Prolonged periods of expiration are characteristic of the condition and would be relieved with treatment.
    ④ Aminophylline does not act directly on secretion production but does dilate airways, making it easier to expectorate secretions. Secretions could appear increased because of easier expectoration.

41. Comprehension, implementation, psychosocial (a)
    ❹ Response shows understanding and allows patient to verbalize feelings.
    ①,②,③ Clichés, advice, and excuses that do not reflect understanding and empathy by the nurse.

42. Comprehension, planning, environment (a)
    ❶ A necessary part of the care of an anorexic.
    ② Frequently offering food may increase anxiety and have a negative effect.
    ③ Pressuring the patient to eat is usually what she has experienced from her family and has a negative impact.
    ④ Medications may have only a limited effect.

43. Comprehension, assessment, environment (b)
    ❷ Not oriented in time, because he thinks it's 1886.
    ① Not oriented in time.
    ③ Although confused, not oriented better describes the patient's state.
    ④ Dishonest may or may not be true but is not relevant.

44. Application, implementation, psychosocial (c)
    ❶ Concrete, short-term solution may resolve crisis.
    ② Long-term therapy not indicated.
    ③,④ Long-term solution not indicated.

45. Knowledge, planning, psychosocial (b)
    ❹ The patient needs to be involved in the care plan and treatment. A conference will let her know that all team members are clear about expectations.
    ① Dwelling on unit rules will cause a "war" between the nurse and patient.
    ② Isolation is inappropriate behavior. Letting the patient continue in this is nontherapeutic.
    ③ One is not to demand or threaten patients, and this is also nontherapeutic.

46. Application, assessment, psychosocial (c)
    ❷ This nursing diagnosis is correctly worded in NANDA format.
    ① Incorrect, because myocardial infarction is a medical diagnosis and cannot be the etiology.
    ③ Incorrect, because chest pain is a symptom and cannot be the etiology.
    ④ Incorrect, because role performance, altered is a nursing diagnosis of its own and cannot be the etiology of a different nursing diagnosis.

47. Knowledge, implementation, psychosocial (b)
    ❹ This is an excellent expected outcome and goal for the nurse and client to work toward.
    ① No negative behavior is an unrealistic outcome.
    ② This is not an expected outcome. This is an ongoing observation process.
    ③ Successful coping with all problems is not a realistic outcome at this time.

48. Application, implementation, psychosocial (b)
    ❷ Most elderly patients exhibit some form of short-term memory loss.
    ① Long-term memory is not normally affected in healthy older adults.
    ③ Most elderly individuals exhibit some short-term memory impairment.
    ④ The underlying physical condition of the patient is not disclosed in the question.

49. Comprehension, assessment, psychosocial (b)
    ❸ It is most important to assess the suicide potential for any patient presenting symptoms of depression. The patient may be asking for medications that could be used for overdosing.
    ① Financial ability is not the first assessment to make. Asking questions about finances at this point could add to her stress and depression.

    ② Determining the patient's living situation is important but does not take precedence over suicide potential.
    ④ Legal problems and all the above areas will eventually need assessment, but the first assessment must be suicide potential.

50. Comprehension, evaluation, psychosocial (b)
    ❹ This behavior indicates a serious risk for suicide.
    ① She has already made the decisions about who gets what.
    ② She is not asking for anything in return.
    ③ These are prized possessions, even if not needed.

51. Comprehension, assessment, psychosocial (b)
    ❸ This is the data collection phase of the nursing process, an essential component of assessment.
    ① This is planning, the second phase of the nursing process.
    ② This is implementation, the third phase of the nursing process.
    ④ This is developing a nursing diagnosis, part of the planning phase of the nursing process.

52. Knowledge, planning, psychosocial (a)
    ❷ This is the American Nurses Association's legal definition of nursing and, therefore, the role of the psychiatric nurse.
    ① Clinical psychologists are PhDs who study mental processes and treat mental disorders.
    ③ Psychiatric social workers hold a master's degree in social work and study social causes of the patient's illness, the environment, and families.
    ④ Psychiatrists are medical doctors who diagnose and treat mental diseases.

53. Knowledge, assessment, physiologic (c)
    ❶ Thiamine replacement is given to prevent this syndrome, which results from malabsorption and the poor dietary intake common in alcohol-dependent patients. Muscular activity coordination impairment, disorientation, confusion, and coma are characteristic of this syndrome. Death is possible.
    ② Patient loses the ability to speak while retaining the ability to understand because of organic brain disorders; not a psychiatric disorder.
    ③ Untoward effect of psychotropic drug therapy.
    ④ Fear of being in an open, crowded, or public place.

54. Comprehension, assessment, psychosocial (b)
    ❹ According to statistics, men commit suicide more often than women. Forty-five years and older is considered a high risk group. Individuals without spouses and with chronic illnesses are also considered high risk.
    ① Not considered high risk.
    ② Although at risk, the 59-year-old divorced male with a chronic disease is still considered a higher risk.
    ③ Not considered a high risk.

55. Comprehension, implementation, physiologic (a)
    ❶ It is not unusual for patients to wish to eat and drink at times other than designated mealtimes.
    ② Inappropriate, as severely depressed patients may hope to die or become sick from not eating.
    ③ Inappropriate, because many patients are likely to eat at other times during the day.
    ④ Depressed patients may not have the physical energy or desire to handle this degree of independence.

56. Knowledge, assessment, physiologic (b)
    ❷ A colostomy accessing the sigmoid colon would produce a soft, formed stool, once or twice per day, mimicking a normal bowel pattern.

① Ileostomies normally produce a continuous liquid stool.

③ Ascending colostomies produce a more liquid stool, which is continuous in nature.

④ Transverse colostomies produce a semisoft stool with an irregular pattern of occurrence.

57. Comprehension, planning, environment (a)
    ❹ Correct dose.
    ①,②,③ Incorrect dose.

58. Knowledge, planning, environment (a)
    ❹ Cellulose is found in the stalks and leaves of plants and in the skins of fruits and vegetables.
    ① Refined cereals have most of the fiber removed.
    ② Milk products are low in cellulose.
    ③ Tender meats are low in cellulose.

59. Knowledge, assessment, physiologic (a)
    ❶ Frequent diarrheic stools result in loss of essential electrolytes, especially potassium.
    ②,③,④ Not relevant assessment for stated situation.

60. Knowledge, assessment, physiologic (b)
    ❶ Normal serum potassium level is 3.5. Symptoms of hypokalemia are muscle weakness and paralysis.
    ② Normal serum sodium concentration: 135 to 145 mEq/L.
    ③ Normal serum potassium concentration.
    ④ Serum sodium concentration low; edema would not be present.

61. Knowledge, implementation, environment (a)
    ❷ A principle of surgical asepsis states that sterile objects only touch sterile objects.
    ① Forceps can be used but they must be sterile. Response does not indicate if forceps are sterile.
    ③,④ Response not relevant to dressing change procedure.

62. Knowledge, assessment, physiologic (b)
    ❸ These are three elements to score in obtaining total for Glasgow Coma Scale.
    ①,②,④ All of these are part of a complete neurologic assessment but not specific for Glasgow Coma Scale.

63. Knowledge, planning, environment (a)
    ❶ Correct procedure for GTT.
    ②,④ Not a procedure for any test.
    ③ Not a procedure for any test, although these are essentially postprandial blood samples.

64. Comprehension, assessment, physiologic (b)
    ❹ During fasting, blood sugar levels should fall, stimulating release of glucagon; glucagon acts to raise plasma glucose levels by increasing glycogenolysis and glyconeogenesis and inhibiting glycogen synthesis; insulin checks this rise in plasma glucose levels in nondiabetic patients; a deficiency in insulin allows the glucose to persist at high levels.
    ① The blood glucose level should be low or normal, not elevated.
    ② Normal plasma glucose levels range between 60 and 110 mg/dl blood, depending on the laboratory method used.
    ③ Plasma glucose levels would be decreased.

65. Comprehension, planning, health (b)
    ❸ In case of an emergency a medical identification tag can indicate the anticoagulant and the dosage being taken.
    ① Not without first consulting with the physician.
    ② Stockings are to be removed for bathing and at night when retiring; they are to be reapplied after bathing and upon awakening in the morning.
    ④ Incorrect since restrictions will apply.

66. Comprehension, planning, environment (b)
    ❶ Causes vasodilation and reduces edema.
    ②,③ Inappropriate treatment for this patient because this would aggravate the condition.
    ④ Coumadin does not dissolve clots, but prevents their formation; may not be an initial treatment.

67. Knowledge, evaluation, physiologic (a)
    ❸ Causes venous stasis.
    ①,②,④ A preventive measure.

68. Application, implementation, environment (a)
    ❹ Proper procedure.
    ①,②,③ Improper procedure.

69. Comprehension, planning, physiologic (b)
    ❸ Irrigating the tube will ensure patency.
    ①,② Inappropriate first action.
    ④ Inappropriate action.

70. Knowledge, assessment, environment (b)
    ❶ Sucking chest wound is a direct threat to airway, breathing, and circulation.
    ②,③,④ Not immediately life threatening.

71. Application, planning, physiologic (c)
    ❷ Vitamin K promotes hepatic formation of active prothrombin.
    ①,③,④ Not applicable.

72. Knowledge, assessment, environment (a)
    ❸ All foods on a soft diet have limited fiber; therefore they are easily digested and require less work by the heart.
    ① Soft diets have no specific caloric restrictions and, in fact, may have more calories.
    ② Although many protein foods can be included in this diet, that is not its primary reason for being given.
    ④ Bland diets are used for gastrointestinal disturbances.

73. Comprehension, planning, safe environment (b)
    ❶ Frequent mouth rinses with warm water decrease the discomfort of a sore mouth.
    ② Use of a soft, not firm, toothbrush is recommended.
    ③ Diet would consist of soft, bland foods.
    ④ ASA may irritate oral mucosa.

74. Application, planning, health (b)
    ❷ The patient with osteoporosis is at increased risk for injury. These patients are usually older and fracture-prone. The home environment should be assessed for hazards and measures discussed for making the home environment safer.
    ① Foods high in calcium should be encouraged. An inadequate intake of calcium is frequently seen in patients with osteoporosis. In addition to increasing dietary intake, supplemental calcium may be necessary.
    ③ Sun protection measures are indicated for the patient with SLE.
    ④ Weight-bearing exercise, such as walking, should be encouraged. Range-of-motion exercises help maintain and increase bone formation.

75. Comprehension, assessment, physiologic (b)
    ❶ Typically a person with a fractured hip lies with a painful, injured leg that is shortened and in a position of external rotation.
    ② The affected leg will be shortened because of a fracture of the proximal end of the femur.
    ③ The affected leg will externally rotate because the fracture causes a nonunion of the joint.
    ④ A patient with a hip fracture will be unable to bear weight on the affected leg and unable to walk.

76. Comprehension, implementation, physiologic (c)
   ❶ A potentially lethal complication resulting from long bone fractures is a fat embolism, which can travel and reach either the pulmonary or cerebral circulation. Patients are at greatest risk for fat embolism 12 hours to 3 days after the fracture.
   ② There is no need to release the traction. This may add to the problem of fat embolism by allowing motion at the fracture site.
   ③ The patient has given no evidence of being confused or disoriented.
   ④ Inappropriate action; the nurse should be thinking about physical complications.

77. Comprehension, planning, physiologic (b)
   ❶ Individuals with hyperthyroidism often have an intolerance to heat. A cool, quiet, nonstressful environment should be provided.
   ② The individual with hyperthyroidism will need a high-calorie diet and feedings between meals as the hyperthyroid patient often experiences weight loss even with an increased appetite.
   ③ Testing for urine glucose is not indicated. Hyperthyroidism is overactivity of the thyroid gland and not related to problems of glucose metabolism.
   ④ The hyperthyroid patient's skin is usually warm and moist with increased perspiration.

78. Application, implementation, physiologic (c)
   ❶ Lying on the side with the neck in a normal position allows secretions to flow out by gravity.
   ② Trendelenburg's position could facilitate aspiration because the lungs are now above the head.
   ③ Prone position in an unconscious patient makes airway management difficult because the head must be supported.
   ④ Hyperextending the neck while in a high-Fowler's position could cause the patient to aspirate.

79. Application, implementation, safe environment (b)
   ❹ Massaging after administering the heparin can cause bleeding in the tissue.
   ① Heparin is usually given subcutaneously.
   ② Aspirating can cause bleeding in the tissue.
   ③ All injection sites should be rotated.

80. Comprehension, planning, physiologic (b)
   ❷ Wiping from front to back will help prevent contamination from the rectal area to the urinary meatus.
   ① Volume of output is not always affected by an infection.
   ③ Antibiotics are ordered at specific intervals, that is, every 4 hours, every 6 hours, and so forth.
   ④ Emptying the bladder completely is more effective than training the bladder to be emptied every 2 hours.

81. Comprehension, implementation, psychosocial (b)
   ❸ This response encourages expression of feelings and validates the nurse's observations about the present situation. This type of response encourages a supportive nurse-patient relationship.
   ① This response is based on unreliable data and offers the patient no choices or opportunity to express concerns.
   ②,④ This response avoids dealing with the patient's feelings and concerns. There is no encouragement for feedback.

82. Comprehension, planning, environment, (b)
   ❷ The individual with Alzheimer's disease has difficulty remembering, even forgetting how or what to do to eat. As motor function becomes impaired, the individual will require more time to complete tasks.
   ① The Alzheimer's patient will become confused and agitated when presented with a variety of choices. Frequent, small feedings with few choices is an appropriate intervention.
   ③ Distractions at mealtime should be eliminated; they tend to confuse and irritate the patient. Quiet surroundings help keep the patient calm.
   ④ Complex tasks should be avoided. The patient with Alzheimer's often cannot remember complex directions, so there is a lack of compliance.

83. Knowledge, planning, health (a)
   ❷ Large amounts of salt are used in canning dill pickles.
   ① Canned peaches contain significant quantities of potassium and sugar.
   ③ Fresh peaches are a good source of carbohydrates.
   ④ Cucumbers are very low in sodium.

84. Comprehension, planning, physiologic (b)
   ❶ NPH insulin is an intermediate-acting insulin preparation. It will have an onset of action within 1 to 2 hours after administration, with a peak action 6 to 12 hours after administration.
   ② This time frame represents the peak action time of NPH.
   ③ This time frame is too late; the onset of action will already have occurred.
   ④ This time frame is too late for NPH; the onset of action will already have occurred.

85. Comprehension, implementation, physiologic (b)
   ❹ Cold acts as a local anesthetic.
   ① Cold constricts superficial blood supplies.
   ② Cold will decrease blood flow to an area.
   ③ Heat helps reduce muscle spasms.

86. Application, planning, physiologic (b)
   ❹ A safety razor may cause profuse bleeding if the patient cuts himself.
   ① Aspirin is contraindicated because it enhances bleeding.
   ② ITP does not affect the leukocytes.
   ③ Orthopnea is usually not associated with ITP.

87. Application, implementation, physiologic (c)
   ❷ Metastasis means the spread of cancer beyond the primary site.
   ① It is no longer just the primary tumor growing.
   ③ Rarely does cancer metastasize to the breast.
   ④ Microscopic tissue examination should reveal that it looks similar to the breast tissue.

88. Comprehension, planning, physiologic (b)
   ❹ These readings show improvement of respiratory status.
   ① A better goal would be to have no cyanosis after ambulation.
   ② Pulse rate should return to baseline within 10 minutes or less.
   ③ Respiratory rates should return to normal within 10 minutes or less.

89. Comprehension, planning, physiologic (b)
   ❷ This should improve bowel elimination.
   ① Not indicated for constipation.
   ③ Does not solve the problem.
   ④ Limited because of fractured hip.

90. Comprehension, implementation, physiologic (b)
    ❷ The resident may eat more if offered small amounts more often.
    ① Not indicated.
    ③ Important but not the number one priority.
    ④ Eating is a social event, so he needs to have others around.

91. Application, planning, physiologic (b)
    ❸ Smoked meats generally contain high levels of the carcinogen nitrite.
    ① Wild rice is a high-fiber grain.
    ② Dietary fat should be reduced.
    ④ Vitamin B is water soluble, so increased intake won't affect cancer risk reduction.

92. Application, assessment, safe and effective care (b)
    ❷ Raising the height of the infusion should increase the rate of flow.
    ① Lowering the bag should slow the rate of infusion.
    ③ Minidrop tubing may make it more difficult to maintain the prescribed rate.
    ④ A 22-gauge needle is smaller than the one being used.

93. Application, implementation, safe and effective care (b)
    ❸ Buck's traction is applied to the skin and may be temporarily removed for hygiene and skin assessment.
    ① Crutchfield tongs are applied to the head to provide cervical traction.
    ② Thomas Pearson's splints are skeletal traction and may not be removed.
    ④ External fixators are skeletal traction and may not be removed.

94. Application, implementation, safe and effective care (c)
    ❹ This site prevents turning the patient unnecessarily.
    ① The operative side should be avoided because of alteration in microcirculation.
    ② This muscle is on the operative side.
    ③ Turning the patient to the operative side could cause dislocation of the new prosthesis.

95. Application, planning, safe and effective care (c)
    ❸ The joints that are still able to move should be exercised to prevent contractures.
    ① This may cause the fracture to dislocate because it is too high.
    ② Strenuous activity should be avoided while the fracture heals.
    ④ Complete range of motion may cause the fracture to dislocate.

96. Application, planning, safe and effective care (b)
    ❶ The abdomen is the safest site.
    ② Intramuscular is not a recommended route of administration for insulin.
    ③ The vastus lateralis is an IM injection site.
    ④ The ventral gluteal is also an IM injection site.

97. Knowledge, assessment, physiologic (b)
    ❷ Cachexia is a state of general ill health and malnutrition.
    ① Ascites refers to the accumulation of fluid in the abdomen.
    ③ Aphasia is inability to communicate verbally.
    ④ Dysphagia refers to difficulty in swallowing.

98. Knowledge, assessment, physiologic (c)
    ❷ The therapeutic range for theophylline is 10 to 20 mg/dl.

① This is subtherapeutic.
③ This level is above the therapeutic range.
④ This level is toxic.

99. Knowledge, assessment, physiologic (b)
    ❶ Aminoglycosides have ototoxicity and nephrotoxicity as side-effects.
    ② Penicillins frequently have anaphylactic-type reactions.
    ③ Cephalosporins frequently have rashes as major side effects.
    ④ Tetracyclines may stain the teeth.

100. Knowledge, evaluation, physiologic (b)
    ❹ Partial thromboplastin time measures the clotting time specific to heparin therapy.
    ① Prothrombin time measures clotting ability specific to warfarin (Coumadin).
    ② Indirect Coombs test is used to diagnose hemolytic anemia.
    ③ Direct Coombs test is used to diagnose hemolytic anemia.

101. Knowledge, evaluation, physiologic (c)
    ❹ An elevated creatinine level may indicate that the vancocin is causing nephrotoxicity.
    ① The hemoglobin is normal.
    ② The sodium is normal.
    ③ The potassium is normal.

102. Knowledge, evaluation, physiologic (b)
    ❸ Oxygen by cannula will allow the patient to maintain oxygen levels.
    ① The patient may be severely dyspneic the rest of her life.
    ② A full liquid diet would allow the patient to expend less energy while chewing, but the selection is very limited.
    ④ This option wouldn't supply enough oxygen to meet the patient's needs.

103. Knowledge, implementation, physiologic (b)
    ❹ Grade determines how different-appearing the cancerous cell is from normal tissue.
    ① Depth of tumor penetration is not measured.
    ② The extent of tumor spread is called metastasis.
    ③ Cancer cells may be present for years before a tumor is large enough to detect.

104. Application, planning, physiologic (c)
    ❸ Small, frequent meals allow for rest in between and decreases frustration caused by difficulty handling and consuming food.
    ① Foods should be soft and easy to chew and swallow.
    ② Protein interferes with the absorption of levodopa (Dopar). Some protein is allowed in the diet, but large amounts should be avoided.
    ④ Untrue statement. Individuals with Parkinson's disease eat regular food with little special preparation.

105. Application, planning, physiologic (c)
    ❸ Campho-Phenique or other drying agents are useful in the relief of pain and pruritus associated with herpes.
    ① Neosporin is an antibacterial ointment. It would be useless and could even do harm by holding in moisture to the area.
    ② The area should be kept clean and dry.
    ④ Condoms are recommended during intercourse whether the virus is active or not, but intercourse would increase the pain.

106. Application, planning, physiologic (c)
    ❶ A high-protein and high-calorie diet will promote healing while giving him the energy calories he requires.
    ② Intestinal stimulants will irritate the intestinal mucosa.
    ③ Food should be chewed well, but pureed foods are generally not necessary at home.
    ④ To promote healing, the patient will need adequate vitamin C.

107. Application, planning, physiologic (b)
    ❷ Cleansing removes resident bacteria and decreases the risk of infection.
    ① Checking the incision daily is often enough.
    ③ Heavy lifting should be avoided. Normal activities should be resumed over a 2- to 3-week period.
    ④ Once the Steri-Strips fall off, there is no need to replace them.

108. Comprehension, application, environment (b)
    ❸ This is an empathetic statement to the visitor and does not break the patient's right to privacy concerning her treatment.
    ① This statement offers empathy, but no action is taken to help the visitor communicate with her friend.
    ② This is not a totally true statement because usually some visitors are permitted.
    ④ This is true, but infringes on the patient's right to privacy concerning her mode of therapy.

109. Application, assessment, physiologic (b)
    ❷ The tube is blocked. The nurse has done all within her scope of practice to clear the blockage. The doctor has to be notified for anything else to be done for the patient.
    ① Intestinal tubes are not taped to the nose because they must be able to progress through the tract by gravity and peristalsis.
    ③ Drainage is to be on low intermittant pressure unless ordered differently. High suction could injure the intestinal mucosa.
    ④ Protocol is to irrigate with 30 ml normal saline, which has already been done.

110. Application, assessment, physiologic (b)
    ❷ Severe pain indicates a complication.
    ① Tylenol might be administered, but it is not the first priority.
    ③ Eye surgery patients are positioned on their back or the nonoperative side, but this is not the priority.
    ④ Eye surgery patients are positioned on their nonoperative side or their back.

111. Application, assessment, health (b)
    ❹ More information is required before making a decision.
    ① This is true but does not clarify whether the patient's problem is related to the vaccine or not.
    ② The nurse might be denying the patient a chance to be immunized if she doesn't give the doctor more information.
    ③ This should be asked after the patient explains the signs and symptoms of the reaction to the previous flu shot.

112. Comprehension, assessment, physiologic (b)
    ❸ This indicates that the patient can swallow and not choke.
    ① Not most important assessment.
    ② May request it but not be able to tolerate it.
    ④ Should have never been absent.

113. Knowledge, assessment, physiologic (b)
    ❶ The correct action in an eye laceration is to loosely patch the eye.
    ② The eye is irrigated with running water in chemical splash accidents.
    ③ A physician's order is needed to administer an eye antibiotic ointment.
    ④ A physician's order is needed to administer eyedrops. Eyelid and lacerations need to be seen first before treatments are ordered.

114. Knowledge, implementation, physiologic (a)
    ❹ The correct rescue breathing rate for adults is 10 to 12 respirations per minute.
    ③ This is an incorrect rate.
    ①,② Because a pulse is present, there is no need for compressions.

115. Comprehension, assessment, physiologic (c)
    ❷ The highest priority because physiological death is impending unless myocardial tissue perfusion is reestablished.
    ① Airway, breathing, and circulation problems take priority over all other problems.
    ③ Alteration in comfort: chest pain is an important nursing diagnosis and must be addressed promptly to decrease myocardial oxygen demand. However, the major focus is relieving ischemia in the myocardium.
    ④ Self-care deficit related to fear of dying in the acute phase of a myocardial infarction is not usually important at this time.

116. Knowledge, assessment, physiologic (a)
    ❹ Congenital heart defects occur at birth and are structural abnormalities.
    ① Congestive heart failure is a complication of other heart problems. Congestive heart failure occurs as a result of myocardial weakness.
    ② Endocarditis is an inflammation of the inner lining of the heart.
    ③ Coronary heart disease is a disease that affects the coronary blood vessels and leads to obstruction of blood flow.

117. Comprehension, implementation, physiologic (b)
    ❸ A more liberal use of carbohydrate, mainly complex forms, is recommended because complex carbohydrates break down more slowly and release available glucose over time, leading to a more stable blood sugar level.
    ① The diabetic diet should consist of 40% complex carbohydrates (starches) and 20% simple carbohydrates (fruits and milk).
    ② Fat consumption should be no more than 25% to 30% of the diet's total calories, and high protein intake is not recommended because of saturated fat content and excess nitrogen content, which stresses renal function.
    ④ People with diabetes can eat out. The recommendation is to choose a restaurant that has appropriate foods available to meet and maintain blood sugar levels.

118. Comprehension, implementation, physiologic (c)
    ❸ Persistent coughing after insertion of a nasogastric tube indicates that the tube is in the patient's lung. The tube should be immediately removed to prevent injury to the lung and possible pneumothorax.
    ① Allowing the patient to rest will not stop the coughing, because the tube has entered the lung.

② Encouraging the patient to swallow will not remove the tube from the patient's lung.

④ Elevating the patient's head and flexing his neck will not stop the coughing, which is caused by the entrance of the tube into the lung.

119. Knowledge, planning, physiologic (c)

❶ Assays of hemoglobin A_{1C} test glucose control over a period of time. The test is performed to ascertain compliance and patient motivation with the prescribed treatment plan.

② The glycosylated hemoglobin test is not used to diagnose diabetes but to monitor the progress of a person who is already a diabetic.

③ The glycosylated hemoglobin test is a blood test, not a urine test.

④ The test does not determine insulin dosing, it determines control.

120. Knowledge, implementation, physiologic (b)

❸ Ventilation has just occurred, so the second rescuer starts with compressions.

② No need to ventilate because the first rescuer just did that.

④ The second rescuer should start with compressions, therefore he should not be at the victim's head.

① The compression ventilation ratio for 2-rescuer CPR is 5:1.

121. Knowledge, evaluation, physiologic (b)

❸ The supportive data are the 30-pound weight loss and the emaciated appearance, which supports the nursing diagnosis.

① The data to support the diagnosis are not available.

② The patient may have feelings related to death; however, there aren't enough data to support the nursing diagnosis at this time.

④ Social isolation often occurs with the AIDS patient because of societal fears and lack of knowledge regarding the disease. No data exist in this situation to support the nursing diagnosis.

122. Application, implementation, safe and effective care (c)

❷ Fowler's position facilitates breathing and decreases swelling of the operative site; sandbags relieve tension on suture lines; frequent monitoring of vital signs allows for early intervention should complications arise.

① A complication of a thyroidectomy is a thyroid crisis, which causes a sudden increase in thyroxine. Signs of thyroid crisis are body temperatures as high as 106° or higher, an increased heart rate of 200 beats per minute or greater, increased respiratory rate, apprehension, and restlessness. If the crisis is not arrested, death may occur.

③ Redness, some swelling, and discomfort at the operative site are expected.

④ Tetany secondary to hypocalcemia is a possible complication of the surgery secondary to accidental removal of the parathyroid glands.

123. Knowledge, evaluation, physiologic (b)

❸ The data support absence of infection with normal physiological responses expected after surgery.

① The data suggest the patient has developed an infection.

② The data suggest the patient has developed an infection, especially with a white blood count of 13,000.

④ A reddened incision site with purulent drainage indicates the presence of an infection.

124. Comprehension, assessment, environment (a)

❶ Many patients experience an aura or unusual sensory perception before having a seizure.

② Hallucinations are auditory or visual and are mental stimuli not based in reality.

③ Petit mal seizures are usually confined to children without an associated aura. Petit mal is classified as a brief loss of consciousness.

④ Has nothing to do with seizure activity.

125. Comprehension, assessment, physiologic (c)

❶ General hypoxia of the tissues causes fatigue and dyspnea especially on exertion, which results in increased demands.

② The compensatory mechanism of the heart to meet oxygen demands is to increase heart rate.

③ The blood pressure is usually increased because of the decreased lumen size of coronary arteries, secondary to the disease process.

④ Coronary artery disease causes general hypoxia, not limited to a single system.

COMPREHENSIVE EXAMINATION 2: PART 2

1. Knowledge, assessment, environment (b)
   ❷ True labor is characterized by regular, forceful contractions, dilation and effacement of the cervix, and descent of the presenting part into the pelvis. Other options refer to signs of impending labor and possible complications (abdominal pain).
   ①,③,④ Incorrect—see rationale for #2.

2. Application, assessment, environment (b)
   ❷ This patient is now in the second stage of labor. All options listed include nursing responsibilities done during this time. Increasing the frequency of monitoring FHTs and maternal vital signs is most critical to maternal-infant well-being.
   ①,③,④ See rationale for #2.

3. Knowledge, planning, physiologic (a)
   ❷ Absence of prenatal care precludes early detection so that condition can be watched and controlled.
   ① Hypertensive drugs were discovered and used for primary hypertension and were adopted for use by obstetricians; poor answer.
   ③ Controversial; recent studies reveal may have no effect.
   ④ PIH may occur at any age; number of pregnancies is of more concern, that is, whether first baby; although PIH is more likely in teenagers or older women, not best possible answer.

4. Comprehension, implementation, environment (a)
   ❸ Because there is danger of bladder rupture if the bladder is full, it is important to be sure the bladder is emptied.
   ① Expected in this situation.
   ② Physician's responsibility.
   ④ Assessing FHS is a normal nursing responsibility before any delivery.

5. Comprehension, implementation, environment (b)
   ❷ Best response; facts are true, and you are suggesting alternatives.
   ① Giving only partial response is not advisable.
   ③ Have not answered anxieties regarding IUDs.
   ④ Unwarranted criticism; unanswered question.

6. Knowledge, implementation, health (b)
   ❸ True and best response.
   ① The physician or nurse should instruct the woman how to determine time of ovulation.
   ② Several days of abstinence are suggested, not 10.
   ④ Cycle must be regular, not necessarily every 30 days; could be every 26 days; the key word is *regular*.

7. Knowledge, assessment, physiologic (b)
   ❸ The zygote is implanted in the uterine wall at about 3 weeks and thus ends the preembryonic stage.
   ① At birth, the fetus becomes a neonate.
   ② The fetal stage is from 9 weeks to birth.
   ④ The embryonic stage occurs from the fourth to eighth week, and consists of rapid growth and differentiation.

8. Application, implementation, physiologic (b)
   ❶ The umbilical cord has two arteries, which return waste from the system, and one vein, through which nutrients pass from the mother to the fetus.
   ②,③,④ This is incorrect. There are 2 arteries and 1 vein in the umbilical cord.

9. Comprehension, planning, health (b)
   ❶ A balance of all nutrients provides a favorable environment for the developing fetus.
   ② An adequate amount of calories is needed for protein utilization and fat metabolism.
   ③ Fluid intake facilitates the clearance of creatinine, urea, and other waste products of fetal and maternal metabolism.
   ④ A well-balanced diet is recommended for adequate metabolism.

10. Comprehension, assessment, physiologic (a)
    ❶ Amenorrhea is a presumptive sign of pregnancy that most women recognize as a need to seek medical attention.
    ② Amenorrhea is only a presumptive sign because it can be caused by many other factors, including disease and stress.
    ③ It is true that there are other changes. However, the woman must get to the doctor before she can notice them.
    ④ This is false. Nausea is found in only 50% of pregnancies, and quickening does not usually appear until 18 to 20 weeks.

11. Comprehension, implementation, psychosocial (b)
    ❶ Acknowledges her feelings and encourages her self-confidence without being unrealistic about her mother.
    ② A partially true statement. However, it ignores the cultural realities that grandmothers do play a major role in raising many children.
    ③ Sarcastic; undermines self-confidence.
    ④ She should go to the class even if her mother is around. The child is her responsibility.

12. Comprehension, implementation, psychosocial (b)
    ❸ Acknowledges her pride in her baby and gives her realistic information without undermining her self-confidence.
    ① This may be true. However, it does undermine her self-esteem.
    ② This is also true. However, it does not deal with the immediate concern of the nurse to provide truthful information.
    ④ The nurse may be aware that it is a very common practice to have grandmothers help. However, this young mother needs to develop her own skills of child care.

13. Knowledge, planning, physiologic (a)
    ❶ Cord pulsations usually cease within seconds after respiration is initiated.
    ② It is important that respirations are initiated and pulsation of the cord stops before the cord is clamped and cut.
    ③,④ Such a lengthy period of time is not necessary before the cord is clamped and cut.

14. Knowledge, implementation, psychosocial (a)
    ❷ This is correct information.
    ① Incorrect; the nurse is not addressing the mother's concern.
    ③ There is no specific treatment required for milia.
    ④ Incorrect information is being given to the mother, as well as a cause for needless concern.

15. Comprehension, evaluation, psychosocial (b)
    ❷ Suits may be brought by patients who believe they have not been actively treated.

① Legal competency does not alter the patient's rights to treatment.

③ Nurses may be called to testify.

④ Patients retain civil rights.

16. Comprehension, assessment, physiologic (c)

❷ Drug users, especially cocaine users, are often in financial difficulty and may be in realistic danger from dealers and others.

① One cannot conclude that he is delusional from the data given.

③ Faulty statement.

④ This is not a specific legal requirement.

17. Analysis, assessment, psychosocial (b)

❷ Projection is assigning one's feelings to others.

① Repression pushes material out of consciousness.

③ Displacement places angry feelings onto a safer object.

④ Rationalization applies logical reasons to guard against feelings.

18. Comprehension, implementation, psychosocial (a)

❸ To allow feedback is essential.

① Logical argument may block communication.

② Questioning may block communication.

④ Advising may block communication.

19. Comprehension, assessment, environment (b)

❷ This is a symptom of the condition.

① Amenorrhea, not dysmenorrhea, is commonly seen in these patients.

③ Bradycardia and hypotension are common, probably because of the state of starvation.

④ Constipation, not diarrhea, is a symptom of anorexia nervosa.

20. Application, implementation, psychosocial (b)

❶ The nurse should promote a positive self-image in a patient with anorexia nervosa because her present self-image is a negative one.

②,③,④ Current measure used in the treatment of a patient with anorexia nervosa.

21. Comprehension, assessment, environment (b)

❶ Scattered thoughts are indicated by rapid frequent topic changes.

② Rapid speech may or may not indicate scattering.

③ Physical appearance is only a general indicator.

④ History is only a general indicator.

22. Application, assessment, psychosocial (c)

❸ Antianxiety drugs decrease physiologic manifestations of anxiety such as elevated blood pressure, pulse, respiration.

① Signs of anxiety.

② Paradoxical reactions.

④ Signs of anxiety.

23. Application, implementation, psychosocial (b)

❸ Allows patient to maintain some independence and dignity while ensuring procedure is done properly.

①,②,④ Inappropriate nursing action.

24. Knowledge, assessment, psychosocial (c)

❹ Compensation is making up for a "deficiency" in one area by excelling or emphasizing another one. This patient is attempting academic excellence to compensate for his short stature.

① This patient is not in denial as he is aware of his problem.

② Conversion is when emotional conflicts are turned into physical symptoms.

③ Projection is when one attributes to others the characteristics that the person does not want to admit possessing.

25. Knowledge, assessment, psychosocial (b)

❸ Identification is when people try to identify with another group.

① Projection is attributing to others character traits that the individual does not want to admit having.

② Compensation is when one makes up for deficiencies by excelling in something else.

④ Rationalization is giving reasons to justify behavior.

26. Application, planning, psychosocial (b)

❹ Behavior modification is a technique based on the theory that behavior must be rewarded or reinforced to continue. Removing a reward for behavior is used to change undesirable behaviors.

① Setting limits does not change or improve behaviors.

② Confronting the client for inappropriate behavior will not necessarily change the behavior.

③ A reprimand gains nothing and may lead to more aggressive behavior.

27. Application, implementation, psychosocial (b)

❸ This is the correct response at this time. The nurse needs to establish a trusting relationship and get a pattern of communication started.

① This is not true. A court order can force one to be admitted to this unit.

② This would not be appropriate at this time; the nurse has not established a good communication relationship with the client, who would probably lie at this point. Ask this question much later.

④ This is not an appropriate response; the nurse has already judged the client and is putting him down by stating that it is for his own good.

28. Application, planning, physiologic (b)

❶ The tracheostomy tray is obtained in the event that the patient develops an obstructed airway. Tracheal edema results from the inhalation of smoke and heat.

②,③,④ Routine for any emergency.

29. Application, planning, environment (a)

❸ Reverse isolation protects the patient and the burn areas from infections transmitted by others.

①,②,④ Not applicable to situation at hand.

30. Application, planning, physiologic (a)

❷ To help him cope with immobility, you can use play therapy and diversional activity to decrease his anxiety. Preschoolers describe objects as real, and by simulating application of Russell traction on his favorite toy you can lessen his feelings of aloneness.

① Short-term diversional activity.

③,④ Inappropriate to situation.

31. Knowledge, implementation, physiologic (a)

❷ Increasing fluids, cellulose, and bulk in the diet will facilitate bowel elimination.

① Not appropriate foods.

③,④ Lacks fluid and large amounts of bulk and/or cellulose.

32. Knowledge, assessment, health (b)

❷ School-age children are in this stage of development.

① Toddlers are in this stage of development.

③ Preschoolers are in this stage of development.

④ Infants are in this stage of development.

33. Comprehension, evaluation, physiologic (b)
   ❶ A change in level of consciousness (LOC) may be one of the first signs of increased intracranial pressure.
   ② Not associated; GI symptoms are nausea and vomiting.
   ③ Pulse rate and respirations are decreased.
   ④ Problems related to glaucoma.

34. Comprehension, assessment, psychosocial (b)
   ❷ Patient's way of expressing anxiety.
   ① Maladjustment may contribute to the stress of pending surgery, but it is the stress that causes her behavior.
   ③ No information regarding prior hospitalization.
   ④ Inadequate preparation may contribute to the stress of pending surgery, but it is the stress that causes her behavior.

35. Knowledge, assessment, environment (b)
   ❸ These are all common symptoms of acute glomerulonephritis.
   ① Severe edema and proteinuria are symptoms of nephrotic syndrome.
   ② These are symptoms of nephrotic syndrome.
   ④ These are not symptoms of acute glomerulonephritis.

36. Application, evaluation, physiologic (c)
   ❸ Not oriented to general season (Thanksgiving being in November).
   ① Not significant; he may not be closely familiar with the hospital.
   ② Orientation to person must be someone he is familiar with.
   ④ Amnesia concerning the accident is common.

37. Knowledge, implementation, environment (b)
   ❸ Corticosteroids are used to reduce the edema seen in nephrotic syndrome, not acute glomerulonephritis.
   ①,②,④ This is commonly used in the treatment of acute glomerulonephritis.

38. Comprehension, assessment, environment (b)
   ❶ Acute glomerulonephritis usually occurs as a reaction to infections, especially streptococcal infections.
   ②,③,④ This does not lead to acute glomerulonephritis.

39. Knowledge, assessment, psychosocial (c)
   ❷ Toddlers are becoming more independent and want to do things for themselves.
   ① An infant normally wants to be cuddled and cries for immediate gratification of its needs, such as hunger or comfort.
   ③ A school-age child may cry when first taken to school but should stop crying quickly. A child who continuously cries has a fear of desertion.
   ④ Children normally begin talking at 2 years of age and by 4 years of age have a fairly large vocabulary.

40. Comprehension, evaluation, health (b)
   ❷ Solid foods need to be stopped and liquids encouraged. Solid foods will stimulate colon and cause more diarrhea.
   ① Liquids only will replace fluids and electrolytes and allow the colon to rest and heal.
   ③ Gatorade may help replace lost electrolytes.
   ④ Dehydration is a serious problem with a young child who has diarrhea. It can be life-threatening.

41. Comprehension, assessment, health (b)
   ❶ Closing one nostril can force bacteria into the ear canal. Leave both nostrils open while blowing.

② Washing hands will decrease spread of infection.
③ Ointment will prevent dry, cracked areas on the nose from frequent blowing.
④ Bacteria can be forced into the ear canal and cause an infection.

42. Application, implementation, physiologic (b)
   ❷ An infant can be overloaded with fluids easily. Monitor IV fluids with a Microset and give fluids slowly.
   ① Rapid infusion of fluids can actually drown the infant.
   ③ Dehydration is very dangerous for the infant. Fluid needs to be given as soon as possible.
   ④ IVs are painful for the infant, but dehydration needs to be treated as quickly as possible. Fluids by mouth take too long to correct the dehydration. Also, the cause of the dehydration may be vomiting, so PO fluids will not stay down.

43. Knowledge, assessment, health (b)
   ❶ The primitive Moro reflex is still present at 3 weeks of age.
   ②,④ Vocalizations and holding head erect are behaviors which can be observed in the 2-month-old infant. This infant does not have the neuromuscular development to perform these behaviors.
   ③ Recognizing familiar faces occurs at approximately 3 months. Before this time, younger infants may start to recognize familiar voices.

44. Comprehension, assessment, health (c)
   ❹ Tight undergarments may result in perineal inflammation, which may inhibit the flow of urine during micturation. If the bladder is unable to empty fully, urine stasis results. Urine stasis is a major risk factor for UTI.
   ① Restriction of fluids at night only will not increase the risk of UTI as long as adequate fluids have been consumed during the day.
   ② Daily tub baths in plain water are not harmful. Tub baths may facilitate keeping the perineal area clean, which reduces the risk for UTI. Adding bubble bath to the water in contrast may increase the risk.
   ③ Because of the short female urethra and the close proximity to the rectum, it is recommended that females use a front to back motion when wiping to decrease the likelihood of *E. coli* contamination from the rectum.

45. Comprehension, planning, health (c)
   ❹ To stimulate the immune system to produce antibodies against the rabies virus, the entire series of HDCV injections must be completed on the exact recommended dosing schedule. Failure to follow this schedule could result in development of rabies in the patient, which is usually fatal.
   ① Although some type of wound care may be ordered, it is not the priority in discharge instructions.
   ② Same as #1. Also in many cases these wounds are not sutured because of the danger of infection by other bacteria, because the wound is usually considered a dirty wound.
   ③ Temperature elevation is a potential side-effect of the injections but again not the priority in discharge instructions.

46. Application, evaluation, physiologic (b)
    ❸ Insertion of the catheter no farther than 0.5 cm beyond the tip of the tube depth will prevent excessive damage to the tracheal mucosa.
    ① Hydrogen peroxide should never be instilled into the trach tube. It can however be used to remove crust externally around the stoma or to clean the inner cannula when removed during tracheostomy care.
    ② The suction gauge should be set at no more than 120 mmHg pressure; greater pressures will result in damage to the tracheal mucosa and possible excess depletion of oxygen, causing hypoxemia.
    ④ Leaving the suction catheter in the tube longer than 5 to 10 seconds may result in depletion of oxygen, resulting in hypoxemia.

47. Comprehension, assessment, physiologic (c)
    ❶ Inhalation of noxious fumes as produced by ammonia may precipitate an asthma attack caused by irritation of respiratory passages.
    ② Emotional upset will not precipitate an asthma attack in children. It may, however, exacerbate an attack if already present.
    ③,④ Cool humidification of respiratory passages as could occur while swimming or when using a humidifier does not usually precipitate an attack. Respiratory passages may be soothed.

48. Application, planning, health (b)
    ❶ Food supplementation is not required; breast milk will supply the infant with all required nutrients the first 4 months of life.
    ② Mothers should pump their breasts and place breast milk in a bottle for the father to use during feeding.
    ③ Solid foods should not be introduced before 4 months of age. The gastrointestinal tract is not mature and infants still have the extrusion reflex before this time.
    ④ Breast milk supplies all nutrients needed for the young infant.

49. Application, implementation, health (c)
    ❸ The pertussis component of the injection frequently causes fever and irritability as adverse reactions.
    ① The single injection does not offer complete immunity. Two additional doses are needed as well as boosters later in childhood. Tetanus boosters are needed at least every 10 years.
    ② Contact with children is not contraindicated because the immunization does not contain live virus/bacteria.
    ④ Seizure activity is a rare adverse effect of the pertussis component (1 in 110,000).

50. Knowledge, assessment, health (b)
    ❶ Development of scoliosis is predominant in preadolescent girls (7:1) at the beginning of the preadolescent growth spurt.
    ② Infants rarely develop idiopathic scoliosis.
    ③ Most college-age females have already achieved their maximum bone growth in relation to height during high school. Idiopathic scoliosis would have already occurred.
    ④ Lordosis, not scoliosis, is a normal finding in the toddler.

51. Knowledge, assessment, physiologic (c)
    ❷ Plethora or reddened complexion occurs with increased red blood cells. A child with a cyanotic heart defect manufactures more red cells as a compensatory mechanism to the hypoxemia.
    ①,③,④ Neck vein distention, peripheral edema, and adventitious breath sounds are more frequently associated with acyanotic defects, which usually involve increased pulmonary blood flow or obstruction to flow from the ventricles. Blood becomes congested in the periphery, particularly coming into the right heart, which produces the symptoms listed.

52. Application, planning, physiologic (c)
    ❸ Infants with bronchiolitis have copious secretions that cannot be expectorated without assistance. Frequent suctioning is indicated. Also, the secretions should be removed before feeding so the infant does not begin coughing and vomit the feeding, risking aspiration.
    ① Infants must receive adequate fluids to keep secretions thin. Fluid requirements may actually be increased because of fever and increased losses from tachypnea.
    ② The RSV virus is found primarily in respiratory passages and on respiratory secretions. Respiratory isolation is usually ordered, as well as gloves for suctioning.
    ③ The infant may aspirate if placed in a prone position after feeding.

53. Application, assessment, health (c)
    ❷ Imitating toileting behaviors indicates potential interest in learning to toilet, a major sign of readiness for toilet training.
    ① Children unable to sit for longer than 2 minutes will probably not be able to sit for a sufficient time to learn to toilet.
    ③ Although not an absolute indicator, children who dislike soiled diapers are more ready to learn toileting skills.
    ④ Children must be dry consistently for long periods of time (i.e., naps) to achieve success with toilet training. Children unable to stay dry may still have an immature bladder/sphincter.

54. Application, assessment, physiologic (c)
    ❹ Research has demonstrated that using an age-appropriate pain scale provides the most objective way of measuring a client's pain. Traditional methods of determining presence and intensity of pain such as observing visual cues are unreliable because of individual client responses to pain and variability in the caregiver's interpretation of cues.
    ① Same as #4.
    ② Although it might be helpful to have the client describe his/her pain, it will be difficult to quantify the intensity with words. We need to quantify the intensity to ascertain if our comfort measures are working.
    ③ Parents can be a wonderful resource when ascertaining pain levels in the preverbal shy child. This patient, however, is an adolescent and should participate actively in her/his own care.

55. Application, assessment, physiologic (c)
    ❷ Combined with the type of injury he had and his symptoms, this patient is experiencing a fat embolus.
    ① Crackles and wheezes are common with many respiratory conditions.
    ③ Absence of a fever is a normal state.
    ④ Falling blood pressure is usually more consistent with hypovolemia.

56. Comprehension, implementation, safe care (b)
    ❹ This will prevent air embolism.
    ① The site may yet be salvageable and there isn't an order to discontinue.
    ② Without purging the air, there is a risk of air embolism.
    ③ This option is unsafe and may cause a clot to form at the insertion site.

57. Knowledge, implementation, health (b)
    ❷ It is the *Staphylococcus* strain that can cause infections in women. These can begin in the vagina during menstruation.
    ① *Chlamydia trachomatis* is a chronic STD, characterized by genital ulcers, swollen lymph nodes, headache, fever and muscle pain.
    ③ *Neisseria gonorrhoeae* (coccus) is a common STD and can progress to pelvic inflammatory disease if not treated.
    ④ Group A beta-hemolytic streptococci can cause rheumatic fever, an inflammatory disease resulting from delayed reaction to a strep infection, and may affect the skin, joints, brain, or heart.

58. Knowledge, implementation, environment (b)
    ❹ The RDA are suggested levels of nutrients known from research to meet dietary needs of most healthy individuals.
    ① Individuals with nutritional deficiencies may need amounts above what the RDA suggest.
    ② They are not the same as the food pyramid guide, yet another guide to proper nutrition.
    ③ This pertains to the U.S. Dietary Goals, another set of guidelines to proper nutrition.

59. Comprehension, assessment, psychosocial (b)
    ❸ A child between the ages of 3 and 6 years is said to be in the phallic stage.
    ① This is the oral stage, with the focus on using the tongue and mouth to deal with anxiety-producing experiences.
    ② This is the anal stage, with the focus on learning muscle control, especially muscles involved with defecation and urination.
    ④ This is the latency stage. Sexual maturity develops and the individual learns to form satisfying relationships with the opposite sex.

60. Comprehension, planning, health (b)
    ❸ Good source of iron with a texture appropriate for an 8 month old.
    ① Good source of iron, but an 8 month old could choke on the tiny pieces.
    ② Source of vitamin A but not iron.
    ④ Provides calcium and protein but not iron.

61. Application, implementation, physiologic (c)
    ❷ Stopping the burning process is the first priority with a burn injury. Cool water will stop the process.
    ① Stopping the burning process is the first priority with a burn injury; petroleum jelly will keep the heat in, causing further damage.
    ③ Stopping the burning process is the first priority with a burn injury; a dry dressing should not be applied initially.
    ④ Although ice will certainly cool an area it also decreases blood flow to the area, which will cause further damage. Ice should not be used.

62. Comprehension, assessment, physiologic (a)
    ❹ The gallbladder secretes bile to emulsify dietary fat.
    ①,②,③ Not classically associated with pain precipitation in gallbladder disease.

63. Application, implementation, physiologic (a)
    ❸ Primary intervention to maintain muscle tone.
    ① Inappropriate to transfer to chair in unconscious state; does not relate to increasing mobility.
    ② Necessary, but not the best.
    ④ Inappropriate position and will promote skin breakdown.

64. Comprehension, assessment, environment (b)
    ❸ Palpation reveals the amount of pitting involved.
    ① No sounds are produced by ankle edema.
    ② Evaluation is a step in the nursing process.
    ④ Percussion is used to assess masses, organs, and body cavities.

65. Comprehension, implementation, physiologic (b)
    ❸ The discarded specimen consists of urine produced before 8 AM of the first day. Urine produced and voided within 24 hours is necessary for the specimen.
    ① Collecting urine from only two voidings during a 24-hour period does not constitute a 24-hour collection.
    ② Discarding the urine produced at 8 AM of the second day would mean that some urine produced within the 24 hours would not be included in the specimen.
    ④ Including the first day's 8 AM urine would mean that the specimen included urine produced during more than a 24-hour period.

66. Application, implementation, physiologic (b)
    ❹ The fall in blood sugar decreases available glucose for cell metabolism, causing the motor and sensory symptoms; because the brain does not store glucose, a depletion of available glucose for metabolism affects the brain cells, rapidly causing the CNS symptoms: irritability, confusion, etc.
    ① Symptoms of hyperglycemia.
    ② Symptoms of thyrotoxicosis.
    ③ Symptoms of hypovolemic shock.

67. Comprehension, planning, physiologic (b)
    ❶ Fresh or frozen beef is permitted. Also fresh fruits and vegetables have very little sodium.
    ② All smoked, processed, and canned meats are high in sodium. Most frozen foods have sodium added.
    ③ Corned beef and dill pickles are high in sodium.
    ④ Ham, cheeses, and regular bread are high in sodium.

68. Comprehension, assessment, physiologic (b)
    ❸ In skim milk much of the fat has been removed. Lean fish and fruit contain little fat.
    ① Whole milk and pastry contain considerable fat.
    ② Fried potatoes and avocado contain fat.
    ④ Ham and creamed peas are high in fat content.

69. Comprehension, planning, physiologic (b)
    ❶ Bowel retraining is easier, and success is usually met in a much shorter period of time.
    ② Both are demoralizing.
    ③ Bowel retraining does not solve urinary incontinence.
    ④ Patient cooperation does not usually vary.

70. Comprehension, planning, environment (a)
    ❶ Correct calculation.
    ②,③,④ Incorrect dose.

71. Application, planning, environment (b)
 ❸ Correct response.
 ①,②,④ Not applicable to this specific situation.
72. Knowledge, assessment, physiologic (c)
 ❷ Cardiac dysrhythmias are associated with hypokalemia.
 ① Tendency toward bleeding is not associated with hypokalemia.
 ③ Nausea and vomiting are associated with hyperkalemia.
 ④ Thirst is not associated with hypokalemia.
73. Knowledge, assessment, environment (c)
 ❷ Autonomic dysreflexia may occur in 85% of all spinal cord–injured patients with lesions at T6 level or above.
 ①,③,④ Given symptoms do not describe this condition.
74. Knowledge, implementation, physiologic (a)
 ❶ All are good sources of potassium.
 ② Good sources of iron.
 ③ Good sources of vitamin C.
 ④ Good sources of vitamin D.
75. Application, planning, environment (b)
 ❶ ADLs before admission can be used as a baseline for ADLs in the hospital and to measure change.
 ②,③,④ Not relevant in development of nursing care plan.
76. Application, implementation, health (a)
 ❶ Weakened cognitive skills need stimulation.
 ②,③ Incorrect, unrelated to cognitive skill improvement.
 ④ Opposite to the goal of cognitive stimulation.
77. Application, planning, physiologic (c)
 ❸ A patient who is comatose may lack many of the body's protective mechanisms such as a cough reflex and gag reflex. As a result the patient is at risk for occluding the airway with secretions. A patent airway is vital for life. Maintenance of a patent airway should therefore be the major priority.
 ① A comatose patient would certainly be at risk for skin breakdown because of an inability to move. Skin breakdown is not an immediately life-threatening problem, however. Airway is still the priority.
 ② A comatose patient would certainly have difficulty communicating. Communication, however, is not immediately a life-threatening problem. Airway is still the priority.
 ④ A comatose patient would certainly be at risk for musculoskeletal problems because of an inability to move. Musculoskeletal problems, however, are not immediately life-threatening problems. Airway is still the priority.
78. Application, planning, health (c)
 ❸ Parkinson's disease affects the brain centers responsible for control and regulation of movement. The three characteristic symptoms are tremor, muscle stiffness, and bradykinesia.
 ① Ptosis and diplopia are symptoms of another neurological disorder, myasthenia gravis (MG). In MG the difficulty is in the transmission of nerve impulses.
 ② Blurred vision and loss of balance are symptoms of another neurological disorder, multiple sclerosis (MS). MS is a chronic degenerative progressive disease of the central nervous system characterized by demyelination of the brain and spinal cord.

 ④ Chorea and slurred speech are symptoms of another neurological disorder, Huntington's disease (HD). HD is a chronic, progressive hereditary disease resulting in dementia and involuntary movements.
79. Comprehension, evaluation, physiologic (c)
 ❸ Repeated exposure to an individual with TB increases the risk of the exposed individual developing the disease.
 ① Following initiation of the chemotherapy for TB, the individual must have sputum specimens examined every 2 to 4 weeks. The individual with TB may return to work after 2 successive sputum cultures are negative.
 ② The chemotherapy course for TB is approximately 9 to 12 months. The individual must take the medication for the entire time to eradicate the disease. Symptoms may subside in a much shorter time period.
 ③ An individual who has had TB will have a positive skin test forever, even when active disease is not present.
80. Knowledge, assessment, physiologic (b)
 ❶ In vasoocclusive crisis, sickled cells become lodged within the vessels, causing tissue hypoxia and resulting in pain.
 ② Jaundice results from accelerated red blood cell destruction as occurs in SC hyperhemolytic crisis, not vasoocclusive crisis.
 ③ Plethora or a "red complexion" occurs in polycythemia or increased red blood cells in the circulation. A patient with SC is usually anemic.
 ④ Hemarthrosis or "bleeding into joints" does not usually occur in sickle cell crisis; occlusion is the problem.
81. Comprehension, planning, safe environment (b)
 ❸ Clients with PD frequently have difficulty swallowing because of dry mouth from medications and disturbances in pharyngeal motility. A semisolid may be easier to tolerate.
 ① Clients with PD frequently have difficulty swallowing because of dry mouth from medications and disturbances in pharyngeal motility. Although increased calories may be needed, a regular diet may not be tolerated.
 ② Clients with PD are frequently embarrassed by their difficulties eating. Placing a client in a public area may exacerbate the problems with eating.
 ④ Clients should be encouraged to remain as independent as possible with daily activities to promote their self-esteem.
82. Comprehension, assessment, physiologic (b)
 ❸ If the patient has stable vitals but irregular pulse, atrial irritability is the cause.
 ① Sinus bradycardia means a slow but regular pulse.
 ② Sinus tachycardia means a fast but regular pulse.
 ④ Ventricular fibrillation will render the patient unconscious.
83. Application, physiologic, health (c)
 ❸ Application of a nasal cannula assures comfortable and adequate administration of oxygen for the duration of the meal.
 ① This would increase dependence and would not adequately oxygenate the patient.
 ② The patient's oxygen would be depleted quickly during the meal and damage could occur while attempting to overoxygenate
 ④ The patient has lung cancer. He needs his oxygen.

84. Knowledge, implementation, physiologic (c)
   ❷ Ketosis and dehydration are caused by a serious deficiency of carbohydrates. To prevent this, one needs a minimum of 50 to 100 grams of carbohydrates daily.
   ① Excess carbohydrate intake leads to obesity.
   ③ Dental problems are caused by excess carbohydrates, leading to plaque. Microbes thrive on sugars.
   ④ Excess gas can be caused by excessive carbohydrate intake.

85. Comprehension, assessment, health (b)
   ❹ These foods all have a high content of dietary fiber, which helps prevent constipation by softening and increasing the size of the stool.
   ① These fruits are very low in dietary fiber and should not be recommended as a good source of roughage.
   ② These foods are processed or refined foods, and contain little, if any, cellulose.
   ③ These meats are not good sources of fiber or roughage.

86. Knowledge, assessment, health (b)
   ❹ A high intake of animal foods is not recommended. Cholesterol is found only in animal tissue, and the mayonnaise used in tuna and ham sandwiches is high in fat content.
   ① Using olive oil is acceptable.
   ② Liquid vegetable oils are recommended for cooking.
   ③ Fruits, oat brans, and legumes bind with cholesterol-containing substances and prevent their reabsorption by the blood.

87. Comprehension, physiologic, intervention (b)
   ❷ Increased temperature is frequently the first sign of atelectasis.
   ① Analgesics will not treat the cause of the fever.
   ③ The doctor should be informed of an elevated temperature, but this doesn't have to be done immediately.
   ④ The dressing should be inspected but left alone until it needs changing.

88. Knowledge, implementation, physiologic (a)
   ❹ The safest way to give medications is to check the patient's identification bracelet. In a pediatric or geriatric unit, some agencies put the ID bracelet or name on the beds because the bracelets fall off the patients.
   ① The danger in asking patients to state their name is that some patients don't know their name and will answer to anything.
   ② The nurse giving the medications should not rely on another nurse to identify a patient. She may be wrong.
   ③ There are too many patients who will answer to any name.

89. Knowledge, implementation, physiologic (b)
   ❹ Thyroid hormone drugs are usually given in single doses, once a day. The best time to take them is before breakfast on an empty stomach to help increase absorption of the drug.
   ①,② The doses are not normally divided and are usually given once a day.
   ③ When patients begin thyroid therapy, their energy level should increase. If it decreases, they need to check with the physician, as the therapeutic effects may not be working.

90. Knowledge, implementation, safe environment (c)
   ❷ The metal object is probably the radiation implant and should not be touched or allowed to stay in the bed. Notify the radiation department for proper handling of the implant. Nurses are generally not trained to handle radiation implants.
   ① The metal object is probably the radiation implant and should not be touched. The hazardous waste box is for blood and tissues. It will not protect one from radium exposure. Every precaution possible should be taken by the nurse against unnecessary exposure.
   ③ The physician should be contacted, but notification of the radiation department is the priority.
   ④ The nurse should never attempt to reinsert an implant. This is not a nursing function and could harm the patient or the nurse.

91. Knowledge, implementation, physiologic (c)
   ❶ The patient is showing early symptoms of anaphylaxis. Benadryl is an antihistamine and will decrease the response to the penicillin.
   ② Vital signs should be taken every 5 minutes to monitor the patient's progress, but they are not the priority. The Benadryl will decrease the allergic response to the drug; so it is the priority.
   ③ Oxygen should be administered if respiratory distress occurs. The Benadryl will decrease the allergic response to the drug; so it should be given first.
   ④ Cool compresses may relieve some itching. This would be a comfort measure. Because the itching is not life-threatening, the Benadryl is given first to decrease the allergic response to the penicillin.

92. Knowledge, implementation, physiologic (c)
   ❶ Hyperreflexia (dysreflexia) is an involuntary response of the sympathetic nervous system to external stimulation, such as bladder or bowel distention, enemas, or rectal examination. It can also occur in response to infections, bladder irrigations, and skin ulcers. It occurs in high spinal cord injuries.
   ② Although the patient may be immobile because of a spinal cord injury, the immobility does not trigger the sympathetic response as discussed in #1.
   ③ Comfort or discomfort is not an underlying cause of dysreflexia. See #1.
   ④ Nutrition is not an underlying cause of dysreflexia.

93. Application, implementation, physiologic (c)
   ❸ Muscle spasms are usually the cause of pain in a laminectomy patient. Relieving the spasms will generally relieve the pain. Because muscles are longer when they are relaxed, the spasms can best be relieved by positioning the patient in such a way as to lengthen the muscles.
   ① Tension in the lumbar area strains the lumbar area and does nothing to relax the cervical area.
   ② The lower leg and the back muscles do not act in opposition. Tension or contraction of the lower leg will have no effect on promoting comfort for the laminectomy patient.
   ④ Muscles of the scapula and neck region are usually stretched, such as with traction, collars, or braces, to promote comfort. Contraction or shortening would increase discomfort.

94. Application, implementation, physiologic (c)
   ❷ Output of less than 60 ml in 2 hours could indicate ureteral obstruction, impending renal failure, or a leak in the urinary diversion. Notify the physician.

① Pain relief is needed, but left flank pain is also indicative of ureteral obstruction.

③ Not a priority in this situation. Should assess if morphine is given.

④ Position of comfort is called for but is not a priority.

95. Application, physiologic, health (c)

❸ Urine pH greater than 6.0 encourages bacterial growth.

① Recommended fluid intake is 8 to 10 glasses per day.

② Teach patient to relax abdominal muscles rather than bearing down to facilitate catheter insertion.

④ With a physician's order, patient is instructed to take 500 to 1000 mg vitamin C daily to increase urine acidity.

96. Application, implementation, physiologic (c)

❷ An increase in output from the T-tube could indicate an obstruction below the T-tube.

① A T-tube is never clamped without an order. As healing progresses, the surgeon may order clamping before meals and unclamping after meals.

③ Tension on the T-tube can dislodge the internal placement of the tube.

④ Normal colored urine and stools indicate that bile is being deposited normally in the gastrointestinal tract.

97. Comprehension, implementation, care environment (a)

❶ Blue food coloring is used to differentiate gastric contents from respiratory secretions if aspiration occurs. When combined with bile, it turns green.

② Green food coloring is not used because it would not change color in the GI tract.

③ Multiple vitamins would change the color of urine to bright yellow. They would not affect the color of the stools.

④ The patient is being tube fed. Also, the color is a unique color for stools and not similar to anything else.

98. Application, implementation, physiologic (b)

❷ Correct. At 50 ml per hour, the feeding will last for 4 hours as recommended safe to avoid spoilage.

①,③ Incorrect. Solutions hung for longer than 4 hours run the risk of spoilage.

④ Incorrect. This would only last 1 hour and would not be time efficient for the nurse.

99. Comprehension, implementation, physiologic (c)

❶ Erythromycin may cause gastric upset. It is tolerated better with food.

② An empty stomach may increase the gastric upset.

③ Only the physician may discontinue a medication order.

④ Milk frequently inhibits the absorption of antibiotics.

100. Comprehension, evaluation, physiologic (c)

❹ Loss of voice may indicate internal bleeding or edema.

① Serosanguineous drainage is a normal finding.

② Slightly increased respiratory rate is normal initially.

③ Cerumen is a normal finding.

101. Comprehension, assessment, physiologic (b)

❷ Typically, HIV presents with fever and chills.

① Cytomegalovirus infections frequently occur once AIDS occurs.

③ *Pneumocystis carinii* pneumonia usually occurs after AIDS develops.

④ MRSA also occurs in patients without AIDS or HIV.

102. Comprehension, assessment, physiologic (b)

❹ The loss of bone density will affect the lower vertebrae. The weight of the body causes compression fractures.

① Tibia fractures occur with trauma or stress.

② Calcaneal fractures usually occur as the result of falls.

③ Rib fractures usually result from trauma or tumors.

103. Comprehension, assessment, physiologic (c)

❷ Fat emboli may travel to the brain, therefore assessment should include level of orientation.

① Assessment of muscle control is not an important consideration with fat emboli.

③ Fatty emboli are usually not painful.

④ Visual acuity is usually not affected by fat emboli.

104. Comprehension, assessment, physiologic (b)

❸ Petechiae and bruising indicate a problem with clotting.

① An increased leukocyte count is usually found with bacterial infections.

② Hypocalcemia may result from malnutrition.

④ An elevated BUN is associated with renal failure.

105. Comprehension, assessment, physiologic (c)

❷ Elevated weight often increases blood pressure and taxes the heart.

① The very young and the very old are at surgical risk.

③ Well-controlled cardiac problems generally pose minimal risk.

④ The patient's potassium level is normal.

106. Comprehension, planning, psychosocial (b)

❹ This opens lines of communication and provides emotional support.

① This forces the patient and family to deal with emotions during a stressful time.

② This is a situational depression and antidepressants aren't recommended.

③ Depression and withdrawal are normal parts of the grieving process.

107. Comprehension, assessment, psychosocial (b)

❶ The patient may continue to grieve for several months.

② Anger is frequently a part of the grieving process.

③ Symptoms of anxiety are usually elevated blood pressure and indecisiveness.

④ Becoming silent and withdrawn are symptoms associated with depression.

108. Comprehension, assessment, psychosocial (b)

❷ Discharge planning should begin on admission.

① Developing good rapport is essential for effective communication to occur.

③ Life-style changes are important to assess because they may indicate the nature of injury to the patient.

④ Determining self-care practices may be helpful at dismissal.

109. Knowledge, planning, safe and effective care (b)

❷ Tylenol #3 has 30 mg codeine in each pill.

① 15 mg codeine is found in Tylenol #2.

③ 45 mg of codeine is not found in Tylenol with codeine prescriptions.

④ 60 mg codeine is found in Tylenol #4.

110. Knowledge, planning, safe and effective care (b)

❸ Freckles are only pigment changes.

① Administration of an anticoagulant would cause more bleeding to occur.

② Scar tissue has poor circulation.

④ Whenever possible, moles should not be irritated.

111. Knowledge, planning, safe and effective care (b)
   ❹ Radiation to the abdominal area may produce nausea, vomiting, and diarrhea.
   ① Stomatitis usually occurs when the head is radiated.
   ② Pelvic or sternal radiation affects the main bone-marrow–producing areas.
   ③ Temporary hair loss occurs with radiation to the head.

112. Knowledge, implementation, safe and effective care (b)
   ❹ Using the formula of 125 ml/hr × 10 gtts/ml/60 min/hr = 21 gtts/ml.
   ① This drop rate delivers 50 ml/hr.
   ② This drop rate delivers 75 ml/hr.
   ③ This drop rate delivers 90 ml/hr.

113. Knowledge, implementation, safe and effective care (b)
   ❷ Positioning the patient on the left side with a suspected air embolism allows the trapped air in the heart to stay in the right side of the heart or go to the lungs.
   ① A steady stream of small bubbles may allow a significant amount of air to accumulate.
   ③ Raising the head of the bed may allow the trapped air to travel to the brain and cause stroke-like symptoms.
   ④ The subclavian site should not be discontinued without a physician's order.

114. Knowledge, implementation, safe and effective care (b)
   ❹ Identifying marks should be left to aid in treatment.
   ① Most lotions contain additives, which would cause thermal burns with the next treatment.
   ② The marks should be left intact until treatment is complete.
   ③ Acetone would remove the treatment marks, requiring more time at the next treatment to remark the site.

115. Knowledge, implementation, safe and effective care (b)
   ❷ Splinting the incisional area supports the muscles and decreases pain.
   ① Coughing and deep breathing rarely induce vomiting.
   ③ Coughing and deep breathing exercises rarely cause rib fractures.
   ④ Early ambulation enhances bowel motility more effectively.

116. Knowledge, implementation, safe and effective care (b)
   ❸ The sciatic nerve may be permanently damaged if given an injection.
   ① The brachial plexus is in the axilla.
   ② The femoral artery is located in the groin.
   ④ The greater saphenous vein is located in the lower leg.

117. Knowledge, implementation, safe and effective care (b)
   ❹ NPO means no food or drink unless specified.
   ① This explanation still allows the patient to drink fluids.
   ② NPO means *N*othing *P*er *O*s or by mouth.
   ③ This explanation still allows the patient to eat food.

118. Knowledge, assessment, safe and effective care (b)
   ❶ Swollen, red, warm IV sites are consistent with thrombophlebitis.
   ② Infiltration produces swollen, pale, cool sites.

③ Symptoms of overload include dyspnea, tachycardia, and frothy sputum.
④ Speed shock occurs when bolus medications are given too quickly.

119. Knowledge, planning, physiologic (b)
   ❷ A small instrument is inserted to visualize the cartilage.
   ① Radiographic dye is not typically used with joints.
   ③ Biopsies are taken if there is a concern about cancer; the patient was injured.
   ④ If there is a question of infection, synovial fluid is collected for culture.

120. Knowledge, planning, physiologic (b)
   ❹ Acetaminophen is a mild analgesic without antiinflammatory properties.
   ① Aspirin is contraindicated because it may cause gastric bleeding.
   ② Ibuprofen may be irritating to the gastric mucosa.
   ③ A side-effect of naproxen is gastric ulcers.

121. Knowledge, intervention, physiologic (b)
   ❸ Chemotherapy drugs are designed to affect different stages of cell reproduction.
   ① It is not known if the blood-brain barrier needs to be crossed in this scenario.
   ② End-stage disease usually requires supportive and comfort care only.
   ④ Adjuvant therapy is recommended with many types of cancer, not just aggressive ones.

122. Knowledge, implementation, physiologic (b)
   ❶ Not taking the medication may cause the bacteria to become resistant to treatment with cephalexin.
   ② Symptoms may actually disappear after a few doses.
   ③ Most antibiotics do not have a cumulative effect.
   ④ Pneumococci are bacteria.

123. Knowledge, implementation, physiologic (b)
   ❸ Warm, moist compresses facilitate the reabsorption of excess fluids.
   ① Ice reduces circulation and slows reabsorption of excess fluids.
   ② Elevating the right hand will not help the left hand.
   ④ A dependent position delays reabsorption of excess fluids.

124. Knowledge, implementation, physiologic (b)
   ❶ Frequent oral care will reduce the risk of bacterial overgrowth.
   ② Stomatitis is internal and doesn't affect body image greatly.
   ③ Antiinflammatory drugs will not reduce oral irritation.
   ④ Additional spices may irritate oral mucosa.

125. Knowledge, planning, physiologic (b)
   ❶ Buck's traction is a temporary skin traction.
   ② Crutchfield tongs are used for spinal traction.
   ③ Bryant's traction is a type of skeletal traction.
   ④ Russell's traction is a skeletal traction.

Index

Copper, 124
Coramine, 85
Corgard, 87, 90
Coricidin, 88
Cornea, 249
Corneal abrasion, 444
Coronary angiography, 170
Corpus luteum, 232, 234
Cortef, 94
Cortef acetate, 94
Cortex, 221
Corticotropin, 212
Cortisol, 94, 212
Cortisone, 212
Cortisone acetate, 94
Cortone acetate, 94
Cortril, 94
Cosmegen, 100
Cost capitation, 44
Coughing, 10, 27
Coumadin, 91
Coumarins, 91
Cowper's gland, 229, 230
Coxsackie, 498
CPD, 322
CPR, 439, 440
Cranial, 145
Cranial nerves, 203
Cream, 71
Creatinine level, 223, 324
Cretinism, 380, 381
Criminal abortion, 332
Crisis, 310
Crisis intervention, 310
Crohn's disease, 195, 389
Cross tolerance, 72
Cruex, 100
Crutches, 420
Cryptorchidism, 348, 378
Crystalline, 92
Crysticillin, 98
Crystodigin, 90, 91
CS, 322
CST, 254
CT scan
   endocrine system disorders, 214
   female reproductive disorders, 235
   gastrointestinal disorders, 190
   musculoskeletal disorders, 150
   neurologic disorders, 204
   respiratory disorders, 161
Cuffed tracheostomy tube, 22
Culdoscopy, 235
Cultural background, 9
Culture and sensitivity, 19, 235
Cushing's syndrome, 219, 220
Cutaneous ureterostomies, 226
CVA, 207, 208
Cyanocobalamin, 92, 102

Cyclandelate, 89
Cyclobenzaprine hydrochloride, 83
Cyclogyl, 86, 96
Cyclopentolate hydrochloride, 86, 96
Cyclophosphamide, 100
Cyclopropane, 82
Cycloserine, 99
Cyclospasmol, 89
Cycrimine hydrochloride, 83
Cyesis, 323
Cylert, 85
Cyproheptadine hydrochloride, 88
Cyst, 245
Cystic fibrosis, 382
Cystitis, 10, 224, 346
Cystocele, 240
Cystoscopy, 224
Cytarabine, 100
Cytologic testing, 324
Cytology, 162
Cytomegalovirus (CMV), 335
Cytomegalovirus infection, 507
Cytomel, 95
Cytoplasm, 145
Cytoplasmic membrane, 145
Cytosar-U, 100
Cytoxan, 100

D

D & C, 235
D-S-S, 94
D-xylose tolerance test, 191
da Vinci, Leonardo, 322
Dacarbazine, 100
Dactinomycin, 100
Daily bath, 29
Dalmane, 84
Danazol, 96
Dance therapy, 312
Dangle, 27
Dantrium, 83
Dantrolene, 83
Dantrolene sodium, 83
Dapsone, 99
Daranide, 96
Darbid, 86
Daricon, 92
Darvon, 80
Darvon-N, 80
Datril, 81
DDAVP, 94
DDH, 379, 380
Death, 310; *see also* Dying
Debridement, 32
Decadron, 94
Decamethonium bromide, 86, 97
Decidua, 325
Decidua basalis, 325
Decidua capsularis, 325

Decidua vera, 325
Deciduous teeth, 187
Decisional conflict, 468
Declomycin, 99
Decubitus ulcer care, 31
Decubitus ulcer formation, 27
Deep breathing, 27
Deep partial thickness burn, 248, 447
Defamation, 41
Defense mechanisms, 299, 304
Deferoxamine mesylate, 92, 102
Dehydration, 23
Delatestryl, 96
Delaxin, 83
Delcoid, 95
Delirium, 203, 421
Delirium tremens (DTs), 308, 454
Delivery of health care, 44
Delivery of nursing care, 39
Delta-Cortef, 94
Delta-Dome, 94
Deltasone, 101
Deltoid, 148, 149
Delusion, 307
Delusions of grandeur, 307
Delusions of persecution, 307
Delusions of sin or guilt, 307
Demecarium bromide, 86, 96
Demeclocycline hydrochloride, 99
Dementia, 421, 422
Demerol, 80
Dendrid, 100
Dendrites, 201
Denial, 304
Denial, ineffective, 468
Dentures, 30
Deodorant, 30
Depakene, 82
Department of Health and Human Services
   (DHHS), 45
Depo-Medrol, 94
Depo-Provera
   antineoplastic agent, as, 101
   birth control, 356
   progestin, as, 95
Depressants
   alcohol, 84
   analgesics, 79-81
   anesthetics, 82
   anticonvulsants, 82
   antiparkinsonian drugs, 83
   effects of, 455
   narcotic antagonists, 81
   sedatives/hypnotics/antianxiety drugs, 83,
      84
   skeletal muscle relaxants, 83
Depression, 423, 424
Depressive disorders, 307
Dermatophytosis, 498, 499

Gracilis, 148, 149
Grafts, 248
Grand mal seizure, 207
Grand multipara, 323
Granuloma inguinale, 507
Graves' disease, 215, 216
Gray matter, 201
Greater trochanter, 146
Greenstick fracture, 155, 450
Grieving, 310
Grieving, anticipatory, 468
Grieving, dysfunctional, 468
Grifulvin-V, 91, 100
Grisactin, 100
Griseofulvin, 91, 100
Gross negligence, 40
Group B streptococcus, 335
Group therapy, 311
Growth and development, 8
Growth and development, altered, 468
Growth hormone, 94
GTH, 94, 212
GTPAL, 322
GTT, 214
Guanethidine monosulfate, 87, 90
Gum karaya, 93
Gustatory hallucination, 307
Gyne-Lotrimin, 100

H

Habitual abortion, 332
HAD test, 328
Hair, 244, 245
Hair care, 30
Hair follicle, 244
Haldol, 93
Hallucination, 307
Hallucinogens, 309, 455
Haloperidol, 93
Haloprogin, 100
Halorex, 100
Halotestin, 96
Halothane, 82, 455
Hamstring group, 149
Hand bladder irrigation, 24
Hand-foot-and-mouth disease, 500
Hand washing, 12
Hard measles, 501
Harmonyl, 90
Harsh colors, 31
Hashish, 309, 455
HAV, 198
Haversian canals, 146
Hay fever, 386
HBV, 198
HCG, 95, 322
HDL, 122
Head injuries, 208, 209, 443, 444
Healing, 10

Health, 8
Health care agencies
  ambulatory care, 46
  DHHS, 45
  geriatric day-care centers, 46
  health service providers, 45
  home care, 45, 46
  hospices, 45
  hospitals, 45
  international agency, 45
  nursing homes, 45
  official agencies (U.S.), 45
  state health departments, 45
  voluntary agencies, 45
Health care team, 38, 39
Health-illness continuum, 8
Health maintenance organizations (HMOs), 46
Healthy People 2000, 119
Health perception-health management pattern, 474
Health Resources and Services Administration, 45
Health-seeking behaviors, 468
Health service providers, 45
Hearing aids, 418
Hearing loss, 254
Heart, 167, 168
Heart attack, 173, 174
Heart beat, 18
Heart rates, 168
Heat applications, 32
Heat exhaustion, 451
Heat stroke, 451
Hegar's sign, 326
Height, 19
Heimlich maneuver, 439-441
HELLP, 322
Helper T-cells, 169
Hemagglutination inhibition (HAD) test, 328
Hematologic conditions
  AIDS, 185-187
  anemia, 182-184
  diagnostic tests/methods, 181, 182
  frequent patient problems, 182
  leukemia, 184, 185
  lymphoma, 187
  nursing assessment, 180, 181
Hematomas, 347
Hematuria, 223
Hemodialysis, 228, 229
Hemoglobin electrophoresis, 181
Hemolytic disease of newborn, 353, 354
Hemophilia, 10, 384
Hemorrhage, 441, 442
Hemorrhoids, 196, 197
Hemostatic agents, 91
Hemothorax, 164, 446

Heparin
  anticoagulants, and, 91
  reaction to blood-thinning drugs, 481
  reaction to ibuprofen, 476
  reaction to salicylates, 476, 482
  reaction to warfarin sodium, 481
Heparin sodium, 91
Hepatic coma, 199
Hepatitis, 198, 500
Hepatitis A, 335
Hepatitis B, 335
Hepatitis C, 198
Hepatotoxicity, 72
Hereditary factors, 10
Hernias, 201
Herniated nucleus pulposus, 154, 155
Hernioplasty, 201
Herniorrhaphy, 201
Heroin, 308, 455
Herpangina, 500
Herpes genitalis, 243
Herpes simplex, 246, 501, 508
Herpes zoster, 246, 498
Herplex Liquifilm, 100
Hesitancy, 223
Heterograft, 248
Heterozygote testing, 324
Hexa-Betalin, 102
Hexadrol, 94
HHNC, 218
Hiatal hernia, 192, 193
Hierarchy of needs, 13, 15
High blood pressure, 172, 173
High calorie diet, 130
High carbohydrate diet, 130
High-density lipoprotein (HDL), 122
High Fowler's, 29
High iron diet, 130
High protein diet, 130
High residue diet, 130
High risk, 323
Hilus, 221
Hinge joint, 147
Hirschsprung's disease, 376, 377
Histamine H$_2$-receptor antagonists, 93
HIV infection, 186; *see also* AIDS
Hives, 245, 387
HMOs, 46
Hodgkin's disease, 187
Holism, 292
Holmes, Oliver Wendell, 322
Holter monitoring, 170
Homapin, 92
Homatrocel, 96
Homatropine hydrobromide, 86, 96
Homatropine methylbromide, 92
Home care, 45, 46
Home maintenance management, impaired, 468